THIRD EDITION

nursing in the
community

DIMENSIONS OF COMMUNITY

HEALTH NURSING

THIRD EDITION

nursing in the
community

DIMENSIONS OF COMMUNITY

HEALTH NURSING

Mary Jo Clark, RN, MSN, PhD
Associate Dean
Associate Professor
Hahn School of Nursing and Health Science
University of San Diego
San Diego, California

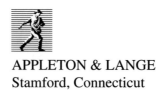

APPLETON & LANGE
Stamford, Connecticut

Notice: The author and the publisher of this volume have taken care to make certain that the doses of drugs and schedules of treatment are correct and compatible with the standards generally accepted at the time of publication. Nevertheless, as new information becomes available, changes in treatment and in the use of drugs become necessary. The reader is advised to carefully consult the instruction and information material included in the package insert of each drug or therapeutic agent before administration. This advice is especially important when using, administering, or recommending new or infrequently used drugs. The author and publisher disclaim all responsibility for any liability, loss, injury, or damage incurred as a consequence, directly or indirectly, of the use and application of any of the contents of this volume.

00 01 02 / 10 9 8 7 6 5 4 3 2

Prentice Hall International (UK) Limited, *London*
Prentice Hall of Australia Pty. Limited, *Sydney*
Prentice Hall Canada, Inc., *Toronto*
Prentice Hall Hispanoamericana, S.A., *Mexico*
Prentice Hall of India Private Limited, *New Dehli*
Prentice Hall of Japan, Inc., *Tokyo*
Simon & Schuster Asia Pte. Ltd., *Singapore*
Editora Prentice Hall do Brasil Ltda., *Rio de Janeiro*
Prentice Hall, *Upper Saddle River, New Jersey*

Library of Congress Cataloging-in-Publication Data

Clark, Mary Jo Dummer.
    Nursing in the community : dimensions of community health nursing
/ Mary JoClark. — 3rd ed.
        p.   cm.
    Includes bibliographic references and index.
    ISBN (invalid) 0-8385-6984-7 (case : alk. paper)
    1. Community health nursing.   I. Title.
    [DNLM: 1. Community Health Nursing.   2. Nursing Process.   WY 106
C594n 1998]
RT98.N88 1998
610.73'43—dc21
DNLM/DLC
for Library of Congress   98-17066
                                                      CIP

Acquisitions Editor: Patricia E. Casey
Associate Editor: Elisabeth Church Garofalo
Development Editor: Patricia Cleary
Production Editor: Angela Dion
Art Coordinator: Eve Siegel
Artist: Academy Artworks
Designer: Janice Barsevich Bielawa

ISBN 0-8385-6984-6

9 780838 569849   90000

PRINTED IN THE UNITED STATES OF AMERICA

*This book is lovingly dedicated
to Phil and Phil
who continue to be the wind beneath my wings
and to all the students
who have taught me to clarify my thinking
and reminded me that there is a reason
for what I do everyday.
Thank you.*

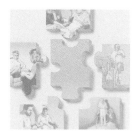

CONTENTS

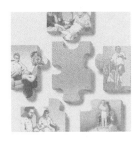

CONTENTS IN DEPTH

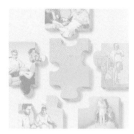

CREDITS

The poetry that introduces each unit in this textbook is from *just who,* a book of poems written by Veneta Masson, a community health nurse in Washington, DC. Some of the poems have been excerpted; however, they appear in their entirety on pages 935 to 941. Mary Jo Clark and Appleton & Lange express our appreciation to the poet for her heartfelt expressions of nursing in the community and for her generosity in permitting us to reprint her work. *just who* was published in 1993 by Crossroad Health Ministries, Inc., which operates a family medical and nursing practice in Washington, DC.

▼ ▼ ▼

The sources of photographs in this third edition of *Nursing in the Community* are John Van-S, Visiting Nurse Association of Boston; New York Visiting Nurse Association, American Red Cross, Washington, DC.

▼ ▼ ▼

A contributor to the second edition who did not participate in the third edition is Kathleen Heinrich, PhD, RN.

▼ ▼ ▼

The ANA Standards for Community Health Nursing listed on page 55 are reprinted with permission from American Nurses Association, *Standards of Community Health Nursing Practice,* copyright 1986 American Nurse Publishing, American Nurses Foundation/American Nurses Association, 600 Maryland Avenue, SW, Suite 100 W, Washington, DC 20024-2571.

Table 11–2 "Standards of Case Management Practice and Related Measurement Criteria" on page 218 is reprinted with permission from Case Management Society of America, 8201 Cantrell Road, Suite 230, Little Rock, AR 72227-2448; www.cmsa.org.

The Standards for Nursing Practice in Correctional Settings listed on page 686 is reprinted with permission from American Nurses Association, *Standards of Nursing Practice in Correctional Facilities,* copyright 1995 American Nurses Publishing, American Nurses Foundation/American Nurses Association, 600 Maryland Avenue, SW, Suite 100 W, Washington, DC 20024-2571.

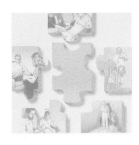

CONTRIBUTORS

Patricia Caudle, DNSc, FNP
Assistant Professor
College of Nursing
University of Arkansas for Medical Sciences
Little Rock, Arkansas

Susan Chen, RN, PHN, CIC
Infection Control Practitioner
San Mateo County Health Services Agency
San Mateo, California

Charlene M. Hanson, EdD, FNP-CS, FAAN
Associate Professor of Nursing
Director of the Center for Rural Health and Research
Georgia Southern University
Statesboro, Georgia

Elizabeth Harper Smith, RN, MSN, PhD
Professor of Nursing, Program Director
Milligan College
Department of Nursing
Milligan, Tennessee
Adjunct Faculty for East Tennessee State University
Johnson City, Tennessee

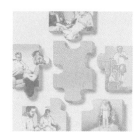

REVIEWERS

Evelyn Cesarotti, PhD, FNP
Assistant Professor
School of Nursing
Arizona State University
Tempe, Arizona

Elizabeth A. Cutezo, RN, MS
Theory & Clinical Instructor
School of Nursing
Pennsylvania State University
University Park, Pennsylvania

Teri Gorman, RN, MS
Associate Professor
Department of Nursing
California State University, Hayward
Hayward, California

Philip A. Greiner, DNSc, RN
Assistant Professor
Director, Health Promotion Center
Fairfield University
Fairfield, Connecticut

Corazon R. Lafuente, DNSc, RN
Associate Professor of Nursing
School of Nursing
Louisiana State University Medical Center
New Orleans, Louisiana

Sara J. Boskovich, RN, DNSc
Practitioner
College of Nursing
Rush University
Chicago, Illinois

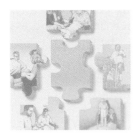

PREFACE

This book reflects more than a century of community health nursing in the United States. The year 1993 marked the 100th anniversary of the founding of the Henry Street Settlement, the beginning of modern American community health nursing practice. Since then, the work of community health nurses has led to improved health among individuals, families, and population groups. In this textbook, the contributors and I have tried to distill the wisdom and expertise of community health nurses who have practiced during the past century and use it to guide and direct future generations of community health nurses.

We are now at a time when health care delivery is increasingly focused on the community. The singular breadth and depth of the specialty requires that community health nurses have a wide knowledge base. They need to know something about everything—from the ethics and economics of health care resource allocation, to the influence of culture on health, to the best means of promoting health and preventing the spread of communicable disease, to treating constipation in a newborn. Knowledge must be theoretically and scientifically sound, yet practical and applicable to changing professional demands. This book has been written to give students a strong, balanced foundation for community health nursing.

Nursing in the Community: Dimensions of Community Health Nursing is written for all students in community health nursing courses and provides a thorough introduction to all aspects of the specialty. The book is designed to prepare nurse generalists who can function in any setting, providing care to individuals, families, and population groups.

Each unit in this third edition is introduced by the poetry of a community health nurse, Veneta Masson. Her verses reflect some of the realities of day-to-day community health nursing practice. The following dialogue between nurse and client is excerpted from one of Ms. Masson's poems and portrays a home visit. Throughout the text the poetry presents other intimate glimpses of individual clients and the profession for the student to ponder.

> Guess what today is Maggie.
>   What is today? I prod
>   tense with expectation
>   as her fingers tighten round her empty
>   wallet.
> Why, I reckon . . . Well, praise the Lord!
>   It must be the first of the
>   month and my check come!
>   No, Maggie, it's Christmas Eve.
>   I came to wish you Merry Christmas.
>   Sorry.
> She fumbles with the stale debris
>   of yesterday's carry-out sandwich.
>   That so? she says, wiping the wreath
>   of crumbs from her month.
>   And here I thought it was the
>   first of the month.

▶ THE APPROACH

A unique feature of this textbook is the Dimensions Model used to structure the discussion of community health nursing, incorporating principles of both public health science and nursing. Use of the Dimensions Model follows the five-step nursing process, but encompasses an epidemiologic perspective in assessing factors that contribute to health or illness and emphasizes the public health concept of levels of prevention. The model consists of three major elements: the dimensions of nursing, health, and health care. The dimensions of nursing element encompasses the knowledge, attitudes, and skills used for community health nursing practice in a variety of settings and with a variety of clients with differing health needs. Specific dimensions of nursing addressed include the cognitive dimension, the interpersonal dimension, the ethical dimension, the skills dimension, the process dimension, and the reflective dimension. Students are introduced to these dimensions as they relate to specific areas of community health nursing practice. For example, advocacy issues relevant to inmates are addressed as an important element of the ethical dimension in the chapter dealing with correctional health care. In the cognitive dimension, educational preparation for effective school health nursing is addressed in the chapter on health care in the school setting.

The dimensions of health element provides an organizational framework for assessing the health of clients (individuals, families, groups, or communities) and the factors that influence clients' health status. The model examines health and illness from the perspective of six dimensions of health: the biophysical, psychological, physical, social, behavioral, and health system dimensions. For example, in the chapter dealing with communicable diseases, students become aware of factors in each dimension that influence the development of childhood diseases, sexually transmitted diseases, hepatitis, tuberculosis, and influenza.

The third element of the Dimensions Model, the dimensions of health care, addresses the levels of primary prevention, secondary prevention, and tertiary prevention. The levels of prevention are used to direct planning, implementation, and evaluation of nursing care. In each chapter, students are acquainted with nursing interventions for each level of prevention relevant to the chapter topic. Again, using the chapter on communicable diseases as an example, students are introduced to primary preventive measures for the control of childhood diseases, as well as secondary and tertiary prevention measures that community health nurses may employ.

The model is introduced in Chapter 5, and each subsequent chapter uses the model to organize content related to the topic. In addition, case studies at the end of each chapter assist students to apply the concepts of the model to typical community health nursing situations. In each chapter, students apply the principles of both public health science and professional nursing to community health nursing practice. Use of the model helps students to observe the melding of the two disciplines. Through the understanding that results, students are prepared to employ the principles of both in practice.

Nursing in the Community: Dimensions of Community Health Nursing is designed to foster critical thinking. The consistent use of the Dimensions Model encourages students to identify links between health problems and contributing factors and to design nursing interventions that are appropriate for each client situation. Critical thinking is fostered by case studies and questions for critical thinking found at the end of each chapter. Students are also given the opportunity to apply skills in critical thinking to nursing research through the presentation of research findings and associated thought questions in each chapter.

▶ ORGANIZATION

Nursing in the Community: Dimensions of Community Health Nursing is organized in six units:

- Contexts
- Processes
- Influences
- Clients
- Settings
- Problems

The first three units address the general concepts of community health nursing practice; Unit IV examines specific client groups; Unit V, specialized settings; and Unit VI focuses on solving commonly encountered community health problems.

Unit I traces community health nursing practice from its historical roots to its current status. Because the health of groups of people is the underlying focus of all community health nursing, the community context is addressed in the first chapter. Readers are introduced to the concept of communities, or population groups, as the recipients of care, rather than individuals or families. The unit proceeds with the historical development of public health practice, the structure of the American health care system, and an examination of the roles and functions of community health nurses. Unit I concludes with a description of the Dimensions Model and an exploration of other nursing and non-nursing models that may be used by community health nurses.

Unit II, The Process Dimension of Community Health Nursing, first explores the *nursing process* in community health nursing practice (Chapter 7) and then fundamental concepts of epidemiology (Chapter 8). Chapter 8 applies the Dimensions Model specifically to health promotion in the community.

The remainder of the chapters in Unit II present other processes essential to community health nursing: health education; the home visit and home health nursing; case management; change, leadership, and group processes, and the political process.

Unit III examines social and environmental influences on the dimensions of health in population groups. Economic factors are an example of social dimension influences (Chapter 14). Community health nurses need to understand how economics influence health and illness, as well as the financing of current and projected modes of health care.

Chapter 15 examines ethics in health care delivery. The ethical decision making that is discussed is related to individuals, families, and groups of people. The emphasis, however, is on the ethical dilemmas that one confronts in providing nursing care for population groups—the dilemmas that occur when values conflict.

The cultural practices of population groups in the United States not surprisingly influence health care delivery. This is illustrated in Chapter 16 where the general principles of transcultural nursing are reviewed. Content focuses on providing community health nursing care for clients from another culture from the perspective of the Dimensions Model.

In Chapter 17, environmental issues of concern in community health are addressed as well as nursing interventions to modify adverse environmental influences.

In **Unit IV**, Care of Clients, the general concepts and principles presented in earlier units focus on target populations. The Dimension Model is applied to families and communities (target groups), children, women, men, the elderly, and the homeless.

Unit V examines how care is provided in specialized settings: schools, workplaces, rural communities, and correctional and disaster settings. Although the principles of practice are the same in all, chapters within the unit elucidate how those principles are modified in different settings.

Unit VI focuses on communicable diseases, chronic physical and mental health problems, substance abuse, and violence.

▶ **SPECIAL FEATURES OF THE BOOK**

National Health Objectives for the Year 2000

Among the continuing features in the third edition of the textbook is a summary listing of the national health objectives that have been specified for the year 2000. The extent of progress toward the objectives is discussed in the evaluation section of relevant chapters.

Chapter Structure

Each chapter in *Nursing in the Community: Dimensions of Community Health Nursing* includes:

- **Chapter Objectives** which summarize important points and assist the reader in identifying key issues discussed.

- **Key Terms** also direct readers' attention to critical issues explained throughout the chapter.
- **Numerous Tables, Figures, and Information Boxes** provide concise compilations of material as well as visual aids in understanding concepts.
- **Assessment Tips** include a series of questions that help the reader to assess the dimensions of health relevant to specific client population and practice settings.
- **Critical Thinking in Research** boxes are designed to enhance readers' abilities to critically evaluate research studies and their implications for community health nursing practice. Questions that follow a brief description of a research study also assist readers to grasp principles of research design and execution.
- **Critical Thinking in Practice: A Case in Point** provides a case study reflecting to the chapter topic followed by questions sure to evoke critical thinking among readers.
- **Testing Your Understanding** includes challenging chapter review questions aimed at stimulating reader thought and discussion of important chapter topics. Each question is followed by page references for quick review.
- **What Do You Think? Questions for Critical Thinking** asks chapter related questions that force the reader to go beyond the content and apply chapter topics to their own community situations.
- **References** include the most up-to-date topics and provide a wide range of supplementary material for the reader.
- **Resource Listings** provide the reader with additional resources of information for more in-depth study of specific chapter topics. Organization names and addresses can put the reader in direct contact with key research and support organizations.

Recommended Readings

Following the final chapter, an extensive bibliography describes pertinent publications not included in the references cited for each chapter. Additional titles are suggested for every chapter.

Appendices

The 21 appendices include assessment tools and other information that can be used by students in clinical practice. Each tool is adapted to the Dimensions Model and reflects the principles of community health nursing discussed in the text. Among the new appendices in the third edition are the summary of national health objectives, recommended screening procedures, special assessment considerations for work and correctional settings, and information on several risk assessment tools. Other appendices include assessment and planning guides for specific client populations, information about selected communicable and chronic diseases, suspected child and spouse or elder abuse report forms, and a Political Astuteness Inventory. Each appendix can also be used by the instructor as the basis for class discussion or clinical learning experiences.

Computer Disk

Nursing in the Community: Dimensions of Community Health Nursing is packaged with a computer disk that includes additional information and tools to apply principles of community health nursing in practice. The disk contains the Chapter Highlights and information needed to answer the questions posed in the Testing Your Understanding section of the textbook. Readers are also presented with a series of multiple choice questions with answers and rationales that test a student's ability to apply principles presented in each chapter.

The disk also contains three global assessment tools for:

- individual clients
- families
- population groups

These tools are designed so students can tailor them to the assessment needs of a particular client. Using the disk, students can design and print a customized assessment tool to fit any practice situation.

▶ THE CHALLENGE OF THE NEXT CENTURY

The overall approach of this book is to convey to nursing students on the brink of the 21st century the excitement and challenge of providing nursing care in the community. As we begin a new era of community health nursing, I believe that well-educated community health nurses can provide a focal point for positive change in the public's health. Early community health nurses changed the face of society, and we can be a strong force in molding the society of the future. I am convinced that when the bicentennial anniversary of community health nursing occurs in 2093, community health nurses will be able to look back on the accomplishments of our second century with as much pride as the first.

▶ TEACHING SUPPORT

The **Instructor's Manual** which accompanies *Nursing in the Community: Dimensions of Community Health Nursing* supplements the teaching supports that are provided in the text itself. The Instructor's Manual will facilitate the use of the text in a variety of community health curricula and maximize student learning. The Instructor's Manual includes the following features:

- **Key Terms** provided in the core text.
- **Chapter Outlines** which pinpoint the main issues discussed throughout the chapter.
- **Learning Objectives** which provide instructors with student goals for each chapter.
- **Suggested teaching strategies** that actively involve students and help bring community health nursing alive.
- **Discussion Topics** which will evoke active student participation in the classroom.
- **Answers to Critical Thinking in Practice: A Case in Point** which help the instructor to moderate class discussions or correct written case analyses by students.
- **Test Questions** provided along with rationales for the correct answers. These questions are also provided on an IBM formatted diskette packaged with the Instructor's Manual.
- **Transparency Masters** of the figures provided in the core text are included in the back of the Instructor's Manual. Each master is specially designed for easy readability on an overhead projector, and the pages are perforated for convenience.

The Instructor's Manual and the test bank are available for faculty upon adoption of *Nursing in the Community: Dimensions of Community Health Nursing.*

▶ ALSO OF INTEREST TO STUDENTS

The *Community Health Nursing Handbook* by Clark is also available from Appleton & Lange. The Handbook is designed to further assist students in translating the theoretical principles presented in the textbook into community health nursing practice. The handbook is a portable, easily accessible reference for students in clinical practice settings and provides additional assessment tools for students to use. The handbook also provides a synopsis of pertinent information students are likely to need in clinical practice.

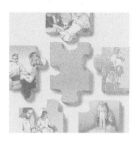

GUIDE TO KEY FEATURES

Key Terms

Key Terms list the important vocabulary covered in each chapter. At the point of introduction within the chapter, each term is set in boldface type.

28
CHAPTER

▶ KEY TERMS

CARE OF CLIENTS IN CORRECTIONAL SETTINGS

detainees
jail
juvenile detention facility
prison
TB prophylaxis

The correctional facility is a relatively new practice setting for community health nursing compared to the settings discussed in previous chapters. Correctional nursing, however, is congruent with the primary focus of community health nursing, the health of groups of people, and offers a challenging position for the community health nurse who wishes to expand the frontiers of nursing practice. Corrections nursing frequently involves challenges not encountered in other community health nursing settings. As noted by one author, "Health in prisons is a product of the demographic characteristics of prisoners and the health behaviors that they bring with them into the prison environment. It is influence within prison by the built environment, the regime, and the organizational culture of the prison, and is dependent on the connections that prisoners maintain with the environment outside" (Squires, 1996).

Correctional nursing takes place in three general types of facilities, prisons, jails, and juvenile detention facilities (American Nurses Association, 1995). *Prisons* are state and federal facilities that house persons convicted of crimes, usually those sentenced for longer than one year. Local or county facilities are usually called *jails* and house both convicted inmates and detainees. *Detainees* are people who have not yet been convicted of a crime. They are being detained pending a trial either because they cannot pay the set bail, or because no bail has been set (Kay, 1991). Juvenile detention facilities may house children and adolescents convicted of crimes and those who are awaiting trial but who cannot be released in the custody of a responsible adult. Jails and juvenile detention facilities tend to be smaller and house fewer inmates than prisons.

Whatever the size of the facility or the terminology used, nurses working in correctional facilities must be committed to the belief that inmates retain their individual rights as human beings despite incarceration and that they have the same rights to health care as other individuals. Society does not categorically deprive any other group of individuals of access to adequate health care. In fact, there are carefully monitored standards of health care in such institutions as nursing homes, mental health facilities, and orphanages. It has only been as recently as 1975, however, that a pro-

Chapter Objectives

Chapter Objectives identify essential learning concepts, stimulate thought and assist students in reviewing chapter content.

686   UNIT V. THE DIMENSIONS MODEL IN SPECIALIZED SETTINGS

Chapter Objectives

After reading this chapter, you should be able to:

- Identify at least three reasons for providing health care in correctional settings.
- Describe at least three elements of the ethnical dimension of nursing in correctional settings.
- Differentiate between basic and advanced nursing practice in correctional settings.
- Identify at least three biophysical dimension elements influencing the health status of inmates.
- Describe at least four major considerations in assessing the psychological dimension of health in correctional settings.
- Discuss at least three aspects of the behavioral dimension that influence health in correctional settings.
- Identify three aspects of primary prevention in correctional settings.
- Describe two approaches to secondary prevention in correctional settings.
- Discuss two considerations in tertiary prevention in correctional settings.

▶ **THE NEED FOR HEALTH CARE IN CORRECTIONAL SETTINGS**

Health care in correctional facilities is an appropriate endeavor for several reasons. First, the right to adequate health care is a constitutionally recognized right arising from the Eighth Amendment which prohibits "cruel and unusual punishment" of those convicted of crimes. Detainees also have a constitutional right to health care under the Fifth and Fourteenth Amendments which prohibit punishment of any kind without "due process" which means conviction through the normal legal processes of the nation. In the case of both convicted inmates and detainees, "deliberate indifference" to serious illness or injury is interpreted as unusual punishment (*Estelle v. Gamble*, cited in Kay, 1991).

In addition to the constitutional right to health care, correctional care is good common sense for a variety of other reasons. Because of poverty, lower education levels, and unhealthy lifestyles that frequently involve substance abuse, inmates may enter a correctional facility with significant health problems (Shields & de Moya, 1997). Because many of these individuals cannot afford to pay for care on the outside, the cost of care will be borne by society. Societal costs for this care will be less if interventions occur in a

timely fashion, before they become severe. Provision of care within the correctional facility also saves taxpayers the cost of personnel and vehicles to transport inmates to other health care facilities. Primary prevention in correctional settings is also cost-effective.

Another possible societal cost of failure to provide adequate health care to inmates lies in the potential for the spread of communicable disease from correctional facilities to the community. Environmental conditions and behaviors within correctional facilities lend themselves to the transmission of communicable diseases such as tuberculosis (Koo, Baron, & Rutherford, 1997), HIV infection (Polych & Sabo, 1995), hepatitis B (National Commission on Correctional Health Care, 1997b), and other sexually transmitted diseases (Beltrami, Cohen, Hamrick, & Farley, 1997). In fact, correctional facilities have been described as a "pocket of risk" for communicable disease (Polych & Sabo, 1995). The more than 22 million admissions and

▶ **STANDARDS FOR NURSING PRACTICE IN CORRECTIONAL SETTINGS**

Standards of Care: The nurse:
- collects client health data
- analyzes assessment data in determining diagnoses
- identifies expected outcomes individualized to the client
- develops a care plan that prescribes interventions to attain expected outcomes
- implements the interventions identified in the care plan
- evaluates the client's progress toward attainment of outcomes

Standards of Professional Performance: The nurse:
- systematically evaluates the quality and effectiveness of nursing practice
- evaluates his/her own nursing practice in relation to professional practice standards and evaluates statutes and regulations
- acquires and maintains current knowledge in nursing practice
- contributes to the professional development of peers, colleagues, and others
- determines decisions and actions on behalf of the client in an ethical manner
- collaborates with the client, significant others, other criminal justice system personnel, and health care providers in providing client care
- uses research findings in practice
- considers factors related to safety, effectiveness, and cost in planning and delivering client care

(Source: American Nurses Association, 1995.)

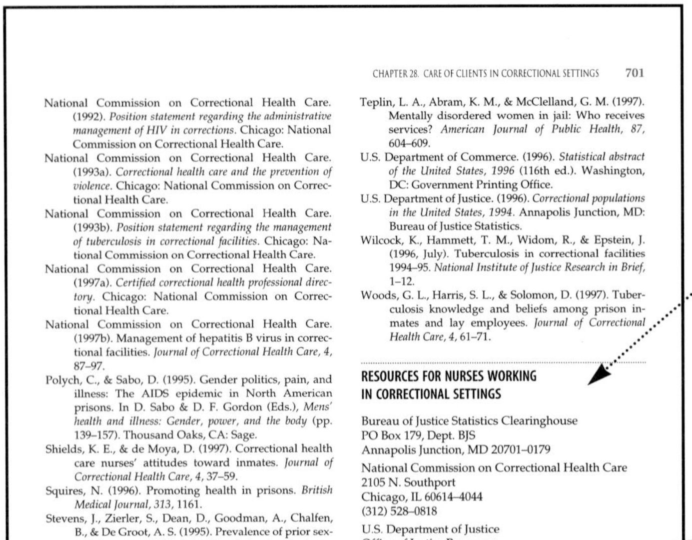

CHAPTER 28. CARE OF CLIENTS IN CORRECTIONAL SETTINGS 701

National Commission on Correctional Health Care. (1992). *Position statement regarding the administrative management of HIV in corrections.* Chicago: National Commission on Correctional Health Care.
National Commission on Correctional Health Care. (1993a). *Correctional health care and the prevention of violence.* Chicago: National Commission on Correctional Health Care.
National Commission on Correctional Health Care. (1993b). *Position statement regarding the management of tuberculosis in correctional facilities.* Chicago: National Commission on Correctional Health Care.
National Commission on Correctional Health Care. (1997a). *Certified correctional health professional directory.* Chicago: National Commission on Correctional Health Care.
National Commission on Correctional Health Care. (1997b). Management of hepatitis B virus in correctional facilities. *Journal of Correctional Health Care, 4,* 87–97.
Polych, C., & Sabo, D. (1995). Gender politics, pain, and illness: The AIDS epidemic in North American prisons. In D. Sabo & D. F. Gordon (Eds.), *Mens' health and illness: Gender, power, and the body* (pp. 139–157). Thousand Oaks, CA: Sage.
Shields, K. E., & de Moya, D. (1997). Correctional health care nurses' attitudes toward inmates. *Journal of Correctional Health Care, 4,* 37–59.
Squires, N. (1996). Promoting health in prisons. *British Medical Journal, 313,* 1161.
Stevens, J., Zierler, S., Dean, D., Goodman, A., Chalfen, B., & De Groot, A. S. (1995). Prevalence of prior sexual abuse and HIV risk-taking behaviors in incarcerated women in Massachusetts. *Journal of Correctional Health Care, 2,* 137–149.
Teplin, L. A., Abram, K. M., & McClelland, G. M. (1997). Mentally disordered women in jail: Who receives services? *American Journal of Public Health, 87,* 604–609.
U.S. Department of Commerce. (1996). *Statistical abstract of the United States, 1996* (116th ed.). Washington, DC: Government Printing Office.
U.S. Department of Justice. (1996). *Correctional populations in the United States, 1994.* Annapolis Junction, MD: Bureau of Justice Statistics.
Wilcock, K., Hammett, T. M., Widom, R., & Epstein, J. (1996, July). Tuberculosis in correctional facilities 1994–95. *National Institute of Justice Research in Brief,* 1–12.
Woods, G. L., Harris, S. L., & Solomon, D. (1997). Tuberculosis knowledge and beliefs among prison inmates and lay employees. *Journal of Correctional Health Care, 4,* 61–71.

RESOURCES FOR NURSES WORKING IN CORRECTIONAL SETTINGS

Bureau of Justice Statistics Clearinghouse
PO Box 179, Dept. BJS
Annapolis Junction, MD 20701–0179

National Commission on Correctional Health Care
2105 N. Southport
Chicago, IL 60614–4044
(312) 528–0818

U.S. Department of Justice
Office of Justice Programs
National Institute of Justice

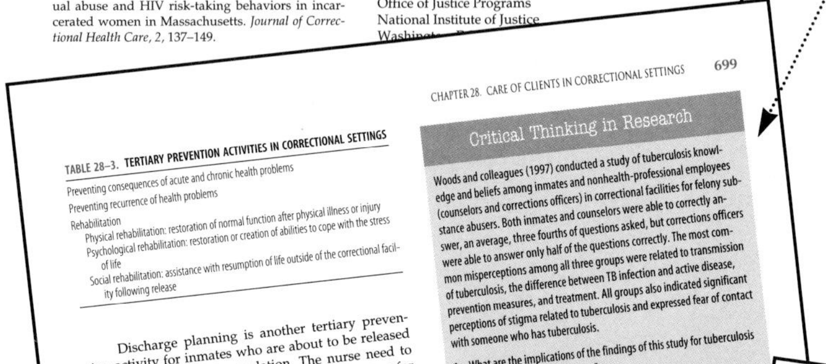

CHAPTER 28. CARE OF CLIENTS IN CORRECTIONAL SETTINGS 699

TABLE 28–3. TERTIARY PREVENTION ACTIVITIES IN CORRECTIONAL SETTINGS

Preventing consequences of acute and chronic health problems
Preventing recurrence of health problems
Rehabilitation
Physical rehabilitation: restoration of normal function after physical illness or injury
Psychological rehabilitation: restoration or creation of abilities to cope with the stress of life
Social rehabilitation: assistance with resumption of life outside of the correctional facility following release

Discharge planning is another tertiary prevention activity for inmates who are about to be released back into the general population. The nurse need to make arrangements for continuing care or arrange for housing or other survival needs. Nurses may also assist clients to anticipate and deal with some of the difficulties that are likely to arise with reintegration into families or communities after prolonged absences. Discharge planning and continuity of care are particularly important for clients experiencing ongoing chronic conditions or communicable diseases such as tuberculosis and HIV infection. Table 28–3 summarizes tertiary prevention emphases in correctional health care.

Critical Thinking in Research

Woods and colleagues (1997) conducted a study of tuberculosis knowledge and beliefs among inmates and nonhealth-professional employees (counselors and corrections officers) in correctional facilities for felony substance abusers. Both inmates and counselors were able to correctly answer, an average, three fourths of questions asked, but corrections officers were able to answer only half of the questions correctly. The most common misperceptions among all three groups were related to transmission of tuberculosis, the difference between TB infection and active disease, prevention measures, and treatment. All groups also indicated significant perceptions of stigma related to tuberculosis and expressed fear of contact with someone who has tuberculosis.

1. What are the implications of the findings of this study for tuberculosis control in correctional settings?
2. What nursing interventions could minimize the effects of misperceptions on TB control efforts? Would the interventions differ for the three groups involved? Why or why not?
3. Do you think the findings of this study would be any different if it was conducted with the general public? Why or why not? How might you go about replicating this study with the general public?

Evaluating Health Care in Correctional Settings

The principles that guide the evaluation of health care in correctional settings are the same as those applied in other settings. The nurse evaluates the outcomes of care for individual clients in light of identified ... Correctional nurses may also be involved in ... ing health outcomes for groups of inmates o... entire facility population, including staff. In ... the nurse examines processes of care and r... ommendations for improvements in terms ... efficiency, and cost-effectiveness.

Critical Thinking in Practice: A Case in Point

You are the only nurse on the night shift in a county jail housing 150 male inmates. A new inmate is admitt... ving under the influence of alcohol. During your initial history and physical, the inmate tells you that he is ... missed his last dialysis appointment which was yesterday. It is Sunday night and your facility does not ha... The dialysis unit at the local hospital does not function on Sundays except in the case of emergencies. Th... in no immediate distress and has normal vital signs and no evidence of edema. He is appropriately alert... odor of obvious alcohol consumption. The watch commander tells you he has no one to spare to transp... pital and if he goes, it will have to be by private ambulance. Your back-up physician is out of town for ... call physician is tied up with an emergency.

1. What are the biophysical, psychological, physical, social, behavioral, and health system factors ...
2. What are your nursing diagnoses? How would you prioritize those diagnoses?
3. What action would you take in this situation? Why?

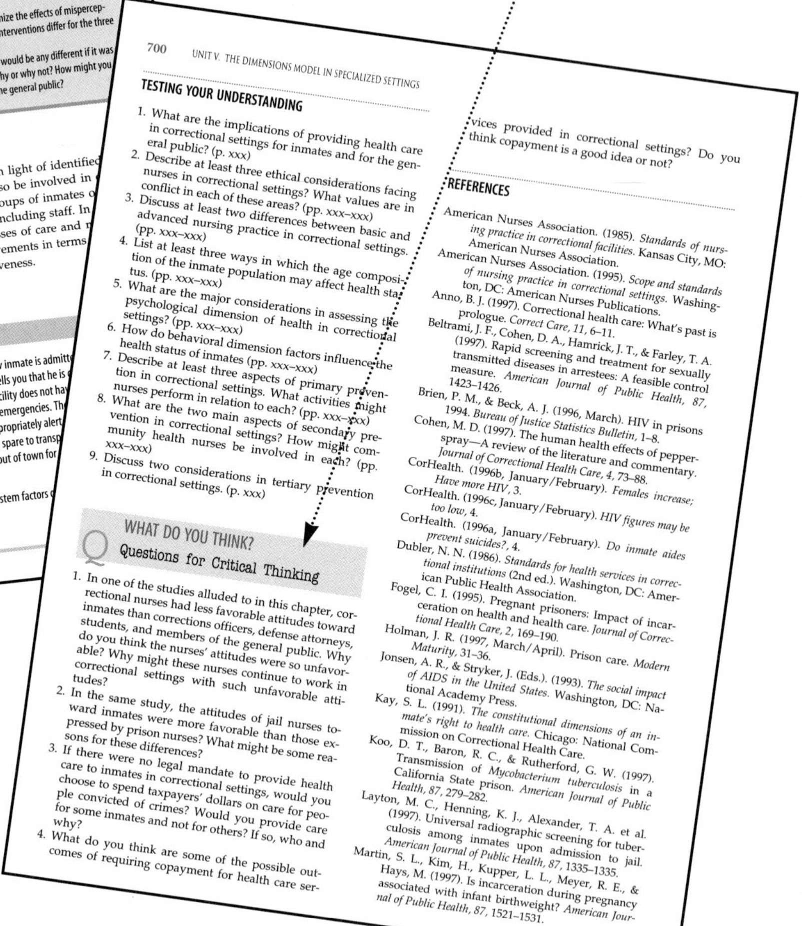

700 UNIT V. THE DIMENSIONS MODEL IN SPECIALIZED SETTINGS

TESTING YOUR UNDERSTANDING

1. What are the implications of providing health care in correctional settings for inmates and for the general public? (p. xxx)
2. Describe at least three ethical considerations facing nurses in correctional settings? What values are in conflict in each of these areas? (pp. xxx–xxx)
3. Discuss at least two differences between basic and advanced nursing practice in correctional settings. (pp. xxx–xxx)
4. List at least three ways in which the age composition of the inmate population may affect health status. (pp. xxx–xxx)
5. What are the major considerations in assessing the psychological dimension of health in correctional settings? (pp. xxx–xxx)
6. How do behavioral dimension factors influence the health status of inmates (pp. xxx–xxx)
7. Describe at least three aspects of primary prevention in correctional settings. What activities might nurses perform in relation to each? (pp. xxx–xxx)
8. What are the two main aspects of secondary prevention in correctional settings? How might community health nurses be involved in each? (pp. xxx–xxx)
9. Discuss two considerations in tertiary prevention in correctional settings. (p. xxx)

WHAT DO YOU THINK? Questions for Critical Thinking

1. In one of the studies alluded to in this chapter, correctional nurses had less favorable attitudes toward inmates than corrections officers, defense attorneys, students, and members of the general public. Why do you think the nurses' attitudes were so unfavorable? Why might these nurses continue to work in correctional settings with such unfavorable attitudes?
2. In the same study, the attitudes of jail nurses toward inmates were more favorable than those expressed by prison nurses? What might be some reasons for these differences?
3. If there were no legal mandate to provide health care to inmates in correctional settings, would you choose to spend taxpayers' dollars on care for people convicted of crimes? Would you provide care for some inmates and not for others? If so, who and why?
4. What do you think are some of the possible outcomes of requiring copayment for health care services provided in correctional settings? Do you think copayment is a good idea or not?

REFERENCES

American Nurses Association. (1985). *Standards of nursing practice in correctional facilities.* Kansas City, MO: American Nurses Association.
American Nurses Association. (1995). *Scope and standards of nursing practice in correctional settings.* Washington, DC: American Nurses Publications.
Anno, B. J. (1997). Correctional health care: What's past is prologue. *Correct Care, 11,* 6–11.
Beltrami, J. F., Cohen, D. A., Hamrick, J. T., & Farley, T. A. (1997). Rapid screening and treatment for sexually transmitted diseases in arrestees: A feasible control measure. *American Journal of Public Health, 87,* 1423–1426.
Brien, P. M., & Beck, A. J. (1996, March). HIV in prisons 1994. *Bureau of Justice Statistics Bulletin,* 1–8.
Cohen, M. D. (1997). The human health effects of pepper-spray—A review of the literature and commentary. *Journal of Correctional Health Care, 4,* 73–88.
CorHealth. (1996b, January/February). *Females increase; Have more HIV,* 3.
CorHealth. (1996c, January/February). *HIV figures may be too low,* 4.
CorHealth. (1996a, January/February). *Do inmate aides prevent suicides?,* 4.
Dubler, N. N. (1986). *Standards for health services in correctional institutions* (2nd ed.). Washington, DC: American Public Health Association.
Fogel, C. I. (1995). Pregnant prisoners: Impact of incarceration on health and health care. *Journal of Correctional Health Care, 2,* 169–190.
Holman, J. R. (1997, March/April). Prison care. *Modern Maturity, 31*–36.
Jonsen, A. R., & Stryker, J. (Eds.). (1993). *The social impact of AIDS in the United States.* Washington, DC: National Academy Press.
Kay, S. L. (1991). *The constitutional dimensions of an inmate's right to health care.* Chicago: National Commission on Correctional Health Care.
Koo, D. T., Baron, R. C., & Rutherford, G. W. (1997). Transmission of *Mycobacterium tuberculosis* in a California State prison. *American Journal of Public Health, 87,* 279–282.
Layton, M. C., Henning, K. J., Alexander, T. A. et al. (1997). Universal radiographic screening for tuberculosis among inmates upon admission to jail. *American Journal of Public Health, 87,* 1335–1335.
Martin, S. L., Kim, H., Kupper, L. L., Meyer, R. E., & Hays, M. (1997). Is incarceration during pregnancy associated with infant birthweight? *American Journal of Public Health, 87,* 1521–1531.

Resource Listings

Resource Listings include names and addresses of agencies and organizations that may provide additional information to students and community health nurses about a variety of topics.

Critical Thinking in Research

Critical Thinking in Research presents a brief summary of findings from research studies followed by questions to critically evaluate the research and its implications for community health nursing.

What Do You Think? Questions for Critical Thinking

What Do You Think? includes several questions that promote critical thinking and insight on the part of the reader.

Critical Thinking in Practice: A Case in Point

Critical Thinking in Practice: A Case in Point presents a case study related to the chapter topic, and helps students to apply community health nursing principles to actual practice situations. Questions follow that stimulate critical thinking.

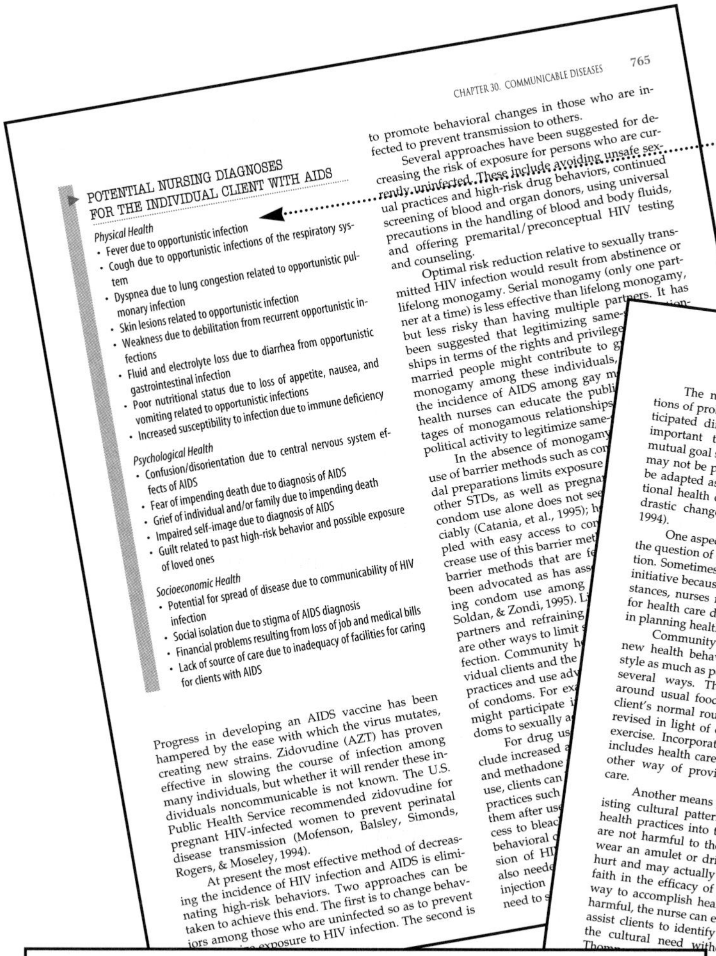

CHAPTER 30. COMMUNICABLE DISEASES 765

POTENTIAL NURSING DIAGNOSES FOR THE INDIVIDUAL CLIENT WITH AIDS

Physical Health
- Fever due to opportunistic infection
- Cough due to opportunistic infections of the respiratory system
- Dyspnea due to lung congestion related to opportunistic pulmonary infection
- Skin lesions related to opportunistic infection
- Weakness due to debilitation from recurrent opportunistic infections
- Fluid and electrolyte loss due to diarrhea from opportunistic gastrointestinal infection
- Poor nutritional status due to loss of appetite, nausea, and vomiting related to opportunistic infections
- Increased susceptibility to infection due to immune deficiency

Psychological Health
- Confusion/disorientation due to central nervous system effects of AIDS
- Fear of impending death due to diagnosis of AIDS
- Grief of individual and/or family due to impending death
- Impaired self-image due to diagnosis of AIDS
- Guilt related to past high-risk behavior and possible exposure of loved ones

Socioeconomic Health
- Potential for spread of disease due to communicability of HIV infection
- Social isolation due to stigma of AIDS diagnosis
- Financial problems resulting from loss of job and medical bills
- Lack of source of care due to inadequacy of facilities for caring for clients with AIDS

Progress in developing an AIDS vaccine has been hampered by the ease with which the virus mutates, creating new strains. Zidovudine (AZT) has proven effective in slowing the course of infection among many individuals, but whether it will render these individuals noncommunicable is not known. The U.S. Public Health Service recommended zidovudine for pregnant HIV-infected women to prevent perinatal disease transmission (Mofenson, Balsley, Simonds, Rogers, & Moseley, 1994).

At present the most effective method of decreasing the incidence of HIV infection and AIDS is eliminating high-risk behaviors. Two approaches can be taken to achieve this end. The first is to change behaviors among those who are uninfected so as to prevent ... exposure to HIV infection. The second is to promote behavioral changes in those who are infected to prevent transmission to others.

Several approaches have been suggested for decreasing the risk of exposure for persons who are currently uninfected. These include avoiding unsafe sexual practices and high-risk drug behaviors, continued screening of blood and organ donors, using universal precautions in the handling of blood and body fluids, and offering premarital/preconceptual HIV testing and counseling.

Optimal risk reduction relative to sexually transmitted HIV infection would result from abstinence or lifelong monogamy. Serial monogamy (only one partner at a time) is less effective than lifelong monogamy, but less risky than having multiple partners. It has been suggested that legitimizing same-... ships in terms of the rights and privilege... married people might contribute to g... monogamy among these individuals, ... the incidence of AIDS among gay m... health nurses can educate the publi... tages of monogamous relationships... political activity to legitimize same-...

In the absence of monogamy... use of barrier methods such as con... dal preparations limits exposure... other STDs, as well as pregna... condom use alone does not see... ciably (Catania, et al., 1995); h... pled with easy access to co... crease use of this barrier met... barrier methods that are fe... been advocated as has ass... ing condom use among ... Soldan, & Zondi, 1995). L... partners and refraining... are other ways to limit ... fection. Community h... vidual clients and the ... practices and use adv... of condoms. For ex... might participate i... doms to sexually a...

For drug us... clude increased ... and methadone ... use, clients can ... practices such ... them after use ... cess to bleac... behavioral ... sion of HI... also neede... injection ... need to s...

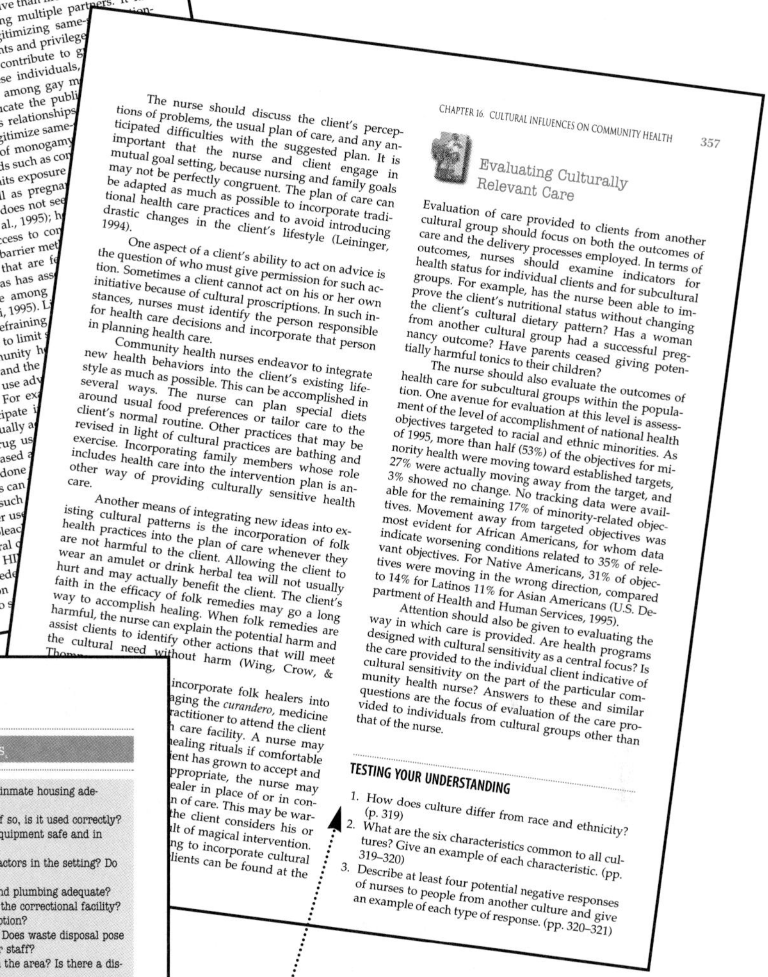

CHAPTER 16. CULTURAL INFLUENCES ON COMMUNITY HEALTH 357

The nurse should discuss the client's perceptions of problems, the usual plan of care, and any anticipated difficulties with the suggested plan. It is important that the nurse and client engage in mutual goal setting, because nursing and family goals may not be perfectly congruent. The plan of care can be adapted as much as possible to incorporate traditional health care practices and to avoid introducing drastic changes in the client's lifestyle (Leininger, 1994).

One aspect of a client's ability to act on advice is the question of who must give permission for such action. Sometimes a client cannot act on his or her own initiative because of cultural proscriptions. In such instances, nurses must identify the person responsible for health care decisions and incorporate that person in planning health care.

Community health nurses endeavor to integrate new health behaviors into the client's existing lifestyle as much as possible. This can be accomplished in several ways. The nurse can plan special diets around usual food preferences or tailor care to the client's normal routine. Other practices that may be revised in light of cultural practices are bathing and exercise. Incorporating family members whose role includes health care into the intervention plan is another way of providing culturally sensitive health care.

Another means of integrating new ideas into existing cultural patterns is the incorporation of folk health practices into the plan of care whenever they are not harmful to the client. Allowing the client to wear an amulet or drink herbal tea will not usually hurt and may actually benefit the client. The client's faith in the efficacy of folk remedies may go a long way to accomplish healing. When folk remedies are harmful, the nurse can explain the potential harm and assist clients to identify other actions that will meet the cultural need without harm (Wing, Crow, & Thomp...

... incorporate folk healers into ...aging the *curandero*, medicine ...ractitioner to attend the client ...h care facility. A nurse may ...ealing rituals if comfortable ...ent has grown to accept and ...ppropriate, the nurse may ...ealer in place of or in con...n of care. This may be war...he client considers his or ...lt of magical intervention. ...ng to incorporate cultural ...lients can be found at the

Evaluating Culturally Relevant Care

Evaluation of care provided to clients from another cultural group should focus on both the outcomes of care and the delivery processes employed. In terms of outcomes, nurses should examine indicators of health status for individual clients and for subcultural groups. For example, has the nurse been able to improve the client's nutritional status without changing the client's cultural dietary pattern? Has a woman from another cultural group had a successful pregnancy outcome? Have parents ceased giving potentially harmful tonics to their children?

The nurse should also evaluate the outcomes of health care for subcultural groups within the population. One avenue for evaluation at this level is assessment of the level of accomplishment of national health objectives targeted to racial and ethnic minorities. As of 1995, more than half (53%) of the objectives for minority health were moving toward established targets, 27% were actually moving away from the target, and 3% showed no change. No tracking data were available for the remaining 17% of minority-related objectives. Movement away from targeted objectives was most evident for African Americans, for whom data indicate worsening conditions related to 35% of relevant objectives. For Native Americans, 31% of objectives were moving in the wrong direction, compared to 14% for Latinos 11% for Asian Americans (U.S. Department of Health and Human Services, 1995).

Attention should also be given to evaluating the way in which care is provided. Are health programs designed with cultural sensitivity as a central focus? Is the care provided to the individual client indicative of cultural sensitivity on the part of the particular community health nurse? Answers to these and similar questions are the focus of evaluation of the care provided to individuals from cultural groups other than that of the nurse.

TESTING YOUR UNDERSTANDING

1. How does culture differ from race and ethnicity? (p. 319)
2. What are the six characteristics common to all cultures? Give an example of each characteristic. (pp. 319–320)
3. Describe at least four potential negative responses of nurses to people from another culture and give an example of each type of response. (pp. 320–321)

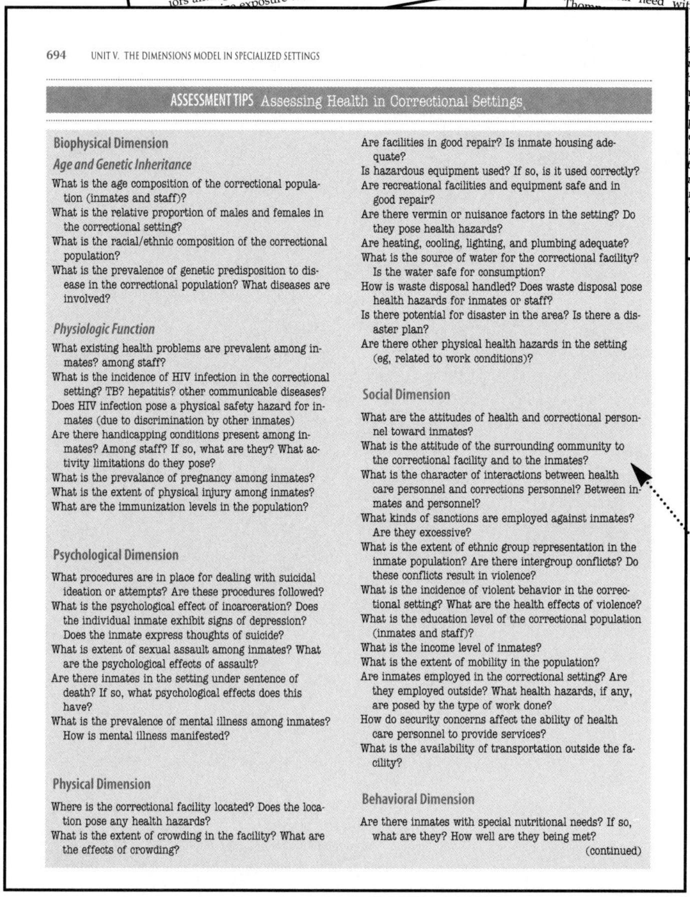

694 UNIT V. THE DIMENSIONS MODEL IN SPECIALIZED SETTINGS

ASSESSMENT TIPS Assessing Health in Correctional Settings

Biophysical Dimension

Age and Genetic Inheritance

What is the age composition of the correctional population (inmates and staff)?
What is the relative proportion of males and females in the correctional setting?
What is the racial/ethnic composition of the correctional population?
What is the prevalence of genetic predisposition to disease in the correctional population? What diseases are involved?

Physiologic Function

What existing health problems are prevalent among inmates? among staff?
What is the incidence of HIV infection in the correctional setting? TB? hepatitis? other communicable diseases?
Does HIV infection pose a physical safety hazard for inmates (due to discrimination by other inmates)
Are there handicapping conditions present among inmates? Among staff? If so, what are they? What activity limitations do they pose?
What is the prevalance of pregnancy among inmates?
What is the extent of physical injury among inmates?
What are the immunization levels in the population?

Psychological Dimension

What procedures are in place for dealing with suicidal ideation or attempts? Are these procedures followed?
What is the psychological effect of incarceration? Does the individual inmate exhibit signs of depression? Does the inmate express thoughts of suicide?
What is extent of sexual assault among inmates? What are the psychological effects of assault?
Are there inmates in the setting under sentence of death? If so, what psychological effects does this have?
What is the prevalence of mental illness among inmates? How is mental illness manifested?

Physical Dimension

Where is the correctional facility located? Does the location pose any health hazards?
What is the extent of crowding in the facility? What are the effects of crowding?
Are facilities in good repair? Is inmate housing adequate?
Is hazardous equipment used? If so, is it used correctly?
Are recreational facilities and equipment safe and in good repair?
Are there vermin or nuisance factors in the setting? Do they pose health hazards?
Are heating, cooling, lighting, and plumbing adequate?
What is the source of water for the correctional facility? Is the water safe for consumption?
How is waste disposal handled? Does waste disposal pose health hazards for inmates or staff?
Is there potential for disaster in the area? Is there a disaster plan?
Are there other physical health hazards in the setting (eg, related to work conditions)?

Social Dimension

What are the attitudes of health and correctional personnel toward inmates?
What is the attitude of the surrounding community to the correctional facility and to the inmates?
What is the character of interactions between health care personnel and corrections personnel? Between inmates and personnel?
What kinds of sanctions are employed against inmates? Are they excessive?
What is the extent of ethnic group representation in the inmate population? Are there intergroup conflicts? Do these conflicts result in violence?
What is the incidence of violent behavior in the correctional setting? What are the health effects of violence?
What is the education level of the correctional population (inmates and staff)?
What is the income level of inmates?
What is the extent of mobility in the population?
Are inmates employed in the correctional setting? Are they employed outside? What health hazards, if any, are posed by the type of work done?
How do security concerns affect the ability of health care personnel to provide services?
What is the availability of transportation outside the facility?

Behavioral Dimension

Are there inmates with special nutritional needs? If so, what are they? How well are they being met?

(continued)

Summary Boxes

Summary Boxes assist students to identify key principles in each chapter.

Testing Your Understanding

Testing Your Understanding asks the important questions to assist students in reviewing chapter content. Page references are provided to cross reference information.

Assessment Tips

Assessment Tips direct students in health assessment with particular clients and specific population groups.

THE ARITHMETIC OF NURSES

S-s-s, S-s-s, S-s-s
Bennie Smith is trying to speak
I am counting out cookies
from a faded blue tin.

S-s-s, S-s-s, S-s-s
Twelve!
Are twelve cookies enough to hold
a sick old man for thirty-six hours?
Twelve cookies and one can of juice?
Twelve cookies wrapped in a towel
tucked under a pillow where roaches
ply a brisk trade in crumbs?

Six!
He blurts it out
face lit up by the restless flicker
of the television screen.
No, twelve, I muse.
Unless someone comes
that's all he'll have
till I get back again.

S-s-six thousand!
He strains under the weight of the words.
Clearly he has something important to say
but I am caught up with my own
    calculations—

The number of minutes
it will take a rivulet of urine
to reach the screaming bedsores
on his back

The number of degrees
his temperature will rise
as infection sets in

I tilt my ear toward his mouth
to catch the stutterings

S-s-six thousand nurses …
on strike today …
Meh- Meh- Meh-Minnesota!

Half his face breaks into a grin
for if there's one thing Bennie understands
it's the arithmetic of nurses
and old, abandoned men.

Excerpted with permission from V. Masson (1993) just who. *Washington, DC: Crossroads Health Ministry.*

THE COMMUNITY HEALTH NURSING CONTEXT

Community health nurses have been crusaders in bringing health care to those most in need. Their history has been one of service and advocacy for underserved populations. Through the years, the practice of community health nurses has been shaped by social and historical influences. Today, the health care system within which community health nurses practice has been minimally responsive to the health needs of the total population and the continuing need for change.

In accomplishing change, community health nurses can be prime movers. Effective change is more certain when community health nurses understand the clients and their needs, as well as the factors that led to the current situation. For community health nurses, a client is a group of individuals or a community, and the goal of practice is to improve the health of the total population and its members.

An historical overview (Chapter 2) traces the major events that influenced the development of the health care system, community health, and community health nursing. Community health nurses can profit from knowing where they have been and how they got where they are today. From this information, previous successes and failures to improve health status and health care delivery will become apparent. By understanding both the positive and negative influences on health, mistakes are pinpointed as are those societal forces that can be manipulated to achieve better health for all people.

The health care delivery system (Chapter 3) is plagued by inequity and inefficiency, and the American public is ready for significant change. To foster effective change, community health nurses must understand the current system and identify where change is needed. That information may be gathered by exploring the organization, focus, and function of various components of the system.

This first unit explores clientele, community, and the goal of community health, historical influences, and health care delivery, providing the groundwork upon which to introduce community health nursing. Community health nursing is defined and the roles of community health nurses explored (Chapter 4). In Chapter 5, we explore a model designed specifically for community health nursing practice, and Chapter 6 examines the application of several other models to this practice specialty.

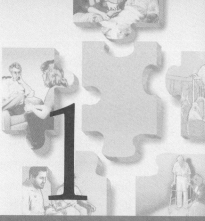

THE COMMUNITY CONTEXT

This book is about community health nursing; however, that does not mean we are going to focus exclusively on the practice of nursing in community settings as opposed to hospitals or other institutions. When we talk about the "community context" of community health nursing, we mean that our primary client is the community itself rather than its individual members.

Sometimes our practice involves individuals and families within the community, but our primary focus is improving the health of the total population group. We want to create healthy communities. When we say that the community is our client, what do we mean? What exactly is a "community"? How can we tell if a community is healthy or unhealthy? What kinds of activities result in a healthy community? The answers to these and similar questions are the focus of this chapter.

▶ Chapter Objectives

After reading this chapter, you should be able to:

- Describe three critical attributes that define a community.
- Distinguish between communities with territorial bonds and those with relational bonds.
- Differentiate among the goals of therapeutic medicine, preventive medicine, and public health practice.
- Discuss the significance of the National Health Objectives for the year 2000.

▶ DEFINING COMMUNITY

Over the years, community has been defined in many ways. Some definitions focus on functions performed by communities. For example, a community has been defined as "a system of formal and informal groups characterized by interdependence and whose function is to meet the collective needs of group members" (Goeppinger, Lassiter, & Wilcox, 1982). Another functional definition describes communities as "wherever the needs of the individual are being met" (Wigley & Cook, 1975).

Other definitions use locale as the basis for community (Harper & Lambert, 1994). For instance, a community is defined as "a social system, a place, and a people" (Josten, 1989). Community is also defined operationally as a group of people in a specific time and place who have a common purpose, the "who," "where and when," and "why and how" of community (Shamansky & Pesznecker, 1981). Another operational definition of community incorporates such components as people, location, social climate, social structure, social activity, and sentiment, as well as the concept of outside influences (Orr, 1992).

The use of place as a defining attribute for community is somewhat problematic, though, if we wish to address certain groups of people as communities. Certainly it would be impractical to consider the aspect of place in defining military veterans as a community, yet we can apply principles of community health to meet the health needs of this group.

In some definitions, the focal point is the existence of commonalities among members of the community. A community has been referred to as "a collection of people who share some important features of their lives or a group of people sharing values and institutions" (Thompson & Kinne, 1990). Similarly, a community has been defined as "a social unit in which there is a transaction of a common life among the people making up the unit" (Green & Anderson, 1986). Some authors define communities as "geographical or interest communities, consisting of relatively small, noninstitutional aggregates of people linked together for common goals or other purposes" (Green & Raeburn, 1990). Other authors take the more eclectic view that community can be "defined in terms of either geography or special interests" (Williams, 1988). The variety of definitions of community is further exemplified in the definition selected by the National Institute for Nursing Research (NINR) Priority Expert Panel (1995) in its report on nursing strategies for community-based practice. This group chose to define community as "a neighborhood, entire town, school, prison, or worksite, or . . . groups of persons that share similar characteristics such as lifestyle, culture, or religion."

Critical Attributes of Communities

Although the definitions of community are diverse, common elements are found. These elements are a group orientation, a bond between individuals, and human interaction. These are the critical attributes that define a group of people as a community.

Group Orientation

Humans form communities because to do so is advantageous. Through group membership, an individual gains access to skills, services, necessities, and amenities of life that one cannot provide on one's own. For the community to continue to provide these services, it must safeguard its survival. For this reason, communities adopt a group orientation in which the group's needs and goals take priority over those of individual members. Because of this group orientation, communities take collective action with regard to common concerns. For example, an individual may benefit from speeding through an intersection, but speeding does not benefit residents who need to cross a busy street. Through collective action, in the interest of the overall good, the community acts to place a stoplight at the intersection, slowing traffic and ensuring safe crossing for all citizens.

Bond Between Individuals

The second defining attribute of a community is some form of bond between individual members. This bond may take many forms. In some communities, the bond is a common lifestyle. The bond may be shared ethnicity or culture or living in a specific geographic location. In other instances, the bond assumes the form of similar interests, goals, or occupations. The type of bond between members determines the type of community.

Human Interaction

The third critical attribute of a community is some type of human interaction. Significant social interaction must occur between individuals for a community to exist. For example, a number of people may live side by side in an apartment building. They have a bond in their way of life as apartment dwellers and in their common residence. They cannot, however, be considered a community unless they interact with one another. Without social interaction they remain a collection of isolated individuals rather than a community. Such interaction might be visiting back and forth, cooperative babysitting, or unified action on some common grievance.

A Working Definition of Community

Bearing in mind these critical attributes of communities, the following definition can be derived for use in community health nursing. A **community** is a group of people who share some type of bond, who interact with each other, and who function collectively regarding common concerns.

A variety of groups, or aggregates, encountered by community health nurses can be viewed as "communities." **Aggregates** are groups of people with some common characteristic. Aggregates may or may not be communities depending on the presence of the defining attributes. For example, all the people in town with arthritis constitute an aggregate. They have a common bond in their shared disease, but because they do not interact with each other or take collective action on common concerns, they are not a community. If, however, they form an association to work for handicapped access to public buildings, the aggregate becomes a community.

Our working definition of community also helps to decrease a frequently encountered tendency to define community health nursing responsibility in terms of specific cases or political jurisdiction. The activities of community health nurses are not confined to a specific locale but are directed to any group or aggregate with health needs. The entity served by the community health nurse is the total group or aggregate, not only those individuals or families referred for services. This aggregate focus is the hallmark of community health nursing.

► TYPES OF COMMUNITIES

As mentioned previously, the type of bond between group members is a major determinant of the type of community. Two basic categories of bonds unite communities: territorial bonds and relational bonds.

Communities With Territorial Bonds

Territorial bond communities have specifically defined boundaries that may be spatial, temporal, or both. Such bonds reflect the "where" and "when" dimension of the definition of community discussed earlier. Inmates of a county jail, security staff, and ancillary personnel would be a community bound by specific spatial boundaries, the walls of the jail. Likewise, the graduates of Nurse University from 1990 to 2000 constitute a community bound by time relationships. The boundary here excludes graduates from Nurse University prior to 1990, graduates of the class of 2001, and graduates from other programs. Several subtypes of communities exist within the territorial bond category: geopolitical communities, communities of identifiable need, and communities of solution.

Geopolitical Communities

Geopolitical communities are probably most familiar to us. They are communities with defined geographic and jurisdictional boundaries such as towns, cities, and counties. A city is defined by its boundaries, the city limits. Either one lives within the city limits or one does not, so it is easy to decide whether or not one is a member of that particular community. A school of nursing could also be considered a geopolitical community because it typically has specific physical boundaries as well as enrollment boundaries.

Communities of Identifiable Need

The second and third types of territorial bond communities are not quite so well defined in terms of specific boundaries but are closely related to each other. A **community of identifiable need** is the locale within which a particular problem exists, the area that encompasses any type of health problem and its contributing factors (Archer, 1979). This type of community frequently cuts across territorial bounds of one or more geopolitical communities. For example, a river may be polluted by chemicals dumped by an industry in one state but affect drinking water in a large city in another state. The area in which the problem and its contributing factors exist is the community of identifiable need; in this case it includes both states.

Communities of Solution

The **community of solution** has been defined by the National Commission on Community Health Services (1967) as the "boundaries within which a problem can be defined, dealt with, and solved." As with the community of identifiable need, the community of solution does not always coincide with the boundaries of a specific geopolitical community. It may coincide with the community of problem ecology, but frequently does not. In the case of the polluted river, the solution may not lie within the affected area but may require the assistance of the federal Environmental Protection Agency (EPA) and the federal courts.

Figure 1–1 illustrates the three types of territorial bond communities for the water pollution example. The areas bounded by solid lines in the figure represent four geopolitical communities, in this instance, four neighboring states. City C is also a geopolitical community. The broken line encompasses the portions of two states involved in the water pollution problem. This area constitutes the community of identifiable need for *this* problem. The green area represents the community of solution, or the area in which the resources necessary to solve the problem are to be found. In this instance, the community of solution goes beyond the boundaries of the states affected by the problem and involves the federal government.

Communities With Relational Bonds

The second major category of communities, *relational bond communities,* includes groups in which the bond between individuals is a common relationship rather than specific boundaries. There are two types of rela-

tional bond communities: communities of interest orientation and feeling communities.

Communities of Interest Orientation

In the *community of interest orientation,* the relational bond is one of shared interests or goals. Examples of this type of community are the state nurses' association, an ostomy support group, or a right-to-life group. In each instance, members of the group share a common interest or concern, and they use the group to advance that interest.

Feeling Communities

A *feeling community* is one in which the relational bond is an emotional feeling of belonging or camaraderie. One feels at home in one's "neighborhood" or with one's own ethnic group. This is the community in which one has "roots." Your nursing class may be an example of a feeling community. Members of the class are bound together by certain emotional ties or feelings of closeness that arise from shared experiences.

The types of communities discussed here are not mutually exclusive. Any group may simultaneously represent more than one type of community. Take, for

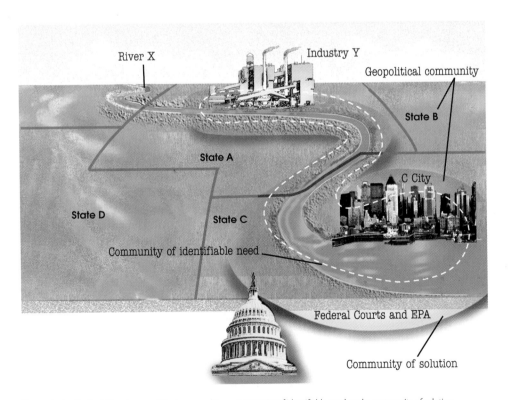

Figure 1–1. Territorial bonds: geopolitical communities, a community of identifiable need, and a community of solution.

example, members of your own nursing class. Certainly you are all part of a community of interest orientation with a common interest in nursing and, more specifically, in graduating from nursing school. At the same time, you are part of a feeling community with emotional attachments resulting from shared experiences. You are also part of a geopolitical community that has specific spatial and temporal boundaries.

▶ DEFINING COMMUNITY HEALTH

The goal of nursing in any form is to maintain or improve the health of the client. In community health nursing, the primary client is the community itself. What does the health of a community entail? What is community health?

Health has been described as "a condition involving a subjective sense of well-being" (Harper & Lambert, 1994) or as an "asset that is a resource for everyday living" (Federal, Provincial, and Territorial Advisory Committee on Population Health, 1994). The health status of a community is a composite of the health of the individuals, families, and groups that constitute the community. Community health, however, is not just the sum of the health status of all community members. More than this, community health relates to the community as a unique entity, a totality in itself. This distinction between the health of its members and the health of the total community is embodied in the phrase "personal troubles—societal issues," coined by sociologist C. Wright Mills in 1959 (Portnoy & Dumas, 1994). Health problems experienced by individual community members constitute personal troubles. When those problems adversely affect the larger community, they become societal issues of concern to all.

What are the health problems of the community as a whole? How can the health of the total community be conceptualized? A decided shift is evident in definitions of community or public health over the last several decades. In the 1920s, community health was defined in terms of longevity and absence of disease (Winslow, 1923). More recently, community health has been defined as "the common attainment of the highest level of physical, mental, and social well-being consistent with available knowledge and resources at a given time and place" (Hanlon & Pickett, 1984) or as successful adaptation to the environment that allows people to live relatively free of disease and to achieve successfully their "biological, psychological, and chronological potential" (Banta, 1979).

Community health has also been viewed as competence in carrying out community responsibilities. These responsibilities include five community functions described by Warren, a public health scientist of the 1970s (English & Hicks, 1992):

1. Production and distribution of goods and services
2. Social control and maintenance of norms of social interaction
3. Promotion of social participation by community members
4. Socialization of community members
5. Mutual support to meet the individual needs of members

These functions are discussed in more detail in Chapter 6.

Florence Nightingale (1860) defined health as "not only to be well, but to use well every power that we have." This definition can be applied to both communities and individuals. A healthy community, then, is one that uses well its powers for the benefit of its members.

In comparing these definitions of community health, one notes a subtle change in emphasis. This shift occurred, in part, because of the decline in mortality due to communicable diseases. As a result, health began to be viewed less in terms of survival and more in terms of quality of life (Harper & Lambert, 1994). Earlier definitions dealt with preventing disease and prolonging life; later ones speak first of attaining the highest possible level of well-being. Outside of nursing, there has been a change in focus over the years from preventing specific diseases in enhancing the quality of life and a greater tendency to deal with death as a part of life. As demonstrated by Florence Nightingale's definition, nursing has always focused on high-level wellness.

This shift to wellness and optimal function are further exemplified in recent descriptions of health and community health by the Ottawa Charter for Health Promotion and the World Health Organization. In 1986, the Ottawa Charter for Health Promotion described health as follows:

> Health is created and lived by people within the settings of their everyday life; where they learn, work, play, and love. Health is created by caring for oneself and others, by being able to make decisions and have control over one's life circumstances, and by ensuring that the society one lives in creates conditions that allow the attainment of health by all its members (Health and Welfare, Canada, 1986).

In a similar vein, the World Health Organization (WHO), in conjunction with the International Epidemiological Association, in 1987 described two aspects of health: balance and potential. *Health balance* reflects a state of equilibrium between person and environment. *Health potential* reflect one's ability to cope with environmental changes to maintain balance (Noack, 1987). Communities, as well as individuals, need to achieve both balance and potential.

Further evidence of the emphasis on quality of life as an element of health lies in the development of the disease-adjusted life-year (DALY) as a measure of the burden of disease. This system combines the previous concept of years of potential life lost (YPLL) due to premature death with a measure of health loss due to disability and suffering to provide a means of assessing quality of life as well as longevity (Foege, 1994).

Given the growing emphasis on wellness, **community health** can be defined as the attainment of the greatest possible biologic, psychologic, and social well-being of the community as an entity and of its individual members. A healthy community displays evidence of biologic, psychologic, and social well-being in itself. For example, a healthy community is economically stable, unpolluted, and able to provide for the needs of its members at adequate levels. In addition, individual members of the community are able to achieve their greatest physical, mental, and social potential (Breslow, 1990).

▶ GOALS OF COMMUNITY HEALTH PRACTICE

Therapeutic medicine, preventive medicine, and public health practice differ in terms of their respective goals. *Therapeutic medicine* is aimed at diagnosing and treating disease. *Preventive medicine* has three aspects: (1) preventing disease (eg, through immunizations and vitamins); (2) preventing consequences of preventable or treatable chronic diseases (eg, preventing complications of syphilis through early diagnosis and treatment); and (3) preventing consequences of nonpreventable and noncurable diseases (eg, preventing contractures in arthritic clients). The goal of both therapeutic and preventive medicine is a negatively stated one, absence of disease.

The goal of *public health practice,* on the other hand, is not stated in terms of disease. Its goal is the promotion of health and the development of maximum potential of individuals, families, and communities. The Institute of Medicine (1988) stated the goal of

public health practice as "assuring conditions in which people can be healthy."

▶ NATIONAL HEALTH OBJECTIVES

The goal of public health practice was operationalized more specifically in several objectives for improving the health of Americans by the year 1990. These objectives were established in 1980 in the publication *Promoting Health/Preventing Disease: Objectives for the Nation* (U.S. Department of Health and Human Services, 1980) and targeted 15 priority intervention areas in three strategic action categories: preventive health, health protection, and health promotion. Preventive health objectives addressed such areas as immunization, family planning, hypertension control, and treatment of sexually transmitted diseases. Objectives related to health protection reflected efforts to control toxic agents, prevent accidents, and ensure occupational safety. Finally, health promotion strategies focused on behavioral changes such as smoking cessation, diet, and exercise (Jamison & Mosley, 1991). Approximately one third of the 226 objectives were met by the target date of 1990 (National Center for Health Statistics, 1992).

A subsequent set of National Health Objectives was established for the year 2000 (U.S. Department of Health and Human Services, 1990). The broad goals for this second set of objectives are: (1) increase the span of healthy life (not just longevity), (2) reduce health disparities among subpopulations, and (3)

Critical Thinking in Research

Community health nurses need to engage in research to define and justify their realm of practice. Some research questions related to material presented in this chapter might be, "To what extent do health care professionals engage in activities directed toward achieving specific National Health Objectives?" or "What is the extent of the general public's involvement in activity directed toward achieving the National Health Objectives?"

1. Why might we want to find answers to these two questions? Who might be interested in those answers?
2. How might you design a study to answer one of these two questions? What type of research would be involved?
3. Where would you look for participants to create a representative sample for your study?

achieve access to preventive health services for all (U.S. Department of Health and Human Services, 1995). The year 2000 objectives differed from those for 1990 in several ways. First, priority intervention areas were increased from 15 to 22 to include cancer screening, HIV infection, and preventive services. Second, the focus of the objectives was moved beyond reduction of mortality to improving the quality of life. A third difference was the special attention given to the needs of high-risk populations such as the elderly and minority groups. Fourth, the year 2000 objectives reflect concern for access to basic health services for all (Jamison & Mosley, 1991). Finally, responsibility for overseeing and monitoring achievement in each priority area was delegated to a specific agency of the U.S.

Public Health Service (U.S. Department of Health and Human Services, 1996). These lead agencies and the areas for which they are responsible are presented in Table 1–1. A summary of the major health objectives for the year 2000 is included in Appendix A.

Community health nurses and other health care professionals are actively involved in efforts to achieve the national health objectives. As of 1995, 50% of the objectives for the year 2000 were moving toward their targeted outcomes. For another 18%, however, movement is occurring away from the target (U.S. Department of Health and Human Services, 1996). These areas, in particular, will require continued effort on the part of community health nurses and others to achieve the desired outcomes.

TABLE 1–1. **HEALTHY PEOPLE 2000: PRIORITIES AND RESPONSIBLE PUBLIC HEALTH SERVICE AGENCIES**

Priority Area	Responsible Agencies
Physical activity and fitness	President's Council on Physical Fitness (202) 272–3421
Nutrition	National Institutes of Health (301) 594–8822
	Food and Drug Administration (202) 205–5483
Tobacco	Centers for Disease Control and Prevention (770) 488–5709
Substance abuse	Substance Abuse and Mental Health Services Administration (301) 443–7790
Family planning	Office of Population Affairs (301) 594–4000
Mental health and mental disorders	Substance Abuse and Mental Health Services Administration (301) 443–7790
Violent and abusive behavior	Centers for Disease Control and Prevention (770) 488–4276
Educational and community-based programs	Centers for Disease Control and Prevention (770) 488–5080
	Health Resources and Services Administration (301) 443–2460
Unintentional injuries	Centers for Disease Control and Prevention (770) 488–4652
Occupational safety and health	Centers for Disease Control and Prevention (800) 356–4674
Environmental health	National Institutes of Health (919) 541–5723
	Centers for Disease Control and Prevention (770) 488–7297
Food and drug safety	Food and Drug Administration (301) 443–1382
Oral health	National Institutes of Health (919) 541–5723
	Centers for Disease Control and Prevention (770) 488–5080
Maternal and infant health	Health Resources and Services Administration (301) 443–2170
Heart disease and stroke	National Institutes of Health (301) 496–1051
Cancer	National Institutes of Health (301) 496–9569
Diabetes and chronic disabling diseases	National Institutes of Health (301) 654–3327
	Centers for Disease Control and Prevention (770) 488–5080
HIV infection	Centers for Disease Control and Prevention (800) 488–5231
Sexually transmitted diseases	Centers for Disease Control and Prevention (800) 227–8922
Immunization and infectious diseases	Centers for Disease Control and Prevention (404) 639–8200
Clinical preventive services	Health Resources and Services Administration (301) 443–2460
	Centers for Disease Control and Prevention (404) 637–7075
Surveillance and data systems	Centers for Disease Control and Prevention (301) 436–3548

Note: The address for the Health People 2000 website is http://odphp.osophs.dhhs.gov/pubs/hp2000/
(Source: U.S. Department of Health and Human Services, 1996.)

Critical Thinking in Practice: A Case in Point

Over the years, several people who have become disenchanted with the modern world have relocated to a small valley in the hills of Tennessee. Residents of the surrounding towns refer to this valley as "Hermit Hollow." The people raise their own fruits and vegetables in small gardens. Many of them make craft items to trade for other items they need in the nearby towns. They are relatively solitary individuals and rarely speak to each other. Indeed, they tend to build their cabins so that they neither see nor can be seen by their neighbors. Each family tends to its own concerns and works to meet the needs of family members.

Medical care is usually sought outside the valley in one of the surrounding towns. Recently, when flooding threatened the homes in the valley, residents packed up their valuables and family members to stay with friends or family outside the area. There are no schools, churches, or stores in the valley itself. Those families that do not educate their children themselves take them to school in one of the surrounding towns.

A number of health problems are common to residents of the valley. These include pinworms and anemia in the children, and tetanus among the working adults (particularly men working in the gardens). Many adults are also obese and have hypertension.

1. Would you consider the residents of Hermit Hollow a community? Why?
2. If Hermit Hollow constitutes a community, what type(s) of community does it represent? If it is not a community, what critical attributes would be needed to view this group of people as a community? If these attributes were present, what type(s) of community would exist?

TESTING YOUR UNDERSTANDING

1. What three critical attributes define a group of people as a community? Give an example of each. (pp. 4–5)
2. Distinguish between communities with territorial bonds and those with relational bonds. Give examples of each type of community. (pp. 5–8)
3. How does the goal of public health practice differ from the goals of therapeutic medicine and preventive medicine? (p. 8)
4. What is the significance of the National Health Objectives? (pp. 8–9)

WHAT DO YOU THINK?
Questions for Critical Thinking

1. What changes in perspective are required when you think of a group of people rather than an individual as your client?
2. Is longer life an objective to be achieved in and of itself? Would it be appropriate to use public health funds to prolong life? Why or why not?

REFERENCES

Archer, S. E. (1979). Selected concepts for community health nurses. In S. E. Archer & R. P. Freshman (Eds.), *Community health nursing: Patterns and practice* (pp. 27–28). North Scituate, MA: Duxbury.

Banta, J. E. (1979). Definition of community health. In *Community health for today and tomorrow.* New York: National League for Nursing.

Breslow, L. (1990). A health promotion primer for the 1990s. *Health Affairs, 9*(2), 6–21.

English, J. C. B., & Hicks, B. C. (1992). A systems-in-transition paradigm for healthy communities. *Canadian Journal of Public Health, 83*(1), 61–65.

Federal, Provincial, and Territorial Advisory Committee on Population Health. (1994). *Strategies for population health: Investing in the health of Canadians.* Ottawa: Health Canada Communications Directorate.

Foege, W. (1994). Preventive medicine and public health. *JAMA, 271,* 1704–1705.

Goeppinger, J., Lassiter, P. G., & Wilcox, B. (1982). Community health is community competence. *Nursing Outlook, 30,* 464–467.

Green, L. W., & Anderson, C. L. (1986). *Community health nursing.* St. Louis: Times Mirror/Mosby.

Green, L. W., & Raeburn, J. (1990). Contemporary developments in health promotion: Definition and challenges. In N. Bracht (Ed.), *Health promotion at the community level* (pp. 29–42). Newbury Park, CA: Sage.

Hanlon, J. J., & Pickett, G. E. (1984). *Public health administration and practice* (8th ed.). St. Louis: Times Mirror/Mosby.

Harper, A. C., & Lambert, L. J. (1994). *The health of populations: An introduction* (2nd ed.). New York: Springer.

Health and Welfare, Canada, Canadian Public Health Association. (1986). *Ottawa charter for health promotion.* Copenhagen: World Health Organization.

Institute of Medicine. (1988). *The future of public health.* Washington, DC: National Academy Press.

Jamison, D. T., & Mosley, W. H. (1991). Disease control priorities in developing countries: Health policy responses to epidemiological change. *American Journal of Public Health, 81,* 15–22.

Josten, L. E. (1989). Wanted: Leaders for public health. *Nursing Outlook, 37,* 230–232.

Noack, H. (1987). Concepts of health and health promotion. In T. Abelin, Z. J. Brzezinski, & V. D. L. Carstairs (Eds.), *Measurement in health and health promotion.* Copenhagen: World Health Organization and International Epidemiological Association.

National Center for Health Statistics. (1992). *Health United States, 1991.* Washington, DC: Government Printing Office.

National Commission on Community Health Services. (1967). *Health is a community affair.* Cambridge, MA: Harvard University Press.

National Institute for Nursing Research Priority Expert Panel. (1995). *Community-based health care: Nursing strategies.* Bethesda, MD: National Institute for Nursing Research.

Nightingale, F. (1860). *Notes on nursing: What it is and what it is not.* London: Harrison.

Orr, J. (1992). Health visiting in the community. In K. Luker & J. Orr (Eds.), *Health visiting: Towards community health nursing* (pp. 73–106). London: Blackwell Scientific.

Portnoy, F. L., & Dumas, L. (1994). Nursing for the public good. *Nursing Clinics of North America, 29,* 371–376.

Shamansky, S., & Pesznecker, B. (1981). A community is. . . . *Nursing Outlook, 29,* 182–185.

Thompson, B., & Kinne, S. (1990). Social change theory. In N. Bracht (Ed.), *Health promotion at the community level* (pp. 29–42). Newbury Park, CA: Sage.

U.S. Department of Health and Human Services. (1980). *Promoting health/preventing disease: Objectives for the nation.* Washington, DC: Government Printing Office.

U.S. Department of Health and Human Services. (1990). *Healthy people 2000: National health promotion and disease prevention objectives.* Washington, DC: Government Printing Office.

U.S. Department of Health and Human Services. (1995, Fall). Healthy People 2000—A mid-decade review. *Prevention Report,* 1–60.

U.S. Department of Health and Human Services. (1996). *Healthy people 2000: Fact sheet.* Washington, DC: Government Printing Office.

Wigley, R., & Cook, J. R. (1975). *Community health: Concepts and issues.* New York: D. Van Nostrand.

Williams, C. A. (1988). Population-focused practice. In M. Stanhope & J. Lancaster (Eds.), *Community health nursing: Process and practice for promoting health* (2nd ed.) (pp. 292–303). St. Louis: C. V. Mosby.

Winslow, C. E. (1923). *The evolution and significance of the modern public health campaign.* New Haven, CT: Yale University Press.

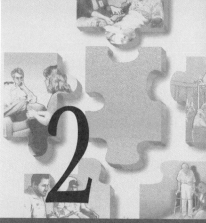

THE HISTORICAL CONTEXT

One work on the history of community health nursing states the "task of the true historian is to so relate the past with the present that our future work is more clearly outlined in the light of former mistakes or seemingly feeble beginnings" (Foley, 1985). Knowledge of past social and political events that have shaped the present allows us to identify factors that promote or undermine the health of the public. Such historical awareness also gives us a sense of the direction that community health nursing should take to achieve its goal—improved health for all people. Historical events that gave rise to a concern for the health of population groups influenced the development of both public health science and community health nursing. As noted by Rear Admiral Julia Plotnick (1994), Chief Nurse of the U.S. Public Health Service:

> The profession of public health nursing was created in response to the social, political, and environmental forces that threatened the health of Americans a century ago. Previous generations of public health nurses saw the need for community-based programs that connected the work of health departments and the people at risk. They led many of the policy revolutions that helped bring family planning, workplace safety, and maternal–child health services to people in need.

This chapter examines some of the forces that shaped community health nursing practice with an eye toward understanding how it is practiced today and how it should be practiced in the future.

▶ **Chapter Objectives**

After reading this chapter, you should be able to:

- Identify the contributions of Florence Nightingale and Lillian Wald to the development of community health nursing.
- Discuss the report that prompted creation of the forerunner of the modern board of health.
- List significant historical events in the development of community health nursing in the United States.
- Describe the influence of diagnosis-related groups (DRGs) on community health nursing.
- Describe evidence for a shift in public health policy toward a greater emphasis on health promotion.

▶ **HISTORICAL ROOTS**

The roots of modern public health and community health nursing practice go far back in history. Early historical records provide evidence of concern for health and prevention of disease in several ancient civilizations. As early as 3000 to 1000 B.C., Minoans and Cretans had established drainage systems and flush sewage disposal (Harper & Lambert, 1994). Around 2000 B.C., Hammurabi, king of Babylonia, codified the laws of that land. Portions of the *Code of Hammurabi* specified health practices and regulated the conduct of physicians (Anderson, Morton, & Green, 1978).

In ancient Egypt there was a well-developed system of sewage disposal and personal hygiene measures were encouraged, while Hebrew Mosaic law addressed many aspects of health. Hebrew segregation of lepers and proscriptions against eating pork are examples of early community health measures. Other aspects of Mosaic law specified personal and community responsibilities for maternal health, communicable disease control, fumigation, decontamination of buildings, protection of food and water supplies, waste disposal, and sanitation of campsites (Benson, 1993).

The early Greeks were more concerned with personal than community health, but they practiced many health-promoting behaviors that are encouraged today. These included emphasis on a healthy diet, exercise, and hygiene. Ancient Rome, on the other hand, emphasized the welfare of the total population and developed a number of regulations related to community health. Roman concern for public sanitation was evident in systematic efforts at street cleaning and rubbish removal and in the construction of

elaborate water and sewage systems. The Romans also regulated building construction, ventilation, and heating, and mandated nuisance prevention and destruction of decaying goods. In 494 B.C., the Roman Office of Aedile was created to supervise health concerns (Winslow, 1923). This official was the forerunner of today's state or county health officer.

Nursing of the sick at this period in history was the function of the women of the family (Bullough & Bullough, 1993). In the case of large and wealthy households, the matron of the family cared for the health needs of both family members and servants or slaves. The care provided, however, was primarily palliative and was only slightly related to today's concept of nursing.

▶ **THE INFLUENCE OF CHRISTIANITY**

The Early Church

The advent of Christianity brought an emphasis on personal responsibility for the corporal and spiritual welfare of others. Care of the sick was seen as one means of fulfilling this responsibility, and early Christians employed their time and monetary wealth ministering to the sick. Such efforts were intended to provide comfort and material goods to the sick and suffering (Brainerd, 1985) and bore little resemblance to modern community health nursing. Such services, although lacking an emphasis on prevention and health promotion or cure, did serve to bring about an awareness of illness within the population.

With the growth of Christianity and charitable giving by Christians, the wealth of the early Christian Church began to accumulate. A large portion of this wealth was used for organized care of the sick and needy through almshouses, asylums, and hospitals rather than through personal visitation of the sick. Hospitals or hospices of this time were not designed exclusively for care of the sick but ministered to all in need, including the sick, the poor, and travelers or pilgrims. The first hospital exclusively for the care of the sick was the Nosocomia or "house for the sick" established by the Roman matron Fabiola in the fourth century (Bullough & Bullough, 1993).

The Middle Ages

The mystical tradition of Christianity during the Middle Ages (500–1500 A.D.) led to a decline in community and personal health status. Castigation and neglect of the body to purify the soul resulted in a number of health problems. Many health promotive activities of antiquity were abandoned in favor of fasting and the wearing of sackcloth and ashes. The need for healthy warriors to fight in the Crusades sparked a slight renewal of interest in health and led to the development of military nursing orders such as the Ancient Order of the Knights of Malta. The function of this order and similar groups was not only military service but also care of the sick and wounded (Kelly, 1981). The creation of these orders was justified in the light of evidence that the majority of casualties suffered in the Crusades were the result of illness rather than battle wounds.

Although European Crusaders took home with them the Byzantine model of hospital care for the sick with the growth of the military nursing orders, they failed to import the concept of paid professionals to care for the sick. Institutional care of the sick had evolved into a paid occupation in the Byzantine Empire as early as the sixth century, but remained a charitable or family function until the nineteenth century in the West. Eastern nurses, both men and women, received a basic education and passed a qualifying examination making them forerunners of today's registered nurse (Bullough & Bullough, 1993).

Following the Crusades, other religious orders were formed to look after the sick. Groups of monks and nuns established hospitals to care for the ill. In many instances, particular orders would focus on the care of specific groups or illnesses. For instance, the Knights Templar cared for pilgrims, travelers, and soldiers, whereas the Lazarists emphasized care of those with leprosy, smallpox, and pustular fevers (Brainerd, 1985). The concept of specialization among health care providers is not as recent as one might believe.

In addition to the religious orders, groups of laypeople also cared for the sick. One such group was the Beguines, an order of laywomen who tended the sick in both the hospital and the home. The Beguines was a forerunner of modern visiting nurse associations and is an early example of political influence by nurses. Because they refused to accept rules for cloistered orders, they were often at odds with the Church hierarchy and were periodically excommunicated. Their exemplary service to the communities, however, allowed them to enlist the aid of wealthy and influential patrons who prevented the Church from disbanding the order (Brainerd, 1985). The focus of nursing care remained the easing of distress rather than therapeutic or preventive activity.

The concept of quarantine, developed in response to repeated epidemics of bubonic plague, was one of the few advances in public health science during the Middle Ages. Venice banned the entry of infected ships in 1348, and quarantine was officially legislated in Marseilles in 1383 (Anderson, Morton, & Green, 1978).

► THE EUROPEAN RENAISSANCE

From 1500 to 1700, the European Renaissance gave rise to the beginnings of scientific thought. Also evident were the development of a social conscience and early recognition of social responsibility for the health and welfare of the population. England enacted the first Poor Law in 1601, making families financially responsible for the care of their aged and disabled members and creating publicly funded almshouses for those with no families.

For most of the population, nursing was performed by family members. In 1610, however, St. Frances De Sales and Madame De Chantal established a Parisian voluntary organization of well-to-do women to care for the sick in their homes, and in 1617, St. Vincent De Paul founded the order of the Sisters of Charity to care for the needs of the sick poor (Byrd, 1995). The activities of this order approximated those of a modern visiting nurse service and incorporated the use of field supervisors for sisters making home visits (Brainerd, 1985).

► A NEW WORLD

The Colonial Period

While new avenues of scientific thought were being opened in Europe, some of the ideas generated were being translated into a new way of life on a new continent. In the early colonial period in America, the health status of those living in the colonies was good compared with that of their European counterparts, and longevity at that time approached today's figures for life expectancy. The relative good health of the population was due primarily to low population density and, interestingly, poor transportation. Communities remained relatively isolated, and the spread of communicable diseases, the major health problem of the era, was curtailed by lack of movement between population groups (Fee, 1997).

Because doctors were few, health care was primarily a function of the family. Nursing care was provided by the women of the family, with assistance from neighbors where this was possible.

Early Public Health Efforts

The growth of population centers led to concern for sanitation and vital statistics, the foci of early public health efforts in the colonies. In 1639, both Massachusetts and Plymouth colonies mandated the reporting of all births and deaths, instituting the official reporting of vital statistics in what would later become the United States. Environmental health and sanitation were also of concern in the early colonies. Evidence of such concern is legislation in 1647 prohibiting pollution of Boston Harbor (Anderson, Morton, & Green, 1978).

Control of communicable disease was another concern as populations increased in size. In 1701, Massachusetts passed legislation regarding isolation of smallpox victims and quarantine of ships in Boston Harbor. For the most part, health was seen as a personal responsibility with little governmental involvement. Temporary boards of health were established in response to specific health problems, usually epidemics of communicable disease, and were disbanded after the crisis had passed. The first such board of health was established in Petersburg, Virginia, in 1780. Similar temporary state boards of health were established in New York and Massachusetts in 1797 (Smolensky, 1982).

Recognition of the need for a consistent and organized approach to health problems was growing, however, and in 1797, the state of Massachusetts granted local jurisdictions legal authority to establish health services and regulations. The following year, Congress passed the Act for Relief of Sick and Disabled Seamen to create hospitals for the care of members of the merchant marine. The group of hospitals created under this act was renamed the Marine Hospital Service in 1871 (Fee, 1997). The act also provided for a systemic approach to quarantine of seaports as one of the first efforts to deal with health problems at a national, rather than a state or local, level.

Nursing during this period remained a function of the family. Although the care given was primarily palliative, the women of the house might also engage in some health promotive practices, such as regular purging with castor oil. Treatment tended to rely on home remedies, and the literature of the era is replete with housewives' recipes for a variety of ailments.

In 1813, the Ladies' Benevolent Society of Charleston, South Carolina, was established. This was the first organized approach to home nursing of the sick in the United States. This organization was initiated in response to a yellow-fever epidemic and was completely nondenominational and nondiscriminatory in an era characterized by widespread racial discrimination. Care was provided to the sick in their homes by upper-class women. Because these women had no background in nursing, care focused on relieving suffering and providing material aid (Brainerd, 1985). With the exception of a 20-year period during and after the Civil War, the Ladies' Benevolent Society provided services until the 1950s.

A similar service was instituted in 1819 in Philadelphia's Jewish community by the Hebrew Female Benevolent Society of Philadelphia. This service was organized by Rebecca Gratz, a Jewish society woman believed to be the model for Sir Walter Scott's Rebecca (Benson, 1993).

Another early attempt at home care nursing also saw upper-class women visiting the homes of indigent women during childbirth. The Lying-in Charity for Attending Indigent Women in Their Homes was established in 1832. The purpose of this organization was to assist poor women during and after delivery. Because of their lack of training, the services provided by these women emphasized social and emotional support for the woman in labor and assistance to her after delivery.

▶ THE INDUSTRIAL REVOLUTION

The *Industrial Revolution* profoundly influenced health in both Europe and United States. Movement on both continents from agricultural to industrial economies led to the development of large industrial centers and the need for a large work force to labor under unhealthy conditions in mines, mills, and factories. The demand for manufactured goods and the necessity to get goods to market prompted advancements in transportation that increased mobility and the potential for spreading communicable diseases. In the United States, rural–urban migration and the presence of large contingents of poor immigrants, who came to escape the poverty of their homelands, created crowded living conditions that further enhanced the potential for disease (Estabrooks, 1995).

The poor were overworked and underpaid. Poor nutrition contributed to increased incidence of a variety of diseases, particularly tuberculosis. Recognition of tuberculosis as a growing problem led to the creation of the first tuberculosis hospital in England in 1840 (Zilm & Warbinek, 1995). The use of children in the work force, coupled with low wages, inadequate food, and hazardous living and working conditions, led to many preventable illnesses and deaths among the children of the poor (Estabrooks, 1995).

The nineteenth century saw a beginning recognition of the effects of these social and economic conditions on health, and the concept of social responsibility for public health began to take root. The growth of this concept was fostered by the publication in the mid-1800s of several landmark reports. The first of these publications was C. Turner Thackrah's treatise on occupational health, *The Effects of Arts, Trades, and Professions . . . on Health and Longevity.* In this document, Thackrah described the effects of working conditions on health. In 1842, Edwin Chadwick's *Inquiry into the Sanitary Conditions of the Labouring Population of Great Britain* provided additional fuel for reformers' efforts to change the working and social conditions that contributed to disease.

While Thackrah and Chadwick addressed the effects of working conditions on health and instigated reforms to prevent disease, Henry W. Rumsey focused on health promotion. Rumsey's *Essays on State Medicine* emphasized health promotion and illness prevention as social obligations of government. His description of the functions of a proposed district medical officer embodied most aspects of modern community health programs (Rosen, 1974).

Similar documents were published in the United States. The Massachusetts Sanitary Commission was established in response to concern over the effects of crowded living conditions, poverty, and poor sanitation on health. In 1850, Lemuel Shattuck drafted the commission's findings, aptly titled the **Report of the Massachusetts Sanitary Commission.** This report included recommendations for establishing state and local health departments, systematic collection of vital statistics, sanitation inspections, and the institution of programs for school health and control of mental illness, alcohol abuse, and tuberculosis. Other recommendations included public education regarding sanitation, control of nuisances, periodic physical examinations, supervision of the health of immigrants, and construction of model tenements. In addition, the report recommended improved education for nurses and the inclusion of content on preventive medicine and sanitation in medical school curricula.

Publication of the *Report of the Massachusetts Sanitary Commission* marks the beginning of community health practice as we know it today. Recommendations of the report form the basis for much of the present work of official state and local public health agencies. The eventual effect of the commission's report was the establishment of state boards of health. The first state board was established in Louisiana in 1855, but has been described as a "paper organization." In 1869, nearly 90 years after the advent of the first temporary boards of health and 19 years after publication of Shattuck's report, Massachusetts established the first working board of health, followed by California in 1870 (Fee, 1997). These first permanent boards, similar to modern boards of health, emphasized six aspects of community health practice: inspection of housing, public education in hygiene, investigation of disease, regulation of slaughterhouses, regulation of the sale of poisons, and health care for the poor (Anderson, Morton, & Green, 1978).

During this period, great strides were being made in the fledgling science of epidemiology. In 1856, without knowledge of the nature of the causative organism, John Snow determined the source of a London epidemic of cholera to be something in the water of the Broad Street pump. It was not, however, until 1877 that Louis Pasteur and Robert Koch, working independently, identified specific bacteria. These and other epidemiologic findings allowed more scientific measures to be applied to the control of communicable disease and contributed greatly to the armamentarium used by later community health nurses in preventing disease.

▶ DISTRICT NURSING IN ENGLAND

The "three great revolutions" of the late eighteenth and early nineteenth centuries—the intellectual revolution, the French and American political revolutions, and the Industrial Revolution—set the stage for the development of community health nursing. In England, the same spirit that motivated industrial and prison reform led to concern for the health of large urban populations and development of nursing practices to address these concerns.

In addition to being the acknowledged founder of modern hospital nursing, **Florence Nightingale** was instrumental in the development of community health or district nursing. Nightingale received her training in nursing at the school for deaconesses established by Theodor Fliedner. Fliedner's second wife, Caroline Bertheau, conceived the idea of extending the nursing services offered in the hospital to the sick in their homes. This concept influenced Nightingale, who endorsed the idea of "health nursing" as well as home care for illness.

In 1859, Nightingale assisted William Rathbone to form the first district public health nursing association in England. The organization was funded by philanthropic citizens and hired trained nurses who were assigned to specific districts in London. Each nurse was responsible for the health needs of the people in her district. The nurses were viewed as social reformers as well as providers of care for the sick, evidence of the early development of the advocacy role of the community health nurse.

The need to standardize community health nursing services was recognized early in the development of the district nursing associations. The East London Nursing Society was established for this purpose but proved ineffective. Subsequently, investigation of the district nursing system revealed a need for a national association. As a result, the Metropolitan and National Nursing Association for Providing Trained Nurses for the Sick Poor was established in 1875. This group fostered employment of educated women in public health nursing as a step toward the professionalization of nursing.

One of the first activities of the association, which was headed by Florence Lees, a protégé of Nightingale, was a study of the needs for public health nursing, the personnel available, and the training required and work done by district nurses. Results of the study of 115 district nurses employed by various organizations throughout London indicated that the work done by those nurses who were trained was effective. Unfortunately, more than half of those studied had no training in public health and were found to be insufficiently prepared for their role in the unsupervised care of the sick. Hospital training was found to be inadequate for district nursing and a recommendation was made that district nurses receive 3 months of training in public health in addition to their year of hospital training (Brainerd, 1985).

The district nursing associations embodied three of the principles of modern community health nursing. The first of these, as noted above, was the need for special training for nurses working in the community. By 1889, this need had been widely recognized. At that time, monies donated to Queen Victoria's Jubilee fund were allocated to Queen Victoria's Jubilee Institute for Nursing (Cohen, 1997). The institute was established to prepare nurses for community health practice and to extend community health nursing throughout the British Empire. A program was instituted to provide an additional 6-month educational experience for community health nurses following the initial 3 years of training in the hospital (Gardner, 1952).

The second principle of modern community health nursing embodied in the district nursing associations was the separation of nursing care from the provision of material goods. As noted earlier, many early efforts at visiting the sick focused on dealing with material needs through the distribution of money, food, or clothing. The district nursing concept eliminated such charitable activities from the role of the nurse and focused on the provision of nursing care per se. This principle was strongly supported by Florence Nightingale as a primary difference between district nurses and "philanthropic visitors" (Montiero, 1987).

The third principle was the prohibition of religious proselytizing by the nurses. Again, because much prior visiting of the sick had been done in the name of Christian charity, visits had been used as an opportunity to encourage supposed sinners to mend their evil ways. Much of this type of activity derived from convictions that poverty, illness, and suffering were punishment for sins and that repentance was needed.

▶ VISITING NURSES IN AMERICA

In the United States, proselytizing was also part of the role of nurses who provided early home care to the sick poor; however, efforts had been made to incorporate the provision of *nursing care* in addition to proselytizing and providing for material needs. In 1877, the Women's Branch of the New York City Mission employed Frances Root as the first salaried American nurse to visit the sick poor. Her role, and that of many *missionary nurses* to follow her, was to provide nursing care and religious instruction for the sick poor (Brainerd, 1985).

In 1878, the Ethical Culture Society of New York employed four nurses in dispensaries, inaugurating the ambulatory care role of the community health nurse. These nurses worked under the supervision of a physician and emphasized health teaching as well as illness care (Brainerd, 1985). In the next few years, *visiting nurse associations* were established in Buffalo

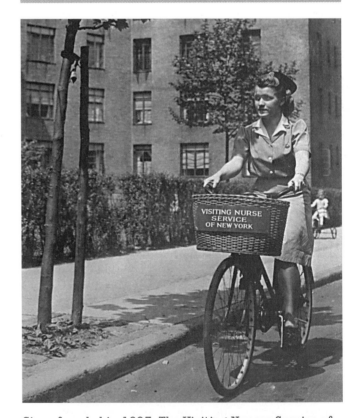

Since founded in 1893, The Visiting Nurses Service of New York has grown to be the largest nonprofit home health service provided in the United States.
Photo courtesy of the Visiting Nurses Society of New York.

(1885), and in Boston and Philadelphia (1886). The Philadelphia agency was the first to institute a nurse's uniform, a fee for services, and the community nursing supervisor. The Boston Instructive Visiting Nurse Association emphasized the community health nurse's educative function as well as her role in the care of the sick, signaling the beginning of the health promotion emphasis that now characterizes community health nursing. Similar events were taking place in Canada with the establishment of the *Victorian Order of Nurses* (VON) in 1897 and the hiring of the first community health nurse in British Columbia in 1901 (Zilm & Warbinek, 1995). By 1890, visiting nurse services were available in 21 American cities (Novak, 1988), and 22 years later, when the National Organization for Public Health Nursing (NOPHN) was founded, there were 3000 visiting nurses in the United States (Winslow, 1993).

▶ NURSING AND THE SETTLEMENT HOUSES

The settlement movement was based on the belief espoused by Arnold Toynbee that educated persons could promote learning, morality, and civic responsibility in the poor by living among them and sharing certain aspects of their poverty. Groups of students from Oxford and Cambridge, acting on this belief, "settled" in homes in the London slums with the idea that their poor neighbors would learn through watching their behavior (Erickson, 1987).

In the United States, the settlement idea was adapted by nurses such as *Lillian Wald,* who believed that the most effective way to bring health care to the poor immigrant population was for nurses to live and work among them. Accordingly, Wald and her associate Mary Brewster established the forerunner of the *Henry Street Settlement* in New York City in 1893. The actual Henry Street establishment was purchased in 1885 and incorporated in 1901. The house on Henry Street differed from many other settlement houses of the era in its incorporation of visiting nurse services (Estabrooks, 1995).

The Henry Street Settlement is usually considered the first American community health agency because of its incorporation of modern concepts of community health nursing. The nurses of the Henry Street Settlement did more than visit the sick in their homes. Health promotion and disease prevention were heavily emphasized, as was political activism. Wald herself was a prime example of the political activist, supporting many changes in social conditions that would benefit the health of the public (Coss, 1989). Other Henry Street nurses like Lavinia Dock were also ac-

tively involved in promoting social change (Estabrooks, 1995).

Other nursing settlement houses patterned on the Henry Street model were established. One particularly inspiring example was the Nurse's Settlement established in 1900 in Richmond, Virginia, by the graduating class of Old Dominion Hospital. These nurses had been exposed to the needs of Richmond's poor during student experiences with the Instructive Visiting Nurse Association of Richmond. The settlement they founded differed from the Henry Street Settlement in that it did not have any wealthy patrons to provide support and was initiated with the limited resources of the graduates themselves. Like Henry Street, the Richmond settlement focused on health promotion and education as well as care of the sick (Erickson, 1987).

▶ EXPANDING THE FOCUS ON PREVENTION

The effectiveness of community health nurses in preventing sickness and death among the poor was recognized and became the basis for visiting nurse services offered by the Metropolitan Life Insurance Company (Hamilton, 1988). This program was begun at the instigation of Lee Frankel and Lillian Wald. Wald convinced the Metropolitan board that providing nursing services to its policyholders would improve the public image of an industry tarnished by economic scandal. The telling argument, though, was evidence that community health nursing reduced mortality and would limit the benefits paid by the company. Services were begun on an experimental basis in 1909 with one of the Henry Street nurses.

The 3-month experiment was such a success that the program was extended and continued to provide services until 1953. This association with the business world was an education for community health nurses who had no conception of marketing or economic bases for programs. The program was finally discontinued because of nursing's failure to grasp economic realities and the realization of diminishing returns by the insurance company (Hamilton, 1989).

The emphasis of community health nursing on health promotion began with health in the home during visits to the poor in large cities. Gradually, however, the concepts of health promotion and illness prevention were expanded to other population groups to include services to mothers and young children, school-age youngsters, employees, and the rural population.

Concern for the health of mothers and children was growing, and the nurses of Henry Street Settle-

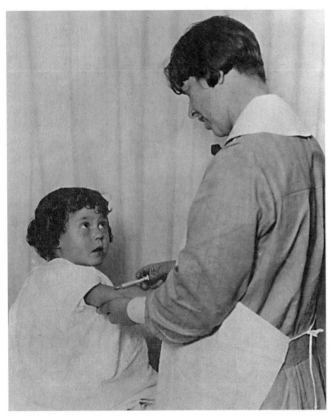

Historical awareness gives us a sense of direction that community health nursing should take to achieve its goal-improved health for all people.

Photo courtesy of the Visiting Nurses Society of New York.

ment and other similar programs spent a large portion of their time in health promotion for this group of clients. Because they recognized that services to individual families would not overcome the effects of poverty, they worked actively to improve social conditions affecting health. Because of the efforts of Lillian Wald and other social activists, the first White House Conference on Children was held in 1909. As a result of the conference, the U.S. Children's Bureau was established in 1912 to develop programs to promote the health of youngsters.

School nursing, another arena for health promotion, actually began in London in 1892 and was introduced in the United States by Lillian Wald of the Henry Street Settlement (Igoe, 1994). The initial impetus for school health nursing was the high level of school absenteeism due to illness. In New York City in 1902, 15 to 20 children per school were being sent home daily. In response, Wald assigned Lina

Struthers from the Henry Street Settlement to a pilot project in school nursing. Because of the overwhelming success of the project, the New York Board of Health absorbed the program and hired additional nurses to continue the work (Jossens & Ferjancsik, 1996).

The concept of school nursing spread to other parts of the country and to Canada. In 1904, Los Angeles became the first of many municipalities to employ nurses in schools (Gardner, 1952). Early school nursing focused on preventing the spread of communicable diseases and treating ailments related to compulsory school life. By the 1930s, however, the focus had shifted to preventive and promotive activities including case finding, integrating health concepts into school curricula, and maintaining a healthful school environment (Igoe, 1980).

The first rural nursing service was established in 1896 in Westchester County, New York, by Ellen Morris Wood and was followed in 1906 with the initiation of a nursing service for both the poor and the well-to-do of Salisbury, Connecticut. Despite her usual sphere of activity in the city, Lillian Wald was also involved in the growth of rural community health nursing. She convinced the *American Red Cross,* founded in 1881, to direct its peacetime attention to expanding community health services in rural America. In 1912, the Red Cross established the *Rural Nursing Service* (later the Town and Country Nursing Service) to extend community health nursing services to rural areas (Brainerd, 1985). In Canada, rural nursing services were provided to large immigrant populations by such organizations as the Victorian Order of Nurses for Canada, the Canadian Red Cross Society, and the Women's Missionary Society (Bramadat & Saydak, 1993).

Other largely rural populations experiencing significant health problems were the Native American population on federal reservations and African Americans in the South. Community health nursing services on the reservations arose out of a 1922 study of health conditions by the American Red Cross commissioned by the Bureau of Indian Affairs (Ruffing-Rahal, 1995). Nurses in this setting often found themselves breaking official rules in order to provide effectively for the needs of their clients (Abel, 1996). To meet the needs of black women in the South, some states coopted local black midwives to work closely with public health nurses. As on the reservations, the rules imposed frequently violated accepted cultural health practices. For example, the nurses "forbade midwives to use any folk medicine or herbal remedies in their childbirth work" (Smith, 1994). In spite of the cultural insensitivity displayed, the partnership between public health nurses and midwives helped to create a modern public health system in the rural South.

Occupational health nursing provides another avenue for health promotion by community health nurses. This specialty area began in 1895 when Vermont's Governor Proctor employed nurses to see to the health needs of villages where employees of his Vermont Marble Company lived (Novak, 1988). In 1897, the Employees' Benefit Association of John Wanamaker's department store in New York City hired nurses to visit employees' homes. These nurses soon expanded their role to include first aid and prevention of illness and injury in the work setting. The number of firms employing nurses increased rapidly from 66 in 1910 to 871 by 1919 (Brainerd, 1985). About this same time, Simmons College offered a certificate program in industrial nursing, acknowledging the need for advanced educational preparation for this specialty area (Golden & Moore, 1986).

Health promotion activities by community health nurses were often combined with advocacy efforts. The work of Margaret Sanger is a striking example. Sanger was instrumental in initiating the National Birth Control League in 1913, and in 1916 opened the first birth control clinic in the United States. Despite serious opposition and her arrest, Sanger persisted. She eventually succeeded in her efforts to make contraceptive information and services available to American women and after World War II founded the International Planned Parenthood Federation to carry on her work (Ruffing-Rahal, 1986).

▶ STANDARDIZING PRACTICE

The need to standardize community nursing practice was recognized in both the United States and England. Early American attempts to standardize visiting nursing services included publications related to public health nursing and development of a national logo by the Cleveland Visiting Nurse Association (VNA). This logo, or seal, was made available to any visiting nurse organization that met established standards. Both the Chicago (1906) and Cleveland (1909) VNAs published newsletters titled *Visiting Nurse Quarterly* to aid attempts to standardize care (Brainerd, 1985).

In 1911, a joint committee of the American Nurses Association and the Society for Superintendents of Training Schools for Nurses met to consider the need for standardization. The result was a second meeting held in 1912. Letters inviting representation were sent to 1092 organizations employing visiting nurses at that time. These organizations included VNAs, city and state boards of health and education,

private clubs and societies, tuberculosis leagues, hospitals and dispensaries, businesses, settlements and day nurseries, churches, and charitable organizations. A total of 69 agencies responded with their intent to send a representative to the meeting. The result of this second meeting was the formation of the *National Organization for Public Health Nursing (NOPHN)* (Brainerd, 1985). The objective of this organization was to provide for stimulation and standardization of public health nursing. This was the first professional body in the United States to provide for lay membership.

The NOPHN was influential in maintaining public health nursing services at home during World War I and in the organization of the Division of Public Health Nursing within the U.S. Public Health Service in 1944. NOPHN also provided advisory services regarding postgraduate education for public health nursing in colleges and universities. NOPHN was incorporated into the *National League for Nursing (NLN)* in the 1952 restructuring of professional nursing organizations.

▶ EDUCATING COMMUNITY HEALTH NURSES

During the 1920s nursing education was under study. The *Goldmark Report, Nursing and Nursing Education in the United States,* published in 1923, dealt with nursing education in general and pointed out the need for advanced preparation for community health nursing. The report recommended that nursing education take place in institutions of higher learning. At the same time, the Committee on Trained Nursing of the American Medical Association recommended university education for management or teaching functions in specialty areas (Krampitz, 1987). As a result, the Yale University School of Nursing and the Frances Payne Bolton School of Nursing at Western Reserve University opened in 1923. Canada's first baccalaureate program in nursing was established in 1919 at the University of British Columbia (Zilm & Warbinek, 1995). The curricula of both U.S. and Canadian programs included community health nursing content.

Prior to the education of nurses in university settings, special postgraduate courses in public health nursing had been established by various agencies. The first of these in the United States was undertaken by the Instructive District Nursing Association of Boston in 1906. In 1910, Teachers' College of Columbia University offered the first course in public health nursing in an institution of higher learning (Brainerd, 1985). In 1949, NOPHN developed criteria for evaluating courses in public health nursing (Golden & Moore,

1986). In Canada, the Canadian Red Cross Society instituted a 14-week certificate course for public health nurses in 1920 (Zilm & Warbinek, 1995).

In addition to witnessing the movement of community health nursing education to institutions of higher learning, the 1920s saw a shift in employment of public health nurses. Before this time, most public health nursing services were provided by voluntary agencies such as the Red Cross and similar organizations. During the 1920s, however, public health nursing services began to be taken over by official governmental agencies such as local and state health departments (Bigbee & Crowder, 1985). In 1937, 67% of all community health nurses were employed in official public health agencies (Winslow, 1993). This same incorporation of public health nurses into governmental agencies began in Canada in the early 1900s (Matuk & Horsburgh, 1989).

The *Brown Report* of 1948, *Nursing for the Future*, reemphasized the need for nurses to be educated in institutions of higher learning so as to prepare them to meet community health needs (Benson & McDevitt, 1976). In 1964, the American Nurses Association (ANA) formally defined the public health nurse as a graduate of a baccalaureate program in nursing. In 1995, the Pew Health Professions Commission Report, *Critical Challenges: Revitalizing the Health Professions*, reinforced baccalaureate education as the entry level for community-based practice. Today, in some states, such as California, only graduates from baccalaureate programs in nursing can be certified as public health nurses. Moreover, there are now master's and doctoral programs with a community health nursing focus.

▶ FEDERAL INVOLVEMENT IN HEALTH CARE

For most of its history the federal government has left health matters to the states. It was not until 1879 that the United States established a National Board of Health in response to a yellow-fever epidemic. This board continued to function until 1883 when it was dissolved. In 1912, the need for a permanent national agency responsible for the country's health was recognized, and the *U.S. Public Health Service (USPHS)* was created out of the reorganization of the Marine Hospital Service (Fee, 1997). In that same year, federal legislation was passed creating the office of the Surgeon General and mandating federal involvement in health promotion. It was not until 1953, however, that the need for advisement on health matters at the cabinet level was recognized in the creation of the De-

partment of Health, Education, and Welfare. This department was reorganized in 1980 to create the present Department of Health and Human Services (DHHS).

Since the beginning of the twentieth century, the federal government has become progressively more involved in health care delivery. Unfortunately, this involvement has been rather haphazard, dependent on the interests and concerns of differing administrations. In the early years of the twentieth century, the health needs of specific segments of the population began to be recognized, resulting in federal programs designed to enhance the health of mothers and children, the poor, those with sexually transmitted diseases, the mentally ill, and others. For example, in 1921 Congress passed the Sheppard–Towner Act to help state and local agencies meet the health needs of mothers and children (Pollit, 1991). In addition to providing funds for maternity centers, prenatal care, and child health clinics, the legislation provided monies to enhance visiting nurse services (Krampitz, 1987). These funds allowed local agencies, for example, the San Diego County Health Department, to hire additional community health nurses known as "Sheppard–Towner nurses" (interview). Later, recognition of the need for federal support of health care research to address the health needs of mothers and children and other special groups led to the development of the National Institutes of Health in 1930.

As a result of the Great Depression of the 1930s, the federal government became even more active in health and social welfare programs. Jobs were created to employ thousands of the unemployed. Nurses were also employed at this time to meet the health needs of the population. The first public health nurse was employed by USPHS in 1934.

Recognition of the economic plight of the elderly led to passage of the *Social Security Act* in 1935, 60 years after the efforts of Lavinia Dock and others to provide health care to the elderly poor. This act established the Old Age Survivors Insurance Program (OASI, better known as Social Security) to improve the financial status of the elderly. In 1966, the Social Security Act was amended to create the Medicare program funding health care for older Americans. Medicaid, a program that funds health care for the indigent, was instituted in 1967. These two programs contributed to increased demands for health care services and resulted in rapid increases in the cost of health care.

World War II also influenced health care delivery. During the war, some 15 million U.S. service members were exposed to quality health care, some for the first time in their lives. Afterward, these veterans began to demand the same quality of care for themselves and their families in the civilian sector. This increased demand for care led to new arrangements for financing health care and a subsequent burgeoning of the health insurance industry. The growth in health insurance was further influenced by the 1954 inclusion of premiums as legitimate tax deductions (Ginzberg, 1985). This development led to the use of insurance benefits as a tax-deductible substitute for higher wages in business and industry. Because such benefits were tax exempt for employees, they were readily accepted in lieu of salary increases by unions and other bargaining agents.

Increased demands for services also led to a lack of adequate facilities, especially in nonurban areas. In 1946, pressured by USPHS officials, congress responded with passage of the Hill–Burton Act to finance hospital construction in underserved areas (Miller, 1992). Hospital construction and insurance coverage for care provided in the hospital further strengthened the national emphasis on curative rather than preventive care and widened the gap between bedside nursing care and health promotion and prevention. In fact, a 1928 Bureau of Indian Affairs (BIA) circular directed BIA public health field nurses that it was "unwise to make bedside care the greatest factor, as the hospital should be used to a larger extent than is customary at present" (Abel, 1996). Hospitals became a major focus for health and illness care. Ironically, during this same period, the first hospital-based home care program was established at Montefiore Hospital (Jonas & Rosenberg, 1986), setting a precedent for the burgeoning home care industry of today. The present emphasis on cost containment has led to a shift away from institutional care and more home and community-based care. This development has resulted in a growing need for community health nurses to provide home health services, a partial return to the practice patterns of a century ago.

Acknowledging the growing demand for health care and recognizing the differing abilities of certain areas of the country to meet those needs, the U.S. federal government responded with the Comprehensive Health Planning Act of 1966 and the National Health Planning and Resources Development Act of 1974. Both pieces of legislation were attempts to organize the planning of health care delivery to meet differing needs throughout the country (Sofaer, 1988). Unfortunately, both efforts failed. One positive effect of the 1974 act was recognition of the contribution of nurse practitioners to the health status of the public, 9 years after the establishment of the first nurse practitioner program in 1965 (Jenkins & Sullivan-Marx, 1994).

The Child Health Act of 1967 and the Health Maintenance Organization Act of 1973 also recommended use of nurses in extended roles. The 1971 publication of a report entitled *Extending the Scope of Nursing Practice* provided additional support for the use of nurses in expanded capacities. Subsequent legislation has led to the increased use of nurse practitioners in a variety of settings. Over the last few years there has been increased use of community health nurses with advanced educational preparation as nurse practitioners providing primary care to selected populations.

While the United States was attempting to decentralize health care policymaking through health planning legislation, efforts were being made elsewhere to focus attention on risk factors for population health problems. The **Lalonde Report,** *New Perspectives on the Health of Canadians,* was published in Canada in 1974 identifying the importance of biological, environmental, and lifestyle risks as determinants of health and recommending greater attention to elimination of risks in each of these areas. In 1978, at an international conference on primary health care, the Declaration of Alma Alta was developed calling for access to primary health care for all. This concept was further developed in the World Health Organization's *Global Strategy for Health for All by the Year 2000* published in 1981 and the *Ottawa Charter for Health Promotion* developed at the First International Conference on Health Promotion, both focusing on social, economic, and political reform and empowerment as strategies for improving the health of the world's populations (Harper & Lambert, 1994).

Reform efforts in the United States have focused more on health care financing and the organization of services than on changes in social conditions affecting health. The **Tax Equity and Fiscal Responsibility Act (TEFRA)** of 1982 has had a profound effect on health care and community health nursing. This act, passed in an effort to reduce Medicare expenditures, led to the development of **diagnosis-related groups (DRGs)** as a mechanism for prospective payment for services provided under Medicare (Harris, 1988). Basically, prospective payment means that health care institutions are paid a flat fee set in advance under Medicare. The fee is based on the client's diagnosis. The effect of this legislation has been earlier discharge of sicker clients and greater demand for home health and community health nursing services. Diagnosis-related groups and their effects have changed the role of community health nurses, who may need to return to the earlier role of care of the sick in their homes, in addition to their roles in promoting health and preventing illness.

Another recent event that will probably have a

significant impact on community health nursing is the development of the Nursing Interventions Classification (NIC) system to categorize nursing services and facilitate their direct reimbursement (McCloskey & Bulechek, 1996). The NIC system should lend itself to direct reimbursement for nursing services under managed care, the new focus of the U.S. federal government. Both Medicare and Medicaid clients are being encouraged to enroll in managed care programs in pilot projects throughout the country. The growth of managed care should lead to a resurgence of the case management role traditionally played by the community health nurse. Community health nurses, however, will need to seize this opportunity with alacrity to prevent encroachment on this area of practice already underway from other professional groups.

Critical Thinking in Research

It is important for community health nurses to understand the forces that shaped their practice in the past and continue to influence community health nursing today. Historical research can provide us with this understanding.

1. What historical events in the development of public health in your local area might be of interest to study? How could information about those events be of use today?
2. Where would you begin to look for information about those events? What documents might provide information? Where might you find those documents?
3. Are there people still living who might be able to shed light on those events? How would you go about finding them? What would you want to ask them? Why?

▶ THE PRESENT AND THE FUTURE

Community health nursing, as practiced today, differs somewhat from the practice arena envisioned by Lillian Wald and her associates. Over the past 100 years, community health nursing practice has changed to meet the changing needs and demands of society. The Henry Street nurses and their contemporaries combined personal care and health promotion services as two aspects of community health nursing practice. When official health agencies began to provide population-based screening and education services, community health nurses employed by these agencies began to emphasize the health promotive and disease preventive aspects of their practice, leaving the provision of personal health services for the sick in their homes to visiting nurse associations (Jenkins & Sullivan-Marx, 1994). More recently, community health nurses have assumed a more clinical, illness-oriented role, downplaying their previous home- and community-based preventive role, as official agencies began to provide more direct clinical care. This shift has occurred, in part, in response to societal need, but also in large part to the reimbursability of these services as opposed to traditional public health services (Plotnick, 1994).

This situation led to what a 1988 Institute of Medicine report on the status of the nation's public health system, *The Future of Public Health*, described as a system in disarray. The report concluded that major reforms will be required to promote and protect the health of the public. Unfortunately, the report did not address at all the contribution of community health nursing to public health. This, in itself, may be

ominous. Community health nursing may not survive as an area of specialty practice if it is not seen as contributing to public health. To forestall this possibility, community health nurses in several areas are engaged in efforts to reframe and reorganize community health nursing in terms of the core functions of public health (Gebbie, 1996; Josten, Aroskar, Reckinger, & Shannon, 1996; Virginia Department of Health, 1996). Some groups, like the Washington State Department of Health, have identified core competencies for health professionals related to the core functions of public health and have instituted specific training to develop those competencies in community health nurses and other public health professionals (Joint Council of Governmental Public Health Agencies, 1996).

There are, however, some indications of greater concern for community health. Growing evidence indicates a shift to greater emphasis on health promotion and illness prevention in national health policy. The national health objectives, published first in 1980 and again in 1990, and discussed in Chapter 1 are one sign of this shift. A second bit of evidence is the 1988 creation of the Center for Nursing Research (now the National Institute for Nursing Research) within the National Institutes of Health. One reason given in Senate testimony favoring the center was the health promotion and illness prevention focus in much of nursing research.

In this chapter we have seen how community health nursing grew to its present state. Some of the events influencing its development are summarized in Table 2–1. The future direction of community

TABLE 2–1. HISTORICAL EVENTS INFLUENCING THE DEVELOPMENT OF COMMUNITY HEALTH NURSING

Date	Event	Date	Event
1601	First Poor Law is enacted in Great Britain.	1906	*The *Visiting Nurse Quarterly* is first published (Chicago).
1639	Massachusetts and Plymouth colonies mandate reporting of births and deaths.		*First postgraduate course in public health nursing is established by Instructive District Nursing Association of Boston.
1647	Massachusetts enacts regulations regarding pollution of Boston harbor.	1909	White House Conference on Children has first meeting.
1701	Massachusetts enacts laws regarding quarantine of ships and isolation of persons with smallpox.		*Metropolitan Life Insurance Company offers visiting nurse services to policyholders.
1780	First local board of health in the United States is established at Petersburg, Virginia.	1910	*First postgraduate course in community health nursing in an institution of higher learning is established at Columbia University.
1797	Temporary state boards of health are established in Massachusetts and New York. Massachusetts grants local jurisdictions the authority to establish local health services.	1912	Children's Bureau is set up to foster child health. First law empowering Surgeon General to promote health is passed.
1798	National Quarantine Act provides a systematic national approach to quarantine of seaports.		Marine Hospital Services becomes U.S. Public Health Service (USPHS). *National Organization for Public Health Nursing (NOPHN) is established.
1813	*Ladies' Benevolent Society is organized in South Carolina as the first home nursing service in the United States.		*Red Cross Town and Country Nursing Service is established.
1819	*Visiting nursing services are organized through the Hebrew Female Benevolent Society of Philadelphia.	1923	*Goldmark Report recommends education for nurses in institutions of higher learning and additional preparation for community health nursing.
1831	Thackrah's treatise on occupational health is published.	1929	*NOPHN establishes criteria and procedures for grading courses in public health nursing, initiating the accreditation process.
1832	*Lying-in Charity for Attending Indigent Women in Their Homes is established.	1930	National Institutes of Health is set up to fund and conduct health research.
1840	First tuberculosis hospital opened in England.	1934	*First public health nurse is employed by USPHS.
1842	Chadwick's *Inquiry into the Sanitary Conditions of the Labouring Population of Great Britain* is published.	1935	Social Security Act establishes Old Age Survivor's Insurance Program (OASI).
1850	Shattuck's *Report of the Massachusetts Sanitary Commission* is published.	1944	*Division of Nursing is established in USPHS.
1856	Rumsey's *Essay on State Medicine* argues for government responsibility for public health.	1946	Hospital Survey and Construction (Hill–Burton) Act provides funds for hospital construction in underserved areas.
	Snow's historic epidemiologic study of cholera is conducted.		Communicable Disease Center established from Office of Malaria Control in War Areas.
1858	National board of health is established in the United States.	1948	*Brown Report reemphasizes the need to educate nurses in institutions of higher learning and to include community health nursing content in curricula.
1869	First modern state board of health is established in Massachusetts.	1952	*NOPHN is absorbed into National League for Nursing (NLN).
1872	American Public Health Association (APHA) established.	1953	U.S. Department of Health, Education, and Welfare is created.
1875	*Metropolitan and National Nursing Association for Providing Trained Nurses for the Sick Poor is established in England.	1954	Health insurance premiums are first allowed as tax deductions.
1877	Pasteur and Koch independently identify specific bacteria.	1964	*Public health nurse is defined by American Nurses Association as a graduate of a baccalaureate program in nursing.
	*Women's Branch of the New York City Mission is first to employ trained nurses for home visiting.	1966	Comprehensive Health Planning and Public Health Services Act is passed.
1878	*Ethical Culture Society of New York City places four nurses in dispensaries.		Medicare program is instituted to fund health care for the elderly.
	Federal Quarantine Act is passed.	1967	*Child Health Act recommends use of nurse practitioners in the care of children.
1881	*American Red Cross is founded.		Medicaid program is instituted to fund health care for the indigent.
1885–6	*Visiting nurse associations are established in Buffalo, Boston, and Philadelphia.	1974	National Health Planning and Resources Development Act is passed in an attempt at systematic health care planning.
1892	*First school nurse is employed in London.	1980	Department of Health, Education, and Welfare is reorganized, creating the Department of Health and Human Services.
1893	*Henry Street Settlement is founded by Lillian Wald.		First National Health Objectives are developed.
1895	*Vermont Marble Company employs first occupational health nurse.	1982	Tax Equity and Fiscal Responsibility Act (TEFRA) is passed.
1896	*First rural nursing service is established (Westchester County, New York).	1983	Prospective payment system based on diagnosis-related groups is instituted under Medicare.
1897	*Victorian Order of Nurses (VON) founded to pioneer community health nursing in Canada.	1988	Institute of Medicine report, *The Future of Public Health*, recommends changes in the U.S. health care system.
1900	*Richmond, Virginia, nurses' settlement house is founded.	1993	*National Center for Nursing Research is established.
1902	*First school nursing program in the United States is established by Henry Street Settlement.	1995	*Pew Health Professions Commission reinforced baccalaureate as entry level for community health nursing practice.
1903	*Henry Street Settlement school nursing program is absorbed by New York City Department of Health.		
1904	*First school nurse is employed by a municipality (Los Angeles).		

*Events affecting nursing directly.

Critical Thinking in Practice: A Case in Point

LILLIAN WALD—"BEST HELPS TO THE IMMIGRANT THROUGH THE NURSE"—1907

The following is an excerpt from a typed manuscript of comments made by Lillian Wald, founder of the Henry Street Settlement.

District nursing today follows the tradition of its earliest conception. It has been used since the beginning of its history to carry propaganda as there has been always an enthusiastic belief in the possibility of the nurse as teacher in religion, cleanliness, temperance, cooking, housekeeping, etc. My argument loses none of its force, I think, if much of this education has seemed to her lost energy because with greater knowledge and wider experience she has learned that the individual is not so often to blame, as she at first supposed. That while the district nurse is laboring with the individual she should also contribute her knowledge towards the study of the large general conditions of which her poor patient may be the victim.

Many of these conditions seem hopelessly bad but many are capable of prevention and cure when the public shall be stimulated to a realization of the wrong to the individual as well as to society in general if (they) are permitted to persist. Therefore her knowledge of the laws that have been enacted to prevent and cure, and her intelligence in recording and reporting the general as well as the individual conditions that make for degradation and social iniquity are but an advance from her readiness to instruct and correct personal and family hygiene to giving attention to home sanitation and then to city sanitation, an advance from the individual to the collective interest. The subject is tremendously important, even exciting, and adds the glamor of a wide patriotic significance to the daily hard work of the nurse. The prevalence of tuberculosis, for instance, brings attention directly to conditions of industry and housing, next to hours of work, to legal restrictions, to indifference to the laws, to possible abuse of the weaker for the benefit of the stronger.

It is splendid vindication of the value of comprehensive education and stimulated social conscience that the district nurses who have had this vision have been the most faithful and hard working and zealous in their actual care of the sick . . . [The] wider vision [of the district nurse] makes for thoroughness as an all important educational, social and humanitarian necessity where the patients are concerned.

These opportunities . . . bear the closest relationship to the immigrants, because they are the most helpless of our population and the most exploited; the least informed and instructed in the very matters that are essential to their happiness. The country needs them and uses them and it is obviously an obligation due them as well as safe guarding of the country itself to give them intelligent conception and education of what is important to their and our interests.

1. Based on this excerpt, what do you think was Lillian Wald's perception of the primary focus of community health nursing practice?
2. What kinds of roles does Lillian Wald envision for community health nurses?
3. Lillian Wald speaks of European immigrants as those most in need of community health nurses' services and advocacy. What groups today take the place of these immigrants in their need for assistance?
4. What do you think would be Miss Wald's perception of the modern world? Would she think it had changed for the better or worse? In what ways? Is there still a need for the type of role she describes for the community health nurse?

Reprinted with permission of Lillian Wald Papers, Rare Books and Manuscripts Division, The New York Public Library, Astor, Lenox, and Tilden Foundations.

---

health nursing will be determined by the community health nurses of today and tomorrow. As noted by one historian of the Henry Street nurses, "We live in times not unlike those of the early Henry Street days. Our inner cities—cities within cities—are frightening, bleak places of despair. I am struck by the similarity of issues—poverty, sanitation, prostitution, pornography, . . . violence, drugs, communicable diseases, hopelessness" (Estabrooks, 1995). It may be time to return to the dual nature of the initial community health nursing role, personal care in conjunction with community-based health promotion and illness prevention. Perhaps then we can achieve the goal, set in 1923 but never accomplished, of one community health nurse to every 2000 Americans (Winslow, 1993).

TESTING YOUR UNDERSTANDING

1. Describe the contributions made by Florence Nightingale to the development of community health nursing. (pp. 17–18)
2. Describe the contributions of Lillian Wald to the development of community health nursing in the United States. (pp. 19–20)
3. What report led to the creation of the forerunner of the modern board of health? List at least five recommendations from this report. (p. 17)
4. List at least four major historical events in the development of community health nursing in the United States. (pp. 18–22)
5. How have DRGs influenced community health nursing practice? Will a similar reimbursement system for ambulatory care services have the same kind of effect on community health nursing? (p. 24)
6. Describe evidence for a shift in public health policy toward greater emphasis on health promotion. (pp. 24–25)

WHAT DO YOU THINK?
Questions for Critical Thinking

1. Would the settlement house concept be appropriate to the health care needs of the U.S. public today? Why or why not?
2. What would the modern equivalent of a settlement house be like?
3. Does public health history reveal any repeated patterns or trends?

REFERENCES

Abel, E. K. (1996). "We are left so much alone to work out our own problems:" Nurses on American Indian reservations during the 1930s. *Nursing History Review, 4,* 43–64.

Anderson, C. L., Morton, R. F., & Green, L. W. (1978). *Community health* (3rd ed.). St. Louis: C. V. Mosby.

Benson, E. R. (1993). Public health nursing and the Jewish contribution. *Public Health Nursing, 10*(1), 55–57.

Benson, E. R., & McDevitt, J. Q. (1976). *Community health and nursing practice.* Englewood Cliffs, NJ: Prentice-Hall.

Bigbee, J. L., & Crowder, E. L. M. (1985). The Red Cross Rural Nursing Service: An innovative model of public health nursing. *Public Health Nursing, 2,* 109–121.

Brainerd, A. M. (1985). *The evolution of public health nursing.* New York: Garland. Reprinted from A. M. Brainerd (1922), *The evolution of public health nursing.* Philadelphia: W. B. Saunders.

Bramadat, I. J., & Saydak, M. I. (1993). Nursing on the Canadian prairies, 1900–1930: Effects of immigration. *Nursing History Review, 1,* 105–117.

Bullough, V. L., & Bullough, B. (1993). Medieval nursing. *Nursing History Review, 1,* 89–104.

Byrd, M. E. (1995). A concept analysis of home visiting. *Public Health Nursing, 12*(2), 83–89.

Cohen, S. (1997). Miss Loane, Florence Nightingale, and district nursing in late Victorian Britain. *Nursing History Review, 5,* 83–103.

Coss, C. (1989). *Lillian Wald: A progressive activist.* New York: Feminist Press.

Erickson, G. (1987). Southern initiative in public health nursing. *Journal of Nursing History, 3*(1), 17–29.

Estabrooks, C. A. (1995). Lavinia Lloyd Dock: The Henry Street years. *Nursing History Review, 3,* 143–172.

Fee, E. (1997). History and development of public health. In F. D. Scutchfield & C. W. Keck (Eds.), *Principles of public health practice* (pp. 10–30). Albany, NY: Delmar.

Foley, E. L. (1985). Introduction. In A. M. Brainerd, *The evolution of public health nursing* (pp. i–vii). New York: Garland. Reprinted from A. M. Brainerd (1922), *The evolution of public health nursing.* Philadelphia: W. B. Saunders.

Gardner, M. S. (1952). *Public health nursing* (3rd ed.). New York: Macmillan.

Gebbie, K. M. (1996). *Preparing currently employed public health nurses for changes in the health system: Meeting report and suggested action steps.* New York: Center for Health Policy and Health Sciences Research.

Ginzberg, E. (1985). *American medicine: The power shifts.* Totowa, NJ: Rowman & Allanheld.

Golden, J., & Moore, P. (1986). The Simmons Harvard graduate program in public health nursing. *Public Health Nursing, 4,* 123–127.

Hamilton, D. (1988). Clinical excellence, but too high a cost: The Metropolitan Life Insurance Company Visiting Nurse Service (1909–1952). *Public Health Nursing, 5,* 235–240.

Hamilton, D. (1989). The cost of caring: The Metropolitan Life Insurance Company's Visiting Nurse Service. *Bulletin of the History of Nursing, 63,* 414–434.

Harper, A. C., & Lambert, L. J. (1994). *The health of populations: An introduction* (2nd ed.). New York: Springer.

Harris, M. D. (1988). The changing scene in community health nursing. *Nursing Clinics of North America, 23,* 226–229.

Igoe, J. B. (1980). Changing patterns in school health and school health nursing. *Nursing Outlook, 28,* 486–492.

Igoe, J. B. (1994). School nursing. *Nursing Clinics of North America, 29,* 443–458.

Interview with Harney M. Cordua, son of Dr. Olive Cordua, San Diego County Medical Officer. San Diego: San Diego Historical Society.

Jenkins, M. L., & Sullivan-Marx, E. M. (1994). Nurse practitioners and community health nurses: Clinical partnerships and future visions. *Nursing Clinics of North America, 29*, 459–470.

Joint Council of Governmental Public Health Agencies Work Group on Human Resources Development. (1996). *Public health improvement plan: Education and training competency model.* Seattle: Washington State Department of Health.

Jonas, S., & Rosenberg, S. (1986). Ambulatory care. In S. Jonas (Ed.), *Health care delivery in the United States* (3rd ed.) (pp. 125–165). New York: Springer.

Jossens, M. O. R., & Ferjancsik, P. (1996). Of Lillian Wald, community health nursing education, and health care reform. *Public Health Nursing, 13*(2), 97–103.

Josten, L., Aroskar, M., Reckinger, D., Shannon, M. (1996). *Educating nurses for public health leadership.* Minneapolis: University of Minnesota.

Kelly, L. Y. (1981). *Dimensions of professional nursing* (4th ed.). New York: Macmillan.

Krampitz, S. D. (1987). The Yale experiment: Innovation in nursing education. In C. Maggs (Ed.), *Nursing history: The state of the art* (pp. 60–73). London: Croom Helm.

Matuk, L. Y., & Horsburgh, M. C. (1989). Rebuilding public health nursing: A Canadian perspective. *Public Health Nursing, 6*, 169–173.

McCloskey, J. C., & Bulecheck, G. M. (Eds.). (1996). *Nursing interventions classification: Iowa Interventions Project* (2nd ed.). St. Louis: Mosby-Year Book.

Miller, D. F. (1992). *Dimensions of community health* (3rd ed.). Dubuque, IA: W. C. Brown.

Montiero, L. A. (1987). Insights from the past. *Nursing Outlook, 35*, 65–69.

Novak, J. C. (1988). The social mandate and historical basis for nursing's role in health promotion. *Journal of Professional Nursing, 4*(2), 80–87.

Pew Health Professions Commission. (1995). *Critical challenges: Revitalizing the health professions for the twenty-first century.* San Francisco: University of California, San Francisco Center for the Health Professions.

Plotnick, J. (1994, March). *Public health components of the Health Security Act.* Paper presented at the meeting of the Public Health Nursing Division, San Diego County Department of Health Services, San Diego.

Pollit, P. (1991). Lydia Holman: Community health pioneer. *Nursing Outlook, 39*, 230–232.

Rosen, G. (1974). *From medical police to social medicine: Essays on the history of health care.* New York: Science History Publications.

Ruffing-Rahal, M. (1986). Margaret Sanger: Nurse and feminist. *Nursing Outlook, 34*, 246–249.

Ruffing-Rahal, M. A. (1995). The Navajo experience of Elizabeth Foster, public health nurse. *Nursing History Review, 3*, 173–188.

Smith, S. L. (1994). White nurses, black midwives, and public health in Mississippi, 1920–1950. *Nursing History Review, 2*, 29–49.

Smolensky, J. (1982). *Principles of community health* (3rd ed.). Philadelphia: W. B. Saunders.

Sofaer, S. (1988). Community health planning in the United States: A postmortem. *Family Community Health, 10*(4), 1–12.

Virginia Department of Health. (1996). *The role of public health nursing in Virginia's changing health care environment.* Richmond, VA: Virginia Department of Health.

Winslow, C. E. (1923). *The evolution and significance of the modern public health campaign.* New Haven, CT: Yale University Press.

Winslow, C. E. A. (1993). Nursing and the community. *Public Health Nursing, 10*, 58–63. (Reprinted from *The Public Health Nurse*, April 1938).

Zilm, G., & Warbinek, E. (1995). Early tuberculosis nursing in British Columbia. *Canadian Journal of Nursing Research, 27*(3), 65–81.

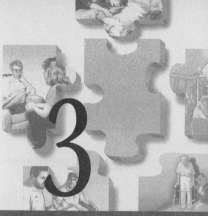

3

THE HEALTH CARE CONTEXT

Community health nursing occurs in the context of the health care delivery system, and the characteristics of that system profoundly influence community health nursing practice. For example, the lack of emphasis on health promotion in the health care delivery system increases the need for health promotion efforts by community health nurses, but simultaneously limits funds available for health promotion activities.

Health and health care are concerns throughout the world, and each jurisdiction (community, state, or nation) has developed a system to address these concerns. A *health care system* is "an organized arrangement to provide specified promotive, preventive, curative, and rehabilitative services to designated persons, using resources allocated for that purpose" (Basch, 1990). Health care systems can be organized in a variety of ways. Although each jurisdiction has its own way of organizing and providing health care, some features are common to all systems.

Exploring the organization of health care delivery can help us understand how these systems developed, how they work, and how and why they sometimes fail to work. Moreover, we can identify factors that positively or negatively influence community health nursing practice. Finally, we can identify areas where change is needed in the health care delivery system to best fulfill our goal as community health nurses, namely, promotion of the public's health. In this chapter we examine the organization of health care delivery in the United States, as well as in other countries, and make comparisons that permit us to see the advantages and disadvantages of various approaches to health care.

▶ Chapter Objectives

After reading this chapter, you should be able to:

- Diagram the organizational structure of the U.S. health care delivery system.
- Discuss three major characteristics of the U.S. health care system.
- Compare and contrast official and voluntary health agencies.
- Identify the core public health functions of official health agencies.
- Describe at least five functions performed by voluntary health agencies.
- Identify the level of official agencies with primary responsibility for the health of the American public.
- Identify the type of health system that exists in the United States.
- Describe at least three alternative types of national health care delivery systems.
- Describe two types of international health agencies.
- Identify major areas of concern in international health.

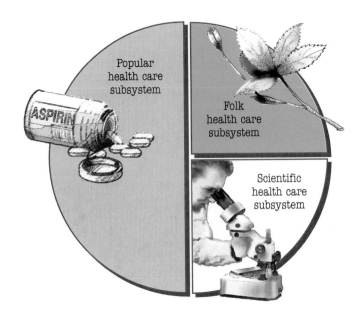

Figure 3–1.   Organizational structure of the U.S. health care delivery system.

▶ HEALTH CARE DELIVERY IN THE UNITED STATES

Health care delivery in the United States has been called a "complex health care nonsystem" (Sofaer, 1988). Indeed, the United States has been described as the only developed country, aside from South Africa, that does not have a true system of health care delivery (Birchfield, Dvorak, Scully, Haas, & Duberly, 1991). Despite the relative accuracy of this description, we can still examine U.S. health care delivery in terms of the hierarchical structure depicted in Figure 3–1.

The health care delivery system in the United States consists of three major elements or subsystems. These subsystems are depicted in Figure 3–1 and include the popular health care subsystem, the folk or traditional health care subsystem, and the scientific health care subsystem.

The Popular Health Care Subsystem

Most health-related care is provided within the *popular health care subsystem.* In fact, it is estimated that worldwide two thirds of illness care is provided outside of the professional system, traditional or scientific (Harper & Lambert, 1994). The popular subsystem component of the health care system includes health care that each of us provides for ourself and our family. When you have a headache, for example, you may

take an over-the-counter analgesic. If you are constipated, you may either increase the bulk, fiber, and fluid in your diet or take a laxative. If your child has a mild fever, you might give him or her acetaminophen or some other antipyretic. All of these self-care or family care practices constitute popular subsystem health care.

Although health care in this subsystem is provided by oneself or by family members, community health nurses have an educational role in the popular subsystem. As we shall see in Chapter 9, one of the purposes of health education is to prepare clients to make informed self-care decisions. For example, a community health nurse might caution a client against overuse of laxatives and suggest dietary approaches in dealing with constipation. Or, the nurse might inform parents about the hazards of giving aspirin to children and recommend a nonaspirin substitute.

The Folk or Traditional Health Care Subsystem

When self-care fails or seems inappropriate, people often turn to other sources of health care. Some of these sources might be folk health practitioners found in the folk or *traditional health care subsystem.* Folk health practitioners are individuals who are believed to have special health-related knowledge or training above that provided to the average member of the society. Examples of folk health care providers are the *curandera* found among Latinos in the northeastern and southwestern regions of the United States and the herbalists found in these and other areas. The role of the community health nurse in the traditional subsystem is to assess the influence of this subsystem on health and to incorporate traditional health practices into the plan of care as appropriate. We discuss the folk health care subsystem in more detail in Chapter 16.

The Scientific Health Care Subsystem

The professional or *scientific health care subsystem* has been defined as "the health services professions and bureaucracies basing clinical practice on highly developed and complex professional health cultures" (Chrisman & Kleinman, 1983). Health care provided in the scientific subsystem is based on knowledge derived from the biologic, physical, and behavioral sciences and includes the services of nurses, physicians, pharmacists, social workers, and other health care professionals. The scientific health care subsystem in the United States is characterized by three major qualities: pluralism, multicentricity, and fragmentation.

Pluralism

The first characteristic of the U.S. scientific health care subsystem, *pluralism,* is defined as tolerance for organizational diversity that may involve both complementary and competing agencies (Rodwin & Sandier, 1993). Rather than one single system, such as is found in Great Britain, Canada, Australia, and elsewhere, many independent systems provide scientific health care in the United States. Personal health care services are separated from community health services, and care may be provided by either public or private organizations (Blendon, Leitman, Morrison, & Donelan, 1990).

Multicentricity

The U.S. scientific health care subsystem is also characterized by *multicentricity;* that is, decisions regarding health care arise at many points within the system. No single agency is totally responsible for determining health care goals and activities for the nation. The multicentric nature of the American health care system often results in conflicting health care goals and little concerted effort to consolidate resources or apply them in an effective and efficient manner.

Fragmentation

The third characteristic of the U.S. scientific health care subsystem, *fragmentation,* arises out of the first two. Because there are multiple foci for decision making, health care delivery is fragmented, resulting in

duplication in some services and gaps in others. Concerted planning efforts have decreased, but not entirely eliminated, fragmentation. A 1988 report by the Institute of Medicine (IOM) indicated that the nation's health care system is ineffective in meeting the needs of the public. The report included findings of a total lack of any local public health care facility in some parts of the nation and ineffective use of resources in all areas. According to the report, health care crises, such as the high cost of health care and the growing AIDS epidemic, are consistently addressed on a short-term basis without considering long-term solutions. There is also inequity in the way in which health care resources are distributed and a lack of response by health officials to the needs of the population. The report concluded that, because of the weaknesses of a fragmented health care system, unnecessary deficits in the public's health continue to exist.

Components of the Scientific Health Care Subsystem

The scientific health care subsystem consists of two sectors that differ primarily in terms of their focus of care. These sectors are the personal health care sector and the community health care sector (American Public Health Association Executive Board, 1995).

The Personal Health Care Sector

The focus of care in the *personal health care sector* is the health of the individual. The primary emphasis in this sector is on cure of disease and restoration of health, although individuals may also receive some health promotive and illness preventive services. Personal health services are provided in office settings, clinics, hospitals, and other places where care is dispensed to individual clients. Institutions that provide personal health care, such as hospitals and clinics, may be either privately or publicly funded. For example, both private hospitals and publicly funded community hospitals are part of the personal health care sector.

The Community Health Care Sector

Although health care services may be provided to individual clients in the *community health care sector,* the primary focus of this sector is the health of populations. Care provided usually centers on promoting health and preventing disease, although some curative care does occur in this sector. Emphasis is on designing health care programs that meet the needs of population groups. Health care services in the community health care sector may be provided by official or voluntary agencies.

Official Health Agencies. **Official health agencies** are agencies of local, state, and national governments that are responsible for the health of the people in their jurisdictions. Official agencies are supported by tax revenues and other public funding. They are accountable to the citizens of their jurisdictions, usually through an elected or appointed governing body. Many of the activities conducted by official agencies are mandated by law. For example, local health departments are required by state law to report cases of certain diseases. We discuss specific functions of official agencies at local, state, and national levels in more detail later in this chapter. Generally speaking, however, all official health agencies are responsible for carrying out what have been called certain "core" public health functions.

The **core public health functions** are essential services required to safeguard the health of populations (Kuss, Proulx-Girouard, Lovitt, Katz, & Kennelly, 1997). The Institute of Medicine (1988) identified three core functions: assessment, policy development, and assurance. Under its **assessment** function, the public health sector is responsible for collecting and analyzing data to identify population health problems. The **policy development** function entails using a scientific knowledge base to provide direction for health program development. Finally, in its **assurance** function, the public health sector is responsible for assuring that the health care services needed by the population are available and accessible to those in need (Miller, Moore, Richards, & Monk, 1994). The kinds of services that are conceptualized under the core functions vary among policy groups, but, as the comparison of the U.S. statement of core functions and the Canadian description of the essential contributions of public health depicted in Table 3–1 indicate, there are striking similarities.

Voluntary Health Agencies. **Voluntary health agencies** are organizations that are formed by groups of people because of their interest in a particular health concern, such as diabetes, child abuse, or environmental pollution. Voluntary agencies are funded primarily by donations. They are accountable to their supporters, and their activities are determined by supporter interest, rather than legal mandate. Their primary emphasis is on research and education, although they may provide a few direct health care services.

Voluntary agencies can be categorized on the basis of their source of funding. The first category consists of agencies supported by citizen contributions, such as the American Cancer Society. The first agency of this type in the United States was the Antituberculosis Society founded in Philadelphia in 1892. The focus of this type of agency frequently changes as

TABLE 3–1. CORE PUBLIC HEALTH FUNCTIONS, UNITED STATES AND CANADA

United States	Canada
ASSESSMENT	
Assess population health needs	Focus on individuals and communities in a societal and global context
Investigate health hazards	
Analyze determinants of health needs	Provide disease surveillance and control
POLICY DEVELOPMENT	
Advocate for public health and build constituencies	Build capacity in individuals and communities to improve health
Set priorities	Advocate for the health of the public
Develop plans and policies to address needs	Influence the orientation of the health system toward health outcomes
	Build partnerships among sectors at the local level
ASSURANCE	
Manage resources and organize care	Facilitate community mobilization through participation
Implement programs	
Evaluate programs	Embrace promotion, prevention, protection
Inform and educate the public	

(Sources: Miller, Moore, Richards, & Monk, 1994; Canadian Public Health Association, 1996.)

health needs change. For example, the Antituberculosis Society is known today as the American Lung Association, indicating its broader focus on a variety of respiratory conditions. The second category consists of foundations established by private philanthropic contributions. An example of this type of voluntary organization would be the Kellogg Foundation, which provides funding for health care research. Today, more than 3000 philanthropic foundations support health efforts. The third category of voluntary agency is funded by member dues. The American Public Health Association and the American Nurses Association are examples of this type of agency. Integrating agencies, such as the United Way, coordinate the fund-raising activities of several voluntary agencies. A fifth type of voluntary agency includes religious organizations that derive their funds from contributions by members of a congregation. These groups often focus on local needs and are particularly effective because of their ability to draw on volunteers (Miller, 1995). The final category of voluntary health agency is the commercial organization that engages in health care activities. For example, the American Dairy Association provides literature and visual aids for nutrition education. Similarly, health insurance companies often put out literature on health promotion and illness prevention.

Voluntary agencies perform eight basic functions within the scientific health care subsystem. The first of these is *pioneering* activities. Voluntary agencies explore areas that are underserved by the other components of the health care system. For example, research that culminated in the development of a vaccine for polio was the early focus of the March of Dimes. Now, polio immunization is largely a function of official agencies.

The second function of voluntary agencies is *demonstration* of pilot projects in health care delivery. For instance, the Planned Parenthood Association instituted clinics for contraceptive services long before most official health agencies became involved in this area of service. *Education* of the public and health professionals is the third function of voluntary agencies. For example, the American Cancer Society has spearheaded educational campaigns on the hazards of smoking. The fourth function of voluntary health agencies is *supplementation* of services provided by official health agencies. Some voluntary agencies provide transportation to clinics, respite care, special equipment, and other ancillary services.

Fifth, voluntary health agencies *advocate* for the public's health. A voluntary agency may campaign against reduction of health care services due to budget cuts. The sixth function, promoting *legislation* related to health, is a closely related function. In Tennessee, the Fraternal Order of Police and the Tennessee Nurses Association were instrumental in getting child car restraint legislation passed.

The seventh function of voluntary agencies relates to health *planning and organization.* Voluntary agencies often assist official agencies in determining health care needs in the population and in planning programs to address those needs. The final function of voluntary agencies is *assisting official agencies* in developing well-balanced community health programs. For example, in 1915 when the San Diego Common Council passed an ordinance creating the position of Municipal Tuberculosis Visiting Nurse, but could not afford to pay her salary, the state Tuberculosis Society agreed to fund the position for one year, allowing the city to hire its first community health nurse (communication from the City Auditor, 1915).

▶ LEVELS OF HEALTH CARE DELIVERY

Health care delivery in the United States takes place on local, state, and national levels. Each level has certain responsibilities with respect to the health of the population. Both official and voluntary agencies exist at each level, but official agencies are the focus of this discussion.

The Health Services Extension Act of 1977 mandated the development of standards for official community preventive health services. This mandate led

to the creation of a Model Standards Work Group composed of representatives of the American Public Health Association (APHA), the Association of State and Territorial Health Officials, the National Association of County Health Officers, and the Centers for Disease Control (CDC). This work group developed the document *Model Standards for Community Preventive Health Services,* first published by APHA in 1979. A second edition of this document was prepared and published in 1985 (Model Standards Work Group, 1985), and a third set of standards, *Health Communities 2000: Model Standards,* is intended as a companion volume to the year 2000 objectives (Mason, 1990).

The model standards identified 34 areas of responsibility for preventive health services by official public health agencies. These areas range from responsibilities for program administration to providing care for special population groups such as the elderly, the poor, and mothers and children. Official agencies are also responsible for environmental and occupational health; control of specific types of health problems such as chronic and communicable disease; and substance abuse, animal control, health promotion, and illness prevention services.

The Local Level

The official agency at the local level is usually the *local health department.* The health department's authority is derived, in part, from responsibilities delegated by the state. For example, the state delegates to the local level the responsibility for collecting statistics on births and deaths. Because this responsibility has been legally delegated, the local health department has the authority to ensure that a death certificate is filed for every death that occurs. The local agency also derives authority from local health ordinances. For instance, local government might pass an ordinance requiring all residential rental units to have functioning smoke detectors. Enforcement of this ordinance might then become the responsibility of the local health department.

Funding at the local level comes from both local taxes and state and federal subsidies. Figure 3–2 depicts the typical organizational structure of a local health department. The staff and programs included will vary from place to place. In some areas, the district health officer might also fulfill the role of administrative officer. Small counties and districts may not be able to afford the full-time services of some types of personnel, and the services of nutritionists, social workers, dentists, and other personnel might be shared by several counties. Nurses and clerical staff would be found in almost any health department. Other personnel who may be available include envi-

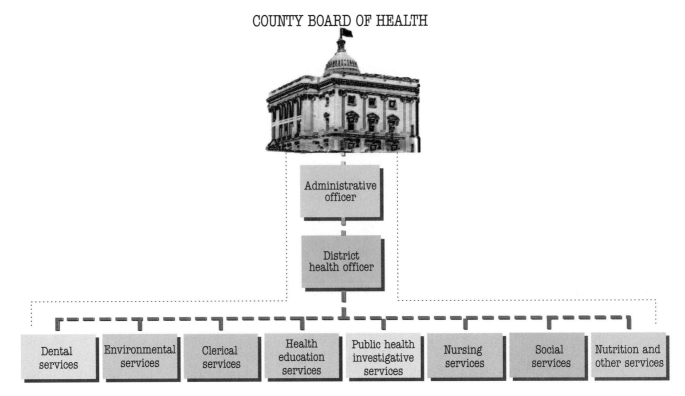

Figure 3–2. Typical organizational structure of a local health department.

ronmental specialists, physical therapists, psychologists, laboratory and x-ray technicians, and pharmacists.

Because delegation of specific responsibilities to local jurisdictions is the function of the state, the responsibilities assumed vary from state to state. Local responsibilities may also vary within regions of a particular state, depending on the local jurisdiction's capabilities and resources. In general, local health agencies are responsible for several basic functions identified by the National Association of County and City Health Officials. These functions include conducting community assessment, controlling epidemics, providing a safe environment, evaluating health services, promoting healthy lifestyles and educating the public, assuring access to laboratory services, and engaging in outreach activities and partnership formation. Additional functions include providing some personal health services, research, and mobilizing communities for action (Rawding & Wasserman, 1997).

The State Level

The official agency at the state level has traditionally been a state department of health. The state, not the federal government or the local jurisdiction, has pri-

mary authority in matters relating to health. This authority is derived from the sovereign powers reserved to the states under the U.S. Constitution. The state retains the ultimate responsibility for the health of the public and possesses essential power to make laws and regulations regarding health.

The state health department derives funding from state tax revenues and may also receive monies from the federal government. A general organizational schema for a state department of health is depicted in Figure 3–3. The various divisions coordinate services at the state level and provide assistance to the local level.

In general, the functions of state health agencies fall into five categories: health information, disease and disability prevention, health protection, health promotion, and improving the health care delivery system (Dandoy, 1997). Specific activities related to the information function include collecting and recording vital statistics and monitoring the incidence of specific health problems. Disease and disability prevention activities focus on screening and treatment services for specific conditions (eg, tuberculosis) or special groups (eg, children with disabilities), immunization, outbreak investigation, and laboratory services. Activities geared toward health protection include pollution control, inspections, and licensing of

STATE BOARD OF HEALTH

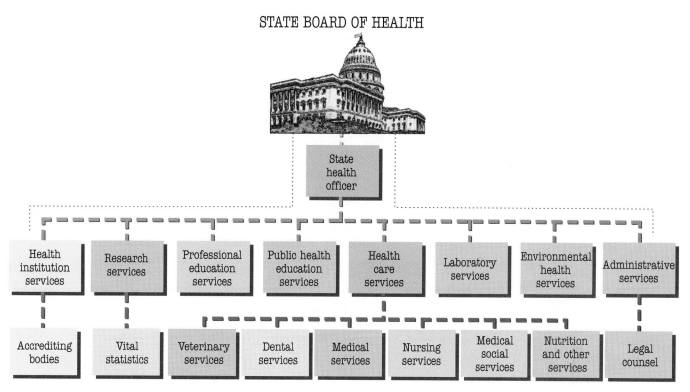

Figure 3–3. Typical organizational structure of a state health department.

health care facilities. Health promotion activities typically focus on providing specific services (eg, family planning and prenatal care) and health education. Finally, activities under the health delivery system function include education of health professionals and policy development.

The National Level

Because the Constitution makes no reference to any responsibilities of the federal government regarding health, the federal government has no direct authority to regulate health-related matters. The authority of the federal government with respect to health is derived indirectly from three constitutional powers. The first of these is the *power to regulate foreign and interstate commerce.* For example, because most cosmetics are transported across state lines, the federal Food and Drug Administration has the authority to establish standards of purity for the manufacture of cosmetics.

The second constitutional source of authority over health matters is the *power to levy taxes and promote the general welfare.* For example, it can be argued that such programs as Medicaid and Medicare promote the general welfare and are therefore within the authority of the federal government. The *power to make treaties* is the third source of federal power in matters relating to health. For example, a treaty with Mexico

might specify that the Mexican government would take specific steps to control the shipment of illicit drugs into the United States.

The official health agency at the national level is the *Department of Health and Human Services (DHHS),* created in 1980 with the division of the former Department of Health, Education, and Welfare into two separate departments. The head of the agency is the Secretary for Health and Human Services, who fills a cabinet post and acts in an advisory capacity to the president in matters of health. The major agencies within DHHS are the Administration for Families and Children, the U.S. Public Health Service, the Health Care Financing Administration, the Social Security Administration, and the Administration on Aging.

Figure 3–4 depicts part of the organizational structure of DHHS. The public health component of the department is the *U.S. Public Health Service (USPHS).* USPHS consists of eight agencies. The *Food and Drug Administration (FDA)* is responsible for establishing and enforcing standards for the manufacture and processing of food, drugs, and cosmetics. It is also responsible for ascertaining the safety of new drugs and other health-related products such as food additives and medical devices. The *Centers for Disease Control and Prevention (CDC)* investigates causes of disease and establishes policies and standards for the prevention, diagnosis, and treatment of a variety of health problems.

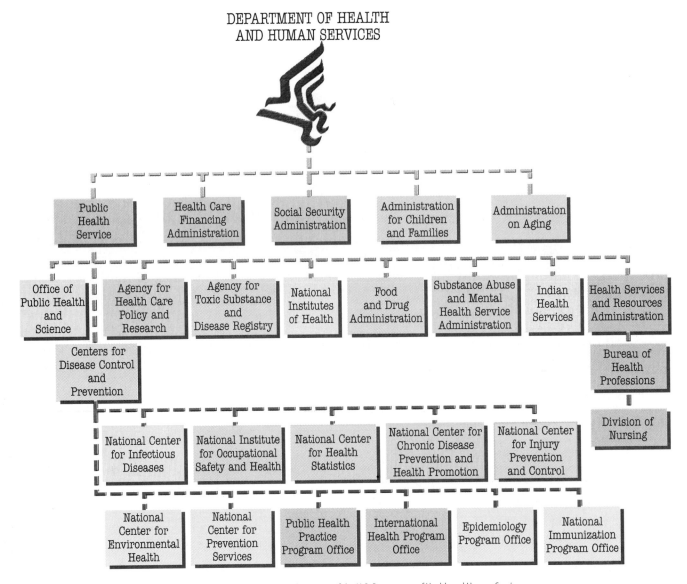

Figure 3–4. Partial organizational structure of the U.S. Department of Health and Human Services.

CDC consists of several component agencies depicted in Figure 3–4. The National Center for Infectious Diseases maintains the original focus of CDC, investigating factors that contribute to communicable diseases, monitoring their occurrence, and developing policies and standards for their control. The National Center for Prevention Services focuses on health promotion and disease prevention activities and provides research and program support for these activities. The National Center for Environmental Health and the National Center for Injury Prevention and Control investigate factors underlying environmentally caused diseases and unintentional injuries and support policies and programs for their control. Control of occupational disease and injury is the focus of the National Institute for Occupa-

tional Safety and Health (NIOSH), and health promotion and prevention of chronic illness are the foci of the National Center for Chronic Disease Prevention and Health Promotion. CDC also houses the Epidemiology Program Office, the International Health Program Office, and the Public Health Program Office. Finally, CDC includes the National Center for Health Statistics, previously a part of the Office of the Assistant Secretary for Health.

The *Substance Abuse and Mental Health Services Administration (SAMHSA)* was created with the reorganization of the Alcohol, Drug Abuse, and Mental Health Administration (ADAMHA). This organization focuses on prevention and treatment programs for mental health problems, including substance abuse, and encompasses three centers: the Center for Substance Abuse Treatment (CSAT), the Center for Substance Abuse Prevention (CSAP), and the Center for Mental Health Services (CMHS). As part of the reorganization of ADAMHA, three research institutes previously housed in this agency were moved to the *National Institutes of Health (NIH)*, another component of USPHS. NIH conducts health-related research and provides some direct service to individuals in the course of that research. With the transfer of the three institutes from ADAMHA, NIH currently houses 26 research institutes, offices, and centers, each focusing on research in a special interest area. The major components of NIH are depicted in Figure 3–5.

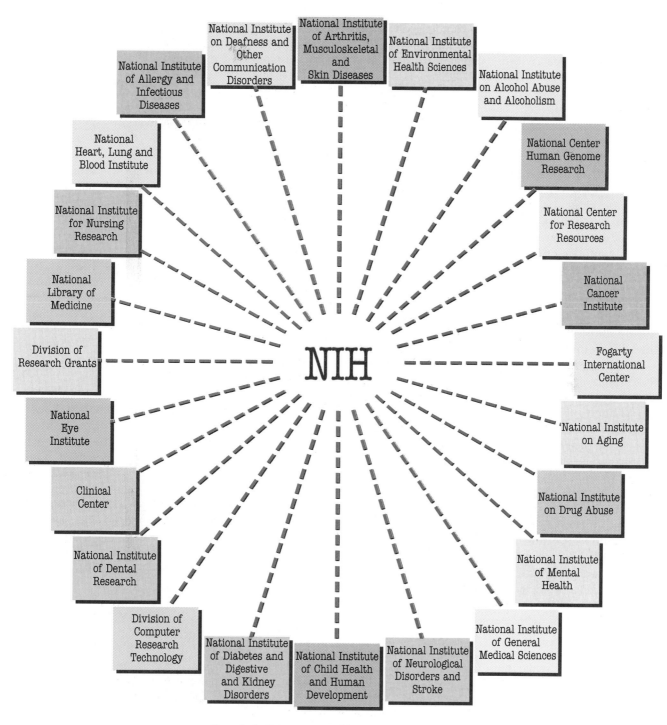

Figure 3–5. Major components of the National Institutes of Health.

The *Health Resources and Services Administration (HRSA)* was created by the merging of the previous Health Services Administration and Health Resources Administration. This combined agency is responsible for training and utilization of health professionals and health resources planning and utilization. Major components of HRSA include the Bureau of Primary Health Care, the Bureau of Health Resources Development, and the Division of Immigrant Health Services. One additional HRSA bureau of interest to community health nurses is the Bureau of Health Professionals, which houses the Division of Nursing.

Other agencies within USPHS include the Agency for Toxic Substances and Disease Registry, the Indian Health Service, and the Agency for Health Care and Policy Research. The *Agency for Toxic Substances and Disease Registry* monitors exposures to toxic substances and the occurrence of disease related to toxic exposures. The *Indian Health Service,* previously housed under the Health Resources and Services Administration, is responsible for providing direct care services for large segments of the Native American population. Finally, the *Agency for Health Care Policy and Research* focuses on generating and disseminating information for use in health policy formation, with emphasis on quality, effectiveness, and cost of health care.

The *Health Care Financing Administration (HCFA)* is responsible for federally funded programs under Medicare and Medicaid. HCFA is responsible for reimbursement under these programs and sets reimbursement rates under the diagnostic-related groups (DRG) system discussed earlier. HCFA is also responsible for quality and utilization control for the programs under its jurisdiction.

The *Social Security Administration* handles the Social Security program, more properly titled the Old Age, Survivors and Disability Insurance program (OASDI). This agency is also responsible for the administration of the Supplemental Security Income for the Aged, Blind, and Disabled program (SSI) and is the administrative agency for the program of Aid to Families with Dependent Children (AFDC).

The *Administration for Families and Children* addresses the health needs of children and families, persons with developmental disabilities, and Native Americans (other than those addressed by the Indian Health Service). The agency consists of the Administration on Children, Youth, and Families; the Administration on Developmental Disabilities; the Administration for Native Americans; the Office of Child Support Enforcement; and the Office of Community Services. The *Administration on Aging* focuses on the needs of the elderly population in the United States

and develops policies, plans, and programs designed to enhance the health of this growing population.

Although DHHS is the agency primarily responsible for national health, other agencies within the federal government are also involved in addressing health issues. For example, the Department of Defense provides health care for military personnel, dependents, and retirees, and the Department of the Interior addresses health concerns related to environmental pollution. Similarly, the Department of Labor is concerned with occupational health as well as other employment concerns, and the Treasury Department is actively involved in efforts to control drugs subject to abuse (Miller, 1995).

Agencies at the federal level provide assistance to state and local agencies in the form of health resources and professional education. Agencies also assist in improving health care delivery and conduct, support, and disseminate findings of health-related research. Additional federal responsibilities related to health include protecting the public against unsafe food and drugs, controlling communicable diseases, and functioning as liaison between the United States and international health organizations or with other countries. Federal agencies also provide direct services to certain population groups such as Native Americans and military personnel, retirees, and dependents. Federal health-related agencies are included in the Resources List at the end of this chapter.

▶ INTERNATIONAL HEALTH CARE

Because of the interdependence among nations and the ability that people now have to travel any place in the world in a matter of hours, there is increasing concern for international health. Increased mobility means increased potential for the spread of disease from nation to nation. This remains true of communicable diseases traditionally spread by travelers from infected to noninfected areas. For example, cholera was reintroduced into South America, after an absence of nearly 90 years, by bilge water from a Chinese freighter (Morse, 1992). In addition, increased global communication and mobility have led to changes in lifestyle that bring the attendant risks of many lifestyle-related chronic illnesses. For example, dietary changes that occur as many developing countries are exposed to Western culture have contributed to a rise in heart disease. Adoption of new lifestyles in many parts of the world has contributed to the development of stress-related disorders. Increased travel and import/export opportunities have increased the potential for trafficking in illegal substances and increased drug use around the world. Alcoholism is another growing concern worldwide. Finally, environmental concerns are now international, rather than local, in scope.

Since 1977, the major emphasis in international health care has been on the achievement of *"health for all by the year 2000,"* the outcome of the World Health Assembly of that year. The following year the International Conference on Primary Health Care held in Alma Alta in what was then the U.S.S.R. produced a report entitled *Primary Health Care,* otherwise known as the **Declaration of Alma Alta.** The central goal of the "health for all" movement is the provision of basic health care to all peoples of the world by the year 2000. Its three main objectives are promotion of healthy lifestyles, prevention of preventable conditions, and therapy for existing conditions (Orr, 1992).

The major strategy to be employed in achieving the objectives is that of primary care. **Primary health care (PHC)** has been described as "both a philosophy of health care and an approach to providing health care resources. Its basic elements are essential health care, socially acceptable and affordable methods and technology, accessibility, public participation, and intersectoral collaboration" (Beddone, Clark, & Whyte, 1993). In 1985, Cuba was recognized as the first country to have achieved health care for all using a PHC strategy (Swanson, 1987). In the Cuban model, community health nurses operating from neighborhood health centers form part of a coordinated care team providing personal care services and community-based health promotion and disease prevention services. This model is reminiscent of the dual focus of early community health nursing in the United States described in Chapter 2.

Health Care Systems in Other Countries

The approach taken to achieve "health for all" varies from nation to nation, and the health care delivery systems of many other countries differ greatly from the U.S. system of health care. These systems can be categorized on the basis of their economic structure and the political system governing their operation. Economic features include a system's source of funding and its payment mechanisms, whereas political considerations reflect the extent to which government is involved in the health care delivery process. The five categories of health systems thus achieved are (1) the free enterprise system, (2) the welfare system, (3) the transitional system, (4) the underdeveloped system, and (5) the socialist system (Roemer, 1977). The

health care system of any given nation, however, may combine features of more than one of these categories.

Free Enterprise Systems

The free enterprise system is exemplified by the United States. In this type of system, health services are delivered primarily in an open market, with comparatively little government intervention or control over supply, demand, or cost of services. Another term for such systems is "demand-side" system, in which consumers decide what services to purchase and how much they will pay (Hsiao, 1992). A free enterprise system usually operates on a fee-for-service basis, although the fee may not be paid directly by the person receiving care. Periodic proposals for a national health system would eliminate the free enterprise system in the United States and would move the nation toward a welfare system of health care delivery.

Welfare Systems

The welfare system emphasizes equal services for all members of the population and is usually financed by some form of social insurance contributions (Basch, 1990). There is considerable government involvement in the delivery of health care, and the government may actually provide the bulk of available health care services. Welfare systems of health care delivery are found in the United Kingdom, France, Canada, Sweden, Norway, and Germany.

In the United Kingdom, the National Health Service provides basic health care to all citizens, but services are separately administered and differ somewhat in each of the four countries (England, Wales, Scotland, and Northern Ireland). Services are relatively comprehensive and are purchased by the responsible administrative agencies (area health authorities or health boards) from provider organizations, most of which are National Health Service hospitals and community health services units (Birt, 1996). Physicians are of two primary types: general practitioners and specialists. General practitioners are paid a basic salary plus a per capita allotment for the number of clients served. Specialists are salaried employees of the hospitals, though many specialists also maintain a part-time, fee-for-service practice. In most cases, hospitalization or specialist services require a referral from a general practitioner.

The Canadian health care system shares many features of the British system, but it also has some features in common with the U.S. model. Mandated features of the Canadian system include universal coverage, comprehensive services, access to all without charge, portability throughout the country, and public administration (Di Marco & Storch, 1995). Initially established as a 50-50 cost sharing venture between the federal and provincial governments, the federal government contribution is now based on population and economic growth within each province. In most provinces, health care is funded through tax revenues, although insurance premiums are charged in two provinces, and employer payroll taxes are assessed in some others. Coverage does not include drugs or dental care, nor does it pay for some extended-care and rehabilitation services; for example, nursing home services are not covered (Spasoff, 1996).

Canadian hospitals have not been nationalized as is the case in Great Britain; they do, however, submit budgets to the government to cover their operating costs. The Canadian system of payment for physicians also differs from the British system. In Canada, as in the United States, most physician services are reimbursed on a fee-for-service basis rather than salary (Spasoff, 1996). Fee schedules are negotiated between medical associations and the government (Miller, 1995).

Transitional Systems

Transitional systems exist in countries where much of the population is poor and rural and where there is a modest government-run structure for providing basic health services coexisting with a growing private fee-for-service health care sector for the affluent. There may be a rudimentary program of social insurance for health care for workers and their families. Many Latin American and Middle Eastern countries have transitional health care systems.

Mexico has a transitional health care system under which the Mexican Institute of Social Security provides health services to both public and private employees, independent businesspersons, and students. Financing is derived from general revenues, premiums paid by employees, and employer contributions. Health care for nonemployees, particularly marginalized rural populations, is provided under the Program of Social Solidarity Through Community Cooperation. Private fee-for-service health care meets the needs of less than 1% of the population. Mexico has been in the process of creating a National Health System since 1982, but this task is complicated by the multiple sources of services, both public and private. In Mexico, hospitals may be either publicly or privately owned (Enciso & Pliego, 1996).

Another transitional system is found in India, where there is a plurality of sources of health care and funding. The Ministry of Health controls a centralized health care system that provides basic services throughout the country. These services are supplemented, however, by those provided on a fee-for-service basis by a variety of practitioners of both Western and traditional medicine. With increasing economic prosperity, the private health care sector in India is growing rapidly (Berman & Kahn, 1993). India has made a concerted effort to integrate some groups of indigenous healers, particularly midwives, into the scientific health care system. Government physicians are salaried and are usually educated at government expense. Following their education, they are usually expected to serve in a rural location within the official system for several years before they are free to establish a private practice. Hospitals may be government-owned or private and provide a wide variety of services based on scientific, homeopathic, and traditional paradigms (Bhat, 1993).

Underdeveloped Systems

Underdeveloped countries have poorly organized systems of health care delivery, particularly in rural areas. There is little government involvement in health care and little funding available for services. In many instances, the health care available is provided by missionary groups and other humanitarian organizations. Many African nations have underdeveloped systems.

Socialist Systems

Socialist systems are characterized by almost complete government control of health care delivery. Examples of such systems are found in Cuba and the People's Republic of China.

The Cuban health care system is based on provision of care in neighborhood clinics. Each clinic serves a group of 120 families (Swanson, 1987). The clinics combine primary health care and community health services and are designed to meet the needs of those who seek personal health services and those who do not seek care. Emphasis is on health education, promotion, and prevention, as well as on primary care for existing conditions. Clinics are staffed by physician/community health nurse teams who have additional specialty resources available at geographically distributed "polyclinics."

All Cuban health care services are provided under the aegis of the Ministry of Health, and all hospitals have been nationalized. The Cuban system emphasizes local participation in health care policy development and includes lay representatives in each of the polyclinics. Unlike India and China, Cuba has made a concerted effort to eliminate health care services provided in a traditional health care subsystem, and folk medicine is officially prohibited (Basch, 1990).

In China, despite revolutionary tenets of health care as a right, services are not free. China's health care system is funded primarily by a health insurance fund to which all employees contribute. There is also some copayment required of some clients and some care provided by charitable organizations. Like India, China mixes both scientific and traditional health services and approximately 95% of western-style hospitals incorporate traditional Chinese medicine units (Ge & Yang, 1996).

As noted by one author, "Developing an optimal structure for a health care system has been an elusive task" (Hsiao, 1992). Each type of health care system discussed here has both advantages and disadvantages. Table 3–2 compares the primary features of the health care systems of several nations with those of the U.S. health care system.

Organization for International Health

On the global level the organization of health services is somewhat less structured than in the national systems discussed above. A number of organizations and agencies are concerned with international health. Organizations addressing international health concerns can be divided into several groups: private voluntary agencies, philanthropic foundations, semiofficial agencies, private industries, and official agencies (Basch, 1990). Private voluntary organizations include both religious and secular groups that provide health assistance at the international level. The efforts of many of the religious organizations are coordinated by the Evangelical Foreign Missions Association or the Church World Service; coordination of secular groups is the function of the International Council of Voluntary Agencies. CARE and Project HOPE are examples of secular voluntary agencies; Catholic Relief Services is an international religious organization providing health assistance to developing countries. Philanthropic foundations are similar to those discussed earlier, but with an international rather than a national focus for their efforts. One example is the Rockefeller Foundation. Private industries such as pharmaceutical companies also provide overseas health assistance.

Official international health agencies include member countries participating via official governmental structures. These agencies can be described as either bilateral or multilateral (Basch, 1990). ***Multilateral agencies*** involve several countries in joint activi-

TABLE 3–2. **COMPARISON OF U.S. AND SOME OTHER NATIONAL HEALTH CARE SYSTEMS**

| System Type | Country | Economic Features | | | Government Involvement | | |
		Source of Funding	Set Fee Schedule?	Physician Payment	Client Payment	Locus of Control	Hospitals	Comprehensive Services?
Free enterprise	United States	Multiple sources	No	Fee-for-service	Variable	Pluralistic	Public and private, profit and nonprofit	No
Welfare	United Kingdom	General revenues and social insurance	N/A	Capitation and/or salaried	Some copayment	Centralized	Nationalized	Yes
	Canada	Provincial health insurance	Yes	Fee-for-service	—	Decentralized	Government supported	No
	Sweden	Health insurance taxes	N/A	Salaried	Some copayment	—	—	Yes
	Norway	Social insurance and general revenues	Yes	Salaried and fee-for-service	Some copayment	Centralized	Nationalized	No
	Germany	Sick fund contributions	Yes	Fee-for-service and salaried	Some copayment	Decentralized	Government support and per diem negotiated with sick fund	Yes
Transitional	Peru	General revenues, Social Security, charity, private pay	No	Fee-for-service and salaried	Variable	Decentralized	Variable	No
	India	General revenues charity, private pay	No	Fee-for-service and salaried	Variable	Pluralistic	Public and private	No
Socialist	Cuba	General revenues	N/A	Salaried	—	Centralized	Nationalized	Yes
	Poland	General revenues	No	Salaried and fee-for-service	None	Centralized	Nationalized	Yes
	People's Republic of China	Health insurance fund	N/A	Salaried	Some copayment	Decentralized	Nationalized	Yes

ties related to health, whereas *bilateral agencies* usually involve only two countries in any single project.

Multilateral Agencies

The primary agency dealing with health concerns at the international level is the *World Health Organization (WHO)*, a multilateral agency. A specialized agency attached to the United Nations by formal agreement, but not subordinate to the U.N., WHO is funded through subscription by member nations and is responsible for monitoring the incidence of disease throughout the world. The organization also sets international standards for sanitation, biologic products, laboratory techniques and procedures, and manufacture of drugs. WHO supports graduate study and research efforts and assists member nations in controlling disease. Further responsibilities are monitoring environmental pollution levels through a program called Earthwatch and providing assistance to underdeveloped countries to prevent or eliminate pollution. The World Health Assembly, held yearly in May, is the arena for policy formation within WHO.

The *Pan American Health Organization (PAHO)* is another multilateral health organization of particular interest. This agency deals with health-related concerns in the Americas and provides an avenue for collective efforts to promote the health status of people in all nations in the Western Hemisphere.

One PAHO program provides profiles of the health assessment efforts of international agencies. The Health Situation and Trend Analysis Program develops health profiles of member nations as part of a continuing effort to identify factors influencing health. National profiles include information on the health status of citizens, the health system within the country, and the environmental context in which the society is evolving. This information provides direction for programs to enhance health status in member nations.

Other multilateral agencies include the health components of the North Atlantic Treaty Organization (NATO) and the Southeast Asia Treaty Organization (SEATO). The United Nations International Children's Emergency Fund (UNICEF) and the United Nations Educational, Scientific, and Cultural Organization (UNESCO) are two other agencies within the United Nations that provide assistance with matters of international health. The Food and Agricultural Organization (FAO) is a multilateral organization designed to enhance the world's food supply. Finally, the World Bank provides both funding and technical assistance in dealing with health problems around the world.

Bilateral Agencies

A number of bilateral organizations with health concerns exist throughout the world. Virtually all developed countries provide some form of health-related aid to underdeveloped countries, with the contribution of some countries far in excess of that provided by the United States. This section focuses on the bilateral organizations involving the United States. Such organizations may be either governmental or nongovernmental. One federal agency concerned with international health is the Agency for International Development (AID), which administers all federally financed projects for foreign development, including those that are health related. This agency is housed in the U.S. State Department.

The Department of Health and Human Services includes the International Health Program Office within CDC. This agency is also concerned with cooperative projects for improving international health. The Fogarty International Center is housed in NIH and focuses on international health. Other branches of NIH (eg, the Geographic Medicine Branch of the Institute of Allergy and Infectious Diseases) are involved in activities that are international in focus, as is CDC. ACTION, the volunteer organization of the federal government, houses both the domestic assistance programs of VISTA (Volunteers in Service to America) and the international programs of the Peace Corps, many of which have a health focus. Federally chartered institutions such as the Institute of Medicine and the National Science Foundation are also concerned with problems of international health, as well as with domestic problems. Names and addresses of several international health organizations are included in the Resource List at the end of this chapter. Similar information on additional agencies is available in the *Encyclopedia of Associations*.

Concerns in International Health

Global health concerns fall into several major categories: infectious and chronic diseases, injury prevention, mental health, nutrition, and environmental health.

Infectious diseases continue to be a major area of concern throughout the world. Much of the infectious disease burden lies in vaccine-preventable childhood illnesses. It has been suggested that a worldwide expenditure of $0.50 per person could provide immunizations to all children and reduce the economic cost of disease by 6% (Foege, 1994). In 1990, the U.N. World Summit for Children established the goal of a 90% immunization rate for the world's children by the year 2000 (UNICEF, 1995). By 1994, immunization levels had risen to 80% and an estimated 3 million child deaths from these diseases were prevented (*The Nation's Health,* 1995a). Despite these gains, childhood diseases remain significant causes of death and disability throughout the world. For example, in 1993, an estimated 10 million people suffered disabilities due to polio (*The Nation's Health,* 1995b). In 1994, a total of 2 million children died from three preventable diseases: measles, tetanus, and pertussis (*The Nation's Health,* 1995a).

In addition to the continuing depredations of vaccine-preventable illnesses, other new and reemerging communicable diseases threaten world health. New diseases include Ebola virus, hepatitis C, Lyme disease, and HIV. Previously well-controlled diseases that are reemerging include tuberculosis, diphtheria, cholera, dengue fever, yellow fever, and bubonic plague. In addition, significant increases in antibiotic resistant strains of bacteria causing gonorrhea, staphylococcus, and malaria have been noted. For example, tuberculosis incidence increased almost 28% from 1984 to 1993 (*The Nation's Health,* 1995c). HIV infection affects more than 21 million of the world's population and further complicates the international health problem posed by tuberculosis. In 1995, tuberculosis was expected to be a factor in the death of more than one third of those infected with HIV (*The Nation's Health,* 1995d).

Some degree of global control has been achieved over certain infectious diseases. The last recorded case of smallpox in the world occurred in 1977, and smallpox was declared eradicated by WHO in 1980 (Centers for Disease Control, 1993). The goal of eliminating poliomyelitis in the Americas appears to be within reach. *Eradication* is the "reduction of the worldwide incidence of a disease to zero as a result of deliberate efforts, obviating the necessity for further control measures" (Centers for Disease Control, 1993). *Elimination* is the same phenomenon on a smaller scale; that is, the disease in question no longer occurs in one area of the world. Diseases currently targeted for worldwide eradication include dracunculiasis (Guinea worm disease), poliomyelitis, filariasis, mumps, rubella, and pork tapeworm. By 1994, cases of wild polio virus had been virtually eliminated from the entire Western hemisphere (UNICEF, 1995).

Although infectious diseases continue to be the primary health concern in several countries, many nations are experiencing a shift in health problems to encompass more chronic disease, injury, mental illness, nutritional problems and environmentally caused disease (Jamison & Mosley, 1991). The rising incidence of chronic diseases in developing countries is a result of rising incomes, dietary changes, changes in exercise and substance use behaviors, and an aging

population due to lower death rates and greater life expectancy. A worldwide report predicts that by 2020 chronic diseases will account for 73% of all deaths (*The Nation's Health,* 1996). In 1993 alone, heart disease killed 5.4 million people, and chronic obstructive pulmonary disease was associated with 2.9 million deaths throughout the world (*The Nation's Health,* 1995b).

Economic growth brings about an increase in motor vehicle use with a concomitant increase in injury rates. Potential for injury from industrial accidents and toxic chemicals also increases with industrialization. Improving economic status increases access to tobacco, alcohol, and other drugs and leads to increased potential for abuse of these substances (Jamison & Mosley, 1991). Chronic mental disorders are frequently thought to occur primarily in developed countries, yet research has indicated no significant differences in the prevalence of mental disorders throughout the world.

Nutritional deficits are another area of significant concern in international health. For example, it is estimated that 655 million people throughout the world suffer from goiter due to iodine deficiency, and vitamin A deficiency affects more than half a million

Critical Thinking in Research

Blendon and associates (1993) conducted a telephone survey of randomly selected physicians in the United States, Canada, and Germany to explore their concerns about health care delivery in their respective countries. Physicians in all three countries identified barriers to care, but the barriers differed from nation to nation. Affordability was perceived as the biggest barrier by U.S. physicians. Long waits for services and nonavailability were problems noted by Canadian physicians, but German physicians noted few problems with access to care. Similar proportions of each group considered the level of use of health care services by clients appropriate, but U.S. and German physicians were more likely to use unnecessary clinical services to avoid litigation than Canadian physicians. Finally, German and U.S. physicians were more likely than Canadian physicians to indicate that more services than were needed were provided to terminally ill clients, but only U.S. physicians had this perception of the appropriateness of services provided to elderly clients.

1. What features of the U.S., Canadian, and German health care systems might be contributing to the findings of this study?
2. Do you think that similar differences in perceptions about the health care system would be found among nurses in these three countries? How would you go about answering this question?
3. What implications do the findings of this study have for the plausibility of initiating a national health care service in the United States?

Critical Thinking in Practice: A Case in Point

Design a health care delivery system that would meet the health needs of the American public. Diagram the organizational structure of the system, making sure that your system addresses the core functions of public health as well as the goals of medical care described in Chapter 1. Address the following questions:

1. What features (if any) would you incorporate from the health care delivery systems summarized in Table 3–2?
2. How would you address the responsibilities of official health agencies discussed in the chapter?
3. How would you fund your system? Would health care providers operate on a fee-for-service basis or be salaried employees of the system? Why?
4. Would you offer comprehensive health care services? Why or why not? What would be included in the basic health services package?
5. How would you address the three levels of prevention in your health care delivery system? Would one level receive priority over the others? If so, why?
6. What changes would be required in the United States for your proposed system to be implemented?

children, more than half of whom die. It is also estimated that 26 of 87 developing countries are unlikely to achieve global goals of reducing protein-energy malnutrition to less than 10% of children by the target date of 2000. In 1990, 40% of women in developing countries were suffering from iron deficiency anemia (UNICEF, 1995).

Environmental concerns are drawing greater concern in international health than ever before. Safe drinking water is a serious area of concern. Despite marked improvements in accessibility, 34% of people living in Southeast Asia, 20% in Latin America, and 58% in Africa still do not have access to safe drinking water. Access to effective sanitation is even more limited with lack of access reported for almost two thirds of the populations of developing nations (UNICEF, 1995).

Health care for a growing elderly population is also of concern throughout the world. It is estimated that the number of individuals over the age of 65 increases by 800,000 every month (Kinsella, 1994); by the year 2025, this group will number 1.2 billion people (Carballo, 1994). Increased population mobility and the decline of the extended family as a social institution have increased the social burden of care for these older adults and many countries are experiencing serious difficulty in providing health care for this population (Hafez, 1994). Specific areas of concern include financial assistance, food, housing, assistive aids such as glasses and hearing aids, adult day care, safety hazards, and social isolation.

A final concern in international health is that of human response to disasters. One can hardly pick up a newspaper without reading of natural or manmade disasters that affect large numbers of people. International efforts coordinated by WHO and the International Red Cross have led to the development of disaster planning groups throughout the world. These groups or collaborating centers provide information, services, research, and training in support of international disaster response. One group in the United States designated as a WHO collaborating center is the Center for Emergency Preparedness and Response at the CDC. The function of this group is to coordinate disaster response and to conduct field research related to disasters. Disaster preparedness and the community health nurse's role in disaster are addressed in some detail in Chapter 29.

International cooperation and effort make a difference in the health status of the world population. The classic example of the benefits of such cooperation is the eradication of smallpox. It took just 13 years of global effort to wipe out a disease that was taken for granted by the populations of two millennia. Similar concerted international efforts in other areas can influence the health of population groups throughout the world.

TESTING YOUR UNDERSTANDING

1. Diagram the organizational structure of the U.S. health care delivery system. (pp. 30–38)
2. What are the three major characteristics of the U.S. scientific health care subsystem? Give an example of each characteristic. (pp. 30–31)

3. Compare and contrast voluntary and official health agencies. (pp. 32–33)
4. What are the three core functions of public health? Describe how each of the essential services relates to the core functions. (p. 32)
5. Describe five functions performed by voluntary health agencies. Give an example of each. (pp. 32–33)
6. What level of official health agencies has primary responsibility for the health of the U.S. public? How is this authority derived? (p. 34)
7. What type of health care delivery system exists in the United States? (p. 39)
8. Describe three alternative types of national health care delivery systems. Identify at least one national health care system that exemplifies each type. (pp. 39–41)

WHAT DO YOU THINK?
Questions for Critical Thinking

1. What are the advantages and disadvantages of a centralized, government-supported health care system for all citizens?
2. How would the American public respond to the type of health care system present in Great Britain or Canada? Why?
3. What gaps do voluntary agencies fill in your community? What advantages do they have in filling these gaps over official public health agencies in your locale? What difficulties do they face?

REFERENCES

American Public Health Association Executive Board. (1995, September). The role of public health in ensuring healthy communities. *The Nation's Health,* 18–19.

Basch, P. F. (1990). *Textbook of international health.* New York: Oxford University Press.

Beddone, G., Clark, H. F., & Whyte, N. B. (1993). Vision for the future of public health nursing: A case for primary health care. *Public Health Nursing, 10,* 13–18.

Berman, P., & Khan, M. E. (1993). Introduction: Paying for India's health care. In P. Berman & M. E. Khan (Eds.), *Paying for India's health care* (pp. 21–30). New Delhi: Sage.

Bhat, R. (1993). The private health care sector in India. In P. Berman & M. E. Khan (Eds.), *Paying for India's health care,* (pp. 161–196). New Delhi: Sage.

Birchfield, M., Dvorak, E. M., Scully, J., Haas, S., & Du-berly, J. (1991). Health systems and policy in the USA and in the United Kingdom: An overseas programme. *Journal of Advanced Nursing, 16,* 1131–1137.

Birt, C. (1996). United Kingdom. In K. Hurrelmann & U. Laaser (Eds.), *International handbook of public health* (pp. 363–377). Westport, CT: Greenwood Press.

Blendon, R. J., Donelan, K., Leitman, R., et al. (1993). Health reform lessons learned from physicians in these nations. *Health Affairs, 12,* 194–203.

Blendon, R. J., Leitman, R., Morrison, I., & Donelan, K. (1990). Satisfaction with health systems in ten nations. *Health Affairs, 9*(2), 185–192.

Canadian Public Health Association, Board of Directors. (1996). Focus on health: Public health in health services restructuring. *Canadian Journal of Public Health, 87,* I1–I26.

Carballo, M. (1994). Emerging needs of the elderly. *World Health, 47*(3), 11–12.

Centers for Disease Control. (1993). Recommendations of the International Task Force for Disease Eradication. *MMWR, 41*(RR-16), 1–38.

Chrisman, N. J., & Kleinman, A. (1983). Popular health care, social networks, and cultural meaning. In D. Mechanic (Ed.), *Handbook of health, health care, and the health professions* (pp. 569–590). New York: Free Press.

Communication from the City Auditor regarding tuberculosis nurse. (August 20, 1915). San Diego, CA: City of San Diego Archives.

Dandoy, S. (1997). The state public health department. In F. D. Scutchfield & C. W. Keck (Eds.), *Principles of public health practice* (pp. 68–86). Albany, NY: Delmar.

Di Marco, M. M., & Storch, J. L. (1995). History of the Canadian Health Care System. In D. M. Wilson (Ed.), *The Canadian health care system* (pp. 5–16). Edmonton, Alberta: Health Canada.

Enciso, G. F., & Pliego, J. P. (1996). Mexico. In K. Hurrelmann & U. Laaser (Eds.), *International handbook of public health* (pp. 247–260). Westport, CT: Greenwood Press.

Foege, W. (1994). Preventive medicine and public health. *JAMA, 271,* 1704–1705.

Ge, K., & Yang, X. (1996). China. In K. Hurrelmann & U. Laaser (Eds.), *International handbook of public health* (pp. 97–108). Westport, CT: Greenwood Press.

Hafez, G. (1994). The "greying" of the nations. *World Health, 47*(4), 4–5.

Harper, A. C., & Lambert, L. (1994). *The health of populations: An introduction* (2nd ed.). New York: Springer.

Hsiao, W. C. (1992). Comparing health systems: What nations can learn from one another. *Journal of Health Politics, Policy, and Law, 17,* 613–615.

Institute of Medicine. (1988). *The future of public health.* Washington, DC: National Academy Press.

Jamison, D. T., & Mosley, W. H. (1991). Disease control priorities in developing countries: Health policy responses to epidemiological change. *American Journal of Public Health, 81,* 15–22.

Kinsella, K. G. (1994). An aging world population. *World Health, 47*(4), 6.

Kuss, T., Proulx-Girouard, L., Lovitt, S., Katz, C. B., & Kennelly, P. (1997). A public health nursing model. *Public Health Nursing, 14*(2), 81–91.

Mason, J. O. (1990). A prevention policy framework for the nation. *Health Affairs, 9*(2), 22–29.

Miller, C. A., Moore, K. S., Richards, T. B., & Monk, J. D. (1994). A proposed method for assessing the performance of local public health functions and practices. *American Journal of Public Health, 84,* 1743–1749.

Miller, D. F. (1995). *Dimensions of community health* (5th ed.). Dubuque, IA: W. C. Brown.

Model Standards Work Group. (1985). *Model Standards: A guide for community preventive services* (2nd ed.). Washington, DC: American Public Health Association.

Morse, S. S. (1992). Global microbial traffic and the interchange of disease. *American Journal of Public Health, 82,* 1326–1327.

The Nation's Health. (November, 1995a). Global immunization of children showing increase, p. 7.

The Nation's Health. (May/June, 1995b). Many deaths preventable, says WHO's first global health survey. p. 17.

The Nation's Health. (November, 1995c). WHO reports on new, re-emerging diseases threatening world health, p. 24.

The Nation's Health. (November 1995d). WHO says dangerous TB treatment practices threaten lives of AIDS patients, p. 6.

The Nation's Health. (October, 1996). Non-communicable diseases to become leading cause of death worldwide, p. 15.

Orr, J. (1992). The community dimension. In K. Luker & J. Orr (Eds.), *Health visiting: Towards community health nursing.* London: Blackwell Scientific.

Rawding, N., & Wasserman, M. (1997). The local health department. In F. D. Scutchfield & C. W. Keck (Eds.), *Principles of public health practice* (pp. 87–100). Albany, NY: Delmar.

Rodwin, V. G., & Sandier, S. (1993). Health care under the French national health insurance. *Health Affairs, 12*(3), 111–131.

Roemer, M. I. (1977). *Systems of health care.* New York: Springer.

Spasoff, R. A. (1996). Canada. In K. Hurrelmann & U. Laaser (Eds.), *International handbook of public health* (pp. 85–96). Westport, CT: Greenwood Press.

Sofaer, S. (1988). Community health planning in the United States: A postmortem. *Family and Community Health, 10*(4), 1–12.

Swanson, J. (1987). Nursing in Cuba: Population-focused practice. *Public Health Nursing, 4,* 183–191.

UNICEF. (1995). *The state of the world's children.* Oxford: Oxford University Press.

····································

RESOURCE LIST OF FEDERAL HEALTH-RELATED AGENCIES

Administration for Families and Children
Cohen Bldg, 4760
370 L'Enfant Promenade SW
Washington, DC 20447
(202) 401–9200

Administration on Aging
330 Independence Avenue, SW
Washington, DC 20201
(202) 401–4541

Agency for Health Policy and Research
2101 E. Jefferson Street
Rockville, MD 20852
(301) 594–6662

Agency for Toxic Substances and Disease Registry
1600 Clifton Road
Atlanta, GA 30333
(404) 452–4111

Bureau of Health Professions
5600 Fishers Lane, 8–05
Rockville, MD 20857
(301) 443–5794

Centers for Disease Control and Prevention
1600 Clifton Road, NE
Atlanta, GA 30333
(404) 639–3311

Division of Nursing
5600 Fishers Lane, 5C-26
Rockville, MD 20857
(301) 443–5786

Food and Drug Administration
5600 Fishers Lane
Rockville, MD 20857
(301) 443–1544

Health Care Financing Administration
200 Independence Avenue, SW
Washington, DC 20201
(202) 690–6726

Health Resources and Services Administration
5600 Fishers Lane
Rockville, MD 20857
(301) 443–2086

Indian Health Service
5600 Fishers Lane
Rockville, MD 20857
(301) 443–1083

National Institutes of Health
9000 Rockville Pike
Bethesda, MD 20892
(301) 496–4000

Social Security Administration
6401 Security Bldg.
Baltimore, MD 21235
(800) 772–1213

Substance Abuse and Mental Health Services
   Administration
5600 Fishers Lane
Rockville, MD 20857
(301) 443–4797

U.S. Department of Health and Human Services
200 Independence Avenue, SW
Washington, DC 20201
(202) 619–0257

U.S. Public Health Service
200 Independence Avenue, SW
Washington, DC 20201
(202) 690–6467

RESOURCE LIST OF INTERNATIONAL HEALTH AGENCIES

Agency for International Development Cooperation
U.S. Dept. of State Bldg.
320 21st Street, NW
Washington, DC 20523
(202) 647–4000

American Association for World Health
1129 20th Street, NW, Ste. 400
Washington, DC 20036
(202) 466–5883

Baptist World AID
6733 Curran Street
McLean, VA 22101-6005
(703) 790–8980

Catholic Relief Services
209 W. Fayette Street
Baltimore, MD 21201
(410) 625–2220

Concern/America
2024 N Broadway, Ste. 104
PO Box 1790
Santa Ana, CA 92702
(714) 953–8575

Direct Relief International
27 S. La Patera Lane
Santa Barbara, CA 93117
(805) 964–4767

Federation of World Public Health Association
c/o American Public Health Association
1015 15th Street, NW
Washington, DC 20005
(202) 789–5696

International Committee of the Red Cross
19, avenue de la Paix
CH-1202 Geneva, Switzerland
22–734–6001

International Emergency Action
10, rue Felix Zeim
F-75018 Paris, France

International Organization for Cooperation
   in Health Care
19, rue de Marteau
B-1040 Brussels, Belgium

International Planned Parenthood Federation,
   Western Hemisphere Region
902 Broadway, 10th Floor
New York, NY 10010
(212) 995–8800

International Union Against Tuberculosis
68, boulevard St. Michel
F-75006, Paris, France
1–46330830

International Women's Health Coalition
24 E. 21st Street, 5th Floor
New York, NY 10010
(212) 979–8500

Mother and Child International
c/o Mrs. Gerda M. Santschi
16, Chemin Grande Gorge
CH-1255 Vevrier, Switzerland
22–7840658

National Council for International Health
1701 K Street, NW, Ste. 600
Washington, DC 20006
(202) 833–5900

OXFAM
274 Banbury Road
Oxford OX2 7DZ, England

Pan American Health Organization
525 23rd Street, NW
Washington, DC 20037
(202) 861–3200

Peace Corps
1990 K Street, NW
Washington, DC 20526
(202) 606–3970

Project Hope (People to People Foundation)
Carter Hall
Milwood, VA 22646
(703) 837–2100

Task Force for Child Survival and Development
Carter Presidential Center
1 Copenhill Avenue
Atlanta, GA 30307
(404) 872–4122

United Nations International Children's
    Emergency Fund (UNICEF)
3 United Nation's Plaza
New York, NY 10017
(212) 326–7000

U.S./Mexico Border Health Association
6006 North Mesa, Ste. 600
El Paso, TX 79912
(915) 581–6645

World Bank
1818 H Street, NW
Washington, DC 20433
(202) 477–1234

World Health Organization
1825 K Street, NW, Ste. 1207
Washington, DC 20006
(202) 466–5883

WHO Collaborating Center on AIDS
c/o Centers for Disease Control
1600 Clifton Road, NE
Atlanta, GA 30333
(404) 329–3311

World Medical Relief
11745 Rosa Parks Boulevard
Detroit, MI 48206
(313) 866–5333

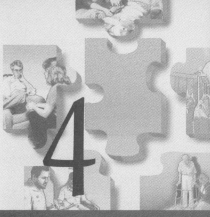

COMMUNITY HEALTH NURSING

► KEY TERMS

advocate
case finding
case management
categorical funding
change agent
client-oriented roles
collaboration
community care agent
community health
  nursing
coordination
corporatization
counseling
delivery-oriented roles
discharge planning
education
index of suspicion
leadership
liaison
population-oriented
  roles
primary care
privatization
referral
researcher
role model

In his 1916 address to Johns Hopkins Hospital Training School graduates, William H. Welch noted that America had "made at least two unique contributions to the cause of public health—the Panama Canal and the public health nurse" (Krampitz, 1987). According to a 1988 survey of registered nurses conducted by the Division of Nursing (1988), community health nurses constituted 11.5% of employed registered nurses in the United States. They practice within the community, historical, and health care system contexts described in the previous chapters. Who are they and what makes their practice unique? In this chapter we explore the features that set community health nursing apart from other nursing specialties and examine the roles and functions performed by community health nurses.

▶ Chapter Objectives

After reading this chapter, you should be able to:

- Define community health nursing.
- Identify at least five attributes of community health nursing.
- Describe the primary focus of community health nursing.
- Summarize the American Nurses Association (ANA) Standards for Community Health Nursing Practice.
- Distinguish among client-oriented, delivery-oriented, and population-oriented community health nursing roles.
- Describe at least five client-oriented roles performed by community health nurses.
- Describe at least three delivery-oriented roles performed by community health nurses.
- Describe at least four population-oriented roles performed by community health nurses.

▶ DEFINING COMMUNITY HEALTH NURSING

Community health nurses, other health care providers, and the public are confused about the definition of community health nursing. There is also debate whether the term *community health nursing* or *public health nursing* best describes the field. Many authors within and outside of nursing use the terms interchangeably.

On the other hand, participants in the Consensus Conference on the Essentials of Public Health Nursing Practice and Education made a distinction based on education rather than practice setting (Division of Nursing, 1985; Keating, 1992). In the view of the conference members, community health nurses possess a standard array of nursing competencies, but they practice nursing in community, rather than institutional, settings. Public health nurses have had specific educational preparation and have received supervised clinical experience in a public health setting. The public health nurse may or may not function in an official public health agency but has the qualifications to do so. An example of this distinction might be the home health nurse who provides care to clients in a community setting, but focuses the care on the individual with no concern for the health of the total population. According to the conference participants, this nurse is a community health nurse, not a public health nurse. The public health nurse, on the other hand, may provide care to individuals and families, but the

primary focus is the health of the larger population group.

Other authors suggest that community health nursing is more than just nursing carried out in non-hospital settings. For example, community health nursing has been described as "the synthesis of nursing theory and public health theory applied to promoting and preserving the health of populations" (Hickman, 1990). In the eyes of some authors, public health nursing is seen as a subspecialty of community health nursing (Josten, Clarke, Ostwald, Stoskopf, & Shannon, 1995; Matuk & Horsburg, 1992) in which public health nurses are defined as those employed by official government agencies versus home health nurses, school nurses, hospice nurses, and other subspecialties of community health nursing (Division of Nursing, 1985). Both community health nursing and public health nursing are terms that have come to be associated with nursing practice focused on the health of populations (Josten, Aroskar, Reckinger, & Shannon, 1996).

In 1996, the Public Health Nursing Section of the American Public Health Association (APHA) defined public health nursing as "the practice of promoting and protecting the health of populations using knowledge from nursing, social, and public health sciences." The section further described public health nursing as a systematic process of assessing populations to identify groups in need of health promotion or at risk for disease, planning for community intervention, implementing the plan, evaluating outcomes, and using the resulting data to influence health care delivery.

The American Nurses Association (ANA) (1986) presented a similar definition, but used the term *community health nurse*, in the introduction to *Standards of Community Health Nursing Practice:*

> Community health nursing practice promotes and preserves the health of populations by integrating the skills and knowledge relevant to both nursing and public health. The practice is comprehensive and general, and is not limited to a particular age or diagnostic group; it is continual, and is not limited to episodic care. . . . While community health nursing practice includes nursing directed to individuals, families, and groups, the dominant responsibility is to the population as a whole.

A number of similar elements are noted in the ANA and APHA definitions of public health nursing or community health nursing. These definitions speak to the combination of elements from nursing science and public health science, and both view population aggregates as the primary focus of care. Both definitions emphasize promoting health and preventing illness. The essential elements of a satisfactory definition of community health nursing or public health nursing describe the relationship between nursing and public health practice, the focus of care, the goal of care, and the methods of achieving those goals.

For our purposes, the terms *community health nurse* and *public health nurse* are used interchangeably within the context of the following definition of community health nursing. **Community health nursing** is a synthesis of nursing knowledge and practice and the science and practice of public health, implemented via systematic use of the nursing process and other processes, designed to promote health and prevent illness in population groups. The focus of care is the aggregate. The goal of care is the promotion of health and the prevention of illness. Health promotion and illness prevention in the population may be achieved through interventions directed at the total population or at individuals, families, and groups that constitute its members. The mode of achieving this goal is the application of principles of both public health and nursing science in the use of the nursing process with clients at all levels—individual, family, group, and community. Community health nursing, as used in this text, is not merely the performance of nursing activities in a community setting.

► SOCIAL FORCES INFLUENCING COMMUNITY HEALTH NURSING

As we noted at the beginning of this chapter, community health nursing is influenced by the community, historical, and health care system contexts in which it is practiced. Community health nursing is also influenced by a variety of social forces. A group of community health nursing experts categorized these influences into seven areas: general social forces, economic changes, government changes, technological changes, health forces, care system changes, and professional changes. General social forces include the move to let market forces determine health care service distribution, greater diversity in client populations, an aging population, globalization of many endeavors including health efforts, rapid change, a litigious atmosphere, and increases in addictive behaviors. Economic forces influencing community health nursing include conflict between demands for health services and lower taxes, economic decisions to scale back services without attention to health risks involved, and an increased emphasis on marketing health services. An increased em-

phasis on **corporatization,** or provision of health care services on a for-profit basis, is another economic factor influencing community health nursing.

Government changes are related to economic ones and include funding cutbacks and failure to acknowledge a growing segment of disadvantaged citizens in need of health care services. **Privatization** of some health department services by contracting them out to private providers is another government change affecting the role of community health nurses in official agencies. Emphasis on revenue generation from traditional public health services is another change reflecting both government emphasis and economic forces. Positive government changes are increasing political activity and input into policy decisions by nurses, increasing state assistance to local jurisdictions in dealing with public health issues, and eliminating categorical funding tied to specific program areas. A final influencing factor in this area is a lack of government understanding of public health practice and issues including those related to community health nursing.

Burgeoning information systems are the primary technological change influencing practice, and increased complexity of health problems addressed by community health nurses, as well as the increased impact of chronic disease, are health and illness forces influencing community health nursing. Other health and illness factors include the health effects of social problems such as adolescent pregnancy and violence and emerging conflicts between individual rights and public health.

Major care systems changes that influence community health nursing include the growth in the uninsured population, the emergence of managed care, increased use of nonlicensed workers, and failure to shift health care from a curative to a promotion and prevention focus. Other system influences include lack of diversity in the health work force coupled with growing diversity in the population and a diminished concern for the values of caring and justice. Positive changes in this area include the focus on outcomes of care and community-based practice with increasing community partnerships and a better informed, more demanding public.

Finally, there are forces specific to the discipline of nursing itself that are influencing practice. Positive forces in this area include movement into nontraditional practice areas such as independent practice and school-based clinics and the reframing of community health nursing education in light of the core public health functions. Movement of other health professionals into a wide variety of community settings, confusion regarding the role and identity of community health nursing, lack of nurses in public health leadership roles, and lack of data on the effectiveness of community health nursing are some of the negative discipline-related forces influencing community health nursing.

▶ GENERALIST OR SPECIALIST

In addition to the controversy over the appropriate title for our specialty, debate is ongoing regarding the general or specialized nature of community health nursing. For several years, the focus of community health nursing had become increasingly specialized in area of focus (eg, maternal–child health, family planning, mental health), developmental stage (eg, young children, school-age children, or the elderly), or setting (eg, health department, school, workplace) (Underwood, Woodcox, Berkel, Black, & Ploeg, 1991). In the United States, this move to specialization was fostered by *categorical funding* (funding specifically targeted for special types of services) approaches at the federal government level (Feagin & Alford, 1990). In Ontario, Canada, specialization in community health nursing was recommended by an ad hoc Generalist/Specialist Committee of the Public Health Branch of the Ontario Ministry of Health as a means of decreasing role strain among community health nurses (Underwood, et al., 1991). In the U.S. experience, such specialization has resulted in fragmentation of care when clients must make multiple visits to an agency to secure the wide variety of services needed. In addition, specialization increased staffing requirements and cost of care provided. From this perspective, then, generalist preparation in community health nursing that permits the community health nurse to address a wide variety of health care needs and to modify roles as needs change is desirable. The generalist perspective also has certain disadvantages. For example, a generalist role tends to be difficult to define, and generalists may have difficulty giving up elements of their practice to acquire newer roles as societal needs change (Reutter & Ford, 1996).

There is growing agreement, however, that there is room for both generalist and specialist practice in community health nursing and that differentiation of the two should be based on educational preparation. From this perspective, the generalist community health nurse would be prepared at the baccalaureate level, and specialist practice is seen as the purview of the community health nurse with graduate preparation (American Public Health Association Public Health Nursing Section, 1996; Josten, et al., 1995; Keating, 1992). Within this view, a community health nurs-

ing generalist is defined as "a licensed professional nurse who has a baccalaureate degree in nursing and has demonstrated expertise in community health nursing" (Hickman, 1990), whereas the community health nursing specialist is defined as "one who practices with a working knowledge of the community, the residents, the organization and distribution of health care services, the population, and the networks of other care providers" (McMurray, 1990). This expertise is demonstrated as advanced skills in community assessment and health program planning, implementation, and evaluation, where the generalist may demonstrate beginning skills in these areas (Dunn & Decker, 1990). These skills must also be demonstrated in abilities to adjust care to meet client needs in four areas: conservation of health, prevention of illness, restoration of health, and amelioration of illness effects (Kelly, 1996).

▶ ATTRIBUTES OF COMMUNITY HEALTH NURSING

Community health nursing is characterized by a constellation of attributes that make it a unique field of nursing practice. These attributes are an orientation to health, a population focus, autonomy, continuity, collaboration, interactivity, public accountability, intimacy, and variability. The attributes of community health nursing are summarized in Table 4–1.

Orientation to Health

A 1988 Institute of Medicine report noted that the mission of public health is that of "fulfilling society's interest in assuring conditions in which people can be

TABLE 4–1. ATTRIBUTES OF COMMUNITY HEALTH NURSING

Health orientation	Emphasis on health promotion and disease prevention rather than cure of illness
Population focus	Emphasis on health of population groups (aggregates) rather than individuals or families
Autonomy	Greater control over health care decisions by both nurse and client than in other settings
Continuity	Provision of care on a continuing, comprehensive basis rather than a short-term, episodic basis
Collaboration	Interaction between nurse and client as equals; greater opportunity for collaboration with other segments of society
Interactivity	Greater awareness of interaction of a variety of factors with health
Public accountability	Accountability to society for the health of the general population
Intimacy	Greater awareness of the reality of client lives and situations than is true of other areas of nursing
Variability	Wide array of clients at different levels, from different ethnic backgrounds, and in different settings

healthy." Promotion of health has also been a nursing function from as far back as the first school of nursing established by Florence Nightingale. At that time, a full year of the nursing curriculum was devoted to the promotion of community health (Laffrey & Page, 1989).

In other nursing specialties, health promotion is a facet of care, but one that is, of necessity, frequently given lower priority than health restoration needs. In community health nursing, on the other hand, the emphasis is on health promotion and maintenance rather than the cure of disease or disability. This health orientation is one of the sources of satisfaction voiced by community health nurses in several surveys (Clarke, Beddome, & Whyte, 1993; Liepert, 1996; Reutter & Ford, 1996). Although community health nurses frequently help clients resolve existing health problems, their major goal is to promote clients' highest level of physical, emotional, and social well-being.

Population Focus

As noted earlier, the primary concern of community health nurses is the health of the general public rather than that of individuals or families. Indeed, this focus on whole populations has been considered the defining characteristic of community health nursing (Gebbie, 1996). Community health nursing practice is designed to gather and interpret data on the health status of groups of people in an effort to identify and resolve health problems common to the population as a whole or to certain subgroups within the population. When care is provided to individuals and families, it is done so primarily as a means of enhancing the health status of the total population. Consequently, it is the needs of the population that determine which individuals or families are to be served.

From its earliest days in the United States, community health nursing has focused on the health of population groups. Even while they provided care to individuals and families, the nurses of the Henry Street Settlement and other similar organizations had as their goal the improved health of the immigrant population, schoolchildren, and the working poor. As noted by one community health nurse "one-to-one contact was often the way you got the community. . . . That's where it [community development] starts" (Liepert, 1996).

Recently, there has been a call for a return to balance among the care provided to individuals, families, and population groups. It has been noted that the separation of sick and well care within public health nursing resulted from economic exigencies and reimbursement policies. Many community health nurses continue to provide significant service to individuals and families, and devaluing this care in favor of "pop-

ulation-based" practice is seen as further dividing community health nurses as a group (Zerwekh, 1992b). As noted in the APHA definition statement, "Public health nurses integrate community involvement and knowledge about the entire population with personal, clinical understanding of individuals and families within the population" (American Public Health Association Public Health Nursing Section, 1996). Community health nurses are encouraged to discover the "extraordinary clinical wisdom developed by going to the people . . . working among them, listening to their stories, and developing the groundwork for individuals and families to help themselves" (Zerwekh, 1992a).

Autonomy

Autonomy, or self-direction, is a twofold attribute of community health nursing. Both the community health nurse and the client tend to be more self-directed than either might be in an institutional health care setting. Although all clients have the right and responsibility to make decisions about their health care, their autonomy in this regard tends to be eroded by the way health care institutions operate. Because community health nursing care is typically provided in the client's home or neighborhood, the client is more likely to demand an active role in health care decision making, a situation the community health nurse should anticipate and foster.

Community health nurses also exercise a considerable degree of professional autonomy. In some situations, community health nurses may be the only providers of health care available. They must then rely on their own judgment to choose an appropriate course of action, usually without the guidance of a physician or supervisor. In this sense, the community health nurse is more autonomous in practice than is the institution-based nurse. Autonomy in practice is a factor that has been consistently associated with job satisfaction for community health nurses (Liepert, 1996; Parahoo & Barr, 1994; Reutter & Ford, 1996; Stewart & Arklie, 1994).

Continuity

Continuity of care is another hallmark of community health nursing. Whatever the setting in which community health nurses work, relationships between nurse and client tend to be of relatively long duration. Practicing community health nurses identified this factor as "being a constant in the community over time" (Family Health Services, 1993). Community health nurses usually have the flexibility to work with most clients until both feel that services are no longer needed. Because of the extended nature of the relationship, community health nurses are able to evaluate long-term as well as short-term effects of nursing interventions. They are also able to provide care for a wider range of client needs than is usually possible in acute care nursing. Problems not addressed today can be dealt with in subsequent meetings, and changing circumstances can be evaluated over time.

Collaboration

Because of the autonomy discussed earlier and the fact that interaction occurs in settings familiar to clients, nurse and client interact on a more equal footing than might otherwise be the case. This equality increases the potential for a truly collaborative relationship between nurse and client.

There is also greater opportunity for interaction and collaboration with other providers of client services linked directly or indirectly to health. In the acute care setting, nurses frequently interact with other health and social services providers. These opportunities for collaboration also arise in community health nursing. In addition, community health nurses have the opportunity to collaborate with a variety of nonhealth-related personnel. Examples of others with whom a community health nurse might collaborate include teachers, police and fire personnel, religious leaders, and government officials.

Interactivity

The community health nursing attribute of interactivity reflects the community health nurse's perspective on factors that contribute to client health problems. Because community health nurses see clients in their own setting, they are able to identify a wide range of factors and interrelationships among factors that lead to health problems. The community health nurse is aware of the fact that health and illness are not isolated events in human existence. Both health and illness result from a complex interaction of multiple factors. This multiplicity of influences must be explored and dealt with if the nurse is to have any impact on the health status of the community. This awareness of interactivity also means that the nurse is cognizant of factors that influence potential solutions to identified client problems.

Public Accountability

Community health nursing also differs from other nursing specialties in the level of accountability involved. Like all nurses, community health nurses are morally and legally accountable for clients for the adequacy of care provided and for reasonable outcomes of care. Community health nurses, like their acute care counterparts, are also accountable to employers and to the nursing profession for the quality of care provided. Unlike most other nurses, however, community health nurses are also accountable to society for the overall health of the public (Kristjanson & Chalmers, 1991).

Because of their focus on the health of population groups, community health nurses need to deal with the public health problems they encounter. This is true whether the nurse is employed by a public agency or institution. For example, the community health nurse working in a well-child clinic who sees the multiple problems that homelessness creates for some of these children needs to work to resolve the problems of homelessness in addition to dealing with the specific needs of children seen in the clinic. Community health nurses are accountable, as well, for providing health promotive and illness preventive care that emphasizes community participation in health planning.

The source of legal authority for nursing practice is another facet of public accountability. The legal authority for nursing actions in the hospital setting is based on institutional policy and the applicable nursing practice act. Authority to perform medically delegated tasks derives from the client's personal physician who closely oversees these dependent functions of the nurse.

Legal authority for the practice of the community health nurse also arises from state nursing practice acts in addition to health-related laws and regulations of a particular jurisdiction. The local health department has the legal responsibility for the health of the community and is one source of the community health nurse's authority. Medical authority is more indirect, and in many cases, clients may not be under the care of a physician at all.

Intimacy

Another difference between community health nursing and other areas of nursing practice is the sphere of intimacy that typifies community health practice settings. Hospitals and other institutional health care environments often modify a client's behavior, thus affecting the accuracy of the nurse's observations of clients, their families, and their problems. Practicing in the community setting, however, the nurse can get a more accurate picture of the factors that affect the client's health. The community health nurse may also become more intimately aware of everyday details of the client's normal life and environment. For example, the community health nurse might discover evidence of spouse abuse that might not be uncovered in other health care settings.

Intrusion into the client's sphere of intimacy may provoke hostility, particularly in instances when care has not been sought but is mandated by circumstances (eg, child abuse) (Kristjanson & Chalmers, 1991). In these cases, community health nurses identified a need for the "courage to care" (Family Health Services, 1993) even though care may pose a threat to the nurse's safety.

Variability

The last characteristic of community health nursing, one that is highly valued by practicing community health nurses, is variability. Community health nurses deal with diverse clients of different levels (individual, family, or population group) and ethnic backgrounds in a wide variety of settings (Liepert, 1996). This variability necessitates a broad knowledge base and provides an exciting area of practice for those willing to accept the challenge.

All of these attributes are evidence of the unique status of community health nursing, which uses principles of both nursing and public health to prevent or alleviate health problems of groups of people as well as individual members of society.

▶ STANDARDS FOR COMMUNITY HEALTH NURSING PRACTICE

One of the hallmarks of a profession is the establishment of standards of practice. Nursing, like other health-related professions, has set up standards for nursing practice and nursing service. The standards for nursing practice are further delineated in standards established for each of several specialty areas in nursing. Among these, and of particular interest to community health nurses, are the American Nurses Association's *Standards of Community Health Nursing Practice.*

Why does a profession need standards? According to the ANA, "standards are developed to characterize, to measure, and to provide guidance in achieving excellence in care" (American Nurses Association, 1986). A set of standards for practice provides a means by which one can evaluate the quality of nursing service provided. The standards for community health nursing practice have been developed within the framework of the nursing process. They relate to the areas of assessment, diagnosis, planning, implementation or action, and evaluation. Additional standards deal with the use of theory as a basis for practice, qual-

▶ ANA STANDARDS FOR COMMUNITY HEALTH NURSING

1. The nurse applies theoretical concepts as a basis for decisions in practice.
2. The nurse systematically collects data that are comprehensive and accurate.
3. The nurse analyzes data collected about the community, family, and individual to determine diagnoses.
4. At each level of prevention, the nurse develops plans that specify nursing actions unique to client needs.
5. The nurse, guided by the plan, intervenes to promote, maintain, or restore health, to prevent illness, and to effect rehabilitation.
6. The nurse evaluates responses of the community, family, and individual to interventions, to determine progress toward goal achievement and to revise the database, diagnoses, and plan.
7. The nurse participates in peer review and other means of evaluation to assure quality of nursing practice. The nurse assumes responsibility for professional development and contributes to the professional growth of others.
8. The nurse collaborates with other health care providers, professionals, and community representatives in assessing, planning, implementing, and evaluating programs for community health.
9. The nurse contributes to theory and practice in community health nursing through research.

Source: American Nurses Association, 1986.

ity assurance, and professional development, collaboration, and research. The ANA standards for community health nursing practice are summarized above. Similar standards for community health nursing have been established in areas such as Ontario, Canada (Registered Nurses Association of Ontario, 1985).

The first ANA standard asserts the need to base community health nursing practice on a sound theoretical foundation. The theoretical concepts underlying community health nursing are derived from nursing, public health, and the physical, social, and behavioral sciences.

The second and third standards address client assessment. Data collection (second standard) regarding the health status of individuals, families, and communities should be systematic, continuous, and accessible, and should be recorded in a way that facilitates communication with others. Data pertinent to individuals and families include health history and physical assessment, growth and developmental data, and information on mental and emotional status and family dynamics. Other individual and family assessment data include economic, legal, political, and environmental factors influencing health; cultural and religious factors; knowledge of and motivation toward health; strengths; and health risk factors. Community-related data to be obtained include information on community resources and power structure, demographics and vital statistics, community dynamics, and socioeconomic, cultural, and environmental characteristics.

The third standard states that nursing diagnoses should be derived from the data collected. Nursing diagnosis includes identification of client needs as well as availability of resources and patterns of health care delivery. A complete nursing diagnosis also necessitates identifying the client's potentials and limitations. The concept of nursing diagnosis is discussed in more detail in Chapter 7.

The fourth standard directs planning to meet client health needs. Plans for nursing intervention should be based on the nursing diagnoses derived from the data collected and should include measurable goals and objectives. Plans should also be based on sound theoretical concepts and should identify an appropriate sequence of activities for achieving the goals specified. Finally, the plan of care should list resources required for its implementation and reflect consideration of the costs involved.

The fifth standard addresses plan implementation. Achieving desired outcomes requires client participation. The client should be provided with sufficient information to make informed decisions regarding health-related activities and the selection of appropriate health care services. During the intervention phase of the nursing process, the community health nurse may serve as direct caregiver, supervisor of other caregivers, coordinator, advocate, educator, and modifier of plans.

Client participation is also required to achieve the outcomes of the sixth standard, which deals with evaluating interventions and their results. Evaluation involves comparing baseline and current data regarding the status of health problems diagnosed by the nurse. Evaluative data must be interpreted and the results of nursing interventions documented. Finally, data must be used to revise priorities, goals, and interventions as needed.

The seventh standard describes the nurse's responsibility for assuring quality care and participating in professional development. In meeting this standard the nurse evaluates the quality of care provided, updates personal knowledge and that of others, and incorporates new knowledge into community health practice.

The eighth standard directs the nurse to collaborate and consult with professional colleagues and community representatives. These activities include joint goal setting, planning interventions, teaching, and research, as well as communicating nursing and public health knowledge to others.

The final standard describes the nurse's responsibility with respect to research. The community health nurse is expected to be a critical consumer of research. He or she should also be involved in identifying researchable problems in community health and should participate in the investigation of these problems.

The ANA also developed criteria to measure the degree to which each of the standards has been achieved. These are divided into structural, process, and outcome criteria. Structural criteria describe the environment and resources required for achieving the standard. For example, a structural criterion related to the standard for use of theory states that resource materials discussing conceptual bases for practice must be available to the nurse. Process criteria describe the activities or processes in which the nurse engages to meet the standards. For instance, a process criterion dealing with data collection details the manner in which the nurse records data. Outcome criteria describe the expected result of the nurse's activities, for example, that data are accurate and current.

The ANA standards for community health nursing apply general principles of nursing to the unique practice of community health. The standards delineate the means by which the nursing process can be incorporated into community health nursing. They provide a mechanism and criteria for evaluating the quality of care given and can be applied throughout the trilevel focus of community health nursing: care of individuals, families, and groups or communities. Application of ANA standards to client assessment, diagnosis, planning, implementation, and evaluation of nursing interventions with respect to family and community clients is addressed in Chapters 18 and 19.

▶ ROLES AND FUNCTIONS OF COMMUNITY HEALTH NURSES

The role of the community health nurse has evolved over the last few years, and it remains in transition, evolving as societal needs change.

Some authors have expressed concern about the proliferation of various specialties that diminish the role of community health nurses. Some examples of this phenomenon are the advent of the "health educator" and the use of nurse practitioners to provide primary care, a function that has historically been part of the community health nurse role. Similar concern has been voiced in England regarding the diminished role of the health visitor (Fatchett, 1990), the British counterpart of the community health nurse. On both sides of the Atlantic, the point is made that there is no need to create new specialties to meet new societal health problems, but only for community health nurses as a group to reassert the fullness of their role. This need to explicitly define the community health nursing role was noted as one of ten priority issues concerning community health nurses in a recent study (Clarke, Beddome, & Whyte, 1993).

The roles most commonly performed by community health nurses are categorized on the basis of their orientation as client-oriented roles, delivery-oriented roles, and population-oriented roles. Because the needs of specific population groups with which they work differ, not all community health nurses engage in each of the roles mentioned here. Some nurses may perform several of the roles and functions discussed, whereas others restrict their activities to a few, depending on the situation and setting.

Client-oriented Roles

Client-oriented roles involve direct provision of client services. These include the roles of caregiver, educator, counselor, referral resource, role model, advocate, primary care provider, and case manager.

Caregiver

The caregiver role involves applying the principles of epidemiology and the nursing process to the care of clients at any level—individual, family, group, or community. Some of the functions entailed in this role are assessing client needs and planning appropriate nursing intervention. Implementing the plan of care may involve performing technical procedures or assuming one or more of the other client-oriented roles. Evaluating nursing care and its outcomes is another function performed in the caregiver role. This role is basic to all client encounters, and its functions are performed whether or not any of the other community health nursing roles are assumed. In a recent survey of community health nurses, 65% of the nurses indicated they often provided such care to individuals and families, and almost 40% often provided care to communities (Chambers, Underwood, Halbert, Woodward, Heale, & Isaacs, 1994).

Educator

Education is the process of providing someone with the knowledge and skills needed to make appropriate choices among alternative courses of action. In the educator role, the community health nurse provides clients and others with information and insights that allow them to make informed decisions on health matters. The educator role may be performed at any client level. In fact, more than 80% of community health nurses in one survey indicated providing frequent educational services to individuals, families, and groups, and more than half often provided community education services (Chambers, et al., 1994). Community health nurses, for example, educate individuals and their families about adequate nutrition. At the same time, they may educate the general public regarding the harmful effects, say, of a high-cholesterol, low-fiber diet.

In the educator role, the nurse assesses the client's need for education and motivation for learning, develops and presents a health lesson, and evaluates the effects of health education. We discuss these functions in greater detail in Chapter 9.

Although the educator role is primarily a client-oriented role, the community health nurse may also serve as an educator for his or her peers or other professionals. The nurse may be involved, for example, in educating student nurses or students in other health-related disciplines. On occasion, the nurse may be called on to educate other health professionals as well. For example, it has been the responsibility of community health nurses in some jurisdictions to assist in educating private physicians regarding appropriate diagnostic, treatment, and reporting procedures for sexually transmitted diseases.

Counselor

Although many people do not distinguish between counseling and education, they *are* different. **Counseling** is the process of helping the client to choose viable solutions to health problems. In educating, one is presenting facts. In counseling, one is *not* telling people what to do but is helping them to employ the problem-solving process and to decide on the most appropriate course of action. In the role of counselor, community health nurses explain the problem-solving process and guide clients through each step. In this way, the nurse is not only helping the client to solve the immediate problem but also assisting in the development of the client's problem-solving abilities. This is true whether the client is an individual, a family, or a community.

Counseling involves several steps on the part of the community health nurse. The first step is to assist the client to identify and clarify the problem to be solved. The nurse and client together examine the factors that contribute to a problem and those that may enhance or impede problem resolution.

At the second step of the counseling process, the community health nurse helps the client identify alternative solutions to the problem. If, for example, the client's problem is lack of money for food, one could suggest applying for food stamps, getting a second job, or establishing a budget.

Assisting the client to develop criteria for an acceptable solution to the problem is the third step in the counseling process. For example, an acceptable solution to the problem of poor nutrition would need to fit the client's budget and might need to conform to cultural dietary patterns.

Next, the community health nurse would assist the client in evaluating each of the alternative solutions in terms of criteria established for an acceptable

solution. The most appropriate alternative is one that best meets the acceptability criteria. This alternative is then implemented. Evaluation is the fifth step of the problem-solving process. If the alternative selected solves the problem, fine! If not, the process begins again. The problem-solving process is depicted in Figure 4–1.

Referral Resource

Referral is the process of directing clients to resources required to meet their needs. These resources may be other agencies that can provide necessary services or

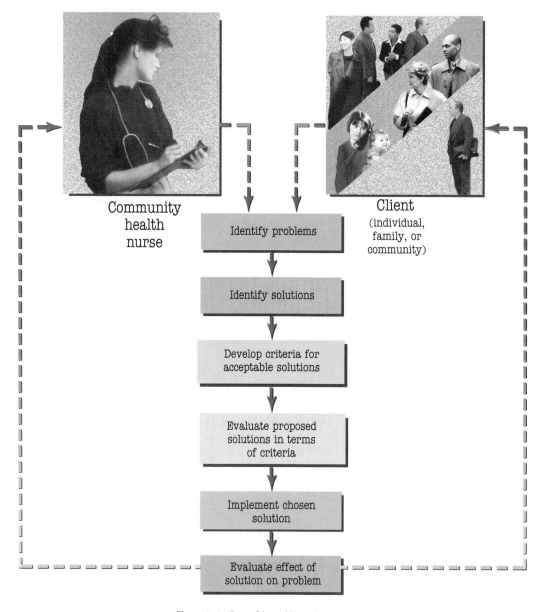

Figure 4–1. Steps of the problem-solving process.

sources of information, equipment, or supplies that the client needs and the community health nurse cannot supply. Referral is one of the key functions of community health nurses. In fact, almost 85% of community health nurses surveyed in one study indicated frequently serving as a referral resource for individual clients and almost three fourths provided these services to groups of people (Chambers, et al., 1994).

A distinction must be made, however, between the functions of referral and consultation. In a referral, the client is directed toward another source of services. On the other hand, in consultation, the nurse may seek assistance or information needed to help the client, but the client does not receive services directly from the consultant. Community health nurses also provide consultation to other professionals and to policy-making bodies. In one study, 72% of community health nurses provided consultation services to colleagues and 15% provided them to government policy makers (Chambers, et al., 1994).

Referral is an important part of the role of the community health nurse in any practice setting. It is the nurse's responsibility to explore available resources and direct clients to them as appropriate. The degree of intervention required in a specific referral varies with the type of referral and the client situation. Sometimes it is sufficient to let a client know that a certain resource exists. On other occasions, the particular agency may require a written referral from the nurse or from a physician.

In some instances, the client may not be capable of following through on a referral. For example, the depressed client may not have the energy to phone for an appointment at the local mental health center, but may be able to keep an appointment made by the nurse. The nurse must determine in each situation the degree of dependence or independence needed by that client at that time, with the goal, of course, of gradually increasing the client's ability to function independently. Specific functions of the community health nurse in the referral role include determining the need for referral, identifying the appropriate referral resources, and making and following up on the referral. The referral process is discussed in more detail in Chapter 11.

Role Model

A *role model* is someone who consciously or unconsciously demonstrates behavior to others who will perform a similar role. Community health nurses serve as role models for a variety of people with whom they come in contact. Through their own behavior, nurses influence the behavior of others. For instance, the community health nurse's ability to deal with crisis without panic provides direction for clients to do the same.

The community health nurse's role as a model is not confined solely to influencing the health-related behavior of clients. The nurse also serves as a role model for other health care professionals. One of the areas in which the role modeling function is of primary importance is in the educational preparation of student nurses. The way the community health nurse treats clients, the type of activity in which the nurse engages, and the level of competence displayed may all influence students' attitudes and practice. This influence can be either positive or negative.

Advocate

Advocacy has been defined as "the process of promoting patients' rights of self-determination" (Zerwekh, 1992b). An *advocate* is someone who speaks on behalf of those who, for whatever reason, cannot speak for themselves. Client advocacy is another of the roles of the community health nurse that may take place at the individual, family, or community level. The nurse may serve as an advocate for the individual client in explaining the client's needs to the family or to other health care providers. For example, the parents of a handicapped child may tend to be overprotective, refusing to allow the child to engage in normal activities out of fear for the child's safety. The nurse can serve as an advocate for the child by explaining to the parents that their behavior is actually detrimental to the child's development. The nurse is intervening here to prevent the child from developing a further handicap, a psychological one, and is speaking for the child who cannot speak for him- or herself.

Community health nurses also engage in advocacy when they act to resolve difficulties encountered by clients in dealing with the health care system. Insisting that a case worker reevaluate a family's application for food stamps because their financial status has changed is an example of advocacy at the family level. In both of these examples, the nurse is engaging in "reactive" advocacy (Snowball, 1996).

"Proactive" advocacy tends to take place at the community level (Snowball, 1996). As mentioned in Chapter 2, this level of advocacy was a primary concern of the early leaders in community health nursing. Helping communities organize and present grievances to the city council is an example of advocacy for aggregates in today's world. Other forms of advocacy at this level include nurses' involvement in political activity at local, state, and national levels. Advocacy via the political process is discussed in Chapter 13.

As an advocate, the community health nurse engages in a number of activities or functions. The first of these is determining the need for advocacy and the factors that prevent clients from acting on their own behalf. Such factors can be quite varied. Some clients, for example, may not know how to go about making their needs known. Fear of reprisal might be another reason why clients do not speak for themselves. Other factors include apathy, feelings of hopelessness, and even language barriers.

A second function of the nurse as advocate is determining the point at which advocacy will be most effective. For example, should the nurse raise concerns of safety violations in rental housing with the landlord, with the housing authority, or with the media? Answers to such questions might be derived from knowledge of what has been tried previously and the effects of prior action. Related questions involve how the case should be presented. Should one ask, for example, for a meeting with interested parties or stage a demonstration?

Collecting facts related to the problem is another advocacy-related function. An advocate is considerably less effective when he or she does not have all the facts about a situation. A community health nurse advocate should get a detailed chronologic account of events related to the problem for which advocacy is needed. The nurse should also try to validate or verify the information obtained to support the claim that a problem exists and action is needed.

The fourth task in advocacy is presenting the client's case to the appropriate decision makers. This function requires tact and interpersonal skill. Threatening or confrontational behavior should be avoided whenever possible, as either can set up an adversarial relationship, rather than a collaborative one, which may be detrimental to the client's cause. When other avenues fail, threats may have to be employed, but nurse and client must be committed to acting on them. For example, if the nurse threatens to report a landlord for safety code violations unless action is taken to remove hazards, he or she should actually be prepared to make the report.

The final function of the nurse as an advocate is to prepare clients to speak for themselves. The activities and functions of advocacy should not be carried out by the nurse alone, but should be a collaborative effort between nurse and client. In this way, clients learn how to develop and present a forceful argument for their own needs and may, in the future, be able to act without nursing intervention.

Advocacy necessitates involvement and commitment. The effective community health nurse cannot be content with the attitude that "I'd like to help, but my hands are tied." Advocacy is not a popular concept. It frequently means frustration and argument. It is the antithesis of complacency and is essential to the practice of effective community health nursing. Community health nurses must speak for those who cannot speak for themselves and articulate their needs to those in power. Nurses must also assist members of the community to learn how to speak for themselves rather than remain dependent on the nurse. Advocacy is a twofold obligation to take the part of others and, in time, to prepare them to stand alone.

A final comment is necessary with respect to advocacy. Because advocacy promotes clients' right to self-determination, community health nurses must be prepared to support clients' decisions even when they run counter to health interests (Gadow, 1990). For instance, the nurse may need to accept a client's unwillingness to agree to cancer therapy and then support the client's decision in interactions with other health care providers.

Primary Care Provider

Many community health nurses have assumed roles as nurse practitioners providing primary care to a variety of clients. *Primary care* is defined as essential health care services made universally accessible to all. It consists of initial care provided to clients at their point of entry into the health care system. The primary care function of most community health nurses involves health promotive and illness preventive interventions such as routine prenatal assessments, well-child care, and immunizations. Community health nurses also routinely deal with minor health problems such as constipation and diarrhea.

Other community health nurses, with advanced educational preparation, provide primary care as nurse practitioners. These nurses have assumed diagnostic and treatment services that were once the exclusive province of physicians. There has been some concern that incursions into medical practice by nurse practitioners might detract from the emphasis placed by community health nurses on health promotion and illness prevention (Fatchett, 1990). Although this is sometimes the case early in a nurse practitioner's career, most practitioners regain their nursing perspective fairly rapidly and provide both curative and health promotive services.

Performance of the primary care role by community health nurses and other advanced practice nurses (APNs) enhances the accessibility and comprehensiveness of health care services available to the general public. Education of nurses as primary care providers costs only one fourth the cost of physician training. Add to this the fact that APNs can provide care for half the cost of physician-provided primary care (Mundinger, 1994) and can meet 60 to 80% of the need for primary and preventive health services, and

APNs become a viable alternative for health care services. In addition, APNs have been shown repeatedly to provide equal or better quality care than physicians in a cost-effective manner (American Association of Colleges of Nursing, 1993).

Case Manager

Although case management is a new concept for many nurses, it has long been an integral component of community health nursing and has even been described as "old hat" (Erkel, 1993). Indeed, *case manager* may be seen as a comprehensive role that encompasses many of the other client-oriented roles described here.

The Case Management Society of America (1995) defined case management as "a collaborative process which assesses, plans, implements, monitors, and evaluates options and services to meet an individual's health needs through communication and available resources to promote quality cost-effective outcomes." The aims of case management include identifying high-risk clients or those with the potential for high-cost service needs, identifying opportunities to coordinate care, selecting appropriate treatment choices, controlling costs, and managing care to achieve optimal client outcomes (Brown, Mayer, & Jackson, 1992).

Case management has been shown to be cost-effective and to result in enhanced health outcomes in many settings. This is also true in terms of fostering client health-promoting behavior (American Association of Colleges of Nursing, 1993). Given this fact and community health nursing's long association with case management, it would seem appropriate to retain case management as an essential part of the community health nursing role. The process of case management will be addressed in more detail in Chapter 11.

Nursing functions in the case manager role and other client-oriented roles are summarized in Table 4–2.

Delivery-oriented Roles

The *delivery-oriented roles* of community health nurses are those designed to enhance the operation of the health care delivery system, resulting in better care for clients. Roles in this category include coordinator, collaborator, and liaison.

Coordinator

Community health nurses frequently care for clients who are receiving services from a variety of sources. Because of their awareness of the needs of the client as

TABLE 4–2. CLIENT-ORIENTED COMMUNITY HEALTH NURSING ROLES AND RELATED FUNCTIONS

Role	Function
Caregiver	• Assess client health status • Derive nursing diagnoses • Plan nursing intervention • Implement the plan of care • Evaluate the outcome of nursing intervention
Educator	• Assess client's need for education • Develop health education plan • Present health education • Evaluate outcome of health education
Counselor	• Identify and clarify problem to be solved • Help client identify alternative solutions • Assist client to develop criteria for solutions • Assist client to evaluate alternative solutions • Assist client to evaluate effects of solution • Make client aware of problem-solving process
Referral resource	• Obtain information on community resources • Determine the need for and appropriateness of a referral • Make the referral • Follow up on the referral
Role model	• Perform the behavior to be learned by clients or others
Advocate	• Determine the need for advocacy • Determine the appropriate avenue for advocacy • Obtain facts related to the situation • Present the client's case to decision makers • Prepare clients to stand alone
Primary care provider	• Assess client health status and identify problems • Plan and provide treatment for problems • Introduce other supportive services as needed • Teach and supervise others • Modify care plan as required • Teach clients self-care • Coordinate health care services • Serve as liaison between client and system
Case manager	• Identify need for case management • Assess and identify client health needs • Design plan of care to meet needs • Oversee implementation of care by others • Evaluate outcome of care

a whole being, community health nurses are in an ideal position to serve as coordinators of care. *Coordination* is the process of organizing and integrating services to best meet client needs in the most efficient manner possible. Unlike the case manager, the coordinator does not plan the care to be carried out by other health care professionals, but organizes that care to meet clients' needs as effectively as possible.

It is the community health nurse who most frequently enters the home or community and sees first hand how the client is responding to a physical therapy program or how effective a roach-control program has been. She or he is also in the best position to transmit to other providers information regarding client needs, attitudes, and progress. The community health nurse is also best able to interpret to the client, in language he or she can understand, the purposes and procedures involved in programs instituted by other health care providers.

The community health nurse serving as a coordinator of client care performs a variety of functions. The first function involves determining who is providing care to the client, where services overlap, and where gaps in care may be occurring. The second function is to communicate with other providers regarding the particulars of the client situation and needs. Communication includes informing providers of other persons and agencies dealing with the client. Except in certain circumstances (eg, child abuse or threat of harm to self or others), communication should be undertaken *only* with the consent of the client.

A simple example of coordinating services might involve arranging for appointments in a prenatal clinic and a child health clinic on the same day, when both services are provided at the same location. Coordinating appointments in this way assists a pregnant woman with a 2-year-old and limited transportation to obtain needed health care for herself and her child without a second bus trip.

One additional function of the community health nurse in a coordinator role might be arranging a case conference to include nurse, client, and other providers of services. For example, the school nurse might arrange a meeting that would include not only the nurse but also the child, parents, teachers, and school psychologist to discuss the child's behavior problems in school.

Collaborator

Collaboration is a process of joint decision making by two or more people. As a collaborator, the community health nurse engages in joint decision making regarding action to be taken to resolve client health problems. Collaboration should always take place between nurse and client or a significant other. Collaborative efforts, however, may also include other providers.

Collaboration is frequently confused with the nurse's coordination role. Coordination is essentially a management function, and involves making sure that efforts to provide services are consistent and occur without gaps or overlaps. Collaboration, on the other hand, entails joint decision making. Both collaboration and coordination, of course, necessitate working with clients and other professionals (and nonprofessionals) who contribute to the health care of clients. This contribution by others may be directly re-

lated to the client's health status, as in the case of physicians, physical therapists, nutritionists, and other health care personnel. It may also be indirectly related to the client's health status, as are the services of police and firefighters, sanitation collectors, and city officials.

Collaboration is not a matter of each health care worker designing and providing a program in his or her area of expertise with a certain amount of coordination between efforts. Rather, it is a joint effort on the part of health care providers *and clients* to set mutual goals and to arrive at a mutually acceptable plan to achieve them. Collaboration is a relatively new function for most nurses and cannot take place without a mutual feeling of respect and collegiality among health team members.

The two primary functions of the community health nurse in a collaborative role are communication and joint decision making. In communicating, the nurse conveys to other team members his or her perceptions of client needs, factors influencing those needs, and ideas for problem resolution. In decision making, the community health nurse participates in joint problem-solving efforts, using the problem-solving process with the health care team to identify and evaluate alternative solutions to client problems and to select an appropriate alternative. Collaboration may also extend to joint activity to implement solutions selected and to evaluate the outcome.

Liaison

The liaison role of the community health nurse incorporates facets of the coordinator and referral resource roles and may even incorporate the advocacy role depending on the client situation. A *liaison* provides a connection, relationship, or intercommunication. The community health nurse working with clients and dealing with multiple health and social agencies may serve as that connection or liaison. In the referral resource role, the community health nurse may function as the initial point of contact between client and agency. The liaison role might involve continued communication between client and other providers via the nurse. Sometimes this communication includes the additional function of interpretation and reinforcement of provider recommendations to the client or advocacy for the client with the provider agency.

A summary of delivery-oriented roles and related functions is presented in Table 4–3.

Population-oriented Roles

The client-oriented and delivery-oriented roles of community health nurses usually relate to the care of

TABLE 4–3. DELIVERY-ORIENTED COMMUNITY HEALTH NURSING ROLES AND RELATED FUNCTIONS

Role	Function
Coordinator	• Determine who is providing care to client • Communicate with other providers regarding client situation and needs • Arrange case conferences as needed
Collaborator	• Communicate with other health team members • Participate in joint decision making • Participate in joint action to resolve client problems
Liaison	• Serve as initial point of contact between client and agency • Facilitate communication between client and agency personnel • Interpret and reinforce provider recommendations • Serve as client advocate as needed

specific clients. At times these roles may be extended to the care of groups of people or communities. For example, the role of coordinator may be applied to the organization of several services provided to groups of people, as when a community health nurse occupies the position of clinical services coordinator for a county health department. More often, though, client-oriented and delivery-oriented roles focus on providing services to specific clients.

As noted throughout this text, community health nurses are concerned primarily with the health of the population, and they perform a number of roles that are exclusively group-oriented. *Population-oriented roles* are those of case finder, leader, change agent, community care agent, and researcher.

Case Finder

Case finding has been described as basic to community health nursing. *Case finding* by the community health nurse involves identifying individual cases or occurrences of specific diseases or other health-related conditions requiring services. Why, then, is this considered a population-oriented role? Despite the fact that case finding involves location of individual cases of a condition, the primary intent is the assessment and protection of the health of the general public. As we will see in Chapter 30, case finding is an important strategy in preventing the spread of communicable diseases in large population groups. Case finding is also a means of monitoring the health status of a group or community. For example, identifying more instances of child abuse may be an indication of a community health problem.

Community health nurses have a relatively close and usually prolonged association with clients and have the opportunity to detect changes in health status or early signs of health problems. This "detecting" has been identified as one of the critical competencies

of expert community health nurses (Zerwekh, 1991). During a visit to a hypertensive client, for example, the community health nurse may discover that the client's teenage daughter is pregnant and in need of prenatal care. Or, the nurse may observe that members of a number of families who obtain water from a common source have had recent episodes of vomiting and diarrhea. If the nurse is dealing with clients as unified entities (whether individuals, families, or communities), he or she is in a position to detect potential or actual health problems early and intervene rapidly. The ability of community health nurses to conduct physical examinations has further enhanced their case finding ability by giving them another avenue for detecting the presence of disease or disability.

Case finding responsibilities include developing an index of suspicion, identifying instances of disease or other health-related conditions, and providing follow-up services. An *index of suspicion* is an estimation of the likelihood that a disease or problem may exist and is based on a broad foundation of knowledge of the signs and symptoms of a variety of health problems and their contributing factors. For example, to identify a potential case of tuberculosis (TB), the nurse must be familiar with the signs and symptoms of TB. The nurse should also be aware of the factors associated with TB. The community health nurse who encounters a client from Asia (where the incidence of tuberculosis is relatively high) complaining of a chronic cough with hemoptysis, weight loss, and night sweats suspects TB.

The case finder role necessitates use of the diagnostic reasoning process to identify potential cases of disease or instances of other health-related conditions (such as pregnancy or the need for immunizations) based on relevant cues. This diagnostic processing of relevant signs and symptoms into a probable diagnosis of the disease is the second function of the community health nurse as case finder. The diagnostic reasoning process is discussed in more detail in Chapter 7.

The third community health nursing function related to case finding is the provision of follow-up care to the person with a specific condition. This usually entails referral for further diagnostic services and for treatment if needed. Community health nurses who are advanced practice nurses might provide these services themselves.

Leader

Leadership in the community health nursing context is a requisite skill for community health nurses. The leadership role of the community health nurse may be enacted both with individual clients or families and with groups and communities; however, because this role demands knowledge of group dynamics as well as interpersonal skills, we deal with leadership as a population-oriented role.

Leadership is the ability to influence the behavior of others. Community health nurses may assume a leadership role with a variety of individuals, including clients, other health care professionals, members of other disciplines, public officials, and the general public. Because of the number of different types of followers that may be involved, the community health nurse as leader must be able to adapt a leadership style to fit the needs of the moment.

Community health nurse functions in the leadership role include identifying the need for action and leadership, assessing the leadership needs of followers, and selecting and executing a style of leadership appropriate to both the followers and the situation. The leadership process and the functions involved are discussed in greater detail in Chapter 12.

Change Agent

Community health nurses also fill the role of change agent. A *change agent* is one who initiates and brings about change. Frequently this role is performed in conjunction with the leadership role. Change is an unavoidable part of human existence, but when change is systematically planned it can be controlled and used to enhance rather than undermine health. Specific functions of the community health nurse in the change agent role include recognizing the need for change, making others aware of the need for change, motivating others to change, and initiating and directing the desired change.

Community health nurses may serve as change agents working with individuals, families, groups, and communities or in health care delivery. For example, change may be required in the dietary patterns of individual clients or families. Or, there may be a need to alter the way a community deals with the homeless or approaches sex education in its schools. Similar changes might be needed in the health care system. For example, services might need to be redesigned to meet the needs of ethnic minority groups moving into the area. Work toward changes in health care delivery to meet evolving societal needs has been an area of strength throughout the history of community health nursing in the United States. If we are to continue to fulfill our role as community health nurses and achieve our purpose of improved health for all, we must renew our efforts as change agents at the aggregate level. The change process and its implications for community health nursing are discussed in greater detail in Chapter 12.

Critical Thinking in Research

Chambers and colleagues (1994) conducted a study of community health nurses' perceptions of their role and activities in light of the Canadian Public Health Association description of the roles and qualifications of community health nurses in Canada. Frequently performed roles reported by the nurses surveyed included caregiver, educator/consultant, social marketer, and collaborator. Less frequently performed roles included those of community developer, policy formulator, researcher/evaluator, and resource manager or planner. Community health nurses indicated a need for further education to be able to effectively perform these latter roles, but anticipated being called upon to perform them in the future.

1. If you conducted a similar study in the United States, do you think the findings would be similar to those described by Chambers, et al.? Why or why not?
2. How would you go about determining whether or not the role perceptions of Canadian and U.S. community health nurses are similar?
3. Would you design your study differently if you were trying to describe what roles U.S. community health nurses perform? If so, how would the study differ?

Community Care Agent

Earlier, we discussed the primary care provider role of community health nurse practitioners and other advanced practice nurses with individuals and families. In their population-oriented role as community care agents, community health nursing clinical specialists work with communities as clients. They diagnose and treat health problems of population groups or communities much as the nurse practitioner diagnoses and treats the health problems of individuals and families. The *community care agent* provides care at an expanded level to communities as clients.

Community diagnosis requires an understanding of the wide variety of factors that impinge on the health of the community. Only a nurse with the theoretical background necessary for community assessment can delineate the interrelationships of these factors and use the information to plan for solutions to community problems. Because of recent changes in educational preparation, a community health nurse is emerging who is capable of gearing extended practice to the needs of communities in general rather than individuals or families. Several years ago, the Pan American Health Organization (1977) delineated four functions that are part of the community care agent role of the community health nurse.

1. Diagnosis of the level of health of the community
2. Decision making regarding solutions to health problems diagnosed
3. Preparation of the community to identify and meet health needs
4. Evaluation of health care delivery

The concept of the community as the recipient of health care is discussed in detail in Chapter 19.

Researcher

A *researcher* explores phenomena observed in the world with the intent of understanding, explaining, and ultimately controlling them. The research role of the community health nurse is sometimes seen as a relatively recent one; however, even at the beginnings of community health nursing in the United States, Lillian Wald and her contemporaries made use of carefully documented data to identify societal needs and fuel social reforms. The community health nurse's current research role may be carried out at several levels. Responsibilities of the community health nurse related to research include critically reviewing relevant research and its application to practice, identifying researchable problems, designing and conducting research studies, collecting data, and disseminating research findings. The research role in community health nursing is discussed in greater depth in Chapter 8. Functions related to the role of researcher and other population-oriented community health nursing roles are summarized in Table 4–4.

TABLE 4–4. POPULATION-ORIENTED COMMUNITY HEALTH NURSING ROLES AND RELATED FUNCTIONS

Role	Function
Case finder	• Develop knowledge of signs and symptoms of health-related conditions and contributing factors • Use diagnostic reasoning process to identify potential cases of disease or other health-related conditions • Provide follow-up care to identified cases
Leader	• Identify the need for action • Assess situation and followers to determine appropriate leadership style • Motivate followers to take action • Coordinate group member activities in planning and implementing action • Assist followers to evaluate the effectiveness of action taken • Facilitate adaptation of group members • Represent the group to outsiders
Change agent	• Identify driving and restraining forces operating in change situation • Assist in unfreezing and creating motivation for change • Assist in implementation of change • Assist group to internalize change
Community care agent	• Diagnose the community's level of health • Develop solutions to identified community health problems • Prepare the community to identify and meet health needs • Evaluate health care delivery
Researcher	• Critically review research findings • Apply research findings to practice as appropriate • Identify researchable problems • Design and conduct nursing research • Collect data • Disseminate research findings

Critical Thinking in Practice: A Case in Point

Ms. Brown, a community health nurse, has received a request to visit Mrs. Jones to inform her of a class II Pap smear from her last visit to the family planning clinic. On her record, Ms. Brown notes that Mrs. Jones is 45 years old, married, and has three children. When Ms. Brown arrives at the home and explains the reason for her visit, Mrs. Jones tells her that Mr. Jones is unemployed and they have no health insurance. She does not know how she will be able to afford to have a repeat Pap smear now.

Mrs. Jones is also concerned because she has not had a period for 2 months. She has been on birth control pills for several years and has had no problems with missed periods until now. Her periods have become rather scanty in the last few months. She has no complaints of urinary frequency or breast tenderness.

Mrs. Jones states that she has been very irritable lately and cannot stand to be around her older daughter, who is 15 years old, because they argue all the time. The problem with her daughter has strained Mrs. Jones' relationship with her husband; he thinks she is being too hard on their daughter. Mrs. Jones suspects the daughter might be pregnant, because she is very moody and has gained several pounds in the last few months. When Mrs. Jones asks her daughter what is wrong, the girl changes the subject.

1. What community health nursing roles will Ms. Brown probably perform in caring for Mrs. Jones and her family? Why are these roles appropriate to this situation?
2. Give examples of some specific activities that Ms. Brown might carry out in performing each role.

TESTING YOUR UNDERSTANDING

1. Define community health nursing. (pp. 50–51)
2. Discuss the seven categories of social forces influencing community health nursing. Give an example of influence in each category. (pp. 51–52)
3. Describe at least five attributes of community health nursing. Give an example of each attribute. (pp. 52–55)
4. What is the primary focus of community health nursing? (p. 53)
5. Summarize the ANA standards for community health nursing practice. (pp. 55–56)
6. Distinguish among client-oriented, delivery-oriented, and population-oriented community health nursing roles. (pp. 56–57)
7. Describe at least five client-oriented community health nursing roles. Give an example of the performance of each role. (pp. 56–61)
8. Describe three delivery-oriented community health nursing roles. Give an example of the performance of each role. (pp. 61–62)
9. Describe at least four population-oriented community health nursing roles. Give an example of the performance of each role. (pp. 62–65)

WHAT DO YOU THINK?
Questions for Critical Thinking

1. Which of the three categories of community health nursing roles are most crucial to achieving the goals of community health nursing? Why?
2. What kinds of clinical learning experiences would best equip community health nurses to carry out the full spectrum of roles in this practice specialty?
3. Should some of the community health nursing roles discussed in this chapter be the focus of practice in specific educational levels in nursing (eg, ADN prepared nurse, BSN, MSN, etc.)? If so, which roles should be performed by nurses at which educational levels?

REFERENCES

American Association of Colleges of Nursing. (March 1993). In search of the advanced practice nurse. *American Association of Colleges of Nursing Issue Bulletin,* 1–4.

American Nurses Association. (1986). *Standards of community health nursing practice.* Kansas City, MO: American Nurses Association.

American Public Health Association Public Health Nursing Section. (1996). *The definition and role of public health nursing: A statement of the APHA Public Health Nursing Section.* Washington, DC: American Public Health Association.

Brown, N. P., Mayer , G. G., & Jackson, L. K. (1992). Case management. In A. E. Barnett & G. G. Mayer (Eds.), *Ambulatory case management and practice* (pp. 363–370). Gaithersburg, MD: Aspen.

Case Management Society of America. (1995). *Standards of practice for case management.* Little Rock, AR: Case Management Society of America.

Chambers, L. W., Underwood, J., Halbert, T., Woodward, C. A., Heale, J. A., & Isaacs, S. (1994). 1992 Ontario survey of public health nurses: Perceptions of roles and activities. *Canadian Journal of Public Health, 85,* 175–179.

Clarke, H. F., Beddome, G., & Whyte, N. B. (1993). Public health nursing's view of their future reflects changing paradigm. *Image, 25,* 305–310.

Division of Nursing, Bureau of Health Professions. (1985). *Consensus conference on the essentials of public health nursing and practice.* Rockville, MD: U.S. Department of Health and Human Services.

Division of Nursing, U.S. Department of Health and Human Services. (1988). *National sample survey of registered nurses.* Washington, DC: U.S. Department of Health and Human Services.

Dunn, A. M., & Decker, S. D. (1990). Community as client: Appropriate baccalaureate- and graduate-level preparation. *Journal of Community Health Nursing, 7,* 131–139.

Erkel, E. A. (1993). The impact of case management in preventive services. *JONA, 23*(1), 27–32.

Family Health Services. (1993). *Making a difference: Public health nursing.* Edmonton, Alberta.

Fatchett, A. B. (1990). Health visiting: A withering profession? *Journal of Advanced Nursing, 15,* 216–222.

Feagin, R., & Alford, R. L. (1990). Public health nursing: Cross-training in core services. *Public Health Nursing, 7,* 52–57.

Gadow, S. (1990). Existential advocacy: Philosophical foundations of nursing. In T. Pence & J. Cantrall (Eds.), *Ethics in nursing: An anthology.* New York: National League for Nursing.

Gebbie, K. M. (1996). *Preparing currently employed public health nurses for changes in the health system: Meeting report and suggested action steps.* New York: Center for Health Policy and Health Sciences Research.

Hickman, P. (Ed.). (1990). *Essentials of baccalaureate nursing education for entry level community health nursing practice.* Louisville, KY: Association of Community Health Nurse Educators.

Institute of Medicine. (1988). *The future of public health.* Washington, DC: National Academy Press.

Josten, L., Aroskar, M., Reckinger, D., & Shannon, M. (1996). *Educating nurses for public health leadership.* Minneapolis: University of Minnesota.

Josten, L., Clarke, P. N., Ostwald, S., Stoskopf, C., & Shannon, M. D. (1995). Public health nursing education: Back to the future for public health sciences. *Family and Community Health, 18*(1), 36–48.

Keating, S. (1992). *Educational preparation of nurses for community settings.* San Francisco: California Association of Colleges of Nursing.

Kelly, A. (1996). The concept of the specialist community nurse. *Journal of Advanced Nursing, 24,* 42–52.

Krampitz, S. D. (1987). The Yale experiment: Innovation in nursing education. In C. Maggs (Ed.), *Nursing history: The state of the art* (pp. 60–73). London: Croom Helm.

Kristjanson, L. J., & Chalmers, K. I. (1991). Preventive work with families: Issues facing public health nurses. *Journal of Advanced Nursing, 16,* 147–153.

Laffrey, S. C., & Page, S. (1989). Primary health care in public health nursing. *Journal of Advanced Nursing, 14,* 1044–1050.

Liepert, B. D. (1996). The value of community health nursing: A phenomenological study of the perceptions of community health nurses. *Public Health Nursing, 13,* 50–57.

Matuk, L. K. Y., & Horsburgh, M. E. C. (1992). Toward redefining public health nursing in Canada: Challenges for education. *Public Health Nursing, 9,* 149–154.

McMurray, A. (1990). *Community health nursing: Primary health care in practice.* Edinburgh: Churchill Livingstone.

Mundinger, M. O. (1994). Health care reform: Will nursing respond? *Nursing & Health Care, 15,* 28–33.

Pan American Health Organization. (1977). *The role of the nurse in primary care.* Geneva: World Health Organization.

Parahoo, K., & Barr, O. (1994). Job satisfaction of community health nurses working with people with a mental handicap. *Journal of Advanced Nursing, 20,* 1046–1055.

Registered Nurses Association of Ontario. (1985). *Standards of nursing practice for community health nurses in Ontario.* Toronto: Registered Nurses Association of Ontario.

Reutter, L. I., & Ford, J. S. (1996). Perceptions of public health nursing: Views from the field. *Journal of Advanced Nursing, 24,* 7–15.

Snowball, J. (1996). Asking nurses about advocating for patients: "Reactive" and proactive accounts. *Journal of Advanced Nursing, 24,* 67–75.

Stewart, M. J., & Arklie, M. (1994). Work satisfaction, stressors and support experienced by community health nurses. *Canadian Journal of Public Health, 85,* 180–184.

Underwood, E. J., Woodcox, V., Van Berkel, C., Black, M., & Ploeg, J. (1991). Organizing public health nursing for the 1990s: Generalist or specialist? *Canadian Journal of Public Health, 82,* 245–248.

Zerwekh, J. V. (1991). Tales from public health nursing true detectives. *American Journal of Nursing, 91,* 30–36.

Zerwekh, J. V. (1992a). Community health nurses—A population at risk. *Public Health Nursing, 9,* 1.

Zerwekh, J. V. (1992b). The practice of empowerment and coercion by expert public health nurses. *Image, 24,* 101–105.

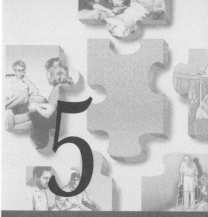

THE DIMENSIONS MODEL OF COMMUNITY HEALTH NURSING

The goal of community health nursing, as described in Chapter 4, is the improvement of the health of populations or groups of clients. Achievement of this goal requires systematic use of nursing knowledge and skills. Models of nursing practice provide a framework for systematic application of knowledge and skills to the resolution of clients' health problems and to efforts to promote or maintain health.

A number of models have been developed within nursing to direct practice. The application of several of these models to community health nursing practice is discussed in Chapter 6. In this chapter we will present the elements of the Dimensions Model developed specifically for community health nursing practice. In the Dimensions Model, community health nursing practice is examined in light of three dimensional elements that influence the interaction of client and nurse in pursuit of the goal of optimal health. These elements are derived from nursing and from public health science, the two disciplines that intertwine to create the unique field of community health nursing. The elements of the model include the dimensions of nursing, health, and health care.

The dimensions of nursing reflect professional nursing practice, and the dimensions of health encompass factors that influence the health of clients whether individuals, families, or groups of people. The dimensions of health are derived primarily from the public health science of epidemiology. The dimensions of health care also arise from the discipline of public health and reflect the three levels of prevention in community health practice.

▶ Chapter Objectives

After reading this chapter, you should be able to:

- Identify the three major elements of the Dimensions Model of community health nursing.
- Describe six dimensions of community health nursing practice.
- Identify the six dimensions of health in the Dimensions Model of community health nursing.
- Distinguish among the three dimensions of health care in the Dimensions Model of community health nursing.

▶ DIMENSIONS OF NURSING

The first element in the Dimensions Model is the nursing dimension which incorporates the elements of nursing practice employed by the community health nurse. The dimensions included in this category include the cognitive, interpersonal, ethical, skill, process, and reflective dimensions.

The Cognitive Dimension

The cognitive dimension of community health nursing practice encompasses the knowledge base used by the nurse to identify client health needs and to plan and implement care to meet those needs. This knowledge base includes an understanding of concepts drawn from myriad disciplines in addition to nursing. In order to interact effectively with client populations, for example, the community health nurse will need knowledge derived from psychology, sociology, physiology, epidemiology, public health, and so on.

The Interpersonal Dimension

The interpersonal dimension of nursing includes affective elements and interaction skills. Affective elements consist of the attitudes and values of the community health nurse that affect his of her ability to practice effectively with a variety of different people. The community health nurse must value health and its promotion among clients. In addition, the nurse must value human dignity and be able to work effectively with people whose values may differ from his or her own or from those of the dominant culture. Because the primary aim of community health is promotion of health, community health nurses must, in essence, work to eliminate the need for their services by facilitating self-care and healthy behavior among clients (National Institute for Nursing Research Priority Expert Panel, 1995). Interaction skills and the abili-

ties to collaborate and communicate effectively with others are additional elements of the interpersonal dimension.

The Ethical Dimension

In the ethical dimension of nursing, the community health nurse acts in accord with moral and ethical principles. Community health nurses must be able to make ethical decisions and be willing to act for the benefit of clients rather than for personal gain. Willingness to advocate for clients is another element of the ethical dimension of community health nursing. Aspects of the ethical dimension influence all of the other dimensions of nursing.

The Skill Dimension

The skill dimension of community health nursing encompasses both manipulative and intellectual skills which are common to all areas of nursing practice. Manipulative skills include the ability to perform such activities as giving immunizations, providing tuberculin skin testing, conducting hearing examinations and physical assessments, and so on. Intellectual skills include capacities for critical thinking as well as abilities to examine data and draw inferences.

The Process Dimension

Community health nurses employ knowledge, attitudes, and skills in the application of several specific processes when providing care to individuals, families, and population groups. The most fundamental of these processes is, of course, the nursing process. Other processes used by community health nurses in their practice are the epidemiologic process, the health education process, the home visit process, and the case management process. Community health nurses also use change, leadership, group, and political processes in their care of clients. Each of these processes is addressed in greater detail in Unit II of this book, The Process Dimension in Community Health Nursing.

The Reflective Dimension

The last of the nursing dimensions in the Dimension Model is the reflective dimension. Within this dimension, the nursing profession engages in activities that promote reflection on the profession itself, its knowledge base, and the care provided by its practitioners. Activities included in this dimension include theory development, research, and evaluation. The creation

▶ THE DIMENSIONS OF NURSING

COGNITIVE DIMENSION
    Knowledge

INTERPERSONAL DIMENSION
    Affective elements
    Interaction skills

ETHICAL DIMENSION
    Ethical decision making
    Advocacy

SKILLS DIMENSION
    Manipulative skills
    Intellectual skills

PROCESS DIMENSION
    Nursing Process
    Epidemiologic process
    Health education process
    Home visit process
    Case management process
    Change process
    Leadership process
    Group process
    Political process

REFLECTIVE DIMENSION
    Theory development
    Research
    Evaluation

of the Dimensions Model is, itself, an example of theory development in community health nursing. The importance of the other elements of the reflective dimension, research, and evaluation of practice, is emphasized in each chapter of this book. The dimensions of nursing are summarized above.

▶ DIMENSIONS OF HEALTH

The dimensions of health are many and reflect the variety of influences that affect human health. The Dimensions Model incorporates six specific dimensions of health: the biophysical dimension, the psychological dimension, the physical dimension, the social dimension, the behavioral dimension, and the health system dimension. These dimensions are based on the work of epidemiologists (Blum, 1974; Lalonde, 1974; Dever, 1991; Evans & Stoddart, 1994) and health advisory bodies (Federal, Provincial, and Territorial Advisory Committee on Population Health, 1994). Factors within each of these dimensions affect health individually and in interaction with each other and form the basis for community health nursing assessment of clients' health status.

The Biophysical Dimension

The biophysical dimension of health includes factors related to human biology that influence health. These factors may be related to age, genetics, and physiologic function. One's age can affect one's propensity for developing specific health problems. For example, pertussis, or whooping cough, is usually confined to unimmunized children under the age of 10, and sexually transmitted diseases are more prevalent among adolescents and young adults than among other age groups. Similarly, the elderly are more susceptible to complications and death due to influenza than people in other age groups. Age-related differences in the probability and effects of disease are seen in many chronic health problems as well (eg, cardiovascular disease and arthritis).

In part, age-related differences in susceptibility to specific health problems may be due to intrinsic aspects of maturation and aging. For example, it is diminished immune system response that occurs with age that puts older persons at higher risk for influenza mortality than their younger counterparts. In other cases, increased risk is a function of behaviors typically associated with certain ages. For example, adolescents are developmentally more inclined to engage in risk-taking behaviors than adults and may, therefore, be at higher risk for accidental injury.

As a biophysical factor, genetic inheritance encompasses gender and racial/ethnic characteristics as well as the specific gene pattern transferred by one's parents. Certain health problems are more frequently associated with some gender or racial/ethnic groups than with others. With respect to gender as a biophysical factor, pregnancy obviously only affects the physiologic status of women, and hemophilia occurs primarily in men. The classic example of race as a biological factor in a specific illness is, of course, sickle cell anemia among African-Americans. African-Americans have traditionally had a higher incidence of hypertension as well. There is evidence, however, to suggest that hypertension in this group may be a byproduct of the stresses resulting from lower socioeconomic status rather than a racial influence.

The presence of certain genetically transmitted traits also increases one's risk of developing some health problems (Baird, 1994). For example, genetic inheritance is known to play a significant role in the development of diabetes, heart disease, and cancer and may be implicated in substance abuse (Kendler, Heath, Neale, Kessler, & Eaves, 1992) and other psychiatric disorders (Comings, 1991). There is even some evidence that genetic makeup may influence one's propensity to smoke (Carmelli, Swan, Robinette, & Fabsitz, 1992) or be divorced (Bower, 1992).

Factors related to complex physiologic function in the biophysical dimension include one's basic state of health as it affects the probability of developing other health problems. Considerations in this area would include the presence or absence of other disease states. For example, HIV infection increases one's chances of developing tuberculosis, and obesity contributes to a variety of health problems including heart disease, diabetes, and stroke. Other physiologic conditions may prevent some health problems from occurring. For example, the teenage girl who does not ovulate is not likely to become pregnant. Lactation, another hormonally controlled process, appears to have a beneficial effect on a woman's risk of premenopausal breast cancer (Newcombe, et al., 1994), and pregnancy seems to result in temporary remission of arthritis symptoms (Fackelman, 1993). Maternal physiology may also affect the health of the fetus; for example, maternal diabetes during pregnancy has been shown to affect later behavioral and intellectual development of the child.

Another aspect of physiologic function that affects susceptibility to disease is the concept of physiologic immunity. Immunity is the ability to resist the influence of an infectious agent and its effects. Immunity can be either general or specific. General immunity consists of the body's normal defenses against the invasion of an agent and includes an intact skin, the normal pH of gastric secretions, and the presence of adequate coping mechanisms. Specific immunity is exemplified by the antigen–antibody responses to immunizing agents. The concept of immunity will be addressed in greater detail in Chapter 8, The Epidemiologic Process.

The Psychological Dimension

The psychological dimension encompasses the health effects of both internal and external psychological environments. Depression and low self-esteem are two factors in one's internal psychological environment that contribute to a variety of health problems including suicide, substance abuse, family violence, and obesity. Internal psychological factors can even contribute to such problems as sexually transmitted diseases if sexual behavior is used as a primary mode of interpersonal interaction.

External psychological factors can also influence the development of health problems. For example, a person who has a great deal of emotional support in a crisis is less likely to attempt suicide than a person who faces a crisis without such support. Stress is another factor in the external psychologic environment that is associated with a variety of health problems. The ability to cope with stress, on the other hand, is a factor in one's internal psychological environment.

The Physical Dimension

While the psychological dimension addresses aspects of one's psychological environment, the physical dimension of health encompasses the health effects of factors in the physical environment. The physical environment consists of weather, geographic locale, soil composition, terrain, temperature and humidity, and hazards posed by poor housing and unsafe working conditions. For example, the presence of a physical environmental factor, such as many swimming pools in a community, increases the potential for drowning accidents among young children. Similarly, high noise levels in the work environment contribute to hearing loss, and the presence of ragweed in the environment contributes to hayfever in susceptible individuals.

Light and heat are other physical environmental factors known to influence health. For example, fewer fatal motor vehicle accidents occur during daylight savings time than during the rest of the year (Ferguson, Preusser, Lund, Zador, & Ulmer, 1995). Heat waves, on the other hand, have been associated with increased mortality due to heart disease and respiratory disease as well as heatstroke (National Center for Environmental Health, 1995). In addition, maternal exposure to heat during pregnancy has been linked to neural tube defects in offspring (Milunski, Ulcickas, Rothman, Willett, Jick, & Jick, 1992).

Other environmental exposures also contribute to health effects. For example, exposure to high fluoride concentrations in water supplies has been correlated with decreased birth rates (Freni, 1994). Environmental exposures also occur in the presence of pathogenic organisms such as viruses and bacteria. For example, Rocky Mountain spotted fever occurs in areas where animals, such as deer and rodents, carry infected ticks (Benenson, 1995). Physical environmental influences on health will be addressed in greater detail in Chapter 17, as well as Chapters 27 and 29.

The Social Dimension

The social dimension of health consists of those factors within the social environment that influence health, either positively or negatively. Elements of the social structure such as employment, economics, politics, ethics, and legal influences all fall within this dimension of health. The social dimension also includes societal norms and culturally accepted modes of behavior. For example, social factors such as employment, education, income, occupation, and marital status have all been shown to have significant influence on mortality and morbidity (Sorlie, Backlund, & Keller, 1995).

Another important factor in the social dimension is prevailing attitudes toward specific health problems. For example, the fear and stigma attached to HIV infection may seriously hamper efforts to control the spread of disease. Substance abuse, mental illness, family violence, and adolescent pregnancy are other examples of health problems in which social attitudes contribute to the problem or hamper the solution. Societal action with respect to health behaviors can also influence health. For example, legislative actions to increase cigarette taxes have been shown to lead to reduced smoking in the populations affected (Office on Smoking and Health, 1996).

The social dimension can also contribute to the development of health problems in other ways. Congregating in large groups, particularly indoors during the winter, enhances the spread of certain diseases such as colds and influenza. Media portrayals of a variety of healthy and unhealthy behaviors are another way in which the social dimension influences health and illness. For example, the communication media's graphic coverage of suicide and other forms of violence are thought to lead to imitative behavior, and their presentation of smoking, drinking, and sexual activity as desirable behaviors may contribute to the incidence of lung cancer, heart disease, substance abuse, and sexually transmitted diseases. One's occupation is another aspect of the social dimension that may influence health. Several aspects of the social dimension of health are addressed in greater depth in Chapters 14 through 16 and Chapters 24 through 28.

The Behavioral Dimension

The behavioral dimension of health consists of those behaviors in which people engage that either promote or impair their health. Behavioral factors are often those most amenable to change in efforts to prevent disease and promote health and, so, are of particular importance in community health nursing practice. Health-related behaviors to be considered include diet, recreation and exercise, substance use and abuse, sexual activity, and use of protective measures.

Nutritional habits can either enhance or undermine health, and both leanness and obesity can predispose one to other health problems. Exercise patterns also influence health status as do smoking, drinking, and drug use. For example, smokers have been found to have a significantly higher risk of developing cataracts than nonsmokers (Christen, Manson, et al., 1992) in addition to the well-known risks of heart disease and lung cancer.

Recreational activities may also pose health risks or provide emotional outlets that promote health. Skiing and hang gliding, for example, increase the risk of serious accidental injury, but regular physical exercise can improve both physical and emotional health. Sexual activity poses risks related to pregnancy and sexually transmitted diseases. Failure to use protective measures such as contraceptives or barrier devices during intercourse can also increase one's chances of health problems. Similarly, not wearing seat belts or motorcycle helmets increases the potential for serious injury.

The Health System Dimension

The final dimension of health to be addressed is the health system dimension. The way in which health care services are organized and their availability, accessibility, affordability, appropriateness, adequacy, acceptability, and use influence the health of individual clients and population groups. Availability refers to the type and number of health services available, and accessibility reflects the ability of clients to make use of those services. Affordability, the ability to pay for services, also influences health outcomes. Service appropriateness refers to a health care system's ability to provide those services needed and desired by its clientele. The adequacy of health services refers to the quality and amount of service provided relative to need, and acceptability reflects the level of congruence between services provided and the expectations, values, and beliefs of the target population (National Institute for Nursing Research Priority Expert Panel, 1995). Finally, the extent to which members of the population actually make use of available health care services will influence health status.

Health system factors can influence health status either positively or negatively. For example, immunization services that are available and easily accessible to all community members promote control of communicable diseases such as measles, polio, and tetanus. Conversely, the failure of health professionals to take advantage of immunization opportunities contributes to increased incidence of these diseases (National Immunization Program, 1994).

Some health care system contributions to health problems stem from the economics of health care delivery. The high cost of health services limits the ability of many to take advantage of them. In other instances, inappropriate actions on the part of health care providers may actually contribute to health

▶ DIMENSIONS OF HEALTH

BIOPHYSICAL DIMENSION
   Age
   Genetics
   Physiologic function

PSYCHOLOGICAL DIMENSION
   Internal psychological environment
   External psychological environment

PHYSICAL DIMENSION
   Physical environment
   Environmental hazards

SOCIAL DIMENSION
   Social structure
   Societal norms
   Societal attitudes
   Social action

BEHAVIORAL DIMENSION
   Dietary practices
   Recreation and exercise
   Substance use and abuse
   Sexual activity
   Use of protective measures

HEALTH SYSTEM DIMENSION
   Availability
   Accessibility
   Affordability
   Appropriateness
   Adequacy
   Acceptability
   Use

problems. For example, inappropriate use of antibiotics has contributed to the development of antibiotic-resistant strains of gonorrhea and syphilis. Failure of health care providers to recognize and intervene with persons at risk for suicide, substance abuse, and family violence has also led to increased incidence of such problems. Elements of the dimensions of health are summarized above.

▶ DIMENSIONS OF HEALTH CARE

The dimensions of health care aspect of the Dimensions Model incorporates the public health concept of

levels of prevention. Prevention is the hallmark of public health practice and community health nursing and takes place at three levels as originally conceptualized in the work of Leavell and Clark (1965). These levels of prevention comprise the dimensions of the health care component of the Dimensions Model. The levels of prevention are primary prevention, secondary prevention, and tertiary prevention.

The Primary Prevention Dimension

Primary prevention was defined by the originators of the term as "measures designed to promote general optimum health or . . . the specific protection of man against disease agents" (Leavell & Clark, 1965, p. 20). Primary prevention is action taken prior to the occurrence of health problems (Maynard, 1996) and encompasses aspects of health promotion and protection (Parrish & Alfred, 1995). In its health promotion aspect, primary prevention focuses on improving the overall health of individuals, families, and population groups. Examples of health promotion activities include eating a well-balanced diet, getting regular exercise, and developing effective coping strategies. Health protection is aimed at preventing the occurrence of specific health problems. For example, immunization is a protective measure for certain communicable diseases. The health protection aspect of primary prevention may also involve reducing risk factors as a means of preventing disease (Centers for Disease Control, 1992).

The Secondary Prevention Dimension

Secondary prevention focuses on the early identification and treatment of existing health problems (Last, 1992) and occurs after the health problem has arisen. In community health practice at this stage, the major emphasis is on resolving health problems and preventing serious consequences. Secondary prevention activities include screening and early diagnosis, as well as treatment for existing health problems (National Institute of Nursing Research Priority Expert Panel, 1995). Screening for glaucoma is an example of secondary prevention. Secondary prevention would also include the actual diagnosis and treatment of a person with glaucoma.

The Tertiary Prevention Dimension

Tertiary prevention is activity aimed at returning the client to the highest level of function and preventing further deterioration in health (Scutchfield & Keck, 1997). In community health nursing, tertiary prevention also focuses on preventing recurrences of the problem. Placing a client on a maintenance diet after the loss of a desired number of pounds constitutes tertiary prevention.

A particular nursing intervention may be viewed as a primary, secondary, or tertiary preventive measure depending on its relationship to the occurrence of a problem. Take for example, nutrition education as a particular nursing intervention. Nutrition education is a primary preventive measure when the nurse is teaching concepts of food nutrition in an effort to promote health and prevent overweight; the in-

tervention is employed prior to the occurrence of a problem. Nutrition education for the client who is already overweight is a secondary preventive measure; the problem has already occurred and the education program is designed to help the client lose weight. Nutrition education may also be a tertiary preventive measure when the client goes on a "maintenance diet" after the weight loss has occurred. Elements of the health care dimension are summarized below.

The interaction among the three elements of the Dimensions Model and their respective dimensions is depicted in Figure 5–1. Factors in the six dimensions

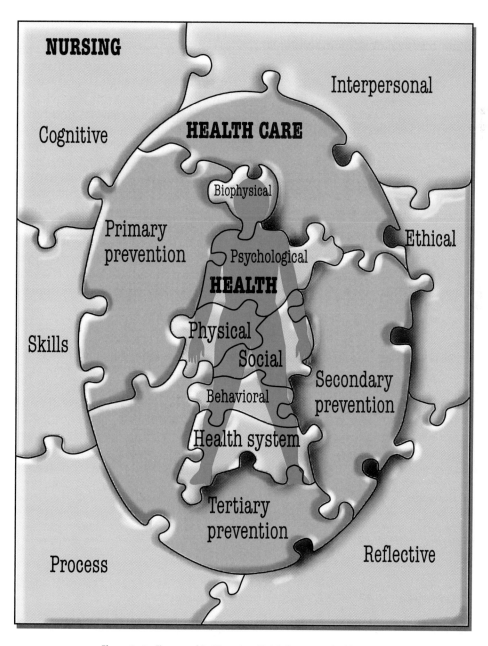

Figure 5–1. Elements of the Dimensions Model of community health nursing.

HEALTH CARE DIMENSION

- Primary prevention
- Secondary prevention
- Tertiary prevention

of health interact with each other to result in a state of health or illness. The interaction among these factors can be influenced by actions in the primary, secondary, and tertiary prevention dimensions of health care. Community health nurses employ the dimensions of nursing to design primary, secondary, and tertiary preventive interventions to promote health, prevent illness, and resolve existing health problems, thereby improving the health status of individuals, families, and communities.

▶ APPLYING THE DIMENSIONS MODEL TO COMMUNITY HEALTH NURSING

Chapter 6 presents several other nursing and non-nursing models that may be used in community health nursing. Each of those models is applied to resolution of the problem of adolescent pregnancy. To facilitate comparison of the Dimensions Model and the models presented in Chapter 6, the Dimensions Model will also be applied to adolescent pregnancy as it affects the three levels of clients in health nursing,

individual, family, and community. The individual involved is the pregnant teenager, the family is her immediate family, and the community is one that is experiencing an increase in the incidence of adolescent pregnancy.

Applying the Dimensions of Nursing

Each of the dimensions of nursing will be applied in the care of the individual, family, and community, but their application will differ somewhat from client to client. Examples of elements within each dimension are presented in Table 5–1. Nursing care at each client level will require somewhat different knowledge in the cognitive dimension. For example, in working with the adolescent the nurse will need to be knowledgeable regarding normal and abnormal physiologic changes in pregnancy as well as knowledgeable of the potential psychological and social effects of pregnancy on an adolescent. Knowledge of family dynamics and groups dynamics and how each might be affected by adolescent pregnancy will be required in work with the family and community, respectively. In the interpersonal dimension, communication skills will be required at each client level, but negotiation skills and collaboration skills will be particularly important in working with the community client.

Advocacy is an ethical dimension element that may be required in caring for each level of client. For example, the nurse may need to advocate with the family for the adolescent who wishes to keep the baby when family members think abortion or adoption are

TABLE 5–1. ELEMENTS OF NURSING DIMENSIONS IN THE CARE OF INDIVIDUAL, FAMILY, AND COMMUNITY CLIENTS

Dimension	Individual	Family	Community
Cognitive	Knowledge of normal and abnormal physiologic effects of pregnancy	Knowledge of family dynamics	Knowledge of group dynamics
Interpersonal	Communication skills	Communication skills	Communication, negotiation, and collaboration skills
Ethical	Advocacy for self-determination	Advocacy for services to family	Advocacy for sexually active adolescents' needs
Skills	Physical assessment skills Analytic skills to identify problems Problem-solving skills	Analytic skills to identify problems Problem-solving skills	Analytic skills to identify problems Problem-solving skills
Process	Nursing process Educational process Home visit process Referral process Change process Leadership process Case management process	Nursing process Educational process Home visit process Referral process Change process Leadership process Case management process	Nursing process Change process Leadership process Group process Political process Epidemiologic process
Reflective	Research Theory development Evaluation of care outcomes	Research Theory development Evaluation of care outcomes	Research Theory development Program evaluation

more appropriate courses of action. Similarly, the nurse may need to advocate for the family to assure that they have access to prenatal care for their daughter. Finally, advocacy may be needed at the community level to ensure the availability of contraceptive and prenatal services for adolescents.

The manipulative skills involved in physical assessment will be required in caring for the pregnant adolescent, whereas analytic and problem-solving skills will be needed with all three client levels. Similarly, many of the same processes will be used at all three levels; for example, the nursing process, change process, and leadership processes will be used with all three client levels. The educational process could also be used with all three clients, but is more likely to be needed with the individual and the family as are the home visit, referral, and case management processes. Political and epidemiologic processes, on the other hand, are more likely to be employed with the community client than with the individual or family.

Each of the three elements of the reflective dimension, research, theory development, and evaluation may be employed with each level of client. The emphasis, however, will vary from level to level. Research with individual clients may explore reasons why adolescents engage in unprotected sexual activity and theory development may proceed along those same lines. With the family, research and theory development might focus on family factors that con-

tribute to adolescent pregnancy; whereas the focus at the community level might be on the effects of high rates of adolescent pregnancy on overall community health. Evaluation at the individual and family level will address the outcomes of care. At the community level, the focus will be on program evaluation.

Applying the Dimensions of Health

Elements of each of the dimensions of health will influence both the development of the problem of adolescent pregnancy and how the problem affects client health. Some examples of factors within each dimension are presented in Table 5–2. Biophysical factors for the individual client include the normal changes experienced with pregnancy, signs of complications, the client's level of physical maturity, and the existence of any other health problems that may affect the pregnancy. The existence of other health problems will also influence the ability of the family and the community to deal with the problem of adolescent pregnancy.

Coping abilities and feelings and attitudes related to adolescent pregnancy are important factors in the psychological dimension for all three client levels. In the physical dimension, only the factor of sufficient space within the home for an additional family member is immediately relevant to the problem of adolescent pregnancy. Social dimension factors of educa-

TABLE 5–2. ELEMENTS OF THE DIMENSIONS OF HEALTH IN THE CARE OF INDIVIDUAL, FAMILY, AND COMMUNITY CLIENTS

Dimension	Individual	Family	Community
Biophysical	Normal physiologic changes in pregnancy Signs of complications of pregnancy Client's physical maturation Presence of other health problems	Health status of other family members	High incidence/prevalence of other conditions
Psychological	Feelings about pregnancy Self-concept Coping abilities	Feelings about pregnancy Coping abilities	Attitudes toward adolescent sexual activity Coping abilities
Physical		Adequate space in home for an additional family member	
Social	Interaction with peers Educational level Cultural values Effects of pregnancy on school performance	Economic status Educational level Cultural values Employment	Economic status Educational levels Cultural values
Behavioral	Use of caffeine, alcohol, other drugs Smoking Dietary patterns Exercise patterns	Family use of alcohol, other drugs Smoking by family members Dietary patterns	Prevalence of substance use in adolescents Access to drugs, alcohol, and cigarettes by adolescents
Health system	Source of health care Attitudes toward health care Insurance coverage	Source of health care Attitudes toward health care Insurance coverage	Availability of services for pregnant adolescents Extent of insurance coverage in community

tional level and cultural values will influence the response of each level of client to the pregnancy. For the individual client, the pregnancy may affect her interaction with peers or her school performance, additional social dimension consideration factors. At the family and community levels, employment status and income will influence their abilities to respond effectively to adolescent pregnancy.

Behavioral dimension factors relevant to the situation include the use of potentially harmful substances by both the individual and family members and access to such substances in the community. Additional factors relevant to the individual client include diet and exercise. Dietary patterns are also relevant to the family. Finally, source of health care and attitudes toward health care, particularly prenatal care during pregnancy, are important health system factors for the individual and family. Insurance coverage for needed services is another factor that will influence their abilities to obtain prenatal care. For the community, the availability of services for care of adolescents and the extent of insurance coverage within the community will influence its ability to respond effectively to the problem of adolescent pregnancy.

Applying the Dimensions of Health Care

Nursing interventions may be employed at the primary, secondary, and tertiary level of prevention with each of the three levels of client (individual, family, and community). Table 5–3 presents some examples of primary, secondary, and tertiary interventions with individuals, families, and community clients. Primary prevention of adolescent pregnancy itself requires use of contraceptives and access to contraceptive services for sexually active adolescents. For the individual and family, referral for prenatal services is a primary prevention activity designed to prevent

---

Critical Thinking in Research

One purpose of research is to assist in the development of theoretical models for practice by testing their applicability in practice. Because the Dimensions Model is relatively new, it has not been extensively tested in practice, although some elements of the model have been tested in its previous form as the Epidemiologic Prevention Process Model.

1. How would you design a study to determine if the dimensions of nursing within the Dimensions Model can incorporate all of the activities performed by community health nurses?
2. What kind of data collection methods would you use to make this determination? What specific information would you collect in your study?

---

complications of pregnancy and ensure a healthy mother and baby. For the community, however, planning of prenatal care services is a secondary prevention activity because it is directed toward "curing" an existing problem, lack of adequate services. Other primary prevention for individual and family revolve around health promotion related to diet and exercise, and, for the pregnant teen, development of child care skills. For the community, additional primary prevention activities might entail planning to prevent adverse effects of a high rate of adolescent pregnancy on other community systems. For example, the community may need to plan for alternative educational programs for adolescents with children in which the adolescents learn both academic subjects and child care skills.

Secondary prevention for the individual client may involve assistance in dealing with the normal discomforts of pregnancy or referral for signs of complications of pregnancy. The family may need financial assistance to obtain prenatal care if they have ex-

---

TABLE 5–3. ELEMENTS OF THE DIMENSIONS OF HEALTH CARE FOR INDIVIDUAL, FAMILY, AND COMMUNITY CLIENTS

Dimension	Individual	Family	Community
Primary prevention	Educate regarding contraceptive use Refer for prenatal care Educate on dietary needs Educate on exercise needs Teach child care skills	Provide anticipatory guidance on adolescent sexuality Refer for prenatal care Help plan healthy family diet Provide anticipatory guidance on family role changes	Ensure access to contraceptive services for teens Plan to prevent harmful effects on other community systems
Secondary prevention	Assist in dealing with discomforts of pregnancy Refer for signs of complications	Assist family to get financial help for prenatal care	Plan for prenatal care services for adolescents
Tertiary prevention	Educate regarding contraceptive use	Educate on need for contraceptives	Plan for access to contraceptive services for teens

Critical Thinking in Practice: A Case in Point

Think of your own family as a potential client for community health nursing intervention. Address the following with respect to your family and its health needs:

1. What factors in the dimensions of health are influencing the health of members of your family? Are there additional factors that are influencing the health of the family as a unit? If so, in which dimensions of health do they occur?
2. What primary, secondary, and tertiary prevention activities might a community health nurse employ to provide assistance to your family? Are activities needed at all three levels? Why or why not?
3. Which of the dimensions of nursing included in the Dimensions Model would come into play in providing care for your family? What areas of knowledge in the cognitive dimension would the nurse need? What attitudes within the affective dimension would make the nurse most effective in dealing with your family? Would elements of the ethical dimension come into play in caring for your family? What particular skills would the nurse need, and what elements of the process dimension would be needed? Finally, how might the reflective dimension influence the care provided to your family by the community health nurse?

---

isting economic problems. Tertiary prevention at all three levels is aimed at preventing additional pregnancies via contraceptive services.

As we have seen, the Dimensions Model can be used to guide care for all three levels of clients encountered by community health nurses. In the next chapter, we will explore the application of several other models to the same problem of adolescent pregnancy to allow the reader to compare the utility of the models presented.

TESTING YOUR UNDERSTANDING

1. What are the three elements of the Dimensions Model of community health nursing? (pp. 70–76)
2. What are the dimensions of nursing incorporated into the Dimensions Model? How does each dimension of nursing influence the health of clients? Give examples of this influence. (pp. 70–71)
3. What are the dimensions of health incorporated in the Dimensions Model? Give an example of how factors in each separate dimension could affect the health status of an individual. Of a population group. Give examples of interactions between dimensions that may influence health. (pp. 71–74)
4. Distinguish among primary, secondary, and tertiary prevention. Give an example of a nursing intervention at each level of prevention. (pp. 74–76)
5. How do the three dimensional elements interact to influence the health of clients? (pp. 76–78)

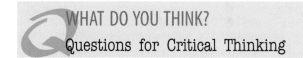

WHAT DO YOU THINK?

Questions for Critical Thinking

1. What advantages does the Dimensions Model have over other nursing models for community health nursing practice?
2. Does the Dimensions Model cover all potential factors that influence health within the six dimensions of health? Or, are there other dimensions of health that are not addressed by the model? If so, what are they?
3. Should community health nurses already in the field use a model to guide their practice? Why or why not? How might you go about persuading them to use the Dimensions Model in practice?

REFERENCES

Baird, P. A. (1994). The role of genetics in population health. In R. G. Evans, M. L. Barer, & T. R. Marmor (Eds.), *Why are some people healthy and others not? The determinants of health of populations* (pp. 133–159). New York: Aldine De Gruyter.

Benenson, A. S. (Ed.) (1995). *Control of communicable diseases manual* (16th ed.). Washington, DC: American Public Health Association.

Blum, H. L. (1974). *Planning for health—Development and application of social change theory.* New York: Human Sciences Press.

Bower, B. (1992). Nature joins nurture to boost divorce rate. *Science News, 142,* 374.

Carmelli, D., Swan, G. E., Robinette, D., & Fabsitz, R. (1992). Genetic influence on smoking—A study of male twins. *New England Journal of Medicine, 327,* 829–833.

Centers for Disease Control. (1992). A framework for assessing the effectiveness of disease and injury prevention. *MMWR, 41,* (RR-3), 1–12.

Christen, W. G., Manson, J. E., Seddon, J. M., Glynn, R. J., Buring, J. E., Rosner, B., & Hennekens, C. H. (1992). A prospective study of cigarette smoking and risk of cataract in men. *JAMA, 268,* 989–993.

Comings, D. E. (1991). The dopamine D_2 receptor locus as a modifying gene in neuropsychiatric disorders. *JAMA, 266,* 1793–1799.

Dever, G. E. A. (1991). *Community health analysis: A global analysis at the local level* (2nd ed). Gaithersburg, MD: Aspen.

Evans, R. G., & Stoddart, G. L. (1994). Producing health, consuming health care. In R. G. Evans, M. L. Barer, & T. R. Marmor (Eds.), *Why are some people healthy and others not? The determinants of health of populations* (pp. 27–64). New York: Aldine De Gruyter.

Fackelman, K. (1993). The nine-month arthritis cure. *Science News, 142,* 266–268.

Federal, Provincial, and Territorial Advisory Committee on Population Health. (1994). *Strategies for population health: Investing in the health of Canadians.* Ottawa, Ontario: Health Canada Communications Directorate.

Ferguson, S. A., Preusser, D. F., Lund, A. K., Zador, P. L., & Ulmer, R. G. (1995). Daylight saving time and motor vehicle crashes: The reduction in pedestrian and vehicle occupant fatalities. *American Journal of Public Health, 85,* 92–95.

Freni, S. C. (1994). Exposure to high fluoride concentrations in drinking water is associated with decreased birth rates. *Journal of Toxicology and Environmental Health, 42,* 109–121.

Kendler, K. S., Heath A. C., Neale, M. C., Kessler, R. C., & Eaves, L. J. (1992). A population-based twin study of alcoholism in women. *JAMA, 268,* 1877–1882.

Lalonde, M. (1974). *A new perspective on the health of Canadians.* Ottawa: Office of the Canadian Minister of National Health and Welfare.

Last, J. M. (1992). Scope and methods of prevention. In J. M. Last & R. B. Wallace (Eds.), *Maxcy-Rosenau-Last public health and preventive medicine* (13th ed.) (pp. 3–10). Norwalk, CT: Appleton & Lange.

Leavell, H. R., & Clark, E. G. (1965). *Preventive medicine for the doctor in his community: A epidemiologic approach* (3rd ed.). New York: McGraw-Hill.

Maynard, M. (1996). Promoting older ethnic minorities' health behaviors: Primary and secondary prevention considerations. *Journal of Primary Prevention, 17,* 219–229.

Milunski, A., Ulcickas, M., Rothman, K. J., Willett, W., Jick, S. S., & Jick, H. (1992). Maternal heat exposure and neural tube defects. *JAMA, 268,* 882–885.

National Center for Environmental Health. (1995). Heat-related illnesses and deaths—United States, 1994–1995. *MMWR, 44,* 465–468.

National Immunization Program. (1994). Impact of missed opportunities to vaccinate preschool children on vaccination coverage levels—Selected U.S. sites, 1991–1992. *MMWR, 43,* 709–711; 717–718.

National Institute of Nursing Research Priority Expert Panel. (1995). *Community-based health care: Nursing strategies.* Bethesda, MD: National Institute of Nursing Research.

Newcombe, P. A., et al. (1994). Lactation and reduced risk of perimenopausal breast cancer. *New England Journal of Medicine, 330* 81–87.

Office on Smoking and Health. (1996). Cigarette smoking before and after an excise tax increase and an anti-smoking campaign. *MMWR, 45,* 966–970.

Parrish, R. S., & Alfred, R. H. (1995). Theories and trends in occupational health nursing. *AAOHN Journal, 43,* 514–521.

Scutchfield, F. D., & Keck, C. W. (1997). Concepts and definitions of public health practice. In D. F. Scutchfield & C. W. Keck (Eds.), *Principles of public health practice* (pp. 3–9). Albany, NY: Delmar.

Sorlie, P. D., Backlund, E., & Keller, J. B. (1995). US mortality by economic, demographic, and social characteristics: The national longitudinal mortality study. *American Journal of Public Health, 85,* 949–956.

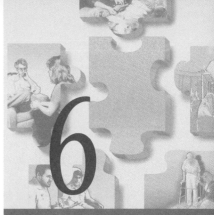

OTHER MODELS FOR COMMUNITY HEALTH NURSING

One of the hallmarks of a scientific profession is the unique body of knowledge that it uses to direct professional practice. This body of knowledge is the result of systematic, scientific inquiry involving the formulation and testing of theory. As is the case with other scientific disciplines, professional nursing practice needs a sound theoretical foundation that describes the interrelationships among key concepts. For nursing, these concepts are client, environment, health, and nursing (Nunnery, 1997).

A nursing theory is a statement that characterizes or explains an event of interest to nursing. Many nurses regard nursing theory and practice as separate professional dimensions that are only vaguely interrelated. In reality, theory and practice are inseparably intertwined. Theory arises out of practice to direct or explain practice.

Community health nursing research has often lacked a theoretical basis. This professional shortcoming has been attributed in part to the lack of a community or aggregate focus in many nursing models developed to date (Koziol-McLain & Maeve, 1993). There are, however, some theoretical models in nursing and in other fields that can be adapted for use in community health nursing.

► KEY TERMS

adaptive modes
behavioral system
behavioral subsystems
cognator mechanism
conservation of energy
contextual stimuli
developmental self-care
family developmental
   tasks
flexible line of defense
focal stimuli
function
health deviation self-care
lines of resistance
normal line of defense
personal integrity
psychic integrity
reconstitution
regulator mechanism
residual stimuli
self-care deficit
set
social integrity
stressor
structural integrity
structure
therapeutic self-care
   demands
universal self-care

► Chapter Objectives

After reading this chapter, you should be able to:

- Apply concepts from the Roy Adaptation Model to community health nursing practice.
- Apply Levine's Principles of Conservation to community health nursing practice.
- Apply concepts of Orem's Self-care Model to community health nursing practice.
- Apply concepts from Johnson's Behavioral Systems Model to community health nursing practice.
- Apply concepts of the Neuman Health Systems Model to community health nursing practice.
- Apply concepts of Pender's Health Promotion Model to community health nursing practice.
- Apply systems theory concepts to community health nursing practice.
- Apply concepts of developmental theory to community health nursing practice.
- Apply concepts of the structural–functional model to community health nursing practice.

► MODELS FOR COMMUNITY HEALTH NURSING PRACTICE

For it to be systematic rather than haphazard, nursing practice requires a framework that arises from a specific approach to the client. This framework is supplied by a nursing model. A *nursing model* is a tangible, schematic, frequently visual representation of the relationships between and among key concepts that explains how something works (Girard, 1993). A model may encompass several theories and give rise to others.

Think of a model in terms of building a house. The model is similar to the blueprint according to which the house is constructed. The blueprint provides the basic outline or framework around which the structure is erected. The materials from which the house is constructed (eg, the bricks and wood) are analogous to the concepts involved in nursing, such as self-image and oxygenation. Theories are the cohesive bond that joins the materials into a unit—nursing practice—just as the mortar and nails join bricks and wood in a house.

To direct practice, nursing models must incorporate three basic components: the client, the goal of nursing intervention, and the activities involved in nursing intervention. First, a nursing model must de-

fine who is the client or recipient of nursing action. Is the nursing client always someone who is ill or can the client be a healthy individual? Furthermore, can the recipient of care be a family or a community rather than an individual? Second, the model must specify the expected outcome of nursing intervention. Different nursing models use different terms to express outcomes, for example, *adaptation, reconstitution,* and *self-care.* The final requisite for a nursing model is a description of the nurse's activities in providing care. Again, depending on the nursing model, these activities may be educative, curative, restorative, supportive, or preventive.

► NURSING MODELS FOR COMMUNITY HEALTH NURSING

Most of the chapters in this book apply one nursing model, the Dimensions Model, to community health nursing. This chapter presents six other nursing models developed by Roy, Levine, Orem, Johnson, Neuman, and Pender. All of these models were developed for use with individual clients but can be adapted for use with families, groups, or communities. Three types of non-nursing theoretical models useful in community health nursing are also presented. These include systems models, developmental models, and structural–functional models.

The Roy Adaptation Model

The adaptation model of Callista Roy conceives of the client as a unified whole adapting to changes in the environment (Tiedeman, 1996). Within the environment, the client interacts with others, including the nurse, and this interaction influences adaptive capabilities.

Concepts of the Roy Model

Three concepts are basic to the Roy model: person or client, adaptation, and nursing. The person or client is viewed as a totality, as an adaptive system interacting with the environment. In adapting the model for use in community health nursing, the "person" or client who receives nursing care can be an individual, a family, a group, or a community.

The goal of the client in interactions with the environment is an adaptive response, a positive response to changes in the internal and/or external environment that promotes the integrity of the system (Andrews & Roy, 1991a). The client's ability to adapt is related to the extent of the change experienced and to the ability to cope with the change. For example, everyone is exposed to various forms of stress each day. Stress causes changes in one's internal psychological environment as well as psychiologic changes. Moderate levels of stress keep one alert and motivated, whereas too much stress causes maladaptation. One's ability to cope with stress also influences one's response. Suppose that two people are exposed to the same level of stress, but that one has good coping skills and one does not. The person with good coping skills will probably be able to adapt positively to the stress encountered; the other person will not.

Families and groups of people can also vary in their ability to adapt to changes in the environment. For example, a family may adapt positively or negatively to a move to another town, whereas a community adapts positively or negatively to the establishment of a new industry in town.

The client's ability to cope, or adaptation level, is influenced by three categories of stimuli: focal stimuli, contextual stimuli, and residual stimuli (Srp & Martaus, 1995). *Focal stimuli* include the environmental change to which the client attends and with which he or she must deal. *Contextual stimuli* are those other stimuli in the situation that influence the client's response to the focal stimulus. In the stress example, the focal stimulus might be a dead auto battery, the current source of stress; other factors such as fatigue and worry about being late for work would be contextual stimuli affecting the client's response to the focal stimulus. *Residual stimuli* are the result of past experiences, beliefs, and values that affect current responses to focal stimuli (Gless, 1995). For example, one might have painful memories about a time when a dead car battery caused one to miss an important appointment. Once residual stimuli are recognized as influencing the situation, they become focal or contextual stimuli (Lutjens, 1995).

Adaptation occurs when the total stimuli impinging on the client fall within the clients' zone of adaptive capability. For the individual, the amount of stress related to the focal stimulus of a dead battery and the contextual and residual stimuli operating in the situation may result in a negative response, or maladaptation. Similarly, if unemployment is the reason for the family's move to another locale, that factor, coupled with the move itself, may place events beyond the family's adaptive capacity. In the same way, a community that is coping with other stressors may not be able to adapt effectively to the advent of a new industry. For example, if roadways are already heavily congested with traffic, the addition of a major new industry may move the traffic problem beyond the community's adaptation level.

Adaptation occurs in four *adaptive modes* or categories of behavioral responses that indicate effective or ineffective responses to environmental stimuli: the physiologic, self-concept, role function, and interdependence modes (Andrews & Roy, 1991a). Responses in the physiologic mode include activities at the cellular, tissue, organ, or organ system level directed toward maintaining physiologic integrity. Physiologic integrity involves adequately meeting needs for oxygen, nutrition, elimination, rest and activity, and protection against trauma, heat, cold, and so on (Gless, 1995). Assessment of adaptation in the physiologic mode includes consideration of how well these needs are met, as well as the level of function of four complex processes that help maintain integrity: sensory function, fluid and electrolyte balance mechanisms, neurologic function, and endocrine function (Andrews & Roy, 1991b). A client's ability to effectively discharge body heat through perspiration is an example of adaptation in the physiologic mode.

Maintenance of *psychic integrity*, or knowledge of oneself as a unified being, is the goal of adaptation in the self-concept mode (Andrews, 1991b). The self-concept model has two perceptual aspects, the physical self and the personal self. Within the physical self-concept, one perceives both body sensation and body image. Body sensation refers to the ability to experience oneself as a physical body with specific feelings such as exhaustion and well-being. Body image is one's view of and attitude toward the physical self as fat, attractive, physically strong, and so on.

The personal self consists of three components: self-consistency, ideal self, and moral–ethical–spiritual self. Activities of the self-consistency component are directed toward maintaining a consistent self-organization and avoiding disequilibrium and reflects one's perceptions of one's actual performance or capabilities (Buck, 1991). The ideal self, on the other hand, incorporates perceptions of how one would like to be. The moral–ethical–spiritual self includes one's beliefs and values that help form one's concept of self (Andrews, 1991b).

The role function mode involves adaptation in interpersonal interactions to maintain social integrity. Within the role function mode, clients engage in two types of behaviors, instrumental behaviors and expressive behaviors (Andrews, 1991a). Instrumental behaviors are activities designed to fulfill the expectations associated with one's social roles. The new mother or father who feeds, diapers, and comforts the infant is engaging in instrumental behaviors related to the parental role. Expressive behaviors reflect the feelings and attitudes of the role occupant about the role. For example, grumbling about having to get up at night to feed the baby is an expressive behavior related to the parental role.

The goal of activity in the interdependence mode is affectional adequacy, or the ability to be comfortable in nurturing relationships with others (Tedrow, 1991). Adaptation in this mode is reflected in the ability to love and respect others, contributive behavior, and to accept love and respect in return, receptive behavior (Andrews & Roy, 1991a). Relationships both with significant others and with other components of one's support system contribute to meeting the need for affectional adequacy (Tedrow, 1991).

Adaptation in each of the four modes is initiated and controlled by one of two coping mechanisms, the regulator and the cognator. The *regulator mechanism* is an innate and automatic coping mechanism that influences behavior within the physiologic mode (Robinson, 1995). Automatic physiologic responses to environmental stimuli, such as the immune response, are mediated by this regulation mechanism. The *cognator mechanism* is cognitive rather than automatic in nature and its activity is directed toward adaptive responses to social and psychological, as well as physiologic stimuli (Ryan, 1996). Its activation reflects one's perceptions of environmental stimuli. For example, if one perceives the growing independence of one's teenage son as a threat to one's self-image as a mother, the cognator will initiate behavior in the self-concept mode to minimize that threat. The types of behavior initiated may be either adaptive or maladaptive. For example, redefining one's self-image as a successful parent would be an adaptive behavior. Restricting the teenager's independence would be maladaptive for both the teen and the family.

Nursing intervention, in the Roy model, attempts to alter stimuli to fall within the client's adaptation level or to alter the client's response to stimuli (Gless, 1995). Nursing action begins with assessment at two levels. First-level assessment involves looking for evidence of maladaptive behaviors. Second-level assessment involves determining the focal, contextual, and residual stimuli influencing the maladaptive behavior (Tiedeman, 1996). The nurse then engages in activity designed to promote adaptive behaviors by altering stimuli or the client's response to them.

Applying the Roy Model to Community Health Nursing

The Roy model can be used to direct nursing care for an individual, a family, or a community as client. All three levels of client must adapt to changes in the environment to survive. Table 6–1 describes a situation involving adolescent pregnancy in which an individual, a family, and a community must engage in adaptive behaviors. This example is used throughout the chapter and is addressed from the perspective of the adolescent client who plans to continue the pregnancy and keep the baby.

Table 6–1 presents an assessment of the potential focal, contextual, and residual stimuli involved for the individual, the family, and the community. The focal stimulus for the individual is the fact of her pregnancy. The daughter's pregnancy is also the focal stimulus for the family. In the case of the community, the focal stimulus is a recent rise in the number of teenage pregnancies. Contextual stimuli for the individual include her overall health status, the extent of family support available, her attitude toward the pregnancy, her relationship with the baby's father, and the availability of prenatal care. All of these factors influence the way in which the teen responds to the fact of pregnancy.

Contextual stimuli for the family include the age of the daughter, family attitudes toward teen sexual

TABLE 6–1. CLIENT ASSESSMENT IN THE ROY ADAPTATION MODEL

Model Concept	Assessment		
	Individual	*Family*	*Community*
Situation requiring adaptation	Unwed pregnancy	Teenage daughter's pregnancy	Increased incidence of teenage pregnancy
Focal stimulus	Pregnancy	Pregnancy of teen	Increased incidence rate for teenage pregnancy
Contextual stimuli	Overall health status Extent of family support Attitude toward pregnancy Relationship with baby's father Access to prenatal care	Age of teenage daughter Family attitude toward teen sexual activity Presence or absence of other family stressors	Availability of contraceptive services Community attitudes toward teen sexual activity
Residual stimuli	Age and maturity of teen Family and cultural attitude toward illegitimacy Attitudes toward children Personal ambitions and goals Income level Education level	Cultural and religious background Family income Education level	Extent of teen population Availability of prenatal and child health services Community attitudes toward illegitimacy and sex education for teens Income levels Education levels

activity, and the extent of other stressors in the family. If the girl is quite young, parents might argue for abortion or adoption rather than keeping the baby. Or, if family members have strong feelings against sexual activity by teens, they might feel compelled to force the girl to leave home. Additional stressors within the family also affect the family's ability to adapt effectively. For example, if parents are unemployed, the addition of another family member will be more difficult than if family income is adequate.

In the case of the community, contextual stimuli might include the availability of contraceptive services and community attitudes toward adolescent sexual activity. Communities with adequate facilities for contraceptive services for teens will have less difficulty adapting to the problem of teenage pregnancy than those with inadequate services. Similarly, community resistance to sexual activity by teens will make it more difficult to deal realistically with the problem.

From the point of view of Roy's model, residual stimuli are less amenable to change than are focal or contextual stimuli. For the individual, residual stimuli include the age and maturity level of the teen, family and cultural attitudes toward illegitimacy, attitudes toward children, personal ambitions and goals, and income and education levels. A very mature teenager will adapt to the reality of pregnancy more readily than an immature girl. Adaptation is also easier in situations in which illegitimacy carries little stigma and in which children are welcomed and cherished. On the other hand, personal goals for college and a career might influence decisions in favor of abortion or adoption. Income and education levels also affect the ease of adaptation by influencing the resources at hand for dealing with the pregnancy.

Residual stimuli for the family are similar to those for the individual client and include the family's cultural and religious background and income and education levels. These factors influence family adaptation in much the same way that they influence the adaptation of the individual. For the community, residual stimuli include the extent of the teenage population, the availability of prenatal and child health services to meet increased demands for care, community attitudes toward illegitimacy and sex education, and community income and education levels. If there are relatively few teens in the total population, the problem is more easily dealt with than if teens constitute a large percentage of the population. Similarly, the existence of adequate health care services allows the community to deal with the problem of increased demands for prenatal and child health care with greater ease than would otherwise be the case. Community attitudes and income and education levels influence community adaptation in much the same way that these factors influence the adaptation of the individual and family.

In Roy's model, when the total of focal, contextual, and residual stimuli falls within the client's adaptation level, adaptation occurs. Table 6–2 presents examples of possible adaptive behaviors on the part of the individual, family, and community in each of the adaptive modes. Again, the situation requiring adaptive behavior is adolescent pregnancy.

Adaptation in the physiologic mode involves maintaining appropriate internal functioning to deal with the problem. For the individual, the body's response to pregnancy includes increased hunger, fatigue, and changes in hormonal levels. These responses stimulate behaviors of eating and rest designed to meet the body's heightened needs during pregnancy. For the family, adaptation in this mode involves activities to provide for the physical needs of

TABLE 6–2. SAMPLE ADAPTIVE BEHAVIORS IN THE ROY MODEL

Model Concept	Adaptive Behaviors		
Mode of Adaptation	*Individual*	*Family*	*Community*
Physiologic mode	Hunger increases to meet baby's need for food. Fatigue increases. Hormonal levels change.	Provisions are made to meet physical needs of teen and baby.	Health care delivery system expands prenatal care and well-child services to meet increased need.
Self-concept mode	Client perceives self as good, deals with guilt over pregnancy.	Parents deal with feelings of guilt and do not see themselves as "failures." Family adjusts to advent of new member.	Community recognizes problem and begins to take action for resolution.
Role function model	Client begins to learn maternal role. Client makes adjustments in student, family, and social roles to accommodate motherhood.	Family recognizes daughter in mother role. Family members prepare for new roles as grandparents, aunts, uncles, and so on.	Community expands its role in provision of sex education by mandating sex education in school curricula.
Interdependence mode	Client is able to accept love and support from family members.	Family members are able to provide love and support to the teenager despite her pregnancy.	Community provides assistance to pregnant teenagers without stigmatizing them.

the teen and the new baby. In the community, adaptation may necessitate expansion of existing prenatal and well-child services to meet increased needs.

Within the self-concept mode, the individual client who is adapting effectively adjusts to the pregnancy without perceiving herself as "bad." Parents must also adapt by accepting the situation without blaming themselves. For the community, adaptation in the self-concept mode entails recognition that a serious problem exists and that action must be taken to resolve it. The community that is not adapting well in this mode might continue to display the attitude that adolescent pregnancy does not occur despite evidence to the contrary.

Changes in the role function mode must be made by clients at all three levels. The individual must begin to learn the mother role and must make adjustments within other roles (eg, student, daughter, single person) to accommodate additional role functions. For example, the girl might enroll in a school that provides child care services on the premises. Dating activities might also be curtailed and scheduled around the baby's needs.

Family members must acknowledge the assumption of the mother role by the teen and must adjust relationships with her in relation to this role. It is sometimes difficult for parents to see their daughter as a mother with responsibility for a child, and parents may need to be encouraged to allow the girl to care for the baby herself. Family members must also adopt new roles as grandparents, aunts, uncles, and so on, which may necessitate other changes in relationships.

The community may need to reshape perceptions of its role in providing sex education and contraceptive services for teens. If these activities have been relegated to families and the private medical sector in the past because of community attitudes toward adolescent sexuality, the community may need to assume a more active role in these efforts. One way to accomplish this might be to mandate the inclusion of sex education in junior high and high school curricula.

In terms of the Roy model, adaptive behaviors in the interdependence mode for all three levels of client would reflect affectional adequacy. For both the individual and the family, affectional adequacy involves the ability to give and receive love and support despite feelings about the pregnancy. Affectional adequacy at the community level would be reflected in the community's ability to provide for the needs of pregnant teenagers without stigmatizing them or castigating them as evil.

Using the Roy adaptation model, the nurse dealing with the individual, family, or community assesses the client's adaptive capabilities in each of the four modes and examines the focal, contextual, and residual stimuli involved. Nursing intervention is indicated whenever the total stimuli lie beyond the client's adaptive capacity. Intervention may involve manipulation of the client or the environment, or both, directed toward a positive response to the situation. Table 6–3 presents sample nursing interventions with the individual client, family, and community in each of the four adaptive modes.

Working with the individual client and family in

TABLE 6–3. NURSING INTERVENTIONS IN THE ROY MODEL

Model Concept	Nursing Interventions		
	Individual	*Family*	*Community*
Physiologic mode	Provide adequate nutrition. Maintain hydration. Encourage exercise. Deal with discomforts of pregnancy. Educate client to meet baby's physiologic needs. Promote rest to allow redirection of energy.	Review family diet to ensure adequate nutrition for mother and baby. Educate family to meet nutrition needs of both teen and baby.	Help expand prenatal and child health services to meet needs of both teens and babies.
Self-concept mode	Allow client to express feelings regarding pregnancy. Help client to deal with guilt over pregnancy. Help client to adjust to bodily changes.	Allow family members to express feelings regarding difficulty posed by pregnancy. Help parents deal with feelings of guilt. Help family adjust to advent of new member.	Help community to recognize existence of problem. Educate community to extent of problem.
Role function mode	Assist client to learn maternal role. Assist client to adjust school, family, and social roles to accommodate motherhood.	Encourage family to allow teen to exercise mother role. Assist family to adapt to changing roles of other members.	Encourage view of community as having responsibility for sex education for teens. Help establish contraceptive services for teens.
Interdependence mode	Encourage client to express love for and seek the support of family members. Refer for counseling as needed.	Encourage family to express love and support for daughter.	Advocate sensitive, nonjudgmental services.

the physiologic mode, the nurse can aid adaptation by acquainting the teen and her family with the nutrition needs of a pregnant adolescent and, later, of a new baby and breastfeeding mother. The nurse might also encourage the teen to get adequate exercise and may provide suggestions for dealing with the discomforts of pregnancy. The nurse also assesses the client's ability to care for the child and educates her and the family to meet the baby's physiologic needs. Manipulation of the environment could include encouraging arrangements for the teen to get adequate rest and assisting in exploring safe sleeping arrangements for the new baby. Manipulation of the community client in the physiologic mode might include the participation of the nurse in plans to expand existing prenatal and child health services to meet increased demands.

Intervention in the self-concept mode might involve allowing the individual client and family to ventilate their feelings about the pregnancy and the difficulties it poses. The nurse can also help the teen and her parents deal with any feelings of guilt related to the pregnancy. In addition, the teen may need help in adjusting to bodily changes that occur with pregnancy, and the nurse can help her to explore and deal with her feelings regarding these changes. Both individual and family may need help in thinking of themselves in new ways necessitated by the assumption of new roles.

For the community client, nursing intervention in the self-concept mode might involve making the community aware of the growing problem of adolescent pregnancy. The nurse might accomplish this by educating the community and policy makers about the extent of the problem and its consequences for those involved and for the community at large. If the community continues to regard itself as not having a problem, adaptation will not occur.

Assistance in the role function mode would include helping the client to learn the maternal role and suggesting ways of modifying old roles to accommodate the assumption of new role functions. For example, the nurse might teach the teen to feed, bathe, and dress the baby or make a referral for a special education program for teens with children. The nurse may also need to encourage the family to allow the teen to exercise her role as the baby's mother and assist family members to learn new roles as grandparents. In the community, the nurse can foster a sense of community responsibility for providing sex education and contraceptive services for teenagers.

In the interdependence mode, both individual and family may require assistance in expressing continued love and support. The nurse might also provide referrals for counseling as needed. The nurse may also need to function as an advocate for the teen, encouraging the family to let her function as the mother of a young child. For the community, the nurse may serve as an advocate for sensitive and nonjudgmental services for pregnant adolescents.

Levine's Principles of Conservation

The nursing model proposed by Myra Levine also addresses the necessity of adaptation to ensure survival. In this model, however, adaptation involves the conservation of energy and the integrity of the client.

Concepts of Levine's Model

Health, in Levine's model, is defined as "wholeness" incorporating structural, personal, and social integrity, and energy (Levine, 1991). Disruption in any of these areas results in health problems. Nursing care is directed toward conservation of these four elements of health, thereby maintaining the unity and integrity of the client. Nursing intervention is based on four principles of conservation: conservation of energy, conservation of structural integrity, conservation of personal integrity, and conservation of social integrity (Artigue, Foli, Johnson, et al., 1994).

Levine maintained that the ability of the individual to function depends on his or her energy potential and the energy available. In the *conservation of energy,* the nurse assesses the extent of the client's energy expenditure in relation to energy resources. Energy must be channeled into those functions most vital to survival when energy demands exceed resources. When the client is unable to conserve energy, the nurse must institute measures to assist in energy conservation.

Changes in structure lead to functional changes. *Structural integrity* reflects normal physiological structure and function. The structural integrity of the client must be maintained so as to ensure adequate function. For example, when a client loses an arm, the structural change results in loss of function. The client must adapt and relearn activities of daily living such as dressing and tying shoes. Similarly, a family must adapt to the structural change involved in death of the mother, whereas a community must adapt to destruction of part of the town by fire. When structural integrity is threatened, the nurse intervenes to assist the client to maintain integrity or to adapt to the change.

Personal integrity relates to the client's self-respect, identity, and individuality. Personal integrity is maintained when clients are assured their rights as unique entities and participate in decisions regarding health care. Maintenance of personal integrity also involves consideration of the client's values and social patterns.

The last of Levine's principles, conservation of *social integrity,* is concerned with the effectiveness of the client's interactions with other people. Ethnic and subcultural considerations as well as interpersonal relationships are elements of social integrity. Maintenance of social integrity involves fostering positive interactions with others.

Nursing, in Levine's model, involves assessing the degree of clients' adaptation to changes in the internal or external environments. Whenever structural, personal, or social integrity or energy use is threatened, the nurse intervenes. Intervention is directed toward conservation of energy and promotion of integrity and can be either supportive or therapeutic. Supportive interventions may maintain the client at the current level of integrity or fail to prevent progressive loss of integrity. Therapeutic intervention influences adaptation to renewed integrity.

Applying Levine's Model to Community Health Nursing

Myra Levine's principles of conservation can be applied to all levels of clients. Table 6–4 presents possible activities by an individual client, a family, and a community for each of the four principles of conservation related to the problem of adolescent pregnancy.

Activities of the individual directed toward conservation of energy in Levine's model include increasing caloric intake to provide for the needs of a growing fetus and maintaining a good balance between rest and exercise. For the family, efforts in the area of energy conservation might involve redirection of family energies to deal with the pregnancy and planning the advent of a new family member. For example, the family might decide to use its savings to build an extra room on the house. Because savings can be considered an expendable commodity, it might be considered a source of family energy. The community might choose to conserve energy by redirecting resources to provide sex education and contraceptive services for teens.

In terms of Levine's model, preventing complications of pregnancy would be one way of conserving structural integrity for the individual teen. The family might take steps to be sure that the daughter's pregnancy did not cause a division of husband and wife, thus threatening the structural integrity of the family. For the community, conservation of structural integrity might involve revising the health care structure to meet the demands of teen pregnancies, or preventing the problem from becoming a divisive issue within the community.

For the individual client, conservation of personal integrity involves maintaining one's self-concept as a productive individual, which may be impaired by guilt feelings regarding the pregnancy. Dealing positively with such feelings helps the individual to maintain personal integrity. Maintaining family cohesion by working as a group to resolve the problems of a teen pregnancy can promote the personal integrity of the family. Promotion of citizen participation in health care decisions can serve the same function for the community.

TABLE 6–4. SAMPLE CONSERVATION ACTIVITIES

Model Concept	Conservation Activities		
	Individual	*Family*	*Community*
Problem	Pregnancy.	Pregnancy of teenage daughter.	Increased incidence of adolescent pregnancy.
Conservation principles			
Conservation of energy	Increase dietary intake to provide needed energy sources. Maintain balance between energy resources and expenditures.	Redirect family energy to deal with pregnancy and advent of new family member.	Redirect community energy and resources to provide sex education and contraceptive services for teenagers.
Conservation of structural integrity	Prevent complications of pregnancy. Maintain bodily functions.	Maintain family function despite pregnancy. Restructure family roles.	Maintain vital community functions related to teenage pregnancy (eg, prenatal and family planning services). Revise community structure to accommodate role in sex education.
Conservation of personal integrity	Maintain self-concept as a productive person.	Maintain family cohesion.	Promote community participation in health care decisions.
Conservation of social integrity	Maintain interpersonal contacts despite pregnancy.	Maintain relations with external support system. Deal with guilt related to daughter's pregnancy.	Maintain relations with the outside world. Promote cooperation of various groups in dealing with the problem.

Conservation of social integrity in the case of the individual client involves maintaining interpersonal relationships and contacts despite the pregnancy. Too often, adolescent girls who become pregnant are removed from school and lose the contact with peers necessary for accomplishing adolescent developmental tasks. If this is a local policy, other opportunities for interpersonal contact need to be provided. Families, likewise, often shut themselves off from others in such situations, fearing the stigma of an illegitimate birth. Dealing with these feelings openly and maintaining external relationships, particularly with support networks, can assist the family to conserve social integrity. Social integrity within the community can be maintained by promoting the cooperation of various groups in the resolution of the teen pregnancy problem. When some groups work in isolation or in opposition to each other, the social integrity of the community is threatened.

Using Levine's model, the nurse working with an individual, family, or community must assess the degree of client adaptation achieved in each of the four areas of conservation. Wherever problems are identified, the nurse plans and implements supportive or therapeutic interventions as appropriate. Table 6–5 lists several nursing interventions with each level of client designed to conserve energy or structural, personal, or social integrity.

Nursing interventions that promote conservation of energy for the individual client include provid-ing an environment conducive to rest, teaching about adequate nutrition, and encouraging an appropriate balance between rest and exercise. The family client can be encouraged to problem-solve with respect to the pregnancy and related problems, rather than to waste time and energy on recriminations. The nurse can help the family focus on the desire to protect the health of the teen and the unborn child. The nurse might also assist the family to reallocate resources to meet the needs of a new baby. Similarly, the nurse might assist the community to allocate resources to provide needed prenatal and child health services. Conservation of community energy might also entail coordinating health personnel and their activities to ensure efficient use of resources in the delivery of care.

Conservation of the structural integrity of the individual in terms of Levine's model might include preventing complications of pregnancy. The nurse would closely monitor the course of the pregnancy, encourage the client in regular prenatal visits, and teach and encourage healthful behaviors such as moderate exercise, adequate nutrition, and not smoking or drinking. The structural integrity of the family could be maintained by encouraging family members to discuss problems and feelings related to the pregnancy and by providing referrals to minimize the stress of the pregnancy on the family. For example, if family income is limited, the nurse might refer the family to an agency providing low-cost prenatal care. At the

TABLE 6–5. NURSING INTERVENTIONS IN THE LEVINE MODEL

Model Concept	Nursing Interventions		
	Individual	*Family*	*Community*
Conservation of energy	Provide environment conducive to rest. Provide adequate nutrition with sufficient energy sources. Encourage appropriate exercise.	Encourage family to deal realistically with pregnancy and not waste energy on recriminations. Help family explore allocation of resources to meet needs of new member.	Coordinate activities of health personnel to ensure efficient delivery of prenatal, child health, family planning, and sex education services. Assist community to allocate resources to meet demands of teen pregnancies.
Conservation of structural integrity	Prevent complications of pregnancy.	Assist family to meet all necessary functions. Refer to outside help as needed. Encourage family to discuss problems presented by pregnancy.	Work to lower teen birth rate to prevent overload of community resources.
Conservation of personal integrity	Encourage expression of anxiety regarding changes in self-image, fears of labor, and delivery. Praise demonstration of appropriate parenting behaviors.	Encourage family to discuss problems and plan to meet needs of the situation. Reinforce positive efforts to deal with problems.	Encourage participation of community members in health services planning. Reinforce positive accomplishments in dealing with problem.
Conservation of social integrity	Provide for interpersonal contacts (eg, return to school, dating).	Function as liaison with outside sources of help. Make referrals to other agencies as needed. Help family maintain normal relationships with outside world as much as possible.	Facilitate cooperative efforts among groups within community. Function as resource and/or liaison with outside agencies.

community level, nursing efforts to lower the teen birth rate, such as providing sex education and contraceptive services for teens, would help to prevent overloading local health resources, thereby maintaining the structural integrity of the community.

From the perspective of Levine's model, activities designed to conserve the personal integrity of the individual might include encouraging ventilation of feelings about the pregnancy such as guilt feelings or fears about labor. The teen may need assistance in adjusting to the bodily changes that occur as the pregnancy advances, maintaining a positive self-image despite an ungainly figure. The personal integrity of the family can be enhanced by encouraging family members to discuss their problems and to plan to meet situational needs. Both the individual and the family can be assisted to conserve personal integrity by praising positive efforts to deal with problems. For the community client, active participation by community members in health care planning and reinforcement of positive accomplishments in dealing with the teen pregnancy problem can help to conserve personal integrity.

The social integrity of the individual and family can be conserved by promoting interpersonal contacts with persons outside the family. In terms of Levine's model, both teen and family should be encouraged to maintain as normal a social life as possible. The nurse can also help maintain relationships with the outside world by making referrals and acting as a liaison with other health care agencies and providers. The nurse can also function as a liaison between the community and other sources of assistance. For example, the nurse might contact a nearby city for information on a successful program to lower the teen pregnancy rate. In addition, the nurse can facilitate cooperative efforts in the community to resolve the problem, thus assisting the community to maintain its social integrity.

Orem's Self-care Deficit Theory of Nursing

Dorothea Orem's model is based on the premise that human beings engage in self-care activities that serve to maintain a state of well-being. Self-care may be performed by the client or by a self-care agent, as when a mother cares for a young child (Orem, 1995).

Concepts of Orem's Model

Orem's self-care deficit theory is actually a hierarchical set of three theories in which each lower level is subsumed within the next higher one (Fawcett, 1993). The most basic element of this theory set is the theory of self-care. Self-care involves activities performed to maintain one's own life and health. Self-care ability is predicated on the existence of three types of capabilities: foundational capabilities and dispositions, power components, and actual self-care operations (Bliss-Holtz, 1996). Foundational capabilities and dispositions include general capabilities that allow self-care to take place. For example, one needs to be cognitively aware to perform self-care. Lack of cognitive function is the basis for self-care deficit in the severely mentally disabled. Similarly, depression may constitute a foundational disposition that impedes self-care. An example of a power component is having the authority to engage in self-care or dependent care. The mother of a toddler who refuses to let the child feed himself is denying a power component necessary for the child to engage in self-care. Finally, the actual ability to engage in self-care procedures may be lacking. For example, the arthritic client may lack the joint mobility required to dress him- or herself.

Self-care operations occur in three stages: an estimative stage, a transition stage, and a production or action stage (Bliss-Holtz, 1996). In the estimative stage, the self-care agent is involved in identifying the need for self-care and possible courses of action. The transition stage consists of decision making regarding the action to be taken, and the action stage involves the actual performance of the self-care activity (Carroll, 1995). Self-care activities are directed toward meeting three types of self-care requisites necessary for continued health and function: universal self-care requisites, developmental self-care requisites, and health deviation self-care (Gast, 1996). These are influenced by basic conditioning factors such as age, sex, health, and so on (Roberson & Kelley, 1996).

Universal self-care includes activities designed to meet the needs of everyday life related to (1) air, food, and water; (2) excretion of body wastes; (3) rest and activity; (4) both solitude and social interaction; (5) elimination of physical, social, or psychological hazards to health; and (6) being "normal" within the context of human social interactions (Orem, 1995). Table 6–6 depicts typical universal self-care activities by the individual, family, or community client.

Developmental self-care involves activities designed to foster achievement of developmental tasks. For example, a mother engages in certain activities designed to help her child achieve the developmental task of becoming toilet-trained.

Health deviation self-care involves activities designed to deal with conditions of defect, disability, illness, or injury or with diagnostic and therapeutic measures related to these conditions. Health deviation self-care requisites include (1) obtaining appropriate medical assistance, (2) dealing with the effects of health deviations, (3) effectively performing medically prescribed measures, (4) dealing with any adverse ef-

TABLE 6–6. SAMPLE UNIVERSAL SELF-CARE ACTIVITIES

Model Concept	Self-care Activities		
Universal Self-care	Individual	Family	Community
Air, food, and water	Ingest food and water needed for life. Maintain oxygen source.	Purchase, prepare, and consume food.	Maintain pure food, air, and water supplies.
Excrement	Maintain elimination processes.	Remove family trash. Dispose of unwanted items.	Dispose of community waste (eg, sewage, solid waste).
Rest/activity	Maintain a balance between rest and activity.	Provide resources for adequate rest for all family members. Provide adequate sleeping arrangements.	Direct community activity into productive channels. Provide avenues for community members to be active in decision making.
Solitude/social interaction	Maintain harmonious interpersonal relations. Develop ability to be comfortable alone.	Maintain harmonious relationships within the family. Provide for both joint and individual activities. Maintain harmonious relationships with those outside the family.	Maintain harmonious relationships among groups in the community and with the outside world.
Elimination of hazards	Repair a broken stair.	Childproof the house.	Purify water supplies. Control noise patterns.
Normalcy	Engage in age-appropriate social interactions.	Foster family participation in actions as expected by society.	Promote "normal" social interactions between and among members.

fects of medical care measures, (5) modifying one's self-concept to incorporate a realistic view of one's current state of health, and (6) adjusting one's lifestyle to promote continued personal development in light of existing health conditions and required treatment measures (Bliss-Holtz, 1996).

Inability to meet any of the three categories of self-care requisites gives rise to self-care deficits addressed in the second of Orem's hierarchical theories, the theory of self-care deficit. A *self-care deficit* is an inability to meet one's own *therapeutic self-care demands* (Roberson & Kelley, 1996), those actions necessary to maintain function and promote development. Persons charged with the care of others (eg, dependent children) who experience difficulty in discharging one or more aspects of their responsibilities are said to have dependent-care deficits (Orem, 1995). A deficit does not reflect a disorder per se, but one's inability to fulfill needs associated with the disorder. The existence of self-care or dependent-care deficits necessitates nursing intervention which occurs in accordance with Orem's third theory, the theory of nursing systems.

Nursing intervention is indicated whenever the client experiences impairment of the ability to engage in universal, developmental, or health deviation self-care. Nursing intervention involves delineating specific activities within one of three nursing systems: the wholly compensatory system, the partly compensatory system, or the supportive/educative system (Gast, 1996).

The choice of system used depends on the needs of the client. In the wholly compensatory system, the client is unable to engage in self-care and the nurse carries out self-care activities on behalf of the client. In the partly compensatory system, the nurse and client share responsibility for self-care activities, whereas in the supportive/educative system, the client carries out self-care activities with assistance from the nurse as needed (Orem, 1995).

Applying Orem's Model to Community Health Nursing

Orem's self-care model can easily be adapted for application to the care of individuals, families, or communities. Table 6–7 presents ways in which an individual, a family, and a community might meet health deviation self-care needs. The area of deviation is that of adolescent pregnancy.

In accordance with Orem's model, the individual client might obtain needed care by enrolling in a prenatal program, while family members might ensure her access to such a program. The community may need to revise its health care structure to provide programs needed to meet the needs of pregnant teens.

Dealing with the effects of the pregnancy for the teenager might involve measures to deal with nausea during the early stages of pregnancy as well as coping with the fatigue that is often felt. Changing dietary habits and buying loose-fitting clothing are other adjustments that may need to be made. For the family, dealing with the effects of the pregnancy might mean providing emotional support for their daughter in the face of community disapproval and dealing with guilt regarding the pregnancy. At the community level, there may be a need for additional child health ser-

TABLE 6–7. SAMPLE ACTIVITIES RELATED TO HEALTH DEVIATION SELF-CARE REQUISITES

Requisite	Individual	Family	Community
Obtaining care	Enroll in prenatal program.	Ensure access to prenatal care.	Provide prenatal care services for teens.
Dealing with effects of the deviation	Take action to control nausea. Get additional rest. Improve diet. Buy loose clothing.	Provide emotional support for teen. Deal with feelings of guilt.	Develop additional child health services. Modify educational systems to meet needs.
Performing prescribed measures	Take prenatal vitamins. Eat recommended food. Practice relaxation.	Provide transportation. Revise family diet. Function as childbirth coach.	Make new budget allocations. Develop new services.
Dealing with adverse effects of treatment	Curtail spending. Cope with bedrest.	Curtail spending.	Cut funding to other programs.
Modifying self-image	Accept pregnancy. Accept mother role.	Accept teen in mother role. Develop new family roles.	View community as having a problem.
Adjusting lifestyle	Date less. Change education plans.	Change family member interactions to reflect new roles.	Establish planning group to deal with problem.

vices to address the needs of children of adolescent parents or modifications in the education system to allow teenage mothers to continue their education while caring for their infants.

Effectively performing related treatments and procedures may require the adolescent to remember to take her prenatal vitamins, to improve her diet, or to practice breathing and relaxation techniques for natural childbirth. Family members may need to provide transportation for prenatal appointments, revise family dietary patterns, or serve as childbirth coaches in order for the teen to comply with health care providers' recommendations. For the community, compliance with health care providers' recommendations for services for pregnant teens may involve rethinking budget allocations and developing new services and facilities.

Dealing with adverse effects of medical treatments may involve curtailing individual or family spending to pay for prenatal care. If complications arise necessitating bed rest, the teen will need to cope with enforced inactivity and boredom. For the community, providing adequate care for pregnant teens and their children may require budget cuts to other programs or increased taxes.

From the perspective of Orem's model, modification of self-image would occur for the individual and family when both are able to accept the pregnancy without giving or accepting blame for its occurrence. Again, the teen needs to adjust to bodily changes occurring with the pregnancy. Self-image is also modified for the teen and other family members as they take on new roles and adjust relationships in existing roles. For example, the teen must accept the new role of mother and the family must allow her to

do so. The community must also modify its self-image to acknowledge the existence of a problem and to accept outside help in its resolution.

In terms of the model, teenage pregnancy requires lifestyle adaptations on the part of the individual, family, and community. The teen may need to date less frequently so as to care for her infant or delay or alter plans for her education. The family needs to change family member interactions to accommodate new roles. For example, mother and dad may not be able to go out as often should they be called on to babysit for their grandchild. The community might also need to make some long-term changes in the ways in which it addresses the health care needs of the adolescent population. It may be necessary to establish a special task force to explore the problem and oversee its solution.

According to Orem's model, whenever the client is unable to engage in effective self-care, nursing intervention is required. Table 6–8 presents possible nursing interventions with the individual, family, and community in each of the three nursing systems. In the *wholly compensatory system*, the nurse acts for the client. If the teen has had a particularly difficult delivery or experienced complications during the pregnancy, the nurse may need to carry out universal and health deviation self-care activities for her—feeding, bathing, and dressing both client and baby.

If the family is likewise disabled by the crisis of the teen's pregnancy, the nurse may need to refer the family to others for help with self-care needs. For example; the nurse might assist the family to obtain a homemaker aide to cook, clean house, or shop for food. The nurse can also arrange for child care, transportation, and other family needs if family members

TABLE 6–8. NURSING INTERVENTIONS IN THE OREM MODEL

| Model Concept | Nursing Interventions | | |
	Individual	*Family*	*Community*
Wholly compensatory system	Nurse carries out all universal and health care functions for the client (eg, feeds and bathes client and baby).	Nurse carries out or arranges for others to carry out family functions related to universal and deviation self-care needs (eg, sends home-maker to cook, care for children, clean house; arranges transportation for visit to physician).	Nurse initiates mandatory sex education in schools.
Partly compensatory system	Client carries out self-care activities with assistance by nurse as needed (eg, client feeds and dresses baby, nurse assists with bath).	Family carries out most of its functions; nurse arranges for child care so teen can return to school.	Nurse assists community in planning to resolve problems, helps set up family planning and prenatal clinics, and encourages other systems in the community to participate as appropriate (eg, schools provide sex education).
Supportive/educative system	Nurse instructs client in self-care and child care measures and provides support as needed.	Nurse assists family to adjust to new member, provides suggestions for child care, and reinforces positive approach to problems.	Nurse educates community on need for sex education and contraceptive services for teens.

are unable to deal with these needs themselves. At the community level, health care personnel may find the teen pregnancy problem warrants mandating sex education in all junior and senior high schools. This can be done, of course, only when such action lies within the jurisdiction of the local health authority.

Once the teen has recovered somewhat from the delivery experience, nursing intervention moves into the *partly compensatory system*, with the client carrying out most self-care activities with some help from the nurse. For example, the client might feed the baby and then dress the infant after the nurse has demonstrated how to give the baby a bath. In the family situation, most functions may be executed by the family, but the nurse may be called on to make a referral for child care. With the community, the nurse facilitates activity to resolve the teen pregnancy problem and may be involved in establishing or expanding family planning and prenatal services or sex education programs. The nurse also encourages active involvement of other segments of the community in resolving the problem. For example, the nurse might organize and instruct school teachers in providing sex education.

In the *supportive/educative system*, the nurse provides support while the client engages in self-care activities. With the individual client, such support might take the form of instruction in child care techniques and information about contraception or immunizations. The nurse might also assist the family to adjust to a new member, providing emotional support and practical suggestions for dealing with problems that arise. For the community client, the nurse may need to educate community members regarding the extent of the teen pregnancy problem and the necessity for sex education and contraceptive services. The commu-

nity, once alerted, could then take steps to deal with the problem with additional supportive input from the nurse as needed.

Johnson's Behavioral Systems Model

Dorothy Johnson defined nursing's contribution to client welfare as "the fostering of efficient and effective behavioral functioning in the patient to prevent illness and during and following illness" (Johnson, 1980). The focus of Johnson's model is the client's behavior—what is done, why it is done, and its consequences.

Concepts of Johnson's Model

A **behavioral system** is "the patterned, repetitive, and purposeful ways of living which characterize each man's life" (Johnson, 1980). One's behavioral system determines the character of one's interaction with the environment. For example, one person's usual behavioral response to stress may be aggression. This will undoubtedly result in continual conflict between the individual and his or her environment.

The behavioral system consists of several **behavioral subsystems** or sets of responses designed to maintain the system and regulate its interaction with the environment (Wilkerson & Loveland-Cherry, 1996). These subsystems are reasonably stable, occur with regularity, and are capable of a certain degree of modification. Each subsystem consists of four structural elements: (1) a drive or goal that motivates behavior, (2) "set," (3) the repertoire of behavioral choices available, and (4) the behavior itself. A drive results from a need that is not being met that provides a stimulus for action, whereas a goal is an outcome sought through action. For example, hunger is a drive resulting from a need for food. "Set" is a predisposition to act in certain ways. For example, one person will typically satisfy the hunger drive by cooking a meal, whereas another may habitually eat in a restaurant. The totality of the behavioral repertoire relates to the alternative choices available to achieve a goal. With respect to the hunger drive, for example, the behavioral repertoire of the first person included the ability to cook. Other alternatives might include stealing food or going home to mother's cooking. The behavior is the implementation of the alternative selected from the repertoire.

The behavioral subsystems common to humanity are (1) the affiliative subsystem, (2) the dependency subsystem, (3) the ingestive subsystem, (4) the eliminative subsystem, (5) the sexual subsystem, (6) the aggressive subsystem, and (7) the achievement subsystem (Connor, Harbour, Magers, & Watt, 1994). Instability in any of these subsystems is demonstrated by disorderly, purposeless, or unpredictable behavior

(Johnson, 1990). Table 6–9 describes the goals of behavioral subsystems for an individual, a family, and a community.

Nursing assessment in Johnson's model involves consideration of the effectiveness of client behaviors in achieving subsystem goals. First-level assessment includes identifying problem areas and the client's ability to cope with them. Second-level assessment is undertaken when problematic behavior exists. This level involves a more detailed analysis of the structure and function of the subsystem involved. The first consideration in the second-level assessment is the behavior itself. The nurse examines when the behavior occurs, what triggers the behavior, and what terminates it. The behavior is also considered in terms of its function and purpose.

Set is also assessed in relation to the identified problem in a behavioral subsystem. What is the client's usual behavior in a given situation? Why is this behavior inappropriate or ineffective? Set may also include perceptions, attitudes, and values that influence behavior.

TABLE 6–9. BEHAVIORAL SUBSYSTEM GOALS IN JOHNSON'S MODEL

Model Concept	Subsystem Goals		
Subsystem	*Individual*	*Family*	*Community*
Affiliative subsystem	Achieve satisfactory interpersonal relations with family, friends, and coworkers.	Maintain harmonious relationships among family members. Meet family members' needs for affection. Maintain satisfactory relationship with kin and others.	Maintain satisfactory and harmonious relationships among community groups. Develop productive relations with outside world.
Achievement subsystem	Achieve mastery and control of one's body and its functions (eg, toilet training, learning to ride a bike).	Achieve family goals (eg, college education for children, a new house).	Maintain appropriate community functions and mastery of environment (eg, educate members about health, dam a nearby river for power).
Aggressive/protective subsystem	Protect self or others from hazards (eg, take care in crossing streets, prevent others from imposing guilt on oneself).	Protect family members from hazardous circumstances (eg, know where children are, meet their friends; install smoke detectors in the home).	Protect community members from hazardous influences (eg, prevent air pollution by local industry, noise control). Protect the community from infringement by outside groups (eg, prevent graft and corruption in a food supplement program).
Dependency subsystem	Maintain environmental resources necessary for survival (eg, food, clothing, housing).	Provide family needs to ensure survival (eg, arrange housing, purchase and prepare food).	Maintain community resources to ensure survival (eg, provide for pure air, provide access to health care, maintain adequate housing).
Ingestive subsystem	Provide energy resources adequate for survival function (eg, eat a balanced diet).	Provide adequate family nutrition resources (eg, prepare well-balanced meals).	Provide community resources for survival and function (eg, provide adequate funds for health programs, establish a food bank).
Eliminative subsystem	Eliminate bodily wastes (eg, urinate and defecate).	Eliminate family wastes (eg, arrange for trash removal).	Eliminate community waste (eg, sewage treatment or disposal of industrial wastes, noise control).
Sexual subsystem	Provide for personal gratification and procreation (eg, use contraceptives as needed).	Maintain satisfactory sexual relationships. Meet family planning needs.	Provide services related to sexuality (eg, family planning). Provide for community expansion and growth (eg, recruit new industry).

The choice of behaviors open to the client in a given situation and the degree of client awareness of choice are other factors that can influence response to a situation. Clients might use maladaptive behaviors because they are not aware of other options.

Following the detailed assessment of problem areas, the nurse develops a nursing diagnosis that reflects the difficulty in effectively accomplishing subsystem goals. Nursing intervention is planned to establish regular behavior patterns that better fulfill these goals (Barnum, 1994). Nursing intervention can involve any of three categories of action: (1) restricting or controlling behavior through external constraints; (2) fulfilling the functional requirements of the subsystem by means of protection from hazards, nurturance, or stimulation of growth; or (3) changing structural components such as the direction or the drive, set, or repertoire of choices to achieve a more desirable behavior (Wilkerson & Loveland-Cherry, 1996).

Applying Johnson's Model to Community Health Nursing

Johnson's behavioral systems model provides a framework for nursing care to individuals, families, and communities. Employing the model, the community health nurse assesses each behavioral subsystem to identify specific problems, then plans interventions for those problem behaviors. Table 6–10 describes a second-level analysis of problematic behavior in the aggressive/protective subsystem. Problematic behavior exhibited by the individual and the family is failure to seek prenatal care for the pregnant teen. For the community, the problematic behavior is failure to provide sex education for teens.

In Johnson's model, the behavior exhibited by each client is intended to accomplish a specific function. For example, the teen may delay seeking prenatal care in an effort to deny the pregnancy and avoid feelings of guilt. The purpose of family behavior in failing to seek care may also be a wish to deny the problem and the need to deal with it. The community may not provide sex education for teens for fear of appearing to condone or encourage adolescent sexual activity.

For the individual and the family, the set, or preferred behavior, seems to be to ignore the problem, resulting in the failure to seek prenatal care. In the case of the community, set also involves ignoring adolescent sexual activity.

With respect to the available repertoire of behaviors, neither family nor individual may be aware of the range of options for obtaining prenatal care open to them. Similarly, community members might not have considered the possibility of encouraging sex education by training parents or church members to educate teens in a more acceptable atmosphere than the school. Other behavioral options may, of themselves, be either adaptive or maladaptive and their potential consequences should be considered. For example, if the community were to rely exclusively on parents to educate their children regarding sexuality, many youngsters would receive no sex education at all.

Other variables involved in the problematic behavior of the individual and the family, from the perspective of Johnson's model, might include lack of

TABLE 6–10. SECOND-LEVEL ANALYSIS OF PROBLEM BEHAVIOR IN JOHNSON'S MODEL

Model Concept	Second-level Analysis		
	Individual	*Family*	*Community*
Problem area: aggressive/protective subsystem	Unwed pregnancy	Pregnancy of teen daughter	Increased teen pregnancy rate
Behavior	Failure to get prenatal care	Failure to get prenatal care for teen	Failure to provide sex education for teens
Function of behavior	Attempt to deny pregnancy and associated guilt	Attempt to deny pregnancy and need to deal with it	Prevent criticism of condoning teen sexual activity
Set	Belief that pregnancy reflects "bad" behavior Knowledge of family disappointment Fear of unknown related to pregnancy, labor, and delivery Continued failure to follow up on referral for prenatal care	Belief that pregnancy reflects failure as parents Failure to follow up on referral for prenatal care for teen	Belief that sex education increases sexual behavior Belief that pregnancy is just punishment for illicit sexual activity Resistance to inclusion of sex education in school curricula
Choice of behaviors	Going to family physician, prenatal clinic, teen clinic, or nurse midwife	Take teen to family doctor, prenatal clinic, teen clinic, or nurse midwife	Provision of sex education by schools, families, or churches
Other variables	Lack of money, transportation, etc. Education level	Family income Education level Family attitudes toward illegitimacy	Community attitudes toward teen sexual activity Religious and cultural composition of community Lack of qualified educators

money for prenatal care, lack of awareness of the importance of prenatal care, lack of transportation, or attitudes toward illegitimacy. Other factors in community behavior might be community attitudes toward adolescent sexual activity, religious and cultural composition of the community, and lack of qualified persons to implement an effective sex education program.

From the perspective of the model, once the factors contributing to the problematic behavior have been identified, the nurse can proceed to plan interventions that restrict or control behavior; protect the client from exposure to stressors; nurture; stimulate growth; or modify drive, set, or behavioral choices to change behavior. Table 6–11 presents sample nursing interventions in each of these categories for the individual, the family, and the community.

Restrictive action by the nurse, in terms of Johnson's model, might involve arrangements to prevent school attendance until prenatal care is obtained. At the community level, the nurse might push for legislation mandating sex education in all state-supported schools.

A protective intervention with the individual client might involve explaining the benefits of prenatal care in protecting the baby from potential harm. If the teen is concerned about her baby, such knowledge might encourage her to obtain care. A similar intervention might be employed with the family by explaining the higher risk of complications of pregnancy in teenagers and the need for prenatal care to protect the teen. It might even be necessary, if the teen is a minor, for the nurse to report the family's failure to obtain prenatal care for their daughter as child neglect. In the case of the community, the nurse can become politically involved to advocate sex education in

schools, presenting to policy makers the dangers in unprotected sexual activity.

In Johnson's model, nurturance can also encourage both family and individual to seek care. The nurse who exhibits concern for the teen and seems genuinely interested in protecting her welfare may be more effective in educating client and family regarding the need for prenatal care. Again, the nurse might want to focus on the client's desires to benefit the baby and the teen herself. Individuals within the community at odds with these aims can be nurtured by being encouraged to participate in the planning of a sex education program that would be acceptable to them. The nurse can also defuse fears about sex education by pointing out research findings that show a positive effect on teen sexual activity.

The last mode of nursing intervention in Johnson's model involves modifying the structural components of the behavioral subsystem. The nurse can accomplish this with the individual and family client by assisting them to make an appointment for prenatal care, making referrals for financial assistance to pay for care, or arranging transportation. Helping to explore compromise plans for sex education in the community that include church leaders and other influential persons can facilitate effective community behavior in providing sex education for teens.

Neuman's Health Systems Model

The model for nursing intervention developed by Betty Neuman involves a client system striving to prevent "penetration" or disruption of the system by a variety of stressors. The client's state of health is dependent on the degree of success achieved in prevent-

TABLE 6–11. NURSING INTERVENTIONS IN THE JOHNSON MODEL

Model Concept	Nursing Interventions		
Categories of Action	*Individual*	*Family*	*Community*
Restriction	Restrict school attendance	Restrict school attendance	Work for legislative mandate for sex education in schools.
Protection	Advocate for baby by encouraging teen to get prenatal care. Educate client about need for prenatal care.	Advocate for teen and baby within family. Report neglect as needed. Educate family about need for prenatal care.	Become politically involved to advocate sex education for teens. Encourage participation of resistant groups in planning.
Nurturance	Focus on desire for healthy baby.	Focus on desire to protect teen.	Point out research findings on sex education and sexual activity by teens.
Changing structural components	Assist client to make appointment for prenatal care. Give positive reinforcement for seeking care. Arrange transportation for prenatal visit. Refer for financial aid.	Assist family to make appointment for care. Give positive reinforcement for seeking care. Arrange transportation. Refer for financial aid.	Develop compromise plan for sex education employing church leaders and others.

ing penetration of the client system by stressors or in effecting "reconstitution" of the system after penetration by stressors. Nursing intervention is indicated whenever the client is unable to prevent penetration or accomplish reconstitution without assistance (Neuman, 1994).

Concepts of Neuman's Model

A *stressor* is a problem or condition capable of causing instability in the system (Bomar, 1996). Exposure to bacteria, for example, is a stressor that might affect the health status of an individual, whereas unemployment might be a stressor for individuals, families, or communities.

In Neuman's model, the client is viewed as a composite of several elements including a basic structure, lines of resistance, and normal and flexible lines of defense (Neuman, 1994). These elements of the client are depicted in Figure 6–1. The client system is protected from penetration by the flexible line of defense. The *basic structure* is the inner core of the client that must be maintained to ensure survival. For example, elements of the basic core of the individual would be a functioning brain and heart. Penetration of the basic structure results in death. Using the example of

an individual client, a cardiac arrest would constitute penetration of the basic structure, much like the ghost towns of the Old West were the victims of stressor penetration of their basic structures. Elements of the basic structure of a community include its physical structure and its members (Haggart, 1993). For a family, the basic structure includes family members and their relationships. Death and divorce are examples of stressors that may penetrate the family's basic structure.

The *normal line of defense* is the client's usual state of wellness or the normal range of response to stressors (Bomar, 1996). For example, a client with diabetes and a client without any specific medical problem both have a normal state of health represented by their normal lines of defense. For the client with diabetes, that normal state of health includes the presence of a chronic disease.

The *flexible line of defense* is a dynamic state of wellness that changes over time and is composed of factors that fluctuate. The flexible line of defense provides a protective cushion that prevents stressors from penetrating the normal line of defense (Reed, 1995). An individual's flexible line of defense, for example, might include his or her level of fatigue at any given time. If the individual is well rested, he or she

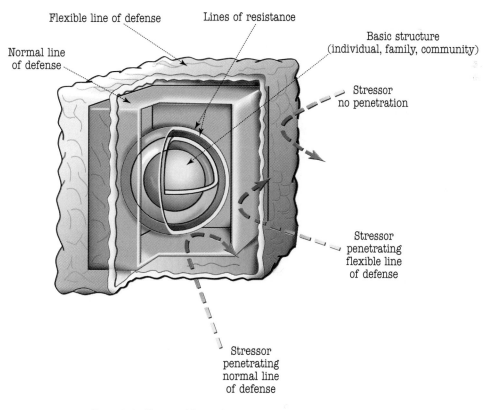

Figure 6–1. Elements of client in the Neuman model. (Adapted from Neuman, 1994.)

may be able to deal effectively with the stress of a noisy child without problems. If the client is tired, on the other hand, exposure to a noisy child might lead to penetration of the normal line of defense and result in a headache. Similarly, unemployment levels might be a factor in a community's flexible line of defense. When unemployment levels are low, the community is better able to withstand the onslaught of a stressor like a flood because people are more likely to possess the resources to rebuild both their homes and their lives.

When the flexible line of defense is incapable of protecting the system, penetration of the normal line of defense occurs. The extent of penetration and the degree of reaction to penetration are influenced by the strength of the normal line of defense and the lines of resistance. *Lines of resistance* are internal factors that protect the client against penetration of the basic structure by stressors. The strength of the lines of resistance influences the degree of the client's reaction to stressor penetration of the lines of defense (Lancaster, 1996). Using the example of someone exposed to a noisy child, if this person can employ relaxation techniques, he or she might be less affected by the stress than might otherwise be the case. The ability to use relaxation techniques minimizes the effects of stressor penetration. Without the use of this element of the lines of resistance, the person might end up in bed with a migraine headache.

The strength of the lines of defense and resistance are affected by developmental, physiologic, psychological, sociocultural, and spiritual variables impinging on the client (Neuman, 1994). Developmental variables relate to the age or developmental level of the client. For example, a new community would probably have fewer resources for dealing with a stressor like a flood than would a well-established community. Physiologic variables reflect physical structure and function. For example, the fact that a client has diabetes affects his or her response to a stressor such as exposure to a communicable disease. Psychological variables include such factors as self-concept and attitudes toward health. For example, individuals who have positive attitudes toward health and engage in health-promoting behaviors like exercise and not smoking are less likely to develop cardiovascular disease than those who do not engage in healthful behaviors. Sociocultural variables are factors such as culture, education level, and income. For example, the better educated client usually has greater knowledge of healthful behaviors that can prevent stressor penetration than someone who is not as well educated. Finally, spiritual variables such as beliefs in divine intervention and punishment for sins may af-

fect client's responses to stressors. This variable has been described as an energy source for the client (Pierce & Hutton, 1992).

Stressors may arise from the internal environment, the external environment, or the created environment. The created environment arises with mobilization of system variables intended to create a protective shield that permits continued system function. The created environment may block awareness of other features of the environment and may increase or decrease wellness (Neuman, 1994). Based on their origin, stressors may be classified as intrapersonal, interpersonal, or extrapersonal. For Neuman, the "person" who receives nursing care is the client system and may be an individual, family, group, or community. From this perspective, then, it is appropriate to think in terms of intraclient, interclient, and extraclient stressors. Intraclient stressors arise from within the client. For example, parental feelings of guilt over a child's illness are an intraclient stressor, whereas increased parental expectations arising from the illness are an interclient stressor. Concerns about paying the child's medical bills constitute an extraclient stressor.

Once penetration of the client system occurs, the system engages in activities aimed at reconstitution. *Reconstitution* involves stabilization of the system and movement back toward the normal line of defense. The normal line of defense may be stabilized at a level either higher or lower than that prior to penetration. For the client system to survive stressor penetration, reconstitution must take place before penetration of the basic structure can occur. For example, when an individual has a heart attack, reconstitution can be accomplished if cardiovascular function can be reestablished (eg, through cardiopulmonary resuscitation) and maintained.

Whenever a client system is unable to prevent penetration by a stressor or to accomplish reconstitution following penetration, nursing intervention is indicated. The nurse assesses the client to identify stressors, the factors involved, and the degree of reaction to penetration. Nursing intervention occurs at three levels: primary, secondary, and tertiary prevention (Neuman, 1994).

Primary prevention involves action taken before stressor penetration occurs and is aimed at preventing penetration by strengthening the lines of defense or decreasing the potential for exposure to the stressor. Secondary prevention takes place after penetration of the lines of defense by the stressor. Activities at this level are geared toward problem resolution and minimization of reaction to the stressor. Tertiary prevention is directed toward reestablishing equilibrium and preventing complications or recurrences of the problem.

Applying Neuman's Model to Community Health Nursing

Components of Neuman's model revolving around the stressor of an unwed teen pregnancy as applied to an individual, a family, and a community are presented in Table 6–12. For the individual, the basic structure consists of the physical body and its characteristics (age, race, sex, etc.) whereas the basic struc-

ture of the family involves its continued existence as a social unit. In terms of the community client, the basic structure consists of the physical structure of the community; locale; community history; age, race, and sex composition of the population; and vital community functions.

The normal line of defense of the individual might include the presence or absence of other health problems. For example, a diabetic teenager who becomes pregnant is at higher risk for complications of pregnancy than a nondiabetic teenager. Other factors

TABLE 6–12. CLIENT ASSESSMENT IN THE NEUMAN MODEL

Model Concept	Client Assessment		
	Individual	*Family*	*Community*
Stressor	Unwed pregnancy	Pregnancy of teenage daughter	Increased incidence of teen pregnancy
Basic structure	Physical body, vital functions, age	Composition of family, typical family roles	Age composition of population, vital community functions
Normal line of defense	Presence or absence of other acute or chronic disease Nutrition level Usual lifestyle and habits (eg, smoking, drinking, exercise) Attitude toward health	Family attitude toward teen sexual activity Family composition Family cohesion	Extent of teen population Education levels Income levels Availability of contraceptive services Usual teen pregnancy rate
Flexible line of defense	Fatigue level Presence or absence of other stressors	Presence or absence of other family stressors	Availability of funding for health programs
Lines of resistance	Attitude toward child Extent of child care skills	Flexibility of family Availability of support system Family income Family education level	Availability and adequacy of health care facilities and services Education and income levels Adequacy of transportation to health care facilities
Developmental variables	Age and developmental stage	Stage of family development	Age composition of population History of action taken in similar situations
Physiologic variables	Current health status Nutritional status Immunization status	Health of other family members	Extent of other health problems
Psychological variables	Self-image Attitudes toward parenthood Personal goals	Family's feelings about pregnancy Religious beliefs and practices Willingness of other family members to assume other role functions	Community attitudes toward teen sexual activity
Sociocultural variables	Cultural influences Income level Extent of child care knowledge	Cultural attitudes toward teen sexuality and illegitimacy Family income	Ethnic and religious composition of population Income and education levels Political structure Sources of funding for health care
Spiritual variables	Personal attitudes toward sin, punishment, and forgiveness	Family attitudes toward sin, punishment, and forgiveness	Community attitudes toward sin, punishment, and forgiveness
Intraclient factors	Presence of juvenile diabetes	Grandmother living in home	Available prenatal and child care services
Interclient factors	Assistance from other family members	Assistance from neighbors and extended family	Existing program for pregnant teens in neighboring city
Extraclient factors	Possession of health insurance	Availability of family counseling to assist in adjusting to daughter's pregnancy	Assistance from federal government with funds for prenatal and contraceptive services for teens
Goal of reconstitution	Healthy mother and baby Development of sound parenting skills Future use of effective contraceptive method	Adjustment of family to new member and related role changes	Provision of sex education and contraceptive services for teens Decrease in teen pregnancy rate

in the normal line of defense for the individual include nutrition level and lifestyle habits. Again, the undernourished or overweight teen or the teen who smokes is at higher risk during pregnancy.

Factors in the normal line of defense for the family might include family attitudes toward teenage sexual activity and illegitimacy, family composition, and degree of family cohesion. From the perspective of Neuman's model, a cohesive family should be better able to adapt to the pregnancy of the teen without threatening its basic structure as opposed to a family that lacks cohesion. If the teen is the only daughter, family response to her pregnancy may be different than if she had several sisters. For example, pregnancy in an older daughter might lead parents to be overly strict with younger girls, driving them to rebellion. Families with decided feelings against illegitimacy are more likely than other families to fail to support the teen in her decision to keep the baby.

Components of the normal line of defense for the community are the extent of the teenage population, community income and education levels, availability of contraceptive services for teens, and the usual teen pregnancy rate. If the teen population is small, the community will be better able to deal with it than if the problem is extensive. In terms of the model, the availability of sex education and contraceptive services could be seen as part of the community's normal state of health, preventing teens from becoming pregnant and thereby preventing the problem of adolescent pregnancy for the community.

Examples of factors influencing the individual's flexible line of defense are the degree of fatigue experienced by the pregnant teen and the presence or absence of other stressors. If the teen has recently broken up with her boyfriend, her pregnancy may be more stressful than would otherwise be the case. If the girl's father is unemployed, this might be an additional stressor that would weaken the family's flexible line of defense and make adaptation to the pregnancy more difficult. The availability of funding for health programs, on the other hand, would strengthen the community's flexible line of defense.

The lines of resistance for the pregnant teenager might include her attitude toward the baby and the extent of her child care skills. According to the model, both factors should affect how well she adapts to pregnancy and motherhood. Flexibility and adaptability within the family as well as the availability of support systems and income and education levels are part of the lines of resistance that affect the family's response to the pregnancy.

For the community, the availability and adequacy of health care services and facilities determine how effectively the community can deal with the problem of teenage pregnancies. Other factors in the lines of resistance for the community include community education and income levels and adequacy of transportation to health care facilities. All of these factors influence the degree to which pregnancy disrupts normal client function and threatens the basic structure of the individual, family, or community.

Developmental variables for the individual client include her age and developmental stage. From the perspective of Neuman's model, an adolescent who has accomplished most of the developmental tasks of adolescence could more easily move on to the tasks of motherhood than one who has not. If the family is a recently constituted stepfamily, the effects of the pregnancy may be more severe than if the family has well-established role expectations and modes of dealing with crisis. For the community, the age composition of the population and a history of action taken in similar situations in the past would affect the community's ability to deal with the problem.

According to the Neuman model, physiologic variables are those related to the physical structure and function of the client. Physiologic variables for the individual include her current health, nutrition, and immunization status. The health of other family members influences family reaction to the pregnancy, and other community health problems affect the extent of concerns caused by widespread teenage pregnancy. For example, high AIDS mortality in the community might overshadow the problem of adolescent pregnancy.

Psychological variables, in terms of the model, include factors such as the client's self-concept and attitude toward health. For the individual, psychological variables might include the teenager's self-image, her attitudes toward parenthood, and her personal goals. If she has always wanted to be a mother, her response to the pregnancy is likely to be more positive than if she views the pregnancy as interfering with personal career goals. Family feelings about the pregnancy, religious beliefs and practices, and the willingness of other family members to assume new roles with respect to the teen and her baby are psychological factors influencing the response of the family to the stressor. Community attitudes toward adolescent sexual activity are a psychological factor for the community. Cultural influences and income and education levels are sociocultural variables that may affect the reaction of the individual, family, or community to the stress of teen pregnancy. Similarly, attitudes toward sin, punishment, and forgiveness are spiritual variables that may influence the response of all three client levels.

Client reaction to stressor penetration is also influenced by intraclient, interclient, and extraclient factors. Intraclient factors are influences within the individual, family, or community that affect reaction to the stressor. In terms of the model, intraclient factors for the individual teen might include the presence of juvenile diabetes. The presence of a grandmother living in the home might be an intrafamily factor that would influence the family's response to the pregnancy. Availability of prenatal and child care services would be an intracommunity factor that could limit reaction to the stressor of teenage pregnancy.

Assistance from other family members, neighbors, and extended family might be interclient factors limiting reaction of the individual and family to stressor penetration, whereas the existence of a successful program for pregnant teens in a neighboring city might aid the community in responding to the situation. Extraclient factors for the individual might include possession of health insurance to pay for prenatal care, while the availability of counseling to help the family deal with the problem of the pregnancy is an extraclient factor for the family. For the community, an extraclient factor might be the availability of federal funding for prenatal and contraceptive services for teens.

Reconstitution is required for each of the three levels of clients. From the perspective of Neuman's model, the primary goals of reconstitution for the individual are a healthy mother and baby and development of sound parenting skills by the teen. An additional goal is the prevention of subsequent pregnancy by the use of an effective contraceptive. Reconstitution for the family entails positive adjustment to the presence of a new member and the role changes involved. For the community, the goal of reconstitution would be sex ed-

ucation and contraceptive services for teens resulting in a decrease in the teen pregnancy rate.

Nursing intervention related to the problem of adolescent pregnancy could take place at levels of primary, secondary, or tertiary prevention for each of the three types of clients. Table 6–13 provides examples of nursing interventions in the Neuman model for an individual, a family, and a community at each of the three levels of prevention.

Primary prevention for the individual client includes general health promotion and encouraging the use of effective contraception to prevent pregnancy. Primary prevention in terms of Neuman's model might also include promotion of a strong self-image to foster resistance to peer pressure for sexual activity. For the family, primary prevention might entail preparing parents to provide sex education to their children and offering assistance in developing communication patterns that foster communication among family members. Such communication encourages teens to come to parents to discuss sexuality issues and may help to prevent later pregnancy. Primary prevention at the community level involves providing sex education and contraceptive services for teens.

From the perspective of the model, secondary prevention for the individual client includes referral for prenatal care, monitoring the course of the pregnancy, and preventing complications of pregnancy. The nurse also educates the client in preparation for labor and delivery and for parenthood. For the family client, secondary prevention might entail activities to assist the family to adjust to a new member, such as helping the family plan role changes, reviewing child care skills, and dealing with feelings about the pregnancy. Secondary prevention for the community in-

TABLE 6–13. NURSING INTERVENTIONS IN THE NEUMAN MODEL

Model Concept	Nursing Interventions		
	Individual	*Family*	*Community*
Primary prevention	Promote health through adequate nutrition, rest, and exercise. Encourage use of effective contraceptive by sexually active teens.	Educate parents to provide sex education for children. Assist development of a climate in which children can discuss sexuality issues with parents.	Provide sex education and contraceptive services for teens.
Secondary prevention	Refer for prenatal care. Monitor course of pregnancy and prevent complications. Prepare for delivery and parenthood.	Assist family to adjust to advent of new member and related role changes.	Assist in development of prenatal and child care services to meet demands.
Tertiary prevention	Encourage use of effective contraception after delivery to prevent recurrence of pregnancy.	Discuss prevention of subsequent pregnancies. Discourage family from overprotection of other daughters.	Educate pregnant teens for future contraceptive use to prevent recurrence of pregnancy. Provide adequate sex education to prevent recurrence.

volves developing programs for prenatal and child health care to meet increased demands for service.

For the individual client, nursing intervention at the tertiary prevention level involves education and encouraging the use of effective contraception to prevent a subsequent pregnancy. The family might also need education regarding contraception. The community health nurse may also find that he or she needs to discourage parents from becoming overly protective or restrictive of other girls in the family in response to their daughter's pregnancy. At the community level, the nurse might develop programs for contraceptive education and services for pregnant teens to prevent subsequent pregnancies.

Pender's Health Promotion Model

Nola Pender has described a nursing model that directs nursing intervention for health promotion. Because health promotion is a major emphasis in community health nursing, Pender's model is presented here even though it addresses only one aspect of community health nursing.

Concepts of Pender's Model

In the health promotion model, behavior is influenced by individual characteristics and behavior-specific cognitions and affect that result in a commitment to action. Commitment to action results in actual behavior but may be modified by competing demands and preferences (Pender, 1996). Individual characteristics include personal biological, psychological, and sociocultural factors that are relevant to the behavior involved. Prior behavior in this area is another individual characteristic that influences health-promoting behavior. For example, a client who was physically active prior to pregnancy, will be more likely to engage in exercise after delivery than one who was not.

Behavior specific cognitions and attitudes include the perceived benefits of and barriers to health-promoting activity as well as one's perceived self-efficacy. For example, the client who does not perceive him- or herself as able to lose weight will probably not even attempt weight loss. Activity-related affect or feeling states related to the behavior, to oneself, or to the situation are also important in motivating health-promoting behavior. Interpersonal and situational influences are additional factors related to cognition and affect that influence behavior. For example, if the client's family members support weight loss, the client is more likely to stick to a diet. Conversely, low income, a situational influence, might adversely affect the client's weight loss options.

Individual characteristics and behavior-specific congitions and affect may lead to a commitment to health-promoting activity. Commitment includes both the intention to act and a specific plan of action. Commitment to action should lead to performance of the actual health-promoting behavior unless there is interference from competing demands and preferences. For example, the client's intention to diet may be subverted by a family member's serious illness and the need to eat in fast food restaurants near the hospital until they are out of danger and the client can return to a more normal lifestyle.

Applying Pender's Model to Community Health Nursing

Pender's model is applicable to individuals, families, and groups or communities. Table 6–14 provides examples of characteristics for the individual, family, or community client using the teenage pregnancy example. Biological factors for the individual would include the existence of other health problems and possible discomforts or signs of complications of pregnancy, all of which might motivate the teenager to seek prenatal care, a health-promoting behavior.

TABLE 6–14. **EXAMPLES OF INDIVIDUAL CHARACTERISTICS INFLUENCING HEALTH BEHAVIORS**

Model Concept	Healthful Behavior		
Characteristic	*Individual*	*Family*	*Community*
Prior related behavior	Vicarious experience of mother's prenatal care: Seeks care	Mother received prenatal care: Seeks care for daughter	Successful resolution of similar problem: Begins planning for adolescent care
Biological factors	Client experiences signs of complications: Seeks care	Father's ill health takes priority: Prenatal care delayed	Increased AIDS incidence takes priority: Plans for adolescent care delayed
Psychological factors	Client feels guilty about pregnancy: Delays seeking care	Family feels guilty about pregnancy: Delays seeking care	Community denies adolescent sexual activity is problem: Delays planning for adolescent care
Sociocultural factors	Client is not allowed to continue regular high school: Tries to hide pregnancy	Family views out-of-wedlock pregnancy as sin: Tries to hide pregnancy	Community views out-of-wedlock pregnancy as sin: Delays plans for care services

These same factors could also influence family efforts to seek care. For the community, the prevalence of other serious conditions may prevent adequate attention to the problem of teenage pregnancy. Psychological factors of guilt and cultural attitudes toward adolescent pregnancy might be similar motivators or impediments to behavior at all three levels. Prior experiences of prenatal care for either the teen or her mother or successful community experiences dealing with similar problems will also influence behavior.

Specific cognitions and attitudes toward obtaining or providing prenatal care for pregnant adolescents will similarly influence behavior at all three levels. Examples of factors related to cognitions and affect are presented in Table 6–15. If clients at each of the three levels, individual, family, or community, perceive that prenatal care will have the benefit of a healthier mother and child as well as reduced expense, the desired health behavior is likely to be enacted. If, on the other hand, prenatal care is perceived as an unnecessary expense, this attitude will pose a barrier to appropriate action. Similarly, if neither the teenager nor her family perceive themselves as able to successfully engage the health care system to obtain prenatal care, they are unlikely to seek care. Perceptions of the community's ability to provide prenatal services to adolescents may also influence the community's willingness to act.

Feelings of guilt on the part of the adolescent or family or outrage on the part of the community are examples of activity-related affect that may hinder health-promoting action, in this case seeking or pro-

viding prenatal care for pregnant teenagers. The attitudes of extended family members or of state health officials may influence the individual/family and community, respectively, in their intention to take health-promoting actions. Finally, situational influences, such as financial status, may affect the commitment of any of the three levels of client to seeking or providing prenatal care.

Even though the individual, family, or community may intend to act to seek or provide prenatal care, action may not occur if competing demands get in the way. For the individual, the demands of finals week at school may delay calling for an appointment for care. Similarly, another family crisis, such as unemployment and loss of health insurance, may prevent the family from seeking care for their daughter, or a natural disaster may disrupt the community's plans to provide prenatal care for pregnant adolescents.

When client characteristics, cognitions, and affect do not lead to a commitment to action, or when competing demands interfere with that commitment, nursing intervention is warranted. Table 6–16 provides some examples of nursing actions to modify contributing factors to promote the desired behavior of individual, family, and community. For example, the nurse might reduce perceptions of cost of services as a barrier to care by discussing with the teenager, family, or community members the higher cost of complications of pregnancy when prenatal care is not received. Or, the nurse might take action to enhance clients' perceptions of self-efficacy by pointing out

TABLE 6–15. EXAMPLES OF BEHAVIOR-SPECIFIC COGNITIONS AND AFFECT INFLUENCING HEALTH BEHAVIOR

Model Concept	Healthful Behavior		
Cognition/Affect	Individual	Family	Community
Perceived benefit	Sees prenatal care as an avenue to healthy baby: Seeks care	Sees prenatal care as an avenue to healthy mother and baby: Seeks care for daughter	Sees prenatal care as less expensive than dealing with problem pregnancies: Develops prenatal care services
Perceived barriers	Client sees exercise as too tiring: Does not exercise	Family sees prenatal care as too expensive: Does not seek care	Community sees teen contraceptive services as too controversial: Does not provide them
Self-efficacy	Client sees self as able to care for child: Learns parenting skills	Parents see themselves as good parental role models: Practice and encourage good family communication patterns	Community views itself as forerunner in teen pregnancy: Seeks innovative ideas for prevention program
Activity-related affect	Client fears going to doctor: Does not seek care	Parents fear social stigma: Do not seek care	Community fears cost of care: Does initiate services
Interpersonal influences	Friends suggest prenatal care: Seeks care	Extended family pushes for prenatal care: Family seeks care	State government mandates care: Develops teen care program
Situational influences	Inadequate funds for care: Does not seek care Unaware of options for care: Does not seek care	Inadequate family funds for care: Family does not seek care Unaware of options for care: Family does not seek care	Inadequate tax funds for care: Does not provide care Unaware of funding options: Does not provide care

TABLE 6–16. NURSING INTERVENTIONS INFLUENCING SELECTED VARIABLES IN THE PENDER HEALTH PROMOTION MODEL

Model Variable	Nursing Intervention
Prior health behavior	Explore client's previous experience with health-promoting behaviors. Determine how previous situation compares and contrasts with current situation. Help client to recognize similarities and differences in situations. Reinforce prior healthful behavior and positive experiences with prenatal care or other successful problem solving.
Biological factors	Point out signs of complications and possible effects on individual, family, or community.
Psychological factors	Assist individual and family to deal with guilt. Educate community members on reality of adolescent pregnancy.
Sociocultural factors	Assist individual to find other education programs. Help family deal with feelings of social stigma. Incorporate religious groups into planning to resolve adolescent pregnancy problem.
Perceived benefit	Educate individual, family, or community on actual benefits of healthful behaviors.
Perceived barriers	Identify potential barriers to healthful behavior. Attempt to eliminate or modify barriers.
Self-efficacy	Enhance client's perception of self-efficacy by praising present abilities and offering opportunities to enhance competence even more. Decrease negative aspects of mastery of skills. Set short-term attainable goals and point out achievement. Point out positive aspects of behavior as well as avenues for improvement.
Activity-related affect	Assist individual and family to voice and deal with fears. Educate community on costs of not providing care.
Interpersonal influences	Reinforce positive influence of others. Educate significant others regarding consequences of unhealthful behavior and incorporate them into care planning efforts.
Situational influences	Assist individual, family, or community to obtain funds for prenatal care. Educate individual and family regarding care options available. Provide referral for other options as needed. Assist community to identify funding sources for adolescent prenatal care.

past successful actions in similar situations. Other potential nursing interventions are presented in Table 6–16.

....

▶ NON-NURSING MODELS

Community health nurses also use a variety of non-nursing theoretical perspectives to direct their practice. Three such perspectives will be presented here: systems theory, developmental theory, and the struc-

Critical Thinking in Research

Robinson (1995) used Roy's model to study the grief responses, coping processes, and social support of widows during their second year of bereavement. She examined the effects of contextual stimuli such as social support, social network, income, education, and spiritual beliefs on cognator function as exemplified in the coping process and their relationship to an adaptive grief response as measured by physiologic, self-concept, role function, and interdependence mode variables. The author found that coping was significantly associated with both social support and social network. Coping was also significantly related to the grief response exhibited by subjects. The variables studied accounted for 18% of the variance in grief response.

1. Using Roy's model, what other contextual stimuli can you think of that might affect subjects' grief responses? What kinds of residual stimuli might operate unconsciously to influence the grief response?
2. How would you characterize this study in terms of its support for Roy's model. What elements of the model does it support? What areas does it not support or not address?
3. How might you frame a similar study in terms of one of the other nursing models described in this chapter? How would you frame the study if you were conducting it from the perspective of one of the non-nursing models?
4. If you wanted to conduct this study using one of the other models, how would you go about finding your subjects?

tural–functional model. Each of these three theoretical models is used extensively with families, but may be applied to the care of individuals and groups or communities as well.

Systems Models

Systems theory has provided the foundation for some of the nursing models already discussed (eg, Neuman and Johnson). Systems theory, however, can itself be used to guide community health nursing practice.

Concepts of Systems Theory

The basic concepts of systems theory are derived from the work of biologist Ludwig von Bertalanffy and sociologist Talcott Parsons working independently to describe biological and social systems, respectively (Friedman, 1998). Systems theory incorporates basic principles that can be applied to any kind of system from an automobile engine, to the human body, to families, to organizations, to communities, and so on (von Bertalanffy, 1973). A system is defined as "a complex of elements in interaction" with each other in which the interaction is ordered rather than random (von Bertalanffy, 1981). The "elements" that make up a system are also known as *subsystems.* Systems are hierarchical in nature with some systems, in turn, constituting subsystems within more complex systems. For example, the cardiovascular system is a subsystem in the human body, a system which is itself a subsystem in the totality of an individual, who is a subsystem in a family system, and so on.

Another concept of systems theory is the *suprasystem* or the context in which a given system functions. The next higher order system in the hierarchy is one aspect of the suprasystem for a lower order system. For example, the family is part of the suprasystem of an individual system, and the community is a suprasystem element for the family system. The concept of hierarchical systems is depicted in Figure 6–2. The system of interest in any given situation is sometimes referred to as the *focal system* and other systems within the suprasystem as *interacting systems* (Friedman, 1998).

Any system is more than the sum of parts or subsystems of which it is made and also incorporates reciprocal interactions among its parts. This system principle means that whatever affects one portion of a system will affect other portions because of their interdependence. The interrelationships between subsystems within the system, between subsystems and the suprasystem, and between the suprasystem and the system as a whole are important determinants of health and are one of the major foci in using a systems approach to community health nursing.

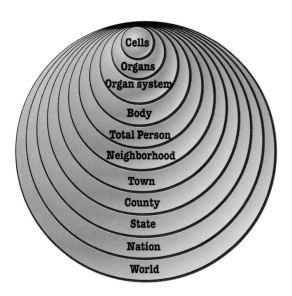

Figure 6–2. Hierarchical systems.

All systems have *boundaries* that define what is part of the system and what is not. For example, a community may have geographic boundaries such as city limits; whereas a family's boundaries are often (but not always) determined by blood and legal ties. The permeability of the system boundary determines whether one is dealing with an open or closed system. An *open system* is one that exchanges matter, energy, or information with the environment; a closed system does not. All of the systems of interest to community health nurses (individuals, families, and population groups) are open systems.

All systems also have two mutual goals: maintenance of a steady state and system growth and engage in three categories of processes designed to accomplish these goals. The first category of processes involves those needed to regulate exchanges with the environment. These processes are the input, throughput, and output processes. *Input* is the process whereby energy, matter, or information enter the system from outside the system's boundaries. *Throughput* is the process in which the material received into the system is transformed in some way, and *output* is what the system discharges back into the environment. As an example, consider the immigration of Southeast Asian refugees to the United States. The input is the refugees entering the U.S. community from the suprasystem. Throughput involves efforts to house and educate the refugees and assist them with other aspects of the transition to a new home. The output of the community system is the incorporation of these new members into the community and the production of new U.S. citizens.

The second category of processes involved in system operation are designed to limit expenditures of system energy, provide for organization, and prevent overload. Using these processes, a system may refuse to accept input. For example, the community may put a cap on the number of refugees that it can absorb. Internal processes, the third category of system processes, include subsystems change processes and adaptive processes. In subsystems change processes, a change in one subsystem results in changes in related subsystems. For example, when the number of refugee children in the community increases, the school system must respond to the increased need for multilingual education.

Adaptive processes, the second type of internal processes, involve the systems concepts of entropy, negentropy, and feedback. *Entropy* is a state of system disorganization resulting from the demands of continual readjustment of subsystem interrelations. A certain level of entropy is necessary for the system to continue to function and to avoid stasis or cessation of activity. However, when entropy rises above optimal levels, the system's ability to work toward its goals decreases proportionately. For example, the advent of a number of refugee families creates entropy forcing the community to grow to meet their needs. If, however, the number of refugees increases beyond the adaptive capability of the community, community function will be impaired.

Negentropy relates to an increase in order and organization, which allows energy to be used to meet system goals. Negentropy is necessary for maintenance of the steady state, but the system must periodically move away from this steady state in order for growth to occur. If, for example, the community refuses to allow any newcomers (including refugees) to reside in the community, it will soon become stagnant and ineffective.

Feedback is the process whereby the system output returns as input. Negative feedback tends to minimize changes in the system and contributes to maintenance of the steady state. Negative feedback, in essence, plays down any discrepancies between the desired state of affairs and circumstances as they are. For example, if feedback from the school system within the community indicates that the system as it currently operates can meet the needs of refugee children, changes in the school system are unlikely to occur. Positive feedback, on the other hand, maximizes discrepancies between what is desired and what is and, therefore, tends to result in system changes contributing to growth.

Applying Systems Models to Community Health Nursing

Table 6–17 provides examples of systems theory concepts as they might be applied to individuals, families, and communities experiencing the problem of adolescent pregnancy. The system in each case is the client. Subsystems for the individual teenager include organ systems, her self-concept, and other facets of the whole person. The subsystems of the family are the family members, and subsystems within the community would include the school system, health care system, governance system, and other subsystems needed to maintain effective community function. Input that necessitates adaptation by each of the systems is the fact of adolescent pregnancy. Income is another element of input that would influence the ability of each system to adapt to the pregnancy.

Effective throughput for the adolescent would include obtaining prenatal care, managing discomforts of pregnancy, learning child care skills, and obtaining contraceptives after delivery. For the family, throughput processes would focus on obtaining prenatal care for their daughter and learning new roles and interaction patterns; community throughput would involve providing prenatal care and contraceptive services for sexually active teens.

If these throughput processes were effective, the desired outputs of each system would be achieved. One desired output for each of the three systems is healthy mothers and babies. Additional outputs desired for the individual adolescent include successful adjustment to the maternal role and prevention of subsequent pregnancies. Another desired output for the family is successful adjustment to the advent of a new member. For the community, a decline in the adolescent pregnancy rate is a desired output.

Because subsystems of any system are interdependent, the fact of adolescent pregnancy will cause multiple interactions between and among subsystems. For example, hormone levels may affect the adolescent's gastrointestinal system resulting in

TABLE 6–17. APPLICATION OF SYSTEMS THEORY CONCEPTS TO INDIVIDUALS, FAMILIES, AND COMMUNITIES

Model Concept	Application		
System	Individual	Family	Community
Subsystems	Organ systems Self-concept, etc.	Family members	School system, health care system, etc.
Input	Pregnancy	Pregnancy of daughter	Increased rate of teen pregnancy
Throughput	Obtaining prenatal care Obtaining contraceptives Learning child care skills	Obtaining prenatal care Learning new roles	Providing prenatal care Providing contraceptives
Outputs	Healthy mother and baby Prevent subsequent pregnancy Adjustment to mother role	Healthy mother and baby Adjustment to new member	Healthy mothers and babies Decrease in adolescent pregnancy
Interactions	Effect of pregnancy on digestive system, self-concept	Tension between parents Restriction of other children	Impact of teen pregnancy on school system, health care system

TABLE 6–18. NURSING INTERVENTIONS USING A SYSTEMS APPROACH

| Model Concept | Nursing Interventions | | |
	Individual	*Family*	*Community*
Input	Education on normal changes of pregnancy	Financial assistance with prenatal care	Assistance in writing grant proposal for adolescent care programs
Throughput	Referral for prenatal care Education for child care	Referral for prenatal care Help renegotiating family roles	Help in planning prenatal and contraceptive services
Interactions	Education for dealing with discomforts of pregnancy, guilt	Assistance with family communication and problem solving	Help in adjusting school system to meet needs of teen parents

morning sickness and uterine enlargement may contribute to constipation. Similarly, the pregnancy may influence the girl's self-concept. For the family client, the daughter's pregnancy may result in tension between mother and father if they blame each other for the pregnancy or in restrictions placed on younger children to prevent similar events. At the community level, increased births to adolescents may necessitate changes in the health care system to provide adequate prenatal care and contraceptive services and changes in the school system to accommodate teenage parents.

Nursing intervention using a systems perspective would focus on assisting the system to adapt to changes in the environment and on accomplishing the dual goals of stability and growth. Table 6–18 presents some possible nursing interventions with individual, family, and community systems experiencing the problem of adolescent pregnancy. Intervention might involve providing system input in the form of education about pregnancy for the teen and financial assistance for obtaining or providing prenatal care for the family and community. Other interventions will be aimed at fostering effective throughput processes through referrals for prenatal care or help in designing prenatal care programs. The adolescent client will also need education for her new role as a mother and the family may need assistance in the process of renegotiating family roles. Finally, intervention may focus on dealing with the adverse subsystem interactions that result from the pregnancy. For the individual client, this may mean helping her to deal with the discomforts of pregnancy caused by the interaction effects on other body systems or aiding her to deal with guilt related to the pregnancy. The family may need assistance to improve family communication patterns or problem-solving skills, and the community may need the nurse's input in planning a program where adolescent parents can bring their children to school and learn parenting skills as well as complete their formal education.

Developmental Models

Developmental models are based on the supposition that human beings and social units develop in a logical fashion with predictable stages or milestones along the way. At each stage of development, the client is expected to accomplish specific tasks that provide a foundation for accomplishing the tasks of the next stage.

Concepts of Developmental Models

Table 6–19 presents some examples of developmental milestones expected of individual clients at selected ages, whereas Table 6–20 presents one conceptualization of the stages of family development. As the individual client ages, he or she would normally pass through a number of different stages similar to those depicted in Table 6–19. Developmental theory related to individuals will already be familiar to most readers from their general education courses in psychology as well as previous nursing courses and will not be belabored here. Family developmental theory may be less familiar so it will be discussed briefly. According to family developmental theory, families pass through predictable developmental or family lifestyle stages first described by Duvall (Duvall & Miller, 1990). According to Duvall, there are differing expectations in each stage of family development. As the expectations change, so do interactions among family members. The terms used for these stage expectations is *family developmental tasks*. The developmental tasks of each stage necessitate certain changes within the family in the roles of its members in order for the family to fulfill its functions.

Duvall divided the family life cycle into the eight stages depicted in Table 6–20. Each stage involves the accomplishment of specific tasks. At the same time that the family is engaged in accomplishing these tasks, individual family members are involved in accomplishing their own individual developmental

TABLE 6–19. DEVELOPMENTAL CHARACTERISTICS OF INDIVIDUAL CLIENTS AT SELECTED AGES

Age		Developmental Characteristic
Birth–1 month	Neurophysical	Newborn reflexes intact, head lag present, follows objects to midline, responds to noise.
	Psychosocial	Regards human face, quiets when picked up.
1–2 months	Neurophysical	Follows objects 180°, holds head up in prone position, head erect and bobbing when supported in sitting position.
	Psychosocial	Vocalizes other than crying, smiles responsively.
2–4 months	Neurophysical	Newborn reflexes diminishing, sits well with support, rolls from side to side, grasps rattle.
	Psychosocial	Laughs aloud, initiates smiling, enjoys play activity.
4–6 months	Neurophysical	Reaches for and gets objects, puts objects in mouth, rolls over completely, supports own weight when standing, tooth eruption.
	Psychosocial	Turns to voice, begins stranger anxiety, strong attachment to mother.
6–9 months	Neurophysical	Sits alone, bounces, stands holding on, thumb-finger grasp.
	Psychosocial	"Mama" or "Dada," plays peek-a-boo and pattycake, imitates speech sounds.
9–12 months	Neurophysical	Pulls to stand, creeps or crawls, walks holding on, sits from standing position, uses a cup with help.
	Psychosocial	Gives toy on request, speaks two to three words, gives affection, indicates wants.
12–18 months	Neurophysical	Scribbles, points to one or more body parts, uses a spoon, climbs and runs, plays ball, beginning bowel training.
	Psychosocial	Likes to be read to, 10-word vocabulary.
18–24 months	Neurophysical	Opens doors, turns on faucets, can throw or kick a ball, walks up and down stairs alone, daytime bowel and bladder control established.
	Psychosocial	Parallel play, 2- to 3-word sentences, imitates household tasks.
2–3 years	Neurophysical	Dresses with help, rides a tricycle, washes and dries hands.
	Psychosocial	Separates easily from mother, uses pronouns, perceives danger, understands sharing and taking turns.
3–5 years	Neurophysical	Dresses with decreasing supervision, hops on one foot, catches bounced ball, heel-to-toe walk.
	Psychosocial	Gives whole name, recognizes 3 colors, draws person with more than 6 parts, tells a story, operates from rules.
5–10 years	Neurophysical	Physical growth slows, motor coordination increases.
	Psychosocial	Begins peer identification, forms friendships, learns more rules, begins sexual identification, increases use of language to convey ideas, begins to understand cause and effect.
11–14 years	Neurophysical	Begins pubertal changes, gawkiness.
	Psychosocial	Importance of peer group conformity, strong identification with sexmates, learning one's role in heterosexual relationships, begins to establish an identity, more abstract thought, negative attitude toward family.
15–18 years	Neurophysical	Completes pubertal changes and adolescent growth spurt, better able to handle the new "body."
	Psychosocial	Develops an independent identity, establishes relationships with members of the opposite sex, adopts an adult value set, moves away from family relationships.
Early to late active adulthood	Neurophysical	Begins manifestation of aging process.
	Psychosocial	Develops and implements career goals, establishes a family, becomes a productive citizen, assists children to become independent, assists older parents, cultivates friendships with age-mates, maintains family relationships and learns new ones with spouses of children, grandchildren, establishes health routines, learns new motor skills, masters complex financial dealings, formulates a philosophy of life.
Late adulthood	Neurophysical	Experiences mobility limitations, sensory impairments, effects of chronic disease may manifest or become worse, appetite decreases.
	Psychosocial	Adjusts to retirement and loss of family members and friends, keeps mentally alert, accepts help graciously, adjusts to reduced income, learns new family roles, preserves friendships, adjusts to declining strength and stamina, maintains social interactions, adapts activities to diminished energy, prepares for death.

tasks which may parellel family tasks or conflict with them. The family must foster accomplishment of both family and individual tasks in order to function as an effective unit. Thus, there may be conflict or stress when the accomplishment of a family task is in direct opposition to task achievement by the individual. The family must develop healthy mechanisms for dealing with this type of conflict when it arises.

Families generally experience some stress as they pass from one stage to the next, since the transition usually involves one or more role changes. The family needs to negotiate these changes and respond by reevaluating roles and goals. Stage I marks the beginning of a new family when the couple separates from their families of origin. The major developmental tasks of this stage focus on establishing the marriage, relating to the expanded kin network, and family planning. The couple must learn to relate to each other in a way that meets the needs of each. Compromise and accommodation become critical elements in meeting the developmental tasks. Changes in relationships occur, not only between husband and wife, but also in relation to their kin. Each partner needs to learn new ways of relating to their family of origin as well as to their in-laws.

Stage II begins with the birth of the first child. At this point the family enters a new stage that necessitates changes in the roles of both husband and wife

TABLE 6–20. STAGES IN FAMILY DEVELOPMENT

Stage	Time Frame	Developmental Tasks
I Beginning family	Marriage to birth of first child	1. Establish mutually satisfying marriage 2. Relate to kin network 3. Family planning
II Early childbearing	Birth of first child plus 30 months	1. Establish stable family unit 2. Reconcile conflict in developmental tasks 3. Facilitate developmental tasks of members
III Family with preschool children	Oldest child 2–5 years of age	1. Integrate second or third child 2. Socialize children 3. Begin separation from children
IV Family with school-age children	Oldest child 6–13 years of age	1. Separate from children to a greater degree 2. Foster education and socialization 3. Maintain marriage
V Family with teenage children	Oldest child 13–20 years of age	1. Maintain marriage 2. Develop new communication channels 3. Maintain standards
VI Launching center family	From time first child leaves to time last child leaves	1. Promote independence 2. Integrate spouses of children into family 3. Restore marital relationship 4. Develop outside interests 5. Assist aging parents
VII Family of middle years	From time last child leaves to retirement	1. Cultivate leisure activities 2. Provide healthful environment 3. Sustain satisfying relationships with parents and children
VIII Family in retirement and old age	Retirement to death	1. Maintain satisfying living arrangements 2. Adjust to decreased income 3. Adjust to loss of spouse

(Source: Friedman, 1998.)

and in their interactions with each other. Major developmental tasks center around adjustment to parenthood and balancing individual with family needs. Stage III consists of families with preschool children. The primary tasks in this stage include nurturing and socializing children, and incorporating other children as they are born. As the number of relationships changes with the expanding size of the family, so do roles. Socialization of children is an important family function and a major task of this stage. Beginning separation of child from parents is also a feature of this stage.

Entry of the oldest child into school initiates stage IV. Critical tasks in this stage are promoting school achievement and encouraging further separation of children from parents as children expand their interactions outside the family unit and begin to respond to other social influences. Because of the multiple directions in which family members may go during this and subsequent stages, maintaining the marriage becomes a critical developmental task and continued communication and trust between the partners is vital.

The stage V family is coping with adolescent children and their developmental need for independence. The primary task at this stage is to balance teenage freedom and responsibility. Conflicts and tension often occur as teens begin to make their own decisions and demand more freedom. The dilemma faced by parents is determining the limits of independence and the extent of parental control warranted. The overall family goal becomes one of loosening family ties in preparation for adult children leaving home which occurs in stage VI. Critical tasks of stage VI are threefold: releasing the children as young adults, developing new interests for husband and wife, and assisting aging parents of the couple. The "empty nest syndrome" that may occur in this stage can pose an identity crisis for many women who have defined themselves in terms of their maternal role. An additional task of this stage may be incorporating children's spouses into the family constellation.

Stage VII, the middle-aged family, lasts from the time the last child leaves home until retirement. Family developmental tasks in this stage center around reestablishing the marital dyad and maintaining links with both older and younger generations. The couple in this stage are often called the "sandwich generation" because of their frequent need to continue to assist children as well as their own parents. Declining health, leisure activity, and preparation for retirement are all important foci in this stage. Stage VIII, the final developmental stage, is that of the aging family. Adjusting to retirement, aging, loneliness, and death of spouse, friends, or other family members become primary tasks.

The developmental approach, as applied to families, seems to address the traditional marital dyad with children. However, it can be adapted and applied to other types of families. Whatever the family structure, the community health nurse assesses the stage of individual or family development and examines the degree to which specific developmental tasks are being achieved.

A developmental approach can also be used with communities. Like individuals and families, effective communities develop in a series of stages or phases that apply to geopolitical communities as well as other entities such as organizations. These stages include: (1) excitement, (2) autonomy, (3) stability, (4) synergy, and (5) transformation (Shaffer & Anundsen, 1993). In the excitement stage, members of the beginning community see the possibilities and benefits of interaction. Developmental tasks in this stage include exploring possibilities and creating a shared vision. The second stage is characterized by "jockeying for power" (Shaffer & Anundsen, 1993), due in part to disillusionment with progress toward shared goals that are not instantly achievable. An important task in this stage is to differentiate individual from community and promote autonomy within the community framework. At this point the community needs to promote individuality and independence before members can become interdependent. Open communication is particularly important at this stage to prevent group dissolution.

In the third stage, that of stability, the group or community settles into defined roles and structures. At this point progress toward group goals is more obvious and expectations are more realistic. Community processes and procedures are established and function virtually automatically. Group roles also become fairly well entrenched. In some groups this stage is never ending or those who routinely perform certain roles become burned out. The end results of these processes may be stagnation or group dissolution. More effective groups or communities progress to the fourth stage, synergy, in which the group is open to new perspectives and ways of doing things and roles and role holders are subject to change. Again, this stage can lead to complacency or to lack of concern with the outside world.

The final stage, transformation, is characterized by a "death and rebirth" sort of phenomenon, when the community or group may expand its boundaries or identity, segment into smaller groups, or, when appropriate, disband in favor of development of other connections. For example, a close knit group within your nursing class will be transformed on graduation and its members will not interact with each other in the same way in the future. The stages of community development and characteristic features are presented in Table 6–21.

Applying Developmental Models to Community Health Nursing

Use of the developmental approach in community health nursing entails identifying the developmental level of the client, individual, family, or community. Intervention focuses on assisting clients at all levels to accomplish the appropriate developmental tasks and on creating an environment in which development is fostered. Sample nursing interventions designed to foster the development of an individual, a family, and a community in the context of adolescent pregnancy are presented in Table 6–22. The pregnant teenager may need help in reconciling the developmental tasks of her infant with her own development. Anticipatory guidance for both client and family regarding infant and adolescent development may assist the teenager to make a more successful transition to motherhood and aid the family to accord the adolescent the independence needed for her to effectively fulfill the maternal role. In the first stage of the development of a community group to deal with the problem of adolescent pregnancy, the nurse may help to generate the enthusiasm that will be needed to bring program plans to fruition. In the power play stage, the nurse can use his or her collaborative skills to keep agency agendas from fragmenting the group and derailing its purpose. Similar interventions might be employed in each stage of client development.

TABLE 6–21. STAGES OF COMMUNITY DEVELOPMENT AND CHARACTERISTIC FEATURES

Stage	Characteristic Feature
1. Excitement	Focus on possibilities, creation of a shared vision, development of tenuous group bonds, establishment of rules and procedures, attempts at total equality.
2. Autonomy	Power struggles, shattering of illusion of unity, attempts to dominate or manipulate others, members develop self-identity separate from group identity, preservation of individual autonomy.
3. Stability	Reaffirmation of group vision; cooperation on group task accomplishment; pursuit of group goals; operation in terms of established behavior patterns and procedures; comfortable roles; may lead to complacency and stagnation, burnout of members, or group polarization.
4. Synergy	Balance between individual and group needs, sense of connection between individual good and group good, periodic changes in leadership without jeopardizing group function, ability to move outside of established roles and rules when appropriate, potential for isolation from larger community and its needs.
5. Transformation	Expansion of boundaries, segmentation into smaller groups, or disbanding if appropriate, outreach to other groups, movement in new or expanded directions.

(Source: Shaffer & Anundsen, 1993.)

TABLE 6–22. SELECTED DEVELOPMENTAL MODEL NURSING INTERVENTIONS FOR ADOLESCENT PREGNANCY

Model Concept	Nursing Interventions		
	Individual	*Family*	*Community*
Stage	Late adolescence: 15–18 years	Family with adolescents	Stability
Tasks	Complete growth and sexual development	Maintain marriage	Reaffirm community vision
	Adjust to "new" body	Develop new communication channels	Avoid stagnation
	Develop an identity	Maintain standards	Continue routines
	Establish relationships with members of opposite sex		
	Adopt an adult value set		
	Achieve growing independence		
Interventions	Ensure adequate nutrition for adolescent growth and pregnancy	Foster effective communication and problem solving regarding pregnancy	Point out that prenatal care for teens fits with community values and vision
	Refer for prenatal care to minimize physical consequences of pregnancy	Explore feelings about pregnancy	Develop modes of adapting to teen pregnancy problem
	Explore relationship with father of child	Discuss effects of pregnancy on family value system and other children	Assess adequacy of current processes for providing needed care
	Assist client to develop child care skills and maternal role	Prevent restriction of other children	
	Assist client to examine values related to pregnancy	Assess degree to which tasks of previous stages were met	
	Assist client to deal with discomforts of pregnancy	Assist family to explore needed role changes to accommodate growing independence of teen	
	Assist client to deal with effects of pregnancy on body image and self-concept		

Structural–Functional Models

A structural–functional approach to community health nursing is based on the principle that all client entities possess structure designed to allow them to perform specific functions. The health of the entity—individual, family, or community—is dependent on performance of these necessary functions.

Concepts of Structural–Functional Models

The two basic concepts of a structural–functional approach are structure and function. *Structure* is the pattern of organization of interdependent parts of a whole. Human anatomy and physiology, for example, reflect the structural make-up of the human body with anatomy reflecting the physical construction of the body and physiology addressing the way that the component parts interact with each other. Comparable elements in the family would be family members and family interaction patterns related to roles, values, communication patterns, and power structure. Community members, organizations, and systems are the components of the physical structure of a community, whereas the interaction patterns between these component parts would be the "physiology" of the community. Structural elements of individuals, families, and communities are presented in Table 6–23.

Structural elements affect clients' abilities to perform functions that contribute to ensure continued survival and influence health. A *function* is one of a group of related actions that lead to accomplishment of specific goals, the goals of interest in community health nursing being client survival and health. Individuals, families, and communities all have necessary functions that must be performed to accomplish these goals. Individual functions can be conceptualized in terms of Maslow's hierarchy of basic human needs (Maslow, 1968). Maslow's hierarchy should be familiar to the reader, but is recapped in Table 6–24 with functions related to each need.

TABLE 6–23. EXAMPLES OF STRUCTURAL ELEMENTS: INDIVIDUAL, FAMILY, AND COMMUNITY CLIENTS

Individual	Family	Community
Anatomic organ systems	Family composition	Government
Physiologic interactions	Values	Education system
Self-concept	Roles	Health care system
Personality	Communication patterns	Business and industry
Mental capacity	Power structure	Welfare agencies
Spirituality		Families and individuals
		Churches
		Clubs and other organizations
		Protective services
		Buildings and environmental features

TABLE 6–24. MASLOW'S HIERARCHY OF HUMAN NEEDS AND RELATED FUNCTIONS

Need	Function
Survival	Provide elements required for human survival: food, water, sleep, oxygen, sexual activity
Safety and security	Protect from physical hazards, provide for emotional security
Love and belonging	Receive affection from others, feel and express affection for others, group identification, companionship
Esteem and recognition	Develop sense of self-worth, achieve recognition of accomplishments by others
Self-actualization	Achieve personal potential
Aesthetic	Achieve order and harmony in life, achieve spiritual goals

(Source: Maslow, 1968.)

Family functions fall into the six categories depicted in Table 6–25. The affective function of the family reflects its ability to meet the emotional and belonging needs of its members. The socialization function is designed to assist family members to become active contributors to the family and to the larger society and includes educating family members as well as transmitting attitudes and values. The reproductive function ensures continuity of the family and of society (Friedman, 1998). Another aspect of this function is control of sexual behavior and reproduction. The goal of the family's economic function is provision and appropriate allocation of family economic resources. This function is intimately tied to the provision of needs function which reflects the family's ability to meet members' needs for food, shelter, health care, and so on. Finally, the coping function reflects family abilities to adjust to changes and environmental demands. The relationship of structural and functional elements in families is presented in Table 6–26.

TABLE 6–25. FAMILY FUNCTIONS AND RELATED GOALS

Function	Goals
Affective	Meet the emotional needs of family members
Socialization	Educate family members as contributing members of society Inculcate family attitudes and values in members
Reproductive	Ensure survival of family and society Regulate sexual activity Provide for sexual satisfaction
Economic	Provide financial resources sufficient to meet family needs
Provision of needs	Meet family member's needs for food, shelter, clothing, health care, etc.
Coping	Allow family to adapt to environmental changes and demands

TABLE 6–26. INTERRELATIONSHIPS AMONG FUNCTIONAL AND STRUCTURAL ELEMENTS IN FAMILIES

Functional Element	Structural Elements
Affective function	*Role:* Who provides support, reassurance, encouragement? *Values:* How, when, and where is affection displayed? *Communication:* How are affective messages conveyed? By whom? *Power:* Do affective bonds confer power? Diminish power?
Socialization function	*Role:* Who socializes children? *Values:* How, when, and where are children socialized? *Communication:* How are standards communicated? Are accepted standards and behavior congruent? *Power:* Is socialization one-way or two-way? Is power maintained or diminished by socialization?
Reproductive function	*Role:* Who engages in reproductive functions? With whom? *Values:* When, where, and how are reproductive functions carried out? *Communication:* How is information about sexuality conveyed? How are sexual desires conveyed? By whom? Does reproductive activity also convey affection? *Power:* Is manipulation of the reproductive function used to confer power?
Economic function	*Role:* Who earns? Who spends? *Values:* How, when, and where are expenditures made? For what? *Communication:* How are economic needs communicated? To whom? *Power:* Who makes economic decisions? How?
Provision of necessities function	*Role:* Who provides what? *Values:* What should be provided? When? Where? How? To whom? *Communication:* How are needs communicated? To whom? *Power:* Who makes decisions about allocation of resources? How?
Coping function	*Role:* Who copes with what? *Values:* What coping mechanisms are acceptable? *Communication:* How is the need for support in coping conveyed? *Power:* Do coping abilities confer power?

As noted in Chapter 1, communites also have specific responsibilities or functions that they are expected to perform. These functions, associated goals, and related community structural elements are presented in Table 6–27. The production, distribution, and consumption function of the community incorporates all community institutions involved in the provision of goods and services necessary for life. Businesses, government, churches, and schools are some of the groups within the community that engage in this function. The socialization function is usually carried out by families, schools, churches, and other similar groups in the community. Socialization involves the transmission of prevailing knowledge, social val-

TABLE 6–27. COMMUNITY FUNCTIONS, GOALS, AND RELATED STRUCTURAL ELEMENTS

Function	Goal	Structural Elements
Production, distribution, and consumption of goods and services	Availability of necessary goods and services to all members	Business, government, churches, schools, health care agencies, welfare agencies, protective services
Socialization of members	Education of members for contribution to community and society	Families, churches, schools
Social control	Regulation of behavior within societal norms	Families, government, police, judicial system
Opportunity for social participation	Active participation of members in community decision making and social interactions	Government, schools, churches, clubs, social groups and organizations
Mutual support	Assistance to members in need	Family, churches, government, welfare agencies, support groups, insurance companies, business and industry

ues, and behavior patterns to members of the community. The third function, that of social control, is the process by which community members' behavior is influenced to conformity with the community norm. This function is usually carried out by such institutions as the family, government, police, judicial system, school, and church. The provision of opportunity for social participation by members of the community is fostered by such groups as churches, clubs, voluntary organizations, and government. The last function, provision of mutual support, was formerly seen as the responsibility of family, neighbors, and churches, but has more recently been assumed as a community function by welfare agencies and insurance companies. Many industries and other community groups are also engaged in voluntary activities to benefit community members. For example, the local utility company may provide electricity to low-income elderly persons at reduced rates.

Applying Structural–Functional Models in Community Health Nursing

Structural elements may influence clients' abilities to carry out required functions, thereby undermining client health. The community health nurse using a structural–functional approach to care first assesses how effectively the client performs expected functions and identifies any problems in functional areas. The nurse then identifies structural elements that are contributing to functional difficulties. Examples of structural–functional problems and nursing interventions related to adolescent pregnancy for the individual, family, and community client are presented in Table 6–28.

Intervention using a structural–functional model is designed to improve functional performance. For example, complications of pregnancy may threaten the individual clients' ability to meet survival needs.

TABLE 6–28. STRUCTURAL–FUNCTIONAL PROBLEMS AND INTERVENTIONS RELATED TO ADOLESCENT PREGNANCY

	Individual	Family	Community
Problem	Morning sickness interferes with dietary intake	Economic function inadequate to afford prenatal care	Community lacks adequate prenatal care services for teens
Intervention	Educate on control of morning sickness	Refer for financial assistance	Help community plan new care programs
Problem	Enlarging uterus leads to constipation	Poor communication patterns impede coping with pregnancy	School system cannot accommodate teens with children
Intervention	Encourage fluids, bulk in diet Encourage exercise	Teach communication strategies	Help to plan alternative education programs
Problem	Guilt over pregnancy interferes with school performance	Teenager's father is father of her child	Teens have little input into community decisions on contraceptive services
Intervention	Assist client to deal with guilt	Refer to child protective services Arrange out-of-home placement	Include teens in planning contraceptive services
Problem	Pregnancy interferes with plans for college	Parents become overly strict with younger daughters	Teen parents receive little emotional support
Intervention	Help client develop alternative education plans Refer for special education programs for single parents	Help foster good communication patterns Discuss adolescents' needs for increasing independence	Help establish support groups for teen parents

Intervention in this case would be directed toward obtaining prenatal care and preventing complications. Similarly, pregnancy may interfere with the client's ability to meet self-actualization needs through achieving career goals, and intervention could encompass referral to an education program designed for teenagers with children. At the family level, ineffective communication patterns and fixed family roles are family structural elements that may interfere with the family's coping function in dealing with the pregnancy. In this case, nursing intervention would focus on improving family communication and redefining roles. For the community, the presence of many teenagers with young children may interfere with the socialization function, and the nurse could assist the community to develop an alternative education program for this population.

Each of the nursing and non-nursing models presented in this chapter can be used by community health nurses to provide care to individual, family, and community clients. Each model organizes client information and focuses on nursing intervention dif-ferently, but each can achieve the same desired outcome, improved client health. The remainder of this book uses the Dimensions Model as the organizing framework for providing community health nursing care, but many of the models discussed here could also be used.

TESTING YOUR UNDERSTANDING

1. Describe three major concepts of the Roy adaptation model. Give an example of how each concept might be applied to an individual, a family, or a community. (pp. 82–87)
2. Describe four major concepts of Levine's principles of conservation. Give an example of how each concept might be applied to an individual, a family or a community. (pp. 87–90)
3. Describe three major concepts of Orem's self-care deficit theory of nursing. Given an example of how each concept might be applied to an individual, a family, or a community. (pp. 90–93)

 ## Critical Thinking in Practice: A Case in Point

Clarksville is a small rural town. Agriculture is the primary industry, and those residents of the area who are not farmers are involved in support services for the farming community. There are a few businesses in town including a grocery store, a hardware store, a grain elevator, a farm machinery dealership, two gas stations, and a bank.

The area recently suffered a severe drought. Several farmers defaulted on loans, and the mortgages on their farms have been foreclosed. Others are barely able to make a living. Because of the failing economy, the businesses in town have also suffered, and the grocery store will close at the end of the month.

Most families have gardens, so they are able to obtain fresh vegetables. Fruits are also available from area orchards, but the yield is small because of the drought. Many of the remaining farm families have been able to raise enough livestock to feed themselves and to have some left over for sale. Chickens have also continued to lay and eggs are plentiful.

Over the years, many young people have left the area and moved to nearby cities where work is available. Last year, the high school was closed because there were not enough students to keep it open. Those few students of high school age are now transported to a school in a nearby town. The grade school is currently open, but several grades have been combined because of the small numbers of students. Elderly residents have remained in their homes, and people over the age of 65 now constitute 60% of the population.

Health problems common in the community include hypertension, cardiovascular disease, anemia, and alcoholism. Tuberculosis and suicide are also prevalent among the elderly. There is one older doctor in town, but he plans to retire in a year or two. There is no hospital in town and no dentist. Consequently, hospital and dental services must be obtained in the nearest city, which is 50 miles away.

1. Select one of the theoretical models presented in the chapter and use the model to assess the community as a client for community health nursing services.
2. Describe the community's problems in terms of the model.
3. What nursing interventions would be appropriate in this situation? How would this intervention be carried out in terms of the model chosen?

4. Describe five major concepts of Johnson's behavioral systems model. Give an example of how each concept might be applied to an individual, a family, or a community. (pp. 93–96)
5. Describe five major concepts of Neuman's health systems model. Give an example of how each concept might be applied to an individual, a family, or a community. (pp. 96–102)
6. Describe three major concepts of Pender's health promotion model. Give an example of how each concept might be applied to an individual, a family, or a community. (pp. 102–104)
7. Describe at least five major concepts of systems models as applied to community health nursing. Given an example of each. (pp. 104–107)
8. Discuss the developmental stages for individual, family, and community clients. Give an example of a nursing intervention designed to promote development at each stage for each level of client. (pp. 107–110)
9. Describe the interrelationships between structure and function in individual, family, and community clients. Give examples of nursing interventions designed to promote function in each level of client. (pp. 111–114)

WHAT DO YOU THINK?
Questions for Critical Thinking

1. What features in a model would make it useful in community health nursing practice? Which of the models presented in the chapter have those factors?
2. Should community health nurses develop their own theories and models, adapt general nursing theories to community health practice (as done in this chapter), or adapt public health models (as is done throughout the rest of the book)? Why?
3. What are the relative advantages and disadvantages of using the models described in this chapter to guide community health nursing practice?
4. Are there other nursing models that could be adapted for use in community health nursing practice? Could they be used with all three levels of client (individual, family, and community)?

REFERENCES

Andrews, H. A. (1991a). Overview of the role function mode. In C. Roy & H. A. Andrews (Eds.), *The Roy adaptation model: The definitive statement* (pp. 346–361). Norwalk, CT: Appleton & Lange.

Andrews, H. A. (1991b). Overview of the self-concept mode. In C. Roy & H. A. Andrews (Eds.), *The Roy adaptation model: The definitive statement* (pp. 269–279). Norwalk, CT: Appleton & Lange.

Andrews, H. A., & Roy, C. (1991a). The essentials of the Roy adaptation model. In C. Roy & H. A. Andrews (Eds.), *The Roy adaptation model: The definitive statement* (pp. 1–25). Norwalk, CT: Appleton & Lange.

Andrews, H. A., & Roy, C. (1991b). Overview of the physiologic mode. In C. Roy & H. A. Andrews (Eds.), *The Roy adaptation model: The definitive statement* (pp. 57–66). Norwalk, CT: Appleton & Lange.

Artigue, G. S., Foli, K. J., Johnson, T., et al. (1994). Myra Estrin Levine: Four conservation principles. In A. Marriner-Tomey (Ed.), *Nursing theorists and their work* (3rd ed.) (pp. 199–210). St. Louis: Mosby.

Barnum, B. S. (1994). *Nursing theory: Analysis, application, evaluation* (4th ed.). Philadelphia: Lippincott.

Bliss-Holtz, J. (1996). Using Orem's theory to generate nursing diagnoses for electronic documentation. *Nursing Science Quarterly, 9,* 121–125.

Bomar, P. (1996). *Nurses and family health promotion: Concepts, assessment, and interventions* (2nd ed.). Philadelphia: W. B. Saunders.

Buck, M. H. (1991). The personal self. In C. Roy & H. A. Andrews (Eds.), *The Roy adaptation model: The definitive statement* (pp. 311–335). Norwalk, CT: Appleton & Lange.

Carroll, D. L. (1995). The importance of self-efficacy expectations in elderly patients recovering from coronary artery bypass surgery. *Heart & Lung, 24*(1), 50–59.

Connor, S. S., Harbour, L. S., Magers, J. A., & Watt, J. K. (1994). Dorothy E. Johnson: Behavioral systems model. In A. Marriner-Tomey (Ed.), *Nursing theorists and their work* (3rd ed.) (pp. 231–246). St. Louis: Mosby.

Duvall, E., & Miller, B. (1990). *Marriage and family development* (6th ed.). New York: Harper College.

Fawcett, J. (1993). *Analysis and evaluation of conceptual models of nursing* (3rd ed.). Philadelphia: F. A. Davis.

Friedman, M. M. (1998). *Family nursing: Research, theory, & practice* (4th ed.). Stamford, CT: Appleton & Lange.

Gast, H. L. (1996). Orem's self-care model. In J. L. Fitzpatrick & A. L. Whall (Eds.), *Conceptual models of nursing: Analysis and application* (3rd ed.) (pp. 111–151). Stamford, CT: Appleton & Lange.

Girard, N. (1993). Nursing care delivery models. *AORN Journal, 57,* 481–488.

Gless, P. A. (1995). Applying the Roy adaptation model to the care of clients with quadriplegia. *Rehabilitation Nursing, 20*(1), 11–16.

Haggart, M. (1993). A critical analysis of Neuman's systems model in relation to public health nursing. *Journal of Advanced Nursing, 18,* 1917–1922.

Johnson, D. E. (1980). The behavioral system model for nursing. In J. P. Riehl & C. Roy (Eds.), *Conceptual models for nursing practice.* New York: Appleton-Century-Crofts.

Johnson, D. E. (1990). The behavioral system model for nursing. In M. E. Parker (Ed.), *Nursing theories in practice* (pp. 23–32). New York: National League for Nursing.

Koziol-McLain, J., & Maeve, M. K. (1993). Nursing theory in perspective. *Nursing Outlook, 41,* 79–81.

Lancaster, D. R. (1996). Neuman's systems model. In J. L. Fitzpatrick & A. L. Whall (Eds.), *Conceptual models of nursing: Analysis and application* (3rd ed.) (pp. 199–223). Stamford, CT: Appleton & Lange.

Levine, M. E. (1991). The conservation principles: A model for health. In K. M. Schaefer & J. B. Pond (Eds.), *Levine's conservation model: A framework for nursing practice* (pp. 1–11). Philadelphia: F. A. Davis.

Lutjens, L. R. J. (1995). Calista Roy: An adaptation model. In C. M. McQuiston & A. A. Webb (Eds.), *Foundations of nursing theory: Contributions of twelve key theorists* (pp. 89–138). Thousand Oaks, CA: Sage.

Maslow, A. (1968). *Toward a psychology of being* (2nd ed.). New York: Van Nostrand Reinhold.

Neuman, B. (1994). The Neuman systems model. In B. Neuman (Ed.), *The Neuman systems model* (3rd ed.). Norwalk, CT: Appleton & Lange.

Nunnery, R. K. (1997). *Advancing your career: Concepts of professional nursing.* Philadelphia: F. A. Davis.

Orem, D. E. (1995). *Nursing concepts of practice* (5th ed.). St. Louis: Mosby Year Book.

Pender, N. J. (1996). *Health promotion in nursing practice* (3rd ed.). Norwalk, CT: Appleton & Lange.

Pierce, J. D., & Hutton, E. (1992). Applying the new concepts of the Neuman systems model. *Nursing Forum, 27*(1), 15–18.

Reed, K. (1995). Betty Neuman: The Neuman systems model. In C. M. McQuiston & A. A. Webb (Eds.), *Foundations of nursing theory: Contributions of twelve key theorists* (pp. 515–560). Thousand Oaks, CA: Sage.

Roberson, M., & Kelley, J. H. (1996). Using Orem's theory in transcultural settings: A critique. *Nursing Forum, 31*(3), 22–28.

Robinson, J. H. (1995). Grief responses, coping processes, and social support of widows: Research with Roy's model. *Nursing Science Quarterly, 8,* 158–164.

Ryan, M. C. (1996). Loneliness, social support, and depression as interactive variables with cognitive status: Testing Roy's model. *Nursing Science Quarterly, 9,* 107–114.

Shaffer, C. R., & Anundsen, K. (1993). *Creating community anywhere: Finding support and connection in a fragmented world.* New York: Putnam.

Srp, F., & Martaus, H. (1995). Case manager outcome reporting and analysis. *Inside Case Management, 2*(7), 3–5.

Tedrow, M. P. (1991). Overview of the interdependence mode. In C. Roy & H. A. Andrews (Eds.), *The Roy adaptation model: The definitive statement* (pp. 385–403). Norwalk, CT: Appleton & Lange.

Tiedeman, M. E. (1996). Roy's adaptation model. In J. L. Fitzpatrick & A. L. Whall (Eds.), *Conceptual models of nursing: Analysis and application* (3rd ed.) (pp. 153–181). Stamford, CT: Appleton & Lange.

von Bertalanffy, L. (1973). *General systems theory.* New York: George Braziller.

von Bertalanffy, L. (1981). *A systems view of man.* Boulder, CO: Westview.

Wilkerson, S. A., & Loveland-Cherry, C. J. (1996). Johnson's behavioral systems model. In J. L. Fitzpatrick & A. L. Whall (Eds.), *Conceptual models of nursing: Analysis and application* (3rd ed.) (pp. 89–109). Stamford, CT: Appleton & Lange.

LADY JANE JACKSON RECEIVES THE VISITING NURSE

Sweetheart, come up.
I'm up here in my chair
But first take a look
around my house.
Do you see the pictures
hung in the stairwell
everyone framed?
That's me as a school girl
me on the arm of one of my beaus
me posing in my wedding dress
me at the church giving a concert
me at my job in the government
I'm a certified graduate
practical nurse
and doctor of divinity.
Go into the kitchen
and look at my pill nook—
medicine boxes and
cups full of capsules
And then on the dresser
there in the bedroom
you'll see my bottles
of perfumes and creams—
the closet won't shut
for all of my gowns.
The bed is arranged
with pillows and dolls.
I haven't slept there
since I don't know when.
I suffered a terrible stroke
you know and I can't
get around like I used to.
But I've been in this house
for thirty years
and everything
is just the way
I want it.

Mrs. Jackson, excuse me
but why are you
sitting there naked?
Do you find it less trouble
than dressing these days?
And you seem to be slipping
out of your chair.
What is that squeaking
under the bed
and those wet stains
on the ceiling?
There are papers and dishes
all over the floor—
Aren't you afraid of falling?
Who do you have
to help you clean up?
I can see you were
very particular, once.
I'm a nurse, you know
and only one person.
You said on the phone
you wanted someone to
check your pressure
once a month.
I wonder somehow
if that's going
to be enough.
I'll have a key made
so you can get in
anytime, night or day
and you don't have
to think about money.
A dollar a visit
is what I pay.

Excerpted with permission from V. Masson (1993). just who. Washington, DC: Crossroads Health Ministry.

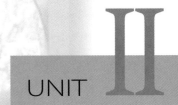

THE PROCESS DIMENSION IN COMMUNITY HEALTH NURSING

The systematic processes that community health nurses employ to promote and safeguard the health of the public include the nursing process as well as the epidemiologic, health education, home visit, case management, change, leadership, group, and political processes. In this unit, each process is discussed as it applies to community health nursing.

The nursing process (Chapter 7) directs the community health nurse in providing care to meet a client's health needs, whether the client is an individual, a family, group, or community. The nursing process, however, does not delineate the kind of data that a nurse should collect to determine a client's health status. Data collection, rather, is directed by the epidemiologic process (Chapter 8). The epidemiologic process is also used to identify factors that influence health and illness in the population.

The health education process (Chapter 9) is a systematic approach to creating a firm foundation of knowledge and attitudes that will permit clients to make positive choices concerning their health. The process is based on the scientific principles of teaching and learning.

Using the systematic process of home visiting (Chapter 10) helps the community health nurse to realize the potential benefits of the traditional home visit. Visits are planned and intervention is focused on meeting identified health needs.

Other processes, such as the case management process (Chapter 11), facilitate movement of clients from one segment of the health care system to another. The community health nurse helps identify and plan for a client's continuing needs for health care and coordinates the provision of care to meet those needs.

Finally, to facilitate change in the health care system, community health nurses implement the change, leadership, and group processes (Chapter 12) and the political process (Chapter 13). These processes enable the nurse to influence changes that will promote client health and prevent illness.

THE NURSING PROCESS

Community health nurses, like nurses in other practice areas, use the nursing process as a framework for nursing care. Community health nurses, however, use the nursing process from a slightly different perspective, incorporating knowledge and principles derived from public health science. In addition, community health nurses apply the nursing process to communities and other client aggregates. Community health nurses work with both sick and well individuals and with people of all ages, applying the nursing process to meet the needs of these different clients. This chapter reviews the attributes and steps of the nursing process as applied in community health nursing practice.

▶ KEY TERMS

actual nursing diagnoses
assessment
collaborative problems
critical path
database
defining characteristics
diagnostic hypothesis
enabling factors
etiology
evaluation
goals
health-promotive
   nursing diagnoses
health status summary
high-risk nursing
   diagnoses
implementation
initial plan of care
nursing diagnosis
nursing interventions
nursing process
objective data
objectives
outcome evaluation
outcome objectives
planning
positive nursing
   diagnoses
problem-focused
   nursing diagnoses
process evaluation
process objectives
progress notes
risk factors
status-oriented record
subjective data
syndromes
variances
wellness nursing
   diagnoses

121

▶ Chapter Objectives

After reading this chapter, you should be able to:

- Discuss components of the nursing process in the context of community health nursing.
- Describe the diagnostic reasoning process.
- Distinguish among categories of nursing diagnoses.
- Write nursing diagnoses that reflect client health needs incorporating appropriate descriptors and etiologic factors.
- Describe four tasks in the planning stage of the nursing process.
- Distinguish between process and outcome objectives for nursing intervention.
- Write nursing interventions for selected community health nursing diagnoses.
- Describe five tasks in implementing the nursing plan of care.
- Differentiate between process and outcome evaluation and develop evaluative criteria for each.
- Identify the components of a SOAP note.

▶ ATTRIBUTES OF THE NURSING PROCESS

The *nursing process* has been described as "an efficient method of organizing thought processes for clinical decision making and problem solving" (Doenges & Moorhouse, 1995). Use of the nursing process involves the planned execution of a series of steps. In 1967, these steps were delineated as *assessment, planning, implementation,* and *evaluation* (Doheny, Cook, & Stopper, 1996). *Diagnosis* was later incorporated as a link between assessment and planning (McFarland, 1996). These steps are performed sequentially and each step depends on adequate performance of prior steps. The process itself is cyclic, and evaluative findings become assessment data in subsequent cycles of the process. All five steps of the process are incorporated in its use, but may overlap to a certain extent.

▶ THE DIMENSIONS OF NURSING

The nursing process is, of course, itself an integral element of the process dimension of nursing in the Dimensions Model. Effective use of the nursing process, however, requires application of several of the other nursing dimensions. The interface between the nursing process and the cognitive dimension necessitates the application of a wide array of knowledge from the physical, social, and behavioral sciences to identify client health problems. The community health nurse must also have a broad knowledge of nursing interventions appropriate to the care of clients at multiple levels. In the interpersonal dimension, the community health nurse will need to be able to collaborate and communicate effectively with clients and with other health care professionals in order to use the nursing process most effectively. Tenets of the ethical dimension of nursing assure that the nursing process is used to the benefit of clients, not to their detriment while guaranteeing that the care provided does not violate client rights to self-determination. Advocacy is frequently an element of nursing care provided.

The use of the nursing process with individuals, families, and groups of clients may also necessitate application of a variety of manipulative and intellectual skills. Certainly, the community health nurse will exercise his or her diagnostic skills in identifying client problems and developing nursing diagnoses. Intellectual skills are also required to design nursing interventions to address those diagnoses. Manipulative skills may be required in the implementation of nursing interventions. In addition to the nursing process itself, other processes might be employed by the nurse in implementing the plan of care. For example, the nurse may need to use the political process to promote access to care for underserved populations. Finally, evaluation is an element of the reflective dimension particularly related to the nursing process.

 Assessing the Dimensions of Health

Client assessment is the first step of the nursing process. Prior to initiating action, the nurse assesses the client to determine the client's health status and the need for nursing intervention. In community health nursing, client needs are many and varied, affecting the biological, psychological, and social well-being of the community and its members.

Assessment involves collection of information in each of the dimensions of health to determine client health status. The data collected may be subjective or objective, current or historical. *Subjective data* are reported by the client or a significant other, and cannot be validated by the nurse. *Objective data,* on the other hand, are observed, described, and verified by the nurse. Historical data are information about the client's past that influence current health status, whereas current data reflect present factors affecting health, either positively or negatively (Doenges & Moorhouse, 1995).

Assessment data may be collected by several methods including interview, physical examination, review of records and diagnostic reports, and collaboration with colleagues. Community health nurses tend to collect a wider array of data than nurses in other specialty areas. For example, the school nurse may need to collect data on crime rates in the area around the school or on the employment level and tax base of the surrounding community so as to plan a school health program that adequately addresses community needs. Community health nurses are also likely to require data on groups of people as well as individuals and families. It is worth noting that the data collection skills used by community health nurses in assessing individuals, families, groups, and communities must also be applied when assessing health policy issues, health care financing issues, and environmental and ethical issues—all of which will be examined in later chapters.

In any given client encounter, the nurse may obtain further assessment data. The amount of data obtained on a first encounter should be as complete as possible, but may be constrained by time or elements of the client situation. Because this is frequently the case, the nurse should attempt to obtain "priority" assessment data related to significant health problems and health risks (Iyer & Camp, 1995). Data regarding educational needs and potential for self-care may also be of primary importance in some client situations. Additional data related to the client's health status can then be obtained in later encounters.

 Diagnosing Client Health Status

Using data obtained through various assessment procedures, the nurse employs diagnostic skills, an element of the skills dimension of nursing, to identify the client's health status and formulate nursing diagnoses. In 1990, the North American Nursing Diagnosis Association (NANDA) redefined *nursing diagnosis* as "a clinical judgment about an individual, family, or community response to actual or potential health problems/life processes" (Carpenito, 1995). Nursing diagnoses reflect client conditions that require nursing intervention. Both positive and negative conditions can necessitate nursing action. Activities of the diagnostic phase of the nursing process include analyzing data and formulating diagnostic statements.

Relationships among these activities are depicted in Figure 7–1.

Data Analysis

To be of value in directing nursing care, assessment data must be processed and analyzed. This analysis involves classification, interpretation, and validation. Data must first be classified or sorted into specific categories. For example, some data may reflect the biophysical dimension, whereas other data relate to the social dimension.

Once data have been classified, they must be interpreted. Data interpretation involves comparison of client-specific data with known norms and standards or diagnostic cues. For example, the community health nurse might note that a particular child has had more injuries than children of that age normally experience. Interpretation also includes clustering cues into recognizable patterns and trends in the data and making inferences based on the data. These inferences may be referred to as *diagnostic hypotheses* (Gordon, 1994).

A ***diagnostic hypothesis*** is a possible explanation for the client's condition and is generated on the

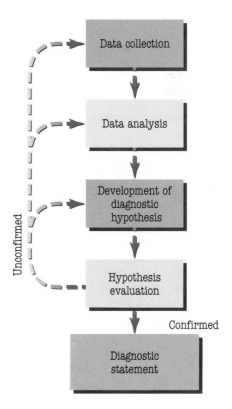

Figure 7–1. Relationships among steps of the diagnostic reasoning process.

basis of data patterns and trends. For example, data may include a history of questionable injuries to a young child with a teenage parent experiencing economic problems and lacking adequate social and emotional support. These data suggest a hypothesis of child abuse to explain a current broken arm.

The last aspect of data analysis is validating inferences or diagnostic hypotheses. This validation process may be referred to as *hypothesis evaluation* (Carnevali, 1993). Because data may generate several diagnostic hypotheses, the community health nurse must prioritize the hypotheses in terms of their likelihood given the cluster of diagnostic cues available (Gordon, 1994). The nurse first evaluates the hypothesis with the greatest probability of fitting the client situation. The hypothesis is tested by collecting additional data that either verify or disconfirm the diagnosis. Using the previous example, the nurse might observe parent–child interaction and question the parent and child more closely about how the broken arm occurred. The nurse might also request an investigation of the situation by the local child protective service to confirm the diagnostic hypothesis of abuse.

If additional data collected fit the diagnostic hypothesis, the hypothesis is verified and a specific diagnosis made. If not, the nurse recycles through the process, collecting data and testing subsequent hypotheses until one is confirmed. Verified hypotheses should be validated by both the client and the nurse (Doheny, Cook, & Stopper, 1996). For example, the nurse might confront the teenage parent with the suspicion of child abuse and evaluate the parent's response.

Formulation of Nursing Diagnoses

Valid inferences or diagnostic hypotheses based on assessment data are formulated as diagnostic statements. Statements of nursing diagnoses may reflect strengths and positive states of health as well as health problems experienced by clients. Guidelines for the development of new nursing diagnoses address four types of diagnostic concepts: actual nursing diagnoses, high-risk diagnoses, wellness diagnoses, and syndromes (Carpenito, 1995). *Actual nursing diagnoses* describe existing health problems experienced by clients. *High-risk nursing diagnoses* reflect the potential for developing health problems because of the presence of identifiable risk factors. *Wellness nursing diagnoses* reflect client states that may be enhanced to a higher level. The diagnoses might be better termed *health-promotive nursing diagnoses*, indicating a need for intervention to actively promote health. Another type of wellness diagnosis identified by community health nurses is *positive nursing diagnoses*. These

include positive client responses in which no change is required and for which nursing intervention consists of reinforcing a current state of affairs. *Syndromes* are clusters of related actual or high-risk diagnoses. Actual and high-risk diagnoses and syndromes are *problem-focused nursing diagnoses;* health promotive and positive diagnoses may be considered wellness diagnoses. This classification schema for nursing diagnoses is reflected in Figure 7–2. Nursing diagnoses may also be labeled "possible" diagnoses. A possible diagnosis is not another category of diagnoses, but a diagnosis suggested by data for which there is insufficient data at present for confirmation (Carpenito, 1995).

The structure of a nursing diagnostic statement varies somewhat depending on the type of diagnosis. All diagnostic statements, however, begin with a description of a client state of health (whether positive or negative) qualified with appropriate modifiers. Using the concept of "parenting" as an example, an actual diagnosis might begin with the phrase "ineffective parenting," where as a high-risk diagnosis might begin "high risk for ineffective parenting." Similarly, a health-promotive diagnosis might reflect "potential for enhanced parenting," whereas a positive diagnosis might indicate "effective parenting."

In addition to the description of a health state or a "problem label," the actual nursing diagnosis includes the etiology of the problem and the presenting signs and symptoms or "defining characteristics" (Gordon, 1994). The *etiology* reflects factors contributing to the problem; the *defining characteristics* are the observable cues or client manifestations that validate the existence of the problem.

Some authors recommend including the defining characteristics of an actual condition in the diagnostic statement itself, usually preceded by the phrase "as evidenced by." The diagnostic statement related to abuse would then be "physical abuse as evidenced by a history of repeated injury and parental explanations incongruent with type and location of injuries." Including the defining characteristics in the actual diagnostic statement, however, often creates a lengthy statement that does not contribute appreciably to an understanding of the client's health status. A more effective approach is to document the presence of defining characteristics using the status-oriented record discussed later in this chapter. An example of an actual diagnosis reflecting both etiology and defining characteristics might be "ineffective parenting due to unrealistic expectations of child, as evidenced by disciplinary action for developmentally appropriate behavior."

Frequently, the phrase "related to" is used to indicate the etiology of a health condition; however, as

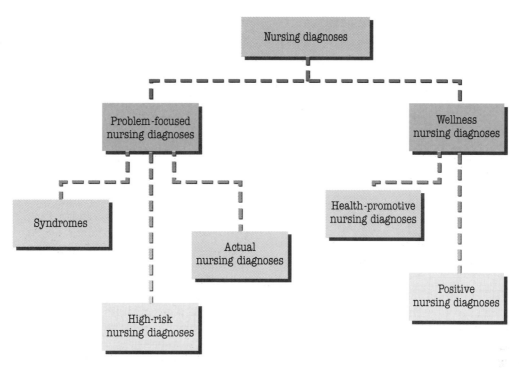

Figure 7–2. Categorization schema for nursing diagnoses.

etiology refers to the "probable factors causing, or maintaining the client's problem" (Gordon, 1994), the phrase "due to" is used in this book. One circumstance might be "related to" another without any connotation of cause and effect. For example, sugar consumption has been found to be significantly related to lung cancer, but certainly does not cause the cancer. But when one states that one event is "due to" another, one implies causality and provides direction for actions to be taken to either change or reinforce a situation. For example, a diagnosis of "ineffective parenting due to lack of parental role models" might be addressed by providing adequate role models. Similarly, when the diagnosis is "effective coping due to use of extended support system," the nurse would encourage continued use of the support system to maintain this healthy state.

High-risk diagnoses are stated somewhat differently than actual diagnoses. Both types of diagnostic statements include a description of the client health state, but, where the actual diagnosis includes etiologic factors, the high-risk diagnosis reflects risk factors present in the client situation (Carpenito, 1995). *Risk factors* are aspects of the situation that increase the client's potential to develop a particular problem. In addition, because the problem does not yet exist, the client does not manifest any defining characteristics. As an example, a community health nurse might diagnose "high risk for ineffective parenting due to high parental stress levels and poor coping skills." For syndromes, the primary etiologic factor is included in the syndrome title. For example, the diagnostic label of Rape Trauma Syndrome suggests a cluster of biological, psychological, and social health problems all resulting from rape (Gordon, 1994).

Unlike other types of nursing diagnoses, wellness diagnoses frequently consist only of the descriptive state (Carpenito, 1995), although some authors suggest including enabling factors (Denner, et al., 1991). *Enabling factors* are actions that could result in an improved state of health. Enabling factors have been included in this wellness diagnosis related to parenting: "potential for enhanced parenting through anticipatory guidance regarding child development." Positive nursing diagnoses should include the description of a positive client health state as well as strengths contributing to the positive state. For example, the community health nurse might diagnose "effective parenting due to adequate coping skills and presence of a strong support system." Including these strengths in the diagnostic statement indicates areas for reinforcement by the community health nurse. In the example given, the nurse would provide positive reinforcement for parental coping and encourage continued use of existing support systems. Components of each of the five types of nursing diagnostic statements are summarized in Table 7–1.

TABLE 7–1. COMPONENT ELEMENTS OF NURSING DIAGNOSTIC STATEMENTS

Type of Diagnosis	Component Elements
Actual nursing diagnosis	• Description of health state with modifiers • Etiologic factors • Defining characteristics
High-risk nursing diagnosis	• Description of health state with modifiers • Risk factors
Wellness nursing diagnosis	• Description of health state with modifiers • Enablers
Positive nursing diagnosis	• Description of health state with modifiers • Strengths
Syndrome	• Common etiologic factor included in diagnostic label

Accepted Nursing Diagnoses

Several "accepted" nursing diagnoses have been developed by nursing groups throughout the nation. Such attempts to generate standardized nursing diagnoses have been criticized by a number of community health nurses because of the concentration of these diagnoses on physical health problems of individual clients and the minimal attention given by psychosocial problems. Many of these diagnoses do not address the myriad social, environmental, and economic problems encountered in community health nursing.

Another criticism of the accepted diagnoses is the absence of diagnoses reflecting positive states of health or client strengths. There is a need for nursing diagnoses that reflect client health status as encountered by community health nurses. This need relates not only to statements of health problems but also to diagnoses related to positive health states.

Some attempts have been made to develop nursing diagnoses applicable to community health nursing. As noted earlier, NANDA has incorporated the concept of wellness diagnoses, a relatively recent development that still fails to address really positive states of health. Another attempt to increase the relevance of nursing diagnoses to community health nursing is the *Omaha Visiting Nurse Association System*, which incorporates the needs of individuals and families in four categories: environmental, psychosocial, physiologic, and health behavior needs (Bowles & Naylor, 1996). The environmental category includes problems related to material resources and physical surroundings and substances. The psychosocial category encompasses problems related to behavior and consumption patterns, relationships, and development, and the physiologic domain reflects difficulties with functional processes that support life, such as circulation and digestion. Finally, the health-related behavior domain reflects activities undertaken by the client to promote or regain health.

In the Omaha system, categories identified are modified by descriptors such as "individual" or "family" and "health promotion," "potential deficit," or "deficit." The health promotion descriptor reflects a wellness diagnosis in the NANDA taxonomy, whereas potential deficit and deficit reflect the high-risk and actual diagnosis categories, respectively.

In addition to the diagnostic categories, the Omaha system also includes an intervention scheme and a problem rating scale for outcomes (Martin, Leak, & Aden, 1992). The intervention scheme incorporates four categories of nursing intervention: health teaching, guidance, and counseling; treatments and procedures; case management; and surveillance (Martin & Sheet, 1992). This scheme directs development of an appropriate nursing care plan. The problem rating scale for outcomes provides a systematic way to measure client health status and change in status over time. The scale addresses three major concepts on a five-point continuum from presence of a serious difficulty to existence of an optimal state. These three concepts are knowledge (assessed from "none" to "superior"), behavior (assessed from "never appropriate" to "consistently appropriate"), and status (assessed from "extreme signs and symptoms" to "none"). The rating scale permits the community health nurse to assess client status in each of these three areas relative to any identified nursing diagnosis and to monitor changes in status with nursing intervention.

Although the Omaha system does address many more of the kinds of client problems encountered by community health nurses than the NANDA taxonomy and provides for health promotion as well as restorative interventions, it fails to address truly positive nursing diagnoses. In addition, as presently structured, its use applies only to the care of individuals and families and not to the care of population groups which is the primary focus of community health nursing.

Some efforts have been made to create nursing diagnoses applicable to population groups within the NANDA taxonomy. Several approaches have been suggested for the development of aggregate-level diagnoses. These include developing a new taxonomy along the lines of the Omaha system, modifying the NANDA taxonomy, adding new diagnoses to the taxonomy, and modifying existing NANDA diagnoses to make them applicable to aggregates (Ridenour, 1992). Whatever the approach taken, the aggregate diagnosis should include the group or aggregate affected, the response or health state identified, contributing factors, and substantiating data (Neufeld & Harrison, 1990). A specific format for developing nursing diagnoses for population groups is presented in Chapter 19. As of the eleventh Conference on Classification of Nursing

Diagnoses of the North American Nursing Diagnosis Association (NANDA) held in 1994, only one potential aggregate diagnosis, "effective community coping," had been submitted for development (North American Nursing Diagnosis Association, 1994).

One further criticism of the current taxonomies of nursing diagnoses is their wordiness, a characteristic that may obscure, rather than clarify, meaning, particularly for clients. For example, clients would probably understand a diagnosis of "constipation." Does the precursor phrase in the related NANDA diagnosis "alteration in elimination, constipation" add clarity? Probably not. What it may do is alienate the typical client of the community health nurse. Nor does such terminology enhance communication with other health care providers.

Although the accepted nursing diagnoses generated thus far leave much to be desired, the community health nurse should make use of the diagnostic reasoning process to generate diagnoses that are meaningful in community health nursing and that accurately reflect client health status. The task is not so much to derive a diagnosis that fits accepted terminology, but to describe client health in terms that are meaningful and provide direction for action.

Collaborative Problems

According to NANDA, client assessment data may give rise to statements of collaborative problems as well as nursing diagnoses. *Collaborative problems* are also clinical judgments or diagnoses, but differ from nursing diagnoses in that the nurse is not responsible for the definitive action to resolve the problem and for the outcomes of actions taken (Carpenito, 1995). In NANDA terms, collaborative problems are complications associated with specific medical diagnoses, the resolution of which requires the collaborative intervention of both physician and nurse. As noted in Chapter 4, however, collaborative efforts by community health nurses go far beyond interactions with physicians to a wide variety of health care and nonhealth care professionals and consumers. In addition, although community health nurses are not completely responsible for resolving a collaborative problem, they are frequently called upon to initiate activity related to the problem. For these reasons, collaborative problems will be treated as nursing diagnoses in the community health nursing context.

Nursing Diagnosis and Community Health Nursing

Community health nurses are likely to develop a broader range of nursing diagnoses than nurses in other fields. In addition to developing diagnoses related to the health of individuals, the community health nurse may also make diagnoses concerning families, groups, or communities. For example, the nurse may make a diagnosis of "inadequate financial resources due to husband's unemployment" for a family unable to afford health care services. A related diagnosis for this family would be "inadequate provision of health care due to limited income."

In a similar vein, the nurse might diagnose health problems found in a community or group of people. A nursing diagnosis at this level might be "inadequate access to health care due to increased unemployment among community members." Such a diagnosis indicates that the problem exists not in one family, but in a sizable portion of the population. Because the problem is widespread, its solution will be more complex. Intervention for a specific low-income family might entail referral for financial assistance, but when the problem involves a group of people, this type of intervention would rapidly deplete the community's economic resources. Effective intervention needs to be directed toward alleviating the problem of unemployment.

Each of these diagnostic statements includes information about the probable cause or etiology of the problem. This component of the diagnostic statement provides direction for problem resolution. Because we know that the family's failure to obtain adequate health care is due to financial limitations, we know what actions are likely to resolve the problem. If the underlying cause of the family's failure to seek health care is lack of motivation, referral for financial assistance will do little to resolve the problem. The same is true in the community situation. If failure to seek health care is due to a low value placed on health, dealing with unemployment will not help. The etiologic portion of the diagnostic statement, then, provides guidance in solving problems. Similarly, factors identified as contributors to positive health states indicate areas for support and reinforcement by community health nurses.

 Planning Nursing Intervention

The next step in the nursing process is planning primary, secondary, or tertiary preventive actions appropriate to the client's diagnosed health conditions. *Planning* was aptly defined several years ago as "a collaborative, orderly, cyclic process to attain a mutually agreed-on desired future goal" (Archer, Kelly, & Bisch, 1984). The plan of care should be developed to provide continuity of care and enhance communication among providers and with the client; to assist in determining priorities for action; and to support the documentation of effective use of the nursing process. In addition, a well-developed plan of care may serve as a learning tool for other providers and for clients in modeling the problem-solving process.

Whether the client is an individual, family, group, or community, the planning component of the nursing process consists of six basic tasks: prioritizing nursing diagnoses; developing goals and objectives for intervention; establishing critical criteria for potential means of achieving goals; selecting appropriate means; designing nursing interventions; and planning for evaluation.

Prioritizing Nursing Diagnoses

Because clients with whom community health nurses come in contact may have multiple health needs, nurses will usually not be able to resolve all of these needs during an initial contact. The nurse, in collaboration with the client, will need to decide which needs must be addressed now and which might be deferred until a later time.

The priority given to a particular condition may be based on the degree to which it threatens health. As a simplistic example, one would certainly want to deal with hemorrhage before worrying about the psychologic trauma that may result from an injury. In this respect, it is useful to consider Maslow's hierarchy of basic human needs as a way of establishing priorities among diagnoses. Problems that impair the client's ability to meet physiologic needs would have a higher priority than those interfering with self-actualization needs.

Priority also may be assigned on the basis of the client's concern about a particular problem. Dealing first with problems of major concern to the client can help to free client energy for dealing with other problems. Addressing the client's concerns first also may improve the nurse's credibility. Clients who see their needs met as they perceive them are likely to be more willing to take action in areas that they may not see as immediate problems.

Another criterion for assigning priorities to specific problems may simply be ease of solution. If a problem can be solved with minimal effort by nurse or client, there are few reasons why that problem cannot be dealt with immediately and "gotten out of the way."

Finally, one diagnosis may be given priority over others because it contributes to other problems. For example, a client may not have a regular source of health care and may also have the problem of unemployment. In this case, if the nurse focused on helping the client to become employed, the lack of health care might resolve itself when the client obtained health insurance through his or her employer.

Developing Goals and Objectives

The second aspect of planning is developing expected outcomes related to identified nursing diagnoses. This involves establishing goals and objectives for each nursing diagnosis. *Goals* are broad statements of outcome, whereas *objectives* are the specific achievements expected to result in goal accomplishment. The community health nurse develops both process objectives and outcome objectives. *Process objectives* are statements of behaviors expected of the nurse in carrying out the plan of care, for example, "teach an anemic client about iron-rich foods." *Outcome objectives* reflect expected changes in the client's state of health or changes in behavior as a result of nursing intervention. Outcome objectives should be client-centered, clear and concise, observable and measurable, and limited in duration. Objectives should also be realistic and jointly established by nurse and client (Iyer & Camp, 1995).

Outcome objectives can reflect either short-term or long-term expectations regarding the effects of nursing care. A short-term outcome objective for the client with anemia might be that "the client will eat at least four iron-rich foods per week" as a result of nutrition teaching. A long-term outcome objective in this situation might be that "the client will achieve a normal hematocrit level within 1 month of initiating nutrition teaching."

A similar set of objectives might be constructed for a community client with the problem of adolescent pregnancy. Process objectives might include the development of a clinic to provide contraceptive services to teenagers. A short-term outcome objective might be that "50% of sexually active adolescents in the community will receive some form of contraceptives within 6 months of opening the clinic." The related long-term objective would be a "50% decline in the rate of adolescent pregnancy within 2 years."

Statements of outcome objectives for nursing care usually include three components: content, modifiers, and time frame for achievement (Carpenito, 1993). The *content component* is a verb and its object, which reflects what the client will be or do as a result of intervention. Using the previous examples, the verbs and their objects were "achieve a hematocrit level" and "eat foods." Modifiers are adjectives and adverbs that qualify the verb and its object. "Normal," "four," and "iron-rich" were modifiers used in the objectives stated previously. The time frames for achieving the short- and long-term outcome objectives for the anemic client are "within one week" (to be able to identify iron-rich foods) and "within one month" (to achieve a normal hematocrit).

Establishing Criteria for Means to Achieve Goals

The next task in the planning phase of the nursing process is establishing criteria by which to evaluate potential nursing interventions. In a given situation several alternative actions may be taken to achieve the desired outcome. In deciding among these alternatives, it is helpful to have criteria for evaluating the relative merit of each option. Criteria to evaluate alternative courses of action should be jointly developed and employed by the nurse and the client. The client best understands the situation in which intervention needs to occur and the effects that specific alternatives might have. The client may, however, not be aware of the consequences of some alternatives, and these consequences may need to be pointed out by the nurse.

Examples of criteria by which to evaluate potential actions might be that the action selected must fit the client's budget and be culturally acceptable to the client. Suppose, for example, that the goal is to reduce adolescent pregnancies in the community by 50% over the next 3 years. Possible alternative actions might include providing sex education programs in schools and referring sexually active teenagers to existing contraceptive services or creating contraceptive clinics in each junior and senior high school. The first alternative is less costly and more apt to be culturally acceptable to the community than the second. Based on the criteria of cost and cultural acceptability, the first alternative would be the most appropriate.

Selecting Appropriate Means to Goals

Once the nurse and client have determined the evaluative criteria to be used, they can generate potential solutions to problems or measures to enhance client health status. The interventions selected might reflect primary, secondary, or tertiary levels of prevention or a combination of levels. Primary prevention would be employed to promote health and prevent illness. This level of prevention is particularly pertinent to clients without identified health problems. Secondary prevention would be warranted when clients have existing health problems, and tertiary prevention would be appropriate to prevent a recurrence of a problem or to return a client to a previous level of function.

Nurse and client evaluate each primary, secondary, and tertiary alternative generated in terms of the evaluative criteria established. Alternatives that come closest to fitting the critical criteria are usually the ones selected for implementation.

For example, a community may be concerned about increased drug abuse reported in other parts of the state. Although the community does not have a drug abuse problem at present, residents may be interested in preventing such a problem from occurring. A variety of primary preventive strategies can be suggested for preventing drug abuse among young people. Those concerned with the issue would probably like to find an alternative that is not too costly, but that has a lasting effect on drug use among the young. Cost and length of effect would then be the criteria used to evaluate potential alternatives. Possible approaches might be an intensive education program for junior high school students, an integrated drug education program throughout elementary and secondary school curricula, or increased police presence to apprehend drug dealers. The costs of the three alternatives might be approximately the same. Education at the junior high level might be effective for a while, but determined drug dealers would be likely to turn, instead, to younger children as buyers. Adding to the police force might also be effective until drug dealers learned to circumvent police efforts. The approach that best fits the criteria of lasting effect is education across all grade levels that helps children refrain from initiating drug use.

Designing Nursing Interventions

When an appropriate alternative has been selected, the nurse develops nursing interventions related to the client condition. *Nursing interventions* are specific statements of actions to be taken to achieve the desired outcome or stated objective. Effective nursing interventions are characterized by consistency with the nursing diagnoses derived from the client assessment and by their basis in scientific principles. Nursing interventions individualize the plan of care to a specific client situation and should reflect appropriate use of resources (Iyer & Camp, 1995). Sample nursing interventions for the problem of inadequate immunization status are listed in Table 7–2. The nursing interventions in Table 7–2 are the activities to be performed to accomplish the stated outcome objectives.

The nursing interventions in Table 7–2 are aimed at primary prevention. When secondary prevention is warranted, nursing interventions focus on activities that relieve symptoms and resolve an existing health problem. Nursing interventions at the tertiary prevention level include activities designed to return the client to his or her previous state of health and prevent a recurrence of the particular health problem. In planning nursing intervention, the nurse and client to-

TABLE 7–2. SAMPLE NURSING INTERVENTIONS FOR THE DIAGNOSIS OF INADEQUATE IMMUNIZATION STATUS

GOAL
Client will be adequately protected against communicable diseases.

OBJECTIVE
Client will receive immunizations appropriate to age.

NURSING INTERVENTIONS
1. Explain to parent the need for immunizations.
2. Explain legal requirement for immunization prior to school entry.
3. Discuss possible side effects of immunizations.
4. Explain how to deal with possible immunization side effects.
5. Give parent information on immunization clinic.
6. Demonstrate how to take child's temperature.

gether establish the expected outcomes and design activities that will lead to their achievement.

Planning to resolve problems typically seen in a given community health nursing setting may result in critical paths. A *critical path* is a set of prescribed activities sequenced at specific intervals designed to achieve established outcomes for a given client population or a specified problem area. A critical path identifies expected outcomes and key activities to be undertaken and the times at which they are to be performed in the course of providing care for a particular type of client. Many disease-specific paths have been developed for the care of hospitalized clients with designated medical diagnoses. For example, the critical path for a client following myocardial infarction might include interventions related to ambulation on the second day or certain laboratory tests initiated on the third day. The concept of critical paths can also be developed for community health nursing clients. For example, a critical path for pregnant clients might include referral for prenatal care if needed on the first encounter, monthly blood pressure checks until the eighth month followed by weekly checks, and contraceptive education in the third trimester. The expected outcomes would be access to prenatal care, normal blood pressure throughout the pregnancy, and prevention of a subsequent pregnancy.

Critical paths are developed for the "typical" client in a particular category and every intervention included may not be appropriate to a given client. Critical paths are considered guidelines rather than standards (Iyer & Camp, 1995) and departures from the typical path are permissible. These departures are termed *variances.* Variances from a critical path should be justified by the client situation (eg, the client has already arranged for prenatal care so a referral is unnecessary), and the variance and rationale adequately documented (Iyer & Camp, 1995).

▶ **TASKS OF THE PLANNING STAGE OF THE NURSING PROCESS**

- Prioritize nursing diagnoses
- Develop goals and objectives
- Establish criteria for means to achieve goals
- Select appropriate means to goals
- Design nursing interventions
- Plan for evaluation

Planning Evaluation

The last task in the planning stage of the nursing process is planning for evaluation. Evaluation of the outcome of nursing care takes place after intervention has occurred. Planning for evaluation, however, should occur while interventions are being planned. If this does not happen, data needed for evaluation may not be available at the time the evaluation is to be conducted. For example, if the objective of an immunization program is to increase measles immunization levels among preschool children by 50% in 6 months, evaluation will focus on comparisons of immunization levels before and after the program. If evaluation procedures have not been planned ahead of time, data on preprogram immunization levels may not be available. If, on the other hand, those planning the program plan for evaluation as well, they will identify the need for these data and take steps to collect the data prior to starting the program.

Considerations to be addressed in planning to evaluate the outcome of nursing intervention include who should conduct the evaluation, what type of data is needed, and how the data should be collected. Both nurse and client should be involved in evaluating nursing effectiveness; others may be involved as well. In the case of the immunization program, evaluation might be conducted by health care providers and community policy makers.

Decisions on the type of data to be collected should be based on the objectives established. Using the immunization example, the objective deals with immunization levels, so data on immunization levels before and after the program will be needed to determine whether or not immunization levels have increased 50%. Decisions on data collection methods depend on the kind of data needed and potential sources of those data. A general estimate of immunization levels among preschool children, for example, might be obtained by examining immunization records in child care facilities and reviewing a sample of client records in the offices of local pediatricians. Planning for evaluation is discussed in greater detail in Chapter 19. Tasks of the planning stage of the nursing process are summarized earlier.

Implementing Nursing Care

Implementation, the fourth stage of the nursing process, is the organizing and carrying out of the plan of care. Tasks involved in this stage of the nursing process include identifying requisite knowledge and skills, designating responsibility for implementation, recognizing impediments to implementation, and communicating the plan to others. Additional tasks are providing an environment conducive to implementation and actually performing the activities required for implementation.

Identifying Requisite Knowledge and Skills

The first task of implementation is identifying the knowledge and skills needed to implement the plan. This information aids in determining the most appropriate person for implementing a specific segment of the plan. For example, knowledge of nutrition and skill in developing menus on a limited budget are required to assist an individual client to adjust to the demands of a diabetic diet on a limited income. Knowledge of contraceptive measures and adolescent development, as well as good interpersonal skills, is needed to implement a plan to increase contraceptive use among sexually active adolescents.

Designating Responsibility for Implementation

The second task of implementation is designating those responsible for carrying out the planned interventions. Responsibility for carrying out the plan of care may be assumed by the community health nurse. Implementation might also entail delegating responsibility to others or making a referral to another source of assistance.

Delegation

To engage in effective delegation, the community health nurse must identify precisely what needs to be done and prioritize the outcomes to be achieved. He or she must then match the tasks required to the appropriate delegate. Decisions about the appropriateness of delegation are based on six areas of consideration: legal considerations, job descriptions, cultural differences, and the competencies, weaknesses, and preferences of the delegate (Hansten & Washburn, 1994). Both legal and job description considerations address authority for implementing the interventions. Nurse practice acts and other state and local regula-

tions may be the determining factor in whether or not delegating a particular intervention to a given individual is appropriate. For example, it would be inappropriate (and illegal) to designate a nurse's aide as the person responsible for giving intravenous medications to a homebound client. As another example, the mayor or police chief would have the authority to initiate community response to a disaster situation and could be assigned responsibility for this aspect of a community disaster plan. Similarly, agency policy may prohibit certain categories of employees from performing specific interventions. For example, in some areas only state-certified public health nurses are permitted to make home visits, while other registered nurses are not.

Cultural differences are another consideration in delegation. The culture of the delegate may prohibit carrying out certain interventions. For example, many Roman Catholic community health nurses are uncomfortable providing abortion counseling to pregnant adolescents and may resist doing so. It would be more appropriate to assign this task to another nurse.

The fourth and fifth considerations in delegation involve the competencies and weaknesses of the proposed delegate. Does the delegate have the requisite knowledge and skills to carry out the interventions needed? Either a nurse or a nutritionist, for example, would have the knowledge and skills to assist a client with a diabetic diet. Many nurses or health educators would also have the knowledge required to teach adolescents about contraceptives. Other competencies that may be needed in a given situation include excellent interpersonal skills for dealing with a difficult client or the ability to speak another language.

Weaknesses of the delegate that may influence the appropriateness of delegation tend to fall into five categories: unclear expectations, inaccurate self-perceptions of performance, lack of knowledge or skills needed, need for supervision or guidance, and poor motivation. The need for specific knowledge and skills was addressed above. Even those delegates who may have the requisite knowledge or skill may not be clear on precisely what is expected in performance of the delegated tasks. Or, they may have an inaccurate perception of their own ability to perform the task. For example, it may not be appropriate to delegate a visit to a new mother and baby to a nurse who recently miscarried, even though she may feel she is capable of functioning effectively. Similarly, persons who require close supervision would not be delegated tasks in situations where supervision is limited. For example, a new graduate who is shaky on the technique for giving intradermal tuberculin skin tests would not be assigned to screen a group of employees exposed to tuberculosis unless a more experienced nurse was available to assist with and supervise the procedure. Finally, delegation may not be appropriate if the delegate does not have the level of motivation required to perform the intervention effectively. Weaknesses do not preclude delegation, but the community health nurse must take action to eliminate the weakness before delegating the tasks involved. For example, the nurse could assist the delegate to develop the required knowledge and skills or find ways to motivate the delegate effectively.

The preferences of the delegate may be related to other considerations such as culture or motivation, but may constitute a consideration in and of themselves. If one nurse enjoys client education and another does not, even though both perform the task effectively, it would be more appropriate to assign an educational intervention to the one who enjoys this activity if at all possible.

Once the choice of the appropriate delegate has been made, the community health nurse needs to communicate the tasks and expectations for their performance to the delegate. This communication usually follows a who, what, when, where, how, and why format (O'Neil, 1994). With respect to who, the community health nurse should clearly identify the delegate and the recipient of the intervention. The what is the task or tasks to be accomplished. Explanation of the task may need to be more or less detailed depending on the expertise of the delegate. The community health nurse should also indicate when the task is expected to be completed, how and when the delegate should contact the nurse following completion, and any prioritization that needs to take place among multiple tasks. The where element might be a client's home, a clinical setting, or under a bridge for a homeless client. The parameters of performance constitute the how element of communicating a delegated task and the community health nurse should be clear about the level of performance expected. Finally, possible resistance to the delegated task will frequently be minimized by letting the delegate know why the task is necessary. Following delegation, the community health nurse should also monitor the delegate's progress toward task accomplishment and provide feedback on his or her performance. The community health nurse should also evaluate the outcome of task delegation for the delegate and the client.

Referral

Referral for outside assistance is another approach that may be used in implementing planned interventions. The nurse should be sure to consider the acceptability of the referral to the client, the client's eligibility for service, and any situational constraints in-

fluencing the referral. Other considerations include providing necessary information to the client and the referral agency and following up on the effectiveness of the referral in solving the client's problem. The referral process is discussed in greater depth in Chapter 11.

Recognizing Impediments to Implementation

The community health nurse must identify any constraints that might impede implementation and take steps to modify or eliminate those constraints. Ideally, limitations of the chosen intervention have been identified during the evaluation of alternative approaches to solving the problem, but it is useful to look again for any constraints that may have been overlooked during the planning stage or that may have arisen in the interim. For example, part of the plan of care might be a referral for financial assistance. At the time the plan was designed, the client may have had adequate transportation. Since that time, however, he or she might have had an accident and be without a car until repairs are completed. In such a case, the nurse would need to assist the client to find another means of transportation so as to implement the planned referral.

Providing an Environment for Implementation

The community health nurse needs to provide an environment conducive to implementing the plan of care. This involves providing the resources needed for implementation, providing for the comfort of the client, and maintaining the client's safety during implementation. Necessary resources can include time, personnel, and equipment. If a staff member is to give a bedfast client a bath, time must be provided within the client's schedule. Or it may be necessary to engage the services of a physical therapist to implement segments of the plan. For some activities, special equipment might be required and the nurse should either obtain that equipment or assist the client to do so. For

> ► TASKS OF THE IMPLEMENTATION STAGE OF THE NURSING PROCESS
>
> • Identify knowledge and skills needed for implementation
> • Designate responsibility for implementation
> • Recognize impediments to implementation
> • Create an environment conducive to implementation
> • Carry out planned activities

example, if preventing an older client from falling necessitates the use of a walker, the nurse can help the family obtain one.

Implementing planned interventions should also allow for both the physical and psychological comfort of the client. For instance, the client might not speak English well and might feel uncomfortable about trying to explain his or her need for financial assistance to social service workers. In this case, the nurse might contribute to the client's psychological comfort by arranging for an interpreter. Or, the plan of care may be implemented in such a way as to diminish fatigue for the older client.

Safety considerations in implementation vary based on the client's age, level of mobility, presence or absence of sensory deficits, and level of orientation. For example, young children would not be expected to take their own medications, or the older person with impaired vision might need color-coded labels on medication bottles to take them correctly.

Carrying Out Planned Activities

The final task in the implementation phase of the nursing process is carrying out the activities included in the nursing interventions. Planned activities are executed by those assigned responsibility for them. These activities may occur at the primary, secondary, or tertiary levels of prevention depending on the needs of the client. Tasks of the implementation stage of the nursing process are summarized on page 132.

Evaluating Nursing Care

The last component of the nursing process, *evaluation,* is a comparison of client's health status with the expected outcomes of care (Iyer, Taptich, & Bernocchi-Losey, 1994). Evaluation can take two basic forms: outcome evaluation and process evaluation. *Outcome evaluation* is the assessment of the outcome of nursing intervention. *Process evaluation,* on the other hand, is the examination of the quality of actions taken and the processes used to achieve that outcome (Doheny, Cook, & Stopper, 1996). Either or both types of evaluation may be involved in evaluating the application of the nursing process to a given community health nursing situation. Evaluation involves several tasks, including conducting the evaluation itself, interpreting findings, and using evaluative findings.

Conducting the Evaluation

Like each of the other steps of the nursing process, evaluation must be planned and executed systematically. Planning for both outcome and process evaluation occurs during the planning stage of the nursing process. Once interventions have been implemented, the planned evaluative procedures are put into effect. Data are gathered (if not gathered throughout the implementation stage) and organized for analysis.

Data should be collected to evaluate both the outcome of interventions and the process used to implement them. Outcome-related data should reflect the stated objectives or expected outcomes for care. Process-related data are obtained by examining how interventions were implemented. If the stated objective was to have the client include at least one iron-rich food in the daily diet, intervention outcomes could be evaluated by asking the client to complete a 3-day diet history and looking for the inclusion of iron-rich foods in each day's diet. Process evaluation might entail examining how well the nurse adapted dietary teaching to the client's education level, culturally determined food practices, and economic situation.

Interpreting Findings

Evaluation always involves comparison of the actual outcome with some kind of standard. These standards are the evaluative criteria developed in planning for evaluation. Once data related to the evaluative criteria have been collected, they must be analyzed and interpreted in terms of the criteria. Has the client included at least one iron-rich food in his or her diet each day? If not, why not? Process evaluation data may provide possible explanations for nonachievement of objectives. In the dietary example, process evaluation may indicate that education about iron-rich foods provided by the nurse focused on foods eaten by members of the dominant cultural group and did not fit the client's food preferences. Or, the nurse may not have suggested food alternatives that were congruent with the client's economic situation. The community health nurse compares the data obtained with the evaluative criteria to determine if set standards were achieved. Judgments on the achievement of these standards form the basis for the third task of evaluation—making further care decisions.

Using Evaluative Findings

Findings of both outcome and process evaluation are used to make decisions about nursing care. Basically, three decisions are possible. First, the evaluation may

TASKS OF THE EVALUATION STAGE OF THE NURSING PROCESS

• Conduct the evaluation
• Interpret data in light of evaluative criteria
• Use evaluative findings to make client care decisions

show that intervention was effective and that objectives were met. Intervention can then be continued or terminated as needed. Second, evaluation findings may indicate that objectives were not met and another approach should be tried. Or, third, the evaluation may suggest that the implementation of the nursing plan was not up to par and the nurse (or other involved party) can make changes in the quality of performance that may lead to the intended outcomes.

Evaluation can also lead to changes in other components of the nursing process. For example, the nurse may find that interventions were not effective because they were based on an inadequate or inaccurate database. If this is the case, the nurse will want to expand the client assessment. Or, the plan of care may not have been sensitive to the constraints of the client situation and modifications can be made in the plan. As we have already seen, evaluation findings might also indicate a need for changes in the way the plan is implemented. Tasks of the evaluation stage of the nursing process are summarized above.

▶ DOCUMENTING USE OF THE NURSING PROCESS

Documentation is a critical feature of all phases of the nursing process. Community health nurses, like their counterparts in other areas of nursing, must carefully document client data and diagnoses, plans and interventions, and their outcomes. Documentation is particularly important in community health nursing because care frequently takes place in settings where witnesses may not be present (Iyer & Camp, 1995). In the assessment phase of the nursing process, documentation focuses on the data on which nursing actions are based. The written diagnostic statements derived from the database document the use of the diagnostic reasoning process. Plans related to each nursing diagnosis are also documented, as is implementation of the plan of care. Finally, the evaluation phase of the nursing process is documented in terms of the outcome of nursing interventions.

Several approaches can be taken to document the use of the nursing process. One of the most effective for use in community health nursing is an adaptation of the problem-oriented record (POR) allowing for positive as well as negative client health states. This adaptation is called the **status-oriented record** (SOR) because it reflects both positive and negative client health status.

The SOR is an organized systematic method for recording client data, nursing diagnoses based on those data, intended outcomes of care, plans for achieving those outcomes, implementation of the plan of care, and outcomes of care. Four basic components of the SOR allow the community health nurse to document each step of the nursing process: the client database, the health status summary, the initial plan of care, and the progress notes. Components of the SOR are depicted in Figure 7–3.

Documenting Client Assessment: The Database

The *database* is a compilation of information about the client obtained in the nursing assessment. Areas included in the database would reflect all aspects of the client's health. Specific information included varies with client and setting. For example, the database in a pediatric clinic would not include the client's work history, whereas that in an occupational setting would. The community health nurse should be involved in the determination of what information will routinely be included in the database used in a given practice setting.

There are several reasons for documenting the database (Iyer, Taptich, & Bernocchi-Losey, 1994). The first reason is the most obvious; the database provides direction for nursing diagnosis and intervention. In addition, the database improves communication between health care providers and provides a baseline for later evaluation of the outcome of intervention. The database also supports both intervention decisions and reimbursement for services (Marrelli, 1996). The database constitutes part of the client's legal record and may be used to determine legal liability for unfavorable client outcomes. Finally, the database may serve as a source of data for later research.

Compilation of the database is not a one-time occurrence. Information contained there should be reviewed and updated as the client's situation changes. Typical components of the database for the individual client include a health history, a physical examination, results of various laboratory and x-ray procedures, and findings of other screening tests. Data obtained about a community client would include information on the physical environment, age composition of the population, common illnesses, and social factors such as unemployment and education levels.

Components of status-oriented record

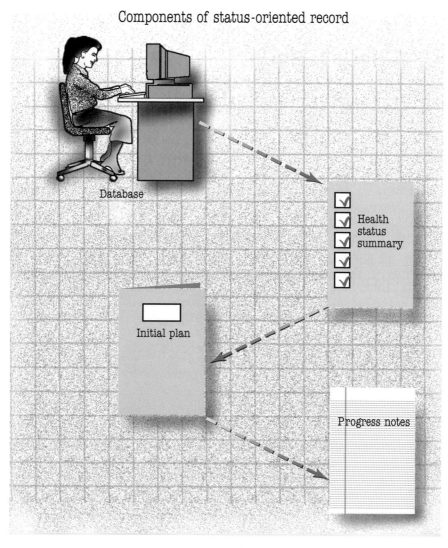

Figure 7–3. Components of the status-oriented record.

The database should be written objectively, without incorporating personal bias or value judgments. Interpretation of data should be supported by specific observations, and generalizations should be avoided. The database should thoroughly describe the client situation and should include both positive and negative findings. Finally, the database should be documented clearly and concisely without irrelevancies, should be legible, and should use correct grammar, spelling, and appropriate abbreviations.

Documenting Nursing Diagnoses: The Health Status Summary

The *health status summary* is a list of abbreviated nursing diagnoses derived from the database. The di-

agnoses are abbreviated in the sense that etiologic factors are not included here. Complete nursing diagnoses, including the statement of etiology, are documented elsewhere in the SOR. Other information in the health status summary includes the date on which a particular diagnosis was established, its assigned number, and the date on which objectives related to the diagnosis were achieved. Table 7–3 is a sample health status summary.

According to the health status summary in Table 7–3, four nursing diagnoses were identified on January 9, 1999. Three are actual diagnoses; the fourth is a positive health state to be maintained. Each diagnosis was given a number and a title that describes the client condition. For example, the first diagnosis was inadequate immunization status. Diagnoses should al-

TABLE 7–3. SAMPLE HEALTH STATUS SUMMARY

Date Identified	No.	Diagnosis	Date Objective Achieved
1–9–99	1	Inadequate immunization status	2–13–99
1–9–99	2	Overweight	
1–9–99	3	Inadequate knowledge of nutrition	
1–9–99	4	Effective coping skills	

ways be referred to by both number and title in subsequent entries in the SOR. Whenever possible, problem-focused diagnoses should be stated in the client's own words.

The status of conditions should be updated on the health status summary as appropriate. As objectives are met, their accomplishment should be noted on the summary sheet. In Table 7–3, diagnosis 1 was inadequate immunization status. At the first encounter with the client, the nurse may have made a referral to an immunization clinic. If the client followed through on the referral and obtained the needed immunizations, inadequate immunization status is no longer a problem for this client. This has been noted on the summary sheet by entering the date of problem resolution in the far right-hand column.

The status of a condition may also be updated through redefinition. For example, an original diagnosis of amenorrhea in an unmarried adolescent may be redefined as unwanted pregnancy following a positive pregnancy test. In this case, the diagnosis would be given a new number and title on the summary sheet and a notation made by the original diagnosis "redefined as diagnosis 5." This is depicted in Table 7–4.

Organization of the health status summary depends on the needs of the agency using the SOR. Diagnoses may be either listed chronologically in the order of identification or organized by categories. For instance, diagnoses might be categorized on the basis of the level of prevention involved. The diagnoses presented in Table 7–3 would then fall into two categories. The diagnoses of inadequate immunization, in-

TABLE 7–4. REDEFINITION OF A NURSING DIAGNOSIS

Date Identified	No.	Diagnosis	Date Objective Achieved
1–12–99	3	Amenorrhea—redefined as diagnosis 5	
1–12–99	4	Conflict with parents	
1–12–99	5	Unwanted pregnancy	

Critical Thinking in Research

Marek (1996) conducted a study to determine the usefulness of nursing diagnoses, medical diagnoses, and demographic variables in predicting clients use of home health care services. The author used retrospective record review to collect data on service use in terms of number of nursing visits and hours of care provided and compared these to demographic variables of age and source of payment, clients' medical diagnoses, and nursing diagnoses based on the Omaha classification system. Findings indicated that nursing diagnoses explained a significant portion of variance in both number of visits needed and hours of care provided over and above that explained by demographic variables and medical diagnoses. Omaha system nursing diagnoses related to income, integument, and vision problems were significant predictors of hours of care provided, accounting for 7% of the variance in this variable beyond that explained by demographic and medical diagnosis variables. These same three diagnoses and sanitation problems accounted for an additional 18% of the variance in hours of nursing care provided. The author concluded that nursing diagnosis models aid in predicting the need for nursing services.

1. Do you have any thoughts on why these particular nursing diagnoses proved to be accurate predictors of the number of hours of care and nursing visits provided?
2. How might you set up a similar study using accepted NANDA diagnoses as predictor variables? Which specific diagnoses might you want to examine as predictors of the need for nursing services?
3. Do you think the NANDA diagnoses would be as accurate in predicting service needs in home health as the Omaha system variables used in this study? Why or why not?
4. How might you go about determining whether or not your supposition is correct?

adequate knowledge of nutrition, and effective coping skills reflect the primary level of prevention, whereas the diagnosis of overweight reflects a need for secondary prevention. Diagnoses might also be organized in terms of the dimensions of health reflected. In this case, inadequate immunization would fall into the biophysical dimension and effective coping skills would reflect the psychological dimension.

Documenting Planning: The Initial Plan

The third component of the SOR is an initial intervention plan for each nursing diagnosis. Each of the diagnoses listed on the health status summary must be addressed, either through action by the community health nurse or through referral to another source of care. The particular agency where the nurse is employed may choose not to provide care for certain

▶ NURSING CARE PLAN FOR THE DIAGNOSIS OF OVERWEIGHT

1–9–99: *Initial Plan*

Diagnosis	Overweight
Goal	The client will reach and maintain optimal weight for height.
Objectives	1. The client will lose 2 pounds per week until goal is achieved.
	2. The client will be eating a well-balanced, nutritious diet by the end of 6 months
S:	States "I have always been fat. I just can't seem to lose weight." Description of typical day's diet indicates predominance of starches, fats, little protein or fiber. Knowledge of adequate nutrition is limited.
0:	Weight 263 lb. Height 5'6".
A:	Overweight due to poor eating habits and inadequate knowledge of nutrition.
P: Diagnostic	1. Obtain a 3-day diet history.
	2. Obtain a list of food preferences.
Treatment	1. Refer to nutritionist for 1500-calorie diet.
	2. Assist client to plan low-calorie meals.
	3. Provide reinforcement of weight loss.
Client education	1. Review basic nutrition.
	2. Discuss hazards of obesity.
Follow-up	1. Recheck weight in 2 weeks.
	2. Obtain a second diet history in 2 weeks.

types of diagnoses. These diagnoses cannot be ignored, however, and some arrangement for providing care must be made. This is essential if the client is to be treated as a whole unit.

The *initial plan of care* for each diagnosis includes the broad goal and specific objectives to be achieved through intervention. The plan of care is then written in the SOAP format taken from the problem-oriented record system. The *S* represents subjective information or data reported by the client or significant others. For example, information from the health history related to a particular diagnosis is included in the *S* component of the initial plan for that diagnosis. The *O* refers to objective data observable by the community health nurse. Objective data might include findings on physical examination, results of laboratory tests, and observations of the home or of client interactions with others.

A refers to the community health nurse's analysis of the situation and a statement of its probable etiology, in other words, the nursing diagnosis. For example, the problem might be a temperature elevation and would be stated in the health status summary as such. The analysis would also include the probable cause, if known, as this information will make a difference in the nursing interventions employed. An expected postsurgical temperature elevation, for example, is treated differently from a fever caused by an infectious process.

The *P* reflects the plan of action or nursing interventions designed to address the diagnosis and includes four components: additional diagnostic measures, treatment measures, client education, and follow-up. In the initial plan of care for a person with a diagnosis of overweight, the goal for intervention is that the client reach a normal weight for her height. The objectives are stated more specifically: "The client will lose 2 pounds per week until goal is achieved" and "The client will be eating a well-balanced, nutritious diet by the end of 6 months."

The subjective data include information that the client has shared with the nurse about her weight problem, typical diet, and knowledge of nutrition. The objective data are the client's height and weight, which indicate that the client is definitely overweight for her height. The analysis includes the nursing diagnostic statement that the client is "Overweight due to poor eating habits and inadequate knowledge of nutrition."

The inclusion of the etiology of the problem in the diagnostic statement provides direction for the intervention plan. If the client's overweight condition

▶ SAMPLE PROGRESS NOTES FOR THE DIAGNOSIS OF OVERWEIGHT

7–11–99: *Progress Notes*

Diagnosis	Overweight
S:	States "I have gone down two whole sizes." Diet history indicates adherence to 1500-calorie diet. States she "uses calorie counter religiously."
0:	Client visited at lunchtime. Found eating well-balanced, low-calorie meal. Weight 225 lb; 38-lb weight loss in 6 months; 2-lb weight loss in last week.
A:	Continued weight loss.
P: Diagnostic	
Treatment	1. Praise client for continued weight loss.
	2. Reinforce new self-image as "not fat."
Education	1. Return visit in 1 month to check weight.
Follow-up	

was due to a metabolic disorder, the plan of care would be quite different. In the situation depicted, the plan of care is based on knowledge that the problem is related to dietary patterns and lack of knowledge about nutrition. Plans are made to obtain additional diagnostic information by having the client complete a 3-day diet history and provide information about food preferences. This allows the nurse to get a better understanding of the client's typical diet and to design interventions that are more likely to be acceptable to the client than might otherwise be the case.

The treatment component of the plan, in this case, involves referring the client to a nutritionist for a 1500-calorie diet and assisting the client to plan low-calorie meals that provide a balanced diet but are as consistent as possible with food preferences. Another aspect of the planned treatment is providing positive reinforcement for the client's progressive weight loss.

The plan for client education focuses on reviewing basic nutrition and discussing the hazards of obesity in terms of self-image as well as physical health. The last element of the *P* in the SOAP mnemonic is the plan for follow-up. The nurse will recheck the client's weight in 2 weeks and obtain an updated diet history at that time.

Documenting Implementation: Progress Notes

The last component of the SOR is the progress notes. *Progress notes* document the current status of health conditions, implementation of the plan, and results of intervention. If for some reason the plan was not implemented, the reason for nonimplementation should also be documented. Progress notes are written in the SOAP format. The sample progress notes on page 137 are related to the diagnosis of overweight.

The subjective data obtained from the client indicate that the plan for dealing with this problem has been implemented, that she is adhering to the 1500-calorie diet, and that she has noticed some results. The nurse's observations included in the objective data also indicate that the client is eating appropriately and has lost weight. The analysis reflects the current status of the particular problem: the client is continuing to lose weight but has not yet achieved the goal of an appropriate weight for her height. At this point, the plan does not include any additional diagnostic interventions because none are needed. Nor is there a need for further educational measures. The plan now focuses on continuing positive reinforcement for weight lost and reinforcing a new self-image. The plan for follow-up is to check back with the client in 1 month.

Progress notes are always numbered and titled,

as well as dated. Someone auditing this client's record would have no difficulty determining the status of diagnosis 2 as of July 1999. Progress notes, as well as plans, should be signed by the person making the entry.

Documenting Evaluation

The SOR also facilitates documenting evaluation of nursing care. Evaluation is documented in several of the components of the SOR discussed earlier. When objectives related to a specific nursing diagnosis have been achieved, their accomplishment is reflected in the progress notes as well as on the health status summary sheet. For example, if the overweight client had reached her desired weight, the objective data in the progress notes would include the client's current weight, and the analysis would reflect that the goal has been achieved and the problem resolved. The nurse would then indicate the date when objectives were achieved in the appropriate column on the health status summary. If the client continues to need support to maintain her weight at this level, the nurse might enter a new diagnosis on the health status summary, "maintenance of desired weight," and develop an initial plan for helping the client to maintain her weight. This diagnosis would reflect a need for tertiary preventive measures designed to prevent the recurrence of the weight problem.

Not every nursing diagnosis is evaluated each time the client is seen. This is particularly true in the case of clients with multiple diagnoses. Therefore, progress notes for any particular client encounter may not include notations about each of the client's diagnoses. The nurse uses his or her judgment to establish priorities, dealing with the most crucial problems first and others as time permits. For example, if the client has made suicidal gestures and also needs new glasses, it is more important to evaluate the status of the emotional problem, if time does not permit exploration of both. The status of the vision problem can be explored at a later date. It is important, however, not to push these secondary problems aside indefinitely, as they need to be addressed and may be contributing factors in the major problems. Therefore, the current status of such secondary problems must be documented as often as appropriate.

When a client no longer requires services and is discharged, progress notes should include a summary of the current status of all diagnoses listed on the health status summary sheet. This summary provides additional evidence of evaluation and that the client's problems are sufficiently resolved for services to be terminated.

Critical Thinking in Practice: A Case in Point

You receive the following request for community health nursing services:

Request for Community Health Nursing

Date: _January 22, 1999_ Source of Request: _Clark Hospital_

Family Name: _Marks_

Address: _8359 Oaks Dr, San Diego_ Phone: _555-1256_

Client(s): _Miranda (birthdate 10-21-78); Jason (1-21-99)_

Reason for referral: _postpartum & newborn follow-up_

Comments: _Has 2 other children at home. Husband is unemployed. No prenatal care. Pregnancy, labor, and delivery uncomplicated._

When you visit the Marks family, you find that mother and baby are doing well. Mother has not yet made an appointment for a postpartum checkup because they have no health insurance, and she does not know how she will pay for the visit. Her husband is a nonunion construction worker. He has been laid off because construction is slow during the winter. He expects to be able to find work in 2 or 3 months, when the weather starts to warm up. Currently, the family is living off his unemployment compensation, which is just sufficient to pay the rent and buy food.

Mrs. Marks is concerned about her 3-year-old son who is fussy and irritable. He has had a fever for 2 days and has not been eating well. Last night he did not sleep well, and now you notice that he is pulling at his ear.

Mrs. Marks also mentions that she and her husband have been arguing about their financial situation. She would like to go back to work as a computer programmer. She feels that the family needs the money. If she were to go back to work for her former employer, the family could obtain health insurance at group rates, and her income would be more stable than her husband's. Her husband thinks that she should stay home and take care of the children.

During your visit, the 6-year-old daughter comes home from school. You note that she is somewhat overweight and looks anemic. In discussing the family's diet with Mrs. Marks, you find that they eat a lot of inexpensive starches, but eat few meats and vegetables because of the cost.

You also note that the baby seems clean, and when Mrs. Marks feeds him during your visit, she uses appropriate feeding and burping techniques. She appears to be knowledgeable about child care and discipline. Despite the fussiness of the 3-year-old, she is patient with him and succeeds in distracting him from pulling on the baby by letting him help hold the baby's bottle.

1. What diagnostic hypotheses are suggested by the data in this situation? Is there evidence of any positive nursing diagnoses in the data presented? How would you go about evaluating your hypotheses?
2. Write a health status summary including at least four nursing diagnoses appropriate to this situation. How would you prioritize your diagnoses? Why?
3. Write one outcome objective for each of your nursing diagnoses. What alternative interventions might achieve these objectives? What criteria might you use to evaluate these alternatives?
4. Using the SOAP format, write an initial plan for addressing one of the nursing diagnoses. How would you evaluate the effectiveness of your interventions?

TESTING YOUR UNDERSTANDING

1. What are the components of the nursing process? Describe how the nursing process might be used somewhat differently in community health nursing than in other nursing specialties. (pp. 122–123)

2. Describe two types of activities involved in developing nursing diagnoses. (pp. 123–125)

3. What are the three components of an actual nursing diagnostic statement? Write an actual nursing diagnosis that incorporates these three components. (p. 124)

4. Describe at least four tasks involved in the planning stage of the nursing process. Give an example of a community health nurse performing each of these tasks. (pp. 127–131)

5. Design a set of nursing interventions for the nursing diagnosis "overweight due to inadequate knowledge of nutrition." (pp. 129–130)

6. Describe at least four tasks in implementing the plan of care. Give an example of the performance of each task. (pp. 131–133)

7. Differentiate between process and outcome evaluation. Give examples of evaluative criteria that might be used for each. (p. 133)

8. Identify the components of a SOAP note. Write an initial plan in the SOAP format for the nursing diagnosis "inadequate access to health care due to financial difficulties." (pp. 137–139)

WHAT DO YOU THINK?
Questions for Critical Thinking

1. Are there situations that you can think of when the accepted NANDA nursing diagnoses would not be appropriate for use in community health nursing? What are they?

2. To be really effective in their care of clients, community health nurses should conduct a thorough assessment of all aspects of clients' health. How would you reconcile this value for holism with some clients' perceptions that nurses should address their physical health problems and do not need information about economic status or interpersonal relationships.

3. When formulating a nursing diagnosis, what are the implications of using the phrase "due to" rather than "related to" to link a client's health state with contributing factors?

4. Why is it especially important in community health nursing to include the client in planning health care?

REFERENCES

Archer, S. E., Kelly, C. D., & Bisch, S. A. (1984). *Implementing change in communities.* St. Louis: Mosby.

Bowles, K. H., & Naylor, M. D. (1996). Nursing intervention classification systems. *Image: Journal of Nursing Scholarship, 28,* 303–308.

Carnevali, D. L. (1993). *Diagnostic reasoning and treatment decision making.* Philadelphia: J. B. Lippincott.

Carpenito, L. J. (1993). *Nursing diagnosis: Application to clinical practice* (5th ed.). Philadelphia: J. B. Lippincott.

Carpenito, L. J. (1995). *Handbook of nursing diagnosis* (6th ed.). Philadelphia: J. B. Lippincott.

Doenges, M., & Moorhouse, M. (1995). *Nurse's pocket guide: Nursing diagnosis with interventions* (5th ed.). Philadelphia: F. A. Davis.

Doheny, M., Cook, C., & Stopper, C. (1996). *The discipline of nursing: An introduction* (4th ed.). Stamford, CT: Appleton & Lange.

Denner, M. L., et al. (1991, May). *Staff nurses using nursing diagnosis.* Paper presented at the meeting of the Toronto Nursing Diagnosis Interest Group, Toronto, Ontario, Canada.

Gordon, M. (1994). *Nursing diagnosis: Process and approach* (3rd ed.). St. Louis: Mosby Year Book.

Hansten, R. I., & Washburn, M. J. (1994). Know your delegate: How can I determine the right delegate for the job? In R. I. Hansten & M. J. Washburn (Eds.), *Clinical delegation skills: A handbook for nurses* (pp. 151–183). Gaithersburg, MD: Aspen.

Iyer, P. W., & Camp, N. H. (1995). *Nursing documentation: A nursing process approach* (2nd ed.). St. Louis: Mosby.

Iyer, P. W., Taptich, B. J., & Bernocchi-Losey, D. (1994). *Nursing process and nursing diagnosis* (3rd ed.). Philadelphia: W. B. Saunders.

Marek, K. D. (1996). Nursing diagnoses and home care nursing utilization. *Public Health Nursing, 13,* 195–200.

Marrelli, T. M. (1996). *Nursing documentation handbook.* St. Louis: Mosby.

Martin, K., Leak, G., & Aden, C. (1992). The Omaha System: A research-based model for decision making. *JONA, 22*(11), 47–52.

Martin, K. S., & Sheet, N. J. (1992). *The Omaha System: Applications for community health nursing.* Philadelphia: W. B. Saunders.

McFarland, G. K. (1996). Nursing diagnosis, the critical link in the nursing process. In G. K. McFarland &

E. A. McFarland (Eds.), *Nursing diagnosis and intervention: Planning for patient care* (3rd. ed.) (pp. 10–20). St. Louis: Mosby.

Neufeld, A., & Harrison, M. J. (1990). The development of nursing diagnoses for aggregates and groups. *Public Health Nursing, 7,* 251–255.

North American Nursing Diagnosis Association. (1994). *Nursing diagnoses: Definitions and classification.* Philadelphia: North American Nursing Diagnosis Association.

O'Neil, T. (Ed.). (1994). *Biomedical ethics: Opposing viewpoints.* San Diego: Greenhaven Press.

Ridenour, N. (1992, April). *Examples of possible approaches to aggregate diagnoses.* Paper presented at the Tenth Conference on Classification of Nursing Diagnoses of the North American Nursing Diagnosis Association, San Diego, CA.

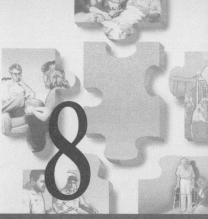

THE EPIDEMIOLOGIC PROCESS

The epidemiologic process is one of the key elements in the process dimension of community health nursing. Epidemiology is a health-related discipline that provides a systematic framework for examining states of health in terms of factors contributing to their development. The primary concern of epidemiology, like community health, is the health of groups of people; however, epidemiologic principles can also direct community health nurses in assessing health-related conditions experienced by both individuals and families. The nursing process indicates the need for client assessment, and the epidemiologic process suggests the types of data to be collected and how they can be organized to facilitate nursing intervention. In this chapter we explore the major elements of an epidemiologic perspective in community health nursing and apply epidemiologic methods to health promotion.

▶ **Chapter Objectives**

After reading this chapter, you should be able to:

- Describe at least two theories of disease causation.
- Identify at least three criteria for determining causality in a relationship between two events.
- Define risk.
- Distinguish between morbidity and mortality rates.
- Identify six steps of the epidemiologic process.
- Differentiate between observational and experimental studies.
- Describe three types of observational studies.
- Identify the three major elements of the epidemiologic triad model.
- Describe the web of causation model.
- Describe the four major components of Dever's epidemiologic model.
- Describe at least three strategies for promoting health.

▶ BASIC CONCEPTS OF EPIDEMIOLOGY

Epidemiology is the study of the distribution of health and illness within the population and the factors that determine the population's health status (Harkness, 1995). This definition encompasses two broad concepts: control of health problems through an understanding of their contributing factors, and application of epidemiologic techniques to health-related conditions other than acute communicable disease.

The purposes of epidemiology are twofold: to search for causal relationships in health and illness, and to control illness through the resultant understanding of causality. The ultimate concern of epidemiology in any of its uses is preventing disease and maintaining health. Specific uses of the epidemiologic process include:

1. Studying the contributing factors, signs and symptoms, effects, and outcomes of a single condition
2. Diagnosing the health status of a specific group of people
3. Evaluating the effectiveness of health programs
4. Establishing indices of risk or the statistical probability of a particular condition occurring
5. Providing information to assist clinical decision making (Gordis, 1996)

The study of factors contributing to communicable diseases was the initial focus of epidemiologic investigation. As the incidence of many communicable diseases declined, epidemiologists directed their attention to chronic disease as a focus of investigation. More recently still, epidemiologic methods have been used to identify factors that promote health.

Three basic concepts underlie epidemiologic investigation of health and illness: causality, risk, and rates of occurrence. Each of these concepts finds direct application in community health nursing.

Causality

To control health problems, epidemiologists and community health nurses must have some idea of causality. The concept of *causality* is based on the idea that one event is the result of another event. Theories about the cause of disease have evolved over time.

Theories of Disease Causation

The first recognized attempt to attribute a cause to illness occurred during the "religious era," which extended from roughly 2000 B.C. through the age of the early Egyptian and Greek physicians to around 600 B.C. During this period, disease was thought to be caused directly by divine intervention, possibly as punishment for sins or as a trial of faith.

Subsequent to the religious era, disease was often attributed to various physical forces, such as miasmas or mists. A rudimentary environmental theory of disease was developed by Hippocrates in his treatise *On Airs, Waters, and Places,* about 400 B.C. The primary belief at that time was that disease was caused by harmful substances in the environment.

The bacteriologic era commenced in the late 1870s with the discovery of specific organisms as etiologic (causative) agents for specific diseases. One of the classic epidemiologic studies demonstrating the probability of some causative organism in communicable diseases was that of John Snow, who deduced that the cause of a cholera epidemic was contaminated water from a specific London well. Subsequently, actual bacteria were isolated and found to be the source of this and other infectious diseases. These discoveries gave rise to theories of a single cause for any specific disease.

Single-cause theories were further supported by the identification of other specific agents as causative elements for certain health problems. For example, lack of vitamin C was found to result in scurvy. The discovery of specific agents responsible for particular diseases did not, however, explain why one person exposed to an agent developed the disease, while another did not, so the evolution of disease theory entered the current era of multiple causation.

The hallmark of the era of multiple causation is the recognition of the interplay of a variety of factors in the development of health or illness. Epidemiology examines this interplay of factors with an eye toward control of a particular health condition. Prevention or control of any disease within population groups depends on knowledge of these factors and determination of the point at which intervention will be most feasible and most effective.

The historical development of theories of disease causation is summarized in Table 8–1. It should be noted that, although the scientific community has accepted the current idea of multiple causation, each of the preceding theories continues to have support among members of the lay population.

Criteria for Causality

With the advent of single cause/single effect theories of disease causation, the scientific community began to look for specific causes for all health problems. Now, however, the concept of causality has become more complicated in view of the recognized interplay of a variety of factors in the development of illness. A factor may be considered causative if the health condition is more likely to occur in its presence and less likely to occur in its absence. Even when these conditions are met, however, a specific factor may not necessarily cause a particular condition. Various authors identify anywhere from four to ten criteria to be used in determining causality (Harkness, 1995; Harper & Lambert, 1994; Tyler & Last, 1992; Timmreck, 1994). Generally, however, they agree on five basic criteria that can be used to attribute causation in both infectious and noninfectious conditions. These criteria are the consistency and the strength of the association, its specificity, the temporal relationship between events, and coherence with other known facts.

Consistency. The first criterion for establishing a causal relationship is *consistency*. The association between the factor in question and the problem must be consistent. The condition in question must occur when the factor is present, not when it is absent. For example, people cannot develop measles without being exposed to measles virus. In addition, the association must always occur in the same direction. Exposure cannot result in disease in one instance, and disease result in exposure to the virus in another.

Strength of Association. The second criterion for establishing causality is the *strength of the association*. The greater the correlation between the occurrence of the factor and the health condition, the greater the possibility that the relationship is one of cause and effect. For example, not every susceptible person who is exposed to measles virus develops the disease, but most of them do. The association between exposure and disease, in this instance, is quite strong and supports the idea that the measles virus causes measles. The strength of the association may reflect a *dose-response gradient* in which the greater the exposure to the presumed cause, the greater the likelihood of developing the problem (Harper & Lambert, 1994). For example, the fact that people who smoke two packs of cigarettes a day are more likely to develop lung cancer than those who smoke one pack is strong evidence for a causal relationship between smoking and lung cancer.

Specificity. *Specificity* is the third criterion for causality. Specificity is present when the factor in question results in one specific condition. For instance, exposure to measles virus results only in measles, not mumps, chickenpox, or any other communicable disease. Specificity is the weakest of the criteria with respect to noninfectious conditions (Harper & Lambert, 1994). For example, smoking not only causes lung cancer, but also contributes to stomach and bladder cancers and heart disease.

Temporal Relationship. The fourth criterion for establishing causation is the *time* (or *temporal*) *relationship* between the factor and the resulting condition. The factor thought to be causative should occur before the condition appears. For example, one is always exposed to measles virus before, not after, one gets measles.

Coherence. *Coherence* with the established body of scientific knowledge is the last criterion for determining causality. The idea that one condition causes another must be logical and congruent with other known facts. For example, it is known that alcohol consump-

TABLE 8–1. HISTORICAL DEVELOPMENT OF THEORIES OF DISEASE CAUSATION

Era	Period	Theory of Causation Prevalent
Religious era	2000–600 B.C.	Disease caused by divine intervention, possibly as punishment for sins or test of faith
Environmental era	Circa 400 B.C.	Disease caused by harmful miasmas, or mists, or other substances in the environment
Bacteriologic era	1870–1900	Disease caused by specific bacteriologic or nutritive agents
Era of multiple causation	1900 to present	Disease caused by interaction of multiple factors

tion increases the time required for voluntary muscles to react to stimuli. Therefore, it is reasonable to consider alcohol consumption as a causative factor in many accidents because this interpretation is consistent with the idea of slowed response to changing driving conditions.

Only the criterion of a correct temporal relationship is absolutely required for attributing causation; however, the greater the number of criteria met, the more credible the idea that the factor in question causes the condition of interest. Criteria for determining causality are summarized in Table 8–2.

Risk

In addition to establishing the causes of health-related conditions, epidemiologists are interested in estimating the likelihood that a particular condition will occur. *Risk* is the probability that a given individual will develop a specific condition. One's risk of developing a particular condition is affected by a variety of physical, emotional, environmental, lifestyle, and other factors. When epidemiologists speak of *populations at risk,* they are referring to groups of people who have the greatest potential to develop a particular health problem because of the presence or absence of certain contributing factors.

The basis for risk may lie in one's susceptibility to a condition or potential for exposure to causative factors. *Susceptibility* is the ability to be affected by factors contributing to a particular health condition. For example, very young unimmunized children are susceptible to, and constitute the population at risk for, pertussis (whooping cough). In this case, the basis for increased risk lies in the increased susceptibility of this group. Persons over the age of 10 and children who have been immunized against pertussis are unlikely to develop the disease and so are not part of the population at risk. Another example of risk based on susceptibility is found in the population of sexually active women of childbearing age who are at risk for pregnancy. Men, children, and older women are not susceptible to pregnancy and, therefore, are not considered part of the population at risk.

Exposure potential is another factor in one's risk of developing a particular condition. *Exposure potential* is the likelihood of exposure to factors that contribute to the condition. For example, those most at risk for sexually transmitted diseases are adolescents and young adults. In this instance, the basis of risk is not increased susceptibility, as in the case of pertussis, but an increased potential for exposure because of more frequent and less selective sexual activity. Another population at risk through increased chance of exposure includes individuals whose occupation brings them in contact with toxic substances.

Members of a population at risk have a greater probability of developing a specific condition than those who are not affected by factors known to contribute to the condition. This difference in the probability of developing a given condition is known as the *relative risk ratio* (Harkness, 1995). This ratio is derived by comparing the frequency of occurrence of the condition in a group of people with known risk factors to that among individuals without these factors. For example, if 50% of smokers develop heart disease versus only 5% of nonsmokers, smokers have a relative risk of 10:1, or have a 10 times greater risk of heart disease than their nonsmoking counterparts. The relative risk ratio is useful in identifying those areas where preventive interventions will have the greatest impact on the occurrence of disease.

When the relative risk is greater than 1:1, there is a positive association between factor and condition suggesting that eliminating the factor may prevent the condition. Similarly, a negative association in which the relative ratio is less than 1:1 (eg, 1:5) suggests that enhancing the factor or causing it to be present may prevent the condition. For example, smoking has a positive relationship with heart disease and regular exercise has a negative relationship, so preventing smoking and promoting exercise should both decrease the incidence of heart disease.

The population at risk becomes the target group for any intervention designed to prevent or control the problem in question. The *target group* includes those individuals who would benefit from an intervention program and at whom the program is aimed. Using one of the previous examples, the target group for an immunization campaign against pertussis would include unimmunized children under the age of 10.

Rates of Occurrence

The rate of occurrence of a health-related condition is also of concern to community health nurses. *Rates of occurrence* are statistical measures that indicate the extent of health problems in a group. Rates of occur-

TABLE 8–2. CRITERIA FOR DETERMINING CAUSALITY

Criterion	Description of Criterion
Consistency	The association between the supposed cause and its effect is consistent and always occurs in the same direction.
Strength of association	The greater the correlation between supposed cause and effect, the greater the possibility the relationship is a causal one.
Specificity	The supposed cause always creates the same effect.
Temporal relationship	The supposed cause always occurs before the effect.
Coherence	The supposition of one event causing another is coherent with other existing knowledge.

▶ BASIC FORMULA FOR CALCULATING STATISTICAL RATES

$$\text{Rate} = \frac{\text{number of events over a period of time}}{\text{population at risk at that time}} \times 1000 \text{ (or } 100,000)$$

For example, in a community with a population of 10,000 females aged 13 to 18 years, there were 200 teenage pregnancies in 1998. What is the rate of teenage pregnancy?

$$\text{Rate of teenage pregnancy} = \frac{\text{200 pregnancies in females 13–18 during 1998}}{\text{10,000 females ages 13–18 in the population at midyear}} \times 1000$$

$$= 20 \text{ pregnancies per 1000 females}$$

rence also allow comparisons between groups of different sizes with respect to the extent of a particular condition. For example, a community with a population of 1000 may report 50 cases of syphilis this year, whereas another community of 100,000 persons may report 5000 cases. On the surface, it would seem that the second community has a greater problem with syphilis than the first; however, both communities have experienced 50 cases per 1000 population. In other words, both have a problem with syphilis of comparable magnitude.

Computing the statistical rates of interest in community health nursing involves dividing the *number of instances of an event* during a specified period by the *population at risk* for that event and *multiplying by 1000* (or 100,000 if the numbers of the event are so small that the result of the calculation using a multiplier of 1000 would be less than 1).

Both morbidity and mortality rates are of concern in community health nursing. **Mortality** is the ratio of the number of deaths in various categories to a given population, whereas **morbidity** is the ratio of the number of cases of a disease or condition to a given population. Mortality rates describe deaths; morbidity rates describe cases of health conditions that may or may not result in death. For example, the number of people in a particular group who die as a result of cardiovascular disease is reflected in the mortality rate; however, the number of people experiencing cardiovascular disease is indicated by the morbidity rate.

Mortality Rates

Mortality rates of interest in community health nursing include the overall or "crude" death rate, cause-specific death rates, infant and neonatal mortality rates, fetal and perinatal mortality rates, and maternal death rate. Each rate is calculated from the number of events during a specified period and the average population at risk during that same period.

Rates are reported in terms of the multiplicative factor used to calculate them. For example, cancer deaths occur in fairly large numbers, so a cause-specific death rate for cancer would be calculated using 1000 as the multiplier. If Community A, with a population of 50,000, had 100 cancer-related deaths, the cause-specific death rate for cancer would be reported as 2 deaths per 1000 population. Deaths from pancreatic cancer, on the other hand, occur relatively infrequently, so 100,000 would be the multiplier used to calculate the pancreatic cancer death rate. For instance, if there were 6 deaths from pancreatic cancer in Community B last year, and Community B has a population of 500,000 people, the annual pancreatic cancer mortality rate would be reported as 1.2 deaths per 100,000 population.

Age-adjusted mortality rates can be calculated to account for differences in age distribution between groups. This allows one to make more accurate comparisons of mortality between groups with widely different age distributions. For example, Community A might have a considerably higher crude death rate for influenza than Community B. If, however, Community A also has a higher proportion of elderly persons in the population, more influenza deaths would be expected, because older people are more vulnerable to this condition. Age-adjusted mortality rates for influenza, on the other hand, allow the community health nurse to compare the effects of influenza on Communities A and B as if they had similar proportions of elderly in the population. If Community A's influenza death rate remains higher when adjusted for age, the nurse would look for other factors in the community to explain this difference.

Morbidity Rates

Morbidity rates reflect the number of cases of particular health conditions in a group or community. Morbidity is described in terms of incidence or prevalence rates. *Incidence* rates are calculated on the basis of the

▶ FORMULAS FOR CALCULATING SELECTED MORTALITY RATES

$$\text{Crude death rate} = \frac{\text{total number of deaths during year}}{\text{total population at midyear}} \times 1000$$

$$\text{Cause-specific annual death rate} = \frac{\text{number of deaths from specific cause during year}}{\text{total population at midyear}} \times 1000$$

$$\text{Annual infant mortality rate} = \frac{\text{number of deaths during year (birth to 1 year of age)}}{\text{number of live births during year}} \times 1000$$

$$\text{Annual neonatal mortality rate} = \frac{\text{number of deaths during year (birth to 28 days of age)}}{\text{number of live births during year}} \times 1000$$

$$\text{Annual fetal death rate} = \frac{\text{number of fetal deaths during year (20 to 28 weeks' gestation)}}{\text{number of live births plus fetal deaths during year}} \times 1000$$

$$\text{Annual perinatal death rate} = \frac{\text{number of perinatal deaths during year (20 weeks' gestation to 1 week of age)}}{\text{number of live births plus fetal deaths during year}} \times 1000$$

$$\text{Annual maternal death rate} = \frac{\text{number of maternal deaths during year}}{\text{number of live births during year}} \times 100,000$$

number of *new* cases of a particular condition identified during a specified period. **Prevalence** is *the total number* of people affected by a particular condition at a specified point in time.

To illustrate the concepts of incidence and prevalence, consider a town with a population of 30,000 in which 15 new cases of hypertension were diagnosed in June. This is an indication of the incidence of hypertension. People who were diagnosed as hypertensive prior to June and who continue to live in the town still have hypertension. These additional cases of hypertension, however, are not reflected in the hypertension incidence rate for June, but are included in the prevalence, the total number of people in the community affected by hypertension. The formulae below are used to calculate annual incidence and prevalence rates. Again, the results of the calculations are reported in terms of the rate per 1000 population.

Case fatality rates and survival rates are also of concern in community health. The **case fatality rate** for a particular condition reflects the percentage of persons with the condition who die as a result of it. For example, at present, many people infected with Ebola virus die because of the lack of an effective treatment. Very few people die of mumps, on the other hand, so mumps has a low case fatality rate.

The converse of fatality is the **survival rate,** the proportion of people with a given condition remaining alive after a specific period (usually 5 years). For example, the 5-year survival rate for women with breast cancer is relatively high compared with the survival rate of those with pancreatic cancer. A related concept is survival time, or the average length of time from diagnosis to death. For example, given current medical technology, the survival time for children with Down syndrome is much longer today than at the turn of the century. Caution should be used in interpreting both survival rate and survival time information. Diagnostic technology has permitted earlier diagnosis of many conditions increasing the time from diagnosis to death, but not appreciably lengthening one's life (Gordis, 1996).

Other rates that may be of interest to community health nurses include marriage and divorce rates, illegitimacy rates, employment rates, utilization rates for health care services and facilities, and rates for alcohol and drug use and abuse.

Community health nurses use morbidity and mortality data in assessing the health status of a community. Community morbidity and mortality rates that are generally high or higher than state or national rates indicate health problems that require nursing intervention. For example, the nurse may note that local morbidity rates for childhood illnesses such as measles and rubella are twice those of the rest of the state. These differences indicate that a significant portion of the local child population is unimmunized.

> **SAMPLE MORTALITY RATE CALCULATIONS USING MULTIPLIERS OF 1000 AND 100,000**

Community A

$$\text{Cancer mortality rate} = \frac{100 \text{ deaths due to cancer, 1998}}{50,000 \text{ population at midyear}} \times 1000$$

$$= 2 \text{ cancer deaths per 1000 population}$$

Community B

$$\text{Pancreatic cancer mortality rate} = \frac{6 \text{ deaths from pancreatic cancer, 1998}}{500,000 \text{ population at midyear}} \times 100,000$$

$$= 1.2 \text{ deaths due to pancreatic cancer per 100,000 population}$$

The nurse then uses these data to begin an investigation of the factors involved in the problem and to plan a solution. Is it a matter of inaccessibility of immunization services, lack of education on the need for immunization, or poor surveillance of immunization levels in the schools? The solution to the problem must be geared to the cause. Statistical data merely serve to indicate the presence of a problem; they do not delineate its specific nature.

Low morbidity and mortality rates do not indicate the absence of health problems in the community, as biostatistics are only one indicator of health status. Many health problems are not reported statistically and their presence in the community is not reflected in morbidity and mortality rates. The nutritional status of the population is one area not addressed by biostatistics such as morbidity and mortality rates. Other indicators that the community health nurse employs in assessing a community's health status are discussed in Chapter 19.

► THE EPIDEMIOLOGIC PROCESS

Epidemiologists use a systematic process to study states of health and illness in an effort to control disease and promote health. The steps of this *epidemiologic process* are:

- Defining the condition
- Determining the natural history of the condition
- Identifying strategic points of control
- Designing control strategies
- Implementing control strategies
- Evaluating control strategies

Determining the natural history of the condition is analogous to the assessment and diagnosis phases of the nursing process. Identifying strategic points of control and designing control programs reflect the planning aspects of the nursing process, and the implementation and evaluation steps are equivalent to similar steps in the nursing process.

Defining the Condition

The first step in the epidemiologic process is defining the health condition requiring intervention. As we will see later, the epidemiologic process can be applied to health as well as illness. In either case, it is necessary to define the state or condition for which intervention is required. Taking a health promotion focus, one needs to define health. With respect to a specific disease or health problem, one must clearly define what is and is not an instance of the problem. For example, to study the factors contributing to sui-

> **FORMULAS FOR CALCULATING ANNUAL INCIDENCE AND PREVALENCE RATES**

$$\text{Annual incidence rate} = \frac{\text{number of new cases of a condition last year}}{\text{total population at risk at midyear}} \times 1000$$

$$\text{Annual prevalence rate} = \frac{\text{total number of cases of a condition last year}}{\text{total population at risk at midyear}} \times 1000$$

cide, one must be able to differentiate suicide from accidental death. Similarly, one must be able to differentiate cases of measles from cases or rubella to study and control either of these diseases.

Determining the Natural History of the Condition

The natural history of a disease or condition is a description of the events that precede its development and occur during its course, as well as its outcomes. Determining the condition's natural history involves identifying factors that contribute to its development, its signs and symptoms, it effects on the human system, and its typical outcomes and factors that may affect those outcomes. For example, crowded living conditions, lack of immunization, and exposure to influenza virus are some factors involved in the development of influenza. The typical course of influenza includes a short incubation period and the rapid onset of respiratory and/or gastrointestinal symptoms. Most cases of influenza resolve after several days, but the eventual outcome depends on such factors as the individual's overall health, age, nutritional status, and personal habits such as smoking. All of these bits of information are part of the natural history of influenza.

The description of the natural history also incorporates information on the frequency of occurrence, severity of outcomes, and geographic distribution of the condition. Information is obtained on time relationships and trends related to the condition. Time relationships refer to the occurrence of the condition at specific times or during particular seasons. For example, influenza occurs primarily in the winter, and the incidence of suicide rises around holidays. Trends refer to patterns of occurrence for the condition. Incidence of hepatitis A, for example, is declining, while patterns of occurrence for family violence indicate increasing incidence.

The natural history of a condition is usually divided into four stages: preexposure, preclinical, clinical, and resolution. In the *preexposure stage,* factors contributing to the development of the condition are present. When exposure to causative factors has occurred, but no symptoms have appeared, the condition is in the *preclinical stage.* The *clinical stage* begins with the onset of signs and symptoms characteristic of the disease or condition. In the *resolution stage,* the condition culminates in a return to health, death, or continuation of a chronic state. These stages are depicted in Figure 8–1.

Determining the factors involved in the natural history of a condition is usually undertaken using a

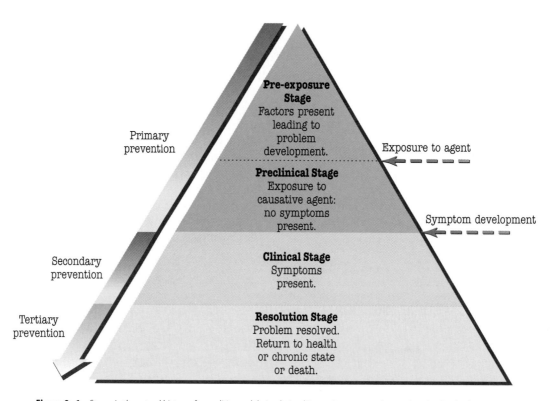

Figure 8–1. Stages in the natural history of a condition and their relationship to primary, secondary, and tertiary levels of prevention.

specific epidemiologic model. Three such models are discussed later in this chapter. The dimensions of health in the Dimensions Model of community health nursing discussed in Chapter 5 also provide an epidemiologic perspective for examining the natural history of a health condition.

Identifying Strategic Points of Control

Knowledge of the natural history of a disease or condition allows epidemiologists to identify strategic points of control. One might, for example, design interventions to eliminate or modify factors contributing to a condition to prevent its occurrence. Similarly, knowledge of factors affecting a condition's course may lead to interventions designed to minimize its effects.

Strategic points of control may involve interventions at the primary, secondary, or tertiary level of prevention. Primary prevention takes place before the problem occurs, during the preexposure and preclinical stages of its natural history. Secondary prevention occurs once the problem appears, during the clinical stage; tertiary prevention may be required during the resolution stage either to prevent lasting effects or to prevent a recurrence of the problem. Figure 8–1 depicts the relationship of levels of prevention to the stages of the natural history of a health-related condition.

Designing, Implementing, and Evaluating Control Strategies

Once strategic points of control for a specific condition have been identified, health care programs can be designed to prevent it or minimize its effects on the health of the population. Programs are then implemented and evaluated in terms of their effects on the occurrence of the particular condition. These steps of the epidemiologic process parallel similar components of the nursing process and are discussed in relation to health care programming in Chapter 19.

▶ EPIDEMIOLOGIC INVESTIGATION

The basic requirement for using the epidemiologic process to control health and illness is information, information on contributing factors as well as on effective control strategies. Information on any given condition is usually obtained over time from multiple epidemiologic investigations. Epidemiologic studies are of two general types, descriptive and analytic.

Descriptive Epidemiology

Descriptive epidemiology is the study of the distribution of a given health state in a specified population in terms of person, place, and time. The person dimension identifies those affected by the condition. For example, who develops arthritis and what features are characteristic of these people? The dimension of place examines where the condition occurs. Does arthritis occur more frequently in some parts of the country than others? What features of those parts of the country might explain these differences? Finally, the time dimension reflects when the condition occurs. For example, measles occurs primarily in the winter. What factors account for this seasonal variation? Information in each of these areas suggests possible causative factors and potential control strategies for arthritis or measles.

Analytic Epidemiology

Analytic epidemiology is the study of factors contributing to health states for the purpose of identifying causal factors and can be divided into two categories of investigations: hypothesis-generating studies and hypothesis-testing studies (Greenburg, 1993). A *hypothesis*, in this context, is a possible explanation for an observed event. In analytic epidemiology we are attempting to develop and evaluate possible explanations for the occurrence of health and illness states in specific populations.

Hypothesis-generating Studies

Hypothesis-generating studies suggest relationships between factors and health states, but cannot establish these relationships as causal. Other items for this type of study are *ecological studies* and *correlational studies*. Ecological studies examine relationships between factors within population groups and compare the incidence of a specific event in population groups with and without a supposed causative factor. For example, ecological studies compared the incidence of dental caries in towns with and without fluoride in the water. The findings of ecological studies may hold true for population groups, but not necessarily for all the individuals who make up a particular group.

Hypothesis-testing Studies

Hypothesis-testing studies examine the relationship between the health state and the supposed cause within single individuals rather than population groups to establish cause and effect. For instance, a researcher could compare the incidence of dental caries in those particular people who obtained their water from the local fluoride-rich water supply and those who drank bottled water that did not contain fluoride. Greater incidence of caries among those drinking bottled water would provide additional support for the hypothesized causal effect of fluoride in decreasing caries.

Hypothesis-testing studies can be either observational or experimental. In *observational studies,* the researcher observes the effects of a naturally occurring event, and contrasts the outcomes in those individuals experiencing the event and those who have not experienced it. For example, the community health nurse who examines the relationship between marital stress and child abuse would conduct an observational study; he or she would not create the marital stress to study its effects. The nurse would compare the incidence of child abuse in families experiencing marital stress with the incidence in families having stable marriages.

In epidemiologic terminology, observational studies can be retrospective, prospective, or cross-sectional depending on the timing of subject selection in relation to exposure to the supposed causative factor and the development of the supposed effect (Timmreck, 1994). *Retrospective studies* are those in which exposure to the supposed cause and development of the effect condition occur prior to the investigation. Retrospective studies are also called *case–control studies* because comparisons are made between people who have the condition (cases) and those who do not (controls) (Valanis, 1999).

In *prospective studies,* some subjects have been exposed to the suspected causative factor and some have not. These two groups or "cohorts" are then followed forward in time to determine the incidence of the condition of interest in those who were exposed versus those who were not. Other terms for this type of study are *cohort study* and *longitudinal study.* An example is a study of the effects of parental smoking on children's decisions to smoke or not to smoke. A cohort of children whose parents smoke and another cohort whose parents do not smoke would be followed for a period of years to determine what proportion of each group starts smoking.

Cross-sectional studies explore the relationship of a health condition to other variables of interest in a defined population at a given time. These studies are also called *prevalence studies* because they aid in determining the prevalence of both condition and potential causative factors at any particular time (Gordis, 1996). A school nurse, for example, might want to study the use of seat belts by children at different grade levels. Differences in findings among grade levels might suggest factors that influence seat belt use (eg, parents may pay more attention to seat belt use by younger children) or suggest particular groups to be targeted for educational efforts related to seat belt use.

Experimental studies involve manipulation of exposure to the supposed causative factor and look for differences in the incidence of the supposed effect. Questions related to the efficacy of primary, secondary, and tertiary prevention would be answered by experimental studies. In such studies, manipulation of the causal variable involves applying an intervention. This application of an intervention by the researcher is called a *trial.* Trials can involve removal of a risk factor or addition of some other factor and can be either prophylactic or therapeutic in nature depending on the timing of the intervention (Valanis, 1999).

In prophylactic trials, the intervention is designed to prevent the occurrence of a health problem. Prophylactic trials can be used to study the effectiveness of either primary or tertiary prevention. In a prophylactic trial of a primary preventive intervention, the dependent variable or supposed effect would be prevention of the event, whereas the dependent variable in a prophylactic trial of tertiary prevention would reflect prevention of the recurrence of a problem. Interventions designed to promote health are also tested in prophylactic trials.

Therapeutic trials, on the other hand, investigate the effects of secondary preventive interventions. In these studies, the researcher exposes a group of subjects to an intervention designed to resolve an existing health problem. The intervention may be either positive or negative. Positive interventions add a factor to the situation being studied, whereas negative interventions reduce or eliminate causative factors. For example, one might explore the effects of teaching parenting techniques (a positive intervention) or reducing environmental stressors (a negative intervention) on the incidence of child abuse by parents who are already abusive.

The relationships among the types of epidemiologic investigations presented here are depicted in Figure 8–2. The selection of a particular investigative approach depends on the purpose of the study to be conducted and the extent of previous research in the area. For example, descriptive studies are appropriate in studying conditions about which little is known. In other areas where there is already evidence of possible relationships between variables, observational or experimental studies might be more appropriate. Choice of an observational or experimental approach depends primarily on whether the situation permits manipulation of variables of interest by the researcher. In some instances, manipulation of variables is not possible; in others, manipulation of the variables involved would be unethical.

Community health nurses may be actively involved in epidemiologic investigations. Some agencies

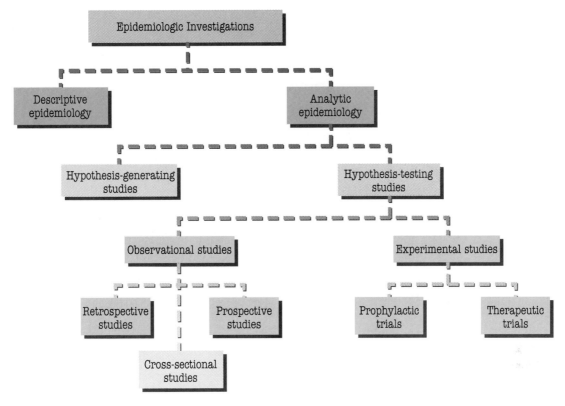

Figure 8–2. Approaches to epidemiologic investigation.

and organizations that support epidemiology and epidemiologic research are listed at the end of the chapter.

► EPIDEMIOLOGIC MODELS

Both nurses and epidemiologists use the epidemiologic process and epidemiologic research findings to direct interventions to control health-related conditions. Determining the natural history of a health condition and identifying control strategies involve collecting large amounts of data about multiple factors that may be contributing to the condition. For this reason it is helpful to have a model or framework to direct the collection and interpretation of these data. We explore three such models: the epidemiologic triad, the web of causation model, and Dever's epidemiologic model. The Dimensions Model of community health nursing discussed in Chapter 5 can also be used in epidemiologic investigations.

The Epidemiologic Triad

Traditionally, epidemiologic investigation has been guided by the epidemiologic triad. In this model, data

are collected with respect to a triad of elements: host, agent, and environment. The interrelationship of these elements results in a state of relative health or illness. The relationship among host, agent, and environment and specific considerations under each are depicted in Figure 8–3.

Host

The **host** is the client system affected by the particular condition under investigation. Community health nursing is concerned with the health of human beings, so, for our purposes, humankind is the host. A variety of factors can influence the host's exposure, susceptibility, and response to an agent. Host-related factors include intrinsic factors (eg, age, race, and sex), physical and psychological factors, and the presence or absence of immunity. These factors are addressed in more detail in the discussion of Dever's epidemiologic model.

Agent

The **agent** is the primary cause of a health-related condition. The causes of some health problems may be so complex that no single agent can be identified. The

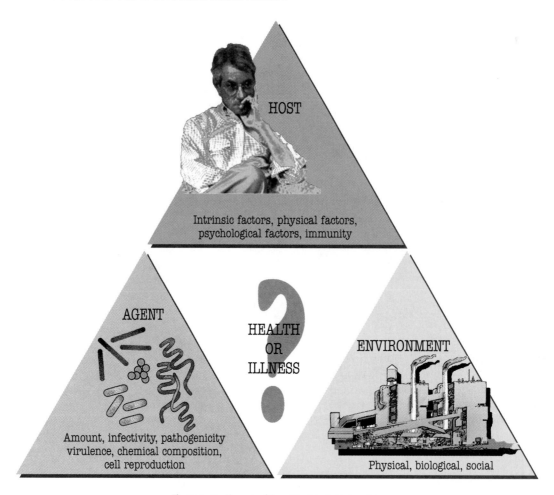

Figure 8–3. Elements of the epidemiologic triad model.

concept of agent, however, remains useful for exploring many health problems.

Agents can be classified into five basic types: physical agents, chemical agents, nutritive elements, infectious agents, and psychological agents. Physical agents include heat, trauma, and genetic mutation. Genetically determined diseases, for example, are the result of physical changes in gene structure, whereas heat is an agent in such conditions as burns and heat exhaustion. Chemical agents include various substances to which people may develop untoward reactions. Some plants such as poison ivy and ragweed can be considered chemical agents because they cause a chemical reaction resulting in an allergic response.

An absence or an excess of a variety of nutritive elements is known to result in disease, as does the presence of and exposure to a number of infectious agents that cause communicable diseases. Finally, psychological agents such as stress can produce a variety of stress-related conditions. The types of agents

and examples of health conditions to which they contribute are listed in Table 8–3.

An agent's characteristics influence whether a given individual develops a particular health-related condition. These characteristics vary somewhat depending on the type of agent involved.

Characteristics of Infectious Agents.   Characteristics that influence the effects of infectious agents include the extent of exposure to the agent and the agent's infectivity, pathogenicity, and virulence. Additional characteristics of infectious agents include chemical composition and structure and cell reproduction. The *extent of exposure* to a disease-causing microorganism, or the *infective dose*, affects the outcome of the exposure. For example, the person exposed to a few *Mycobacterium tuberculosis* is unlikely to develop tuberculosis (TB). The greater the number of these microorganisms inhaled, however, the greater the likelihood of developing TB.

Infectivity is the ability of an agent to invade the host system. Infectivity is determined, in part, by the

TABLE 8–3. AGENTS AND SELECTED HEALTH PROBLEMS TO WHICH THEY CONTRIBUTE

Type of Agent	Example	Problems
Physical	Heat	Burns, heat stroke
	Trauma	Fractures, concussion, sprains, contusions
	Genetic change	Down syndrome, Turner's syndrome
Chemical	Medications	Accidental poisoning, suicide
	Chlorine	Poisoning, asphyxiation (in gas form)
	Poison ivy	Rash and pruritus
Nutritive	Vitamin C	Scurvy (in absence of vitamin C)
	Iron	Anemia (in absence of iron)
	Vitamin A	Poisoning (in excess)
Infectious	Measles virus	Measles, measles encephalitis
	HIV	AIDS
	Varicella virus	Chickenpox
	Influenza virus	Influenza
Psychological	Stress	Ulcerative colitis, heart disease, suicide, asthma, alcoholism, drug abuse, violence

agent's portals of entry and exit. The **portal of entry** is the means by which the agent invades the host; the **portal of exit** is the avenue by which the agent leaves the host. The portals of entry and exit also influence the **mode of transmission,** or means by which the agent is transmitted from one host to another. Portals of entry and exit and modes of transmission are addressed in greater detail in Chapter 30. Measles virus, for example, has a higher infectivity than does tetanus bacillus. The measles virus enters the body quite easily through the respiratory system, whereas tetanus gains entry through a break in the skin, usually a deep puncture wound. **Pathogenicity** is the ability of the agent to cause disease. In terms of infectious agents, measles virus causes disease in most susceptible infected individuals. *Mycobacterium tuberculosis*, on the other hand, produces disease in only a small portion of individuals infected. Therefore, the measles virus has a higher pathogenicity than *M. tuberculosis.*

Another epidemiologic concept closely related to pathogenicity is that of **attack rate,** which is the proportion of those exposed to the agent who develop the disease. As is the case with pathogenicity, measles has a high attack rate, whereas tuberculosis has a low attack rate.

Virulence is a term used to describe the severity of the health problem caused by the agent. Rubeola or measles has a low virulence because uncomplicated measles is not a serious illness. Tetanus, on the other hand, is extremely virulent because it results in fatality unless treatment is instituted. The virus that causes AIDS is another infectious agent with a very high virulence. Virulence is frequently confused with pathogenicity, but the two terms refer to different agent

characteristics. For example, cold viruses that cause disease in infected individuals are highly pathogenic, but have a low virulence because the diseases caused are relatively minor. Virulence is closely related to case fatality rates.

The *chemical composition and structure* of a microorganism can also influence the effects of an infectious agent on a host. It is the composition of bacterial cell walls, for instance, that makes penicillin and similar antibiotics effective against several microorganisms. Similarly, the composition of many viruses makes it necessary for them to attach to specific protein structures in human cells to gain entry.

Another important factor that influences the effect of an infectious agent is its *reproductive cycle.* The rate at which an infectious agent reproduces can influence the body's ability to kill invading organisms before they are able to overwhelm bodily defense mechanisms. An organisms' reproductive cycle influences the incubation period of the disease caused. The **incubation period** is the length of time from exposure to the agent to the development of symptoms. Organisms' reproductive cycles can also affect their ability to cause disease or prompt interventions to control them, both of which affect the natural history of disease. For example, knowledge that the reproductive cycle of *Plasmodium* occurs in the *Anopheles* mosquito prompted efforts to control malaria by eradicating this mosquito. These and other factors influencing infectious agents are addressed in more detail in Chapter 30.

Characteristics of Noninfectious Agents. Noninfectious agents share some of the characteristics of infectious agents. For example, the extent of exposure to the agent affects its ability to cause health problems. Ingesting moderate amounts of alcohol or aspirin does not cause problems, but excessive consumption does. The amount of stress to which one is exposed can also affect the development of stress-related illness.

The concept of infectivity can also be applied to other types of agents, although the term was developed in relation to communicable diseases. For example, asbestos, which can be inhaled, has a higher "infectivity" than over overdose of aspirin, which must be ingested. Stress, as an agent of illness, also has a high infectivity because it is an everyday factor impinging on people. All of us are "infected" by stress.

Stress can also be viewed in terms of its ability to cause disease. Although everyone experiences some degree of stress, not all people develop stress-related illnesses. Stress, therefore, has a relatively low pathogenicity. Noninfectious agents may vary in terms of their virulence as well. Stress can produce a mild stomach upset in some individuals and drive others to suicide. In the first instance, stress has a low virulence, and in the second, a high virulence.

Chemical composition is a relevant factor for many noninfectious agents. For example, it is the chemical composition of a poisonous substance that produces chemical reactions in the human body that result in poisoning. Similarly, it is the chemical composition of poison ivy that causes a pruritic rash.

Although noninfectious agents do not have reproductive cycles, they may have similar properties. For example, a physical agent such as radiation has a half-life that influences its ability to cause damage. Similarly, noninfectious conditions do not have incubation periods, but frequently exhibit a delay between exposure to causative factors and symptom development termed an induction period, or latency period (Valanis, 1999).

Environment

The third element of the epidemiologic triad includes factors in the physical, biological, and social *environment* that contribute to health-related conditions. The physical environment consists of such factors as weather, terrain, and buildings. A variety of physical environment factors can influence health. For example, air pollution contributes to respiratory disease as well as other physiologic and psychological effects in human beings. Similarly, the temperature and humidity of tropical areas are associated with increased incidence of hyperthyroidism.

The biological environment, in the triad model, consists of all living organisms, other than humans. Components of the biological environment include plants and animals as well as microorganisms, all of which can influence health.

The social environment includes factors related to social interaction that may contribute to health or disease. For example, cultural factors, which are part of the social environment, can influence health behaviors. In a similar fashion, social norms may influence health and illness. For example, societal views of alcoholism and drug abuse as character weaknesses have hampered efforts to control these problems.

The Web of Causation Model

The "web of causation" is a second model for understanding the influence of multiple factors on the development of a specific health condition. In this model, factors are explored in terms of their interplay, and both direct and indirect causes of the problem are identified. The web of causation approach allows the epidemiologist to map out the interrelationships among factors contributing to the development (or

prevention) of a particular health condition. This approach also assists in determining areas where efforts at control will be most effective.

The web of causation for the problem of adolescent pregnancy is depicted in Figure 8–4. It is obvious from the complexity of Figure 8–4 that multiple factors contribute to adolescent pregnancy. The interplay of these factors determines whether or not the problem occurs. The most direct causes are those linked directly to the pregnancy outcome: sexual activity and inconsistent or no use of contraceptives. Numerous other factors, however, contribute to the adolescent's decision to engage in sexual activity without effective contraception.

Factors influencing sexual activity and contraceptive use include motivation, perceptions regarding sexuality, knowledge, and factors related to contraceptive services. The motivation to be sexually active without adequate contraception, and even intentionally to become pregnant, may derive from still other factors. The teen may be motivated by a desire to get away, by a desire to love and be loved (either by the partner or by a child), by peer pressure, or by low personal aspirations. Desires to get away and for someone to love may be influenced by a poor home situation and a poor self-concept, both of which have their roots in family interaction patterns and other factors depicted in Figure 8–4.

Perceptions regarding sexuality in general are the result of perceptions about sexual activity, perceptions of pregnancy and parenthood, and perceptions of contraception and abortion. Sexual activity may be seen as a way to interact with others (particularly for the teen with a poor self-concept), as a means of demonstrating "adulthood," or as what one does to be popular. Similarly, the teen may have unrealistic perceptions of pregnancy and parenthood, expecting both to be rewarding experiences devoid of frustration or problems. The adolescent may also perceive contraceptives as dangerous, a nuisance, or evidence of immorality. Or, the adolescent may see abortion as an easy way out if pregnancy does occur.

These perceptions arise out of a number of other factors and are influenced by peer communication, family exposure to pregnancy and parenting roles, and media messages. These factors, in turn, are influenced by community attitudes toward adolescent sexual activity, which also affect factors influencing the teenager's knowledge.

Knowledge factors influencing sexual activity and contraceptive use include information about sexuality and its consequences, knowledge of contraceptive methods, and knowledge of contraceptive availability and accessibility. All of these are influenced by family communication, health services communica-

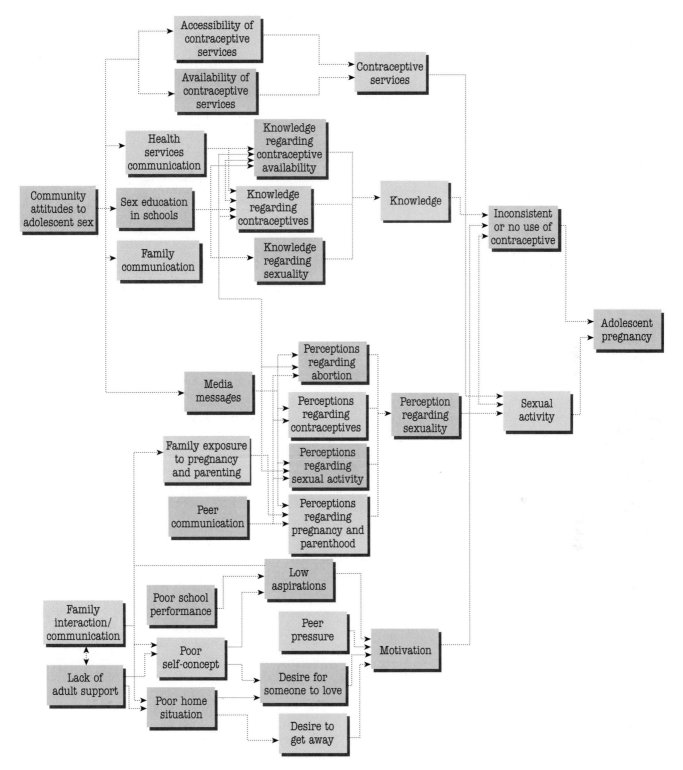

Figure 8–4. The web of causation for adolescent pregnancy, indicating the interplay between multiple direct and indirect causative factors.

tions, and the extent and openness of sex education at home and in the schools. These, in turn, are influenced by community attitudes toward sexuality and adolescent sexual activity. Community attitudes also influence the availability and accessibility of contraceptive services for adolescents, another major factor in decisions to engage in unprotected sexual activity. For example, a community that perceives provision of contraceptive services to teens as condoning sexual activity will resist such services. When this occurs, contraceptives may not be available even to those teens who would use them.

Dever's Epidemiologic Model

Dever's epidemiologic model provides a third approach to conceptualizing the interplay of factors involved in the development of a particular condition. The model, based on prior work by Lalonde and on the work of Blum, was developed as an approach to formulating health care policy for the state of Georgia. The model has been used extensively in Georgia to determine health care priorities and to design programs to address those priorities. G. Alan Dever was a health policy analyst with the Georgia State Department of Health at the time of the model's development. The model itself consists of four basic elements: human biology, environment, lifestyle, and the health care system (Dever, 1991). The elements of Dever's model and specific considerations related to each are depicted in Figure 8–5.

Human Biological Factors

Human biological factors in Dever's model are similar to the host-related factors of the epidemiologic triad and the biophysical dimension of health in the Dimensions Model. Biological factors include genetic inheritance, the functioning of complex physiologic systems, and maturation and aging.

Genetic Inheritance. Genetic inheritance encompasses the influence of human features that are genetically determined such as race, gender, and predisposition to certain types of health problems. As noted in Chapter 5, some health conditions are more prevalent in some racial or ethnic groups than in others and some occur more frequently in men than in women. Genetic predisposition to disease is seen in a variety of conditions including several cancers, heart disease, and diabetes. There is also growing evidence that genetic factors may be operating in some mental illnesses and in other types of conditions.

Complex Physiologic Function. One's state of health and physiologic functional status also influences the de-

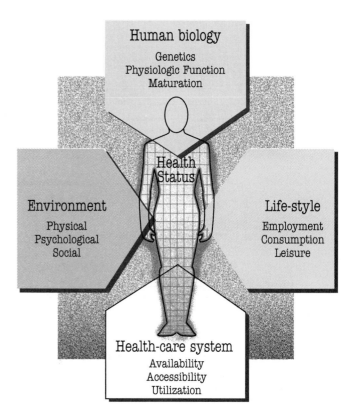

Figure 8–5. Elements of Dever's epidemiologic model.

velopment of other health problems. For example, fatigue and malnutrition are both physiologic states that may predispose one to developing an illness such as influenza. Preexisting disease may also contribute to other health problems. For example, depression may be a factor in child neglect in the same way that hypertension contributes to cardiovascular disease and stroke.

Immunity is another element of one's physiologic state that influences susceptibility to disease. Physiologic immunity is based on the presence of specific antibodies to disease and is described as passive or active depending on the role of the host in developing those antibodies. In *active immunity*, the host is exposed to the antigen, either through having the disease or via immunization with active antigens (eg, diphtheria/tetanus/pertussis [DTP] vaccine). Active immunity is relatively long lasting, waning over several years if at all. In *passive immunity*, externally produced antibodies are provided to the host by way of immunization (eg, hepatitis immunoglobulin) or transfer (eg, from mother to fetus across the placenta).

Cross-immunity occurs when immunity to one agent also confers immunity to a related agent. This type of immunity was operating when Edward Jenner inoculated people with material from cowpox lesions to prevent smallpox. Another concept related to physiologic immunity that has relevance for groups of people is herd immunity. **Herd immunity** is generalized resistance to disease within a population that arises because most of the people have specific immunity to the condition, decreasing the potential for exposure among those few people who do not have immunity.

Maturation and Aging. The third element of Dever's human biology component is the influence of maturation and aging on the development of health problems. The very young and the very old, for example, are often more vulnerable to the effects of abuse than other age groups because of their dependence on the abuser. Similarly, adolescent development which is characterized by a sense of personal invulnerability may lead to risk-taking sexual and drug use behaviors contributing to the development of health problems.

Environmental Factors

The environmental component of Dever's model consists of physical, psychological, and social environments. These categories are comparable to the concepts of physical and social environment and host psychological factors in the epidemiologic triad model. In the Dimensions Model, environmental categories identified by Dever are subsumed within the physical, psychological, and social dimensions of health.

Two aspects of the physical environment form key concepts in communicable disease epidemiology: reservoirs and intermediaries. A **reservoir** is the environment in which a microorganism exists and multiplies. A reservoir does not merely transmit the agent but is actually infected by the agent. For example, humans can acquire bovine tuberculosis from cows or rabies from dogs or other diseased animals. In the first instance, the reservoir is the cow; in the second, it is the dog. An organism that merely transmits the agent is not a reservoir, but an **intermediary.** For example, the *Anopheles* mosquito transfers the *Plasmodium* that causes malaria from an infected person to an uninfected person, but does not have the disease. The reservoir for malaria is infected humans not mosquitoes.

Reservoirs can be human, animal, or environmental. Diseases acquired from animals are called *zoonoses.* Examples of diseases acquired from animal reservoirs include ringworm from cats, anthrax from sheep, and rabies and bovine tuberculosis as previously mentioned.

Human reservoirs may be divided into two categories: cases and carriers. A **case** is an individual who actually has the disease (eg, the person with a cold who coughs in your face). A **carrier** is an individual who harbors the agent without actually having symptomatic disease at the time. Carriers may be classified as incubationary, convalescent, chronic, or transient.

Incubationary carriers are individuals who are in the process of developing the disease. Thus, the susceptible person exposed to chickenpox is an incubationary carrier prior to the development of symptoms. People recuperating from communicable diseases who continue to harbor the agent for a period after clinical symptoms have subsided are **convalescent carriers.** Convalescent carriers continue to be capable of transmitting the disease to others.

Occasionally, a convalescent carrier continues to harbor the agent beyond the usual convalescent period. These people become **chronic carriers** who persist in carrying the infectious agent and may communicate it to others over a prolonged period. Chronic carriers are usually restricted from certain forms of employment, called sensitive occupations, based on the mode of transmission for the particular disease. The concept of sensitive occupations is discussed in greater detail in Chapter 30. Chronic carriers are frequently associated with staphylococcal and streptococcal illness or typhoid.

The last category of human carrier to be considered is **transient carriers.** These persons carry the agent for a limited period but never exhibit signs or symptoms of the illness. For example, someone who has a "subclinical case" of a disease is a transient carrier.

A third type of reservoir involves free-living agents. Hookworm is an example of a free-living agent for which soil is the reservoir. Plants may also be considered free-living agents of health problems.

As noted earlier, an **intermediary** provides the means of transmitting certain agents from reservoir to host. Intermediaries can be either living or nonliving. Living intermediaries are **vectors.** An example of a vector is the flea that transmits *Yersinia pestis,* the bacterium that causes bubonic plague, from infected rodents (the reservoir) to humans (the host). As previously mentioned, the *Anopheles* mosquito functions as an intermediary in malaria, transmitting *Plasmodium* from infected to uninfected individuals.

A nonliving intermediary is called a **vehicle.** Another term that may be used for this type of intermediary is *fomite.* Scabies is frequently transmitted by means of a vehicle. Clothing worn by the infested person contains eggs of the mite. When the clothing is worn by another person, the eggs hatch and infest the other person as well. Food and water also serve as common vehicles for several communicable diseases.

Lifestyle Factors

Dever (1991) contended that lifestyle factors are the greatest contributors to most health problems and provide the best avenue for control of those problems. Lifestyle factors include employment, consumption patterns, and leisure activity and associated risks. Employment or occupation may influence health in several ways including the potential for exposure to hazardous conditions. The fact of being employed (or unemployed) may influence access to survival necessities as well as to health care. Consumption patterns include dietary and exercise patterns as well as the use or abuse of substances like tobacco, caffeine, and alcohol and other drugs. Finally, recreational aspects of lifestyle may influence health either in their presence or absence. Absence of recreational opportunities or leisure activities may influence the effects of stress on health. Certain types of recreation, on the other hand, may contribute to health problems. For example, for the person whose primary mode of recreation is watching television, cardiovascular disease is enhanced. Similarly, persons who engage in mountain biking or skiing encounter injury risks.

Health Care System Factors

Factors within the health care system and the attitudes and activities of health care providers also contribute to health and illness. For example, studies indicate that specific messages from personal health providers influence clients' health promotive behaviors (Hunt, Kristal, White, Lynch, & Fries, 1995). The health care system may also exert negative effects on health. Invasive medical procedures, for example, may increase the risk of HIV or hepatitis infection, or health care providers may miss, or even ignore, evidence of spouse, elder, or child abuse.

Each of the three epidemiologic models presented here can be used to organize information related to client health status, to identify health problems, and to direct intervention. The epidemiologic triad is the most familiar of the three models, but may be somewhat difficult to use in describing health problems that have no identifiable agent or that arise from the complex interaction of multiple factors. The web of causation model addresses the complexity of factors influencing health and illness, but its very complexity may limit its utility. In using the model, one could potentially go on at length examining causative factors. This model is useful, however, in identifying points at which intervention is likely to eliminate or control a health problem. Neither of these two models acknowledges the influence of the health care system on the health of populations, nor do they highlight lifestyle factors that are some of the greatest

influences on health and illness. Dever's model incorporates these elements, but fails to address other aspects of health behavior, such as use of safety measures, that may influence health. For these reasons, the Dimensions Model which incorporates the dimensions of health as outlined in Chapter 5 will be used to provide an epidemiologic perspective throughout the remainder of this book.

► THE DIMENSIONS MODEL AND AN "EPIDEMIOLOGY OF HEALTH"

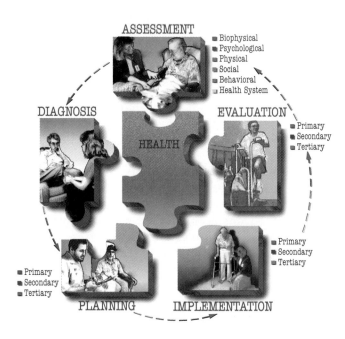

To this point, epidemiology has been discussed primarily in relation to problems of ill health. In addition to considering factors that contribute to or prevent specific problems, community health nurses should investigate and identify those factors that promote health. It has been suggested that the health care professions should focus on an "epidemiology of health."

From its beginning, community health nursing has been engaged in health promotion, and this should remain a primary focus of community health nursing practice. Recently, other health care providers have become aware of the need for promoting health in addition to treating or even preventing specific diseases. This recognition is coming slowly, however, and community health nursing has the advantage of already being the forerunner in this area.

Interest in health promotion has occurred as a result of the shift from infectious to chronic disease as the major cause of death. This shift has been accompanied by increased cost for medical care, changes in payment sources, and research indicating that individual behavior may contribute to chronic illness. These factors have encouraged consumers and funders of health care services to turn to health promotion and behavior modification as means of decreasing costs.

Health promotion has been defined by the World Health Organization (WHO) as the "process of enabling people to increase control over and to improve their own health" (cited in Harkness, 1995). According to the Canadian Public Health Association (1996), health promotion is characterized by an interactive perspective that recognizes the interplay of individual behavior and environmental forces in determining health. Health promotion supports a holistic approach to health in all its facets and focuses on long-term gains. Decisions for health promotion are both centralized and decentralized and true health promotion requires activity within multiple sectors of society and the cooperative efforts of a variety of disciplines. Finally, health promotion is characterized by an emphasis on public accountability for health outcomes. Health promotion differs from health protection or illness prevention in that health protection is directed toward decreasing the probability of illness, whereas health promotion focuses on increasing one's level of well-being (Pender, 1996).

Health promotion entails responsibilities for clients, health care professionals, and society. Clients need to pursue health and health care actively by means of health-related behaviors, while professionals facilitate healthy behavior by clients. Community health nurses do this by preparing individuals to make behavior choices that maximize their health potential. Such preparation may occur on a one-to-one basis or with groups of clients. Societal responsibilities in health promotion include providing access to health promotive services for all people and creating an environment that enhances health.

Critical Dimensions of Nursing in Health Promotion

Elements of each of the dimensions of nursing within the Dimensions Model are required for effective health promotion by community health nurses. In the cognitive dimension, community health nurses must have knowledge of factors that enhance health-promoting behavior in selected populations (eg, young children or members of an ethnic minority group). In addition, the nurse must be aware of actions that promote health and those that do not. Interpersonal dimension skills of communication and collaboration are also needed to motivate clients to engage in health promoting behaviors. In the ethical dimension, community health nurses may need to modify the empha-

sis on personal behaviors and promote awareness of environmental aspects of health promotion that must be addressed at the societal, rather than individual, level. The intellectual skills of diagnostic reasoning and analysis from the skills dimension will enable the nurse to identify client and community needs for health promotion, and virtually all of the processes in the process dimension of nursing can be brought to bear on health promotion efforts. For example, the nurse may need to employ the political process to assure the availability of health promotion services to the public. Finally, research and program evaluation skills in the reflective dimension will provide the knowledge base used for health promotion and program planning.

Identifying the Dimensions of Health

To promote health, the community health nurse must have a solid grasp of factors that lead to optimal health. Using the epidemiologic process with *health,* rather than a health problem, as the focus is one means of identifying these factors. Using the dimensions of health as a framework, community health nurses can examine the biophysical, psychological, physical, social, behavioral, and health system factors that promote health.

Factors in the biophysical dimension that promote health include the absence or control of existing physical health problems, a healthy gene pool, and activities that promote normal growth and development. Activities designed to prevent or control illness lie in the realms of health protection, illness prevention, and secondary prevention and do not reflect health promotion per se. Genetic inheritance can be manipulated to promote health at the population level when genetic counseling regarding the probability of disease in offspring leads to contraceptive decisions. Knowledge of genetic factors may also serve as a motivating factor in promoting healthier behavior by people who have a predisposition to heart disease and other conditions. Perhaps the aspect of the biophysical dimension in which health promotion efforts can have the greatest impact is that of growth and development. Adequate nutrition and opportunities that facilitate development can contribute to health in this area.

Factors that promote health also arise in the internal and external psychological dimension. Adequate coping skills and abilities to adapt to environmental changes without diminishing health are internal factors that promote health. Environments that are relatively free of stress promote health in the external psychological dimension, as does the availability of emotional support.

Physical dimension factors that promote health include an environment free of safety hazards and environmental pollutants. Adequate housing and aesthetic surroundings also promote health in this dimension. Opportunities for social interaction and participation in social policy making are factors that promote health in the social dimension. A social environment that emphasizes healthy behaviors and downplays those that are unhealthy is also conducive to health. Health promotion efforts have focused extensively on the behavioral dimension in efforts to influence health status. Lifestyles that include adequate rest and exercise, nonsmoking, adequate nutrition, and consistent use of safety measures promote health and prevent health problems. Refraining from caffeine and tobacco consumption and engaging in moderate to no use of alcohol are other health promotion factors in the behavioral dimension.

Health system factors that promote health include the availability and accessibility of health promotion services. Health education and emphasis on promotion by health care professionals are other factors promoting health in this dimension. Health professionals who serve as role models in health promotion behaviors can also enhance the health of the population.

Unfortunately, although there is evidence to support the beneficial effects of health promotion activities related to each of the dimensions of health, the extent to which most of these activities are performed by the general public is minimal. Some progress has been made, but many people continue to eat high-fat diets, maintain sedentary lifestyles, use ineffective coping styles, and fail to use seat belts and other protective measures. It is obvious that health promotion efforts have not yet become an inseparable element of life or of health care delivery.

Employing Health Promotion Strategies

By their very nature, strategies to promote health occur within the primary prevention dimension of health care. There are five categories of health promotion strategies: health education, health appraisal, lifestyle modification, provision of a healthy environment, and development of effective coping skills. Health education will be discussed in detail in Chapter 9.

Health Appraisal

Health appraisal is the process of identifying factors that influence the health of an individual or a group. From the perspective of health promotion, a thorough health appraisal can identify healthy behaviors to be reinforced and indicate areas in which health-promot-

---

Critical Thinking in Research

A study conducted by Lusk, Kerr, and Ronis (1995) examined health-promoting behaviors among U.S. blue-collar, skilled trade, and white-collar workers using the Health-Promoting Lifestyle Inventory (HPLP). Significant differences were noted among the three groups on the self-actualization, exercise, nutrition, and interpersonal support subscales of the HPLP, but not on the stress management and health responsibility subscales. White-collar workers scored significantly higher than other groups on self-actualization, exercise, and interpersonal support, and blue-collar workers scored significantly lower than the other groups on nutrition and overall health-promoting lifestyle. When education level was controlled, differences between groups were eliminated suggesting that education level, rather than job category per se, influences health-promoting behaviors.

1. What are the implications of study findings for fostering health promotion behaviors in the American public?
2. Are there other possible explanations for the differences noted between groups in their health-promoting behaviors? If so, what might they be?
3. How would your approach to health promotion differ if your alternate explanation proved to be correct?

---

ing behaviors are not being performed. By conducting health appraisals, community health nurses can help clients identify areas for behavior change to enhance and promote health. They can also identify healthy behaviors currently performed and encourage clients to continue these behaviors. For example, the nurse might encourage an older client to continue daily walks as a form of exercise. Appendix B provides information on several health-risk appraisal tools that can be used to assess client lifestyles and health promotive behaviors.

Lifestyle Modification

The health appraisal provides direction for the next health promotion strategy, lifestyle modification. This strategy involves action in regard to health behaviors rather than just identification provided by the health appraisal. An attempt is made to motivate clients to make lifestyle changes that promote health. For example, a relatively sedentary individual would be encouraged to exercise.

Providing a Healthy Environment

Another health promotion strategy, providing a healthy environment, involves consideration of a client's physical, psychological, and social environments. Safety hazards can be eliminated from the physical environment. For example, a home with small children can be "child proofed," and safety precautions can be taken in handling hazardous substances in the workplace. Other approaches to providing a healthy physical environment include the use of protective devices such as seat belts, hearing protection in high-noise-level areas, mandatory motorcycle helmet use, and legislation and engineering efforts to curb environmental pollution, and so on.

Attention should also be given to the psychological environment. For example, many businesses are attempting to reduce employee stress levels as a means of promoting health. Interventions designed to enhance self-esteem, especially among children, also create a more healthful psychological environment.

Changes in the social environment can also foster health. Positive attitudes to healthy behaviors such as exercising, not drinking, and not overeating can create peer pressure to engage in such behaviors. For example, campaigns to make exercise the "in thing to do" change public attitudes toward exercise and promote exercise by individuals. Social and economic changes can also enhance client access to health promotion services. Providing exercise facilities in the workplace is another example of a social environment change reflecting changes in employer attitudes toward health promotion that influence the behavior of individual employees.

Developing Coping Skills

The last category of strategies for health promotion involves developing effective ways of coping with stress. People who can deal adequately with life's stresses experience fewer stress-related physical and psychological problems. Community health nurses can assist clients to identify sources of stress in their lives. Efforts can then be undertaken to identify coping strategies that allow the particular client to deal with these sources of stress. For example, one client may be encouraged to engage in physical activity to reduce the effects of stress, whereas another might be taught relaxation techniques. Or, the client may be assisted to develop more positive approaches to problem solving as a way of dealing with stress.

The community health nurse should be knowledgeable about health promotion strategies and have expertise in their implementation. Nurses and clients may obtain information about health promotion from a variety of agencies and organizations. Some are listed at the end of this chapter.

TESTING YOUR UNDERSTANDING

1. Describe at least two theories of disease causation. During what periods of history were these theories prevalent? (pp. 144–145)

Critical Thinking in Practice: A Case in Point

Janie, a 14-year-old girl, lives with her mother and grandmother. Janie's parents are divorced and she sees her father only during the summer because he lives in another state. Janie has been having occasional sexual intercourse with her steady boyfriend, Jim, for about a year. She started having sex with him because he told her he would find another girlfriend if she didn't. Most of Janie's girlfriends are also sexually active.

Janie is not using contraceptives. She feels guilty about her sexual activity and keeps telling herself that she isn't going to have sex with Jim any more. Janie's mother and grandmother both work, so Janie is home alone after school until her mother gets home about 5 P.M. Jim usually walks Janie home from school on days when he doesn't have football practice. He frequently stays and has dinner with Janie and her family.

Last week Janie found out that she is pregnant. She is afraid to tell her mother and comes to you, the nurse at her school, for assistance.

1. What factors in the biophysical dimension influenced Janie's pregnancy?
2. What factors in the psychological dimension contributed to Janie's pregnancy?
3. What social dimension factors contributed to Janie's pregnancy?
4. What behavioral dimension factors are involved in this situation? How have they influenced Janie's pregnancy?
5. What factors in the health system dimension might be involved in this situation?
6. What primary, secondary, and tertiary prevention measures might influence this situation?

2. Identify at least three criteria for determining causality in a relationship between two events. Give an example of each. (pp. 145–146)
3. Define risk. Identify at least two risk factors for cardiovascular disease. Who are among the population at risk for cardiovascular disease? (p. 146)
4. Distinguish between morbidity and mortality rates. Give an example of each. (pp. 147–149)
5. Distinguish between incidence and prevalence rates. Give an example of each. Which would give you more information about the effects of a primary prevention program? Why? (pp. 147–148)
6. What are the six steps of the epidemiologic process? (pp. 149–151)
7. Differentiate between experimental and observational studies. Give an example of each. (p. 152)
8. Describe the three types of observational studies. (p. 152)
9. Describe the three major elements of the epidemiologic triad. Identify at least two considerations related to each. (pp. 153–156)
10. Describe the web of causation model. (pp. 156–158)
11. What are the four major components of Dever's epidemiologic model? Identify at least two considerations related to each component. (pp. 158–160)
12. Describe at least three strategies for health promotion. Give an example of each. (pp. 162–163)

WHAT DO YOU THINK?
Questions for Critical Thinking

1. Trace the natural history of a specific health condition. What factors would affect the outcome of this condition? How could these factors be altered to achieve a better outcome?
2. What health promotion activities could be used to modify social factors contributing to disease in the general population?
3. Does the media have a role in health promotion? If yes, what should that role be?
4. How might an individual's level of risk for a specific condition differ from that of the population at large for the same condition?

REFERENCES

Canadian Public Health Association. (1996, July). *Action statement for health promotion in Canada*. Ottawa, Ontario: Canadian Public Health Association.

Dever, G. E. A. (1991). *Community health analysis: A global analysis at the local level* (2nd ed.). Gaithersburg, MD: Aspen.

Gordis, L. (1996). *Epidemiology*. Philadelphia: W. B. Saunders.

Greenburg, R. S. (1993). *Medical epidemiology*. Norwalk, CT: Appleton & Lange.

Harkness, G. A. (1995). *Epidemiology in nursing practice*. St. Louis: Mosby.

Harper, A. C., & Lambert, L. J. (1994). *The health of populations: An introduction* (2nd ed.). New York: Springer.

Hunt, J. R., Kristal, A. R., White, E., Lynch, J. C., & Fries, E. (1995). Physician recommendations for dietary change: Their prevalence and impact in a population-based sample. *American Journal of Public Health, 85,* 722–725.

Lusk, S. L., Kerr, M. J., & Ronis, D. L. (1995). Health-promoting lifestyles of blue-collar, skilled trade, and white-collar workers. *Nursing Research, 44,* 20–24.

Pender, N. J. (1996). *Health promotion in nursing practice* (3rd ed.). Stamford, CT: Appleton & Lange.

Timmreck, T. C. (1994). *An introduction to epidemiology*. Boston: Jones and Bartlett.

Tyler, C. W., & Last, J. M. (1992). Epidemiology. In J. M. Last & R. B. Wallace (Eds.), *Maxcy-Rosenau-Last public health and preventive medicine* (13th ed.) (pp. 11–39). Norwalk, CT: Appleton & Lange.

Valanis, B. (1999). *Epidemiology in health care* (3rd ed.). Stamford, CT: Appleton & Lange.

EPIDEMIOLOGIC RESOURCES

American College of Epidemiology
PO Box 10639
Rockville, MD 20849

International Epidemiological Association
c/o Norman Naah
KCSMD
Department of Public Health and Epidemiology
Bessemer Road
London SE5 9RJ England

Society for Epidemiologic Research
c/o Dr. Joseph L. Lyon
Department of Family and Preventive Medicine
50 N. Medical Drive IC26
Salt Lake City, UT 84132

RESOURCES FOR HEALTH PROMOTION

Action on Smoking & Health
2013 H Street, NW
Washington, DC 20006
(202) 659–4310

American College of Sports Medicine
PO Box 1440
Indianapolis, IN 46206–1440
(317) 637–9200

American College of Preventive Medicine
1660 L. Street, Ste. 206
Washington, DC 20006–5603
(202) 466–2044

American Hospital Association Center for Health Promotion
American Hospital Association
1 N. Franklin, Ste. 27
Chicago, IL 60606
(312) 422–3000

National Eldercare Institute on Health Promotion
601 E. Street, NW. Fifth Floor, Bldg B
Washington, DC 20049
(202) 434–2200

National Center for Chronic Disease Prevention and Health Promotion
4770 Buford Highway, NE
Mailstop K13
Atlanta, GA 30333
(770) 488–5080

President's Council on Physical Fitness and Sports
701 Pennsylvania Avenue, NW, Ste. 250
Washington, DC 20004
(202) 272–3424

Wellness Associates
21489 Orr Springs Road
Ukiah, CA 95482
(707) 937–2331

A Wellness Center, Inc.
145 West 28th Street, Room 9R
New York, NY 10001
(212) 465–8062

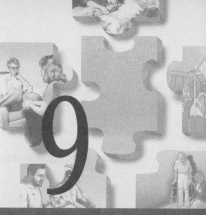

9

THE HEALTH EDUCATION PROCESS

Much of the practice of community health nursing involves educating people about healthier lifestyles. As a primary preventive measure, health education is directed toward promoting health and preventing illness. The health education process also can be used at the secondary and tertiary levels of prevention. As a secondary prevention measure, community health nurses might teach clients about self-care related to specific health problems. Teaching clients to minimize the consequences of health problems or to prevent their recurrence is the object of health education at the tertiary prevention level. Whatever the level of prevention involved, the health education process used remains the same.

The health education process includes two components: learning theory derived from the behavioral sciences, and information content derived from the health sciences. *Health education* has been described as the use of a variety of learning experiences to facilitate changes to more healthful behaviors (Green & Kreuter, 1991) and as a process that frees people to make health-related decisions based on full knowledge of the consequences of their choices (Greenberg, 1991). Learning experiences that free people to make appropriate decisions are created using a systematic health education process, one element of the process dimension of community health nursing.

► Chapter Objectives

After reading this chapter, you should be able to:

- Describe three types of health-related decisions facilitated by health education.
- Describe at least two barriers to health education.
- Assess learning needs in terms of the six dimensions of health.
- Identify five levels of educational diagnosis.
- Distinguish between process and outcome learning objectives.
- Describe five components of learning objectives.
- Classify learning objectives according to the domains of learning involved.
- Define a focusing event.
- Describe the use of formative evaluation in a health education encounter.
- Describe at least four guidelines for developing health education programs.

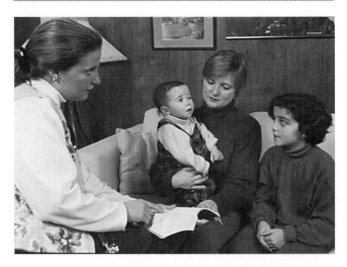

Much of the practice of community health nursing involves educating people about healthier lifestyles. Health education will help the client to make appropriate health decisions for themselves and their families.
From: Berger, K., & Williams, M. (1999). Fundamentals of nursing: Collaborating for optimal health (2nd ed.). Stamford, CT: Appleton & Lange.

► PURPOSE OF HEALTH EDUCATION

The purpose of health education is to assist clients in making appropriate health-related decisions. Clients can make three types of decisions: decisions about personal health behaviors, decisions about use of available health resources, and decisions about societal health issues (Pew Commission, 1995).

Personal Health Behaviors

Health education enables people to make decisions regarding personal behaviors that promote health or prevent or cure illness. Should I smoke? Should I change my diet? Should I exercise? Should I have my child immunized? How should I deal with stress? How should I discipline my child? Should I take my blood pressure medication? Should I stay off my ankle like the nurse told me to? All of these questions require decisions that can be influenced by health education.

Health education has been perceived as a means of freeing people from factors that "enslave" them to unhealthy behaviors (Greenberg, 1991). Unhealthy behavior, in this perspective, is believed to arise from a need to conform that results from poor self-esteem, alienation, guilt, hostility, anger, low assertiveness, inability to communicate effectively, and isolation. The purpose of health education, then, is to improve self-esteem, clarify values, reduce alienation and isolation, and improve clients' understanding of their own mo-

tivations to free them to make appropriate health decisions. As we can see, health education involves more than imparting knowledge and skills, but includes changing and creating attitudes conducive to healthful behavior.

Resource Use

The second type of health decision that people make relates to their use of health resources. Am I sick enough to go to the doctor? Should I see a nurse practitioner or a physician? Should I use the emergency room for care or find a regular health care provider? Health education can help people become aware of the health care resources available to them and help them make decisions regarding what type of resources to use and when to use them.

Health Issues

The third type of decision that can be influenced by health education includes decisions related to societal health issues. Health education, for example, can help people determine whether they should vote for or against mandatory screening for AIDS in the general population, or whether they should contribute funds to the local heart association. Health education can also aid in decisions regarding the merits of motorcycle helmet laws, banning of smoking in public places, or development of a nuclear power plant. Health education can create an informed public prepared to make thoughtful decisions on major health issues.

► BARRIERS TO LEARNING

Prior to planning health education, the community health nurse must recognize that barriers to learning need to be overcome if health education is to be effective. Barriers may be internal or external. Internal barriers can be physical, social, or psychological. Physical barriers such as pain, fever, and visual disturbances, could interfere with clients' abilities to focus on concepts presented. Social barriers to learning may include the client's education level, language barriers, and incongruence of client beliefs and values with those of the health system. Psychological barriers include anxiety, depression, denial, and inability to accept or, occasionally, overacceptance of the sick role. Other psychological barriers might be previous negative experiences with illness or the health care system and lack of readiness to learn.

External barriers to learning may arise from the learning environment (eg, noise, distractions) or from the learning situation. Factors related to the learning situation that may create barriers include the timing of educational efforts, the method of teaching used, the level of material presented, or the quality of interaction between nurse and client. In using the educational process, the community health nurse identifies potential barriers in a given client situation and circumvents these barriers by planning appropriate interventions.

Another potential barrier to desired behavior arising from health education is the *double bind in science policy* (Stein, 1992). This term refers to health education offerings that present conflicting messages. For example, one might attempt to educate adolescents that sexual abstinence is a desired behavior, telling them at the same time to use condoms when they do have sex. Such conflicting messages can undermine the effectiveness of health education efforts and confuse the learner regarding which of the two incompatible behaviors is desired. Some of the confusion in health education may arise from the multicentric and fragmented nature of the health care system (Bastable, 1997a).

One final barrier to desired behavior as a result of health education has been called iatrogenic health education disease (Greenberg, 1991). *Iatrogenic health*

education disease is disease or adverse response caused or made worse by health education. For example, when one teaches a client about possible side effects of medications, the power of suggestion may create those side effects. Similarly, routine education about child safety for new parents may cause them to be overprotective and hinder the child's development. The nurse should remain alert to the potential for such responses to health education and take action to minimize or avoid this type of response.

► THEORIES OF LEARNING

An understanding of how learning occurs helps the community health nurse educator to facilitate learning and behavior change among clients. A variety of learning theories provide that understanding. The theories addressed here include behavioral, cognitive, social, psychodynamic, and humanistic theories (Braungart & Braungart, 1997).

Behavioral Learning Theory

In the behavioral perspective, learning is the result of conditioning in which the learner's behavior is reinforced, either positively or negatively, until the desired behavior becomes the habitual response. Teaching, from this perspective, is a matter of arranging stimuli to elicit the desired response and then reinforcing that response (Babcock & Miller, 1994). For example, a group of young children may be presented with a set of pictures of different foods spread on a table and asked to select foods that contain vitamins. Each correct selection is verbally approved and the child gets to put the picture in the "vitamin" box. A negative verbal comment is made each time a child selects an incorrect food item, and the child is told to replace the picture on the table. Through repeated performances and reinforcement, the children should learn to correctly distinguish vitamin-rich foods from other foods.

Cognitive Learning Theory

According to cognitive learning theory, learning involves a complex process of information recognition, classification, coding, storage, and retrieval for use at the appropriate time (Braungart & Braungart, 1997). This type of learning is also known as information processing (Babcock & Miller, 1994). Behavior based on the information arises as a result of expected consequences valued by the learner (Fleury, 1992). Operating from this perspective, the teacher presents content in a fashion that allows it to be easily integrated into the learner's existing network of information after determining how that network is organized and what prior information it contains (Babcock & Miller, 1994). As an example, the community health nurse educator might determine what a group of high school students knows about communicable diseases in general and then introduce content related to HIV infection by comparing and contrasting the new content with prior knowledge. Behavior to prevent HIV infection would occur when students perceive and value the expected outcome of not being infected.

Social Learning Theory

Social learning theory, developed by Bandura, combines aspects of behavioral and cognitive learning theories (Redman, 1993). The learner attends to new behaviors as modeled by others, including the consequences of the behavior (reinforcing factors), integrates the observations into an existing network, stores and retrieves information to reproduce the behavior, and receives reinforcement through experiencing the expected and valued consequences (Braungart & Braungart, 1997). Returning to the example of the children learning about vitamin-rich foods, children in the group would learn not only from the results of their own food selections, but from observing the outcomes of classmates' selections as well.

Psychodynamic Learning Theory

In the psychodynamic perspective, emotional motivations influence learning. These emotions are derived from past experiences. Suppose, for example, that a nursing student was forced as a child to eat some food he or she abhorred. He or she may later have difficulty learning about the nutritional content of that food. Conversely, fear of becoming a burden to family members may motivate a client to relearn self-care skills following a stroke.

Humanistic Learning Theory

Humanistic learning theories focus on internal motivation for learning rather than on external consequences that figure in behavioral, cognitive, and social theories. One of the most well known of these theories is probably already familiar to you and is based on Maslow's hierarchy of human needs (Braungart & Braungart, 1997). From this perspective, learning is motivated from within by one's need to become self-actualized. In this perspective, both cognitive (informational) learning and affective (attitudinal) learning

are important (Gleit, 1998). Teachers operating from this perspective encourage learners to identify and pursue their own needs for learning. Thus, the role of the teacher becomes one of responding to learners' requests (Babcock & Miller, 1994). As an example, a nurse educator might ask a group of clients enrolled in a parenting class what aspects of parenting are most problematic for them and what areas they would like the class to address.

▶ PRINCIPLES OF LEARNING

Each of the theories of learning presented here conveys some understanding of how learning occurs and what kinds of activities influence learning. This understanding, in turn, gives rise to several principles of learning or statements about conditions that facilitate learning. The community health nurse educator uses these principles to create situations and experiences conducive to learning. Several general principles of learning are listed in Table 9–1.

The first few principles relate to the learner. People vary with respect to their need for information and their perception of its relevance. This variability

TABLE 9–1. GENERAL PRINCIPLES OF LEARNING

LEARNER
- People learn best what they perceive to be most relevant.
- Motivation to learn enhances learning.
- People learn in different ways.

LEARNING SITUATION
- The context of the learning situation influences learning.

PRESENTATION OF CONTENT
- Relevance of content to the learner enhances learning.
- Individualization of presentation to the learner promotes learning.
- Multiple modes of presenting content enhance learning.
- Focusing the learner's attention facilitates learning.
- Content presented first is learned best.
- Logical organization of content facilitates learning.
- Progression from simple content to more complex content promotes learning.
- Association of new material with previous learning enhances learning.
- Presentation of positive, rather than negative, behaviors facilitates behavior change.
- Active participation by the learner facilitates learning.
- Imitation promotes learning.

REINFORCEMENT AND RETENTION
- Repetition enhances learning.
- Positive reinforcement is more effective than negative reinforcement.
- Prompt and accurate feedback enhances learning.
- Recency of learning influences retention.
- Application of information in several contexts promotes generalization of learning.

results in differing levels of motivation or willingness to learn which, in turn, influences learning. People also vary in the modes by which they learn best. For example, some people learn what they see (visual learners), whereas others learn what they hear (auditory learners). Still others learn kinesthetically, by physical manipulation of objects, for example, writing down what they see and hear (Kitchie, 1997).

Learner differences are one aspect of the context of the learning situation that affects learning. Other factors within that context may include psychological factors, such as the degree of trust the learner has for the teacher, or aspects of the physical environment that affect the learning situation.

Variability among learners and learning situations means that various modes of presenting health-related materials will be more effective with some people than with others. Despite this variability, however, there are some general principles related to the way in which material is presented that apply to most health education encounters. These are included under Presentation of Content in Table 9–1. Because of the differences among learners, the more a health-related presentation is tailored to the needs and capabilities of individual learners, the more effective it will be. People learn in a variety of ways, so presenting content in several ways creates greater opportunity for learning. First, however, learners must attend to the presentation, so the nurse educator attempts to focus their attention. Because people tend to learn best what is presented first, the educator may want to present the most important material immediately after gaining the learners' attention.

Content that is logically organized and that associates new material with prior learning facilitates the integration of new concepts into learners' existing cognitive frameworks. Progressing from simple concepts to more complex content creates a sense of mastery that increases the motivation to learn. Similarly, focusing on desirable behaviors facilitates behavior change more effectively than focusing on behavior to be eliminated. For example, a health education message to "use condoms" encourages a positive behavior, whereas the negatively worded message "don't have unprotected sex" leaves learners wondering what they should do.

People learn from doing. From this perspective, it is easy to see why it is important for learners to participate actively in a learning encounter. One form of participation is imitation of the desired behavior which also promotes learning.

Once a behavior has been learned, it needs to be reinforced before it becomes a habitual response for the learner. Principles of learning related to reinforcement and retention of learning are listed last in Table

9–1. Both repetition and reinforcement enhance learning. In this regard, positive reinforcement is more effective than negative reinforcement. Negative reinforcement can create psychological effects such as anxiety that may impede learning. Prompt and accurate, rather than delayed, feedback on the learner's performance also reinforces learning whether the feedback is positive or negative. Positive feedback creates a sense of success and increases motivation to learn; negative feedback, if it includes suggestions for improving performance, can allay anxiety by providing direction.

Material learned recently is more easily retrieved from stored memory than material learned some time ago. This suggests that if current content is to build on prior learning, a review of prior content may be helpful to reinforce that prior learning and provide readily accessible associations for integrating new material. In a similar way, application of learning in several contexts reinforces learning at the same time it promotes generalization to new situations (Breckon, Harvey, & Lancaster, 1994).

▶ THE DIMENSIONS MODEL AND HEALTH EDUCATION

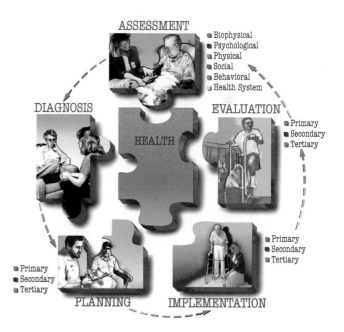

The community health nurse uses the Dimensions Model to design a health education encounter. The education process consists of assessing the learner and the learning setting in terms of the dimensions of health, diagnosing learning needs, and planning, implementing, and evaluating a health education presentation within the dimensions of nursing and health care. A tool to assist in applying the educational process is included in Appendix C.

Critical Dimensions of Nursing in Health Education

Several of the dimensions of nursing enter into effective use of the health education process, which is itself an element of the process dimension. In the cognitive dimension, the community health nurse requires knowledge of principles of teaching and learning as well as content knowledge in the area to be taught. Communication skills, an element of the interpersonal dimension, are critical to effective health education for clients at all levels, individual, family, or community. Motivation skills are another important element in the interpersonal dimension. In the skills dimension, the effective health educator possesses good organization and planning skills as well as the diagnostic skills required to identify clients' learning needs and preferred styles of learning. The change, leadership, and group processes are elements of the process dimension that may be brought into play in the health education encounter. For example, the nurse may need to bring about changes in clients' attitudes for health education to result in behavior changes. Finally, the most important element of the reflective dimension in a health education situation is evaluation. The community health nurse must be able to evaluate the effectiveness of health education.

 Assessing the Learner and the Learning Setting

The health education process begins with an assessment of the learner, his or her learning needs, and the learning environment. When the client is a group or a community, the first task in assessment is to identify the target audience for the educational effort. Selection of the target audience may be based on level of need, resources available, or probability of success. Assessment then proceeds to identifying characteristics of the client that influence the learning situation. The assessment can be conducted in terms of the six dimensions of health: the biophysical, psychological, physical, social, behavioral, and health system dimensions.

The Biophysical Dimension

Human biology influences both the learning needs and the learning capabilities of the client. Areas for consideration include skills and needs related to the client's level of maturation and adequacy of the client's physiologic function.

Skills and Needs Related to the Level of Maturation. To learn effectively, the client needs to have the skills appropriate to his or her level of maturation. In educational terms this is called developmental readiness. For example, small children who have not yet developed abilities for abstract thought will need concrete examples of concepts to be learned. Similarly, a child who still has poorly developed eye–hand coordination will have difficulty learning insulin injection techniques, so teaching will necessarily involve parents as well.

Age or maturation level also affects the client's need for education. For instance, a preschool child does not need information about menstruation, but a preadolescent girl does. In addition, the client's maturation level may influence his or her existing knowledge of a particular subject. For example, a group of third graders will probably have a broader knowledge of nutrition concepts than preschoolers.

Physiologic Function. Assessing a client's physiologic function may reveal special needs for health education or impediments to learning. For example, a young girl with recurrent urinary tract infections may require education on appropriate hygiene, and a diabetic client may require information and assistance with diet, exercise, medication, foot care, and other self-care measures. Inadequate physiologic function can also give rise to impediments to learning. For example, a group of hearing-impaired youngsters or visually impaired older people require specialized approaches to health education to facilitate their ability to learn.

The Psychological Dimension

Elements of the psychological dimension can profoundly influence the client's willingness and ability to learn. Attitudes toward health and health behaviors can either enhance or detract from the motivation to learn. Among clients attending a series of parenting classes, for example, those parents who attend only because of a court mandate related to child abuse usually benefit less than those who attend because they perceive a need for help. Motivation to learn begins with an awareness of a need to learn, and the first task of the community health nurse may be assisting the client to become aware of that need (Falvo, 1994).

Psychological factors such as stress and anxiety can also impede learning, even for those who are motivated to learn. Nurses can limit the negative effects of the psychological dimension by actions designed to decrease stress and anxiety. For example, the nurse can create a climate in which the client does not feel threatened and in which the nurse educator is seen as a source of support rather than a threat. The nurse who has children and who teaches parenting classes for abusive parents might create such a climate by beginning the first session with a description of the frustration the nurse sometimes feels as a parent.

Other psychological factors that motivate healthy client behaviors can be reinforced to enhance learning. For example, if saving money motivates a smoker, the nurse might focus on the cost savings to be expected when the client stops smoking.

The Physical Dimension

Conditions in the physical environment often give rise to the need for health education. For example, families living in older housing painted with lead-based paint need to be taught how to prevent lead poisoning. Similarly, a client using crutches whose apartment is upstairs needs to learn stair climbing with crutches.

The physical environment should also be considered in terms of its effects on learning. Is there adequate lighting for the tasks to be accomplished? Is there too much noise? Will clients be distracted by other activities occurring in the learning environment? During a home visit, for example, it might be wise to turn off the television before attempting to educate a hypertensive client about his or her medication.

The Social Dimension

The social dimension is particularly influential in shaping attitudes about health and health-related behaviors. For example, in one study, perceptions of peer attitudes toward sexual practices strongly influenced adoption of safe sex practices (Castro, Valdiserri, & Curran, 1992).

Elements of the social dimension can also influence one's exposure to health-related information. People with lower education levels are less likely than those with more formal education to have been exposed to prior health education. A client's education level necessarily influences the nurse's choice of teaching strategies and content to be presented.

The client's primary language is another social factor that might hamper learning abilities unless the nurse allows for language differences in planning health education. In conducting the client assessment, the nurse determines the client's fluency in the dominant language (usually English in the United States) as well as the language usually spoken by the client. When educating clients who speak other languages, community health nurses should keep in mind that educational materials translated directly from English may not convey the intended message or may be unintelligible to the client. Interpreters can

be used, but again it is important to use interpreters who speak a form of a language familiar to the particular client. Other important considerations in the use of interpreters include the interpreter's degree of familiarity with health terminology, difference in social background between client and interpreter, incorporation of possible personal bias by the interpreter, and issues of confidentiality (Falvo, 1994). Other social dimension elements that may give rise to learning needs or influence clients' abilities to learn include the attitudes and values of significant others, cultural beliefs and practices, and religious influences. A client's occupation is another social dimension factor that can influence specific learning needs. Trash collectors, for example, might require education related to body mechanics and techniques for lifting heavy objects, whereas nurses require information about how to handle contaminated needles and other equipment.

The Behavioral Dimension

Behavioral dimension factors influence client needs for health education. For example, the client who overeats will probably need dietary education, and those who do not use seat belts need safety education. Other health-related behaviors may also give rise to health education needs. Smokers may need help with smoking cessation and education on alternative ways to meet needs satisfied by smoking. Similarly, sexually active clients may need education regarding contraceptives and safe sexual practices.

The Health System Dimension

In the health system dimension, health care recommendations may precipitate a need for health education. For example, clients may need to be educated on the correct use of medications or how to keep a sprained ankle immobilized to promote healing. Elements of the health care regimen may also influence clients' abilities to learn. For example, the community health nurse may need to consider the effects of pain medication on learning abilities and either time education interventions when pain is controlled but the client is alert or educate a family member along with or instead of the client.

The degree of emphasis placed on health education by health care providers and providers' expertise in using the health education process are health care system factors that influence clients' health-related knowledge and attitudes. Health care providers who engage in health education need a strong background in both educational principles and health content. Community health nurses designing health education

ASSESSMENT TIPS: Assessing the Health Education Situation

Biophysical Dimension

Age

What is the age of the learner(s)?

What learning needs arise from the age and developmental level of the learner(s)?

How will the developmental level of the learner(s) affect the ability to learn?

How will the developmental level of the learner(s) influence teaching strategies and methods?

Physiologic Function

Do physical health problems give rise to the need for health education?

Does physiologic function pose any impediments to learning?

Will teaching strategies need to be modified to accommodate sensory deficits or other physical limitations of the learner(s)?

Psychological Dimension

Is the learner aware of the need for health education?

What is the learner's level of motivation to learn?

What factors will motivate clients to learn healthful behaviors?

Will the learner's attitudes toward health and health behaviors enhance or detract from learning ability?

Does the learner exhibit levels of stress or anxiety that are likely to interfere with learning?

Physical Dimension

Are there conditions in the learner's physical environment that give rise to a need for health education?

What effects will the physical environment have on learning?

Are there elements of the physical environment that will distract learners?

Social Dimension

What effects will the learner's peers have on motivation to learn?

What is the current education level of the learner? What prior exposure to health information has the learner received?

How will the learner's education level influence teaching strategies and content?

What is the learner's primary language?

Are there cultural beliefs and practices that are likely to influence learning?

Does the learner's occupation give rise to a need for health education?

Are there other facets of the learner's social situation that may influence the health education session (eg, a need for child care during the presentation)?

Behavioral Dimension

Is there a need for education related to special dietary needs or other consumption patterns?

Is there a need for education related to rest and exercise?

Does the learner's sexual activity give rise to health education needs?

Do other current health behaviors give rise to a need for health education?

Health System Dimension

Does the learner's regular health care provider emphasize health education?

Does the learner have a need for education regarding the use of health care services?

Do health care recommendations give rise to a need for health education?

Are there elements of the health care regimen that may influence learning abilities (eg, medications)?

Will the learner's attitudes to health care services and providers influence the ability to learn?

offerings assess their ability to employ principles of education and take the steps needed to enhance that ability.

An assessment tool such as the Educational Planning and Implementation Guide (Appendix C) can be used to direct the community health nurse's assessment of the client and the learning situation. Completing the tool also documents assessment findings. In addition, the tool can be employed to document the other elements of the health education process discussed later in this chapter.

Diagnostic Reasoning and Educational Needs

Several years ago, noted health educator Lawrence Green and his colleagues (1991) developed the PRE-CEDE model for educational diagnosis. The acronym PRECEDE stands for *p*redisposing, *r*einforcing, and *e*nabling *c*auses in *e*ducational *d*iagnosis and *e*valuation and addresses five levels of educational diagnosis:

1. Social diagnosis: assessment of learner's quality of life
2. Epidemiologic diagnosis: identification of health problems
3. Behavioral and environmental diagnosis: identification of behavioral and environmental risk factors
4. Educational diagnosis: identification of predisposing, reinforcing, and enabling factors
5. Administrative and policy diagnosis: assessment of administrative and organizational resources and capabilities

In the first level of diagnosis, the community health nurse educator assesses clients' quality of life, problems encountered, and clients' priorities for resolving those problems. Epidemiologic diagnosis, the second level, consists of identifying health-related problems that are contributing to social problems identified in level 1. Third-level diagnosis addresses the environmental and behavioral risk factors underlying these health problems and targeted for intervention.

The educational diagnosis level involves identifying predisposing, reinforcing, and enabling factors that facilitate change to the desired health behavior (Richards, 1997). *Predisposing facts* are factors internal to the client that influence motivation for healthy behavior. These factors include knowledge, attitudes, and values related to the target behavior. *Reinforcing factors* are external forces that affect the client's motivation to act in a healthy way. Reinforcing factors include perceived rewards resulting from the behavior and feedback from significant others about the behavior. When the consequences of the behavior are perceived favorably and feedback from others is positive, the behavior in question is reinforced. For example, when freedom from HIV infection is valued and peers express positive attitudes toward condom use, use of condoms as a healthy behavior is fostered. *Enabling factors* are also external to the client and include other factors in a given situation that influence clients' abilities to act in a healthy manner. Using the previous example, the accessibility of condoms to sexually active adolescents is an enabling factor that influences condom use.

The final level of educational diagnosis in the PRECEDE model is administrative and policy diagnosis. At this level, the health educator assesses administrative and organizational resources and capabilities for developing a health education program to promote the targeted behavior. Incorporating all five levels of educational diagnosis, the community health nurse would develop a diagnostic statement expressing the client's learning needs. Such a diagnosis would be based on information derived from the assessments of the learner and learning setting. A sample diagnosis might be "Need for education regarding effective modes of discipline appropriate to child's age due to limited knowledge of child development, poor parental role models, and poor stress management skills." Reflected in this diagnosis are the social problem of potential child abuse related to parental disciplinary behaviors and the underlying factors contributing to the behavior. Subsumed in the diagnosis is the nurse's assessment of his or her organizational capability to address this need.

Since its development, the PRECEDE model has been linked to a PROCEED model in which the community health nurse educator proceeds to develop, implement, and evaluate a health education program related to the desired health behavior. PROCEED stands for *p*olicy, *r*egulatory, and *o*rganizational *c*onstructs for *e*ducational and *e*nvironmental *d*evelopment. The PROCEED model consists of four steps, the first being implementation of the educational plan and the last three reflecting process, impact, and outcome evaluation of the educational encounter (Richards, 1997). Execution of each of these steps in the health education process is guided by the educational assessment and diagnosis and is addressed in detail in the remainder of this chapter.

Planning the Health Education Encounter

Several tasks are to be accomplished in planning a health education encounter. These tasks include establishing priorities for health education, identifying goals and the level of prevention involved, developing and classifying objectives, and selecting content and teaching strategies. Reviewing or developing educational materials and planning evaluation are two additional tasks in planning a health education encounter.

Prioritizing Learning Needs

The first task in planning health education is prioritizing learning needs. A client may exhibit several unrelated learning needs. Because clients can assimilate only a certain amount of information at a time, the community health nurse and client need to decide which learning needs should be addressed first. Other needs can be addressed later, as time permits.

One approach to prioritizing educational needs begins with a list of clients' current unhealthful behaviors (Lorig, 1995). The second step in prioritization involves determining the relative effects of these behaviors and the benefits to be achieved by changing them. A third consideration is the ease with which specific behaviors can be changed. For example, one client may not use seat belts, get too little exercise, and not conduct monthly breast self-examinations. A change to using seat belts would result in the most immediate and dramatic benefit to the client and be the easiest of the three behaviors to change. For these reasons, the community health nurse might begin health education efforts in this area.

Identifying Goals and Levels of Prevention

Goal identification involves specifying the broad purpose of the lesson (Anspaugh & Ezell, 1994). The goals of a presentation on AIDS, for instance, might be to broaden learners' understanding of AIDS and to decrease fears of the disease. For an educational program on parenting, the goal would be the development of good parenting skills.

Identifying goals for an educational encounter also enables the community health nurse to identify the level of prevention to be addressed. For example, a goal of reducing the incidence of adolescent pregnancy indicates that education will be directed toward preventing teenage girls from becoming pregnant and involves primary prevention. The goal of preparing clients to give CPR in emergency situations, on the other hand, reflects secondary preven-tion—dealing with an existing problem—whereas an educational program directed at preventing further abuse of children by abusive parents reflects tertiary prevention.

Developing Learning Objectives

Developing specific learning objectives is the next activity in planning health education. *Learning objectives* are statements of specific behaviors expected in the health education encounter.

Objectives for learning encounters are of two types: process objectives and outcome objectives (Lorig, 1995). Process objectives are statements that define the process of client education and describe the actions to be taken by the nurse in educating the client. Outcome objectives are statements of behaviors the client is expected to perform as a result of the health education encounter.

Well-constructed process and outcome objectives for learning incorporate five components (Anspaugh & Ezell, 1994). The first component is the identification of the learner or actor, and the second is an action to be performed. The third component is the learning requirement or object of the action. For example, the nurse educator may be expected to "present content on iron-rich foods," and the client may be expected to "list foods high in iron." In the first example, the *nurse educator* is the actor, *present* is the action, and *content on iron-rich foods* is the learning requirement. In the second example, the actor is the *client*, the action is to *list*, and the learning requirement is *foods high in iron*. The objectives should also include conditions for the performance of the action. Using the previous example, the nurse might discuss iron-rich foods "consistent with the client's cultural preferences." The client, on the other hand, might be expected to list iron-rich foods "from memory." The final component of learning objectives is the criteria for judging the accomplishment of the objectives. This component of the objective reflects its measurability. In the dietary iron example, the complete objective for the nurse might read, "The nurse educator will present 20 iron-rich foods consistent with the client's cultural preferences." The expected outcome of the presentation might be that "the client will list at least 5 foods high in iron."

Classifying Objectives

Outcome objectives may be classified according to the learning domain to which they relate and the level of task within the domain (Bastable & Sculco, 1997). A *learning domain* reflects the type of learning desired as a result of the health education encounter. The four domains of learning developed thus far are the cognitive, affective, perceptual, and psychomotor domains (Bloom, Englehart, Furst, Hill, & Krathwohl, 1956). The cognitive domain encompasses intellectual skills related to factual information and its application. In the affective domain, the focus of learning is on attitudes and values. Emphasis in the psychomotor domain is on the learning of physical manipulative skills. Finally, in the perceptual domain, emphasis is on learning to perceive and extract information from stimuli. Another, as yet undeveloped, domain of learning that may be of concern to community health nurses is the social skills domain.

Taxonomies of learning tasks classify tasks within each of the established domains in a hierarchical fashion. In the cognitive and psychomotor domains, learning tasks are arranged in order of increasing complexity of intellectual or physical skill involved. For example, it requires greater intellectual skill to apply a fact to a particular decision-making situation than simply to recall the fact. Similarly, less skill is required to follow printed knitting instructions than to create one's own pattern. Hierarchies of learning tasks in the cognitive and psychomotor domains are presented in Table 9–2.

Tasks in the affective domain are organized in terms of the degree to which an attitude or value has been internalized by the learner (Krathwohl, Bloom, & Masia, 1964). For example, the student who consistently displays empathy for clients is operating at a higher level of internalization than one who merely discusses the importance of empathy in nursing. The taxonomy of the affective domain is also presented in Table 9–2.

Finally, learning tasks in the perceptual domain are arranged in terms of the extent to which the learner is able to extract information from a situation by way of perceptual skills. For example, a nursing student might notice a few salient characteristics of a client during a preliminary encounter, whereas an experienced community health nurse would derive much more information from the same encounter. The levels of a proposed taxonomy for the perceptual domain are listed in Table 9–2.

It is helpful to classify the outcome objectives developed for a specific health education encounter in terms of the domain of learning and the level of task involved (Redman, 1993). This classification helps to refine the precision of outcome objectives and ensure that objectives are realistic. Generally speaking, if an objective cannot be classified according to domain and level, it is not precise enough and needs to be reworded. For example, the previous objective regarding the client's ability to list at least five iron-rich foods is clearly a cognitive objective at the rudimentary level of knowledge recall. It would be difficult,

TABLE 9–2. TAXONOMY OF LEARNING TASKS IN ESTABLISHED DOMAINS

COGNITIVE DOMAIN

Knowledge	Recall of facts, methods, or processes
Comprehension	Basic understanding of the meaning of facts
Application	Use of abstractions in concrete situations
Analysis	Breakdown into constituent parts
Synthesis	Combination of parts into a new pattern or whole
Evaluation	Judgment about the value of information and processes for specific purposes

PSYCHOMOTOR DOMAIN

Perception	Awareness of objects and relationships among them
Set	Physical, mental, and emotional readiness to act
Guided response	Performance of an action with instructor input and guidance
Mechanism	Performance of the task as a habit
Complex overt response	Performance of task with a high degree of skill
Adaptation	Adjustment of the skill to meet the needs of the situation
Origination	Creation of new acts or ways of manipulating materials

AFFECTIVE DOMAIN

Receiving	Sensitization to the existence of a phenomenon
Responding	Low level of commitment to behaviors embodying a value, performance of the behavior because of outside constraint
Valuing	Ascribing worth to a thing, behavior, or value accompanied by fairly consistent performance of related behaviors
Organization	Organization of values in hierarchical relationships
Characterization	Persona can be characterized by consistent behavior in keeping with a specific set of values

PERCEPTUAL DOMAIN

Sensation	Awareness of differences, or change, in stimuli
Figure perception	Awareness of an object or phenomenon as a distinct entity
Symbol perception	Identification of pattern or form, ability to name or classify an object or phenomenon
Perception of meaning	Awareness of significance of symbols, ability to interrelate symbols
Perceptive performance	Complex decisions with multiple factors, ability to change behavior based on its effectiveness

however, to classify an objective such as, "The client will list five iron-rich foods and state which of them best meets dietary needs for iron." As written, this objective contains some elements related to the knowledge level of the cognitive domain and some related to the evaluation level (using criteria to judge which food is "best"). The objective would be better written as two separate objectives dealing with each level of behavior independently.

Classifying objectives by domain and taxonomic level also allows them to be compared with a client's current level of performance and aids in the development of more realistic objectives. For example, if the client is currently in need of learning at the basic level of factual knowledge, it is unrealistic to expect a given health education encounter to raise him or her to the level of being able to apply evaluative criteria. More concretely, if you are just learning how to recognize specific communication techniques, you are not capable of critically evaluating communication techniques employed by staff nurses in your clinical site.

Finally, classifying objectives by level of difficulty within taxonomic domains can bring to light unrealistic expectations in the breadth of accomplishments expected. Generally speaking, objectives for a health education encounter should cluster in similar levels in a given domain. If your objectives address too many different levels within the domain, they may not be realistic given the client's current capabilities in that area. For example, your instructors would not expect you learn research terminology and develop the ability to critique a research article during the same class session.

Selecting and Sequencing Content

The next task is planning the health lesson is selecting and sequencing the content to be presented. Because the nurse usually has greater knowledge of a particular topic than can or should be presented in a health education encounter, the nurse needs to select content that is most appropriate and relevant to clients' needs and that is most likely to result in accomplishing the stated learning objectives. Once content has been selected, it must be organized in a logical sequence so that new learning is based on previous learning. Content may be sequenced from simple to complex, from most important to least important, or from familiar to less familiar.

Selecting Teaching Strategies

Selection of teaching strategies depends on the characteristics of the clients, the characteristics of the nurse, the type of learning tasks and content involved, and the availability of resources needed to implement specific strategies. Several general principles guide selection of teaching strategies (Anspaugh & Ezell, 1994). First, the strategies chosen should contribute to total learning, not just knowledge acquisition. Second, strategies should foster learner participation in the encounter. Third, the more complex the content, the greater the number and variety of activities needed to learn it. Application of this third principle also permits adaptation of the lesson to a variety of learning styles. The fourth principle is that the strategies chosen should reflect simple activities at first, followed by more complex activities. Finally, audiovisual aids should be used whenever possible to promote learning. These principles are summarized in Table 9–3. The teaching strategies selected should be appropriate to the age, developmental level, and educational level of the audience (Bastable, 1997b). Strategies should be

TABLE 9–3. GENERAL PRINCIPLES FOR SELECTING TEACHING STRATEGIES

- Strategies should contribute to total learning.
- Strategies should incorporate learner participation.
- The more complex the content, the more activities needed.
- Strategies should graduate from simple to complex.
- Strategies should incorporate audiovisuals whenever possible.

chosen that maintain the interest of the learner and adequately address the content to be presented. Another consideration here is clients' preferred modes of learning. Some people, for example, learn best when content is presented visually; others tend to learn what they hear.

Certain learning tasks lend themselves to particular teaching strategies (Fitzgerald, 1997). For example, discussion and role playing are effective methods for creating awareness of personal values, whereas lecture is more appropriate to knowledge acquisition. Problem-solving skills, on the other hand, are best learned through exercises in problem resolution. Table 9–4 presents several commonly used teaching strategies and the learning tasks for which they are best suited.

Preparing Materials

Any materials needed for the health education encounter must be either developed or obtained. Materials selected should be appropriate to the client audience and to the content presented. For example, if the audience is a group of young children, a coloring book might be an effective teaching aid in a lesson on nutrition. A coloring book would not be appropriate, though, for a group of adolescents.

Nurses planning health education may use existing materials and teaching aids. This is appropriate when these materials have been thoroughly reviewed and found to be appropriate to the client audience. Materials used need to convey information at a level that can be understood by clients. They should also be sensitive to client cultural beliefs, attitudes, and values. For example, materials on sexually transmitted diseases (STDs) that picture only persons from minority groups imply that only members of these groups get STDs. Such an implication is not only erroneous but also discriminatory and offensive to members of minorities who might be part of the client audience.

Problems with written materials occur when members of the client audience have low literacy skills. Recent studies of written information on a variety of health topics, for example, indicate that most are written at reading levels above that of many

TABLE 9–4. COMMONLY USED TEACHING STRATEGIES

Strategy	Description	Learning Task Applicability
Case study	Use of a detailed account of an actual or hypothetical situation to help learners apply principles learned or to make them aware of attitudes and values and enhance the potential for change	Application, analysis Responding, valuing Perception
Computer-assisted instruction	Use of computers to present content	Knowledge Analysis Perception
Demonstration	Teacher performance of a skill or process to be learned, usually followed by a return demonstration (see below)	Motor skills development
Discussion	Verbal exploration of an idea or concept, attitude, value, etc, with participation by learners and teacher	Application, analysis Synthesis, evaluation Valuing Perception of meaning
Lecture	Formal oral presentation of information by teacher	Knowledge Comprehension
Media	Use of auditory or visual media presentations (ie, audio-tapes, filmstrips) to present content	Knowledge, comprehension Analysis Valuing, perception Motor skills development
Readings	Presentation of content in written form, frequently followed by discussion	Knowledge, comprehension Valuing
Return demonstration	Learner performance of a learned skill or process	Motor skills development
Role modeling	Teacher performance of a behavior to be adopted (ie, sensitivity to the needs of others)	Valuing
Role playing	Acting out the role of another to get a different perspective, usually followed by discussion	Valuing
Supervision	Teacher-guided performance of desired behavior by learner	Motor skills development Analysis Evaluation
Visual aids	Use of visually oriented materials (ie, pictures, posters) to present content	Knowledge, comprehension Motor skills development

clients. In fact, in one study of several populations, 26 to 83% of some client groups were unable to understand such written health-related communications as medication instructions, appointment slips, and informed consents (Williams, Parker, Baker, et al., 1995). In another study, the average readability level of HIV/AIDS education materials was slightly higher than a seventh grade reading level (Johnson, Mailloux, & Fisher, 1995). For clients with low literacy levels, pictorial materials, videotapes, or filmstrips are more appropriate teaching aids than are written materials.

Problems also arise for audiences who are literate in other languages when materials written in English are translated literally. Translated materials should be reviewed for their consistency with local idiomatic language.

Other considerations in selecting teaching aids and other materials to be used include the need for special equipment (eg, projector and screen for filmstrips), currency of content, and ease of use. Constraints may be imposed by the type of setting in which the learning occurs. For example, if a class is to be conducted outdoors, filmstrips are inappropriate. Or, if education is being provided to a family who lacks a television set, a videotape will not be useful. A final consideration in selecting visual aids is the ability of the client to see the materials. If overhead transparencies are used, for example, the print must be large enough to be read by all those in the back of the room. Similarly, when demonstration is used, all clients in the group need to be able to see what is being demonstrated.

Planning Evaluation

The last task of the planning stage of a health education encounter is developing a plan to evaluate the lesson. Criteria for evaluating the outcomes of health education are derived from the stated outcome objectives for the encounter. Criteria for evaluating the performance of the nurse and the educational process used arise from process objectives. The nurse also wants to identify mechanisms for *formative evaluation,* which involves assessing the effects of the presentation as it is given. Formative evaluation includes determining whether clients understand what is being presented and whether the presentation maintains their interest. The nurse would also be alert to cues that indicate client response to the content presented. For example, the nurse might note that description of discrimination against a person with AIDS generates anger in the listeners. If the nurse was trying to make clients aware of attitudes toward AIDS, such a response would indicate success.

Formative evaluation also reflects the quality of the presentation. For example, frenzied note taking by learners would indicate that content is being presented too rapidly. The tasks involved in planning a health education encounter are summarized next.

▶ **TASKS INVOLVED IN PLANNING A HEALTH EDUCATION ENCOUNTER**

Identifying the Goal
Specifying the broad purpose to be accomplished

Developing Objectives
Stating specific behavioral outcomes expected as a result of the encounter

Classifying Objectives
Identifying the learning domains to be addressed

Selecting and Sequencing Content
Determining what will be taught and the order in which it will be presented

Selecting Teaching Strategies
Determining approaches to be used in presenting content

Preparing Materials
Developing any teaching aids to be used in the presentation

Planning Evaluation
Determining criteria and processes to be used for formative, outcome, and process evaluation

 Implementing the Health Education Encounter

Several key points must be kept in mind in implementing a health education encounter. The first is to speak the client's language. This refers not only to using a foreign language or an interpreter for non-English-speaking clients, but also eliminating medical and nursing jargon. The second recommendation is to be specific; the third is to keep the message short. Key points should be presented early in the lesson for emphasis and to enhance recall. Verbal headings will help clients keep track of material presented and recognize transitions from one topic to another. Finally, repetition, particularly of important points, will enhance learning and recall.

The Focusing Event

The lesson itself begins with a *focusing event,* which is a specific strategy designed to gain the attention of the audience and to focus that attention on the material to be presented. A focusing event in a presentation on child abuse might involve showing several slides of abused children or giving statistics on the incidence of child abuse in the community.

Content Presentation

Following the focusing event, the lesson is presented as planned with formative checks during the course of the lesson to determine the need for on-the-spot revisions. The presentation of content should include audience participation whenever possible. Learning theory indicates that the greater the learner's involvement with the material, the greater the learning that results. Client participation can be facilitated by such activities as group discussion, case studies, and role playing. The nurse can also encourage participation by asking thought-provoking questions or questions that serve to summarize and synthesize previous content.

Lesson Summary

The lesson should close with a summary that reinforces pertinent points. In summarizing, the community health nurse recaps and highlights the major concepts covered. He or she should also attempt to synthesize content in a few major themes that the client needs to remember.

▶ **CONSIDERATIONS IN IMPLEMENTING A HEALTH EDUCATION ENCOUNTER**

Focusing Event
A teaching strategy designed to attract attention to the topic

Presentation of Content
Actual presentation of planned content, encouraging learner participation as much as possible

Summary
Restatement and reinforcement of the most important points of the presentation

 Evaluating the Health Education Encounter

As noted earlier, evaluation takes place throughout the presentation and as the last step of the educational process. Three types of evaluation are done: formative, outcome, and process.

Formative Evaluation

During presentation of the lesson, the community health nurse periodically assesses the lesson and its effects as it is being presented. The nurse uses client feedback to determine whether the content of the lesson is being effectively communicated. For example, if clients' facial expressions indicate confusion, the nurse might infer that they do not understand the material being presented. Similarly, the nurse might ask questions on material offered earlier in the lesson as a formative evaluation strategy. If clients are able to answer these questions correctly, the lesson has been effective thus far. Again, formative evaluation might also include assessing client emotional responses to content presented.

Outcome Evaluation

After the lesson, the nurse evaluates the presentation in terms of its effects. Effects can best be measured in terms of the degree to which the outcome objectives were met. Were the learners able to perform the stated behaviors at the expected level of performance?

In evaluating outcomes, the nurse should remain alert to other outcomes of the educational program in addition to the intended outcomes or objectives. Health education may result in serendipitous outcomes. These results should not be overlooked or underestimated and may be reason for continuing a program even when intended objectives are not accomplished.

Process Evaluation

The nurse also evaluates the presentation in terms of the use of the educational process. Were the process objectives established for the encounter met? Was one as well prepared as desired? Did the lesson maintain the interest of the audience? Were the teaching strategies, materials, and content selected appropriate to the

---

Critical Thinking in Research

Williams, et al. (1995) examined the functional literacy related to health communications among clients seen at two urban public hospitals serving predominantly indigent and minority clientele. They assessed clients' abilities to read and understand medical instructions and health care information on prescription bottle labels, appointment slips, and informed consent forms. Over 35% of English-speaking clients, 61% of Spanish-speaking clients, and 81 to 82% of English and Spanish-speaking elderly had difficulty with one or more of these literacy tasks. Overall, 41% of clients did not understand medication instructions on prescription bottle labels, 26% did not understand when their next appointment was scheduled, and 59.5% could not comprehend a standard informed consent document.

1. What are the implications of these findings for health education with indigent and minority group clients?
2. What other tasks might reflect functional illiteracy related to health matters?
3. If you wanted to replicate this study in your community, where would you go to find a comparable subject sample?
4. Do you think your findings would be different if this study was conducted with non-nursing student groups on your campus? Why or why not?

---

learning needs of the clients? The answers to such questions allow the nurse to make any necessary modifications in the lesson plan for future use. Considerations in evaluating the health education encounter are summarized on this page.

▶ DEVELOPING HEALTH EDUCATION PROGRAMS

Health education may involve single presentations to specific individuals, families, or groups. More often, however, health education by community health nurses is structured as an organized ongoing program designed to meet specific community health goals.

Guidelines for Health Education Programs

An Ad Hoc Work Group of the American Public Health Association (1987) issued the following guidelines for developing health promotion and health education programs:

1. Health promotion programs should address one or more carefully defined, measurable, and modifi-

---

CONSIDERATIONS IN EVALUATING A HEALTH EDUCATION ENCOUNTER

Formative Evaluation
An evaluation conducted periodically during the presentation to detect a need for immediate modification

Outcome Evaluation
Evaluating the encounter to determine whether stated outcome objectives have been met

Process Evaluation
Evaluating the performance of the community health nurse in the light of established process objectives

able risk factors that are prevalent among the target groups selected.

2. The program should be designed to reflect the special attributes, needs, and preferences of the target group.
3. Programs should present interventions that clearly reduce the identified risk factors and that are appropriate for the group.
4. Programs should implement interventions that make the best possible use of resources.
5. Programs should be specifically designed to allow for evaluation of program effects and operation.

Elements of Health Education Programs

Four essential elements describe a health education program or campaign: purpose, target, time, and activity (Backer, Rogers, & Sopory, 1992). The purpose of any campaign is ultimately to influence the behavior of the target audience. Levels of influence vary, however, and the type of influence desired within the hierarchy of educational campaign effects should be determined beforehand and should direct program development.

The effects of programs can be arranged in a hierarchy (Backer, Rogers, & Sopory, 1992):

- Audience is exposed to the health issue.
- Audience is aware of the issue.
- Audience is informed about an issue.
- Audience is persuaded with regard to the issue.
- Audience intends to change behavior.
- Audience changes behavior.
- Audience maintains behavior change.

For example, health educators may want initially to expose the public to the existence of a health issue such as child abuse and then make them aware of the extent of the problem. When this has been accomplished, the public should then be informed of signs of abuse and how to report suspected abuse and should be persuaded that reporting abuse is appropriate. Once people are persuaded, they develop intentions to report abuse should they encounter it. Thus, they would actually report suspected abuse when they see it, and would continue to report child abuse. Most health education campaigns attempt to achieve more than one level of effect, but the specific levels chosen depend on the target audience's current status with respect to the health issue.

The second element of a health education campaign is the audience targeted. This is usually a fairly large group of people to increase the cost-effectiveness of the campaign. The target audience may be segmented based on attitudes, values, and beliefs related to the health issue, rather than on demographic variables, and different communication strategies may be applied to each segment.

Time is the third element of the health education campaign. Campaigns should have a defined time limit within which program objectives can reasonably be expected to be achieved. Finally, a health education campaign consists of a set of well-defined communication activities designed to convey the campaign's message to the audience. Some of the activities selected may reflect what is known as the *entertainment–education approach* (Backer, Rogers, & Sopory, 1992). Health educators make use of entertainment media such as music, television, and comic books to educate people about health. For example, in Mexico several health issues have been purposefully incorporated into the scripts of existing popular soap operas. Other research has indicated that the use of celebrities to convey health education messages can be an effective approach if care is taken to select appropriate role models to avoid sending inappropriate messages.

Effectiveness of Health Education Programs

Health education is an effective means of changing health-related behaviors. It has promise for creating an epidemiology of health. For example, health education campaigns coupled with legislation have been found to increase bicycle helmet use (Macknin & Medendorp, 1994) and decrease smoking (Hu, Sung, & Keeler, 1995) more than legislation alone. In another instance, the use of a video-based education program on sexually transmitted diseases increased condom use, and discussion following the video presentation increased use even further (O'Donnell, San Doval, Duran, & O'Donnell, 1995). In another study, a series of educational campaigns to promote exercise was found to be redundant (Owen, Bauman, Booth, Oldenburg, & Magnus, 1995) underscoring the delicate balance between effective educational campaigns and "overkill."

Numerous instances can be found of the effectiveness of health education in changing health-related behaviors. Health education is an effective tool for the promotion of health. It is also one of the community health nurse's most frequently used tools, whether with individuals, families, or groups of clients. To provide effective health education, however, nurses should engage in systematic planning as described here. Additional sources for information about health education are listed at the end of this chapter.

Critical Thinking in Practice: A Case in Point

You have been asked by a private elementary school principal to give a presentation on AIDS to the Parent/Teacher Group and, afterward, to make a presentation to students in the seventh and eighth grades on the same topic. The school is run by a nondenominational Christian foundation. Students in the school come from an upper-middle-class neighborhood and most of their parents are professional people. The students are above the national average in all areas of standardized testing, and English is the primary language spoken by both parents and students.

Recently, in a nearby public school, there was a tremendous parental outcry when it became known that one of the children in the school had AIDS. Parental response in that school was such that the parents of the child with AIDS were finally asked to accept a home-study program for their child rather than keep him in school.

So far, similar problems have not occurred in this school, but school officials are interested in avoiding potential problems should a child with AIDS be admitted. Parents of children in this school have already begun to ask about policies related to children with AIDS.

1. Using the Educational Planning and Implementation Guide in Appendix C, document the assessment data that would be available to you. What additional assessment data might you want to obtain? How would you obtain these data?
2. What are your goals for the two presentations?
3. Develop two or three specific outcome objectives that you would expect learners to accomplish as a result of your presentation.
4. What learning domains are involved in the presentations? Would the learning tasks involved differ between the student and parent groups? Why or why not?
5. Would content presented differ between your two audiences? What would you present and why? Would you sequence content any differently? Why or why not?
6. What teaching strategies might be most effective with each group? What type of teaching aids or materials would you need? Where might you obtain these teaching aids?
7. What type of focusing event would you use for the student group? For the parent group? How would you encourage learner participation in the two groups? Would you use similar or different approaches to stimulate learner participation?
8. What key points would you be sure to include in the summary of your presentation? Would these be the same or different for the two groups of learners?
9. How would you conduct formative evaluation during your presentation? How would you evaluate the presentation in terms of client outcomes and your performance?

TESTING YOUR UNDERSTANDING

1. What three types of health-related decisions can be facilitated by health education? Give an example of each type. (pp. 168–169)
2. Describe at least two barriers to health education. Give an example of each and describe how a community health nurse might circumvent them. (p. 169)
3. Compare and contrast the source of motivation to learn in the behavioral, cognitive, and humanistic theories of learning. (pp. 169–170)
4. Distinguish between process and outcome objectives for a learning encounter. (p. 176)
5. Describe the four established domains of learning. Give an example of a learning task within each domain. (pp. 176–178)

6. What is a focusing event? What is the purpose of the focusing event? (p. 180)
7. Give two examples of how formative evaluation might be used in a health education encounter. (pp. 180–181)
8. Describe at least four guidelines for developing health education programs. Give examples of programs that might meet these guidelines. (pp. 181–182)

WHAT DO YOU THINK?
Questions for Critical Thinking

1. What effects do the media have on health education for the general public? What role should the media play in health education, if any?

2. Do you think that a certain level of stress and anxiety promote learning? Why or why not?
3. What types of learning tasks did your nursing instructor expect you to accomplish in relation to this chapter?
4. If you were making a presentation to a group of nursing students on the teaching learning process, what would you use as a focusing event to get their attention?

REFERENCES

Ad Hoc Work Group of the American Public Health Association. (1987). Criteria for the development of health promotion and education programs. *American Journal of Public Health, 77,* 89–91.

Anspaugh, D. J., & Ezell, G. (1994). *Teaching today's health* (4th ed.). Boston: Allyn & Bacon.

Babcock, D. E., & Miller, M. A. (1994). *Client education: Theory and practice.* St. Louis: C. V. Mosby.

Backer, T. E., Rogers, E. M., & Sopory, P. (1992). *Designing health communication campaigns: What works.* Newbury Park, CA: Sage.

Bastable, S. B. (1997a). Overview of education in health care. In S. B. Bastable (Ed.), *Nurse as educator: Principles of teaching and learning* (pp. 3–15). Boston: Jones & Bartlett.

Bastable, S. B. (1997b). Teaching strategies specific to developmental stages of life. In S. B. Bastable (Ed.), *Nurse as educator: Principles of teaching and learning* (pp. 91–123). Boston: Jones & Bartlett.

Bastable, S., & Sculco, C. (1997). Educational objectives. In S. B. Bastable (Ed.), *Nurse as educator: Principles of teaching and learning* (pp. 237–260). Boston: Jones & Bartlett.

Bloom, B. S., Englehart, M. D., Furst, E. J., Hill, W. F., & Krathwohl, D. R. (1956). *Taxonomy of educational objectives: The classification of educational goals: Handbook 1: The cognitive domain.* New York: David McKay.

Braungart, M. M., & Braungart, R. G. (1997). Learning theory and nursing practice. In S. B. Bastable (Ed.), *Nurse as educator: Principles of teaching and learning* (pp. 31–52). Boston: Jones & Bartlett.

Breckon, D. J., Harvey, J. R., & Lancaster, R. B. (1994). *Community health education: Settings, roles and skills for the 21st century* (3rd ed.). Gaithersburg, MD: Aspen.

Castro, K. G., Valdiserri, R. O., & Curran, J. W. (1992). Perspectives on HIV/AIDS epidemiology and prevention from the Eighth International Conference on AIDS. *American Journal of Public Health, 82,* 1465–1470.

Falvo, D. R. (1994). *Effective patient education: A guide to increased compliance.* Gaithersburg, MD: Aspen.

Fitzgerald, K. (1997). Instructional methods: Selection, use and evaluation. In S. B. Bastable (Ed.), *Nurse as educator: Principles of teaching and learning* (pp. 261–286). Boston: Jones & Bartlett.

Fleury, J. (1992). The application of motivational theory to cardiovascular risk reduction. *Image, 24,* 229–239.

Gleit, C. J. (1998). Theories of learning. In M. D. Boyd, B. A. Graham, C. J. Gleit, & N. I. Whitman (Eds.), *Health teaching in nursing practice* (2nd ed.). Stamford, CT: Appleton & Lange.

Green, L. W., & Kreuter, M. W. (1991). *Health promotion planning: An educational and environmental approach* (2nd ed.). Mountain View, CA: Mayfield.

Greenberg, J. S. (1991). *Health education: Learner-centered instructional strategies* (2nd ed.). Dubuque, IA: Wm. C. Brown.

Hu, T., Sung, H., & Keeler, T. E. (1995). Reducing cigarette consumption in California: Tobacco taxes vs an anti-smoking media campaign. *American Journal of Public Health, 85,* 1218–1222.

Johnson, M. E., Mailloux, S. L., & Fisher, D. G. (1995). *Readability of HIV/AIDS educational materials to injection drug users and cocaine smokers.* Paper presented at the 123rd Annual Meeting of the American Public Health Association. San Diego, CA.

Kitchie, S. (1997). Determinants of learning. In S. B. Bastable (Ed.), *Nurse as educator* (pp. 55–89). Boston: Jones and Bartlett.

Krathwohl, D. R., Bloom, B. S., & Masia, B. B. (1964). *Taxonomy of educational objectives: The classification of educational goals: Handbook 1: The affective domain.* New York: David McKay.

Lorig, K. (1995). *Patient education: A practical approach* (2nd ed.). Newbury Park, CA: Sage.

Macknin, M. L., & Medendorp, S. V. (1994). Association between bicycle helmet legislation, bicycle safety education, and use of bicycle helmets in children. *Archives of Pediatric and Adolescent Medicine, 148,* 255–259.

O'Donnell, L. N., San Doval, A., Duran, R., & O'Donnell, C. (1995). Video-based sexually transmitted disease patient education: Its impact on condom acquisition. *American Journal of Public Health, 85,* 817–822.

Owen, N., Bauman, A., Booth, M., Oldenburg, B., & Magnus, P. (1995). Serial mass media campaigns to promote physical activity: Reinforcing or redundant? *American Journal of Public Health, 85,* 244–248.

Pew Health Professions Commission. (1995). *Critical challenges: Revitalizing the health professions for the twenty-first century.* San Francisco: University of California, San Francisco Center for the Health Professions.

Redman, B. K. (1993). *The process of patient education* (7th ed.). St. Louis: C. V. Mosby.

Richards, E. (1997). Motivation, compliance, and health behaviors of the learner. In S. B. Bastable (Ed.),

Nurse as educator: Principles of teaching and learning (pp. 124–144). Boston: Jones & Bartlett.

Stein, Z. A. (1992). Editorial: The double bind in science policy and the protection of women from HIV infection. *American Journal of Public Health, 82,* 1471–1572.

Williams, M. V., Parker, R. M., Baker, D. W., et al. (1995). Inadequate functional literacy among patients at two public hospitals. *JAMA, 274,* 1677–1682.

RESOURCES FOR HEALTH EDUCATION

American Council for Healthful Living
c/o Jane Westlake
Elite Graphics
285 Cambridge Road
Pine Brook, NJ 07058
(201) 882–9769

Association for the Advancement of Health Education
1900 Association Drive
Reston, VA 22091
(703) 476–3437

Center for Chronic Disease Prevention and Health Promotion
Centers for Disease Control
4000 Rhodes Bldg., Kroger Center
Chamblee Tucker Road
Atlanta, GA 30341
(404) 488–5401

Center for Medical Consumers & Health Care Information
237 Thompson Street
New York, NY 10012
(212) 674–7105

Center for Prevention Services
1600 Clifton Road
Atlanta, GA 30333
(404) 639–1800

Council on Health Information & Education
2272 Colorado Blvd., No. 1228
Los Angeles, CA 90041

Do It Now Foundation
PO Box 27568
Tempe, AZ 85285
(602) 491–0393

Health Education Resources
4733 Bethesda Avenue, Ste. 700
Bethesda, MD 20814
(301) 656–3178

Health Education Services
A Division of Health Research, Inc.
PO Box 7126
Albany, NY 12224
(518) 439–7286

International Union for Health Promotion and Education
North American Regional Office
PO Box 2305
Station D
Ottawa, Ontario, Canada KIP5KO

National Center for Health Education
72 Spring Street, Ste. 208
New York, NY 10012
(212) 334–9470

Office of Disease Prevention and Health Promotion
U.S. Public Health Service
330 C Street, NW
Washington, DC 20201
(202) 205–8611

Society for Public Health Education
2001 Addison Street, Ste. 220
Berkeley, CA 94704

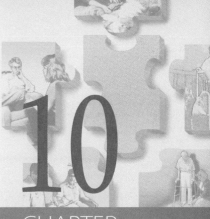

10

CHAPTER

THE HOME VISIT PROCESS AND HOME HEALTH NURSING

► KEY TERMS

certificate of need
distractions
fiscal intermediary
governmental
   agencies
home health care
home visit
hospice agencies
institution-based
   agencies
intermittent care
Medicare-certified
   agencies
preparatory
   assessment
proprietary agencies
respite care
voluntary home health
   agencies

Historical photographs of community health nurses often show them caring for clients in their homes. Indeed, home care was the initial focus of community health nursing. The home was where most clients were to be found and where community health nurses had to go to reach them. Today, the home is only one setting where community health nurses encounter their clients. Despite the broadening of community health nursing over the years to encompass many other places and settings, the home visit process remains a strategic tool for health care delivery. A home visit by a nurse is different from a social visit that might be made by friends or relatives. A ***home visit,*** as conceptualized in community health nursing, is a formal call by a nurse on a client at the client's residence to provide nursing care. The process used to conduct that visit is the subject of this chapter.

187

▶ Chapter Objectives

After reading this chapter, you should be able to:

- Describe at least three advantages of a home visit as a means of providing nursing care.
- Identify at least three characteristics of successful home visiting programs.
- Identify four challenges encountered by community health nurses making home visits.
- Describe the relationship between home health nursing and community health nursing.
- Identify at least three types of home health agencies.
- Describe at least four aspects of planning a home visit.
- Identify at least four tasks in implementing a home visit.
- Identify three types of potential distractions during a home visit.
- Discuss the need for both long-term and short-term evaluative criteria for the effectiveness of a home visit.

▶ ADVANTAGES OF HOME VISITS

Why do community health nurses make home visits? It would seem to be more cost-effective for clients to come to the nurse. More clients might be seen in a given period if the nurse did not have to consider travel time or time wasted being lost in unfamiliar areas. What is there about a home visit that outweighs these obvious disadvantages?

The advantages of home visits can be viewed in terms of six major dimensions: convenience, access, information, relationship, cost, and outcomes. Within the convenience dimension, many clients would prefer to be seen in their homes rather than clinics or other health care settings. Home visits permit health care services to be integrated into the client's usual routine. Moreover, during a home visit, clients are not subjected to the need to find transportation or to the long waits for service that frequently occur in other settings.

The access dimension of home visiting has two aspects. First, clients who are immobile or lack transportation and cannot reach other care settings have access to care that might otherwise be unavailable to them. Similarly, community health nurses may gain access to clients who would not present themselves, for whatever reasons, for services provided in other settings (Liepert, 1996). Second, home visits provide community health nurses with opportunities to identify other clients in need of services (Cowley, 1995).

In the information dimension, the nurse making a home visit has opportunities to obtain a variety of information that is less easily obtained in other settings. The nurse gets a complete picture of the client, whether individual or family, and of the client's environment (Reutter & Ford, 1996). The nurse can see firsthand the effects of physical, psychological, and social environmental factors on a client's health status. A home visit provides the nurse with information about possible resources and hazards that can influence a client's health. The interaction of family members during the visit might suggest the extent of a client's support network and the ability of family members to provide care. Similarly, detecting potential health hazards in a home, such as loose throw rugs in the home of an older client, can provide the stimulus for health education to promote physical safety.

In the home the nurse can better assess the client's ability to perform activities of daily living. Finally, frequent contact in the client's home may permit the nurse to identify minor health changes for which clients would not seek help. The nurse may then act to prevent major problems.

Because the community health nurse has a more complete picture of a client, the nurse has a better understanding of the client's needs and can better design interventions. Finally, during a home visit, the nurse is better able to monitor and evaluate the effects of interventions. For example, the client may tell the nurse in the clinic that he or she is adhering to a low-sodium diet as planned. If the nurse visits at home, however, and finds the client munching potato chips, it is readily apparent that dietary instruction has not been as effective as desired.

The relationship dimension of home visiting has the advantage of the client exercising autonomy and control. In the client's home the nurse is a guest; the client controls the situation. Effective community health nurses build on this aspect of control to foster a client's sense of empowerment. The nurse also acts as an enabler, assisting clients to find resources to take action on their own, and as an enhancer, helping clients build on personal strengths. These actions by the nurse lead to a collaborative atmosphere in which the client is fully involved in planning interventions which, in turn, enhances the probability of successful implementation.

Another advantage to the relationship dimension of a home visit is the privacy and sense of intimacy created. Clients often feel freer to raise sensitive issues in the privacy of their own homes than in more alien health care settings. Thus, the community health nurse may gain more private insights into the client's situation.

The last aspect of the relationship dimension that frequently operates during a home visit is the continuity of the relationship itself. Often, community health nurses make several visits to an individual or family. This continuity intensifies the effects of the information dimension and other aspects of the relationship dimension, particularly intimacy. On occasion, however, the long-term nature of many home visiting relationships may contribute to challenges that are addressed later.

The cost dimension of home visiting is one reason this mode of delivering health care services has experienced a resurgence. It is estimated that the $300 million (Canadian) annual expenditure for home care in Canada saves $2300 million in institutional costs (Sorochan & Beattie, 1994). In addition, several studies demonstrated reduced medical expenses as a result of home visiting programs for mothers and children (Barnett, 1993).

The final dimension of a home visit that contributes to its value is client outcomes. A growing body of evidence suggests that clients recover more rapidly after hospitalization with home visitation (Barnett, 1993) and that well-designed home visiting programs targeted to high-risk children and their families produce healthful outcomes (Cooper, 1996; Olds & Kitzman, 1993; Starn, 1992).

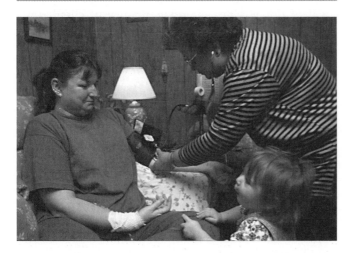

Because community health nurses see clients in their own settings, they are able to identify a wide range of factors that effect the client's health.

From: Berger, K., & Williams, M. (1999). Fundamentals of Nursing: Collaborating for optimal health (2nd ed.). Stamford, CT: Appleton & Lange.

► CHALLENGES OF HOME VISITING

Despite the many advantages of home visits, this mode of health care delivery is not without challenges. Some of these challenges arise out of the diversity of clients and the multiplicity of their problems. Clients differ in age, ethnic background, culture, health status, and attitudes toward health and health providers. They do not usually experience isolated problems, but are faced with multiple problems that impinge on their health. The diversity of clients and the problems encountered in home visiting require the community health nurse to have a broad knowledge base to understand and deal with the variety of factors that may influence clients' health. The multiplicity of problems coupled with the diversity of clientele creates a variety of service demands that can seem overwhelming and lead to a great deal of stress for the visiting nurse.

Maintaining Balance

Other challenges in home visiting derive from the community health nurse's need to maintain balance in his or her interactions with clients. Areas in which a delicate balance is required are depicted in Figure 10–1 and include a balance between intimacy and professional distance, assisting and devaluing clients, dependence and independence, altruism and realism, creativity and inadequacy, risk and safety, cost containment and quality, and, in some cases, health restoration and health promotion services.

As noted earlier, home visits create a sense of intimacy between nurse and client that is not found in other health care settings. This intimacy, while advantageous in some respects, can make it difficult for nurses to maintain an appropriate professional distance in order to be most therapeutic. Although the home visit is not a social visit, a certain amount of socialization is necessary to establish rapport with clients. Nurses making home visits may disclose more about themselves than they would in other settings. Such self-disclosure can help establish rapport and a collaborative relationship with clients, but the nurse must be careful to determine what level of self-disclosure is appropriate to the situation. In addition, the nurse will sometimes have to make difficult decisions: Should hospitality or gifts be accepted? The client's offering them may have cultural overtones and refusal to accept may damage the nurse–client relationship. Often the nurse may feel that the client cannot afford to give what is being offered.

Another challenge arises out of the need to assist clients without conveying that clients are inadequate,

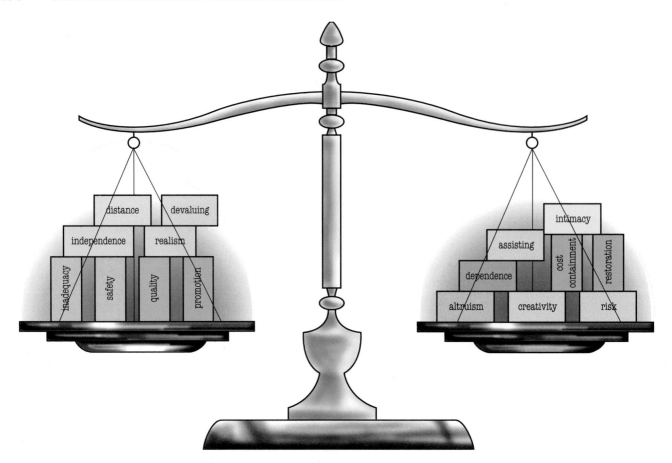

Figure 10–1. Maintaining balance in home visiting.

that is, without devaluing them. Too often, when people are required to accept the help of others, they begin to perceive themselves as inadequate. This is where a collaborative relationship can be very beneficial. In a collaborative relationship, nurse and client work together to resolve problems and the input of both is valued. Within this relationship, the nurse should convey a sense of self-efficacy that prevents clients from feeling inadequate to meet difficulties on their own.

The balance between assisting and devaluing clients affects self-determination. Clients have the right to determine for themselves whether they are going to comply with health providers' suggestions. Because of the relationship engendered in the home visit situation, nurses may feel tempted to trade on the relationship to subtly coerce clients into actions that are "in their best interest." In a truly collaborative relationship, however, client and nurse together determine goals and the actions to achieve them. The nurse must always keep in mind that veto power lies with the client.

Another area in which balance is required is the

level of dependence or independence of client function. The goal of a home visit is to promote client self-sufficiency; however, many clients may not reach this level until well into a series of home visits. One means of promoting client independence is limit setting, not allowing clients to depend on the nurse for action they are capable of taking for themselves. Nurses can be very explicit in saying that they feel the client can do certain things for themselves (Stulginsky, 1993b). Again, collaborative relationship conveys the expectation that clients will do what they can, with assistance from the nurse as needed.

Because of the sometimes overwhelming nature of clients' problems, community health nurses making home visits must also maintain a balance between altruism and realism. The nurse cannot resolve all of the client's problems and must focus on those problems that are amenable to nursing intervention (Stulginsky, 1993a). Nurses must also recognize that they will not be completely successful with all clients. The nurse, therefore, must learn to be satisfied with incremental progress rather than the dramatic improvements in clients' health status that may be seen in other health care settings. Having a realistic sense of what can be accomplished, given the resources available to client and nurse, will diminish the stress of insurmountable client problems.

Balance is also required between creativity and inadequacy. In the home situation, community health nurses frequently have to deal with a lack of materials and resources that would be taken for granted in other settings. Community health nurses have thus learned to exercise their creativity and "make do" with whatever resources are available. The nurse, however, must recognize when "making do" is no longer feasible but, rather, is contributing to inadequate care. In this situation, the nurse must seek other avenues to obtain the resources necessary to provide adequate client care.

The need for balance in the area of risk and safety affects both nurse and client. The nurse must decide what level of risk is acceptable without unduly jeopardizing the safety of the client or his or her own safety. The nurse may need to weigh the relative risks of changing a potentially hazardous environment versus the disruption to the client's life that will result from the change. For example, a visiting nurse may have to help a family decide the best alternative for caring for an older family member no longer capable of self-care. Should the older person live with family members, seek a companion, or be placed in a nursing home?

The risk–safety balance issue affects the nurse as well. Nurses need to be aware of and minimize potential risks to their own safety in making home visits (Stanhope & Knollmueller, 1996). Basic safety precautions frequently prevent risk situations. Table 10–1 lists several suggestions for risk reduction in this area. On occasion, the nurse may need to balance client safety against his or her own safety. In this case, the decision of the nurse will be based, of necessity, on the factors operating in the particular situation and the relative risk to self and client.

Cost containment and quality must also be balanced (Stulginsky, 1993b). As noted earlier, one of the advantages of home visits is their cost-effectiveness. Providing care in the home is not inexpensive, however, and agencies that engage in home visiting need to be reimbursed for their services. Too often, at present, reimbursement is based on provision of technical care services rather than on clients' health needs. Frequently, nurses are not reimbursed for services such as health education. Until reimbursement policies are changed, community health nurses need to continue to provide these services within the context of reimbursable services while continuing to maintain productivity levels that ensure the fiscal viability of the parent agency.

The ability to meet client and family needs effectively must also be considered in balancing cost containment and quality. Sometimes the question is one of "cost containment for whom?" For example, it may cost society less to provide care in the home, but it may cost the family more. Family costs may include higher out-of-pocket costs for items not covered in the home setting by health insurance or lost wages if a family member needs to stay home to provide care (Sorochan & Beattie, 1994).

The final balance that needs to be achieved in many home visit situations is related to the cost containment–quality issue. Because health promotive services are frequently not reimbursable in many home visit programs (particularly home health programs), nurses may need to maintain a balance between the provision of illness-related health restoration care and health-promotive care, the true focus of community health nursing. Again, community health nurses may need to "sneak" these kinds of services in while providing reimbursable acute care services.

Effective community health nurses are able to maintain balance in each of the areas addressed here. In maintaining that balance, nurses provide effective holistic care and yet maintain their own integrity and sanity.

TABLE 10–1. PERSONAL SAFETY CONSIDERATIONS IN HOME VISITING

APPEARANCE
- Wear a name tag and a uniform or other apparel that identifies you as a nurse
- Do not carry a purse or wear expensive jewelry
- Leave any valuables at home or lock them in the trunk of the car

TRANSPORTATION
- Keep your car in good repair and with a full tank of gas
- Carry emergency supplies such as a flashlight and blanket
- Always lock your car and carry keys in hand when leaving the client's home
- Park near the client's home with your car in view of the home whenever possible
- Avoid the use of public transportation if possible
- Get complete and accurate directions to the home

THE SITUATION
- Call ahead to alert the client that you will be coming
- Ask clients to secure pets before your visit
- Walk directly to the client's home, without detours to local shops or other places
- Keep one arm free while walking to the client's home
- Avoid isolated areas, especially late in the day or at night
- Knock before entering the client's home, even if the door is open
- Make joint visits in dangerous neighborhoods or situations or employ an escort service if needed
- Listen to the client's messages regarding potential safety hazards
- Make home visits at times when illicit activity (such as drug transactions) is less likely to occur or when potentially dangerous family members will not be present
- Carry a whistle that is easily accessible
- Become familiar with personal defense techniques
- Leave any situation that appears to hold a risk of personal danger
- Stay alert and observe your surroundings

Three other challenges may arise in home visiting. The first may stem from client and family response to services. Clients are often unaware of referrals to community health nurses or may perceive them as unwarranted or intrusive (Kristjanson & Chalmers, 1991). Because of this, community health nurses may be faced with the challenge of building rapport in an initial contact to permit a therapeutic interaction between nurse, client, and family. This task may be particularly difficult when clients do not have the option of refusing services, as in the case of suspected or confirmed child abuse.

Another challenge in home visiting is the ambiguity of the client situation. Visiting nurses repeatedly refer to the need to shift gears or move from a preconceived agenda to address more pressing needs identified in the family (Cowley, 1995). Frequently, the nurse needs to accomplish this shift within relatively restrictive service parameters of a given agency. Finally, community health nurses may be challenged by the need to avoid client abandonment when services continue to be needed, but funding sources have been exhausted (Gunther, 1996). Avoiding abandonment may require very creative problem solving by nurse and client to ensure receipt of needed services.

► CHARACTERISTICS OF SUCCESSFUL HOME VISITING PROGRAMS

Research has indicated that successful home visiting programs share several characteristics (Gomby, Larson, Lewit, & Behrman, 1993; Olds & Kitzman, 1993). One such characteristic is focusing on a broad spectrum of goals rather than a single area. Single-focus programs have a tendency to produce modest, short-term effects rather than lasting gains in health status. Similarly, programs that use professional staff as home visitors are more effective than those that use paraprofessionals or laypersons. Indeed, nurses have been shown to be one of the most effective groups to make home visits because of their broad knowledge base and ability to link clients with other aspects of the health care system. More research is needed, however, to identify the appropriate mix of staff in most home visiting programs.

Effective programs also differ from less effective ones in terms of the intensity and duration of services. Generally speaking, a single home visit does not accomplish much, but gains in health status can be seen with a series of visits. Finally, home visit programs are more successful when they are targeted to high-risk populations with multiple needs (Deal, 1994). These

PRINCIPLES FOR HOME VISITING PROGRAMS

- Participation in home visiting programs should be voluntary and client–visitor relationships should be collaborative.
- Home visiting programs should foster client progress toward personal goals in addition to program goals.
- Home visiting programs should address multiple goals and should encompass long-term as well as short-term gains in health status.
- Home visiting programs should permit flexibility in the intensity and duration of services provided.
- Home visiting programs should be sensitive to the diversity of clients and needs served.
- Home visiting programs require a well-trained staff.
- Expected outcomes of home visiting programs should be realistic.
- Evaluation of home visiting programs should focus on client outcomes, cost-effectiveness, and processes used in intervention.

characteristics of successful home visiting programs give rise to the principles summarized above.

► PURPOSES OF HOME VISITING PROGRAMS

An array of health-related agencies conduct home visits, either as the major component of service or in addition to other services. Each agency has its own goals for the home visit program, but generally the purposes of visits can be grouped into three categories: case finding and referral; health promotion and illness prevention; and care of the sick, which includes health restoration and maintenance. Any given agency may incorporate all three types of purposes within a home visiting program, but will usually emphasize one purpose over the others.

Case Finding and Referral

Some agencies engage in home visiting primarily to identify clients in need of additional services. These clients are then referred to appropriate sources of services to meet those needs. In this type of program, a minimum number of visits are usually required. In fact, the visitor frequently makes only a single visit to identify and deal with clients' needs. In other cases, the visitor might return to the home to follow up on referrals made.

Health Promotion and Illness Prevention

Health promotion and illness prevention are the primary focus of many visits made by community health nurses, particularly those employed by official public health agencies. For example, in many jurisdictions, community health nurses routinely make home visits to new mothers. Community health nurses working in special projects that focus on prenatal and child health also emphasize health promotion and illness prevention in their visits. For instance, special prenatal health projects frequently employ home visits as well as regular clinic appointments as a means of promoting maternal and child health. Similarly, home visiting programs to foster child development focus on health promotion and prevention of health problems.

Care of the Sick

Specific "home health" agencies are primarily geared to meeting the needs of the sick in their homes. ***Home health care***, in this context, refers to the delivery of services in the home for purposes of restoring or maintaining the health of clients.

Home Health and Community Health Nursing

A number of authors distinguish between home health nursing and community health nursing. The distinction arose from the early split between personal health care services and public health services when official health agencies began to emphasize population-based screening and health promotion services. Authors who make this distinction base it on the fact that home health nursing is primarily illness-focused and that it deals with individuals rather than population groups. Other authors, however, point out that home health nurses do deal with aggregate needs within an "assigned microcosm" or miniature community (Keating & Kelman, 1988). From this perspective, home health nurses identify populations at risk and in need of home health services and define the role of home health nursing in meeting the needs of individual clients and the larger community. The community focus in home health comes in the planning of systems of care based on an assessment of community needs, characteristics, and resources.

Still other authors suggest that illness is both an individual or family problem and a community experience. This was the perspective of early community health nurses (Lent, 1993) who provided personal health services in clients' homes and simultaneously campaigned to improve social conditions. These nurses and their supporters believed that the conditions of the sick in their homes influenced the health of society in general.

Although today home health nurses work primarily with ill individuals, they continue to employ the knowledge of environmental, social, and personal health factors. That knowledge is a combination of public health science and nursing practice and is the hallmark of community health nursing. It would seem, then, that the distinction between community health nursing and home health nursing is an artificial one and that home health is actually a subspeciality within community health nursing in which the primary, but not sole, focus is health restoration. Effective home health nurses who provide holistic nursing care employ principles of community health nursing with the segment of the population that is ill. This perspective is supported by both the *Statement on the Essentials of Home Health Care* by the American Nurses Association (1988) and the *Essentials of Baccalaureate Nursing Education for Entry Level Community Health Nursing Practice* of the Association of Community Health Nurse Educators (1990).

Types of Home Health Agencies

Home health agencies providing health restoration home visit services can be classified into several types including public or governmental, voluntary charitable, proprietary, institution-based, and hospice agencies (Rice & Smiley, 1996; Schulmerich, 1996). ***Governmental agencies*** are publicly funded units of government, usually health departments, that provide home health services. Governmental agencies are funded by tax revenues and occasionally by third-party payment. This type of agency frequently operates in areas where there are few other providers of home health services (eg, the rural southeastern United States) or where financially strapped local governments have attempted to generate revenue by providing reimbursable home health services. Some policy makers suggest that this last activity is an inappropriate focus for official health agencies. Others, however, contend that in underserved areas or areas where private sector services are economically unstable, official health agencies provide a reliable source of care (Cherry, 1988).

Voluntary home health agencies provide home health services on a nonprofit basis. These services are usually funded by charitable donations, fundraising, third-party payment, and some private payment. Visiting nurses' associations are examples of agencies in this category. Both voluntary and governmental agencies tend to care for large numbers of indigent clients with no other source of care, and many voluntary agencies have been forced to reduce service eligibility because of the drain on limited resources posed by this clientele.

Proprietary agencies are independent home health agencies owned by individuals or corporations that operate on a for-profit basis. Their funding sources include third-party insurance payors and private fee-for-service payments. *Institution-based agencies* provide home health services under the auspices of a larger health organization, usually a hospital or health maintenance organization. Their funding often comes from a combination of proprietary and voluntary payment sources. Finally, *hospice agencies* provide home services to the unique population of terminally ill clients. Hospice agencies may be independent voluntary agencies or affiliated with a larger proprietary agency or institution.

Any or all of the home care agencies described here may qualify as Medicare-certified agencies and may provide services under the Medicaid program as well. *Medicare-certified agencies* are home health agencies that have been approved by the federal Health Care Financing Administration (HCFA) to provide specific home health services directly reimbursable, under Medicare, the federal insurance plan for the elderly and disabled. Each year Medicare spends approximately $20 million on home health care services (National Center for Injury Prevention and Control, 1994).

Agencies that wish to be designated Medicare-certified agencies must comply with federal, state, and local standards for home health agencies and be licensed by the appropriate state or local body. In addition, clients who receive services reimbursed under Medicare must meet certain eligibility requirements in addition to being eligible for social security benefits (Schulmerich, 1996). These requirements include certification of the need for care and a care plan developed by the client's physician. Periodically, this plan of care must be reviewed and updated with recertification of need for services. In addition, eligible clients must be homebound and need at least one of the following services: intermittent skilled nursing care; physical, speech, or occupational therapy; skilled observation and assessment; or case management and evaluation. *Intermittent care* is defined as up to 28 hours of skilled nursing and home health aide services per week (Bishop & Skwara, 1993). Medicare may also provide indirect reimbursement for services provided by noncertified agencies that contract with Medicare-certified agencies (Schulmerich, 1996).

In 1989, HCFA removed restrictions on the number of home visits permissible under Medicare and included the need for case management or skilled observation as certifiable needs for care in the absence of other needs. These changes opened the door to provision of long-term maintenance care for persons with chronic illnesses who require these services, in addition to short-term care for clients recovering from acute episodes of illness. These changes further led to massive increases in Medicare home health spending amounting to $5.4 billion in 1991 (Bishop & Skwara, 1993) and may result in further revisions of eligibility policies in the future.

Licensing of Home Health Agencies

Licensure of home health agencies is state or locally controlled depending on where the agency is located. In California, for example, licensing is a state regulatory function. Some areas require a "certificate of need" prior to licensing a home health agency. A *certificate of need* is a statement providing evidence of the need for home health services in that area that are not being met by existing agencies. The trend appears to be toward increasing regulation of licensure for home health agencies; thus, the reader is encouraged to seek out licensing requirements for agencies in his or her own area.

▶ CLIENTS SERVED BY HOME VISITING PROGRAMS

As noted earlier, home health agencies generally provide services to a wide variety of clients who are ill and require nursing care to restore or maintain health. There is no "typical" client requiring nursing care in the home. The client may be a mother and a newborn infant referred from a short-stay hospital unit who require follow-up care. The client may also be the elderly person requiring skilled care or monitoring after surgery for a hip fracture or the adolescent with poorly controlled diabetes. In short, the client can be any individual or family in need of professionally supervised nursing care in the home.

With increasing frequency, clients requiring nursing care at home are receiving complex therapies or using high-technology equipment that was formerly restricted to acute care hospital settings. More chemotherapy patients, for example, are now receiving treatment at home as new technology allows safer infusion of therapeutic agents. Pain management for those with end-stage cancer or chronic disease is also achieved in the home with good results. Clients on ventilators or who require continuous or intermittent oxygen can also be maintained at home and children born with respiratory disease syndrome frequently go home with respiratory monitors.

Many home nursing clients are elderly persons with multiple high-acuity needs. These clients may be bedridden or have restricted activity levels requiring assistance with the tasks of daily living. Typical health problems experienced by home health agency clients include circulatory disorders, cancer, diabetes, and sequelae following unintentional injury. Other clients who frequently receive home visits are pregnant women and children with a variety of handicapping conditions or who are victims of abuse. Indications of a potential need for home visit services are summarized in Table 10–2.

► THE DIMENSIONS MODEL AND HOME VISITING

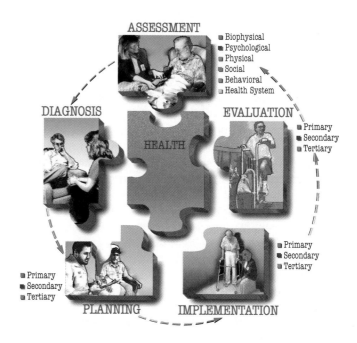

Although home visits have some distinct advantages over care provided in other settings, to be effective, home visits must be focused, purposeful events. Like any other nursing intervention, the home visit should be a planned event with specified goals and objectives. The Dimensions Model provides a framework for systematically organizing the home visit to make it an effective nursing intervention.

The decision to provide services in the home should be based on several considerations (Davis, 1996). First, the home setting should be adequate for providing the services needed and should not jeopardize the safety of client or nurse. Areas that should be considered include the availability of electricity and telephone services, cleanliness, family attitudes toward maintaining the client in the home, and abilities to call for emergency services if needed. Second, the services needed should be within the scope of the agency to provide. Finally, the client should meet eligibility requirements for services (eg, meet Medicare eligibility criteria).

Critical Dimensions of Nursing in Home Visiting

In executing a home visit, the community health nurse will employ elements of several dimensions of nursing. In the cognitive dimension, the nurse must have

TABLE 10–2. CLIENTS WHO MIGHT BENEFIT FROM A HOME VISIT

Indication	Type of Client
Physical needs and conditions	• Pregnant clients • Ill, disabled, or frail elderly clients living alone or with others whose health is impaired • Clients with physical or emotional problems that make it difficult to carry out activities of daily living • Clients discharged from hospitals or nursing homes with continuing health needs • Clients who need special procedures that family members cannot perform or need help in performing • Clients who require periodic monitoring of chronic conditions • Terminally ill clients and their families • Clients with certain communicable diseases (eg, HIV/AIDS, hepatitis, tuberculosis) that require care over time • Clients who need rehabilitation services • Clients who are recovering from work-related injuries • Postpartum clients who experienced perinatal difficulties
Emotional needs	• Clients with chronic mental health conditions • Clients who are anxious about their condition or their ability for self-care • Families undergoing crises • Clients who have experienced the death of a child • Clients who are at risk for suicide or who have experienced a recent suicide in the family
Family role changes	• Adolescent parents • First-time parents and their newborns • Caretakers who need assistance or reassurance • Caretakers who miss work frequently to provide care to family members • Families with multiply handicapped children • Families in which caretakers are experiencing stress
Health education needs	• Clients who have significant knowledge deficits regarding health promotion, an existing conditions, or its treatment
Psychosocial needs	• Clients who live in unsafe physical environments • Children who are experiencing difficulty in school • Clients who have no regular source of health care
Other needs	• Clients who are noncompliant with health recommendations • Clients who need periodic review of medications • Clients who are at risk for abuse or who have experienced abuse • Children with a history of fetal drug exposure • Children with attention deficit disorder or developmental delay

knowledge related to the wide variety of health problems likely to be encountered in home situations as well as knowledge of appropriate nursing interventions for those problems. Skills in the interpersonal dimension will be particularly important for developing the rapport required and to defuse any hostility expressed by clients who may not desire services or feel a need for them.

Elements of the ethical dimension come into play when the nurse encounters unsafe conditions in the home that warrant nursing advocacy even when this may violate a client's wishes. For example, the nurse who discovers that an elderly client is being abused, may report the abuse to the authorities even if the client does not want a report made. Ethical considerations also arise when clients continue to need services but funding for services has been exhausted.

In the skills dimension, the nurse may need to employ diagnostic skills with limited information available in the preparatory assessment phase in order to prepare adequately for the visit. Care in the home may also require creativity in the execution of a variety of technical skills such as catheter care, intravenous infusion, ambulation, and irrigations. Circumstances in the home setting may place constraints on the way in which a typical plan of care must be implemented. For example, if the nurse is visiting a client who does not have running water, he or she will need to help the client find ways of complying with instructions to apply warm compresses.

Initiating the Home Visit

Home visits by community health nurses are initiated for a variety of reasons. Many times the nurse receives a request for a visit from another health care provider or agency. Reasons for such requests include health care needs related to specific health problems or needs for health-promotive services. For example, many hospital obstetrics units refer all first-time mothers for home visits by community health nurses to provide assistance in parenting and to promote a successful postpartum course and adjustment to parenthood. Or, a physician might request a home visit to educate a hypertensive client about prescribed medications.

Home visits might also be initiated by clients themselves. For example, a mother concerned about her child's recurrent nightmares may call and request a home visit by a community health nurse. Friends and family might also initiate a home visit. A neighbor might inform the nurse that he or she thinks the children next door are being abused. Or, a mother may request a home visit to help her daughter deal with the loss of a child. Finally, the community health nurse may initiate a home visit. The nurse might note

that a child seen in the well-child clinic is developmentally delayed and decide to visit the home to see if environmental factors are contributing to the delayed development.

 ## Conducting a Preparatory Assessment of the Dimensions of Health

Before the home visit the nurse conducts a ***preparatory assessment*** to review existing information about the client and his or her situation. Previously acquired client data should be reviewed and factors influencing client health status defined. If the client is already known to the nurse or the agency, a certain amount of data is available in agency records, notes from previous visits, and other material. Such data may be used by the nurse to refresh his or her memory regarding the client's health status.

If the client is new to an agency, data available will most probably be limited to that received with the request for services. In such a case, the nurse needs to look for general cues that suggest client strengths and potential problems. For example, if the home visit is requested for follow up on a newborn and his adolescent mother, the nurse knows that infant feeding, sleep patterns, maternal knowledge of child care, bonding, involution, maternal coping abilities, and family planning are areas that may need to be addressed with this family. Similarly, if the referral is for an elderly woman with uncontrolled hypertension, the nurse will identify areas related to diet, medication, safety, and exercise for investigation during the visit.

All aspects of the client's life should be reviewed to detect strengths, existing problems, and potential problems that may need to be addressed during the visit. Using the dimensions of health as a framework, the nurse reviews available information on biophysical, psychological, physical, social, behavioral, and health system factors that influence the client's health status. By assessing client factors in each of these areas, the nurse enters the client's residence better prepared to deal with the wide variety of client needs likely to be encountered.

The Biophysical Dimension

A client's age and race provide clues to health needs that might be encountered during the home visit. For example, if the client is a child, the nurse may want to assess the child's development; assessing for constipation, on the other hand, is appropriate for both children and elderly clients. Ethnic minority clients frequently have less access to health care; consequently, more health problems are apt to be encountered during home visits to these individuals.

One area of concern in any home visit is the development of the client and other family members. Are developmental tasks being accomplished? Is there evidence of developmental lag? What are possible factors involved in the lag? Table 10–3 summarizes functional, interpersonal, and psychosocial developmental tasks to be accomplished at particular stages of development. Functional tasks reflect the development of physical abilities that allow one to perform the functions and activities of everyday life. Interpersonal tasks relate to the development of abilities to interact effectively with others, and psychosocial tasks reflect development of a personal self and abilities to function effectively in the social environment.

The nurse would assess each member of the household with respect to accomplishment of expected developmental tasks and identify needs for health promotion or problem resolution related to development. For example, if a toddler is present in the home, the nurse might want to focus on anticipatory guidance for toilet training or the diminished appetite common in this age group. Or, if the home includes older family members, attention may be given to the older persons' adjustment to retirement, decreased mobility, and income reduction.

The nurse also considers information about the physiologic function of the client and other family members. Does the mother of a handicapped youngster have asthma? How has the child's problem affected the mother's health status? Does the older client have arthritis? What does this mean in terms of ability to perform activities of daily living? Does someone in the family have other chronic health problems that may affect the health status of the client or the family? Are client or family members taking any medication? What effect, if any, does medication have on ability to function? For example, the child who takes antihistamines for allergies may exhibit poor school performance due to drowsiness.

Normal physiologic states may also give rise to a need for nursing intervention. If the client is pregnant, for example, the nurse will want to address normal physiologic changes in pregnancy, adequate nutrition, and signs of impending labor.

Another consideration to be made by the nurse is the possible interplay between maturation and physiologic function. For example, it may be more difficult for an adolescent with diabetes to adhere to a diabetic diet than an older or younger client because of the pressure to conform to peer group norms, including dietary norms. Similarly, pregnancy poses more of a risk for an adolescent or a middle-aged woman than for a young adult woman.

The Psychological Dimension

Knowledge of the client's psychological environment can also help to identify potential health problems. What was the client's cognitive and emotional status on previous visits? Does the client or any member of the family have a history of substance abuse or mental illness? In recent years, for example, community health nurses have received increasing numbers of requests for home visits to newborns with fetal exposure to drugs. Information regarding past maternal drug use included in the referral alerts the nurse to assess carefully the infant's development and look for evidence of neglect if the mother continues drug use.

Family dynamics also contribute to a positive or negative psychological environment. What is known about family interaction patterns? Coping skills? Is there a history of violence within the family? If the client is debilitated and requires care by family members, what emotional support is available for caretakers? Is respite care available if needed? *Respite care* is the voluntary or paid services of a person who assumes care responsibilities of a homebound person on a temporary basis. The nurse would also look for evidence of client and family strengths. Do extended family members serve as a support system for the client?

The Physical Dimension

Where does the client live? Is the neighborhood safe? Are there adequate services and facilities close to the client's home? For the elderly client, age, distance to shopping facilities, and lack of transportation may contribute to poor nutrition because of diminished opportunity to obtain food.

What is the condition of housing in the client's neighborhood? Is this likely to contribute to health hazards for the individual client or family members? For example, young children in a family living in an older neighborhood may be at risk for lead poisoning from lead-based paint used on older dwellings. Or, if an older client lives in an apartment, he or she may have to deal with stairs or other impediments to mobility.

Review of the client's record prior to the home visit might provide information about known safety hazards in the home. Is the home of a family with young children childproofed? Are there loose rugs in the home of an elderly client? Community health nurses may want to complete the *home safety assessment guides* in Appendix D when children or older persons are living in the home the nurse plans to visit.

Safety concerns may also be directly related to providing nursing care in the home setting. Equipment and preparations that present minimal safety

TABLE 10–3.   LIFE-STAGE-RELATED FUNCTIONAL, INTERPERSONAL, AND PSYCHOSOCIAL DEVELOPMENTAL TASKS

Life Stage	Functional Tasks	Interpersonal Tasks	Psychosocial Tasks
Infant (0–1 yr)	• Achieve physiologic equilibrium • Achieve increased wakefulness • Display neurologic responses appropriate to age • Vocalize • Localize sound • Develop motor skills • Develop beginning mobility	• Develop self-awareness and recognition of others • Develop feelings of trust and affection • Develop rudimentary social interactions • Begin to adjust to expectations of others • Indicate needs and wishes • Develop and resolve stranger anxiety • Begin to say a few words	• Develop awareness of social environment • Understand and control physical world via exploration
Young child (2–6 yr)	• Develop increased physical independence • Become toilet-trained • Refine motor skills • Dress self with decreasing supervision • Feed self	• Give and share affection • Interact increasingly with agemates • Increase language use • Develop team abilities • Express emotion in healthy ways • Increase communication with a wider variety of people	• Follow directions • Learn to obey without supervision • Identify with male/female role models • Display increasing concern for others • Imitate adult behavior • Develop a routine • Function as a family member • Display initiative tempered by conscience • Lay foundations for a philosophy of life
School-age child (6–12 yr)	• Increase motor skills • Display independence in physical hygiene • Increase neuromuscular strength	• Converse with peers and adults • Display increased need for privacy • Form peer friendships • Learn to belong • Display increased interaction with same-sex peers • Verbalize and handle emotions effectively	• Learn math, reading, writing skills • Seek heroes and role models • Begin separation from family • Accept responsibility at home • Develop a sense of humor • Give increasing attention to personal appearance • Become more self-directed in learning • Make logical decisions with help • Be influenced more by peers and less by family • Seek socially acceptable ways of earning money and saving • Develop positive attitudes to self and others and differences noted
Adolescent (13–18 yr)	• Develop secondary sex characteristics • Develop sexual capabilities • Learn to handle a changing body	• Learn appropriate role in heterosexual relationships • Develop mutual affectional bonds with someone of opposite sex • Verbalize value conflict	• Accept self • Display strong sexual identification • Prepare self as a responsible citizen • Display increased influence by peers, then increased self-direction • Become aware of world and national events • Develop abilities to generate alternatives • Take increased financial responsibility • Increase independence from parents
Young adult	• Establish healthy routines of eating, rest, and exercise	• Find means to express love outside sexual activity • Establish an intimate relationship	• Develop adult value set • Become financially independent • Establish a vocation • Establish and manage a home • Decide on having a family • Establish a philosophy of life and value system • Become an involved citizen • Learn a husband/wife role
Middle adult	• Maintain healthy routines • Learn new motor skills as needed for leisure and other pursuits • Accept and adjust to bodily changes of middle age	• Develop interdependence with others • Establish new ways of relating to children and grandchildren • Cultivate and maintain friendships	• Assist children to be independent • Deal with aging parents • Develop a reasonable balance of activities • Carry a socially adequate role • Develop leisure pursuits
Older adult	• Accept and adjust to decreased mobility • Adapt interests to reduced strength and energy • Develop ways to deal with physical illness and disability as needed	• Accept help graciously • Learn new affectional roles with children and grandchildren • Establish and maintain friendships • Be a good companion for an aging spouse	• Establish satisfactory living arrangements • Adjust to retirement • Adjust to reduced income • Adjust to loss of spouse and friends • Maintain social interaction • Maintain integrity and values despite disappointment • Prepare for death

risks in a hospital setting can present considerable, but controllable, risks when used in the client's home. For example, an IV stand becomes a safety hazard when the home has scatter rugs or is particularly crowded. Grounding of electrical outlets is a safety issue for clients requiring infusion pumps. Injectable and other medications can be dangerous in the hands of infants and children.

Continuous chemotherapy infusions are successfully administered in homes, but they present unique safety hazards. For example, some agents are extremely toxic to skin tissue. Needles and other equipment used to administer these agents also present contamination and injury hazards.

Infection control is another safety issue related to provision of health care in the physical environment of the home. Infection control in the home has a dual focus: protecting the client and family and protecting the nurse. The nurse should adhere to the agency's standards of practice, incorporate universal precautions for preventing the spread of disease, and educate clients and family members in infection control measures.

Community health nurses change dressings for infected wounds, change intravenous sites, provide central line care, transfuse clients, and work with clients diagnosed with many communicable diseases. Continuous assessment of the environment for established infection control standards and outcome criteria is a necessary function of the community health nurse in the home setting. In the preparatory assessment, the community health nurse alerts him- or herself to the potential for problems related to infection control within the client's home environment.

Infection control procedures in the home are similar to those employed in other health care settings, but may require more creativity on the part of the nurse working in the client's home. For example, one community health nurse made an early morning visit to change an indwelling urinary catheter in a remote rural area 60 miles from the health department. Because the nurse knew he would be visiting the client before going to the public health center, he put the necessary supplies in his care the day before. Unfortunately, the temperature dropped during the night, and when the nurse went to inflate the bulb to keep the new catheter in place, the fluid was frozen in the syringe. The nurse did not have another catheterization set and could not return to the health center to get one, so he used the warmth of his sterile-gloved hand to thaw the syringe while maintaining a sterile field and keeping the catheter in place in the client's urethra.

The primary infection control measure in any setting is adequate handwashing before and after giving any direct care to clients. Hands should be thor-oughly washed with soap and running water. Again, this may require some creativity on the part of nurses or family members in homes without running water. For example, the nurse may wet his or her hands, apply soap, and lather thoroughly, then ask a family member to pour clean water over the hands to rinse them. The nurse can also make a habit of carrying paper towels on home visits to avoid using towels that were used previously. The nurse may also identify a need to instruct family members in the importance of handwashing in the care of the client and as a general measure for preventing the spread of disease.

Infection control in the home, as in other settings, involves the use of sterile precautions in any invasive procedures, appropriate disposal of bodily secretions and excretions, and isolation precautions as warranted by the client's condition. Nurses working in the home with clients who have bloodborne diseases such as AIDS and hepatitis should use universal blood and body fluid precautions. These precautions apply to any body fluids, including blood, semen, vaginal secretions, cerebrospinal fluid, synovial fluid, pleural fluid, peritoneal fluid, pericardial fluid, and amniotic fluid, and feces, nasal secretions, sputum, sweat, urine, or vomitus that contains visible blood. Identification of the possible need for universal precautions during the preparatory assessment allows the community health nurse to plan effectively to promote personal safety and that of the client and family. Universal precautions to be taken by the nurse to prevent the spread of bloodborne disease are summarized on page 200.

Care should also be taken in the disposal of secretions and excretions of clients with other conditions. For example, sputum from clients with active tuberculosis should be handled with care, and the feces of chronic typhoid carriers should be disposed of in a municipal sewer system.

Nurses and significant others caring for clients with certain conditions may need to be immunized. For example, household contacts to chronic typhoid carriers should be immunized against typhoid, and both family members and nurses caring for clients with hepatitis B should receive immunizations. When the nurse's preparatory assessment indicates client and family needs in these areas, the nurse can plan effective interventions related to them. Careful attention to infection control measures in the home can minimize risks for clients and their families as well as for the nurse.

The Social Dimension

Knowledge of the client's social environment assists the nurse to identify factors contributing to client

▶ **UNIVERSAL PRECAUTIONS**
FOR PREVENTING THE SPREAD
OF BLOODBORNE DISEASES

1. Use appropriate barrier precautions (eg, gloves) to prevent skin and mucous membrane exposure when contact with human blood or other body fluids is anticipated.
2. Wash hands and other skin surfaces immediately after contamination with blood or other body fluids.
3. Take precautions to prevent injuries stemming from needles and other sharp instruments during or after procedures, when disposing of used equipment, or when cleaning used equipment.
4. Do not recap, bend, or break used needles; place them in a puncture-proof container for disposal.
5. Keep mouthpieces, resuscitation bags, or other ventilation devices at hand when the need for resuscitation is predictable.
6. Refrain from direct care of clients and from handling client care equipment when you have exudative skin lesions or weeping dermatitis.
7. Implement these precautions with all clients, not just those known to be infected with bloodborne diseases.

Source: Recommendations for prevention of HIV transmission in health care settings. (1988). *MMWR, 36*(Suppl 2), 35–185.

health status as well as factors that influence nursing intervention. Areas for consideration include the client's education level, financial status, and social network. Other considerations include the influence of religious beliefs on the client's health and clients' access to transportation. Other social factors to be considered include the employment status and occupation of family members. What are the occupations of client and family members? How do these occupations influence health? If the client's condition has interfered with his or her employment or that of family members, the nurse will want to assess the potential for a return to work. For example, the client may have a need for physical or occupational therapy in order to return to his or her previous occupation. If the client is not able to return to a former occupation because of the consequences of illness or injury, the nurse can assist the client to determine the potential for other avenues of employment. Or, if the client is not able to return to work at all, there may be a need for assistance in filing disability claims. Prior knowledge of these needs gleaned from the preparatory assessment allows the nurse to make the home visit prepared to meet these needs.

In a similar vein, the community health nurse preparing for a home visit would assess factors that may influence the ability of family caretakers to return to work. For example, the mother of a handicapped child may require assistance in making appropriate child care arrangements so she can return to work. Or there may be a need for a companion for an elderly client with Alzheimer's disease to free family caretakers for employment.

The Behavioral Dimension

Assessment considerations in the behavioral dimension include nutrition and other consumption patterns, recreation, and health-related practices.

The client record may provide information about family nutritional practices. Are these appropriate to the growth and development needs of family members? Other considerations related to consumption patterns include the presence or absence of substance abuse problems and the influence of such problems on health.

Tobacco use by people in the home is another important consideration in a previsit assessment. If family members smoke, for example, second-hand smoke might further impair the health of an older client with a chronic respiratory condition or a child with asthma. In addition, smoking by either client or family members could pose a serious safety hazard if the client is receiving oxygen therapy. Use or abuse of other substances by the client or family members may also pose health hazards.

One area of assessment that is particularly important in relation to a home visit is a functional assessment. Areas to be addressed in a functional assessment include client abilities to meet needs related to mobility, cognition, eating, toileting, dressing, hygiene, shopping, cooking, and managing money. All of these areas influence client lifestyle.

The Health System Dimension

Information about client interaction with the health care system also assists the community health nurse to prepare for an effective home visit. Where does the client/family usually receive health care? Is access to care limited by the client's financial status or lack of health insurance? What health care providers are working with the client? Is there any coordination between provider activities?

How does the client/family interact with health care professionals? Are they open to recommendations? Are they hostile or suspicious of the motives of providers? This and other information assists the nurse to plan an approach to the client that leads to rapport and a therapeutic relationship.

ASSESSMENT TIPS: Assessing the Home Visit Situation

Biophysical Dimension

Age

What are the ages of persons in the home?

Do the age and developmental level of persons in the home give rise to specific health needs?

Are age-appropriate developmental tasks being accomplished by persons in the home?

Physiologic Function

Do any persons in the home have existing physical health problems?

Does anyone in the home have difficulty in performing activities of daily living?

Do persons in the home exhibit other physiologic states that necessitate health care (eg, pregnancy)?

Psychological Dimension

What is the emotional status of persons living in the home?

How effective are coping strategies used by persons living in the home?

Is there a history of mental illness in anyone living in the home?

If there is a newborn in the home, has the baby been exposed to drugs in utero?

Do persons in the home interact effectively with one another?

Is there a history of violence in the home or evidence of current abuse of persons living in the home?

Physical Dimension

Where is the home located?

Is the neighborhood safe? Are there environmental pollutants in the neighborhood?

Are there physical health hazards in the home?

Is the home in good repair? Does it have the usual amenities (eg, running water, heat, electricity, refrigeration, cooking facilities)?

Does the home environment accommodate the age-related safety needs of persons living there?

Is the home equipped to meet special needs of persons living there (eg, safe administration of oxygen, etc.)

Does the home situation pose a risk for infection for persons living there?

Social Dimension

Education Level

What is the education level of persons living in the home?

What is the extent of their health knowledge?

How does their education level affect their health?

Financial Status

What is the economic level of persons living in the home?

What is their usual source of income?

Is their income sufficient to meet needs?

How do those living in the home finance health care?

Employment

Are persons living in the home employed?

Does occupation pose any health risks for persons living in the home?

Does employment contribute to other needs (eg, child care)?

Social Network

What is the extent of social support available within the home and from outside the home?

What are the attitudes of members of the social support network to health care providers and services? What effects do these attitudes have on the health of persons in the home?

Culture and Religion

Do persons living in the home subscribe to any particular religious beliefs or affiliation?

Does religious belief or affiliation influence health behavior by persons living in the home?

Are there cultural practices in the home that influence health? Is this influence positive or negative?

Behavioral Dimension

Dietary Patterns

What are the dietary needs and habits of persons living in the home?

Are dietary patterns in the home adequate to meet developmental nutritional needs of those living there?

How are foods usually prepared in the home?

What meal patterns are typical of those persons living in the home?

(continued)

Other Consumption Patterns

Does anyone living in the home smoke? What are the potential health effects of smoking on persons living in the home?

Is there evidence of substance abuse in the home?

Do any of those living in the home use medications on a regular basis? If so are they used and stored appropriately?

Do persons living in the home use other substances that may have adverse health effects (eg, caffeine)?

Rest/Exercise

What opportunities for exercise are available to those living in the home?

Is the extent of exercise obtained by persons living in the home adequate?

Are there adequate sleeping accommodations for persons living in the home?

Leisure Activity

What leisure activities are pursued by persons living in the home?

Do leisure activities pose health hazards for those living in the home?

Safety Behaviors

Do persons living in the home engage in appropriate safety measures?

Sexual Activity

Who in the home engages in sexual activity?

Are sexual relationships in the home appropriate?

Are contraceptives used appropriately within the home if needed?

Health System Dimension

Where do persons living in the home seek health care?

Is health care utilization by persons living in the home appropriate?

Are there barriers to access to health care services for persons living in the home?

Diagnostic Reasoning and the Home Visit

Based on the data available in the preparatory assessment, the nurse makes nursing diagnoses related to health conditions to be addressed during the home visit. These diagnoses may be positive diagnoses, health-promotive diagnoses, or problem-focused nursing diagnoses.

The diagnostic reasoning process discussed in Chapter 7 is used. The nurse examines data available and develops diagnostic hypotheses that seem to explain the data. Hypothesis evaluation takes place when the nurse actually makes the home visit and obtains additional data to confirm or disconfirm the diagnostic hypotheses. The diagnostic hypotheses generated from the preparatory assessment, however, give the nurse some direction for planning nursing interventions to be performed during the home visit.

Positive nursing diagnoses reflect client strengths evidenced in the preparatory assessment.

For example, available data may indicate "effective coping with the demands imposed by a handicapped child due to a strong family support system." This diagnosis suggests that the nurse will reinforce family support as a factor contributing to effective coping.

Problem-focused nursing diagnoses may reflect actual problems for which there is evidence in the preparatory assessment data or potential problems. For example, an existing problem of "ineffective contraceptive use due to inadequate knowledge of contraceptive methods" may have been documented on a previous home visit. Unless there is also an indication that this problem has been resolved, the nurse will probably address it during the subsequent home visit. Preparatory assessment data may suggest potential problems as well. For example, the request for services might indicate that the client's husband is in the Navy and is due to leave on extended sea duty. This information would suggest a nursing diagnosis of "potential for ineffective coping due to loss of spousal assistance."

Nursing diagnoses might also reflect the need for health-promotive services. For example, there will soon be a "need for routine immunizations" for a newborn child. Similarly, the mother has a "need for postpartum follow-up due to recent delivery."

 ## Planning the Home Visit

Based on the preparatory assessment, the community health nurse makes plans for a home visit to address the health needs most likely to be present in the situation. Tasks to be accomplished in planning the visit include reviewing previous interventions, prioritizing client needs, developing goals and objectives for care, and considering client acceptance and timing. Other tasks of this stage include delineating activities needed to meet client needs, obtaining needed materials, and planning evaluation.

Reviewing Previous Interventions

The first step in planning is to review any previous interventions related to client health needs and the efficacy of those interventions. This information allows the nurse to eliminate interventions that have been unsuccessful in the past and to identify interventions that have worked.

Prioritizing Client Needs

The next task is to give priority to identified client needs. Client care needs may be prioritized on the basis of their potential to threaten the client's health, the degree to which they concern the client, or their ease of solution (see Chapter 7 for a more complete discussion of criteria for prioritizing health needs). It is often impossible to address all of the client's health problems in a single visit, so the nurse must decide which needs require immediate attention. For example, if the wife has been admitted to an alcohol treatment center and there is no one to care for the children while the father works, provision of child care and dealing with the children's feelings about the mother's absence may be the only things that can be accomplished on the initial visit. Other problems, such as poor nutrition habits and need for immunizations for the toddler, can be deferred until a later visit.

Developing Goals and Objectives

After determining which client needs will be addressed in the forthcoming visit, the nurse develops goals and objectives related to each area of need. Goals are generally stated expectations, whereas objectives are more specific. In the previous example, the nurse's goal might be to enable the family to function adequately in the mother's absence. In this instance, an outcome objective might be that adequate child care will be obtained so the father can return to work.

The health care needs that will be addressed during a home visit may reflect the primary, secondary, and tertiary level of prevention. When health care needs occur in the realm of primary prevention, goals and outcome objectives reflect positive health states or absence of specific health problems as expected outcomes of care. For example, a goal for primary prevention might be "development of effective parenting skills." A related outcome objective might be that the client "will display effective communication skills in relating to children."

Goals and objectives related to needs for secondary prevention focus on alleviation of specific problems. For example, a goal for a hypertensive client might be "effective control of elevated blood pressure," and the related outcome objective might be a blood pressure that is "consistently below 140/90." Similarly, goals and objectives for tertiary prevention reflect client achievement of a prior level of function or prevention or recurrence of a health problem.

Considering Acceptance and Timing

In planning a home visit, the nurse should consider the client's readiness to accept intervention as well as the timing of the visit and introduction of intervention. The nurse may find, for example, that a relatively minor problem with which the client is preoccupied must be addressed before the client is willing to deal with other health needs.

Timing is another important consideration in planning an effective home visit. If the visit interferes with other activities important to the client, the client may not be as open to the visit as would otherwise be the case. Other activities that compete with a home visit for the client's attention might be the visit of a friend, an upcoming doctor's appointment, getting the children ready for an outing, or even something as mundane as a favorite soap opera. Prescheduling or rescheduling home visits can make the visit a more effective intervention if something else is interfering.

Timing also relates to the degree of rapport established between client and nurse. Clients need time to develop trust in the nurse before intimate issues can be addressed. For example, a pregnant adolescent may feel too uncomfortable and threatened by the nurse during early visits to admit to prior drug use and ask about its effects on the baby. The nurse should judge the appropriateness of the timing in bringing up intimate issues for discussion and wait, if possible, until rapport is established with the client.

Delineating Nursing Activities

The next aspect of planning the home visit is the planning of specific nursing activities for each nursing diagnosis to be addressed. The activities planned reflect the nurse's assessment of health care needs and the factors influencing them. For example, referral to a Head Start program may provide assistance with child care, but only if the children involved are of the right ages. If the youngsters are of school age, the appropriate nursing intervention might be to help the father explore the possibility of an afterschool program, of one is available, or have the children go home with the parents of a friend until the father can pick them up after work.

Nursing activities can focus on both health promotion and resolution of health-related problems. For example, the community health nurse might provide the parents of a toddler with anticipatory guidance regarding toilet training or assist parents to discuss sexuality with their preteen daughter. Other positive interventions might focus on providing adequate nutrition for a young child or promoting a healthy pregnancy for the pregnant female.

Specific interventions employed by the nurse include referral, education, and technical procedures. For example, the nurse might refer a family to social services for financial assistance, teach a mother about appropriate nutrition for the family, or check a hypertensive client's blood pressure. The actions selected should be geared to achieving the goals and objectives established while taking into account the constraints and supports in the individual client situation.

Obtaining Necessary Materials

One aspect of planning the home visit that does not apply to many of the other processes discussed in this unit is obtaining materials and supplies that may be needed to implement planned interventions. Because the nurse is going to be in the client's home, one cannot assume that necessary supplies will be available there. If the nurse plans to engage in nutrition education, he or she might want to leave a selection of pamphlets with the client to reinforce teaching. If planned activities involve weighing a premature infant, the nurse will want to take along a scale.

Equipment and supplies may also be needed for other procedures such as dressing changes, catheterizations, injections, and blood pressure checks. Because the nurse frequently does a physical assessment of one or more clients, additional equipment such as a stethoscope, percussion hammer, tongue blade, flash-light, and otophthalmoscope will need to be obtained prior to setting out for the visit.

Planning Evaluation

As with every other process employed by community health nurses, the planning phase of the home visit process concludes with plans for evaluation. The nurse determines criteria to be used to evaluate the effectiveness of the home visit. Criteria for evaluating client outcomes are derived from the outcome objectives developed for the visit. Because the outcome of nursing interventions undertaken during a home visit may not be immediately apparent, the nurse needs to develop both long-term and short-term evaluative criteria. Short-term criteria are likely to be based on client response to interventions. If, for example, the nurse makes a referral for immunizations, the mother cannot follow through on the referral and receive immunizations on the spot. The nurse, however, can evaluate the mother's response to the referral. Does the mother seem interested? Does she indicate that she will follow through on the referral? On subsequent visits, the nurse would employ long-term outcome criteria to evaluate the effects of interventions. In this instance, criteria would include whether the client had her child immunized.

Outcome evaluation addresses the level of prevention of nursing interventions. Evaluative criteria for primary preventive measures, for example, reflect health promotion or the absence of specific health problems. For example, criteria for interventions to foster immunity to childhood diseases would include whether immunizations were obtained and the presence or absence of immunizable diseases such as measles. If the client develops measles, primary prevention of this disease obviously was not effective.

Evaluation of secondary preventive measures focuses on the degree to which an existing problem has been resolved. For example, a client's hypertension may have been uncontrolled because of poor medication compliance. Evaluative criteria in this instance would include the degree of compliance achieved and the client's blood pressure measurements. Criteria to evaluate tertiary preventive measures reflect the degree to which a client has regained a prior level of health or prevented recurrent health problems. For example, have passive range-of-motion exercises helped a client recovering from a broken arm to regain strength and mobility? Or, has parenting education by the nurse prevented further episodes of child abuse in an abusive family?

The nurse also develops criteria to evaluate implementation of the planned home visit. These criteria are derived from process objectives developed for the visit. For example, was the nurse adequately prepared to address the health care needs encountered during the visit? Were the appropriate supplies available for implementing planned interventions?

Implementing the Planned Visit

The next step in the home visit process is conducting the visit itself. Several tasks are involved in implementing the planned visit. These include validating the health needs and diagnoses identified in the preparatory assessment, identifying additional needs, modifying the intervention plan as needed, performing nursing interventions, and dealing with distractions.

Validating Assessment and Diagnoses

The first task in implementing the home visit is to validate the accuracy of the preparatory assessment. Problems identified from the available data may or may not exist when the nurse actually enters the home. For example, the nurse may find that the family's poor diet is not the result of lack of knowledge about nutrition, but stems from a lack of money to purchase nutritious foods. Or the nurse may find that what appeared to nurses on the postpartum unit to be poor maternal–infant bonding was not actually the case. Similarly, the nurse may discover that expected strengths or positive nursing diagnoses do not accurately reflect the client's actual health status. For example, a mother who appeared to be coping effectively with her child's handicap may really have been exhibiting denial of the condition.

Identifying Additional Needs

During the visit, the nurse collects additional data related to biophysical, psychological, physical, social, behavioral, and health system factors to identify additional health care needs. For example, when the nurse arrives to visit a new mother and her infant son, the nurse may find that the client's father has recently had a heart attack and been taken to the hospital. The client may be much more in need of assistance in finding child care for her new baby so she can spend time at the hospital than in discussing immunization and postpartum concerns. Or, the nurse may find that, in addition to having a new baby, the client's husband is out of work and the 12-year-old has been skipping school.

Modifying the Plan of Care

Based on what the nurse finds in the course of the home visit, the initial plan of care may need to be modified. The nurse shares with the client the initial goals established for addressing health needs identified in the preparatory assessment, as well as additional problems identified, and together they set or revise goals. In doing this, the nurse might find a need to restructure priorities based on new data and client input. For instance, if the 2-year-old has cut her arm and is bleeding profusely when the nurse arrives, this problem takes precedence over the nurse's plan to discuss with the mother the potential for sibling rivalry. In other words, the nurse can either implement interventions as planned or modify the plan as the client situation dictates.

Performing Nursing Interventions

Once the plan of care has been modified as needed, the nurse performs whatever nursing interventions are warranted by the client situation. As noted earlier, these activities may include primary, secondary, and tertiary preventive measures. For example, the nurse working with a new mother might discuss parenting skills as a means of preventing child abuse (primary prevention), give the mother suggestions for dealing with the infant's spitting up (secondary prevention), and discuss options for contraception to prevent a subsequent pregnancy (tertiary prevention).

Any or all of the three levels can be emphasized depending on the situation encountered. For example, if the mother is inexperienced and concerned about child care skills in feeding, bathing, and parenting, the emphasis would be on primary prevention. Conversely, if the nurse arrives to find a baby screaming with gas pains, emphasis is placed on making the infant more comfortable and relieving the mother's anxiety. Once this has been accomplished, the nurse can focus on suggestions to prevent a recurrence of the problem.

Dealing with Distractions

One important consideration in implementing a home visit is dealing with distractions. Distractions are generally of three types: environmental, behavioral, and nurse-initiated (Pruitt, Keller, & Hale, 1987). Environmental distractions arise from both the physical and social environments and may include background noise, crowded surroundings, and interruptions by other family members or outsiders. The occurrence of such distractions during the home visit can give the nurse a clear picture of the client's environment and the way in which the client and family interact among themselves and with others. For example, if mother and child are continually yelling at one another during the visit, this suggests the existence of family communication problems. On the other hand, positive interactions between a mother and her young child provide evidence of effective parenting skills.

Despite the information that can be gleaned from these distractions, their negative effects on the interaction between client and nurse need to be minimized. Requesting that the television be turned off during the visit or moving the client to a more private area can minimize some distractions. Or, the nurse may ask an intrusive younger child to draw a picture to allow parent and nurse to talk with fewer interruptions. If there are too many distractions that cannot be eliminated or overcome, the nurse can ask the client if there is a better time for the visit, when fewer interruptions will occur, and reschedule the visit for a later date. For example, subsequent visits might be planned to coincide with the toddler's nap.

Behavioral distractions consist of behaviors employed by the client to distract the nurse from the purpose of the visit. Again, the use of such distractions can be a cue for the nurse that certain topics are uncomfortable for the client or that the client does not quite trust the nurse or may feel guilty about something. The nurse can benefit from the distraction by exploring the reasons for the client's behaviors and working to establish trust with the client.

The last category of distractions originate with the nurse. These distractions create barriers to relationships with clients. Fears, role preoccupation, and personal reactions to different lifestyles can distract the nurse from the purpose of the home visit. Nurses may fear bodily harm, rejection by the client, or the lack of control that is implicit in a home visit. In today's violent society, fear of bodily harm is understandable and nurses making home visits should employ the precautions discussed earlier in this chapter.

Community health nurses may also create distractions by being so preoccupied with their original purpose that they fail to see the need to modify the planned home visit. No planned intervention is so important that it cannot be postponed if more important needs intervene. Nurses who continue to pursue predetermined goals in the light of other client needs reduce their credibility with clients and create barriers to effective intervention. For example, the nurse who insists on talking about infant feeding when the client just had an argument with her husband and fears he will leave her is not meeting the client's needs.

Finally, community health nurses may be put off by the contrast between their own lifestyle and that of the clients they are visiting. In dealing with feelings engendered by such differences, it is helpful to understand that one's own attitudes are the product of one's upbringing and that clients derive their attitudes in the same way. In dealing with lifestyle differences, the nurse must be aware of personal feelings and their impact on nursing effectiveness. The nurse must also determine what aspects of the client's lifestyle may be detrimental to health and focus on those, while accepting other differences in attitude or behavior as hallmarks of the client's uniqueness. Being thoroughly informed about cultural and ethnic differences also minimizes negative reactions by the nurse to such differences. Some of these differences are discussed in Chapter 16.

Evaluating the Home Visit

Before concluding the visit, the nurse evaluates the effectiveness of interventions in terms of their appropriateness to the situation and client response. This evaluation is conducted using criteria established in planning the visit. It may not be possible, at this point, to determine the eventual outcome of nursing care. The nurse can, however, examine the client's initial response to interventions. Was the mother interested in obtaining contraceptives? Is it likely that she will follow through on a referral to the immunization clinic? Did the client voice an intention to reduce salt intake? Could the client accurately demonstrate the correct technique for breast self-examination?

Evaluating the ultimate outcome of interventions may occur at subsequent visits. For example, on the next visit, the nurse might determine whether the mother obtained contraceptives. If she called, but was unable to get an appointment, the nurse would determine the reason. Based on information obtained, there may be a need for advocacy on the part of the nurse. If the client did not seek contraceptive services, the nurse should determine the reason for her behavior. Was the client distracted by crises that occurred in the meantime, but plans to call for an appointment next week? Did she not have transportation to the clinic? Or, maybe she does not really want contraceptives. If the client lacks transportation, the nurse might help her explore ways of getting transportation. If the client does not really want contraceptives, the nurse can either explore why and work to change her attitude or accept the client's wishes.

As noted earlier, evaluation of nursing intervention during a home visit should reflect the level of prevention involved. The nurse examines both short-term and long-term effects of interventions at the primary, secondary, and tertiary levels of prevention, as

Critical Thinking in Research

Braveman and associates (1996) examined the effects of nursing home visits on health service use among healthy newborns discharged before and after the implementation of a nursing home visit follow-up program for early discharge. Comparisons were made between early discharge newborns whose mothers received follow-up home visits and telephone calls and those whose mothers did not. Outcome variables examined included acute care visits, rehospitalization, and well-baby visits. Acute care visits, rehospitalization, and missed well-baby appointments were less likely to occur among the home visit group. Babies in this group had a twofold reduction in acute care visits, a significant finding. Differences in the extent of missed well-baby appointments were not significant, but favored the home visit group. The number of rehospitalizations was not large enough to permit testing for statistical significance, but again favored the home visit group.

1. Given the relative costs of longer hospital stays and the expenses of home visiting new mothers and babies, do the findings of this study support the cost-effectiveness of newborn home visit programs?
2. What other outcome variables might you want to examine to support the effectiveness of nursing home visits to new mothers and babies?
3. How might you go about collecting data on these variables?

appropriate. For example, if the home visit focused on secondary prevention, evaluation will also be focused at this level. If several levels were addressed during the visit, evaluation will focus on the effects of interventions at each level.

The nurse also evaluates his or her use of the home visit process. Was the preparatory assessment adequate? Was information available that the nurse neglected to review, resulting in unexpected problems during the visit itself? For example, did the nurse ask about the husband's reaction to the new baby when the record indicates the client is not married? Did the nurse miss cues to additional problems during the visit? Was the nurse able to plan interventions consistent with client needs, attitudes, and desires? Was the nurse able to deal effectively with distractions? If not, why not? Answers to these and similar questions allow the nurse to improve his or her use of the home visit process in subsequent client encounters.

▶ DOCUMENTATION AND REIMBURSEMENT

Documentation is the last stage of the home visit. It is particularly important in home health care precisely because care is given in that setting (Iyer & Camp,

1995). In the home there are frequently no witnesses other than the nurse, the client, and possibly family members. In the event of an adverse effect of care, without adequate documentation, it may be the nurse's word against that of the client or family member. Accurate documentation is also required for reimbursement and for research to support the effectiveness of home care. Finally, when services are provided by a multidisciplinary team, good documentation facilitates coordination and continuity of care. In documenting the home visit, the nurse must accurately record the client's health status, the nursing interventions employed, and the effectiveness of interventions. The nurse documents validation of diagnoses made in the preparatory assessment, as well as additional needs identified, by recording both subjective and objective data obtained during the visit. Goals and objectives established for addressing client health needs are also recorded. In addition, the nurse documents actions taken, client response to those actions, and the outcome of interventions if known. Also included in documentation are future plans and recommendations for subsequent home visits. A chart entry for a nursing home visit using the status-oriented record format might look like the sample presented in Figure 10–2. Client assessment and health status summary would be documented separately and are not included in the figure.

The entry reflects problems identified in a routine postpartum visit to an adolescent with a new baby. The S and O notations reflect subjective and objective assessment data, respectively. Subjective data are provided by the client or other informant, whereas objective data are observed directly by the nurse. The A notation refers to the nurse's analysis of the situation or the nursing diagnosis, and P is the plan of care for addressing the particular health need. A brief narrative statement evaluates the effects of intervention. In subsequent visits, evaluative comments would be reflected in the subjective and objective data related to the current status of the health care need.

A special note about documentation in home health agencies is needed. Agency reimbursement frequently depends on an accurate portrayal of the client's condition and progress and the nature of service provided.

General Considerations in Home Health Documentation

Most agencies design forms to meet the needs of their clientele and their funding sources. Separate forms may be used for initial evaluation visits and for the progress notes on subsequent visits. Most agencies use specific forms to communicate with the physician about the client's status and to document communica-

NURSING PROGRESS NOTES

Date

7-9-99 H.V. for routine PP & newborn eval as requested by La Paloma Hosp.

   Client is 17 yo unwed Hispanic girl c̄ a normal full-term baby boy born 7-5-99. Lives c̄ parents and two sisters

   ages 13 and 8.

Diagnosis #1: Inadequate family income

   Goal: Provide family income adequate to needs

   Objective: Obtain food stamps, AFDC, & Medicaid assistance.

   S. Client states was unable to afford PN care, has no funds for PP check or well-child care. Family has no health

      insurance, unable to pay hospital bill

   O. Ø

   A. Inadequate family finances due to low income and educational level

   P. 1. Determine eligibility for financial assistance programs

      2. Refer for Medicaid, foodstamps, AFDC

      3. Revisit in 2 wks to f-u on referrals

   Eval: Referrals made, family seemed accepting. Grandmo states will apply for aid next week.

Diagnosis #2: Overprotection of 13 yo girl

   Goal: Provide environment conducive to normal development

   Objective: Parents will be less restrictive of 13 yo's activities

   S. Grandmo states husb will not let 13 yo date or go out c̄ girl friends due to older sister's pregnancy. 13 yo states

      she is not sexually active & resents restrictions

   O. 17 yo unwed mother in home

   A. Potential for inadequate development of 13 yo due to father's overprotectiveness

   P. 1. Explore family attitudes to unwed pregnancy, sexual activity, etc.

      2. Discuss developmental tasks of adolescence with parents

      3. Encourage parents to foster responsible decision-making by 13 yo

      4. Follow-up discussion c̄ family in 1 mon.

   Eval: Grandfather states he'll allow 13 yo to go out c̄ girl friends but not to date 'til age 16.

Diagnosis #3: Inadequate child care skills

   Goal: Improved child care skills

   Objective: 1. Client will be able to adequately feed, bathe, diaper, clothe child

      2. Client will maintain safe environment for child

      3. Client will provide adequate health care for child

   S. Client states she has little experience c̄ child care, no baby-sitting experience. Grandmo states it has been a

      long time since there was a baby in home.

   O. 17 yo girl with newborn son, asking many questions re: child care

   A. Inadequate child care skills due to lack of experience

   P. 1. Assess extent of child care knowledge

      2. Demonstrate child care skills of feeding, burping, diapering, bathing , and clothing over next several visits

      3. Discuss infant nutrition

      4. Discuss infant safety & immunization

      5. Discuss care of minor illnesses

      6. Provide educational material on child care, immunization, growth & development, etc.

      7. Suggest addtl literature from public library

      8. Return visit g 2-3 wks to continue teaching as needed

   Eval: Client eager to learn, accepted educational materials to be read by next visit. Able to exhibit correct bottle-

   feeding & burping technique p̄ demonstration.

                                                                        M. Clark, R.N., P.H.N.

Client name: Flores, Maria   Record No.   567-8359

Figure 10–2. Sample documentation of a nursing home visit.

tions. Each agency has a protocol for documenting the plan of care, case conferences, care given, client outcomes, and discharge from home nursing services. Examples of agency forms for documenting nursing assessments and home care are contained in Appendix E.

Medicare Documentation and Reimbursement

Reimbursement for services provided under Medicare is made by a fiscal intermediary. A *fiscal intermediary* is an agency designated by HCFA to act as a reimbursing agent and deal directly with home health care agencies. For example, in certain portions of Southern California, the Blue Cross–Blue Shield Insurance Company acts as a fiscal intermediary for home health agencies. In other parts of the country, private insurance carriers such as Aetna Life and Casualty and Traveler's Insurance Company serve as intermediaries. Home health agencies are reviewed periodically by representatives of the fiscal intermediary for adherence to Medicare guidelines related to services, documentation, and billing practices.

Fiscal intermediaries for Medicare reimbursement monitor agency documentation via periodic audits of nursing notes submitted with billing forms and on-site review visits. If inconsistencies or inappropriate statements are found, it is possible for reimbursement for all Medicare services to be denied, even those unrelated to the audited notes.

Specific information is required on the original certification and plan of treatment form, along with an estimation of the number and frequency of visits to be provided. This information is derived from the initial evaluation form completed by the nurse at the time of the evaluation visit.

Recertification of the client's condition and eligibility for services must occur at specific intervals, and the physician must be periodically notified of the client's progress. Copies of both the original Medicare certification form and the recertification form are included in Appendix E.

▶ TERMINATION

The community health nurse may terminate home visiting services to a particular client when the goals and objectives established for care have been accomplished, when the duration of services surpasses allowable limits, when clients refuse continued services, or when a client dies. Other possible reasons for terminating services include safety concerns for the client or nurse, noncompliance with the treatment

plan, needs that go beyond the capability of the agency to meet them, institutionalization, and repeated failure to find the client at home (Davis, 1996). In many of these instances, however, services should not be terminated until reasonable efforts have been made (eg, to promote compliance or locate the client).

Obviously, it is less stressful for the nurse to terminate services to clients who no longer require them. Even then, though, the intimacy of the nurse–client relationship developed over a series of encounters makes it difficult for both nurse and client to "let go." In the case of agency moratoria on additional visits, clients with yet unmet needs may feel abandoned unless the nurse has made careful preparation for termination. Client refusal of services may be perceived by the nurse as a personal rejection and the nurse will need to work through feelings of frustration and come to an acceptance of the client's decision without loss of self-esteem. Even in the case of a client's death, the nurse may find it difficult to terminate relationships developed with the client's family.

Effective termination actually begins with the initial home visit. The nurse should recognize and make clients aware that the relationship is necessarily time-limited. It may be helpful at the outset of the relationship to specify a predetermined period during

TABLE 10–4. ELEMENTS OF A HOME VISIT

Preparatory assessment	• Review available client data to determine health care needs related to biophysical, psychological, physical, social, behavioral, and health system dimensions
Diagnosis	• Develop diagnostic hypotheses based on preparatory assessment
Planning	• Review previous interventions and their effects
	• Prioritize client needs and identify those to be addressed during the visit
	• Develop goals and objectives for visit and identify levels of prevention involved
	• Consider client acceptance and timing of visit
	• Specify activities needed to accomplish goals and objectives
	• Obtain needed supplies and equipment
	• Plan for evaluation of the home visit
Implementation	• Validate preparatory assessment and nursing diagnostic hypotheses
	• Identify other client needs
	• Modify plan of care as needed
	• Carry out nursing interventions
	• Deal with distractions
Evaluation	• Evaluate client response to interventions
	• Evaluate long-term and short-term outcomes of intervention
	• Evaluate the quality of implementation in the home visit
Documentation	• Document client assessment and health needs identified
	• Document interventions
	• Document client response to interventions
	• Document outcome of interventions
	• Document future plan of care

which services will be provided. The period designated may be mandated by agency policy or by mutually determined estimates of the time needed to accomplish established goals and objectives. As time passes, the nurse may need to remind the client that the time for termination is drawing near. When the time for termination actually arrives, the nurse and client can review goal accomplishment and the nurse can provide clients with continuing needs or surviving family members of deceased clients with referrals for sources of continued assistance. Some resources that may help community health nurses in making home visits are listed at the end of this chapter. Other resources that address the needs of clients with chronic physical and emotional health problems are included in Chapters 31 and 32.

The Dimensions Model provides a context for structuring home visits to provide health care to individuals and their families. The components of a home visit within the context of the model are summarized in Table 10–4.

TESTING YOUR UNDERSTANDING

1. What is the relationship between community health nursing and home health nursing? (p. 193)
2. Describe at least three advantages of home visits as a means of providing nursing care. (pp. 188–189)
3. Describe at least four challenges faced by community health nurses making home visits. (pp. 189–192)
4. List three characteristics of effective home visiting programs. Describe the principles for developing successful programs related to each of the characteristics chosen. (p. 192)
5. Identify three purposes for a home visit program. How might programs differ with respect to purpose? (pp. 192–193)
6. Identify at least three types of home health agencies. In what ways do they differ? (pp. 193–194)
7. Identify at least four aspects of planning for a home visit. Give an example of each. (pp. 203–205)
8. Describe at least four tasks in implementing a home visit. Give an example of the performance of each task. (pp. 205–206)
9. Identify three types of potential distractions during a home visit. Give an example of each and describe actions by the nurse that might eliminate the distraction. (pp. 205–206)
10. Why is there a need for both long-term and short-term criteria for evaluating the effectiveness of a home visit? Give examples of the use of both types of criteria. (pp. 206–207)

WHAT DO YOU THINK?
Questions for Critical Thinking

1. How would you respond to a situation in which there is a threat to your own safety, but leaving would endanger your client?
2. What kind of home visit distractions might arise from your own personal behavior? What could you do to prevent this kind of distraction?
3. What are the implications of different types of home health agencies for the practice of community health nursing?
4. Under what circumstances should a home health agency discontinue services to a client? Is an agency ever justified in terminating services because the client cannot pay for them? Is an agency justified in refusing to begin services for clients who have no source of payment?

Critical Thinking in Practice: A Case in Point

You are a community health nurse working for the Clark City Health Department. Your supervisor took the following request for nursing services by phone and passed it on to you because the address is part of your district. You know that this address is in an older residential area with a large Hispanic population.

Clark City Health Department
Request for Nursing Services

Source of Request: La Paloma Hospital Maternity Unit

Date of Request: 7-7-99

Client: Maria Flores   Date of birth: 10-21-79

Address: 8359 Marlboro Way, Marquette, AL 36019

Head of household: Juan Flores (client's father)

Reason for referral: Delivered 5lb 7oz baby boy on 7-5-99. Client had no prenatal care. Lives with parents & 2 younger sisters, ages 8 & 13. Both parents work, but family income insufficient to pay hospital bill. Family does not have insurance or Medicaid. Request routine postpartum/newborn evaluation.

---

1. Based on the information you have, what health care needs related to the biophysical, psychological, physical, social, behavioral, and health system dimensions would you identify in your preparatory assessment? List your diagnostic hypotheses.
2. What nursing interventions would you plan for the health needs you are likely to encounter in a visit to this client? Identify your planned interventions as primary, secondary, or tertiary preventive measures.
3. What materials might you need on this home visit?
4. How would you go about validating your preparatory assessment and diagnostic hypotheses?
5. What additional assessment data would you want to obtain during your visit?
6. What evaluative criteria would you use to conduct outcome and process evaluation of care provided to this client and her family?
7. On what basis would you make the determination to terminate services to Maria?

REFERENCES

American Nurses Association. (1988). *Statement on the essentials of home health care nursing.* Kansas City, MO: American Nurses Association.

Association of Community Health Nurse Educators. (1990). *Essentials of baccalaureate nursing education for entry level community health nursing practice.* Louisville, KY: Association of Community Health Nurse Educators.

Barnett, W. S. (1993). Economic evaluation of home visiting programs. *The Future of Children, 3*(3), 93–112.

Bishop, C., & Skwara, K. C. (1993). Recent growth of Medicare home health. *Health Affairs, 12*(3), 95–110.

Braveman, P., Miller, C., Egerter, S., et al. (1996). Health service use among low-risk newborns after early discharge with and without nurse home visiting. *Journal of the Board of Family Practice, 9,* 254–260.

Cherry, N. M. (1988). The role of official tax-supported agencies in home care. *Nursing Clinics of North America, 23,* 431–434.

Cooper, W. O. (1996). Use of health care services by inner-city infants in an early discharge program. *Pediatrics, 98,* 686–691.

Cowley, S. (1995). In health visiting, a routine visit is one that has passed. *Journal of Advanced Nursing, 22,* 276–284.

Davis, S. T. (1996). Patient admission, discharge, transfer, and nonacceptance. In S. C. Schulmerich, T. J. Riordan, & S. T. Davis (Eds.), *Home health care administration* (pp. 257–266). Albany, NY: Delmar.

Deal, L. W. (1994). The effectiveness of community health nursing interventions: A literature review. *Public Health Nursing, 11,* 315–323.

Gomby, D. S., Larson, C. S., Lewit, E. M., & Behrman, R. E. (1993). Home visiting: Analysis and recommendations. *The Future of Children, 3*(3), 6–22.

Gunther, R. W. (1996). Selected legal issues in home health care. In S. C. Schulmerich, T. J. Riordan, & S. T. Davis (Eds.), *Home health care administration* (pp. 61–73). Albany, NY: Delmar.

Iyer, P. W., & Camp, N. H. (1995). *Nursing documentation: A nursing process approach* (2nd ed.). St. Louis: Mosby.

Keating, S. B., & Kelman, G. B. (1988). *Home health nursing: Concepts and practice.* Philadelphia: J. B. Lippincott.

Kristjanson, L. J., & Chalmers, K. I. (1991). Preventive work with families: Issues facing public health nurses. *Journal of Advanced Nursing, 16,* 147–153.

Lent, M. E. (1993). The fundamental importance of bedside care in public health nursing. *Public Health Nursing, 10,* 263–266. Reprinted from *Public Health Nurse,* September, 1920.

Liepert, B. D. (1996). The value of community health nursing: A phenomenological study of the perceptions of community health nurses. *Public Health Nursing, 13,* 50–57.

National Center for Injury Prevention and Control. (1994). Medical-care spending—United States. *MMWR, 43,* 581–586.

Olds, D. L., & Kitzman, H. (1993). Review of research on home visiting for pregnant women and parents of young children. *The Future of Children, 3*(3), 53–92.

Pruitt, R. H., Keller, L. S., & Hale, S. L. (1987). Mastering distractions that mar home visits. *Nursing & Health Care, 8,* 344–347.

Ruetter, L. I., & Ford, J. S. (1996). Perceptions of public health nursing: Views from the field. *Journal of Advanced Nursing, 24,* 7–15.

Rice, R., & Smiley, D. V. (1996). Historical perspectives. In R. Rice (Ed.), *Home health nursing practice: Concepts and application* (2nd ed.) (pp. 3–15). St. Louis: Mosby.

Schulmerich, S. C. (1996). General information. In S. C. Schulmerich, T. J. Riordan, & S. T. Davis (Eds.), *Home health care administration* (pp. 10–19). Albany, NY: Delmar.

Sorochan, M., & Beattie, L. (1994). Does home care save money? *World Health, 47*(4), 18–19.

Starn, J. A. (1992). Community health nursing visits for at-risk women and infants. *Journal of Community Health Nursing, 9*(2), 102–110.

Stanhope, M., & Knollmueller, R. N. (1996). *Handbook of community and home health nursing* (2nd ed.). St. Louis: Mosby.

Stulginsky, M. M. (1993a). Nurses' home health experience. Part I: The practice setting. *Nursing & Health Care, 14,* 402–407.

Stulginsky, M. M. (1993b). Nurses' home health experience. Part II: The unique demands of home visits. *Nursing & Health Care,* 476–485.

SUPPORT AGENCIES FOR HOME NURSING

Home Care

American Association for Continuity of Care
638 Prospect Avenue
Hartford, CT 06105–4250
(860) 586–7525

American Federation of Home Health Agencies
1320 Fenwick Lane, Ste. 100
Silver Spring, MD 20910
(301) 588–1454

National Association for Home Care
519 C Street, NE
Stanton Park
Washington, DC 20002
(202) 547–7424

Sick Kids Need Involved People
216 Newport Drive
Severna Park, MD 21146
(410) 647–0164

Visiting Nurse Associations of America
3801 East Florida Street, Ste. 900
Denver, CO 80210
(303) 753–0218

Hospice

Children's Hospice International
1850 M Street N, Ste. 900
Washington, DC 20036
(703) 684–0330

Hospice Nurses' Association
211 N. Whitfield Street, Ste. 375
Pittsburgh, PA 15206
(412) 361–2470

National Hospice Organization
1901 North Moore Street, Ste. 901
Arlington, VA 22209
(703) 243–5900

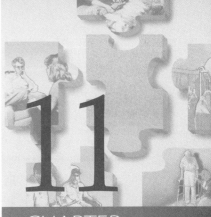

11

THE CASE MANAGEMENT PROCESS

► KEY TERMS

abandonment
case management
comorbidity
coordination of
 benefits (COB) rules
critical path
extracontractual
 benefits
managed care
negligent referral
referral
situational constraints
utilization review
variances

Case management is the recent focus of a great deal of attention, primarily because of its effects on minimizing health care expenditures as managed care becomes a growing emphasis in health care delivery. Recent interest notwithstanding, community health nurses have been doing case management since the beginning of their practice more than a century ago. What is case management? What are the elements of the case management process? What is its relationship to community health nursing? These questions are the focus of this chapter.

▶ Chapter Objectives

After reading this chapter, you should be able to:

- Identify five goals of case management.
- Describe three characteristics of effective case management programs.
- Identify at least five characteristics of effective case managers.
- Discuss the standards of case management practice.
- Describe legal issues related to case management.
- Identify criteria for selecting clients in need of case management.
- Assess the need for case management in terms of the dimensions of health.
- Discuss at least two considerations in developing a case management plan.
- Identify at least three aspects of initiating a referral.

▶ DEFINING CASE MANAGEMENT

A variety of definitions of case management can be found in the literature of several disciplines, including nursing and social work. These definitions are often based on a particular model of case management and so may appear remarkably different (Powell, 1996). In the New England model, case management is a process designed to "achieve standardized outcomes within designated lengths of stay with appropriate use of resources, while promoting professional development and satisfaction of RNs" (Anderson-Loftin, Wood, & Whitfield, 1995). This definition suggests that case management is a process unique to institutional settings. The Case Management Society of America (CMSA) (1995) defined case management as "a collaborative process which assesses, plans, implements, coordinates, monitors and evaluates options and services to meet an individual's health needs through communication and available resources to promote quality cost-effective outcomes." This definition seems to imply a broader area of practice for case managers and implies certain goals of the process. According to the broker model, case management is a process that "focuses on identifying client needs, matching appropriate health and community resources in a timely, cost-effective fashion, and monitoring the results of the match between the client's needs and the provided resources" (Conti, 1996). Again, this definition describes some of the activities and parameters expected in case management.

Case management must be differentiated from care management or managed care. *Managed care* is defined as the "systems and mechanisms used to control, direct, and approve access to the wide range of services and costs within the health care delivery system" (Mullahy, 1995). By contrasting the definition of managed care with the definitions of case management provided above, we can see that case management is concerned with quality of care and acceptable care outcomes as well as with cost containment. Because community health nurses are concerned with services at all levels of prevention and not just management of care to clients with existing health problems, we will adapt the CMSA definition of case management for use in this book. *Case management,* as practiced by community health nurses, is a process of identifying needs for and arranging, coordinating, monitoring, and evaluating quality, cost-effective primary, secondary, and tertiary prevention services to achieve designated health outcomes.

Within the context of this definition, case management can take place in two areas, internal case management and external case management (Newell, 1996). In internal case management, the case manager is employed by the organization providing care and is responsible for overseeing and coordinating the different facets of care provided to the client within the organization. Internal case management may take place in a hospital or in a managed care plan that includes a variety of services. In external case management, the case manager is not a part of the provider organization, but arranges and coordinates services provided by several agencies. Community health nurses may engage in either internal or external case management, although employees of official health agencies are more likely to be involved in external case management coordinating services provided by a variety of other agencies, a traditional role of community health nurses.

▶ THE IMPETUS FOR CASE MANAGEMENT

Why is the concept of case management of such interest in today's health care delivery system? The answer to this question lies in the advantages posed by a case management approach for both the client and the health care industry. For the client, case management assures effective coordination of care and helps to reduce the confusion and complexity of the health care system. The case manager can assist the client to obtain needed services in the most acceptable and affordable settings. Case management, if effectively performed, should also result in improved client health outcomes in most instances. Effective case management also results in attention to all of the client's health needs to minimize the development of other health problems.

TABLE 11–1. BENEFITS OF CASE MANAGEMENT FOR CLIENTS
AND FOR HEALTH CARE DELIVERY SYSTEMS

Beneficiary	Benefits
Client	Better coordination of care
	Assistance in negotiating a complex health care system
	Access to acceptable and affordable health care services
	Attention to multiple health care needs
	Improved health outcomes
Health care delivery systems	Reduced cost of care
	Minimization of hospitalization
	Prevention of rehospitalization
	Elimination of service duplication

Case management also emphasizes service delivery in the least expensive setting possible, thereby limiting the overall costs of health care. Effective case management minimizes hospitalization for needs that can be dealt with in community practice settings. For those clients who do need hospitalization, case management may prevent rehospitalization when continuing health care needs are adequately addressed after discharge. The cost of health care is also minimized when case management eliminates duplication of services. Benefits that create an impetus for case management are summarized in Table 11–1.

▶ GOALS OF CASE MANAGEMENT

As noted earlier, case management focuses on meeting the needs of clients as well as on containing the costs of care. This dual focus leads to multiple goals of case management services. These goals include providing quality health care, achieving designated health outcomes, decreasing fragmentation of services, increasing quality of life or providing for death with dignity, and decreasing costs by making the most efficient use of resources (CMSA, 1995; Flarey & Blancett, 1996). Simultaneous achievement of these multiple goals often requires a delicate balance similar to the concept of balance discussed in Chapter 10. The community health nurse must attempt to provide clients with the type and quantity of services that meet their needs to achieve optimal health outcomes in the most cost-effective manner possible.

Effective case management programs share several characteristics (Mundt, 1996; Flarey & Blancett, 1996). To achieve the goals described above, case management systems must be:

- *Client- and family-centered.* The primary emphasis is on improving the health status of the client, but the needs of family members are also considered and addressed in the development of a case management plan. For example, home care is generally considered more acceptable to clients, as well as less expensive, than hospitalization. If, however, home care will mean that a family member must quit work to care for the client, home care might not be the best option for this client.
- *Coordinated.* Case management involves managing client contacts across multiple settings and with multiple providers (Rice, 1996). In other words, case management provides a multidisciplinary, multiservice approach along a continuum of care (Trella, 1996). This continuum is particularly relevant in community health nursing case management, where care may begin with essentially well clients and continue through illness episodes as they arise.
- *Collaborative and cooperative.* The multidisciplinary nature of case management requires cooperation among various disciplines participating in the client's care. For example, effective care of a pregnant woman may involve prenatal care from the local health department as well as perinatal services provided by the community hospital. After delivery, continuity of care may necessitate home visits by a community health nurse.
- *Outcome-oriented.* Case management is geared toward achievement of specifically defined outcomes.
- *Resource-efficient.* Case management seeks the least expensive mode of care that will meet the client's needs and achieve the desired outcomes.

▶ STANDARDS OF CASE MANAGEMENT PRACTICE

Standards of case management practice have been developed by the CMSA (1995). Measurement criteria have been identified for each standard. Both the standards and related measurement criteria are depicted in Table 11–2. The standards of practice are similar to those for community health nursing presented in Chapter 4.

▶ LEGAL ISSUES IN CASE MANAGEMENT

Although many of the legal issues in case management are common to other aspects of community health nursing, there are some that warrant special attention. These issues include confidentiality, abandonment, negligent referral, and the use of controversial or experimental treatments. The issue of confidentiality has two aspects in case management. The first is the need for client permission to make contacts and

TABLE 11–2. STANDARDS OF CASE MANAGEMENT PRACTICE AND RELATED MEASUREMENT CRITERIA

Standards of Care

STANDARD

The case manager appraises the need for intervention through gathering and critical, objective evaluation of relevant data.

CRITERIA

1. The case manager evaluates proactive triggers to identify clients needing case management services.
2. The case manager seeks authorization for case management services.
3. The case manager conducts a thorough assessment of the client's status.
4. The case manager assess elements of the treatment plan including resource use, cost management, diagnosis, treatment course, prognosis, goals, and provider options.

STANDARD

The case manager selects a case load of clients for whom outcomes can be positively influenced.

CRITERIA

1. The case manager identifies opportunities for intervention.
2. The case manager helps to determine what patterns of care give rise to needs for case management.

STANDARD

The case manager identifies immediate, short-term, and long-term needs, sets appropriate and agreed upon goals and time frames for their achievement, and assures resources needed to achieve goals.

CRITERIA

1. The case manager gathers information as a factual base to formulate a case management plan.
2. The case manager demonstrates understanding of diagnosis, prognosis, care needs, and goals of care.
3. The case manager demonstrates understanding of cost-containment strategies.
4. The case manager is able to identify barriers to goal attainment.

STANDARD

The case manager monitors and documents the quality of care, services, and products provided to determine goal achievement and continued appropriateness of goals.

CRITERIA

1. The case manager maintains effective communication with the client and family to facilitate monitoring.
2. The case manager maintains a collaborative relationship with members of the treatment team to foster review, monitoring, and modification of care plan.
3. The case manager maintains regular communication with all providers; ascertains that goals are appropriate, understood, documented and achieved; and advises providers of changes in the plan of care.
4. The case manager compares client outcomes to established critical pathways.

STANDARD

The case manager evaluates the client's response to services, the effectiveness of the plan, and the quality of services provided.

CRITERIA

1. The case manager reassesses client health status and progress toward goals.
2. The case manager determines reasons for a demonstrated lack of progress and encourages adjustments in the plan of care to promote better outcomes.
3. If the outcome of care is guarded or expected to be terminal, the case manager emphasizes maintaining environmental stability for client and family.

STANDARD

The case manager identifies and coordinates changes in practice patterns and treatments that promote appropriate care and cost-effective outcomes.

CRITERIA

1. The case manager establishes goals that meet client needs with use of appropriate resources.
2. The case manager establishes measurable goals that facilitate evaluation of the cost and quality of care.
3. The case manager plans with client and family a goal-oriented care plan that moves the client toward health, wellness, adaptation, or habilitation.
4. The case manager reports quantifiable impact, quality of care and/or quality of life improvements related to case management goals.
5. The case manager focuses on accountability for care and cost–benefit consistent with expectations of consumers, providers, and payers.

(Source: CMSA, 1995.)

---

arrangements for services on the client's behalf (St. Couer, 1996). The case management plan should be presented to and agreed upon by the client before any further action is taken. The second aspect of confidentiality relates to unauthorized disclosure of information about the client (Nichols, 1996). To avoid a breach of confidentiality in this area, the community health nurse case manager should inform clients of the need to share information with others and obtain client authorization before doing so.

Abandonment occurs when the case manager terminates services to a client with continuing needs without notifying the client or arranging for services from another provider (Nichols, 1996). Although community health nurse case managers may encounter

situations in which services need to be terminated (eg, in the face of client failure to comply with the treatment plan), the nurse should make every effort to avoid abandonment. It may be helpful to develop a contract with clients indicating both case manager and client responsibilities with respect to the case management plan. In addition, the case manager should carefully document both positive and negative aspects of the client's response to case management services and continued efforts to enlist client cooperation.

Nurse case managers may be held legally liable for negligent referrals. A *negligent referral* may be (1) a referral that results in harm or injury to the client because the case manager has not adequately assessed the competency of the provider or (2) a failure to make a referral when one is warranted (Nichols, 1996). Case managers can prevent negligent referrals by investigating the providers or agencies to which they refer clients in terms of licensure and relevant accreditation, client outcomes data, billing practices, insurance coverage, and malpractice information. A second tactic to prevent negligent referrals is to provide the client with several provider options rather than making a single referral. Finally, the case manager should follow up on the outcomes of referrals made (Mullahy, 1995).

The last legal issue to be addressed has ramifications for the client and for the health care system. When clients are facing a terminal condition or treatment options are extremely limited, it may be appropriate to suggest experimental interventions (St. Couer, 1996). Generally speaking, however, clients should not be referred for controversial therapies or experimental treatments. The lack of data to support the effectiveness of such treatments or their safety may place clients at risk, result in expenditures of time and money for ineffective interventions, or lead to unfounded hope or neglect of more effective treatment options. At the health system level, expenditures for unproven therapies are not an effective use of available resources.

► CRITERIA FOR CASE SELECTION

Not all of the clients encountered by community health nurses will need case management services, so the nurse must identify those clients who do need services and can benefit most from them. These clients can be identified on the basis of possible indicators similar to those used to determine clients in need of home health services. These indicators can be categorized as personal indicators, health-related indicators, and social indicators. Personal indicators may include diminished functional status, a history of substance abuse or mental illness, prior noncompliance with treatment plans, age over 65 years, experience of a major life change or significant change in self-image, or unrealistic expectations of the potential for a return to health. Health-related factors include the presence of specific medical conditions or diagnoses (eg, Alzheimer's disease, AIDS, dehydration, eating disorders, severe burns, trauma), recent or frequent hospital readmissions or emergency department use, intentional or unintentional drug overdose, and involvement of multiple health care providers or agencies. Social indicators are living alone or with a person who is disabled, being uninsured, evidence of family

violence, homelessness or an unhealthy home environment, lack of support systems or financial resources, single parenthood, or living in an area where services are lacking (Powell, 1996). Presence of one or more of these indicators does not necessarily mean that the client is in need of case management services, but should alert the community health nurse to that possibility. The nurse would then further explore the client situation to determine an actual need for services.

► THE DIMENSIONS MODEL AND CASE MANAGEMENT

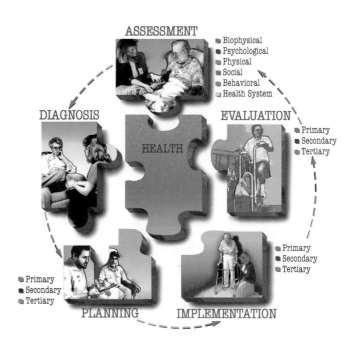

Community health nurses can employ the Dimensions Model to direct their case management activities.

Critical Dimensions of Nursing in Case Management

Attributes desired in a case manager reflect several of the dimensions of nursing and may be categorized in terms of personal characteristics and requisite skills (Mullahy, 1995; Powell, 1996). Personal characteristics that describe effective case managers include commitment, perseverance, self-confidence, flexibility, creativity, attention to detail, resourcefulness, accountability, self-direction, assertiveness, and a sense of humor. In addition, the case manager must have clinical expertise and a thorough knowledge of insurance issues, community resources, and legal and practice standards. Clinical expertise and knowledge of insurance issues, resources, and standards reflect the cognitive dimension of nursing. Case managers who have clinical expertise in areas related to client problems often have a better idea of potential consequences of those problems, treatment options, and resources available than those without such expertise. General knowledge of insurance plans and services covered and of community resources allows the case manager to plan a combination of services that are feasible. Planning for services for which the client is not eligible or which are not available in the community will necessitate extensive modification of the plan of care and may entail considerable frustration for both nurse and client.

In the interpersonal dimension, case managers should be skilled in communication, diplomacy, collaboration, and team building. These skills will enable the case manager to "sell" the plan of care to all concerned parties: client, family, providers, and payers. The nurse will need to communicate effectively and collaborate with the client and family as well as with other health care professionals. The nurse may also need to collaborate with a variety of others not in the health care business per se (eg, government officials or protective services personnel).

The legal issues of confidentiality and abandonment discussed earlier have ethical components as well. It would be unethical as well as illegal for the nurse case manager to disclose client information inappropriately or to abandon a client without recourse to needed services. Another significant element in the ethical dimension is the balance that may be required between the goals of quality care and cost containment. Community health nurse case managers may need to advocate for meeting client health needs even when this means increasing health care costs.

Specific skills required of effective case managers include prioritization, critical thinking, assessment, organization, and personnel management skills (Powell, 1996). Case managers must be able to prioritize client needs and address the most pressing needs first. In part, the ability to prioritize, as well as the ability to assess needs and plan for their fulfillment, rests on the case manager's critical thinking skills. The case manager must be able to interpret client information and recognize the implications for client health and for the services required to promote or restore health. Organization and management skills, on the other hand, will contribute to the accomplishment of the goals of decreased fragmentation of services and increased cost-effectiveness.

Elements of the process dimension that may be employed by the nurse case manager include the change, leadership, and health education processes. Case managers may expend considerable energy on motivating clients, families, and providers to imple-

ment the case management plan. The nurse may also need to educate the client and his or her family in order for them to carry out the plan effectively. Depending on the case management situation, the nurse may also need to use the home visit process.

Finally, research and evaluation are critical elements from the reflective dimension of nursing needed in case management. The nurse uses research findings as one basis for developing the case management plan and conducts evaluation to determine the effectiveness of the plan in accomplishing identified client care goals.

Assessing the Dimensions of Health in Case Management

In order to develop an effective case management plan, the community health nurse case manager must identify factors in the client situation that affect health and are likely to affect the plan and achievement of planned health outcomes. Assessment of these factors involves consideration of each of the six dimensions of health: biophysical, psychological, physical, social, behavioral, and health system dimensions.

The Biophysical Dimension

Biophysical dimension factors of age and physiologic function influence case management needs and the case management plan. The client's age may be a factor in eligibility for services as well as the appropriateness of specific services. For example, a younger person with a traumatic injury may do better in a rehabilitation unit that serves a variety of age groups than one that serves primarily older clients. Similarly, an adolescent with a new baby is likely to need more intensive postdischarge follow up than a more mature woman.

Physiologic function can profoundly influence the level and types of care needed by the client. The nature of medical diagnoses, *comorbidity* (the presence of other disease processes), functional ability to carry out activities of daily living, and abilities to implement a health treatment plan will suggest possible health care needs that the case manager will need to address. For example, the client with decreased functional abilities may need referral for help with household chores, and the client with diagnoses of cardiovascular disease and diabetes will require careful monitoring. Based on physiologic status, some clients may require skilled nursing care or specialized treatments such as intravenous infusions, oxygen administration, or physical therapy.

The Psychological Dimension

Psychological factors may also influence clients' health care needs. A client experiencing a psychiatric disorder, for example, may require referral for continued therapy as well as social and emotional support. The presence of mental illness may also complicate the treatment plan for other conditions. For example, a severely depressed client may be unable to engage in the level of self-care required for managing their diabetes. In this instance, the case manager may arrange for frequent home health visits or transfer to an assisted living facility until the client is able to function effectively at home.

The Physical Dimension

Elements of the physical dimension may also need to be addressed in the case management plan. For example, self-care at home may necessitate the use of assistive devices or equipment, and the case manager would arrange for the client to receive this equipment. Or, the home may require physical modification to accommodate the client's health status. For instance, clients with limited mobility may need to have a ramp installed or change sleeping arrangements to avoid climbing stairs. Other physical dimension factors to be considered include the availability of running water, electricity, adequate heat or air conditioning, space for special equipment, and distance of the home to health care and other services (Hester, 1996). Environmental factors such as the presence of pollutants should also be considered. For example, a child who is being treated for lead poisoning will need environmental accommodations to prevent reexposure to lead.

The Social Dimension

Social dimension factors will also influence the types and extent of services to be included in the case management plan. Some social factors to consider are the client's education level, support systems, economic status, occupation, transportation, and cultural beliefs and behaviors. For example, clients who live alone and have few social supports may require referrals for assistance with self-care or housekeeping, or institutional placement may be appropriate until the client can effectively engage in self-care.

The client's economic status can profoundly influence the case management plan. Clients may need financial assistance to meet basic survival needs as well as help with health care needs. For example, a homeless client will need assistance with housing and possibly with food, clothing, and health care services. Occupation is closely related to economic status and may also influence clients' health needs. The nurse will need to obtain information about the client's em-

ployment status and usual occupation. Is a return to work a relevant goal? If so, what must be accomplished for the client to be able to return to work? Will modifications be required in the work setting or in the tasks performed?

Transportation is another social dimension factor that may influence the client's access to planned health services. Clients who are not able to get to provider agencies may be unable to avail themselves of services needed to meet identified goals. For example, the parent of a handicapped child may recognize the need for medical follow-up, but lack the means to get to the physician's office or specialty clinic. In this situation, the case management plan would incorporate transportation arrangements as well as links to health care providers.

The Behavioral Dimension

Elements of the behavioral dimension that may affect case management include consumption patterns related to diet and substance abuse, rest and exercise, sexual activity, and other health-related behaviors. The nurse would assess special dietary needs that the client might have as well as the client's ability to meet those needs and willingness to do so. Clients with substance abuse problems may need referrals for treatment services in addition to services to meet other health care needs. If the substance abuse problem is not addressed, the client may be unable to follow through on other portions of the case management plan.

Rest and exercise behaviors may also indicate areas of service requirements. Does the client need a referral for an exercise program to lose weight or is there a need for physical therapy services to regain strength or range of motion? Or, does the client have difficulty sleeping or need to arrange their daily activities to accommodate periodic rest periods. Similarly, the nurse would assess the effects of the client's condition on sexual function. If problems are noted, what services might be needed to deal with them? For example, a woman who has had a mastectomy might need the assistance of the Reach to Recovery program to deal with self-concept and body image issues. Finally, the nurse would assess the extent to which the client's condition poses special safety needs as well as the extent to which the client engages in routine safety measures such as seat belt use.

The Health System Dimension

Information related to the other dimensions of health helps the community health nurse identify the types of health care services that the client is likely to need. In the health system dimension, the nurse assesses the

Biophysical Dimension

Age

What is the client's age?

Will the client's age be a factor in eligibility for needed services?

Are services tailored to the client's age group available locally?

Physiologic Function

Does the client have any existing physical health problems?

Do existing health problems interact? If so, how?

Is the client limited in his or her ability to accomplish activities of daily living?

Does the client require specialized treatments or interventions?

Is the client taking any medications? If so, what are their effects, their side effects?

What is the client's level of understanding of physical health problems, recommended treatments, etc.?

Psychological Dimension

Does the client have any existing mental illness?

Is the client confused?

Does the client have the intellectual capacity needed to implement the management plan?

Physical Dimension

Will the client's residence require modification to meet client needs or maintain safety?

Will the client need assistive devices at home?

Does the home have adequate heat, light, water, refrigeration, ventilation, and so on?

Does the home have adequate space and utilities to accommodate special equipment?

Is the distance from the client's residence to shopping or medical facilities able to be negotiated by the client?

Are there pollutants in the environment that will adversely affect the client's health?

Social Dimension

What is the client's education level?

Is the client's income sufficient to meet his or her needs, including health care needs?

Where does the client live? Will living accommodations require modification to meet the client's needs?

Does the client live alone? If so, is the client capable of self-care or will assistance be needed?

What is the extent of the client's support system? Will available support be sufficient to meet the client's needs for assistance?

Is the client responsible for the care of other family members? Is the client capable of providing the care needed?

Is respite needed for family members who care for the client?

Is the client employed? Is a return to work a relevant goal of care?

What is/was the client's occupation? Does his or her occupation pose any health risks or give rise to any specific health needs?

Does the client have transportation? Are there special transportation needs?

Behavioral Dimension

Consumption Patterns

Does the client have special dietary needs? If so, does the client adhere to dietary restrictions?

Does the client abuse alcohol or other drugs?

Does the client use tobacco or caffeine? Does the use of these substances have specific health implications for this client?

Rest/Exercise

Does the client have special needs for rest or exercise?

Does the client have a regular form of exercise?

Does the client have problems with sleeping or waking?

Sexual Activity

Is the client sexually active?

Does sexual activity pose any particular health risks for the client?

Other Health-related Behaviors

Does the client use routine safety measures (eg, seat belts)?

Does the client have any special safety needs? Are these adequately addressed in the home?

Health System Dimension

Does the client have a regular source of health care?

Does the client seek health care services when needed?

What types of health services does the client need?

Are needed health services available and accessible to the client?

Does the client have health insurance? What services does his or her insurance cover?

What are the client's attitudes to health care services? Do these attitudes interfere with his or her ability to obtain needed care?

availability of those services in the client's community as well as influences related to the type and level of insurance coverage the client has. In addition, the nurse assesses the client's attitudes to health care services and providers. If there are needs for services that are not available locally, it may be necessary to transfer the client to a specialized facility elsewhere. This may necessitate arrangements for transportation, housing for the client or significant others, and admission to the new facility. Is home care an appropriate and cost-effective treatment option for this client? What service alternatives are covered by the client's insurance plan if he or she has one?

Client attitudes to the health care system and health care providers are another important consideration in assessing a case management situation. Clients may feel that they do not need or want any additional help or may prefer to receive care from a provider of an ethnic background similar to theirs. Clients may also resist certain types of services because of the emotional overtones attached to them. For example, an elderly client may refuse placement in a skilled nursing facility out of fear that they will never be able to return home. In some cultural groups, nursing home placement is viewed as abandonment of elderly parents and may be resisted by the family. By assessing these attitudes, the case manager will be able to plan for services that are acceptable to the client thereby facilitating plan implementation and goal accomplishment.

Diagnostic Reasoning and Case Management

Once the client's need for and acceptance of case management have been established and factors influencing the client's health status identified, the case manager uses the assessment data to diagnose specific client health care needs. The preliminary diagnosis may reflect the need for case management and the factors contributing to that need. For example, the community health nurse case manager may diagnose a "need for case management due to limited self-care abilities." Secondary diagnoses would address specific areas of focus in developing the case management plan. These areas may be related to the biophysical, psychological, physical, social, behavioral, or health system factors influencing the client's health. For example, in the social dimension the nurse might diagnose a "need for housekeeping assistance due to shortness of breath on exertion" for the client with emphysema. Similarly, a "need for home modification

due to limited mobility and potential for falls" might be diagnosed in the physical dimension.

Developing the Case Management Plan

The case manager works with the client, family, payers, and potential providers to develop a case management plan that meets the client's identified health care needs in the most efficient and cost-effective manner possible. Developing the case management plan involves two basic activities: determining levels of prevention within the health care dimension and selecting resources.

Determining Levels of Prevention

Planning may involve arranging for services at any or all of the three levels of prevention as appropriate to the client's situation. For example, the case manager may arrange for well child and family planning services for the adolescent with a newborn. He or she may also refer the adolescent to a parenting class and a teen parent support group and arrange for enrollment in an education continuation program. All of these interventions would be aimed at primary prevention.

When secondary prevention services are needed, the case manager may devise a case management plan in keeping with a critical path. A *critical path* is an established sequence of operational activities designed to achieve designated outcomes in specific health problems. Critical paths are usually developed for commonly encountered diagnoses and reflect the typical plan of care for that diagnosis. In addition to specifying a particular activity sequence the critical path identifies the time frame within which activities are to be performed and specifies client outcomes to be achieved. Critical paths are diagnosis-specific not client-specific (Newell, 1996), and although the case manager may use a critical path as a foundation for developing a case management plan, the final plan should be tailored to the needs of the individual client. In critical path terminology, these deviations from the typical path are called *variances.* Most critical paths have been established to direct care for clients with specific medical diagnoses, addressing secondary prevention needs. A few agencies, however, have developed critical paths for primary prevention activities with selected groups of clients. For example, one health department has developed a critical path for prenatal care, specifying activities to be accomplished in each trimester and the expected outcomes of those activities. A critical path at the tertiary level of prevention might detail a typical rehabilitation plan following myocardial infarction.

Selecting Resources

The second aspect of developing the case management plan involves selecting the resources, providers, and services to meet clients' identified health needs. Selection decisions will be based on considerations of appropriateness, quality, and cost. The health care services selected should be appropriate to the client's needs as well as to other aspects of the client situation. For example, it might be necessary to find a health care provider who speaks Hmong or who has office hours congruent with the client's work schedule. The appropriateness of the setting for care should also be considered. For example, while periodic home care might be appropriate for a client who is relatively self-sufficient or who has a supportive family, an assisted living situation might be more appropriate for another client.

The quality of services provided is another consideration in the selection of resources. The case manager should be conversant with the competence of providers to whom he or she refers clients and the quality of care should be monitored once the referral is made. Client complaints should be investigated and action taken to ensure provision of high quality services.

Cost is the third area of consideration in developing the case management plan. In many instances, the services available to a given client are constrained by economic considerations and what may or may not be covered by their insurance plan. The case manager has to be conversant with a wide variety of insurance plans and the services that they cover. In most instances, services should be provided in the least costly setting that will meet the client's needs. The vagaries of insurance coverage, however, sometimes mean that services will only be reimbursed if they take place in certain types of settings. For example, under some plans, intravenous infusions are not covered unless they are provided in an inpatient setting.

The nurse case manager should also be familiar with two other concepts related to reimbursement for services: coordination of benefits (COB) rules and extracontractual benefits. *Coordination of benefits rules* designate the responsibility of payers when a client is covered by more than one form of insurance (Newell, 1996). For example, when clients have both Medicare benefits and a supplemental insurance policy, Medicare first pays its share of the cost of services. Then the supplemental plan is billed for remaining costs. The case manager should be familiar with the succession of responsibility among insurance plans in order to develop an effective case management plan. When clients need services that are not covered under an existing plan, the community health nurse case manager may be able to negotiate *extracontractual benefits,* or reimbursement for uncovered services. This is usually only possible when no covered alternative is available and the nurse can demonstrate that the additional coverage will prevent a greater expense to the payer (St. Couer, 1996).

Implementing the Case Management Plan

Implementation of the case management plan involves communicating the plan, initiating referrals, and monitoring plan implementation.

Communicating the Plan

Clients and their significant others need to be informed of arrangements made for care and expectations of them in following through on the management plan. For example, clients may need to call to make a specific appointment with a provider even though care has been arranged by the case manager. Clients will also need to know about any payments required and the names of contact persons in agencies to which they have been referred. Additional information to be conveyed to clients relates to the expected duration and outcome of services.

The case manager also needs to communicate the case management plan to the providers who will be giving the necessary care. Client needs and expectations of the provider should be addressed as well as any previous plans and their effects, expectations for continued care, and any other information relevant to the client's situation. Again, the case manager should be careful to obtain the consent of the client before providing such information. Finally, the payer should be informed of and approve the management plan.

Initiating Referrals

Referral is the process of directing a client to another source of information or assistance. Referrals to a variety of health care and related services may be part of case management for an individual client and his or her family. Four basic considerations enter into the decision to refer a client to a particular provider, agency, or service: the acceptability of the referral to the client, client eligibility for services, constraints operating in the situation, and community resources available.

Acceptability to the Client.   The first consideration in making a referral is the acceptability of the referral to the client. Some clients may be unwilling to obtain help if they perceive it as "charity." In other cases, clients may have philosophies different from those of the referral resource. For example, a Southern Baptist client may be reluctant to accept assistance from an agency supported by the Roman Catholic Church. Barriers to acceptability of a specific referral may include fear of a strange agency or provider, prior negative experiences, lack of faith in the referral resource, failure to acknowledge a problem requiring referral, and concerns about costs. Finally, reaching out for assistance may be counter to the client's culture or frame of reference or following up on a referral may be preempted by other client concerns with higher priorities (Belliston, 1995).

Client Eligibility for Service.   The second consideration in referral is the client's eligibility for the service provided. There are many types of determinants of eligibility for service. Sometimes eligibility is based on financial needs, and clients may need to provide evidence of income and expenditures. In other instances, eligibility might be based on residence within a particular jurisdiction or membership in a particular group. For example, nonresidents are not usually eligible for state-supported medical assistance. Or, a particular agency may only provide services to members of a specific religious or ethnic group. Eligibility can also be based on age. As an example, senior citizens' groups usually do not provide services for anyone under the age of 55. Finally, eligibility is sometimes based on the existence of a particular condition. For instance, shelter services might be available only to abused women rather than to homeless people in general.

Situational Constraints.   The presence of **situational constraints,** or factors in the client's situation that would prevent him or her from following through on a referral, is a third consideration. For example, does the client have transportation available to go to the appropriate place of care? If clients do not speak English, will they be able to find an interpreter to help them? The nurse making the referral should assess any situational constraints present and then take action to eliminate or minimize the effects of those constraints.

Availability of Resources.   Information related to each of the three previous referral considerations will be readily available if the nurse has thoroughly assessed each of the dimensions of health prior to developing the case management plan. Resource availability information,

on the other hand, will be obtained through assessment of the community. The community health nurse case manager needs to be familiar with health care and other support services available in the community. Information on community resources can be obtained in a number of ways. Two major sources of information are the local health department and the yellow pages. Other resources are neighborhood information and referral centers, local government offices and chambers of commerce, and police and fire departments. The local library is also a source of information and may even have a directory of local resources.

It is not sufficient for the community health nurse to merely be aware of the existence of community resources. The nurse must know where these resources are located, and understand the requirements for referral to each resource. The nurse should systematically collect information on the types of services a referral resource provides, criteria for eligibility for services, and whether any fee is involved. Information to be sought also includes indicators of the quality of services provided and the credentials and competencies of providers as noted earlier. The community health nurse case manager may want to establish a **resource file** or database in which to systemically organize and store information on area resources. Figure 11–1 depicts a sample resource file entry. A copy of the Resource File Entry Form is included in Appendix F.

The file could be organized according to categories of resources as in the following example:

- Developmental assessment
- Drug abuse
    Diagnosis and treatment
    Prevention
- Environmental services
    Protection
    Sanitation
- Family planning services
    Contraception
    Infertility
- Family services
    Counseling
    Family advocacy
    Marital counseling
    Parenting classes

A particular agency with more than one type of service could be entered in several different categories or a cross-reference system could be used. The resource described in Figure 11–1 deals with transportation.

Resource category: __Transportation__   Funding source: __Voluntary__

Agency name: __St. Martha's Catholic Church__

Address: __3710 Montebank Rd, Otenada, Mississippi__

Phone number: __817-3421__   Business hours: __Mon-Fri 8-4__

Contact person: __Mrs. Jefferson__   Title: __receptionist / secretary__

Source of referral: __self or other__

Eligibility: __anyone without Transportation - need not be members of church__

Fee: __none__

Services: __Provides Transportation To church services as well as other services such as Dr.'s office, grocery shopping, etc. on periodic basis__

Access: __call To arrange Transportation__

Other comments: __1.) Do not provide Transportation on long-Term basis, i.e., To work or school__
__2.) depends upon availability of volunteer drivers__
__3.) drivers Trained To assist disabled riders__

Figure 11–1. Sample resource file entry.

Information about the resource's funding source can be useful in tracking service availability. For example, if tax revenues have declined in the area, the community health nurse case manager may want to contact agencies funded by public money to determine whether services have been cut prior to making a specific referral. Also, it may be important to some clients to know that the services they receive from an agency are provided by tax dollars rather than "charity."

Of course, the resource file entry includes the referral resource's full name, address, and telephone number. The business hours notation may refer to when the agency is open or times when a particular service is offered. For example, the entry might read "Family planning: Monday, 9:00 A.M.–12 noon, Prenatal: Tuesday, 1:00–4:00 P.M."

It is helpful to have the name of a contact person in the agency as well. Referrals are facilitated when agency personnel are familiar with the person making the referral. Unfortunately, it is often true that some

agency employees are more inclined to accommodate professional colleagues than clients. When the case manager refers a client to an agency and gives that individual the name of a contact person who knows the nurse, the client who mentions that he or she was referred by the nurse may get a more prompt response than the client who does not have a specific person to contact. Having a specific contact person within the agency may also facilitate requests for services when the request is made by the nurse case manager rather than the client.

"Source of referral" in Figure 11–1 refers to the preferred originator of the referral. Some agencies accept referrals only from specific persons, usually physicians. If a professional referral is required, the nurse should specifically inquire about the acceptability of referrals from nurse practitioners, if they are available in the area. In the example in Figure 11–1, no specific referral source is required. Clients may request services on their own or be referred by anyone else.

As noted previously, information related to the eligibility of clients for service is very important. To make appropriate referrals, the nurse must know who is eligible for a particular service and who is not. This helps to minimize client frustration in being referred for services for which they do not qualify. The importance of a notation regarding fees is obvious. Clients need to know beforehand if they will be charged for services provided by the referral resource. The nurse should also be familiar with the types of insurance coverage accepted by the resource. For example, does the agency accept clients covered by Medicaid but not CHAMPUS. An additional notation might indicate whether or not the agency can help clients with financial arrangements for out-of-pocket expenses. The nurse should also know whether payment is expected at the time of services or if the client will receive a bill later.

Notation should also be made regarding the types of services provided by the resource. The entry regarding access refers to the means by which the client gains entry to the system. In the example in Figure 11–1, the client needs to call ahead for an appointment. Additional information under this entry would indicate any supporting documentation the client must provide to be eligible for services. Should he or she bring health insurance papers or just the policy number? Will the client need proof of residence, monthly expenditures, or medical expenses?

Finally, the nurse should obtain and store information regarding the competency of providers to whom referrals are made. Information about the credentials of providers, prior client complaints, malpractice actions, and so on can be recorded in the comments section as indicated in the third comment in Figure 11–1.

The type of information included in the sample resource file entry allows the community health nurse case manager to make appropriate referrals that do not waste clients' time and energy. It also allows the nurse to prepare clients for what they will encounter in following through on a referral. The file should be updated on a regular basis and as circumstances in various agencies change. Having a specific contact person in each agency may help to ensure that the nurse is notified of program changes. Experiences and reactions of clients following the use of a particular resource can also be used to update resource information and to evaluate the quality of service provided.

Monitoring Plan Implementation

Monitoring is another important aspect of implementing the case management plan. Once the plan is developed, the community health nurse case manager does not simply let the plan proceed to unfold on its own or close the case to case management services. Rather, the nurse case manager monitors the implementation of the plan and progress toward achievement of identified goals. Specific areas to be addressed at this stage include monitoring changes in the client's medical status (either positive or negative), social circumstances, and the quality of care provided; observing for changes in functional ability or mobility; and identifying evolving educational needs. In addition, the nurse will assess the effectiveness of pain management if relevant and monitor changes in client or family satisfaction with services and their outcomes (Powell, 1996).

Evaluating the Process and Outcomes of Case Management

Evaluation is an integral component of the case management process. The community health nurse case manager focuses on three areas in evaluating case management: client outcomes, quality of care, and the case management process itself.

Evaluating Primary, Secondary, and Tertiary Intervention Outcomes

The community health nurse case manager evaluates client responses to health care services and the outcomes achieved. Did the client follow through on any referrals made? Has the client consistently performed

---

Critical Thinking in Research

Anderson-Loftin, Wood, and Whitfield (1995) conducted a study of the effects of case management on length of hospital stay, cost, and quality of care in a rural hospital setting. Before implementation of nursing case management, the average length of stay was 8.2 days compared to 6.5 days after implementation. Increased length of stay was associated with older patient age and lower socioeconomic status and with certain physicians, but was not associated with time of year. The reduction in length of stay contributed to estimated savings of almost $66,000 over a 16-month period.

1. How might this study be replicated with a community health focus rather than an inpatient focus? What outcome variables would you substitute for length of stay and cost of hospitalization?
2. What other outcome variables would you want to examine in determining the effectiveness of a case management program in a community health setting?
3. Would your study focus on the effects of case management for specific categories of clients? Why or why not?

the exercises recommended by the physical therapist? Outcome evaluation would focus on the degree of progress made toward identified goals. These goals may reflect primary, secondary, or tertiary prevention. Evaluation of primary prevention would assess whether or not health was promoted or specific problems were prevented. For example, the case management plan for a client with emphysema and hypertension might have included referral for influenza and pneumonia immunization. Evaluative questions would focus on whether the client received the recommended immunizations and remained disease-free.

A secondary prevention goal might be control of the client's hypertension through education on correct medication dosage and administration. The client's blood pressure would be the criterion used to evaluate goal achievement in this case. Evaluation of tertiary prevention endeavors might focus on the client's ability to resume housekeeping chores and other functions after an exercise training program.

When desired client outcomes are not achieved, the community health nurse evaluates factors that may be affecting goal accomplishment. The case management plan would then be revised to modify or eliminate the effects of these factors. Difficulties in goal accomplishment may stem from an inappropriate case management plan, poor quality services, failures in plan implementation (on the part of providers or clients), or changes in the client situation. For example, the case management plan might include weekly physical therapy at a local outpatient facility. If the client's car breaks down and the client has no other source of transportation, the plan may not be implemented as designed and modifications will be needed.

Evaluating the Quality of Services

As noted earlier, the case manager is responsible for monitoring and evaluating the quality of services provided in implementing the case management plan. To obtain evaluative data in this area, the nurse might periodically visit providers to observe and discuss the quality of care given. For example, the nurse might ask an oncologist about the breadth of options usually presented to women with breast cancer. An oncologist who only presents one option to clients may not be the most appropriate referral for the case manager to make. The community health nurse case manager might also contact clients or family members to obtain their perceptions of the quality of services provided. The nurse should be particularly alert to situations in which clients discontinue services from one or more providers before goals are achieved. Exploration of the client's reasons for discontinuing services may indicate poor quality of care.

Evaluating the Case Management Process

The third aspect of evaluation is the assessment of the case management process itself. Was the client really a candidate for case management services? Was the initial assessment accurate and complete enough to permit effective planning? Was the case management plan appropriate to the client's needs? Were the referrals made appropriate? Could the case management process have been carried out more effectively, more efficiently, or in a more timely manner? The answers to these and similar questions will permit the community health nurse to revise the case management plan for a given client in a more effective way and will also enhance the nurse's overall case management ability.

Some case managers may be involved in one other aspect of evaluating case management, utilization review. *Utilization review* is a process of monitoring the necessity of care and the resources used and may involve preadmission review, concurrent review, retrospective review, or telephonics (Powell, 1996). In a preadmission review, the nurse case manager determines the appropriateness of the requested services before they are given. Areas for consideration include the need for the service and the appropriateness of the setting and level of services provided. For example, the case manager may determine that a requested nursing home admission is not appropriate because the client can be effectively cared for at home for far less cost. Concurrent review takes place while services are being provided to determine client progress toward goals and the need to continue services. Telephonics is a form of concurrent review in which the information

---

TABLE 11–3. STEPS IN THE CASE MANAGEMENT PROCESS

- Case selection
- Assessing the dimensions of health in the case management situation
  The biophysical dimension
  The psychological dimension
  The physical dimension
  The social dimension
  The behavioral dimension
  The health system dimension
- Deriving nursing diagnoses to guide the case management plan
- Developing the case management plan
  Determining the level of prevention
  Selecting resources
- Implementing the case management plan
  Communicating the plan
  Initiating referrals
  Monitoring plan implementation
- Evaluating the process and outcomes of case management
  Evaluating primary, secondary, and tertiary intervention outcomes
  Evaluating the quality of care
  Evaluating the case management process
  Utilization review

Critical Thinking in Practice: A Case in Point

Mrs. Davis is 67 years old. She was admitted to the hospital a week ago with a broken ankle. It is believed that she fractured her ankle stepping off a curb. Her bones are very fragile because of osteoporosis.

Mrs. Davis is retired and receives Social Security benefits. She lives with her son and 5-year-old grandson. Mrs. Davis's son is employed in heavy construction. Because of the recent rains, he has not been able to work consistently, and they have little savings. Mrs. Davis confides that she does not know how they will pay for the portion of the hospital bill that Medicare does not cover. Mrs. Davis usually takes care of her grandson when her son is working. She also does the housework, although her son does most of the heavy work around the house.

Mrs. Davis will be discharged later today. She has a follow-up appointment with the orthopedist in a week, but does not know how she will get there if her son is working that day. Mrs. Davis has been taught how to use a walker and will need to continue its use for several weeks.

1. Is Mrs. Davis a candidate for case management? Why or why not?
2. What are Mrs. Davis's health needs? How do biophysical, psychological, physical, social, behavioral, and health system factors influence those needs?
3. What desired outcomes would you establish in Mrs. Davis's case management plan? Do these outcomes reflect primary, secondary, or tertiary prevention?
4. How would you involve Mrs. Davis in developing the case management plan? Who else should be involved?
5. What referrals would be appropriate for Mrs. Davis? What is the expected outcome of these referrals? How would you go about making the referrals?
6. How would you evaluate the case management plan for Mrs. Davis? Be specific about the evaluative criteria you would use and how you would obtain the information to evaluate her care.

---

needed to determine the appropriateness of service continuation is obtained by telephone. In retrospective review, the case manager is determining the need for and appropriateness of services after they have been provided with the intent of approving or denying reimbursement for those services (Newell, 1996). Utilization review is generally performed by case managers who have an identified role in reimbursement decisions and may or may not be required of community health nurse case managers. The elements of the case management process, including aspects of evaluation and utilization review are summarized in Table 11–3.

TESTING YOUR UNDERSTANDING

1. List at least three goals of case management. Give an example of each. (p. 217)
2. Describe two characteristics of effective case management programs and three characteristics of effective case managers. Discuss how each might influence the effectiveness of case management services. (pp. 216–217)
3. Discuss three ways in which a community health nurse case manager could prevent being accused of a negligent referral. (pp. 218–219)

4. What are the stages of the case management process? How do they relate to the nursing process? (pp. 220–223)
5. List one element of data collection in each of the six dimensions of health. Describe how each might influence the case management situation. (pp. 220–223)
6. Discuss two considerations in selecting resources in the development of a case management plan. (pp. 223–224)
7. What are the three aspects of implementing the case management plan? Give an example of each. (pp. 224–227)
8. Describe three areas for consideration in evaluating case management. Give an example of each. (pp. 227–228)

WHAT DO YOU THINK?
Questions for Critical Thinking.

1. Is case management more appropriate for some clients than others? Why or why not? If so, what categories of clients should be targeted for case management?

2. What do you think is the most important goal of case management? Why?

3. Why are community health nurses better prepared to be client case managers than physicians or social workers?

4. What is the role of the community health nurse case manager with respect to other health care providers?

REFERENCES

Anderson-Loftin, W., Wood, D., & Whitfield, L. (1995). A case study of nursing case management in a rural hospital. *Nursing Administration Quarterly, 19*(3), 33–40.

Belliston, M. (1995). *Barriers to accessing referrals.* Unpublished manuscript.

Case Management Society of America. (1995). *Standards of practice for case management.* Little Rock: Case Management Society of America.

Conti, R. M. (1996). Nurse case manager roles: Implications for practice and education. *Nursing Administration Quarterly, 21*(1), 67–80.

Flarey, D. L., & Blancett, S. S. (1996). Case management: Delivering care in the age of managed care. In D. L. Flarey & S. S. Blancett (Eds.), *Handbook of nursing case management: Health care delivery in a world of managed care* (pp. 1–22). Gaithersburg, MD: Aspen.

Hester, L. E. (1996). Coordinating a successful discharge plan. *American Journal of Nursing, 86,* 35–37.

Mullahy, C. M. (1995). *The case manager's handbook.* Gaithersburg, MD: Aspen.

Mundt, M. H. (1996). Key elements of nurse case management in curricula. In E. L. Cohen (Ed.), *Nurse case management in the twenty-first century* (pp. 48–54). St. Louis: Mosby.

Newell, M. (1996). *Using nursing case management to improve health outcomes.* Gaithersburg, MD: Aspen.

Nichols, D. J. (1996). Legal liabilities in case management. In D. L. Flarey & S. S. Blancett (Eds.), *Handbook of nursing case management: Health care delivery in a world of managed care* (pp. 424–442). Gaithersburg, MD: Aspen.

Powell, S. K. (1996). *Nursing case management: A practical guide to success in managed care.* Philadelphia: Lippincott-Raven.

Rice, R. (1996). Case management and leadership strategies for home health nurses. In R. Rice (Ed.), *Home health nursing practice: Concepts and application* (2nd ed.) (pp. 119–138). St. Louis: Mosby.

St. Couer, M. (1996). *Case management practice guidelines.* St. Louis: Mosby.

Trella, B. (1996). Integrating services across the continuum: The challenge of chronic care. In E. L. Cohen (Ed.), *Nurse case management in the twenty-first century* (pp. 87–104). St. Louis: Mosby.

RESOURCES FOR CASE MANAGEMENT

Alliance of Information and Referral Systems
PO Box 3546
Joliet, IL 60434
(815) 744–6922

American Association for Continuity of Care
638 Prospect Avenue
Hartford, CT 06105–4250
(860) 586–7525

Case Management Society of America
8201 Cantrell, Ste. 230
Little Rock, AR 72227–2448
(501) 225–2229——Fax (501) 221–9068

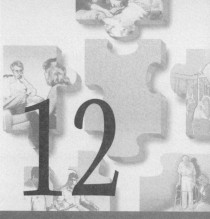

THE CHANGE, LEADERSHIP, AND GROUP PROCESSES

Reading about the accomplishments of early leaders in community health nursing, for example, Lillian Wald and her compatriots, one may wonder how these women came to exercise such influence. The answer lies in their knowledge and use of the change, leadership, and group processes. They knew how to use their leadership abilities to influence individuals and groups of people to achieve desired changes in society and in the health care system. Using these same processes, today's community health nurses can change health care and the health of those they serve.

The change, leadership, and group processes are interrelated. Community health nurses who seek to bring about change must exercise leadership, but leadership without systematic use of the change process may not achieve the desired outcome. Changes often result from the actions of a group of people rather than those of a single individual. Community health nurses exercise leadership skills to direct group activities that will accomplish desired changes. Having knowledge of these three interrelated processes is essential for effective community health nursing practice.

▶ Chapter Objectives

After reading this chapter, you should be able to:

- Discuss the influence of driving forces and restraining forces in change.
- Describe four major considerations in planning for change.
- Identify three approaches to bringing about change.
- Describe the three stages of implementing change.
- Describe the relationship of follower maturity to leadership style.
- Identify three functions of the leader in implementing leadership.
- Discuss the tasks involved in each of the five stages of group development.
- Describe two tasks in implementing the group process.
- Discuss two aspects of evaluation applicable to the change, leadership, and group processes.

▶ CRITICAL DIMENSIONS OF NURSING

Community health nurses use similar elements of the nursing dimensions in executing the change, leadership, and group processes. In the cognitive dimension, the nurse must have sound knowledge of the processes used as well as the outcomes to be accomplished in their use. For example, if the nurse wishes to provide leadership in initiating a change to computer documentation, he or she will need to be conversant with information technology and its applications to nursing practice. All three of the processes described in this chapter involve motivating others to engage in certain behaviors and will require the nurse to use communication and collaborative skills in the interpersonal dimension. In the ethical dimension, the nurse needs to assure that change does not violate the rights of clients or personnel and that the nurse's leadership style acknowledges and supports those rights. A variety of intellectual and manipulative skills may be needed within the skills dimension of nursing. Using the computer example, the nurse may need specific computer skills. Diagnostic and organizational planning skills are required in the execution of all three processes. As noted in the introduction to this chapter, these three processes may be used concurrently, and the nurse may also need to employ other processes from the process dimension of nursing. Finally, as is true of all of the processes discussed thus far, the community health nurse employs the re-

search and evaluation components of the reflective dimension in applying the change, leadership, and group processes.

▶ THE DIMENSIONS MODEL AND CHANGE

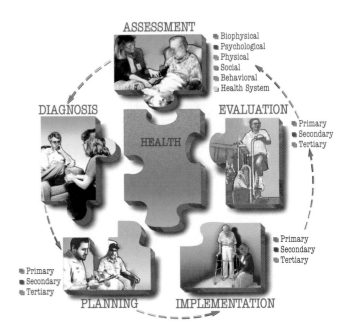

Change as a process used by community health nurses involves a series of definitive activities directed toward an identified goal. The change is planned and directed rather than spontaneous and unguided. Although we know that change does occur spontaneously and without direction, in this chapter change is explored as a planned process over which the community health nurse (and others) can exercise control. Conscious, deliberate, and intentional actions are designed to produce change.

The need for change engineered by community health nurses may arise in several different areas: knowledge, skills and abilities, attitudes and values. For example, an adolescent client newly diagnosed with diabetes may need to increase her or his knowledge of nutrition to be able to adhere to a diabetic diet or to develop the skills required to administer insulin injections. Other changes required of this client may be a change in attitude regarding injections or an alteration in the priority the adolescent gives to group conformity versus health. The ultimate purpose for change in any of these areas is a change in the client's behavior or in the conditions that affect the client's health. Alterations in each of these areas requires active use of the change process by the community health nurse.

Changes in behavior or circumstances are influenced by a variety of forces acting in any given situation. According to *force field theory,* there are always two types of forces that affect the likelihood of change in any situation: driving forces and restraining forces (Lewin, 1951). These two types of forces work in opposition, and it is the relative strength of each that determines whether change will occur (Lewin, 1989b).

Driving forces are those factors that favor or facilitate change. *Restraining forces,* on the other hand, impede change. For example, staff frustration with cumbersome charting procedures may be a driving force that motivates a change to computerized record-keeping. In this situation, feelings of inadequacy regarding computer use and concern for depersonalization of clients may be restraining forces working against change.

Promoting change is a matter of manipulating the driving and restraining forces present in the situation. Community health nurses can increase driving forces, decrease restraining forces, or do both to bring about change. It has been suggested, however, that weakening restraining forces may be a more effective approach (Skinner, 1994). Strengthening driving forces too much can result in precipitous and undirected change in an undesirable direction. When driving forces are stronger than restraining forces, change occurs. In the change agent role, the community health nurse can use the Dimensions Model to assess and modify driving and restraining forces that influence change in a given situation.

 ## Assessing the Dimensions of Health in a Change Situation

To bring about change, the community health nurse must first identify a need for change. Factors related to the biophysical, psychological, physical, social, behavioral, or health system dimensions may give rise to a need for change. For example, in the biophysical dimension a diagnosis of diabetes or heart disease requires a number of alterations in a client's life, and an increase in the number of elderly persons in the population necessitates changes for a community. Physical or social dimension factors such as a flood or a rise in the unemployment rate also contribute to needs for change by individuals, families, and communities. Similarly, factors in the behavioral dimension, such as the number of people who drive while under the influence of alcohol or other drugs, give rise to the need for legal changes and other community activities to curb the problem. Finally, health care system factors, like inequity in access to care or the emphasis on cura-

tive care at the expense of prevention, influence the need for change in the health care delivery system itself. In assessing the change situation, the community health nurse must identify all the forces in the "field" that influence the situation (Lewin, 1989b). The Dimensions Model provides a useful framework for this assessment.

The Biophysical Dimension

Biophysical factors can serve as driving or restraining forces for change. Parents may wish that their small child would outgrow the need for diapers, but until the child develops the muscle control to be toilet-trained, the desired change will not occur. In this instance, the child's age and developmental level are factors restraining change. For an adolescent son or daughter, however, developing an interest in the opposite sex—another maturational event—may lead to positive changes in hygiene practices the parents have been trying to encourage for years. In this case, age and developmental level are forces driving change.

In a similar vein, physiologic status can either enhance or restrain the prospect of change. For example, a recent heart attack may motivate a person to quit smoking, and visual impairment may diminish a diabetic client's ability to change self-care patterns to include insulin injections.

The Psychological Dimension

Factors in the psychological dimension can profoundly affect the potential for effective change. For example, the psychological stresses of a recent divorce may impede the client's ability to attend to the nurse's recommendations for dietary changes necessitated by a new diagnosis of diabetes. Community health nurses functioning as change agents should be aware that people may have different emotional responses to change as they progress through the change process. Generally, people experience seven psychological stages with respect to change, each with its own typical emotional responses (Manion, 1995). These stages and the attendant responses are presented in Table 12–1. The first stage is one of losing focus, being uncertain and anxious about what can be expected as a result of the change. Typical responses in this stage include confusion and disorientation, and difficulty making decisions. Because one tends to dwell on the change, one may also become forgetful. Stage II involves attempts to minimize the impact of the change. Responses in this stage typically include denial of the significance of the change and its effects. The third stage is labeled "the pit" because this is usually the

TABLE 12–1. PSYCHOLOGICAL STAGES AND EMOTIONAL RESPONSES IN CHANGE

Stage	Emotional Response
I. Losing focus	Confusion, disorientation, forgetfulness, difficulty making decisions
II. Minimizing impact	Denial, pretending
III. The pit	Anger, resentment, discouragement, resistance
IV. Letting go of the past	Acceptance, future orientation, renewed energy
V. Testing limits	Willingness to use new skills, optimism
VI. Searching for meaning	Confidence, willingness to help others with change, recognition of positive effects of change
VII. Integration	Change seen as a normal part of life

lowest ebb in feelings about the change. Emotions experienced in this stage include anger, resentment, discouragement, and resistance.

Stage IV begins the return to emotional equilibrium as the end of change seems to be in sight. Responses include letting go of the past, accepting the change, and preparing for the future. A renewed sense of energy may also be noted. Depending on other life circumstances and events, people may cycle back into the pit stage one or more times before moving on to stage V. Stage V, testing limits, is characterized by optimism and a willingness to try out the new skill. People in stage V often want to talk about the change, recounting their experiences with it. This type of response continues in stage VI, in which the person searches for meaning in the change and recognizes what has been learned from the change. Emotional responses at this point include confidence and a willingness to help others experiencing the same change. By stage VII, the change has been fully integrated and become a regular part of life.

Because of the dynamic nature of life, clients may experience several changes at the same time and be in different stages of emotional response with respect to each change. The community health nurse, as change agent, should assess emotional responses to change as a basis for promoting effective change in clients, other health care providers, and health care delivery systems.

The Physical Dimension

Elements of the physical dimension may precipitate the need for change or influence the direction of or ability to change. For example, a residential fire will necessitate a number of changes in clients' lives. Similarly, a large fire may necessitate major changes for a community. Buildings may need to be reconstructed and services reinstituted. Less dramatic changes may also bring about the need for change at the individual or community level. For example, an increase in the size of the population will require expanded health and other services.

Physical dimension factors may also serve as driving or restraining forces in change. For example, the community health nurse may recommend changes in hygiene practices to prevent the spread of lice among family members via contaminated sheets. If the family does not have access to a washing machine, however, it may be difficult for them to wash the sheets as recommended. Or lack of space in the home may preclude acceptance of recommendations for separate sleeping quarters for parents and baby.

The Social Dimension

Social dimension factors might also act as forces driving or restraining change. For example, low education or income levels may prevent a client from making needed changes in housing arrangements for the family. On the other hand, support from significant others for a desired change serves as a driving force. Social factors in the form of legislation often bring about change. For example, increasing the tax on tobacco has significantly decreased smoking in Great Britain.

The Behavioral Dimension

Driving and restraining forces may also be related to the behavioral dimension. Substance abuse, for example, may be a restraining force in efforts to alter interaction patterns in violent families. On the other hand, substance abuse might be a driving force in a divorce.

Other consumption patterns may also create driving or restraining forces in a change situation. For example, adherence to a traditional cultural dietary pattern may make it difficult for a client to accept dietary changes necessitated by heart disease.

The Health System Dimension

Health care system factors may also drive or restrain change. For example, active resistance by some health care providers to health care delivery reforms such as prospective payment and to national health insurance have impeded efforts to lower the cost of health care. On the other hand, political support by health care providers has often resulted in legislative changes,

---

ASSESSMENT TIPS: Change

Biophysical Dimension

Are there developmental factors in the situation that give rise to a need for change?

Do physiologic conditions give rise to a need for change?

How will developmental and physiologic factors affect the ability to implement the desired change?

Psychological Dimension

Are there psychological dimension factors that give rise to a need for change?

What psychological factors are operating in the change situation?

What psychological factors underlie current behaviors that require change?

Will psychological factors enhance or detract from motivation to change?

What stage of psychological response to the need for change is exhibited by the client? How will this affect the change?

Physical Dimension

Are there factors in the physical dimension that give rise to a need for change?

Will physical dimension factors affect the ability to implement change? In what way?

Social Dimension

Do social dimension factors give rise to a need for change?

Will educational level influence motivation for or ability to implement change?

What level of support exists in the social network for making the desired change?

Will economic factors influence the ability to implement change?

Will external societal forces influence the ability to bring about change?

Do occupational factors give rise to a need for change?

How will occupational factors influence the desired change?

Are religious or cultural factors operating in the change situation? If so, how will they affect the desired change?

Behavioral Dimension

Do consumption patterns give rise to a need for change?

Are there substance abuse factors that will influence the change?

Does sexual activity give rise to the need for change?

Do other health-related behaviors give rise to the need for change?

Health System Dimension

Does the health care system give rise to a need for change?

How will the health care system influence the change process?

---

such as mandatory seat beat laws, that protect the public.

 Diagnostic Reasoning and Change

Nursing diagnoses related to change can be developed at several levels. There may be a need for change in the behavior of an individual client or a family. Ex-

amples of diagnoses at these levels are "need for change in dietary patterns due to pregnancy" and "need for change in family decision-making patterns due to increasing maturity of children."

Diagnoses of needed change might also be made in relation to groups or communities. For example, a community may have a high measles mortality rate in children under 1 year of age. Children are usually immunized against measles at 15 months of age. In this instance, however, there is a need to immunize at an earlier age to decrease both measles incidence and mortality. The community health nurse's diagnosis, in this case, might be a "need to change the routine immunization schedule due to increased measles mortality in infants."

Finally, the community health nurse may diagnose a need for change in the health care delivery system itself. An example of such a diagnosis is "need to provide low-cost health services due to high unemployment rates and low levels of health insurance." Another example of change needed in the health care system may involve more effective recruitment and retention of qualified nurses, especially in community health nursing.

 Planning Change

Change may occur with or without planning. In the absence of systematic planning, however, the change that occurs may not be desirable. As change agents, community health nurses approach change through planned and goal-directed intervention. If change is to be effective, the community health nurse and client both must participate in planning the change. When those who are being asked to change are expected to be resistant to the desired change, having them participate in planning the change engages them in *counterattitudinal behavior,* behavior not in keeping with their established attitudes and values. This counterattitudinal behavior results in *cognitive dissonance,* a state of psychological discomfort created by inconsistencies between one's attitudes and values and one's behavior. One way to decrease the resulting discomfort is to modify one's attitudes to be congruent with behavior. By planning a change not in keeping with one's present attitudes, one may begin to adjust those attitudes to reestablish consonance with behavior. In other words, participating in the planning of a change may result in decreased resistance to that change.

Tasks to be accomplished in planning change include establishing goals and objectives, evaluating alternative approaches to change, delineating activities leading to change, and planning to evaluate the change.

Establishing Goals and Objectives

The first aspect of planning change is determining what change should accomplish. This entails setting both broad goals and specific objectives. Suppose a community health nurse wants to improve immunization levels among community residents. Increasing immunity in the population would be the broad goal, and immunizing 95% of children over 1 year of age against measles would be a specific outcome objec-

tive. In this instance, the goal and objective reflect primary prevention, and primary preventive measures would be indicated to achieve them.

Goals and objectives for change may also reflect secondary or tertiary prevention. At the secondary prevention level, for example, change in an obese client's dietary patterns would be desirable. In this instance, the goal would be a balanced diet for the client. Specific outcome objectives might include a decrease in caloric intake to 1800 calories per day, inclusion of at least one iron-rich food in the diet daily, and adequate intake of vitamins and minerals. Similarly, a change to more effective coping strategies by an abusive parent would be the goal of tertiary preventive measures planned in an abusive family situation. A related outcome objective might be a decrease in the amount of alcohol consumed as a coping mechanism.

In developing outcome objectives for change, it is frequently wise to proceed incrementally, with achievement of a few objectives setting the stage for accomplishment of later changes. In this way, the nurse keeps the change at a manageable level that does not overwhelm the client and create resistance to the change (Jellison, 1993).

Selecting an Approach to Change

Generally speaking, there are three approaches the community health nurse might take to bring about change: the empirical–rational approach, the normative–reeducative approach, and the power–coercive approach (Harkness, 1995). Each is appropriate in some change situations. The choice of approach depends on the type of change to be achieved and the willingness and ability of those who require the change.

The Empirical–Rational Approach. The *empirical–rational approach* to change assumes that people act reasonably and follow the promptings of rational self-interest when the need for change is revealed to them (Tacetta-Chapnick, 1996). In short, an awareness of a need for change results in change. Change is accomplished by providing information about the need for change and how to bring it about. The change agent informs those who need to implement the change of an unfavorable condition and a desirable course of action, and those individuals carry out the change (Clark, 1994).

This approach to change is effective in situations when it is clear where one's self-interest lies, when few restraining forces are operating, and when the change does not pose a threat to those who must implement it. For example, school officials made aware of hazards posed by damaged playground equipment will probably take steps either to repair or to remove the equipment. They can see the potential harm to the children and the possibility of lawsuits resulting from injuries, and they have no vested interest in retaining damaged equipment.

The Normative–Reeducative Approach.   Unfortunately, human behavior is not always rational and is often heavily influenced by attitudes, values, and emotions (Clark, 1994). For example, a mother may know that her child needs immunizations but hesitates because she does not like to see her child hurt by the injection. Rather than trying to increase the mother's awareness of the need for immunization, the community health nurse as change agent could employ a ***normative–reeducative approach*** to change using educational strategies directed toward changing the mother's attitude. For example, the nurse might focus on how much greater the hurt would be if the child developed diphtheria, tetanus, or one of the other diseases preventable by immunization.

As another example, teenagers often see unrestrained drinking as evidence of adulthood. By using a normative–reeducative approach the teens would be helped to see that refraining from drinking to excess is more characteristic of adult behavior than going on a Friday night binge. The approach to behavioral change in this instance focuses on their attitudes to drinking.

The normative–reeducative approach would be used in situations in which those who need to make changes have a vested interest in maintaining the current situation or in which there are emotional and attitudinal restraining forces at work, but where attitudes are open and amenable to change.

The Power–Coercive Approach.   Some people, however, cannot be brought to change behavior by rational argument or attempts to change attitudes. In these situations, the ***power–coercive approach*** to change may be effective. This approach uses power to dispense reward and punishment to force change. As an example, children of parents who refuse to have them immunized are denied school entry unless there are religious or health reasons for nonimmunization. Using another example, empirical–rational strategies and normative–reeducative strategies have been somewhat effective in motivating people to use automobile seat belts. Others, however, do not use seat belts. For these individuals, laws mandating seat belt use are a power–coercive strategy to force a change in behavior.

Information obtained by the community health nurse in assessing the change situation indicates the driving and restraining forces that are operating.

When restraining forces are related to misconceptions and lack of knowledge about the need for change, the change itself, or its consequences, the nurse would select the empirical–rational approach to bring about the desired change. When restraining forces include attitudes unfavorable to the desired change but amenable to modification, the normative–reeducative approach may be chosen. When the assessment indicates strongly rooted attitudes and values that impede change or strong resistance to change, the power–coercive approach may be used. This approach is also appropriate in situations where the need for change is immediate and there is no time for explanation or persuasion.

It should be remembered, however, that the power–coercive approach may result in temporary change and that those who are coerced may return to their previous behaviors as soon as coercion is removed. For these reasons, the power–coercive method is the least desirable of the three approaches to change. This approach generally is not used, except in situations in which clients' behaviors are clearly dangerous to themselves or others as in the case of a client threatening suicide, child abuse, failure to obtain necessary medical care for a minor, or someone with a communicable disease who refuses to refrain from infecting others.

The power–coercive approach may be warranted, however, in advocacy situations and other similar occasions. For example, the community health nurse may find that the only way to motivate a landlord to comply with building safety codes is to threaten to report violations to the authorities. Or, health care providers who discriminate against certain types of clients may be motivated to change their behavior if threatened with the loss of their jobs.

Delineating Activities Leading to Change

The next step in planning change is to delineate specific activities required to accomplish the desired change. These activities would reflect process objectives for the change situation and may involve primary, secondary, or tertiary preventive measures. For instance, if an alteration is needed in an infant's diet to accommodate the slowed rate of growth normal at the end of the first year of life, dietary education for the mother would be a primary preventive measure directed toward this change. Similarly, providing clean syringes and needles for intravenous drug users might motivate them to stop sharing needles and prevent exposure to hepatitis and HIV.

Examples of secondary preventive strategies for change might include suggestions to minimize side effects of antituberculosis drugs to resolve the problem of noncompliance, or assisting teenage alcoholics to explore their reasons for drinking. Educating a parent on the role of bottle propping in recurrent middle ear infections in an infant might be a tertiary preventive measure designed to produce behavior changes in the parent that prevent a recurrence of otitis media in the child.

Planning to Evaluate Change

The last step in planning change is to plan to evaluate the effects of the change and the process used to achieve it. Consequently, the community health nurse needs to determine how the change will be evaluated, what data will be collected, and what data collection procedures will be used. In planning to evaluate change, criteria need to be developed that reflect the levels of prevention involved in the changes planned. If desired changes involve primary prevention, evaluative criteria will focus on the promotion of health and prevention of specific health problems. The emphasis in secondary prevention would be on criteria that reflect resolution of existing client problems. Evaluative criteria related to tertiary preventive measures would address prevention of complications or recurrence of problems. As an example, an objective for change at the level of primary prevention might be increased use of condoms among sexually active adolescents to prevent HIV infection. Evaluative criteria for the achievement of change would focus on the proportion of adolescents who use condoms consistently. In summary, the following points must be considered in planning change:

1. Establish goals and outcome objectives for change
2. Evaluate and select an appropriate approach to change
   - *Empirical–rational approach:* focuses on awareness of the need for change
   - *Normative–reeducative approach:* focuses on attitudes toward the change
   - *Power–coercive approach:* uses power over rewards and punishments to enforce change
3. Delineate activities leading to change
4. Plan to evaluate the change

 Implementing Change

Whatever the approach to change selected in the planning stage, implementing it occurs in three stages: unfreezing, moving, and refreezing (Lewin, 1989a). All three stages apply to changes of all kinds, including those in individuals, families, and groups or commu-

nities as well as changes in nursing practice or in the health care system.

Unfreezing

Unfreezing is the process of creating an awareness of the need to change and developing motivation for the change. Unfreezing may be approached somewhat differently in each of the three approaches to change discussed earlier. In the use of the empirical–rational strategy, the community health nurse as change agent may use a tactic known as disconfirmation to motivate others to change. *Disconfirmation* is an awareness that reality does not conform to the desired state of affairs. Creating disconfirmation involves presenting the client or target group with information to make them aware of differences between a desired state and reality. This awareness creates a feeling of discomfort with the current situation and fosters a willingness to change. For example, the community health nurse might present figures on the number of adolescent pregnancies occurring in a specific school to make parents aware of a need for sex education. The desired state is an absence of teenage pregnancies, but, as the community health nurse makes clear, this is definitely not the reality of the situation.

A second tactic used in unfreezing is introducing guilt. This tactic might be used in the normative–reeducative approach to change. When people are made to feel guilty about a current situation, they may be more likely to reexamine attitudes and institute change. For instance, the community health nurse might point out what poor role models smokers are for their children and what the effects of secondhand smoke might be on children's health. Guilt over possible damage to their own children's health might motivate some smokers to quit.

Providing a climate of psychological safety is another tactic used in unfreezing in the normative–reeducative approach to change. Using the change to computerized charting as an example, the community health nurse might assure the group that they will receive detailed instruction and demonstration of the system and will have opportunities to practice and receive feedback before the new system is implemented. These activities lessen fears of making mistakes and decrease restraining forces working against the change. In the power–coercive approach to change, unfreezing may be accomplished by presenting information on the need for change and the sanctions that will occur if the change does not take place.

Another important feature of unfreezing is dealing with resistance, some of which may have already been eliminated by creating a climate of psychological safety. Other steps, however, may be needed. Change, even when desired, produces stress. Stress creates discomfort, and people are often unwilling to experience even temporary discomfort in return for future gains. From this perspective, change is seen as "punishment" and constitutes a force restraining the desired change.

Resistance can be minimized by changing the person's perceptions of the consequences of change, that is, changing restraining forces to driving forces. The community health nurse can foster change by setting up the change situation such that the person(s) expected to change receives benefits that outweigh the "punishment" involved. This can sometimes involve a "trade." For example, a politician may be motivated to change his or her stance on an issue in return for election support from nurses. Similarly, a client who sees changing dietary patterns after a myocardial infarction as burdensome may be brought to see the advantages this will create in preventing another heart attack.

Moving

Moving is the actual process of implementing or carrying out the planned change and involves "moving" to the next level of behavior (Lewin, 1989a). Functions of the community health nurse as change agent during this stage include introducing new information needed to bring about the change; modeling and/or encouraging performance of the new behavior; allowing ample time to practice the behavior; and providing a supportive climate and opportunities to voice feelings of fear, anxiety, frustration, and anger. Other functions include giving feedback on progress in implementing the change and acting as an energizer to maintain the momentum of the change.

Dividing the change into smaller segments and setting up effective communication channels can assist in the actual implementation of the change. The activities needed to implement the change may be delineated so that incremental change is possible. For example, if community health nurses are asked to convert all existing client records to a computerized charting system, they may feel overwhelmed. If, however, the change begins with newly opened records only, the change can be accomplished in manageable increments. As services to previously enrolled clients are terminated, there will be fewer and fewer records that have not been computerized.

Ongoing data collection is needed during the moving stage to monitor the change process. Providing avenues for those involved in the change to communicate regarding problems experienced will smooth the implementation process. Communication permits evaluation of the implementation of change on an ongoing basis and allows modification of the planned change or the activities required to implement it, thus resulting in more effective change.

Refreezing

Refreezing is the process of internalizing the change so it becomes part of the normal routine. In the computerization example, refreezing occurs when the change to computerized charting has become internalized to the point that staff members wonder how they ever managed to chart the old way. Functions of the change agent at this stage include providing continuing motivation, directing the new behavior, and delegating greater responsibility for the change to others. Stages in implementing change and functions of the community health nurse as change agent are presented in Table 12–2.

 Evaluating Change

Evaluating change involves assessing the change itself and the process used in achieving it. In evaluating change itself, the first question is whether the desired change was achieved. Has the individual client, family, or target group made the expected change in health-related behaviors? Are they now, for example, engaging in more effective communication patterns or eating a more appropriate diet? Is charting now done on the computer?

The second consideration in evaluating change is its effects. It may be that even though the change has been achieved, it has not had the desired effect. For example, the client may have changed his or her dietary patterns and still not be losing weight. Or,

TABLE 12–2. STAGES IN IMPLEMENTING CHANGE AND FUNCTIONS OF THE NURSE AS CHANGE AGENT

Stage	Function of the Nurse
Unfreezing	• Create disconfirmation • Introduce guilt • Provide a climate of psychological safety
Moving	• Introduce new information required for change • Encourage performance of new behavior • Allow time to practice new behavior • Provide supportive climate for change • Provide opportunities to voice feelings about change • Give feedback on progress of change • Serve as an energizer • Deal with resistance
Refreezing	• Continue energizing activities • Continue to direct new behavior • Delegate greater responsibility for change to client or target group

more immunization clinics may have been established without appreciably raising immunization levels.

In addition, change may have unanticipated effects that may or may not be desirable. For instance, the change to computerized charting may provide avenues for violation of client confidentiality because the computer increases access to client records. Or, nurses may spend more time correcting computer errors than they spent doing handwritten charting.

Another aspect of evaluating change is the assessment of the process used to achieve the change. Were the need for change and the driving and restraining forces accurately identified? Was the change well planned? Was the appropriate approach to change selected given the factors involved? Was resistance adequately addressed? What activities were involved in unfreezing, changing, and refreezing? Were these activities appropriate to the situation? Answers to these questions provide direction for action if the desired change has not yet been achieved and further attempts are warranted. They also assist the community health nurse as change agent to use the change process more effectively in the future. Components of the change process are summarized in Table 12–3.

▶ THE DIMENSIONS MODEL AND LEADERSHIP

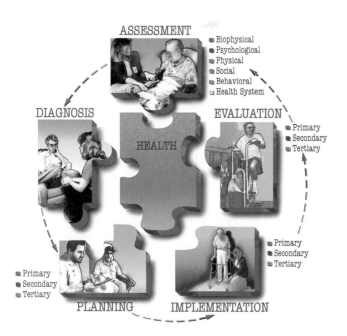

Initiating and directing change require leadership on the part of the nurse. The 1988 Institute of Medicine report, *The Future of Public Health*, noted a lack of leadership in public health. For this reason, community health nurses should prepare to provide leadership in

TABLE 12–3. COMPONENTS OF THE CHANGE PROCESS

Assessment	• Assess the change situation in terms of:
	Factors giving rise to the need for change
	Forces driving change
	Forces restraining change
Diagnosis	• Diagnose the need for change
Planning	• Establish goals and objectives for change
	• Evaluate approaches to change and select an appropriate one
	• Delineate activities leading to change
	• Plan evaluation of change
Implementation	• Facilitate unfreezing
	• Facilitate movement toward the desired behavior
	• Facilitate refreezing
Evaluation	• Evaluate extent to which change has been accomplished
	• Evaluate effects of the change
	• Evaluate use of the change process

the process of designing a health care system that will meet the health needs of the public. In this age of rising costs and diminishing resources, there is a particular need for leadership to ensure that health resources are adequate to meet those needs.

Leadership Competencies

Leadership is defined as an intentional process in which one person attempts to influence the behavior of others to reach a specific goal (Pointer & Sanchez, 1997). To carry out this process effectively, in the health care arena, community health nurses must possess certain specific competencies. These competencies are described in different ways by nursing authors (Josten, et al., 1996; Misener, et al., 1997; Porter-O'Grady, 1995), but fit within the nursing dimension in the Dimensions Model. Competencies required in the cognitive dimension encompass a broad knowledge base in areas like marketing, principles of finance and economics, law, and information technology. Affective dimension skills for leadership include collaboration and communication abilities and the ability to motivate and involve others. The negotiation and conflict management skills required of effective leaders also lie in this dimension. Abilities to lead effectively while maintaining moral and ethical principles and to advocate for the welfare of clients are competencies required in the ethical dimension. Skill dimension competencies include critical thinking and problem-solving skills, pattern recognition and synthesis skills, and the ability to see the whole picture. Other skill dimension competencies include community development and strategic planning skills. Leadership competencies needed in the process dimension of nursing include knowledge and skill in the politi-

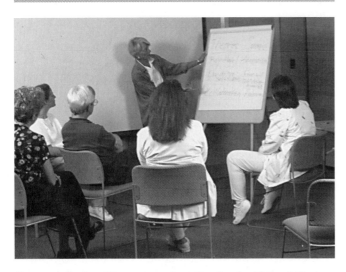

Community health nurses exercise leadership skills to direct group activities that will accomplish desired changes.

From: Berger, K., & Williams, M. (1999). Fundamentals of nursing: collaborating for optimal health (2nd ed.). Stamford, CT: Appleton & Lange.

cal, change, and group processes. Finally, in the reflective dimension, effective leadership requires the ability to evaluate health programs and their effects.

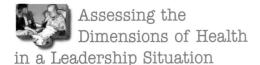

Assessing the Dimensions of Health in a Leadership Situation

Over the years, a variety of theories have arisen to explain effective leadership. Early theories focused on personal traits of effective leaders and later on the leader's behavior. Motivational theories examined the factors that motivated followers and how leaders could influence those factors. Each of these types of theories failed to explain satisfactorily why some leaders were effective and some were not. More recently, contingency theories have suggested that effective leadership is *contingent* on interactions among the leader, the followers, and the situation in which leadership occurs (Fiedler, 1993). The task of the community health nurse leader is to identify the patterns of interaction among these three elements and to choose a leadership approach that is congruent with followers and with the leadership situation. To begin this process, the nurse assesses him- or herself, followers,

and the leadership situation in terms of the six dimensions of health. The resulting information guides the selection of a leadership style appropriate to the situation.

The Biophysical Dimension

One major consideration in leadership is the maturity of one's followers with respect to the task at hand. Maturity is a combination of expertise related to the task and motivation to perform the task (Pointer & Sanchez, 1997).

Age and developmental level can influence both leader and follower maturity. Children usually have less expertise related to many tasks than do adults, although this is not always true. For instance, a school-age child may have had more exposure to computers than many adults. If the task to be accomplished requires computer skills, the youngster may be more mature relative to the task than the inexperienced adult.

Physiologic function can also influence followers' abilities to complete necessary tasks. If, for example, one is trying to provide leadership in a disaster situation and all of one's followers are injured, their ability to perform the required tasks will be influenced by the type and extent of their injuries. Biological factors can also influence the effectiveness of the leader. For example, an ill or injured leader might inspire less confidence on the part of followers than a strong and forceful one.

The Psychological Dimension

The psychological dimension affects both leader and followers. Followers' motivation to act is a function of their psychological environment. For example, followers may be unwilling or unable to act in the manner desired by the leader if incapacitated by emotions such as fear, anxiety, and grief. In assessing the leadership situation, the nurse as leader needs to identify psychological factors motivating current behavior and those that might motivate followers to desired behaviors.

The resulting knowledge allows the nurse to provide the types of motivation needed to promote desired behavior and task accomplishment by followers. For example, if followers are motivated by monetary considerations, monetary rewards might bring about the desired behavior. For other followers, presentation of a challenge might be a motivator.

Psychological dimension factors can also influence the leader and his or her effectiveness. For example, lack of trust of the leader detracts from effectiveness in a leadership situation. Hesitancy on the part of the leader may also lessen follower confidence and willingness to act as directed. Lack of leader attention to the psychological needs of followers may likewise inhibit effectiveness.

Another aspect of the psychological dimension is time and the resulting pressure for decision and action. Time constraints influence of the type of leadership style appropriate to the situation, as we shall see later in this chapter.

The Physical Dimension

The physical environment can give rise to the need for leadership or factors that influence that need. Potential for a flood, for example, might require leadership in the evacuation of local residents.

If followers are physically distant from the leader, the distance may influence how leadership is exercised. For example, if a community health nursing student is making a home visit without his or her instructor and encounters difficulties, the instructor may need to provide leadership and direction by phone rather than in person, and the approach taken to leadership in this situation might be different from the approach that might be used on-site. If there are other incoming telephone calls, for example, the instructor might just tell the student to take specific action rather than assist the student with problem solving.

In addition, the physical environment may or may not contain the materials needed for task accomplishment. This lack of necessary materials might hamper the effectiveness of the leader and followers in accomplishing a given task. Suppose that the task to be accomplished is feeding a group of disaster victims. If no food is available because transportation has been curtailed, it will be difficult to accomplish this task no matter how experienced the leader and followers are.

The Social Dimension

Social dimension factors also influence the leadership situation. Social factors such as low education level and lack of exposure to similar situations can affect follower expertise and their ability to accomplish necessary tasks. In such cases, the followers are said to be "immature" with respect to the task to be accomplished. Occupation is a social dimension factor that may influence followers' expertise relative to the task to be accomplished. For example, if computer expertise is required for task accomplishment, followers who use computers extensively in their jobs would be considered mature in this situation.

Another aspect of the social dimension is the position of the leader with respect to the followers. It is helpful, but not absolutely necessary, if the leader is in a position of authority vis-à-vis the followers. This position of authority gives the leader a certain amount of influence over followers. Followers' perceptions of the leader as being more knowledgeable than themselves regarding the task at hand also contribute to leader influence. Such perceptions might be attributable to the leader's education level, social status, or other social dimension factors.

The Behavioral Dimension

Factors in the behavioral dimension also influence follower experience and expertise related to the task to be accomplished. For example, leisure pursuits may provide followers with experiences relevant to a given leadership situation. Someone who uses computers for recreational purposes may have the skills needed for a computer-related tasks, and an experienced hunter may have the tracking skills required to find a lost child. These skills increase the task-related maturity of followers.

Similarly, life experiences might influence the leadership ability of the nurse leader. Functioning as a leader among coworkers should help prepare the nurse for leadership roles in other areas. For example, the community health nursing supervisor who applies leadership principles to direct the activity of staff members would use the same principles to assist abusive parents to form a self-help group.

The Health System Dimension

Health care system factors also contribute to the effectiveness of the nurse leader. For example, the typical hierarchical arrangement of the health care team, which traditionally acknowledges physician leadership, may make it difficult for the nurse to assume a leadership role. This same traditional hierarchy may make it difficult for health care consumers to act as leaders in health-related situations even when their leadership is warranted. In such circumstances, the nurse or consumer leader needs to pay particular attention to psychological factors motivating follower behavior.

Consumer perceptions of health care providers and their intentions can also influence the ability of the nurse to lead in a situation in which health care consumers are the followers. If health care providers are perceived as intent on serving their own interests, their credibility and influence with followers will be minimal. If, on the other hand, providers are seen to be acting altruistically, they may have more influence on consumer behavior in a leadership situation.

ASSESSSMENT TIPS: Leadership Situations

Biophysical Dimension

Do followers have the developmental capability to execute the desired task?

Do followers have the physical capability to execute the desired task?

Will physiologic factors affect the ability of the leader?

Psychological Dimension

What is the followers' level of motivation to execute the desired task?

What rewards or sanctions will motivate followers to execute the desired task?

Are there psychological factors that will detract from followers' abilities to execute the desired task (eg, fear)?

Do followers have sufficient trust in the leader to do as directed?

Does the leader give sufficient attention to the psychological needs of followers?

Is the leader's usual leadership style congruent with followers' levels of task maturity?

Are there time pressures or other constraints operating in the situation that will affect task accomplishment?

Physical Dimension

Are there factors in the physical dimension that give rise to a need for leadership?

Are leader and followers separated by physical distance? If so, what means can overcome the effects of this distance?

Does the physical environment contain the materials needed to execute the desired task?

Social Dimension

Do social dimension factors give rise to a need for leadership?

Do followers' education levels influence task maturity?

Does the leader have support in the social network necessary for task accomplishment?

What is the quality of interaction between leader and followers? How will this affect task accomplishment?

Are there cultural factors that will influence the leadership situation? If so, how?

Will occupational factors influence task accomplishment? If so, how?

Behavioral Dimension

Will consumption patterns influence the leadership situation?

Will followers' leisure pursuits influence the leadership situation? If so, how?

Health System Dimension

Does the health care system give rise to a need for leadership?

How will followers' perceptions of health care providers influence the leadership situation?

Will interactions among health care providers influence the leadership situation? If so, how?

 Diagnostic Reasoning and Leadership

The community health nurse derives nursing diagnoses from data obtained in assessing the leadership situation. There are two aspects of nursing diagnosis related to leadership: diagnosing the need for action and leadership and diagnosing follower maturity.

Diagnosing the Need for Leadership

The first type of nursing diagnosis involves identifying a need for action and for leadership to promote action. Very often, this is also a diagnosis of a need for change. For example, in assessing a community's health needs, the community health nurse may note a high incidence of pedestrian fatalities at a particular intersection. Action is needed in the form of a traffic signal to permit safe pedestrian crossing; however, local residents have no idea how to go about arranging for installation of a traffic signal. In this instance, the nurse has identified both a problem that requires action and a need for leadership to bring about that action. The nursing diagnosis derived might be a "need for leadership in preventing traffic fatalities due to community members' lack of experience with group action."

Diagnosing Follower Maturity

The second aspect of nursing diagnosis in leadership is the diagnosis of follower maturity. Based on the assessment data obtained, the community health nurse should have an idea of both follower expertise and motivation regarding the action to be taken. Examples of possible diagnoses in this area are "adequate follower expertise related to task but poor motivation due to anxiety," and "adequate motivation for action, but lack of expertise due to low education level."

 Planning Leadership

Planning leadership involves two considerations: selecting an appropriate leadership style and preparing followers for action. Other aspects of planning, such as delineating specific activities, are based on the general principles of planning discussed in Chapters 6 and 19.

Selecting a Leadership Style

A successful leadership outcome is a function of the interaction among the characteristics of the community health nurse as leader, the followers, and the task to be accomplished. In planning leadership, the community health nurse must select a style of leadership appropriate to all three of these components of the leadership situation.

One of four leadership styles that balance task-oriented and relationship-oriented behaviors by the leader may be appropriate to different leadership situations (Hersey & Blanchard, 1996). These four styles of leadership also reflect a continuum of follower maturity and range from "telling," which is used with the least mature followers, to "selling" and "participating," used when moderate levels of follower maturity are evident, to "delegating," which is used with mature followers. The community health nurse's expertise and comfort with each of the four styles also influence the style selected in a given situation. Ideally, the nurse as leader will have developed the ability to use each of the four styles as needed in a given situation.

Telling.   For a situation in which task accomplishment is a priority and relationship concerns are less important, or followers have limited expertise or motivation, *telling* may be an appropriate leadership style. The nurse as leader tells the follower what to do and how to do it. For example, if the community health nurse encounters a client in cardiac arrest, he or she would direct one family member to call for emergency assistance and order another to assist with CPR. There is no time to explain why certain things must be done or to worry about offending family members. Immediate action is required.

Another situation may not be as urgent, but the followers may lack the experience required to determine what needs to be done or how to do it. In this instance, a "telling" or directive approach is also appropriate. For example, when people first begin to use computers, one focuses on telling them the exact steps to take to accomplish a task rather than on the principles behind computer operations. As they become more familiar with the use of computers, one might then change the approach to one that explains as well as tells what to do.

Selling.   The second leadership style, **selling,** is used in situations in which both task accomplishment and interpersonal relationships are important. The leader works to persuade followers that a specific course of action should be taken (Hersey, 1993). For example, the community health nurse might want to persuade school officials and parents that a school-based adolescent clinic is a good solution to health problems identified in this age group. The nurse as leader is not in a position to *tell* these people what to do, but must persuade them.

Participating.   **Participating** is the third leadership style on the maturity continuum. A participative leadership style might be used by the community health nurse who is assisting parents of handicapped children to form a support group. In this instance, the nurse as leader would want to emphasize interpersonal relationships with less attention to the need to accomplish specific tasks. This leadership style is appropriate with a group of followers who are mature with respect to the group's goal, but need some guidance in reaching that goal. Leader and followers share in decision making, and the role of the leader is largely facilitative.

Delegating.   The fourth leadership style is **delegating.** Followers are quite mature and can accomplish the group's goals with little or no direction from the leader. The nurse as a delegative leader places little emphasis on either task or relationship dimensions, but merely presents followers with a desired goal and leaves its accomplishment to them. For example, nursing faculty might delegate to the student organization the task of planning a graduation dinner, expecting students to take care of all the details with minimal input from the faculty. The four leadership styles discussed here are summarized in Table 12–4.

TABLE 12–4. LEADERSHIP STYLES

Style	Characteristic Features
Telling	• Emphasis on task accomplishment rather than interpersonal relationships • Entails specific directions or orders given to followers without explanation • Appropriate in emergency situations • Appropriate when followers do not have expertise or motivation to act on their own
Selling	• High emphasis on both task accomplishment and interpersonal relationships • Entails persuasion of followers to take the desired course of action • Appropriate when followers have expertise but not the motivation to act on their own
Participating	• Emphasis on interpersonal relationships rather than task accomplishment • Entails allowing and encouraging follower input into decisions on action to be taken • Appropriate when followers have some expertise and are motivated to act but need some direction • Appropriate when time is not a factor
Delegating	• Low emphasis by leader on both task accomplishment and interpersonal relationships • Entails informing followers of task to be done and leaving them to accomplish it • Appropriate when followers are highly motivated and have the necessary expertise

Preparing Followers

The second aspect of planning leadership is preparing followers for action. This can involve either enhancing their abilities to accomplish the task involved or improving their motivation to act.

Enhancing Followers' Abilities. Enhancing followers' abilities to perform a desired action might involve teaching new skills or providing opportunities to practice previously learned ones. For example, if the action required of followers involves use of interpersonal skills, the leader may plan to review principles of group dynamics and interpersonal communication with followers. Or, if the task involves use of computers, plans may need to be made to teach computer skills to followers or to broaden existing skills to encompass the desired action.

Improving Motivation. Because leadership is almost always directed to some type of action for change, improving followers' motivation to act may involve manipulation of the driving and restraining forces described earlier in relation to the change process. The community health nurse may need to plan to reduce restraining forces, enhance driving forces, or both.

These forces may reflect the psychological motivators for behavior discussed earlier.

Different people may be motivated by different things. For example, some followers may act to get a traffic signal installed at a dangerous intersection out of fear of injury to themselves or their loved ones. Others may be influenced to act by altruistic motives or because they like the challenge presented by a tussle with city hall.

Knowledge of what motivates a specific individual permits the use of motivators that will reduce restraining forces and enhance driving forces, increasing the potential for accomplishing the desired action. For example, if action is needed to improve the quality of nursing care provided, some followers may be motivated by threats of job loss, whereas others will be better motivated by recognition of a job well done. The community health nurse who has thoroughly assessed the leadership situation will be able to plan rewards and sanctions that motivate specific followers to action.

 ## Implementing the Leadership Plan

Two aspects of implementing a leadership plan are performance of designated activities by followers and performance of leadership functions by the leader. The first aspect is based on general principles of implementation discussed in Chapter 7 and is not reiterated here. The second aspect of implementation is the performance of specific leadership functions by the nurse as leader. These functions include carrying out plans for follower preparation, coordinating and directing follower activity related to task accomplishment, and representing followers to outsiders.

Plans for preparing followers need to be executed. In this phase of implementation, the community health nurse provides whatever education is needed by followers to carry out the desired actions. The nurse also puts into operation planned rewards and sanctions designed to motivate followers.

In addition, the nurse coordinates group members' activities in planning and implementing the desired course of action. The amount of coordination required depends on the maturity of the group, their need for assistance, and the leadership style employed. For example, if the task was appropriately delegated to a mature group of followers, there will be little need for extensive coordination by the nurse as leader. If, on the other hand, the nurse selected the "telling" style of leadership, the leader might need to engage in quite a bit of coordination of follower activities.

Finally, the community health nurse as leader serves as the group's spokesperson. He or she supports group decisions and defends those decisions to outsiders when necessary. For instance, if the task remains unaccomplished because of a lack of necessary materials, the nurse as leader may need to explain difficulties in task completion to policy makers or supervisors.

Evaluating Leadership

As was true in the change process, evaluation in a leadership situation addresses the outcome of leadership as well as the process used. Was the desired action or change brought about? Was the leadership style selected appropriate to the task and to the level of follower maturity? Were followers adequately pre-

Critical Thinking in Research

Misener and colleagues (1997) conducted a Delphi study to identify leadership competencies needed in community health nursing. After five rounds of review by community health nurse leaders and non-nurse leaders in public health, 57 competencies were identified. These competencies clustered in four categories: political competencies, business acumen, program leadership, and management capabilities. Examples of political competencies included client advocacy, community development, use of information systems to develop community diagnoses, and participating in policy development. Competencies involved in business acumen included strategic planning, marketing, use of information systems to manage human and financial resources, and ensuring service reimbursement. Examples of program leadership competencies included development of health promotion programs based on epidemiologic and research principles and implementing strategies for policy change. Finally, sample competencies from the management category included problem-solving skills, conflict resolution, interdisciplinary interaction, and management of staff.

1. To what extent is your nursing education preparing you to display these leadership competencies?
2. How would you go about determining what educational experiences best prepare community health nurses for positions of leadership?
3. Do you think the competencies required to be an effective change agent would be similar to those required of an effective community health leader? Why or why not? How would you design a study to determine whether or not you are correct?

TABLE 12–5. COMPONENTS OF THE LEADERSHIP PROCESS

Assessment	• Assess the leadership situation in terms of: Factors giving rise to the need for leadership Factors influencing the leadership situation
Diagnosis	• Diagnose the need for leadership • Diagnose follower maturity
Planning	• Select an appropriate leadership style • Plan to prepare followers for action • Delineate actions to be taken
Implementation	• Enhance follower abilities • Improve follower motivation • Coordinate follower activities • Represent group to outsiders
Evaluation	• Evaluate actions accomplished • Evaluate use of the leadership process

pared for action? Components of leadership in the context of the Dimensions Model are summarized in Table 12–5.

▶ THE DIMENSIONS MODEL AND THE GROUP PROCESS

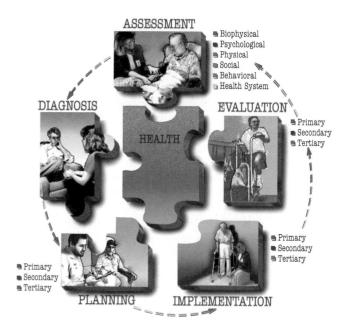

Change is often accomplished by group action. This is particularly true of changes that occur in the health care delivery system. Many of the problems that affect population groups cannot be solved by the action of one health care provider, and cooperative activity by a group is required. Community health nurses are often called on to initiate and direct group problem-solving activities; consequently, they must be conversant with the processes that govern the formation and operation of groups. Group process skills are needed by community health nurses who are members, as well as leaders, of groups.

Group action has a number of advantages over actions taken by individuals. The greater range of knowledge and expertise of group members provides a broader base from which to derive solutions to health problems. For example, if community health nurses are concerned about drug abuse among elementary school children, to address the problem they might form a group that includes school officials, police, child psychologists, and parents. Each member of the group has expertise that can contribute to solving the problem. Police personnel have knowledge of means by which drugs are circulated. School officials and parents can speak to factors in the school setting that contribute to drug traffic. The child psychologist can provide input into ways to motivate young people to refrain from using drugs. Working together, the group can generate a solution to the problem that is realistic and effective.

Another advantage to group activity is the increased efficiency realized by using each member's expertise and by eliminating duplication of effort. When people act cooperatively, those best suited to a particular function can perform that function. When one acts independently, one must carry out all the required functions despite one's level of expertise in those areas. In the drug abuse example cited earlier, school officials and teachers can work on curriculum aspects of a drug abuse prevention program while police concentrate on eliminating drug dealers from school grounds. Furthermore, group action also eliminates duplication of effort. For example, there is no point in the school system and the police department developing independent drug education programs when drug education can be done more effectively and efficiently as a cooperative effort.

Finally, group action promotes communication among members of the group that may enhance problem resolution. Improved communication through group work can also lead to collaborative effort in other areas, which increases the resource network of each of the group's members.

The role of the community health nurse in group action to solve problems frequently involves initiating the group and directing its activity. In other instances, community health nurses are asked to serve in groups formed by others. In either case, knowledge of the group process assists the nurse to make a greater contribution to the group effort.

In working with groups, community health nurses can use the Dimensions Model to direct group efforts. The model can be used both in group develop-ment and in the group's efforts to resolve health problems.

Group development occurs in a series of stages: orientation, accommodation, negotiation, operation, and dissolution. These stages parallel the components of the nursing process. Specific tasks must be accomplished during each stage of group development for the group to function effectively. Each stage of group development with its related tasks is discussed in the context of the nursing process component to which it relates.

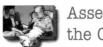

Assessment and the Group Process

Assessment in group work has two components: assessing the problem and assessing the group. The problem to be solved is assessed from an epidemiologic perspective, considering the biophysical, psychological, physical, social, behavioral, and health system factors that influence the problem and its solution.

Ideally, group members are selected because they have characteristics that enable them to contribute to the group. Unfortunately, that is not always the case, and the community health nurse working with a group needs to assess group members to identify their strengths and weaknesses. One potential barrier to effective group action is lack of knowledge of the abilities and characteristics of group members that could enhance or undermine group effort. Careful assessment of group members by the community health nurse can help to eliminate this barrier.

The Biophysical Dimension

Biological factors often influence the group and its ability to function. Age and developmental level may determine the type of life experiences group members have had, and this, in turn, affects their ability to generate solutions to problems. The physical health status of group members may influence their ability to contribute. If one group member is pregnant, the group needs to carry on in her absence if she goes into labor at a crucial time in the group's activity. For example, one group of community health nursing students who were organizing a health fair assigned the pregnant member tasks that could be completed prior to the fair (eg, publicizing the fair) in case she went into labor early.

The Psychological Dimension

The psychological dimension poses several barriers to effective group work that arise out of the personal characteristics of group members. Members who are personally insecure or fiercely independent may feel threatened by the interdependence required in group work. Suspicion and lack of trust in other members may also hamper group effort. For example, in a community experiencing racial unrest, it may be difficult for members of different ethnic groups to work together.

Personal philosophies, values, and goals also impede group effectiveness. It is important for the community health nurse to encourage group members to express their personal beliefs and attitudes both to the problem that needs resolution and to working as a group. It is vital for effective group function that all group members understand and accept the group's purpose and goals. For this reason, it is important that purposes and goals be developed jointly. When philosophical differences are identified early in the group's existence, those differences can be acknowledged and compromises achieved that would not be possible when such differences go unrecognized.

Paradoxically, another psychological barrier to effective group function arises out of commitment to the group on the part of its members. This commitment entails group loyalty that may prohibit group members from acknowledging any weaknesses of the group, thus promoting a possible tendency to cover up any mistakes made. Another possible problem occurs when group loyalties supercede client needs (Griffiths & Luker, 1994).

The tendency of health care providers to adopt a paternalistic attitude to health care consumers is another psychological barrier to effective group work. This can be a serious problem for community health nurses who frequently work in groups that include laypeople and consumers. In such situations, the community health nurse may need to function as an advocate for these individuals to ensure that their input is recognized by the group.

The interpersonal skills of each member also influence the group's ability to work harmoniously. In groups whose members have good interpersonal skills, differences of opinion are dealt with more easily and the group can function more effectively. In groups whose members have poor interpersonal skills, the community health nurse may have to exercise his or her interpersonal skills to aid the group to work as a cohesive unit. The nurse may also need to foster interpersonal skills among group members.

The Physical Dimension

Elements of the physical dimension can influence group activity. If great distances separate group members, for example, much of the group's work may need to be done by e-mail or telephone. Similarly, if group members live in different parts of town, attention needs to be given to a centralized meeting place.

The Social Dimension

The social environment can give rise to barriers to effective group function. Some of the major barriers in this area relate to concepts of authority, power, status, and autonomy. For example, health care policy makers may feel that their authority and power are threatened if health care consumers are included in health planning groups. Or, group members of lower socioeconomic status may resent those from higher socioeconomic levels and have difficult working with them. On the other hand, members from higher socioeconomic groups may have difficulty understanding the needs of those of lower status.

Culture is another social environmental factor that may affect the way a group functions. Cultures differ with respect to their ability to work in groups and commitment to group goals. They may also differ with respect to concepts of group leadership. For example, individuals from traditional Asian cultures may be very committed to working for group goals, but may be reluctant to advance ideas for problem resolution, expecting direction to come from the group leader. Members of various occupational groups and health disciplines also have unique cultures that might influence their ability to work in a group. For example, the use of medical and nursing jargon may be confusing to computer programmers in the group and vice versa.

Differences in education levels among group members can be barriers to effective group function. The community health nurse may find that group members need to be educated about both the problem and the group process. The need for education may be experienced by professional as well as lay members of the group. Although professional members often have an understanding of the health implications of a problem and some idea of how to solve it, very few health professionals have been educated regarding the group process.

The final social dimension consideration in working with groups is the fact that a group is a social system, and whatever affects one part of the system affects the entire system. For example, if a member who has assumed responsibility for gathering data needed by the group becomes ill or has a family emergency, the group needs to make other arrangements for gathering data. All group members must carry out assigned responsibilities adequately if the group is to function effectively. This means that group members must be concerned about the well-being of fellow members and their ability to function. It also means that there must be a mechanism for integrating new members into the group in a way that their lack of familiarity with the group causes the least possible disruption in group function.

The Behavioral Dimension

Behavioral dimension factors affect group function in two ways. First, leisure interests influence group members' areas of expertise. Members' recreational activities may give them specialized knowledge and skills that can be used by the group. For example, a member whose hobby is writing programs for computer games might help the group design a computer-assisted educational program on substance abuse for school-aged children.

The second way in which lifestyle influences group function is the effect of people's schedules on group activity. For instance, if members work and have several other responsibilities, it may be difficult for the group to schedule meeting times. This problem is particularly relevant in many groups with which community health nurses work. For example, the nurse may be helping single parents form a support group. But because of group members' other responsibilities, the nurse as group leader may have to coordinate schedules so the group can meet. He or she may also need to coordinate group members' activities when assigned responsibilities are carried out independently.

The Health System Dimension

Health care system factors influence group function. Professional territoriality is one such factor that may hamper effective group function. **Professional territoriality** is the tendency of a discipline to regard certain activities as the sole province of their discipline and to resent others outside the discipline who engage in those activities. Because some health professions (and other disciplines) are not well defined, some health care roles overlap, and group members may easily infringe on each other's sense of territory. Robert Merton, a sociologist who has studied health professional groups, aptly described the problem of role ambiguity in the following words: "Every profession is to some degree surrounded by a zone of ambiguity—The trouble with this zone of ambiguity is not that it is a no man's land, but that it seems to be everyman's land. And sometimes this leads to undeclared war between adjacent occupations" (Merton, 1958). Role ambiguity and professional territoriality may result in conflict that is detrimental to group effort.

Differences between health care professionals and other professionals in terms of their orientation to time, styles of interpersonal interaction, methods of organization, and value systems can also result in barriers to effective group action. Health care system factors that impair group function may also relate to concepts of authority and autonomy. Traditionally, physicians have been perceived as leaders in groups dealing with health. In many instances, however, this may not be appropriate. It may be difficult for physicians and other health care providers to see someone other than a physician as a legitimate leader in health-related groups.

Professional autonomy can also hamper group function. The joint effort required in group work decreases personal independence in favor of interdependence. Interdependence creates the potential for challenges or criticism of one member's beliefs or actions by other group members, a situation that may be threatening to the individual member. Again, use of good interpersonal skills by the community health nurse can create a climate in which group members do not feel threatened by interdependence.

Diagnostic Reasoning and the Group Process

Based on the assessment of group members, the community health nurse diagnoses group strengths and weaknesses. Diagnoses might also relate to group members' expertise and motivation relative to the problem to be solved. For example, the community health nurse might diagnose a "need for conflict resolution due to different perceptions of group goals by group members." Or, the nurse might derive a diagnosis of "effective group function due to successful accomplishment of tasks of group development." A third possible diagnosis might be a "need to educate members for group work due to inexperience with group dynamics."

Planning the Group Process

There are two aspects to planning group work. One reflects the efforts of the group to resolve the problems in question. This aspect of planning uses the general planning principles discussed in Chapters 7 and 19. The second aspect involves planning the operation of the group itself and includes determining group modes of decision making, conflict resolution, communication, and role negotiation. These activities are

ASSESSMENT TIPS: Group Process

Biophysical Dimension

What are the ages of group members?

What are group members' developmental levels?

How will members' ages and developmental levels affect their ability to work effectively as a group?

What influence, if any, will group members' physiologic status have on the group's ability to function effectively?

Psychological Dimension

Do elements of the psychological dimension pose barriers to effective group work? If so, how?

What is the level of emotional security exhibited by group members? Will this affect their ability to work together effectively?

What is the character of interaction among group members?

Will the personal philosophies, goals, and values of group members provide impediments to effective group work?

Is there evidence of overcommitment to the group on the part of group members?

What is the attitude of health care providers to other members of the group?

Physical Dimension

Are group members separated by physical distance? If so, what effect will this have on group function?

What modes of communication are available to overcome the effects of distance?

Social Dimension

How will concepts of authority, power, status, and autonomy influence members' abilities to function effectively as a group?

Are there cultural factors operating in the situation that will influence the group's ability to work together?

Do group members represent different occupational cultures? If so, what effect will this have on group communication and function?

Will differences in education levels among group members affect their ability to function effectively?

How will changes in group membership affect group function?

Behavioral Dimension

Will group members' consumption patterns affect group function?

Will differences in group members' schedules affect their ability to work together?

Will group members' leisure pursuits affect group task accomplishment?

Health System Dimension

Do group members exhibit professional territoriality that will impede effective group function?

Will emphasis on professional autonomy influence group members' abilities to work together?

Will differences in professional values, styles of interaction, and orientation to time influence group function?

---

carried out during the accommodation and negotiation stages of group formation.

Selecting a Method of Decision Making

Group action requires group decisions, and decisions must be made after careful consideration by group members. To facilitate decision making, group members should agree on the method by which decisions will be made. Because most people are not familiar with group processes or the deliberate need to select a decision-making strategy, the community health nurse may need to guide the group in this task.

Decisions can be made in one of six ways: by default, by the leader, by a subgroup, by majority vote, by consensus, or by unanimous consent. Decisions made by default result from a lack of response by the group. For example, if a class of senior nursing students is invited by faculty to plan a graduation reception but fails to respond, they have, in fact, decided not to have a reception.

The second method of decision making, in which decisions are made by the leader, is appropriate when a decision cannot wait on the slow-moving democratic process (eg, when there is an emergency). The group may decide to give the group leader authority to make independent decisions in certain circumstances, but should decide in advance what circumstances warrant such independent decisions. In an effective group, this is not the method used for making most of the group's decisions.

In the third approach to group decision making, group decisions are made by a subgroup. This might involve "railroading," in which the subgroup uses its power and influence to force a decision on other group members. Or, the larger group may purposefully delegate the making of decisions to a subgroup. Many nursing organizations, for example, delegate authority to an executive board for decisions regarding everyday operation and only make major decisions as a total group.

Majority vote by group members, the fourth method of decision making, is frequently used in many groups with which community health nurses work. The fifth method involves consensus or agreement by all group members despite reservations that individual members might have. Finally, decisions may be made by unanimous consent in which all group members agree without reservation. In both the consensus and unanimous consent methods, the group may take a relatively long time to reach a decision because of the need for all members to agree. For the purposes of true collaboration in a group, majority vote, consensus, and unanimous consent are the most appropriate methods for group decision making.

Developing Mechanisms for Conflict Resolution

Breakdowns in the decision-making process are one source of conflict within the group. Other potential sources of conflict are incompatible goals, differences of opinion on the allocation of resources or rewards, and perceived threats to individual members' personal identities or rights. Conflict is a normal component of group effort and is to be expected. In fact, many group behavior theorists include a conflict stage in describing the development of groups over time (Mullen, 1987). If the group has developed mechanisms for conflict resolution before conflicts arise, conflict can often be a positive rather than a divisive experience for the group.

Recognition of conflict as a normal phenomenon is essential if the group is to plan ahead for conflict resolution. Again, many groups do not anticipate conflict, and when conflict occurs they are unprepared to deal with it. Strategies for resolving conflict constructively involve creating a climate conducive to discussion, identifying and eliminating sources of conflict, capitalizing on areas of agreement, and rationally considering alternative solutions to conflict. The commu-

nity health nurse can explore these approaches to conflict resolution with members of the group and assist members to select the most appropriate approach.

Creating a climate in which disagreement is acceptable can minimize or resolve conflict. Conflict resolution requires that all parties be fully able to express their perspectives through open communication. Open communication cannot take place when there is pressure to conform and lack of acceptance of different opinions. Lack of communication contributes to conflict as well as hampering conflict resolution. As a group leader, the community health nurse may need to encourage group members to express thoughts and opinions that may not be congruent with those of other group members. Through the use of interpersonal skills, the nurse can ensure that communications within the group are not accusatory, but deal with issues rather than personalities.

Recognizing the existence of conflict and identifying its sources and possible solutions are strategies for constructive use of conflict. A conflict that is ignored in the hope that it will resolve itself is likely to become worse. The community health nurse can encourage other group members to acknowledge that a conflict exists and help them explore the reasons for conflict. Again, the nurse should be alert to covert signs of conflict and bring them to the attention of the rest of the group. For example, a nurse working with a group trying to determine budget allocations among health care programs within the county may notice that representatives of programs for the elderly are maintaining a stony silence during the discussion. The nurse may comment on the fact that they have not participated in the discussion and ask why. In the ensuing discussion, it may be learned that these group members feel that too much money is being allocated to maternal–child health programs and that the elderly are being shortchanged. Once this conflict has been exposed, the group can begin work to resolve it.

Another strategy for resolving conflict involves identifying small areas of trust and agreement between group members that can be expanded. For example, although two group members may disagree on the "appropriate" approach to a problem, they can capitalize on their shared concern for clients' welfare. Finally, rational consideration of alternative solutions to a particular conflict using the group's decision-making process and the problem-solving process can result in conflict becoming a valuable learning experience in group problem solving. The community health nurse can assist the group to explore a variety of alternative solutions to a conflict and to select an approach that is agreeable to all members.

Developing Communication Strategies

Developing group communication strategies is another task in planning group operation. The importance of an effective communication network cannot be overemphasized. The group must develop a common language that facilitates communication, and members should refrain from using jargon familiar only to members of their own discipline. When it is necessary to use terminology unfamiliar to others, efforts should be made to translate it into the common language. The nurse in this situation can either play the part of the translator or ask other members for clarification. For example, some members of a group may use acronyms unfamiliar to others, such as AFDC. The nurse should then explain to the group that this stands for Aid to Families with Dependent Children. If the nurse does not recognize the acronym, he or she would ask for an explanation of its meaning.

The group should also agree on the form that communication will take. For example, communications may be verbal, written, or a combination of both depending on the situation. Perhaps the group will decide that communication with sponsoring institutions should take the form of formal written memoranda, whereas communications between group members should be more informal verbal messages.

Consideration should also be given to the fact that communication takes place outside of regular group sessions. The content of these informal encounters between group members should not undermine group function or provide a forum for airing grievances or denigrating other members. The community health nurse who encounters unproductive communication outside of group meetings can bring relevant issues to the attention of the entire group so open discussion can take place and conflict can be avoided or resolved.

Establishing a climate in which group members feel respected and in which differences are accepted contributes to an effective communication network. This means that all group members should be encouraged to participate and should receive positive reinforcement for their contribution whether or not others agree with it. In the beginning of the group's operation, the nurse group leader may need to ask reluctant group members for their ideas and opinions. As their participation is received positively, they will begin to volunteer remarks.

Negotiating Roles

Another task to be accomplished in forming an effective group is role negotiation. As mentioned earlier, professional roles tend to overlap, and role negotiation is crucial to effective group function. When two or more group members possess similar skills, the group must decide who will be responsible for exercising those skills. These decisions may be made as a general rule of thumb, so that one member always has responsibility for certain activities, or may change with the needs of the situation. For example, both teachers and nurses have educational skills. A group developing a health education program for the school system may decide that teachers will be responsible for general health education related to nutrition and hygiene, while the nurse will deal with more complex health topics such as substance abuse and sexually transmitted diseases.

One particular group role that must be negotiated is the role of leader. This position incorporates functions related to group administration, liaison with outside groups, teaching, and coordination of group effort. The leadership role may be assigned to one member, may shift with the situation, or may reside with the group as a whole. In the last instance, no one member acts as the leader, and leadership functions are performed by the group as a unit. In many instances, community health nurses fulfill the leadership role within the group, particularly in groups composed largely of nonprofessionals. In other cases, the nurse may need to help the group identify who is best suited to lead the group, based on the needs of the situation.

Implementing the Group Process

Implementation of the group process involves actually assigning responsibilities for tasks required to achieve group goals and performing assigned tasks. Tasks are assigned on the basis of decisions made in the role negotiation phase of planning. Actual implementation of tasks is based on the general principles of implementation discussed in Chapter 7.

Planned group operating procedures are also executed during the implementation stage. Decisions are made using the method of decision making selected and communication networks are established along lines determined by the group. If conflict should arise during group operation, the group will employ the conflict resolution strategies selected during group formation.

Evaluating the Group Process

Throughout the section on group process, we have alluded to stages of group development that coincide with the nursing process. The final stage of group development, the dissolution stage, is related to the evaluation component of the nursing process. Group tasks in this stage center around evaluation of both the outcome of group activity and the process used to plan and execute group action. Tasks of this stage actually begin during planning and prior to implementation of group actions. The group identifies outcome criteria and plans mechanisms for evaluating the effects of group effort in terms of those criteria. Group members' responsibilities in evaluation should be negotiated in the same manner as other group roles and assigned on the basis of competency. For example, if the group has implemented a school nutrition program, teachers may evaluate students' knowledge of nutrition, while the community health nurse evaluates indicators of nutritional status such as height, weight, and hematocrit. The evaluation process itself is discussed in detail in Chapters 7 and 19.

In evaluating use of the group process, the effectiveness of group decision making, conflict resolution, communication, and role negotiation strategies may be addressed. Were roles allocated in a way that facilitated group goal achievement? Was communication between group members effective? Were conflicts within the group adequately resolved? Answers to these and similar questions can assist the group to work together more effectively in the future and can prepare group members to function effectively in other groups.

In some instances, the results of evaluation actually culminate in dissolution of the group. This may occur either because the group's purpose has been accomplished or because the group is not able to achieve its purpose. Tasks of the dissolution stage of group development, as well as tasks of other stages, are summarized in Table 12–6 in conjunction with the phases of the nursing process during which they occur.

The Dimensions Model can be used to facilitate group process in a variety of groups with whom community health nurses work. Community health nurses may use the model to assist a group of clients to achieve common goals. It can also be used with groups of health care providers and policy makers to facilitate group process and achieve group goals. The components of the group process applied in the context of the Dimensions Model are summarized in Table 12–7.

TABLE 12–6. TASKS OF GROUP DEVELOPMENT BY STAGE AND RELATED NURSING PROCESS COMPONENT

Nursing Process Component	Stage of Group Development	Group Development Tasks
Assessment	Orientation	1. Selection of group members 2. Training for group participation 3. Identification of goals and purposes
Diagnosis		
Planning	Accommodation	1. Establishment of modes of decision making 2. Development of mechanisms for conflict resolution 3. Development of communication network 4. Development of climate conducive to group collaboration
	Negotiation	1. Negotiation of member roles 2. Development of methods of task assignment
Implementation	Operation	1. Assignment of specific tasks to accomplish group goals 2. Performance of actions to accomplish goals
Evaluation	Dissolution	1. Planning of evaluative mechanisms for outcomes of action taken 2. Assignment of member roles and tasks in evaluation 3. Data collection 4. Analysis of evaluative findings 5. Possible group dissolution

TABLE 12–7. COMPONENTS OF THE GROUP PROCESS

Assessment	• Assess the problem to be addressed by the group
	• Assess the members of the group in terms of factors influencing group function:
	  Biophysical dimension
	  Psychological dimension
	  Physical dimension
	  Social dimension
	  Behavioral dimension
	  Health systems dimension

Diagnosis	• Diagnose group strengths and weaknesses, expertise, and motivation

Planning	• Plan achievement of group goals
	• Plan group operation in terms of:
	  Methods for group decision making
	  Mechanisms for conflict resolution
	  Methods of communication
	  Role negotiation

Implementation	• Implement activities designed to reach the group goal • Implement group operation procedures
Evaluation	• Evaluate outcome of the group action • Evaluate use of the group process

Critical Thinking in Practice: A Case in Point

In assessing the town of Clarkston, you, as a community health nurse, note that infant and maternal mortality rates are high. Part of the explanation lies in a lack of prenatal care for large numbers of pregnant women. The local health department prenatal clinic is always full, and clients may have to wait 3 months or longer for an initial appointment. Because many of the pregnant women in the community do not seek care until their pregnancies are fairly for advanced, they may deliver before they can be seen. Seven physicians with private practices in town provide obstetric care, but their services are underutilized. This is primarily because most of the pregnant population come from low-income families and are on Medicaid, which these physicians do not want to accept. Because they are on the obstetrics staff of the local community hospital that accepts indigent clients, four of these physicians deliver many of the women who have not had prenatal care. Two physicians have been sued as a result of complications experienced by these indigent women.

1. What changes or course of action might improve this situation?
2. What would be the objective of your change? Be specific.
3. What biophysical, psychological, physical, social, behavioral, and health system factors are acting as driving and restraining forces in this situation?
4. As the leader in this change situation, who are your followers? How would you describe the maturity level of your followers?
5. What leadership style would be appropriate in this situation? Why?
6. How would you unfreeze this situation? What would you do to bring about the desired change? How would you promote re-freezing?
7. How would you evaluate the outcome of the change and your leadership as a change agent?

Nurses using the Dimensions Model in the context of the change, leadership, and group processes may want additional information about the processes. The agencies and organization listed at the end of this chapter may be appropriate resources.

TESTING YOUR UNDERSTANDING

1. Describe the influence of driving and restraining forces in a change situation. Give examples of each type of force. (p. 233)
2. What are the four major considerations in planning change? Give an example of each. (pp. 236–238)
3. What three approaches may be taken to bring about change? Describe situations in which each approach might be appropriate. (pp. 236–237)
4. Describe the three stages in implementing change. How might you facilitate movement through these stages? Give specific examples related to a change situation with which you are familiar. (pp. 238–239)
5. Describe the relationship of follower maturity to leadership style. (pp. 241–244)
6. What are the three functions of a leader in implementing leadership? Give an example of the performance of each function. (pp. 245–246)

7. Describe the five stages of group development. Give an example of a task to be accomplished in each stage. (pp. 247–253)
8. Discuss two tasks in implementing the group process. Give an example of the performance of each. (p. 252)
9. What are the two aspects of evaluation applicable to the change, leadership, and group processes? Give examples of evaluative criteria for each aspect in each of the three processes. (pp. 233, 246, 253)

WHAT DO YOU THINK?
Questions for Critical Thinking

1. How might effective leadership after a natural disaster differ from effective leadership in your student nurses' organization?
2. Think of some effective leaders you have known. What made them effective? Would they have been equally effective in other kinds of situations? Why or why not?
3. What are some of the potential consequences when health-related groups fail to accomplish tasks of group development?

REFERENCES

Clark, C. C. (1994). *The nurse as group leader* (3rd ed.). New York: Springer.

Fiedler, F. E. (1993). The leadership situation and the black box in contingency theories. In M. M. Chemers & R. Ayman (Eds.), *Leadership theory and research: Perspectives and directions* (pp. 1–28). San Diego: Academic Press.

Griffiths, J. M., & Luker, K. A. (1994). Intraprofessional teamwork in district nursing: In whose interest? *Journal of Advanced Nursing, 20,* 1038–1045.

Harkness, G. A. (1995). *Epidemiology in nursing practice.* St. Louis: Mosby.

Hersey, P. (1993, February). *Situational leadership.* Paper presented at the University of San Diego, San Diego, CA.

Hersey, P., & Blanchard, K. H. (1996). *Management of organizational behavior: Utilizing human resources* (7th ed.). Englewood Cliffs, NJ: Prentice-Hall.

Institute of Medicine. (1988). *The future of public health.* Washington, DC: National Academy Press.

Jellison, J. M. (1993). *Overcoming resistance: A practical guide to producing change in the work place.* New York: Simon & Schuster.

Josten, L., Aroskar, M., Reckinger, D., Shannon, M. (1996). *Educating nurses for public health leadership.* Minneapolis: University of Minnesota.

Lewin, C. (1951). *Field theory in social science: Selected theoretical papers.* New York: Harper & Row.

Lewin, C. (1989a). Changing as three steps: Unfreezing, moving, and freezing. In W. L. French, C. H. Bell, & R. A. Zawacki (Eds.), *Organizational development: Theory, practice and research* (p. 87). Homewood, IL: BPI Irwin.

Lewin, C. (1989b). The field approach: Culture and group life and quasi-stationary processes. In W. L. French, C. H. Bell, & R. A. Zawacki (Eds.), *Organizational development: Theory, practice and research* (pp. 85–86) Homewood, IL: BPI Irwin.

Manion, J. (1995). Understanding the seven stages of change. *American Journal of Nursing, 85*(4), 41–42.

Merton, R. (1958). Issues in the growth of a profession. In *Proceedings of the 41st annual convention of the American Nurses Association* (pp. 295–306). Atlantic City, NJ: American Nurses Association.

Misener, T. R., Alexander, J. W., Blaha, A. J., et al. (1997). National Delphi study to determine competencies for nursing leadership in public health. *Image: Journal of Nursing Scholarship, 29,* 47–51.

Mullen, B. (1987). Introduction: The study of group behavior. In B. Mullen & G. R. Goenthals (Eds.), *Theories of group behavior* (pp. 1–19). New York: Springer-Verlag.

Pointer, D. D., & Sanchez, J. P. (1997). Leadership in public health practice. In F. D. Scutchfield & C. W. Keck (Eds.), *Principles of public health practice* (pp. 87–100). Albany, NY: Delmar.

Porter-O'Grady, T. (1995). *The leadership revolution in health care: Altering systems, changing behaviors.* Gaithersburg, MD: Aspen.

Skinner, M. D. (1994). Getting to X. *Nursing Administration Quarterly, 14*(3), 58–63.

Taccetta-Chapnick, M. (1996). Transformational leadership. *Nursing Administration Quarterly, 21*(1), 60–66.

RESOURCES FOR THE LEADERSHIP, CHANGE, AND GROUP PROCESSES

American Humanics
4601 Madison Avenue
Kansas City, MO 64112
(816) 561–6415

American Organization of Nurse Executives (AONE)
American Hospital Association Building
One N Franklin, 34th Floor
Chicago, IL 60606
(312) 422–2800

Center for the New Leadership
2641 Mann Court
Falls Church, VA 22046
(703) 573–1217

Research Center for Group Dynamics
c/o Marlene Smith
University of Michigan
Ann Arbor, MI 48106
(313) 764–8363

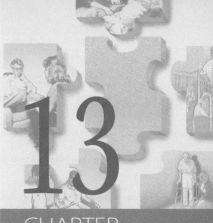

THE POLITICAL PROCESS

Elizabeth Harper Smith

The change, leadership, and group interaction skills described in the preceding chapter are frequently used in the context of the political process. The political process encompasses more than voting and legislation. The political process is all of the activities that result in the formation of policies that guide societal behavior.

Policy guides and directs action in all spheres of social interaction including the provision of health care services. For example, national defense policy determines the size of a standing army as well as the number and types of weapons that will be developed. Environmental policy guides decisions on the use of parklands, prohibition of off shore drilling, and disposal of hazardous wastes. In the same vein, health care policy directs decisions and actions taken in the provision of health care services. When nurses apply the change, leadership, and group processes to the development of health care policy, they engage in the political process.

► KEY TERMS

allocative policies
bill
campaigning
community
  organization
electioneering
health care policy
laws
legislative proposals
lobbying
macropolicy
pocket veto
policy
policy making
political process
politics
power
power base
public health policy
regulation
regulatory policies

▶ Chapter Objectives

After reading this chapter, you should be able to:

- Identify at least three levels at which health policy formation occurs.
- Describe at least five factors affecting nurses' ability to influence health policy formation.
- Identify four strategies for developing a power base for political influence.
- Describe at least four approaches to creating support for a proposed health policy.
- Outline the legislative process at the state and federal levels.
- Describe the regulatory process.
- Identify four criteria for evaluating a proposed health policy.

▶ NURSING AND POLICY FORMATION

Florence Nightingale has been described as a "consummate politician" (Meyer, 1992). She and other early community health nurses were adept at using the *political process* to develop policies to promote the health of the population. These early leaders in community health nursing knew that the only way to make lasting changes in the social factors influencing health was to become involved in the formation of health care policy at all levels. Nursing action to foster changes in sanitary conditions, to promote health legislation, and to change child labor laws are some examples of the early political activities by these nurses. They were active, as well, in many other social movements such as women's suffrage. They realized that the political process was a means of achieving their goal of improved health for all and that, because of its focus on the health of population groups, community health nursing is, by definition, political in nature. Nursing leaders have called for a return to sociopolitical strategies similar to those employed by early community health nurses.

Over the years, many nurses became uncomfortable with the idea of political involvement, with the possible exception of exercising the right to vote. Politics had an unfavorable aura that was seen as incompatible with nursing's altruistic philosophy. More recently, nurses have begun to realize the need to influence health care policy decisions.

There is a need for nursing input in health care policy that affects not only the health of the population but also nursing practice. This need is apparent at all levels of government, but particularly at the federal level. The need for nursing influence at the federal level is underscored by the recommendations of the Secretary's Commission on Nursing (1988) that policy making, regulatory, and accrediting bodies should foster nursing participation in decision activities and that employers of nurses should promote their participation in organizational governance.

Nurses, as a group, can have a tremendous impact on health care policy formation. There are over 2 million registered nurses in the United States and one of every four women registered to vote is an RN. Nurses are politically active with respect to voting; 98% of nurses are "perennial voters" (Brydoff, 1996). Unfortunately, because we are less active in other spheres of political activity, we have less influence than we might otherwise have. As noted by Marla Salmon (1995), former director of the Division of Nursing, "Never before in the history of the United States has the relationship between public policy and the health of the American people been more apparent or more important." Community health nurses, who are responsible for the health of society at large, must become involved in the formation of health care policy.

▶ HEALTH CARE POLICY

Policy is the aggregate of principles directing activity toward a designated goal (Mason & Leavitt, 1993). *Policy making* is the process of synthesizing those principles and the values, interests, and concerns that underlie them in response to an identified problem (Stimpson & Hanley, 1991). Policy is typically concerned with complex issues, and its formation involves the use of the political process. *Health care policy* is a defined set of principles used to guide activities to safeguard and promote the health of the public. Health policies may be allocative or regulatory. *Allocative policies* direct the distribution of resources among members of a society. *Regulatory policies*, on the other hand, are designed to control the actions or decisions of specific people.

Public policy is a direction or course of action undertaken by a government or an official governmental agency. A public policy is a decision made by a society or its elected representatives that has material effects on members of the public. Public policies determine the parameters for individual and collective social behavior in allocating and distributing resources. A *public health policy*, then, is the way a society or its elected representatives allocate and distribute political and economic resources to meet the health needs of the populace.

All policies are values-based; values determine the policy issues that arise, how they are resolved, and by whom. When the values held by different groups in a society vary, the need for politics arises (Mason & Leavitt, 1993). *Politics* is the process or accumulating power and exerting influence over events or the actions of others (Mason & Leavitt, 1993; Skinner, 1994).

Levels of Health Care Policy

Policy can be made in any setting or organizational system where values are at issue, and policy formation takes place at many levels in society: family, community, institution, state, nation, even the international level. Institutional goals and purpose shape policy decisions at the level of the health care agency or institution. Examples of institutional policy related to community health would be decisions to create new programs or to expand or discontinue current ones. Decisions by local health departments to charge fees for previously free services such as immunizations are another example of institutional policy that affects the health of the public. Community health nurses need to be involved in the development of these and similar institutional policies to safeguard the interests of the public.

Health care policy decisions at the community level may be reflected in budget allocations for health care programs, disaster preparation, and housing codes. At the state level, health care policies focus on provision of health care and may include health programming decisions as well as policies related to licensure of health care professionals and regulation of health care institutions. At both the state and local levels, policies may also be formulated in legislation that regulates health-related behaviors by citizens. State laws and local ordinances that limit smoking in public places are examples of such policies.

National policy focuses on issues of concern to the society at large and is exemplified by health-related legislation and regulations that are developed by federal agencies. Although there are a number of health-related policies generated by the federal government, there is, at present, no single coherent policy that directs provision of health care across the country. During the 1994 legislative session, Congress debated the establishment of a national health care policy for the first time.

The United States has allocated financial resources to create special programs that provide limited health care services to selected populations of Americans. The provision of limited health care services to small, select, underserved populations does not, however, constitute a national health care policy. National health care policy at this level is called *macropolicy,* policy that shapes the entire health care delivery system either by controlling funding resources or by controlling the actions of key groups or individuals (eg, insurers or providers) (Longest, 1994).

The current lack of any comprehensive national policy related to health arises from a variety of factors. First, as noted in Chapter 3, there is no constitutionally mandated responsibility for health care decision making at the national level. Up to now the health care function has been viewed as a state responsibility, and the states have no authority to develop policies that apply to the nation as a whole.

The wide variety of health needs experienced by different segments of the population also contributes to the complexity of the debate concerning health care reforms at the national level. It has been argued that a single national health policy generated at the federal level cannot meet the health care needs of the total population. It was this type of argument that led to the creation of regional health systems agencies, discussed below.

Historically, the lack of a definitive national health care policy has resulted in the creation and demise of numerous health-oriented services and programs. Approaches and programs have changed as frequently as the members of the federal administrations that created them. Consequently, efforts to provide health care services to targeted populations have been sporadic and poorly organized. Large gaps and costly overlaps in services have arisen from uncoordinated health care programs. In addition, a pattern of inequitable distribution of resources and services has emerged. In some instances, one federal program has counteracted the effects of another. An example of this is building large medical facilities in major metropolitan areas while simultaneously designing and implementing programs to attract health care providers to rural areas. Excellent programs have often been well designed and instituted, but have not been provided with adequate funding for continued operation when a new administration shifted attention to other issues and concerns.

An example of federal programming intended to assist health care policy development in all regions of the country was the Health Planning and Resources Development Act of 1974 (P.L. 93-641). Variations in health care needs were to be addressed by regional health systems agencies (HSAs) that were created by the act. Each HSA was to assess area health needs, engage in systematic policy formation, and plan for the resources required to meet the specific health needs of the population served. The intent of the bill was to increase access to health care, increase the quality of health care, and decrease overall costs of health care.

During the operation of the HSAs, nursing was in a position to help achieve this policy agenda and to contribute to its own development as a profession. Nurse practitioner programs and clinical practice settings were developed. In addition, legislative changes occurred that supported reimbursement for nurse practitioner services. In some regions of the country, however, there was little coordination with existing state planning agencies. In many of these regions, program overlap and competition occurred. Furthermore, the Health Planning and Resources Development Act provided no specific federal guidelines for the operation of HSAs, and individuals with expertise in systematic planning were not widely available to assist with HSA program development. Following changes in administration policies related to health, federal funds for HSA operations were eliminated. As a result, HSAs are no longer functioning as regional planning agencies directing health care policy development and health care delivery in their designated areas.

Health-oriented organizations such as the American Public Health Association (APHA) have long campaigned for a well-defined national health care policy. APHA's landmark call for a national health program was first made more than 50 years ago. Since that time, the federal government has periodically made tentative efforts to develop a national health care policy. Such efforts have not been sustained and each tentative effort has been lost in the priority changes of successive administrations.

Business and industry, consumers, and, recently, Congress have recognized that the United States is experiencing a health care crisis that can no longer be tolerated. Although efforts have been unsuccessful to date, nurses and other providers must continue their efforts to promote a meaningful national health care policy.

··

▶ AVENUES FOR FORMULATING AND IMPLEMENTING PUBLIC HEALTH CARE POLICIES

Health policy formation may take one of three major forms in the public sector: legislation and health programs created by legislation, rules and regulations implementing legislation, and judicial decisions (Longest, 1994). The first two are open to greater influence by community health nurses and are the focus of this chapter.

Legislation

Laws are public policy decisions generated by the legislative branch of government at the federal, state, or local level. Laws are created in a social system to ex-

press the collective values, interests, and beliefs of the society that generates them. As a society develops, so do its beliefs, values, and interests. Eventually some laws enacted in earlier periods of a society's evolution become obsolete. Sometimes laws are created or revised to address new problems that surface as society changes. Modifications or changes in laws are legislative attempts to correct discrepancies that may have arisen between past and current social practices. Although this description of the function of legislation is highly simplified, the point is that laws reflect societal needs and values and are subject to revision.

Policy formation via the legislative process is very similar at the federal and state levels. Figures 13–1 and 13–2 depict the typical progress of a bill through the state and federal legislative processes. The asterisks in each of the figures indicate points in the process at which community health nurses might influence legislation.

Legislative proposals are statements of beliefs or interests that have been brought to the attention of a legislator. These interests may come to the legislator's attention through his or her constituents, personal experiences, or involvement on a legislative subcommittee dealing with specific issues. Community health nurses can influence the legislative process at this point by making lawmakers aware of the need to develop policy or to modify existing policies (Sharp, 1993). After due consideration, constituents' beliefs or interests are drafted in a *bill*, which is a formally worded statement of the desired policy. Once a bill has been drafted, the sponsoring legislator submits it for identification, meaning that the bill will carry the legislator's name as sponsor. It is not unusual for a proposed bill to have multiple sponsors. Approximately 10,000 bills are introduced in Congress each year; only about 600 of them ever become law (Mittlestadt & Hart, 1993).

At the congressional level, the bill is assigned a number and listed by the House or Senate clerk and sent to a general committee for review. The committee may revise the language of the bill or amend it. In the normal course of events, the bill would then be sent on to the House or Senate floor for its "first reading." A first reading usually consists of a reference to the bill by number and title. The title may address the bill's content or the name(s) of its sponsor. The entire bill is not read at this time.

After its first reading, the bill might be referred to the appropriate committee for hearings. At the congressional level there are six committees that deal with most health-related legislation: (1) the Senate Finance Committee, which establishes policy related to health programs supported by taxes and trusts, such as Medicare and Medicaid; (2) the House Ways and

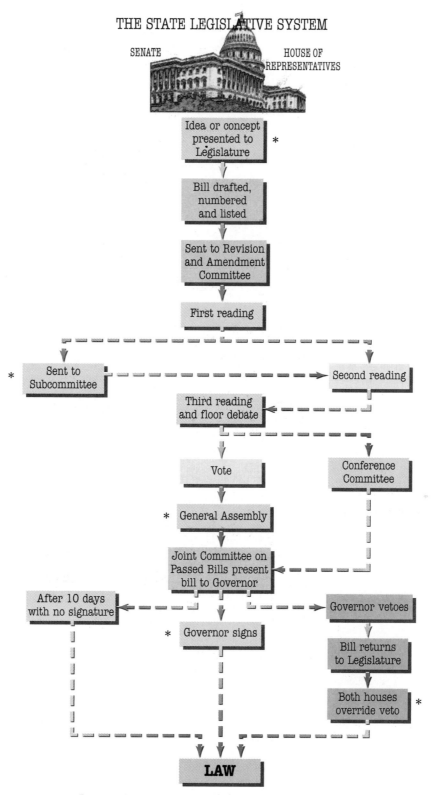

Figure 13–1. A typical state legislative process.

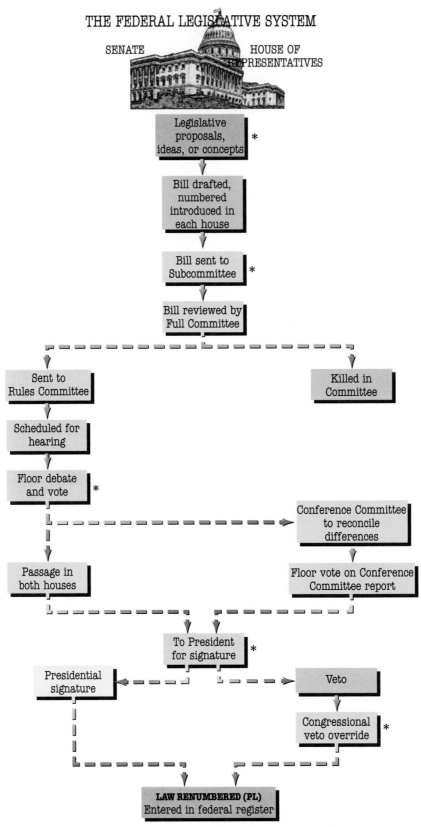

THE FEDERAL LEGISLATIVE SYSTEM

SENATE   HOUSE OF
                REPRESENTATIVES

* Points at which community health nurses can best influence the process

Figure 13–2. The federal legislative process.

Means Committee, which oversees similar legislation for the House of Representatives; (3) the Senate Labor and Human Resources Committee and (4) the House Energy and Commerce Committee, both of which address matters related to programs administered by the Department of Health and Human Services; (5) the House Appropriations Committee; and (6) the Senate Appropriations Committee. The first four of these committees are enabling committees that deal with legislation establishing, modifying, or discontinuing health care programs. The House Appropriations and Senate Appropriations committees are responsible for allocating the funds for the various federal programs. Similar committees exist at the state level.

Community health nurses can influence the legislative process at this point by contacting lawmakers and making their views known on legislation pending before them. The Resource List at the end of this chapter includes some congressional committees and other agencies and organizations that may assist nurses in influencing health care policy.

Committee members considering a particular piece of legislation can either review and modify a bill or decide not to report the bill out of committee, thus effectively killing it. Legislation can also bypass assignment to a committee and advance directly to a second reading on the House or Senate floor. The bill may then proceed to a third reading, be referred back to committee, or be sent to another committee for review and revision before advancing to the third and final reading. Following the third reading, the proposed legislation is placed on the calendar for floor debate and, finally, voted on. At this point in the legislative process, community health nurses can contact their own representatives and try to persuade them to support nursing's position on a particular bill.

If the legislation is passed in the chamber of Congress where it originated, it is sent to the other chamber for approval. In many cases, when a bill has advanced to this point, it is passed by the second chamber without further modification. The bill can, however, be sent to another committee for review and modification. Once a bill has passed the second chamber, it is returned to the house or chamber where it originated for final approval. At the state level, a bill must be signed by the leaders of both houses of the legislature as well as the secretary of state before it is forwarded for the governor's signature. After the bill is signed by the governor, it is renumbered according to the appropriate lawbook code number and filed with the secretary of state, and becomes law. A similar process occurs at the federal level after a bill is signed by the president.

In most states and in Congress, if the two chambers of the legislature cannot agree on a similar version of a given bill, a special committee composed of members of both chambers is formed. The purpose of this *joint conference committee* is to develop a compromise bill. It is highly unusual for a joint committee recommendation not to be passed. If, however, the committee cannot reach agreement, the bill dies. Once the compromise bill has passed both houses of the legislature, it is sent to the executive branch of the government (governor or president) for final approval.

The chief executive (governor or president) can either sign the bill or hamper its progress by not signing it or vetoing it. If the chief executive does not sign the bill, it automatically becomes law after ten days unless the legislative session ends in the interim. In that case, the bill dies. Holding a bill unsigned until the end of the session is called a *pocket veto* (Longest, 1994). Lobbying may also be used at this point to influence the chief executive's disposition of a particular bill. If the executive vetoes a bill, it is returned to the legislature. The legislature is then required to meet a constitutionally prescribed majority vote (usually a two-thirds majority) to override the veto and enact the bill into law. Any bill that does not complete the legislative process during the legislative session in which it is introduced is dead, and it must be reintroduced in a subsequent session if it is ever to become law.

Regulation

Policy decisions enacted as legislation are usually implemented by regulatory agencies charged with implementing specific types of legislation. For example, federal policies related to environmental issues are implemented by the Environmental Protection Agency (EPA); state health-related policies are usually implemented by a state board of health or a comparable agency.

These agencies develop regulations that determine how legislation will be implemented. A *regulation* is a rule or order having the force of law that deals with procedures to be followed in implementing a piece of legislation. Regulations are intended to promote individual accountability for actions and to protect the public health and welfare. Regulations specify how policies are realized in actual behavior.

Regulatory agencies exert a great deal of control over health-related activities by both professionals and the general public. State agencies such as boards of nursing, for example, regulate who may practice nursing and how nursing licensure is granted. These same agencies might also be responsible for determining which health care providers can write prescriptions for medication in those states where such practices are authorized for personnel other than physicians.

When a piece of legislation authorizing an activity such as prescription writing is passed, the legislature usually designates an existing agency or creates a new agency to implement the legislation. This agency develops the regulations that govern implementation of the law. In the case of prescription writing privileges, the regulatory agency would determine who can write prescriptions and what additional qualifications might be required of those persons. For example, in California, nurses who are certified by the state as nurse practitioners may write prescriptions, but only if they have completed an approved course in pharmacology. Other regulations specify who is eligible for certification as a nurse practitioner in the state.

Another example of regulations that implement legislation is the procedures for handling hazardous substances in the workplace, which were developed by the Occupational Safety and Health Administration (OSHA). The enabling legislation mandated protection of employees from exposure to hazardous substances, but regulations developed by OSHA specify how certain substances should be handled. For example, certain types of ventilatory equipment are required in manufacturing processes using hazardous aerosols to minimize the risk of exposure to employees.

Regulations instituted by various agencies may dramatically influence the actual impact of a law. For example, when prescription writing by nurse practitioners was first instituted in Tennessee, one proposal was to restrict the privilege to nurse practitioners prepared at the master's level. As this requirement would have excluded many nurse practitioners in rural counties where physicians were scarce, it would have undermined the intent of the enabling legislation—to provide greater access to health care for underserved populations.

Community health nurses can have input into regulations that affect their professional practice as well as into the legislation that shapes public health policy. When a regulatory agency is in the process of formulating regulations, the public is informed that the process is being initiated. Generally, the agency formulates some preliminary regulations that are published for public review and comment. At the federal level, proposed regulations are published in the *Federal Register* as a *Notice of Proposed Rulemaking* (NPRM); similar registers exist in each state. Interested parties are then allowed to comment on the proposed regulations and suggest changes.

When regulations deal with particularly sensitive areas, the regulatory body involved may hold public hearings to solicit input from interested parties. Community health nurses may either comment on proposed regulations in written communications to the regulatory agency or provide testimony at public hearings. The regulatory agency can then use the input received to refine the regulations. Regulations are published in the appropriate state or federal publication and promulgated among individuals affected by them. For example, schools of nursing in California were informed in writing of changes requiring educational content on child abuse for public health nursing certification in the state.

▶ INFLUENCING HEALTH CARE POLICY FORMATION AND IMPLEMENTATION

Community health nurses can influence health-related policies at all levels. To do so, however, they must be conversant with the political process and its use. The ability of community health nurses to influence policy formation is affected by their education and their skill in setting an agenda, defining and evaluating choices, obtaining data, developing a power base, and creating support for a particular policy or direction.

Education

It is important for community health nurses to understand the various processes involved in policy formation. Lack of educational preparation for political activity has been cited as one factor contributing to nursing's inability to influence health policy formation significantly.

In addition to educating themselves for political activity, community health nurses can educate policy makers regarding the needs of the public. Policy makers rarely have backgrounds related to health and may be largely unaware of health issues or lack a sound understanding of their implications for the health of the public. It is the task of community health nurses and other health care providers to educate policy makers in this regard. It is particularly important that these individuals be apprised of the findings of nursing research related to health care delivery, as uninformed policy makers may profoundly influence the health care delivery system.

Setting an Agenda

Community health nurses need to decide on a policy agenda that they wish to support (Hanley, 1993). There are many policy issues on which community health nurses may wish to have input, including issues related to the needs of the profession as well as those of the public. Choices among these issues must be made carefully to enhance the credibility of community health nurses with policy makers.

As noted earlier, health care providers are often perceived by health care policy makers as self-serving. For this reason, it is important for community health nurses to focus more on health policy issues that concern the public and less on issues of concern only to nursing's professional status aspirations. One aspect of the health care policy agenda that must be promoted by community health nurses is the issue of health promotion and illness prevention. In spite of significant savings in terms of money, mortality, and suffering for prevention over treatment of existing problems, national spending for core public health functions was less than 2% of the $903 billion cost of health care in the United States in 1993 (Division of Public Health Systems, 1995). Additional expenditures for preventive services in the private sector are still only a fraction of total national health care expenditures.

Defining and Evaluating Choices

To influence health care policy decisions community health nurses must be able to define and evaluate policy alternatives. Many avenues can be taken in the development of health care policies. Community health nurses have a responsibility to identify and evaluate alternative directions for health policy and to make policy makers aware of potential advantages and disadvantages of various alternatives. This means that community health nurses must keep abreast of issues and developments that affect the health of the public as well as potential approaches in dealing with health-related issues.

Obtaining Data

To be an effective influence on health care policy makers, community health nurses must generate relevant and persuasive data. Community health nursing research can be geared to obtaining data needed to influence health policy decisions. Factors that have hindered nurses' efforts in this area include the failure of nurses to replicate research and to develop cumulative findings that support specific policy directions and the failure to disseminate research findings beyond the professional community. Research is also needed to define the role of community health nurses in health care delivery and to support their inclusion in policy decisions.

Developing a Power Base

Power generates influence, and community health nurses who wish to influence health care policy need to develop a power base from which to do so. *Power* is the ability to influence the conduct of others without having one's own behavior modified. A *power base* is the resources that allow one person to influence another. Several strategies can be used to enhance one's power base. These include coalition building, bargaining, posturing, and increasing visibility.

In building coalitions individuals or groups with common interests form a temporary alliance to work toward a common goal. The efforts of 18 major nursing organizations, including the American Nurses Association, American Association of Colleges of Nursing, and National League for Nursing, to present a nursing proposal for a national health care plan is an example of coalition building.

Bargaining, or trade-off, is another means of building a power base. In this strategy, individuals or groups relinquish something they want or provide something desired by another group, thus creating a mutual debt. For example, nursing might agree to support a policy direction favored by the American Medical Association (AMA) in return for support of a nurse-sponsored initiative.

In posturing or bluffing, the individual or group building a power base asks for more than should be expected and then falls back to a predetermined position beyond which the individual or group will not retreat. This tactic is frequently employed in contract negotiations.

To increase visibility, individuals or groups purposefully engage in activities that place them in positions where they will be noticed for the right reasons. Increased visibility also involves collaborative efforts among groups to gain favorable media attention. For example, when nurses choose to go on strike, reasons presented to the media usually deal with client-centered issues that gain public support and increase nursing's power and ability to influence policy makers. Strategies for developing a power base are summarized in Table 13–1.

Creating Support

To influence health care policy decisions, community health nurses must create support for the policy alternatives they favor. Support may be created through indirect or direct political participation activities (Walt, 1994). Indirect activities influence the selection of policy makers and issues and include voting, community organization, and campaigning. Direct partici-

TABLE 13–1. **STRATEGIES FOR DEVELOPING A POLITICAL POWER BASE**

Strategy	Description of Strategy
Coalition building	Creating a temporary alliance among individuals or groups to work toward common goals
Bargaining	Trading or giving up something desired by another individual or group in return for support for one's own position
Posturing	Asking for more than one expects to get, with a subsequent retreat to a predetermined position
Increasing visibility	Purposefully engaging in activities that draw attention to an issue and to one's position on the issue

pation activities involve face-to-face interaction with policy makers and include lobbying, presenting testimony, and holding office. These strategies for creating support form the basis for the Political Astuteness Inventory (Appendix G).

Voting

Voting is perhaps the easiest means of influencing health care policy formation at governmental levels. Nurses can themselves vote and motivate others to vote to support policy directions that enhance public health. One vote alone may not seem important, but it may be a key factor in determining the outcome on an important issue. Because lawmakers in the United States are elected, they are susceptible to the power their constituents hold through the ballot box. Thus, voting is a vital component of the political process in which all nurses can participate.

In addition to voting, nurses can educate others regarding the need to vote. Legislative networks among nurses are intended to keep members informed of health-related issues and the need for support or lack of support of certain policy directions. Nurses can also educate the general public on legislative issues that come up for public vote. Finally, nurses can participate in voter registration programs that motivate the general public to exercise their constitutional right to do so.

Community Organization

Another way community health nurses create support for policy directions is community organization. *Community organization* is the process of mobilizing community resources in support of planned change within the community. It is a systematic process of assessment, analysis, and planning, conducted within the context of the political process. Steps in the community organization process include establishing legitimacy, defining the problem to be addressed, as-

sessing and analyzing the problem, selecting goals, planning to obtain these goals, marketing, and evaluating.

Members of the community are involved in each step of the process and provide the motivating force behind the movement. The first step, however, is probably the most critical in creating support for health policy. Legitimizing the project requires development of authority to act. This may involve requesting officials to create a special task force to address a problem or including government officials in the planning body of the community organization structure. Subsequent steps of the community organization process are similar to those of the nursing process and need not be reiterated here. It should be remembered, however, that the steps are carried out by members of the community rather than by the nurse.

Community organization can create a mechanism to influence policy makers in several of the ways discussed earlier in this chapter. Community groups can generate and evaluate policy alternatives and can collect data for presentation to policy makers. In addition, the organization provides avenues to educate voters and motivate their participation in policy decisions affected by voting.

Campaigning

Campaigning is a process designed to influence the public to vote in a particular way on an issue or a candidate. An issue or candidate is presented in a favorable light with the intent of influencing voters. Campaigning can be implemented via media presentations, in group meetings or rallies, or in face-to-face contacts with the public.

Campaigning for an issue involves presenting information related to the issue that persuades people to support nursing's position. Campaigning for a specific candidate can help ensure election of policy makers who support nursing's position on important issues. Campaigning is an opportunity for nurses to become personally known to a candidate and other campaign workers. It is also an opportunity to become known as a reliable source of information about health and health care issues. Campaigning for a candidate also creates a debt on the part of an elected official that may result in future support for a position promoted by community health nurses.

Much of the work of political action committees (PACs) is designed to support the candidacy of specific individuals. The American Nurses Association Political Action Committee (ANA-PAC) was created in response to nursing's perceived lack of influence in the formulation of health care policy. The purpose of ANA-PAC is to promote constructive national health care legislation through the political "electioneering" process. *Electioneering* is the active process of endorsing candidates and contributing time and money to their campaigns. ANA-PAC and similar political action committees supported by nurses seek to enhance the political influence of nurses by supporting the election of candidates who back the profession and its position on significant health-related issues.

Lobbying

Lobbying is a concerted effort to influence legislators to take certain positions on prospective bills, and it is another means of creating support for policies promoted by community health nurses. Individuals may lobby independently, or as groups of people with common interests. For example, health-related organizations, such as APHA, and professional organizations, such as ANA and AMA, employ lobbyists at both federal and state levels. Their function is to acquaint legislators with the position of the organization on a particular issue and to attempt to persuade them to back that position.

Individuals who lobby do so by contacting a legislator and making their position on an issue known. It is not sufficient to acquaint a legislator with one's position, however. That position must be supported by data that persuade the legislator to adopt a similar position. Whether lobbying is done by individuals acting on their own or with an organized group, there are strategies that influence the effectiveness of lobbying. These strategies, as well as approaches to be avoided, are summarized in Table 13–2.

It is important for community health nurses to know both the legislative process and the legislators involved. Legislators can be observed and their statements studied to provide information on their positions on issues influencing community health. Their voting records on significant issues can also be examined.

Once legislators' positions are known, they and their staff can be contacted to establish influential interpersonal relationships. Personal contact through visits followed by telephone calls and follow-up letters or telegrams has been found to be an effective means of influencing lawmakers. Some observers believe that one should not focus exclusively on legislators from one's own political party, but should contact members of both major parties. Legislators who support one's position can be encouraged in that support, and those who do not may be persuaded to change their position.

In addition to knowing a legislator's position on specific issues, nurses should be aware of which legislators serve on committees that deal with health care issues. These legislators, along with one's own elected representatives, are appropriate targets for lobbying efforts. Knowledge of the legislative structure and committee assignments can assist nurses to target lobbying efforts in areas where they will be most effective.

Community health nurses also need to be conversant with the issues they are addressing and with arguments on both sides of particular issues. Research related to health policy issues can be presented to lawmakers and can be persuasive in promoting their support of a position. In discussing an issue, one should acknowledge the nature, source, and extent of possible opposition to one's position. The community health nurse should present the legislator with brief, factual, and documentable data related to the issue. It is usually preferable to provide legislators or their staff members with these data in written form and to include documentation.

Generally speaking, individuals who lobby on their own should focus their efforts on legislators elected from their own districts. Legislators are usually more inclined to listen to constituents than to nonconstituents. Nurses need to network with each other so that several legislators are contacted by their own constituents regarding nursing's position on an issue.

Approaches to legislators that should be avoided when trying to exert influence include making threats regarding loss of voter support and making promises of support; pretending to have influence; repeating one's message too frequently; and demanding a commitment from a legislator before an issue has been completely explored. Such tactics can result in a loss of credibility and decrease one's ability to influence a legislator's behavior.

It is important to acknowledge a legislator's support or lack of support for a given piece of legislation. This action helps legislators realize that their actions

TABLE 13–2. LOBBYING TECHNIQUES

Do	Don't
• Become familiar with the legislative process	• Make threats about loss of votes
• Become familiar with legislators	• Make promises that cannot be kept
• Know the issues	• Pretend to have influence
• Know your lobbying power	• Repeat the message too frequently
• Work through your own representatives	

are indeed monitored. When a legislator does not support nursing's position on a particular bill, a note indicating regret for that nonsupport and the hope that "perhaps, next time we can work together" is the best approach.

Presenting Testimony

Policy makers sometimes hold public hearings or meetings to gather background information on an issue before attempting to draft legislative proposals or regulations. On occasion, such meetings are held by legislative subcommittees to explore the potential impact of a proposed piece of legislation. Writing and presenting testimony in a public hearing is another method community health nurses can use to influence policy makers.

Testimony presented by community health nurses should specifically address the issue in question and be brief, factual, and well documented. Legislative representatives are not health care providers, so in giving testimony, community health nurses need to avoid medical jargon and be clearly understandable. A copy of the testimony should be given to the legislative representatives and staff either immediately preceding or at the time of the hearing. Documentation of sources of data permits later verification by legislators or their staff members.

TABLE 13–3. **STRATEGIES TO CREATE SUPPORT FOR A PROPOSED POLICY**

Strategy	Description of Strategy
Voting	• Exercising one's personal right to vote • Encouraging others to vote • Participating in voter registration drives
Community organization	• Mobilizing community resources in favor of planned change or a proposed policy • Establishing the legitimacy of the organization • Defining the issue • Assessing and analyzing the issue • Selecting goals • Planning to reach goals • Marketing • Evaluating effort
Campaigning	• Providing endorsements or monetary support for specific policy proposals or candidates with the intent of influencing voters' responses
Lobbying	• Engaging in personal communications with policy makers in an attempt to influence their actions in policy decisions
Presenting testimony	• Providing information on an issue to policy makers at a public hearing
Holding office	• Assuming a position as a policy maker by virtue of election or appointment to a specific office

Holding Office

A final means of creating support for policy directions promoted by community health nurses is to become a policy maker oneself. This may involve running for elective office or being appointed to a specific position. In either case, the community health nurse must first become politically active in some of the other ways described in this chapter to be sufficiently well known to be elected or appointed to a policymaking position.

One may also work in the background in policy making by becoming a legislative staff person or a lobbyist for an organized group. Again, such positions require familiarity with the political process and well-developed interpersonal relationships with legislators and other policy makers. Strategies to create support for a policy position are summarized in Table 13–3. Factors affecting nurses' ability to influence health care policy formation are listed in Table 13–4.

► THE DIMENSIONS MODEL AND THE POLITICAL PROCESS

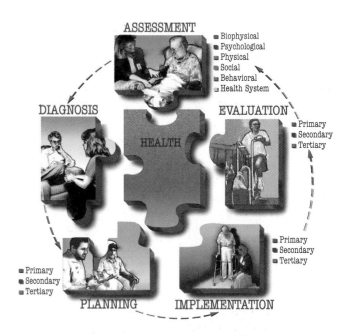

The Dimensions Model can be used to direct community health nurses' involvement in public health policy formation at all levels of society. Community health nurses working in specific organizations can assess the influence of institutional policies on the health of members of the organization. They can also adapt strategies for policy formation to plan, imple-

TABLE 13–4. FACTORS AFFECTING NURSES' ABILITY TO INFLUENCE HEALTH CARE POLICY FORMATION

Education	• Educate community health nurses regarding the political process
	• Educate policy makers regarding the health needs of the public
Setting an agenda	• Decide on a direction to be taken in health care policy formation
Defining and evaluating choices	• Identify alternative directions for health care policy
	• Evaluate advantages and disadvantages of health care policy alternatives
Obtaining data	• Conduct research related to policy formation
	• Collect data related to specific policy issues
Developing a power base	• Create a power base from which to influence health care policy decisions
Creating support	• Develop and implement strategies to mobilize support for a proposed policy

ment, and evaluate programs that enhance rather than undermine health. In a similar fashion, community health nurses can use the Dimensions Model to assess and influence health care policies at the local, state, and federal level.

Critical Dimensions of Nursing in Policy Formation

Political competencies required for effective community health nursing participation in policy formation reflect several of the dimensions of nursing in the Dimensions Model. In the cognitive dimension, nurses need to have knowledge of the political process and of current policy issues. They also should possess scientific knowledge related to those issues. Interpersonal dimension elements relevant to political activity include effective communication skills to influence policy makers (Leavitt & Barry, 1993). The ethical dimension demands that community health nurses use their political influence to advocate for the good of the public rather than for self-gain, a criticism often made of the political activity of other professional groups. Skill dimension elements include analytical, organizational, and critical thinking skills. The political process itself is an element of the process dimension of community health nursing. Other related processes that the community health nurse might employ in policy formation are the change, leadership, and group processes discussed in Chapter 12. Finally, the research and evaluation capabilities included in the reflective dimension will help develop the scientific knowledge base needed for effective policy formation.

 Assessing the Dimensions of Health in Health Care Policy Formation

Assessment of the health status of a community or population group may reveal the need for health policies. In addition, assessment may indicate areas in which existing policies impede achievement of the goals of public health.

Once a need for health policy has been identified, the community health nurse can examine the situation in terms of the dimensions of health to identify factors that influence the direction that policy should take. For example, recent biophysical data indicate that a growing portion of the homeless population is young children, so policies dealing with the problem of homelessness need to address the needs of this age group.

Other biological factors can also influence a given policy situation. If we use the homeless as our example, information on the types of health problems common in this population will influence the direction that policies should take. For example, provisions should be made for tuberculosis control and treatment of mental illness, two health problems frequently encountered among the homeless.

Physical dimension factors also affect policy formation. Again, using the homeless as our example, weather conditions in the Northeast make policies for this population more critical than might be the case elsewhere, whereas the milder climate of the Southwest may encourage homeless individuals to migrate to these areas, thus compounding the problem of homelessness for particular geographic regions.

Factors in both the psychological and social dimensions also affect policy formation related to homeless populations. Because mental illness is prevalent among this group, issues of treatment must be addressed in any effective policy related to the homeless. Social factors such as unemployment and the lack of affordable housing also need to be addressed if a policy for the homeless is to meet their needs on a long-term basis.

Behavioral issues related to nutrition and sleep patterns as well as other consumption patterns affect policies designed to meet the needs of a homeless population. Policy development will have to consider avenues for feeding the hungry and for creating employment opportunities that permit the homeless person to afford housing.

Finally, health care system factors influence the ability of homeless persons to receive necessary health care. Lack of access to care and appointment schedules that rely on possession of a timepiece are two factors that impede adequate health care for the homeless. Policy needs related specifically to the homeless population are addressed in more detail in Chapter 24.

Diagnostic Reasoning and Health Care Policy Formation

Based on the outcome of his or her assessment, the community health nurse might arrive at diagnoses of the need for health care policies to address issues raised. An example of such a diagnosis related to the homeless is "need for a policy to address provision of health care for homeless individuals due to large numbers of homeless and lack of present access to health care in this population." Another diagnosis might be a "need for special programs to house homeless women with children due to growing numbers in

this population and their increased vulnerability to victimization."

Planning the Dimensions of Health Care Policy

The community health nurse might then proceed to initiate or participate in plans to develop appropriate health care policies. Planning policies to meet the needs of the homeless population might include primary, secondary, or tertiary preventive measures. For example, the local health department might suspend its fee policy for immunizations for homeless children in the state or the state Medicaid program might adopt a policy authorizing Medicaid benefits for homeless individuals without the proof of residence usually required for eligibility. Or, action might be taken to collaborate with existing community-based agencies and groups to initiate the development of a

---

ASSESSMENT TIPS: Policy Formation

Biophysical Dimension

Do existing physiologic conditions in the population give rise to the need for health policy?
What age group is affected by the policy being considered?

Psychological Dimension

Do factors in the psychological dimension give rise to the need for health policy?

Physical Dimension

Are there factors in the physical dimension that give rise to a need for health policy?
How will physical dimension factors influence the development of health policy?
How will factors in the physical dimension influence the ability to effectively implement health policy?

Social Dimension

Do social dimension factors give rise to a need for health policy?

How will economic factors influence the development and implementation of health policy?
Are there religious or cultural factors that will influence the development and implementation of health policy?
What effect will social interaction factors (eg, racial tension) have on the development and implementation of health policy?
What societal groups are likely to resist the desired health policy change? How powerful are these groups?

Behavioral Dimension

Do consumption patterns in the population give rise to a need for health policy?
How will health policy influence consumption patterns in the population?
What other health-related behaviors will influence the development of health policy (eg, sexual activity)?

Health System Dimension

Do health care system factors give rise to a need for changes in health policy?
To what extent do health care providers support the desired health policy change?

policy creating jobs for homeless individuals within the local government and business community to enable them to become self-supporting and to prevent recurrent homelessness.

Whatever the level of prevention involved in planning health care policies, the community health nurse will consider certain criteria that are characteristic of effective policies. These criteria include the adequacy of a proposed policy in meeting the health needs of the public, safeguards for the rights of individuals, equitable allocation of resources, and the capacity for implementation. The second and third criteria reflect ethical considerations that are addressed in greater detail in Chapter 15.

Adequacy in Meeting Health Needs

Health policies must be developed that effectively address the health needs of the affected population. For example, a local government policy allowing homeless persons to sleep in city-owned buildings addresses only one small part of the plight of the homeless population. In this case, a more comprehensive policy that addresses both short-term and long-term solutions to the problems of homelessness is needed.

Safeguards for Individual Rights

Safeguarding individual rights is another criterion for sound health care policy development. As an example, a policy that would require homeless individuals to surrender personal belongings to meet communal needs when admitted to a shelter would violate their property rights. There are circumstances, however, in which the good of society supersedes individual rights. For example, homeless persons may be prohibited from smoking in a shelter to prevent exposure of others to smoke or to prevent a fire. Whenever possible, though, health policies should be written so that they do not violate the rights of individuals affected by them.

Equitable Allocation of Resources

Health care policies should also promote equitable distribution of health care resources. This means that policies should not discriminate against certain subgroups within the population. For example, open housing policies in homeless shelters may inadvertently discriminate against women and children who may be subjected to force to make them give way to adult males who desire shelter. Sex-segregated shelters that ensure access for both males and females provide for a more equitable allocation of resources.

Capacity for Implementation

For a specific health policy to be effective in promoting health or preventing illness, it must be capable of being implemented or enforced. For example, a local government might adopt a policy encouraging houses of worship to provide overnight shelter for homeless individuals. But, unless the houses of worship are willing to cooperate, the policy cannot be implemented.

Community health nurses planning to influence health care policy formation should assess proposed policies or modifications of existing policies in light of these four criteria. Policies that do not meet the criteria should be redesigned, if possible, before they are presented to policy makers. If a proposed policy continues not to meet one or more criteria, its supporters should be prepared to justify the need for the policy. For example, nurses should be prepared to convince policy makers that a smoking ban in shelters for the homeless is warranted despite the violation of the individual's personal freedom of choice.

 Implementing the Dimensions of Health Care Policy

Implementing planned policies often involves mobilization of support for the policy as well as actually putting the policy into operation. Community health nurses who desire to influence policy decisions should identify groups within the population who are likely to support the proposed policy. They should then develop specific strategies to elicit that support.

Critical Thinking in Research

In the past, nurses as a professional group have been less politically active than members of other groups. In today's society, political astuteness and involvement are critical to the development of health care delivery systems that support the primary goal of community health nursing: improved health for the public.

1. What contribution might research make to understanding nursing's traditional lack of political involvement?
2. What is the role of research in policy making?
3. How would you go about determining what factors promote political activity by community health nurses?
4. If you wanted to conduct a study of the extent of political activity among certain groups of students on your campus, what groups would you include? Why? How would you design your study?

This may mean educating the general public regarding the issues and proposed policy or contacting health-related agencies and soliciting their support. Other community groups are also a source of support for policies that affect them directly or indirectly. In the case of programs related to care of the homeless, support might be derived from area churches and synagogues or business people on whose doorsteps homeless individuals are sleeping. Concerned health care providers and educational institutions might also be sources of support for implementing health policies related to the homeless population.

Evaluating Health Care Policy

In the evaluation phase, the community health nurse might be actively involved in assessing the effects of health care policies on meeting the needs of the partic-ular target group, in this case, the homeless population. Community health nurses could assist in collecting data related to the outcomes of programs put into operation. For example, data might be gathered on the incidence of specific health problems among the homeless to evaluate the effects of policies designed to promote primary and secondary prevention. In addition, information could be collected regarding the number of persons who continue to be homeless despite assistance from established programs.

Finally, community health nurses would evaluate the effectiveness of the strategies used in policy development. For example, were insufficient funds allocated to implement established programs? Were nurses successful in motivating policy makers to address the problem of homelessness in a comprehensive fashion, or did the policies developed deal with only portions of the problem? The answers to these and similar questions can guide community health nurses' future efforts at influencing policy decisions not only on the issue of homelessness but the entire gamut of health-related issues.

Critical Thinking in Practice: A Case in Point

Nurses in a southern state were concerned about the high incidence of motor vehicle fatalities in children under the age of 4. The state involved was largely rural with poorly maintained roads, and many accidents occurred in outlying regions or in crowded inner-city areas. Fatalities were particularly prevalent among low-income African Americans in the cities, and among low-income whites and African Americans in the rural areas. Few families had child safety seats in their cars, and few adults used seat belts themselves. Many automobiles, especially in rural areas, were older models that did not even have seat belts. The state's population was about evenly divided between African Americans and whites, and the education levels in both groups were well below those of the rest of the nation.

The state nurses' association, in conjunction with the state Fraternal Order of Police, approached a newly elected state assemblyman who was willing to sponsor a bill requiring the use of approved car seat restraints for all children under the age of 4. Both organizations mobilized their memberships in support of the bill. The state nurses' association represented approximately 10% of registered nurses licensed in the state, whereas the Fraternal Order of Police represented nearly 85% of the state's police officers. Neither of the two organizations approached members of the committees that would be reviewing the bill to enlist their support. Very little effort was made to educate the general public regarding the issue. Prior to their involvement in this cause, neither organization had been very active politically.

The bill was soundly defeated in the legislature. Some of the reasons given by various legislators for voting against the bill included the belief that use of a child safety seat is a parental, rather than a governmental, decision, the belief that government already regulated too much of people's lives, concerns about the difficulties and costs of enforcing such legislation, and concerns about the cost of car seats for many poor families in the state.

1. What were the biophysical, psychological, physical, social, behavioral, and health system factors operating in this situation?
2. What are some of the reasons the nurses and police officers were ineffective in influencing policy formation in this situation?
3. In what ways did the proposed policy meet or fail to meet the criteria for effective health care policy?
4. How might the nurses and police officers have developed a stronger power base to influence legislation?
5. What strategies could have been used to bring about a more positive outcome in this situation?

TESTING YOUR UNDERSTANDING

1. Identify at least three levels at which health care policy formation takes place. (p. 259)
2. List and describe at least five factors affecting nurses' ability to influence health care policy formation. Give an example of the influence of each on the participation of community health nurses in policy formation. (pp. 264–265)
3. Identify four strategies for developing a power base for exercising political influence. Give an example of the use of each strategy. (pp. 265–266)
4. Describe at least four approaches to creating support for a proposed health care policy. (pp. 265–268)
5. Outline the legislative process at the state and federal levels. Identify points at which community health nurses might influence the process. (pp. 260–263)
6. Describe the regulatory process. How might community health nurses influence this process? (pp. 263–264)
7. Identify four criteria for evaluating a proposed health care policy. (pp. 271–272)

WHAT DO YOU THINK?
Questions for Critical Thinking

1. Why are nurses not more actively involved in policy formation? What strategies could facilitate their involvement?
2. What coalitions exist between nursing and other groups in your community interested in policy issues? What coalitions might enhance nursing's position on specific issues?
3. What legislators in your area are sympathetic to nursing's position on health-related issues? What could you, as a nurse, do to elicit the support of other legislators who are not currently sympathetic to nursing?

REFERENCES

Brydoff, C. (January 8, 1996). Nurses can make a difference by becoming politically active. *NURSEweek*, 1, 7, 26.

Division of Public Health Systems. (1995). Estimated expenditures for core public health functions—Selected states, October 1992–September 1993. *MMWR, 44*, 421, 427–429.

Hanley, B. (1993). Policy development and analysis. In D. J. Mason, S. W. Talbot, & J. K. Leavitt (Eds.), *Policy and politics for nurses* (2nd ed.) (pp. 71–87). Philadelphia: W. B. Saunders.

Leavitt, J. K., & Barry, C. T. (1993). Learning the ropes. In D. J. Mason, S. W. Talbot, & J. K. Leavitt (Eds.), *Policy and politics for nurses* (2nd ed.) (pp. 47–67). Philadelphia: W. B. Saunders.

Longest, B. B., Jr. (1994). *Health policy making in the United States.* Ann Arbor, MI: AUPHA Press.

Mason, D. J., & Leavitt, J. K. (1993). Policy and politics: A framework for action. In D. J. Mason, S. W. Talbot, & J. K. Leavitt (Eds.), *Policy and politics for nurses* (2nd ed.) (pp. 3–17). Philadelphia: W. B. Saunders.

Meyer, C. (1992). Nursing on the political front. *American Journal of Nursing, 82*(10), 56–64.

Mittelstadt, P. C., & Hart, M. A. (1993). Legislative and regulatory processes. In D. J. Mason, S. W. Talbot, & J. K. Leavitt (Eds.), *Policy and politics for nurses* (2nd ed.) (pp. 399–411). Philadelphia: W. B. Saunders.

Salmon, M. E. (1995). Public health policy: Creating a healthy future for the American public. *Family and Community Health, 18*(1), 1–11.

Secretary's Commission on Nursing. (1988). *Final Report,* Vol. 1. Washington, DC: Department of Health and Human Services.

Sharp, N. (1993). The path of legislation: Best opportunities for nurses' input. *Nursing Management, 24*(9), 28, 30, 32, 34.

Skinner, M. D. (1994). Getting to X. *Nursing Administration Quarterly, 14*(3), 58–63.

Stimpson, M., & Hanley, B. (1991). Nurse policy analyst: Advanced practice role. *Nursing & Health Care, 12*(1), 10–15.

Walt, G. (1994). *Health policy: An introduction to process and power.* London: Zed.

RESOURCES FOR NURSES CONCERNED WITH HEALTH CARE POLICY ISSUES

American Nurses Foundation
600 Maryland Avenue, SW, Ste. 100W
Washington, DC 20024–2571
(202) 554–4444

Center on Human Policy
805 S. Crouse Avenue
Syracuse, NY 13244–2280
(315) 443–3851

Health Policy Advisory Center
47 West 14th Street, No. 300
New York, NY 10011
(212) 627–1847

International Health Policy and Management Institute
c/o Paul Detrick
Christian Health Service Development Corporation
10133 Dunn Road, Ste. 400
St. Louis, MO 63136
(314) 355–0095

National Health Federation
P.O. Box 688
Monrovia, CA 91017
(818) 357–2181

National Health Policy Forum
2021 K Street NW, Ste. 800
Washington, DC 20052
(202) 872–1390

U.S. Department of Health & Human Services
Health Resources & Services Administration
5600 Fishers Lane
Rockville, MD 20857
(301) 443–2086

U.S. House of Representatives Committee
  on Ways & Means
Subcommittee on Health
1114 Longworth House Office Bldg.
Washington, DC 20515
(202) 225–7785

U.S. House of Representatives
  Energy and Commerce Committee
2125 Raeburn House Office Bldg.
Washington, DC 20515

U.S. Senate Committee on Finance
Subcommittee on Health
SD-205 Dirksen
Washington, DC 20510
(202) 225–0130

U.S. Senate Labor and Human Resources Committee
275 Hart Senate Office Bldg.
Washington, DC 20510
(202) 224–7675

MAGGIE JONES

Just
who do you think you are, Maggie Jones
following me home from work
insinuating yourself into my evening
shading my thoughts?

Just
who do you think you are
lying flat as a pancake in the middle of your
    bed
your world ranged round you in brown
    paper bags?

(Rather like a dead Pharaoh in his tomb, I'd
    say
buried with all his treasure)

So you fell one day and had to be taken
to the hospital
You didn't break any bones, after all.
You came home in a taxi
climbed the steep flight of stairs to your
    room
took to your bed and stayed there.
That was three years ago, Maggie
Three years with only one thing to look for-
    ward to—livin'

I'm here by the hand of the Lord, you always
    say when I come
though the hand of the Lord didn't smite
    the rat
that bit your foot
that cold winter day last year
as it foraged in your sheets for bread and
    jelly.
I guess it'll be all right
you said in your genteel way
looking up at me with soft does eyes as I
    dressed
the wound that brought us together.

Why don't you go to a home? we ask,
    shocked
to see the condition you're in
(the church ladies, the social worker,
your niece, your nephew, and I)
Because I still have my right mind
you say simply.
A nursing home is no place
for someone who still has their mind.

But now your gas is cut off
until you come up with $700.
You're lucky it's not freezing and there's an
electric
coffee maker we can use
to heat water to wash you.
I guess the money will come from some-
    where
you say, looking at me steadily.

How can you lie there and say, serenely, you
    guess
things will work out?
Your room is cold
your sheets are soaked with urine
your skin is bleeding from bedsores
you don't know where your next meal is
    coming from
you're a poor old lady
hidden away
in a falling-down house
in a no-good neighborhood.
And you have expectations?

You told your niece not to worry about you
the nurse was coming.
Hey, Maggie Jones, don't wait for me, don't
    count on me.
I'll bathe you
Dress your wounds
treat your minor ailments
even do your laundry and bring you food
once in a while
But save you?
God alone—the hand of the lord—can save
    you.

I see you now in my mind's eye and wonder
as I sit
after dinner
in my warm house
on a safe street
in a good neighborhood

Just
who do you think you are, Maggie Jones?

Excerpted, with permission, from V. Masson (1993). just who. *Washington, DC: Crossroads Health Ministry.*

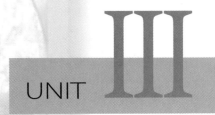
INFLUENCES ON COMMUNITY HEALTH

A population's health is influenced by both individual behavior and societal factors, which include economic, ethical, cultural, and physical environmental influences. The interventions of community health nurses often must address these factors.

Economic influences affect clients' access to goods and services that promote, maintain, and restore their health, for example, nutritious food and adequate housing. Similarly, the economics of a community may limit its provision of services related to health, sanitation, and protection. Community health nursing is also concerned with the high cost of health care and diminished access to care for some segments of the population. Chapter 14 examines these concerns, the mechanisms for financing health care, and the role of the community health nurse.

All nurses must make ethical decisions such as those concerning the care of a child with a life-threatening illness whose parents refuse medical assistance, or the use of technology to prolong life. In community health nursing, however, ethical decisions are also required at the group or aggregate level, for example, the allocation of scarce resources among primary, secondary, and tertiary preventive measures. Chapter 15 focuses on ethical decisions at the group level.

Culture guides and directs behavior, including health-related behaviors. Consequently, community health nurses must understand the cultural basis for behavior. Chapter 16 describes the basic premises of culture, focusing on the health-related behaviors of six diverse groups in the United States—Native American, Arab American, Asian, African American, Latino, and the Appalachian population.

Environmental influences on health are discussed in Chapter 17. In recent years, the declining quality of the environment and its adverse effects on health have been of growing concern. Environmental conditions (for example, air and water pollution, noise, and radiation) affect health directly and indirectly (aesthetically). Community health nurses can intervene to control environmental influences on individuals, families, and other groups of people, for example, by educating families about waste disposal or lead poisoning or by assuming leadership in policy making to reduce pollution. By understanding the environmental as well as economic, ethical, and cultural influences on health, a community health nurse can modify factors to more effectively promote the health of target populations.

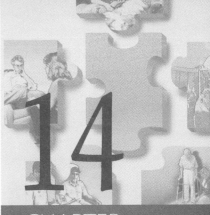

ECONOMIC INFLUENCES ON COMMUNITY HEALTH

► KEY TERMS

Economic factors influence the health of individuals, families, and groups or communities. For individuals and their families, economic factors affect their ability to provide necessities, such as food and shelter. One's income also influences the ability to obtain health care. The general economic climate influences health at the aggregate level. For example, a declining economy contributes to high levels of unemployment. Unemployment, in turn, leads to reduced incomes and a reduced tax base to finance government-supported health and welfare programs. In addition, unemployment is usually accompanied by loss of employer-provided health insurance benefits. Finally, economic factors that contribute to inflation further impair the ability of the public to obtain necessities and health care.

Relationships between economic factors and health (Fig. 14–1) are of concern to community health nurses because they influence the health of the individuals, families, and communities. Although community health nurses cannot significantly influence the overall economic climate, they can help to mitigate its adverse effects. For example, the nurse can assist clients to budget their resources effectively or make referrals to financial assistance programs. Or the community health nurse can use the change, leadership, and political processes to influence policies related to economic issues, particularly funding for health care services. To do so, some understanding of current and proposed mechanisms for financing health care is essential.

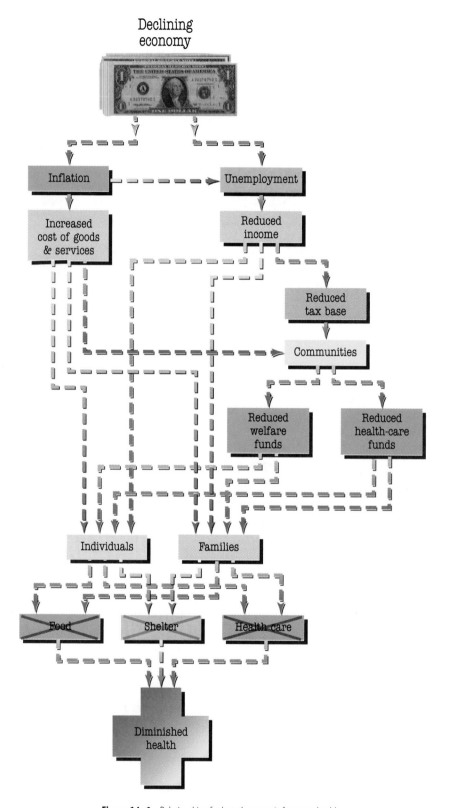

Figure 14–1. Relationship of selected economic factors to health.

▶ Chapter Objectives

After reading this chapter, you should be able to:

- Describe at least three relationships between economic conditions and health status.
- Identify two economic issues of particular concern to community health nurses.
- Differentiate between retrospective and prospective reimbursement.
- Identify three forms of publicly funded health insurance.
- Describe at least three mechanisms for reimbursing health care providers.
- Describe features characteristic of managed care programs.
- Identify at least four requisites for an effective health care reform proposal.
- Describe at least three considerations in evaluating a national health care plan.

▶ ECONOMIC CONCERNS FOR COMMUNITY HEALTH NURSES

Economics is the social science that addresses the production, distribution, and consumption of goods and services. Two basic tools of economics are of interest in providing health care services: optimization and determination of equilibrium situations. *Optimization* is the process of determining criteria to be used in making resource allocation decisions that minimize the cost of achieving specific desired outcomes, in other words, making optimal use of limited resources. *Determination of equilibrium situations* is predicting the impact of changes in demand for services by means of supply and demand analysis.

These tools facilitate making three economic decisions related to health care organization (Feldstein, 1993). The first decision is the total amount of money to be expended for health care and the composition of services to be purchased with that amount. The second decision is determining the best approach to producing those services (eg, fee-for-service practice, managed care). The final decision relates to the best means of distributing these services among the population. To date, we have not really made these crucial decisions at the national level, although states like Oregon and Minnesota have begun to make them at the state level. Failure to systematically make these decisions has led to two major areas of economic influence that are of concern to community health nurses. The first is the increasing cost of health care;

the second is decreased access to care brought about both by rising costs and by reduced income experienced by some segments of the population.

Rising Health Care Costs

Despite cost containment efforts over the last decade, health care costs have continued to rise at an alarming rate. *Cost containment* refers to action designed to slow this rise (Duerksen, 1993). Recent figures show the ineffectiveness of cost containment actions to date. In 1960, for example, the United States spent $26.9 billion on health, including medical research and facility construction. This amount represented 5.1% of the gross domestic product (GDP) (U.S. Department of Commerce, 1996). The *gross domestic product* is the total monetary value of all goods and services produced by the nation in a given period (usually a year). By 1994, total health care expenditures had increased to $949 billion, consuming 13.7% of the GDP (U.S. Department of Commerce, 1996). It is estimated that 19 to 24% of annual health care expenditures are unnecessary (Bodenheimer & Grumbach, 1995). At the current rate of increase, projected annual health care costs by the year 2000 could rise as high as $1.7 trillion or 18% of the GDP (Longest, 1994).

Many factors contribute to higher costs for health care in the United States. The most obvious is population changes over time. Population growth leads to increased demand for and total cost of services. From 1970 to 1995, for example, the U.S. population increased by more than 29%. Increase in the number of people receiving health care, however, does not explain the rise in per capita expenditures. *Per capita expenditures* reflect the average amount spent on health care per person per year. In 1960, per capita spending for health amounted to $143 per person. By 1994, this figure had increased to $3,510 per person (U.S. Department of Commerce, 1996).

Part of the increase in per person spending is due to the increasing proportion of elderly in the population. Older persons use proportionally more health care resources than younger persons because of infirmities related to age and longstanding chronic diseases. In 1970, persons over 85 years of age constituted less than 1% of the U.S. population. By 1995, the size of this subpopulation had doubled, and it is expected to double again before the year 2025 (U.S. Department of Commerce, 1996). The need for long-term care as well as other personal health services in this fragile group will greatly add to health care costs.

One reason for the growth in the elderly population is the ability of "high-tech" medicine to prolong life. Advanced technology is expensive and adds to the cost of health care services. In addition, special-

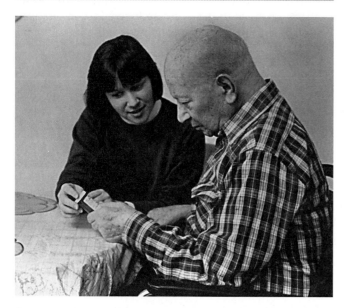

Because of greater incidence of chronic disease among the elderly, they use proportionally more health care resources than younger persons.

Photo courtesy of Visiting Nurses Society of New York.

ized technology contributes to specialization among health care providers, which also adds to cost. In many instances, care is provided by highly specialized providers at high cost, but that care could be provided as effectively by other providers at lower costs (Nichols, 1996). For example, education for nurses as primary care providers consumes one fourth the cost of medical education, and nurses provide comparable care at half the cost of physicians (Mundinger, 1994). Yet, reimbursement policies make it difficult, in the present health care system, for nurses to receive third-party payment for their services. Currently, federal policy mandates reimbursement for services provided only by pediatric and family nurse practitioners and nurse–midwives (Aiken, et al., 1993), and as of 1994, two states (Illinois and Ohio) remained noncompliant with even these limited reimbursement mandates (NURSEweek, 1994).

Not only is care provided by more expensive providers, it is also frequently provided in the most expensive settings, particularly the hospital. In a Rand Corporation study, for example, 23% of hospital admissions were for services that could have been provided in a doctor's office or other ambulatory setting. An additional 17% of surgeries could have been performed on an outpatient basis (Ludlam, 1992). In addition, it is estimated that one fourth of all procedures

and hospital days are unnecessary, as are approximately 40% of the medications prescribed in the United States (Bodenheimer & Grumbach, 1995). Elimination of prescription waste alone could save over $15 billion per year (National Center for Injury Prevention and Control, 1994).

Advanced technology contributes, in part, to overuse, and thus waste, of health care resources. High-tech medical equipment tends to be used more frequently than necessary to justify its cost. Consequently, more expensive diagnostic and treatment procedures may be chosen when less expensive ones might be equally effective. Overuse of high-tech procedures may also be explained as "defensive medicine" in a society where health care providers feel a need to protect themselves from malpractice litigation.

Another factor that contributes to the high cost of health care is the emphasis on cure rather than prevention of illness. As one nurse policy analyst noted, "The American health care system is illness focused. It rewards sickness and frequently pays out only when sickness has been successfully achieved" (O'Grady, 1994). Greater attention to prevention could lead to marked reductions in health care costs. For example, influenza immunization for the elderly may save as much as $1 million in excess hospital costs annually (National Immunization Program, 1994). The relative costs of prevention and cure are exemplified in the fact that the amount of money spent by Humana Hospitals on the artificial heart equals the amount needed to eradicate smallpox worldwide (Lamm, 1990).

Paradoxically, both availability and lack of health insurance have contributed to increased health care costs. When both providers and clients can be assured of payment for health care services by private or government insurance programs, neither has any incentive to contain costs. On the other hand, a large segment of the population is uninsured or underinsured (approximately 41 million people in the United States [Karpatkin & Shearer, 1995]), resulting in large amounts of "uncompensated care" provided by health care institutions and providers. *Uncompensated care* is that proportion of care for which the provider receives no reimbursement. In 1986 alone, U.S. hospitals provided $7 billion worth of uncompensated care (Perkins & Perkins, 1992). Uncompensated care leads to a phenomenon known as *cost shifting*, the passing on of the cost of uncompensated care to those who do pay for care, either those who pay out-of-pocket or those covered by health insurance.

Cost shifting leads, in turn, to higher insurance premiums and higher overall costs for health care. In 1991 alone, businesses expended $152.7 billion in insurance premiums, and private citizens purchased $52.2 billion worth of health insurance. In addition, out-of-pocket spending for services not covered under health insurance amounted to $144.3 billion (U.S. Department of Commerce, 1993). It is estimated that in 1990 costs to business and industry for insuring employees amounted to 62% of corporate profits before taxes (Kerr, 1996). From 1990 to 1991, U.S. wages increased by less than 1%; in that same time period, health benefits costs increased more than 200-fold (Kerr, 1996). A significant portion of insurance costs is attributable to the cost of program administration. An estimated 13% of premiums for private insurance is diverted to pay administrative overhead, whereas slightly less than 3% of the Medicare and Medicaid budgets is spent on program administration (Young, 1993).

A final source of increased health care costs lies in what the Clinton administration labeled as irresponsibility and, sometimes, outright fraud. Insurance companies are charged with selecting only the healthiest persons as eligible for health insurance coverage and with excessive profiteering. Pharmaceutical companies are also accused of charging higher prices for drugs to American than to foreign consumers. Health care fraud is estimated to cost more than $80 billion a year (White House Domestic Policy Council, 1993).

Diminishing Access to Care

The second economic area of particular concern to community health nurses is decreased access to care among some segments of the population. Rising health care costs, coupled with low income, have reduced access to care for many Americans.

The effects of escalating costs of health care have resulted in cutbacks in many services. In many areas, traditional community health programs that promote health and prevent illness have been reduced or eliminated completely. For example, decreased funds are available to prevent sexually transmitted diseases such as syphilis because of the increased costs of AIDS prevention.

There has been an emphasis in community health, as in other areas of health care, on providing services that generate revenues. For example, in some parts of the country, local health departments give preference for well-child care to clients covered by Medicaid (a government program providing medical care for the poor) because the department can be reimbursed for its services by the Medicaid program. This policy effectively limits access to services for clients who are not covered and who cannot afford to seek health care from private providers.

The reverse may be true for clients with Medicaid who seek care for illness. Because of the cumbersome administrative structure of the Medicaid program, reimbursement of providers for services rendered takes time and is less than other payment schedules, prompting some providers to refuse to see these clients (Regan, 1994; Rowland & Salganicoff, 1994). These clients are then forced to seek care in expensive settings such as emergency rooms or to go without care.

Rising costs have also prompted some health departments to institute fees for formerly free services such as immunizations. Although many departments set fees on a sliding scale based on clients' income, such fees continue to deter clients who have no money to pay for health care and do not realize that a sliding scale exists.

Diminished access to health care is also the result of lack of health insurance for many American families. From 1987 to 1994, the number of Americans without private health insurance increased by 28% (U.S. Department of Commerce, 1996). In 1995, approximately 41 million people in the United States, including 11 million children, were uninsured (Karpatkin & Shearer, 1995), and an additional 100,000 people become uninsured each month (Vladek, 1996). Two major reasons for noninsurance include job loss or change with subsequent permanent or temporary loss of benefits or part-time employment that does not include health insurance benefits. Other barriers to health insurance coverage include high premiums that make health insurance for employees unaffordable to small businesses. This is particularly true when premiums are derived from *experience ratings*, a process of rate setting based on usual use data for an occupational group. Some occupational groups are even "blacklisted" by insurance companies due to the high-risk nature of their work. Finally, insurance premiums may be prohibitive for individuals with some existing health conditions; some other conditions make people medically uninsurable at any cost (Bodenheimer & Grumbach, 1995).

Economic status is a significant factor in access to health care over and above one's ability to afford health insurance coverage. In 1994, 14.5% of the U.S. population had incomes below poverty level, and nearly one fifth had incomes less than 125% of poverty level, yet less than 8% received any form of public assistance (U.S. Department of Commerce, 1996). Medicaid, a federal- and state-funded program to provide health care for the indigent, serves only a portion of those in need. For example, in states like Florida and Texas where large segments of the population are medically needy, Medicaid covered only one fourth of those in need (Davis, 1996).

In addition to those without any health insurance, another large segment of the American population is underinsured. These people, as well as those who are uninsured, are some of the 13% of the American public who needed medical care in 1993, but were unable to obtain it, or the 30% who postponed needed care (Davis, 1996). The uninsured and underinsured are not only found among lower socioeconomic groups. Indeed, nurses who work on a per diem basis are often uninsured.

It would seem obvious from the figures cited here that current economic mechanisms for funding health care services are inadequate. Community health nurses can be influential in bringing about changes in funding policies, but first they must have some understanding of current and proposed funding mechanisms.

▶ MECHANISMS FOR FINANCING HEALTH CARE

Traditional means of funding health care have been retrospective in nature. *Retrospective reimbursement* is payment for services rendered based on the cost of those services; cost is determined after the fact. In 1983, the federal government instituted prospective reimbursement for services provided under Medicare. *Prospective reimbursement* is payment at a predetermined, fixed rate for a specific health care program or set of services.

Prospective payment for services provided under the Medicare program is based on clients' diagnoses, with set fees for care of clients who fall into specific diagnosis-related groups (DRGs). *Diagnosis-related groups* are categories of client diagnoses for which typical costs of care have been calculated, based on the cost of specific services required. In the DRG system, providers are paid a set fee based on clients' diagnoses and the typical costs of care for someone with that diagnosis. Prospective reimbursement systems are also a feature of some alternative modes of health care delivery such as health maintenance organizations (HMOs) and preferred provider organizations (PPOs), both of which are discussed later in this chapter.

Retrospective reimbursement has the disadvantage of encouraging health care providers to give services that may not be necessary, merely because they are reimbursable. A provider who can be reimbursed for each office visit may be tempted to see a client three times, when two visits would suffice. Or, tests and treatments may be given that are not strictly necessary. For example, a surgeon might suggest a hysterectomy to a woman when other less expensive measures would be equally effective.

Prospective reimbursement eliminates the incentive to overtreat clients. Because providers are paid at a fixed rate, extending the services provided to a client does not result in additional revenue. Indeed continued service may be to the provider's disadvantage if the costs of service exceed the fixed rate paid for them. Providers, then, have an incentive to minimize the costs of care.

Prospective payment systems also have disadvantages. Health care institutions may attempt to avoid caring for the very sick or provide inadequate care to minimize costs. For example, under the DRG system, a hospital would be paid the same rate for Medicare recipients hospitalized for diabetes, whether their hospital stays were 3 days or 30 days. Those who are very ill and who require more than the average stay for their diagnostic group may be discharged from services before they are actually ready for discharge. In the long run, such practices may lead to subsequent readmissions and to increased health care costs.

Prospective reimbursement has also been criticized as detrimental to provider–client relationships. Because providers may be pressured by hospitals and other institutions to minimize the cost of client's care and maximize revenues, they may put the needs of the institution before those of the client and discharge clients before they are ready for discharge. Or, physicians may mislabel clients' diagnoses to put them into groups with higher reimbursement rates.

Reimbursement Systems

Current approaches to financing health care can be either retrospective or prospective in nature, and several different systems of reimbursement are to be found within the U.S. health care system. Among these are the two-party and third-party reimbursement systems, per case prospective reimbursement, and per capita prospective reimbursement.

Two-party Reimbursement

In two-party reimbursement, the client pays the health care provider directly—the traditional fee-for-service approach. Until this century, it was the only way of paying for health care services beyond charitable care.

The amount of direct payment by clients steadily declined over the years until the majority of health care expenses have begun to be met by public or private third-party payments. In 1960, for example, private, out-of-pocket payment for services constituted almost half of health care expenditures. In 1994, out-of-pocket expenses accounted for only 18% of health-related spending. The amount of direct payment varies considerably with the type of service provided, with consumers paying less than 3% of the costs of hospital care, 19% of the cost of physicians' services, and 62% of medication costs (U.S. Department of Commerce, 1996).

Two-party reimbursement has the advantage of giving consumers some degree of control over the health care they receive. If one is unsatisfied with the care given, one can refuse to pay the bill for services or seek care from another health care provider. Consumers also have a wide choice among providers.

Both providers and consumers are conscious of cost factors in a two-party system. Consumers do not wish to pay too much for the services received, and providers do not want to drive clients away by charging higher fees than competing providers. Unfortunately, because of the high cost of health care, care for serious illness could bankrupt most individuals and families if they had to pay for everything themselves. The two-party reimbursement system is depicted in Figure 14–2.

Third-party Reimbursement

Third-party reimbursement mechanisms were designed to protect the average citizen from the financial devastation of serious illness and to supplement two-party payment. In a third-party reimbursement system, payment for health care services is made by someone or some agency other than the individual receiving service, usually some form of public or private insurance.

Private Health Insurance.   Third-party reimbursement can take place under either public or private auspices. The private component of the third-party reimbursement system consists of voluntary health insurance and includes the Blue Cross and Blue Shield nonprofit insurers and commercial health insurance companies such as Aetna and Prudential. Blue Cross covers hospitalization costs; Blue Shield covers the cost of physician's services. Both Blue Cross and Blue Shield programs are controlled by providers. Commercial insurers operate on a for-profit basis, provide many different benefits packages with coverage for a variety of services, and are outside of provider control.

In 1994, roughly 32% of health care service payments were made by private insurance companies—$266.8 million worth of care. During that same year, the American people paid $313.2 million in insurance premiums (U.S. Department of Commerce, 1996). Insurance premiums may be paid by the individual (Fig. 14–3) or by employers (Fig. 14–4). In both instances, premiums are paid to an insurance company that may pay the provider directly (solid arrows in Figs. 14–3 and 14–4) or reimburse beneficiaries who make payments to providers (broken arrows) (Bodenheimer & Grumbach, 1995). Employment-based group insurance has the advantage of lower premiums compared to individually purchased private health insurance. This is due to increased purchasing power when large numbers of employees are involved. Employment-based health insurance coverage also has the disadvantage that coverage is lost when employment is terminated. In part, this disadvantage is minimized by the Consolidated Omnibus Budget Reconciliation Act (COBRA) which permits employees to continue coverage up to 18 months if they assume up to 102% of the insurance premium costs normally paid by the employer (Powell, 1996).

As noted earlier, employer costs for health insurance benefits for their employees have risen rapidly, and many employers have begun to take several measures to decrease their costs. Some of the strategies used are reducing illness through preventive and health-promotive efforts, shifting greater responsibility for payment to employees, using less costly health

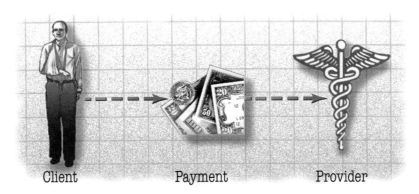

Figure 14–2. Two-party reimbursement.

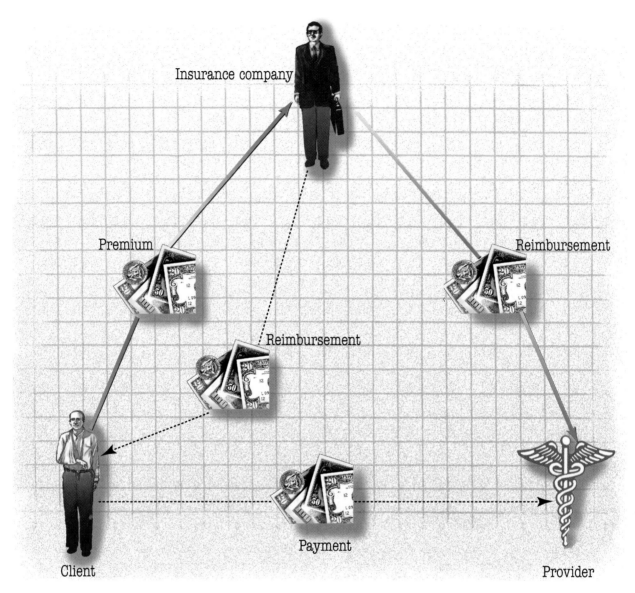

Figure 14–3. Third-party reimbursement—Individual private insurance.

care services, negotiating for discounted prices on health care through preferred provider agreements, and self-funding insurance coverage for employees (Rooney, 1990). Use of preventive efforts, less costly services, and preferred provider arrangements is discussed later in this chapter.

In an effort to make employees more conscious of health care costs and to reduce their own expenditures, employers are shifting the cost of health insurance premiums to their employees through copayments and increased deductibles. Unfortunately, such an approach discourages employees from seeking preventive health services and may, in the long run, increase the overall cost of health care by promoting a tendency to let health problems reach crisis proportions before care is sought.

Many employers are also turning to self-insurance plans to reduce their health-related costs (Rooney, 1990). All 50 states have some form of legislation that mandates certain benefits when insurance is provided by private insurance companies. Because these laws do not apply to employers who self-insure their employees' health care coverage, employers can provide basic coverage at a cost far less than they paid previously to purchase health insurance from private insurance carriers. In addition, self-funded employer health insurance programs are exempt from state taxes, which average 2 to 3% of the premium.

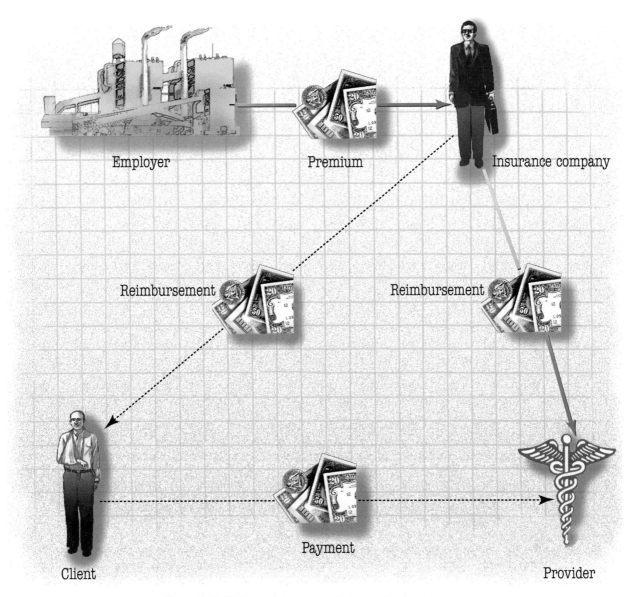

Figure 14–4. Third-party reimbursement—Employment-based group insurance.

More employers are taking this option to provide health care coverage for their employees. Because employers are not required to offer mandated insurance benefits, the coverage provided is less than would be the case under private insurance and, again, health may suffer, resulting in higher societal costs for health care in the long term.

Publicly Funded Health Insurance Programs. Publicly funded health insurance programs are the second component of the third-party reimbursement system in the United States. Government funding accounts for a much lower portion of health care financing in the United States than elsewhere in the world, just over 43.5% compared with 86% for the United Kingdom,

72% for Australia, 75% for Canada, and nearly 98% for Norway (U.S. Department of Commerce, 1996; Gale & Steffl, 1992). The public component of the third-party system consists of the Medicare and Medicaid programs and the Civilian Health and Medical Programs of the Uniformed Services (CHAMPUS).

MEDICARE. Medicare is part of the social insurance program arising from provisions of the Social Security Act. Under Medicare, people over 65 years of age who are eligible for Social Security benefits receive partial coverage of health services. Certain other individuals, such as the disabled, are eligible for Medicare coverage before age 65. In 1996, for example, more than 33 million individuals over the age of 65 and more than

4.5 million disabled people were covered by Part A of the Medicare program (U.S. Department of Health and Human Services, 1996).

Medicare Part A, the Hospital Insurance Program, covers inpatient services. Part B is a Supplemental Medical Insurance Program that covers services by a physician or a nurse or other health care professional working under the direction of a physician. In the case of Rural Health Clinics, nursing services can be reimbursed with or without physician authorization.

Part A coverage is available to all participants in the Social Security program and is provided without additional premiums. Funding for Medicare Part A is derived from nonvoluntary Social Security taxes. Part B coverage is optional and entails payment of an additional premium similar to that paid for private health insurance, but much less costly. Approximately 96% of persons eligible for Part A Medicare benefits also receive Part B benefits (U.S. Department of Health and Human Services, 1996). Under both components of the program, the client is responsible for a deductible and also pays a percentage of the cost of care (usually 20%) for services provided under Part B (Melillo, 1996).

Part A covers hospitalization and related services including payment for a semiprivate room, laboratory and x-ray procedures, nursing care, meals, medications provided by the hospital, medical supplies and appliances, and the cost of operating room and recovery room services. Blood transfusions are also covered with an additional deductible. Care in a skilled nursing facility may also be provided, but the client pays a coinsurance payment after 21 days of care. Beyond 100 days, Medicare pays nothing; thus long-term nursing home care is not covered (Melillo, 1996).

Medicare Part A also covers home health services from nurses or physical, occupational, or speech therapists for homebound clients on a physician's order. Coverage also includes 80% of the cost of home equipment needs. Hospice care is available for clients who are terminally ill.

Part B benefits include payment of 80% of allowable fees for physician care. Clients pay the additional 20% as well as any charges in excess of the allowable amount (Newell, 1996). Other benefits include outpatient clinic and emergency room services, physical and occupational therapy, outpatient psychiatric care, laboratory and ambulance services, and very limited coverage for medications. Part B coverage has been extended to cover routine mammography screening (Melillo, 1996).

Medicare is administered at the federal level by the Social Security Administration. Information on benefits, eligibility requirements, deductibles, and co-payments for Medicare Part A and Part B is summarized in Table 14–1.

As noted earlier, the Medicare program instituted a prospective payment system based on DRGs in 1983. At present the DRG system applies only to hospital costs covered under Medicare Part A. A fee schedule based on a resource-based relative value scale (RBRVS) is used for Part B payments to physicians and other providers. Under this system, providers are paid for care based on fee schedules determined for each specialty area (Newell, 1996).

Because of escalating Medicare costs, the federal government has been trying to recoup some funds by billing other sources for services whenever appropriate. These sources then become primary payers with Medicare as a secondary payer to pay any uncovered costs. Some of the agencies which may function as primary payers in this regard include liability insurers, worker's compensation, the Black Lung program, and the Veterans Administration (Harris, 1996).

Medicare has provided access to health care for many older and disabled persons who could otherwise not have afforded care; however, Medicare deductibles and increasing premiums for Part B coverage still make health care unaffordable for some older persons. All Medicare enrollees pay the same deductibles and premiums, whatever their income. The original premium when Part B coverage was instituted was $3 per month (Miller, 1995). By 1996, the cost of Part B premiums had increased to $42.50 per month, while Part A deductibles increased to $736 for each benefit period (U.S. Department of Health and Human Services, 1996). A benefit period begins with hospitalization and ends 60 days after discharge from all covered institutions, so a beneficiary could be responsible for more than one deductible payment during a calendar year (Powell, 1996). Because of these out-of-pocket expenses, approximately 20% of low-income elderly Americans also require assistance under the Medicaid program (Feldstein, 1993).

MEDICAID. In the past, Medicaid has been an *entitlement* program in which the federal government mandated certain benefits for all people who met federally specified eligibility criteria. Under the program, the federal government paid at least half of the costs of health care to these designated populations with matching funds from the states. The federal government has established eligibility criteria for the *categorically needy,* those who because of membership in certain categories (eg, recipients of Aid to Families with Dependent Children [AFDC]) are automatically eligible for Medicaid, and the *medically needy,* per-

TABLE 14–1. MEDICARE BENEFITS, DEDUCTIBLES, COPAYMENTS, AND REQUIREMENTS, 1991

Benefit	Deductible	Copayment	Requirements for Care
PART A			

Hospital services (150-day maximum)
  Semiprivate room
  Laboratory tests
  X-rays
  Nursing services
  Meals
  Drugs provided by hospital
  Medical supplies
  Appliances
  Operating room services
  Recovery room services
	$763/benefit period	None until day 61
		Days 61–90 $184/day
		Day 91–150 $368/day
			Hospital admission

Blood transfusion	Additional	Cost of replacing first 3 pints	Need for more than 3 pints of blood
Skilled nursing (100-day maximum)	None	None until day 21 Days 21–100 $92/day	Hospitalized for at least 3 days Provided in a Medicare-approved facility, need certified by physician, facility accepts client
Home health care	None	20% of allowable charge for medical equipment plus excess charges if any	Care provided by a Medicare-certified agency; client is homebound; client requires intermittent skilled nursing; physical, speech, or occupational therapy; care is ordered and reviewed periodically by physician
Hospice care (210-day maximum)	None	$5 or 5% of cost of pain-relief drugs if needed	Physician certification of terminal illness
Inpatient psychiatric care (190 days lifetime maximum)			
PART B			
Physician's services	$100 for all Part B care	Monthly premium $42.50; 20 % of allowable charges plus excess charges	Physician accepts client
Outpatient hospital services	No additional		
Emergency services	No additional		
Blood transfusion	No additional	20% of allowable charges plus cost of replacing first 3 pints of blood	None
Physical and occupational therapy	No additional	$600	Physician prescribed treatment plan with periodic physician review
Outpatient psychiatric services	No additional	50% of drug charges	None
Laboratory fees	No additional	None for tests subject to fee schedule	Performance of tests in Medicare-certified labs
Ambulance services	No additional	20% of allowable charges plus excess charges	Medical need, ambulance meets Medicare standards, other forms of transport could endanger client's life

(Source: U.S. Department of Health and Human Services. 1996.)

sons whose health care needs are beyond the scope of their income, but who are otherwise able to maintain themselves financially. The Medicaid program has been administered by the states, but must provide a minimum set of federally defined benefits. In this system, states have had the prerogative to expand the eligible populations, to increase the services covered, and to establish mechanisms for provider reimbursement (Leibowitz & DuPlessis, 1996).

Recent federal policy changes, called by some the *new fiscal federalism,* have initiated a move from entitlement status for Medicaid to a block grant type of program as one aspect of plans to shift responsibility for social action from the federal government to the states (Hosek & Levine, 1996). A *block grant* is a lump sum made available to the states by the federal government to be used as each state sees fit within certain broadly defined parameters. The *Medigrant program,* as the block grant program to cover welfare, health, and training funds is being called, would provide the states with a specific sum of money for use to meet these three social needs. Reconfigured as a block program, there would no longer be any categorical eligibility and the states would have the ability to define eligibility criteria, services to the provided, and how services would be financed. Funds received from the federal government would be less than in the past Medicaid program, but the states would have greater latitude in how that money would be spent. In 1996, the National Governors Association proposed some modifications of the Medigrant proposal that would retain some entitlement provisions, but still allow states more flexibility than they have had in the past. It remains to be seen what the eventual outcome of these changes in Medicaid will be, but initial projections are an increase of 8 million people among the uninsured (Vladek, 1996).

CHAMPUS.   CHAMPUS is a program that provides payment for medical services for the dependents of active duty or retired military personnel. CHAMPUS is usually used to pay for inpatient services not available through a uniformed services medical facility (eg, a naval hospital or an army medical center). CHAMPUS may also be used to finance outpatient services to dependents. Although care provided through a uniformed services medical facility is free (except for a small daily fee for inpatient services), there is a deductible for outpatient services provided under CHAMPUS. Under CHAMPUS, nonmilitary hospitals are reimbursed for services at DRG rates (Powell, 1996).

As noted in previous chapters, the federal government also provides direct care services that are not associated with the publicly funded health insurance programs described here. These services are provided through the Department of Defense, the Veterans Administration, the Indian Health Service, and the National Institutes of Health.

Reimbursing Providers

Whether payment is provided by private or public funds, a number of mechanisms have been developed for actually paying providers for the care given. These include fee-for-service payment, per case payment, per diem payment, capitation, and global reimbursement. Fee-for-service payment is based on the unit of service as a single visit to a provider or a single procedure. Under traditional insurance plans, a physician would be paid for each visit a client made to the office whether that visit was related to a new complaint or a continuing one. Under payment by illness episode, the provider would receive a flat rate for each episode for which care was given. For example, if the client had three sinus infections this year, his or her provider would be paid for each of the three no matter how many visits resolution of each episode involved. The DRG system is another example of a payment by episode system. Under this system, hospitals are paid a flat rate for each admission based on the client's diagnosis, no matter how long the client was hospitalized. In a per diem system, the unit of service

is usually a day. Per diem reimbursement is usually used for institutional providers such as hospitals, skilled nursing facilities, and long-term care facilities. With capitation, health care providers receive a lump sum payment for each client enrolled in the program. The net effect is a fixed budget for the program which must cover all services provided. Finally, in global reimbursement, providers receive a lump sum for all care provided to all clients. Canadian hospitals and salaried physicians or nurse practitioners receive global reimbursement. Methods of provider reimbursement are summarized in Table 14–2.

Managed Care

Whatever the method used to reimburse providers, public and private health care funding sources are increasingly looking toward managed care as a means to minimize costs. For example, as of 1994, 43 states had at least one managed care option for Medicaid clients (Centers for Disease Control, 1995). As noted in Chapter 11, managed care is a system of health care delivery and financing that provides necessary services in an efficient manner with as little cost as possible. Managed care plans share several features. First, clients select a primary care provider who serves as a "gatekeeper" for access to specialized services. Second, managed care plans employ utilization review to determine the appropriateness of care. Utilization review is a prospective, concurrent, or retrospective review of the need for and cost of services provided with the intent of either denying reimbursement or selecting the least costly modes of care. Third, plans incorporate networks of providers who agree to discounted fee schedules in return for access to plan members. Fourth, care is managed by case managers, and, finally, there is an emphasis on prevention as a way to minimize health care costs (MacLaren, 1994).

TABLE 14–2.   **METHODS OF PROVIDER REIMBURSEMENT, UNITS OF SERVICE, AND CHARACTERISTIC FEATURES**

Method	Unit of Service	Characteristic Features
Fee for service	Visit or procedure	Retrospective, based on actual cost of services
Episode	Illness episode	Prospective, includes all services rendered in the care of a single episode of illness, based on type of episode
Per diem	Day	Retrospective or prospective, usually used for institutional services, flat rate
Capitation	Person enrolled	Prospective, lump sum payment for all covered services, flat rate
Global	All services to all persons	Prospective, lump sum, flat rate

Managed care may be provided in a variety of formats including health maintenance organizations, independent physician associations, preferred provider organizations, exclusive provider organizations, and point of service plans.

Health Maintenance Organizations

A *health maintenance organization (HMO)* is an organized health care delivery system providing a wide range of health services to a voluntary enrolled population for a fixed prepaid fee. Under the Health Maintenance Organization Act of 1973, federally designated HMOs must exhibit four characteristics: (1) an organized system to provide health care in a particular geographic area, (2) an agreed-on set of services for health maintenance and treatment, (3) a voluntarily enrolled membership, and (4) rates based on those for similar services in the surrounding community. HMOs may be freestanding or a part of a Blue Cross–Blue Shield or commercial insurance system (MacLaren, 1994).

HMOs can be either public or private agencies and all are regulated under the HMO Act of 1973. The act specified the minimum types of service to be provided, the organization of the HMO, and a mechanism of initial federal support for development. It also specified that industries subscribing to an HMO must offer employees the option to choose either membership in the HMO or more traditional health insurance coverage. In addition, one third of the governing board of an HMO must be health care consumers.

Several different models of HMO organization are based on the arrangement between the HMO and health care providers. The types of arrangements include the staff, group, network, independent practice association, and direct contract models (Centers for Disease Control, 1995). Providers are salaried employees of the HMO in the staff model. This type of provider relationship is becoming more common. In fact, the proportion of physicians employed by organizations increased from 24% in 1983 to 42% in 1994 (Kletke, Emmons, & Gillis, 1996). In the group model, the HMO contracts with a multispecialty group of providers to obtain care for plan enrollees (Raymond, 1994). In this and other remaining models, providers may also see clients from outside the HMO. The network model HMO may contract for services with several provider groups. An *independent practice association (IPA)* is a group of independent health care providers who join together to contract with an HMO to provide services for enrollees. The HMO pays the IPA a capitated amount based on the number of enrollees involved. The IPA, in turn, reimburses individual providers on a fee-for-service basis. Finally, in the direct contract model, the HMO enters contractual agreements with multiple independent providers to obtain services for enrollees (Powell, 1996).

Preferred Provider Organization

A *preferred provider organization (PPO)* is a negotiated association between a funding source (usually an employer, although the source may also be an insurance company) and health care providers, whereby providers give discounted services to a defined group of people (eg, employees). The discount may be as much as 20% of the usual fee for services (Dunham-Taylor, Marquette, & Pinczuk, 1996). When employees use these "preferred" providers, the employer usually covers the bulk of charges. When someone chooses to use other providers, their out-of-pocket costs are higher than if they choose a preferred provider. For example, the client may pay only 10 to 20% of the cost of care from a preferred provider, but as much as 50% for care from an outside provider.

For providers to remain on the preferred list, they must provide quality services at a reasonable cost, thus encouraging efficiency, but not at the risk of quality. In a PPO, providers are paid for specific services on a per case basis at a predetermined fee, and providers are independent of the reimbursement system. PPOs decrease the per visit cost of health care, but, if the number of visits increases, may not reduce the overall cost of health care to the employer or to society.

Consumer choice exists both within and outside of the PPO. Consumers enrolled in the plan have a choice among several providers within the plan and can also choose between in-plan and out-of-plan providers. The final characteristic of PPOs is more expeditious reimbursement of providers than is often the case with other forms of third-party payment.

Exclusive Provider Organizations

An *exclusive provider organization (EPO)* is an offshoot of the preferred provider organization concept. The two are similar except in the matter of choice of providers. In an EPO, consumers are restricted to obtaining care from providers within the plan. If clients choose to use outside providers, they must pay the entire cost of care out-of-pocket. Both EPOs and PPOs frequently use a "gatekeeper" approach to minimize the costs of care. This means that clients have access to specialist providers only on approved referral from their primary care provider, a physician or nurse practitioner who provides for their routine health care needs.

Point of Service Plans

A *point of service plan* (POS) is a combination of an HMO and traditional insurance coverage in which the client chooses whether to use an in-plan provider or another provider. This choice can be made with each episode of health service. For example, a client might elect to see an in-plan provider for gynecologic services, but continue to see an out-of-plan pediatrician liked by her children. Out-of-plan provider use, however, may require a deductible and a 20 to 50% copayment. Specialist referrals must be made by the primary provider to be covered, whether the specialist is a part of the plan or not (Raymond, 1994).

Because most managed care plans are capitated and operate on a prospective payment basis, more services result in greater costs to the organization. This arrangement creates a potential for attempts to minimize costs by skimping on needed care. Research findings are somewhat equivocal on whether or not this actually occurs. For example, HMOs (a type of managed care plan) have been shown to diagnose some cancers at earlier stages (Kerr, 1996; Riley, Potosky, Lubitz, & Brown, 1994), but produce poorer health outcomes for the elderly (Ware, Bayliss, Rogers, Kosinski, & Tarlov, 1996) than fee-for-service practice. In addition, HMO enrollees receive approximately twice as many preventive services as their fee-for-service counterparts (Kerr, 1996). Advantages and disadvantages of managed care approaches are compared to those of fee-for-service and indemnity insurance approaches in Table 14–3.

Proposals for Health Care Reform

As noted earlier in this chapter, current mechanisms for financing health care services leave 41 million Americans without access to care. Despite massive expenditures for health care, the health status of the American people is no better, and in some respects is worse, than that of nations that spend far less. For this reason, many people have called for a new approach to providing health care services.

Several legislative proposals for health care reform have been advanced in recent years. The basic intent of all of these proposals is to contain health care costs while insuring universal access for those in need of care. *Universal access* is availability of health care services for everyone (Hart, 1995). Attempts at health care reform have been undertaken since the beginning of the twentieth century, when the American Association for Labor Legislation advocated state insurance programs to cover all nonwork-related medical services (Miller, 1995). Unfortunately, the social climate has rarely been such that reform was possible. The

TABLE 14–3. **ADVANTAGES AND DISADVANTAGES OF SELECTED APPROACHES TO HEALTH CARE FINANCING**

Approach	Advantages	Disadvantages
Fee-for-service	Unlimited choice of providers	Personal responsibility for all costs No quality control mechanisms except licensure No external review process
Indemnity insurance	Wide choice of providers No gatekeeper	Deductibles, coinsurance Potential for excessive use High-cost premiums No quality control of providers except licensure No external review except state insurance board
Managed care (general)	"Credentialled" providers promote quality control External review process (eg, HEDIS) promotes quality	
HMO	Comprehensive care No deductible or coinsurance Lower premiums than indemnity insurance	Gatekeeper Restricted to plan providers Copayment Potential for lower quality care to minimize costs
PPO	Greater selection of providers than HMO Expedited provider reimbursement Lower premiums than indemnity insurance	Gatekeeper Additional cost for out-of-plan provider use Potential for lower quality care to minimize costs
EPO	Greater discount on services Lower premiums than indemnity insurance	Restricted to in-plan providers Gatekeeper Potential for lower quality care to minimize costs
POS	Most flexibility Comprehensive services within plan	Deductible and 20–50% coinsurance for out-of-plan provider use Referral by primary provider required for services to be covered

only exception was the institution of the Medicare and Medicaid programs in the 1960s.

Requisites for Effective Reform Proposals

A number of requisites have been suggested for effective health care reform proposals. Requisites suggested by Marla Salmon (1995), former director of the Division of Nursing, include universal coverage, a payment system that rewards prevention and health promotion, a national performance monitoring system, and an adequate health work force. Additional elements required include research support, an organizational structure that supports delivery of comprehensive services to underserved populations, and adequate support for core public health functions. Other desirable elements of a reformed health care system suggested by the Clinton administration and others are simplicity and standardization of reimbursement procedures, cost-effectiveness, and mechanisms to assure provision of high-quality health care. Finally, system reforms should foster acceptance of responsibility for health in all segments of society (White House Domestic Policy Council, 1993). For example, insurance and drug company profits should not be exorbitant and frivolous malpractice suits should be eliminated.

Types of Reform Proposals

Recent health care reform proposals can be categorized into two major groups: financing reform plans and system reform plans. Financing reform plans change the bases for financing health care without changing the basic organization of health care delivery. System reform plans change the structure of the health care delivery system.

Financing Reform Plans. Several approaches have been suggested to increase financial access to health care for the population. One suggested approach is to expand Medicaid eligibility criteria to include those most in need while also allowing those with incomes above the eligibility level to pay sliding scale premiums for care based on income. A second approach is to mandate insurance coverage for all workers by their employers, with government subsidization for those who are not employed and cannot afford to pay for insurance. Some plans suggested under this approach are referred to as "pay-or-play" proposals. Under these plans, employers would have the option of "playing" by purchasing health insurance for their employees or "paying" a state tax per employee to cover health care services (Citizen Action, 1994).

A third suggestion is to change the tax treatment of insurance benefits by making employment insurance benefits taxable. Currently, the amount paid by one's employer for health insurance is not taxable income. This change would have the effect of generating more tax revenues that could be used to pay for care for those without employer-provided insurance, while discouraging overuse of health care services by the insured.

Other proposals include legislative mandates requiring all individuals to purchase health insurance in return for refundable tax credit. In this approach, employers who currently pay part or all of employees' insurance premiums would be required to add the amount of the premium to the individual's salary. Medicare and Medicaid would be continued as separate programs to address the needs of the indigent. This type of plan would not resolve the problem of those who are currently uninsured and unemployed, but who have incomes below eligibility levels for Medicaid.

System Reform Proposals.   System reform proposals may include some or major changes in the organizational structure of health care delivery. Managed competition proposals would create some changes in the health care system, but would not result in total health care restructuring as would single-payer proposals. ***Managed competition*** is an approach to health care financing that forces insurers or groups of providers and institutions to compete for large-scale contracts with networks of employers, individuals, and government agencies (National League for Nursing, 1993). Proposals calling for this type of approach would create alliances or cooperatives composed of employers and individuals that, because of their size and purchasing power, could demand favorable premium rates from insurers. Most of the managed competition plans proposed to date would eliminate part or all of the Medicaid program. These plans also contain provisions for government subsidies for low-income persons who cannot afford even discounted premiums available through the alliances (Citizen Action, 1994).

The most sweeping health care reform proposals are those that call for a single-payer system. Under a ***single-payer system***, insurance coverage for basic health and medical services would virtually be eliminated, although individuals might be able to purchase insurance to cover additional services under some proposals. Health care financing would be a government responsibility, and universal access would be ensured. Under such a system, health care would most likely continue to be provided by a variety of private and public sector providers and institutions, but would be reimbursed by the federal government in a system similar to that in place in Canada. An even more radical possibility is provision of care by government-employed providers as occurs in the United Kingdom. Financing for a single-payer system would come from a variety of sources including payroll taxes for employers, corporate and personal income taxes, and "sin" taxes. *Sin taxes* are heavy taxes on products that contribute to unhealthful behaviors such as drinking and smoking.

Public support for a single-payer plan is widespread. Unfortunately, the public's desire for any type of health care reform will probably not be met in the near future. In large part, the failure of all of the bills introduced in Congress has been attributed to the economic influence of several special interest groups such as the insurance industry; the American Medical, Dental, and Hospital associations; and big business such as United Parcel Service, AT&T, and General Electric. This influence came primarily in the form of $46 million in campaign contributions, most of which went to key members of House and Senate committees dealing with health care reform issues (Jordan, 1994).

► THE DIMENSIONS MODEL AND HEALTH CARE REFORM

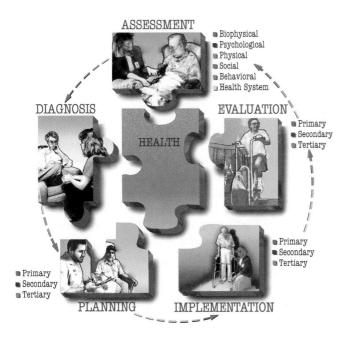

A tremendous potential exists for shaping economic influences on health care, particularly for influencing mechanisms of health care financing. Because community health nurses are concerned for the health of the total population, they should be intimately involved in the development of delivery systems and funding mechanisms that best meet the health care needs of the public. In the following discussion the

Dimensions Model is applied to the development of a reformed national health care system that meets those needs.

Critical Dimensions of Nursing in Formulating a National Health Care Plan

Elements of each of the dimensions of nursing in the Dimensions Model have a bearing on national health care reform. In the cognitive dimension, effective community health nursing action related to health care reform will require knowledge of the current health care system and how it functions as well as an understanding of the health needs of the population. Nurses also need knowledge of basic principles of health economics. Interpersonal dimension elements of communication and collaboration, used in conjunction with the change, leadership, group, and political processes in the process dimension, can help to bring about health care reform. Advocacy for the health needs of underserved populations is a requisite element of the ethical dimension, and analytical and organizational skills will be required in the skills dimension. As always, research and evaluation are the elements from the reflective dimension that will be needed to direct actions for health care system reform.

 Assessing the Dimensions of Health Care Reform

Assessment in the development of a reformed national health care system should focus primarily on identifying the groups of people to be addressed by the system and the types of services that need to be covered. Information related to biophysical, psychological, physical, social, and behavioral dimensions, as well as the current health care system can provide answers to these questions of coverage.

The Biophysical Dimension

Considerations of maturation and aging suggest that certain subgroups within the population should receive priority, even in a national health care system that will eventually address all members of the population. Many health reform proposals give priority to vulnerable groups such as pregnant women and young children. Access to health care for young children is a serious concern in the United States. Failure to promote health and prevent illness in the young contributes to chronic health problems and escalating health care costs in later life.

From 1992 to 1994, more than 4% of children under 18 years of age had no form of health insurance.

The number of children growing up in poverty and with reduced access to health care is increasing. In 1970, just under 15% of children lived in families with incomes below the poverty level. By 1994, more than 21% of children were part of families with incomes below this level (U.S. Department of Commerce, 1996).

The elderly are another population group that need access to health care services often denied in the present system. The elderly expend a greater percentage of their income on health care services than do other age groups. Despite advances in incomes for the elderly due to Social Security, more than 11% of those over the age of 65 remained below the poverty level in 1994 (U.S. Department of Commerce, 1996).

The size of the elderly population is expected to continue to expand, placing additional strain on available health care resources. In 1995, the elderly constituted approximately 13% of the U.S. population. By the year 2025, the elderly will constitute 18% of the population. Because of increased rates of chronic diseases in this age group, the elderly consume an inordinate proportion of health care resources relative to their numbers.

The growing number of retirees in the population has increased the health care cost burden for business and industry. Many employers are responding to this financial drain by reducing health care benefits for retirees and increasing retiree responsibility for a greater portion of the health care services they receive.

Funding for long-term care for the elderly and chronically ill is another area of concern related to both biologic aging and physiologic function. Medicare does not cover long-term nursing home care, and Medicaid coverage begins only after clients have exhausted all personal resources.

The relationship between physiologic function and health care is a dual one. Those who have physiologic abnormalities require more health services than those who do not. Conversely, lack of access to illness preventive and health-promotive care contributes to more illness.

A special area of concern in terms of physiologic function is the cost of care for persons with AIDS. Currently, 25 to 40% of states' Medicaid budgets are spent on care for those with AIDS. In 1992, this was almost $2 billion. Total federal government appropriations for AIDS from 1984 to 1992 was $8.6 billion (U.S. Department of Commerce, 1993).

The Psychological Dimension

A psychological dimension factor that influences the development of a national health care reform program is the prevalence of mental health problems. In 1995, Medicaid alone disbursed $2.1 million for inpatient mental health care (U.S. Department of Health and Human Services, 1996). It is estimated that more than 29 million Americans suffer from some form of mental disorder and that more than 20% of them, including 2 million seriously disturbed children, receive no care for their illness (Rooney, 1990). Clearly, effective national health reforms need to address problems of mental illness.

The Social Dimension

Elements of the social dimension influence health care reforms. The effects of poverty and unemployment on health and access to health care have already been addressed, but these are the types of social environmental factors that community health nurses would need to consider in influencing the direction to be taken by health care reform. Any such reform would need to include mechanisms for providing health care to the poor and those who are not covered by any form of health insurance.

A generally depressed economic climate, another social environmental factor, suggests that a health program based exclusively on employer contributions would not meet the health needs of the population. Business and industry are adversely affected by a declining economy and could not bear the added burden of completely funding a national health care system. In addition, as already noted, not all people without health insurance coverage are employed. These individuals would be left out of any plan that relies exclusively on employer contributions.

The Behavioral Dimension

Behavioral factors contribute to a variety of illnesses in today's society, thereby adding to the overall costs of health care. Primary prevention programs related to diet, exercise, and smoking, for example, can modify behaviors that affect health.

Substance abuse significantly influences health care expenditures. In terms of related health care costs, alcohol abusers receive more medical care than nonabusers, are absent from work more often, and have more accidents than nonabusers. Factors contributing to substance abuse and its control are addressed in Chapter 33.

The Health System Dimension

The potential effects of national health care reform on the health system and the quality of care provided should also be considered. Many health-related groups are actively supporting some form of health care reform. Others are resistant to changes in health care financing that could affect their practice. Because of the longstanding independence of health care

---

ASSESSMENT TIPS: Formulating a National Health Plan

Biophysical Dimension

Should certain age groups receive priority for coverage under a national health plan? If, so which age groups should receive priority?

What kinds of services should be covered under a national health plan for specific age, ethnic, or gender groups?

Should emphasis in a national health plan be placed on preventing physical health problems or dealing with existing health problems?

What specific kinds of health problems should receive emphasis in a national health plan?

Psychological Dimension

Should a national health plan cover mental health services? If so, what services should be covered?

Social Dimension

How will a national health plan address services to the poor?

How would a national health plan be financed? Would funding and coverage be tied to employment?

What cultural considerations should be included in designing a national health plan?

Would participation in a national health plan be voluntary or mandatory?

What would be the response of the general public to a national health plan?

What would be the response of major employers to a national health plan?

Behavioral Dimension

How would a national health plan address education for health behavior change?

Would a national health plan provide coverage for substance abuse treatment services?

Would participation in a national health plan be contingent on changing unhealthful behaviors?

Health System Dimension

To what extent would health care providers support the national health plan proposed?

How would provider reimbursement be handled under a national health plan?

Would all services be provided under the national health plan, or would people be able to contract for additional services if desired?

How would quality of services be assured under a national health plan?

---

providers in the United States, a system in which all providers were salaried employees of government agencies would probably be unpalatable. For this reason, a viable national health care program would most likely have to incorporate both salaried and independent modes of practice.

Diagnostic Reasoning and Health Care Reform

Based on the assessment of factors influencing health care funding and health care needs within the population, the community health nurse would develop nursing diagnoses to guide the development of national health care reform. Diagnoses would reflect the population to be covered as well as the types of services to be provided. For example, the nurse might di-

agnose a "need for a national health care reform program to provide a basic set of standardized services to all Americans due to lack of access to care among some segments of the population." A related diagnosis is a "need for attention to the health care needs of special target groups such as the very young and the very old due to their increased vulnerability to health problems." In a similar vein, the nurse might diagnose a "need for special funding programs to meet the needs of the poor, the uninsured, and the uninsurable due to their increased risk of disease and decreased access to health care."

Nursing diagnoses might also reflect the directions to be taken by national health care reform in the types of services provided. For example, the community health nurse might identify a "need for coverage of primary preventive activities for chronic and communicable diseases and for mental illness due to the high incidence, cost, and preventable nature of many of these conditions." Such a diagnosis suggests that reform plans should cover primary preventive services as well as curative and restorative services. Additional diagnoses include the "need for secondary and tertiary preventive services due to the incidence of existing health problems and the cost to society of problems left untreated."

Planning the Dimensions of Health Care Reform

Planning for health care reform should incorporate all three of the dimensions of health care—primary, secondary, and tertiary prevention; and should involve input from community health nurses who are conversant with the health care needs of the general public. Community health nurses should communicate the needs of the public to policy makers and influence the development of health care financing policy through the change and leadership processes discussed in Chapter 12 and the political processes discussed in Chapter 13.

Areas to be considered in planning national health care reforms include basic services to be covered, mechanisms for paying for care, who will provide care, where care will be provided, and relationships among providers, the health care system, and funding agencies. An effective national health care reform program needs to address plans for services at all three levels of prevention, with an emphasis on primary prevention designed to minimize the occurrence of health care problems and, thereby, reduce the overall cost of care. Primary preventive measures covered would include illness preventive services such as immunizations and education on risk factors for specific illnesses, as well as general health promotive interventions such as counseling on basic nutrition, exercise, and coping strategies.

Secondary preventive activities covered under an effective reform plan would emphasize early detection and treatment of existing physical and emotional problems to prevent exacerbation and higher costs later on. Routine screening services as recommended by the U.S. Preventive Services Task Force (1995) would be incorporated into the basic services provided under the plan (see Chapter 31 for a discussion of recommended screening procedures). The reform plan would also emphasize treatment in the least expensive setting, and treatment facilities would be made easily available to members of the population.

Tertiary prevention would also be provided, but with less emphasis than primary and secondary prevention. If primary and secondary preventive efforts are successful, there is less need for tertiary prevention.

Funding is another area to be addressed in national health care reform. As noted, proposals incorporate funding from, for example, employer contributions, individual contributions, and tax revenues. A combination of these funding sources would probably be most effective in the United States, but the reform plan would need to spell out how each aspect of funding would be handled and provide strategies to control administrative costs.

Questions of who should provide care and in what settings should be resolved by a broad range of consumer choice of providers and setting. Any reform proposal should include incentives to use cost-effective providers (eg, nurse practitioners rather than physicians for routine primary care) and to seek care in the least expensive setting possible. Community health nurses can contribute in this area through research on cost-effective modes of health care delivery.

A final consideration is that of the relationship of providers to funding sources and to the health care system in general. Should providers be independent practitioners, members of practice associations, or salaried employees? Community health nurses influencing the planning of a national health care reform program can acquaint policy makers with various options for provider–funding source relationships and the utility of independent practice by nurses. To summarize, the considerations that need to be addressed in planning health care reform include:

- Basic services covered under the plan
    Primary preventive services
    Secondary preventive services
    Tertiary preventive services
- Mechanisms for financing health care services
- Providers of health care services
- Settings in which health care services will be provided
- Relationships between health care providers and funding agencies

Implementing the Dimensions of Health Care Reform

Implementing a health care reform program includes developing sufficient support in Congress to pass the required legislation, educating both health care providers and consumers about the reform plan, and planning for incremental implementation of the plan. As noted earlier, certain vulnerable populations such as

Critical Thinking in Research

Every and associates (1995) compared resource utilization in the treatment of myocardial infarction in health maintenance organization (HMO) and fee-for-service hospitals. Outcome measures examined included use of invasive procedures and length of stay. Clients admitted to fee-for-service hospitals were 1.5 times more likely to have coronary angiography as HMO clients and twice as likely to undergo coronary revascularization. Utilization of procedures was associated with greater availability of on-site catheterization facilities at fee-for-service hospitals. Average length of stay was almost 1 day shorter in fee-for-service hospitals than in HMO hospitals.

1. What do these findings suggest about the relative cost of services in HMO and fee-for-service hospitals?
2. The findings reported above only address measures of resource utilization. How would you study the effects of these differences in resources utilized on client health outcomes?
3. What comparable measures of resource utilization might you want to study in relation to the delivery of community health services?

young children, pregnant women, the elderly, and the poor should receive priority for plan implementation.

Several strategies have been suggested for nursing to exercise its influence in plans for health care reform. Among them are unifying nursing support for reform plans; increasing visibility in campaigns for good health; marketing nursing services in health promotion; identifying the types and numbers of nurses that will be needed to implement the plans; and educating nurses, other health care providers, and policy makers about proposed plans. Nurses can also seek positions as policy makers and use political strategies discussed in Chapter 13 to develop a power base to influence legislators toward national health care reform.

Evaluating Health Care Reform

Evaluation of the effects of health care reform would be undertaken from a variety of perspectives. One evaluative criterion would be the extent to which reforms ensure access to necessary services for the entire population. Are people, particularly those who have been underserved in the past, able to receive the health-promotive, illness-preventive, curative, and restorative services needed to achieve optimal health?

A second area for evaluation would be the effects of reform on the overall cost of health care. Has the reform plan reduced expenditures or merely shifted them to other areas? Have expenditures actually increased because of the plan? If so, is this a temporary phenomenon to be replaced by long-term gains, or will health care costs continue to rise?

A third general area for evaluation would be the effects of reforms initiated on the quality of care provided. Have cost considerations lowered the quality of care provided? If so, what effect has this had on the health status of the American public? In addition, one would look at consumer satisfaction with the care received under any national health care system.

Finally, one would evaluate the outcomes of the program for those served. Here, emphasis would be placed on the effectiveness of primary, secondary, and tertiary preventive components of the program in improving the overall health of the population. Have primary preventive efforts decreased the incidence of illness? Have health-promotive efforts enhanced the health status of the population? In the area of secondary prevention, one would examine the effects of the program on morality rates and disability due to existing health problems. Are secondary preventive services provided under the plan contributing to reduced mortality from cardiovascular disease or greater longevity for persons with AIDS? Are those with existing chronic diseases better able to function adequately with less disability because of services provided? With respect to tertiary prevention, one would examine the extent to which services offered under reforms have prevented recurrent health problems and minimized complications of existing problems.

Community health nurses could be actively involved in all of these areas of evaluation. They could participate in identifying evaluative criteria, gathering evaluative data, and interpreting findings through research in these areas. Nurses should also be involved in using evaluative findings to revise or modify reform plans as needed through their use of the change, leadership, group, and political processes. To summarize, the considerations that need to be addressed in evaluating health care reform include:

- Extent to which the reform provides access to care for all people
- Effect of the reform on the overall cost of health care services
- Effect of the reform on the quality of care provided and consumer satisfaction with care
- Effect of the reform on the health status of the population in the areas of:
  Primary prevention
  Secondary prevention
  Tertiary prevention

Critical Thinking in Practice: A Case in Point

You have been appointed to the mayor's task force on health care in the midsize community in which you work as a community health nurse. The assessment of community health and economic status conducted by the task force indicates that the bulk of the population's health care needs are adequately met at all three levels of prevention. The exception to this, however, is the population of the migrant farm camp at the edge of town.

This group consists of primarily male Mexican workers who have entered the United States on legal work visas. Very few of the workers have brought their families with them. Most of this population receive no health care except for emergency treatment in the emergency room of the community hospital. Usually this case is provided for work-related injuries or serious illness. Members of this group receive no primary preventive care and do not seek care for minor illness because of their inability to pay.

Because most of these people are in the United States legally, they would be eligible for county medical assistance; however, very few have applied for this program because of language barriers, lack of transportation to the social services office, and inability to afford to take the time off work to submit an application. Even if they did receive assistance, they would be unlikely to find a regular health care provider who has a contract with the county to provide services. Only one community clinic and one independent nurse practitioner, in addition to the community hospital, have county contracts. Local physicians receive adequate income from private paying clients and those with private health insurance. Because of the extended time between provision of services and receipt of reimbursement, these physicians no longer accept county assistance clients.

The rest of the population is well off compared with state and national average incomes. With the exception of the migrant workers, most residents are employed by three large industries and receive salaries that are quite adequate to meet the cost of living. Because of the industry present in the community, the local tax base is more than adequate. The community does not budget any public funds for health care as the majority of the population are adequately served by private providers. There is no local health department, but the country offers public health services in a town 50 miles away.

1. What biophysical, psychological, physical, social, behavioral, and health system factors are influencing the health status of the migrant group?
2. How would you go about arranging to finance health care for this population group?
3. What kind of funding mechanisms might be most appropriate for providing care to the migrant population? Why?

TESTING YOUR UNDERSTANDING

1. Describe at least three ways in which economic conditions may influence the health status of the population. (pp. 280–281)
2. What two economic issues are of particular concern to community health nurses? (pp. 281–284)
3. What is retrospective reimbursement? How does it differ from prospective reimbursement? (p. 284)
4. Identify three forms of publicly funded health insurance. Describe the beneficiaries of each. (pp. 287–290)
5. Describe at least three mechanisms for reimbursing health care providers. (p. 290)
6. Identify at least four requisites for effective health care reform proposals. (p. 293)
7. Describe at least three considerations in planning for health care reform. (p. 297)

8. Describe at least three considerations in evaluating the effects of health care reform. (p. 298)

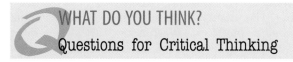

WHAT DO YOU THINK?
Questions for Critical Thinking

1. If you were going to receive direct reimbursement for community health nursing services provided to clients, would retrospective or prospective payment be more advantageous for you?
2. Which do you think is the more appropriate approach to health care reform, financing reform or systems reform? Why? Which approach is more likely to be acceptable to health care consumers? To insurers?

3. Why has more effective health care reform not been achieved before now, given the obvious need for reform?

REFERENCES

Aiken, L. H., Lake, E. T., Semaan, S., et al. (1993). Nurse practitioner managed care for persons with HIV infection. *Image, 25,* 172–177.

Bodenheimer, T. S., & Grumbach, K. (1995). *Understanding health policy: A clinical approach.* Norwalk, CT: Appleton & Lange.

Centers for Disease Control. (1995). Prevention and managed care: Opportunities for managed care organizations, purchasers of health care, and public health agencies. *MMWR, 44*(RR–14), 1–12.

Citizen Action. (1994, January). Comparison of key Congressional health care reform bills—1993. *The Nation's Health,* 14–16.

Davis, K. (1996). *Medicaid: The health care safety net for the nation's poor.* New York: The Common Wealth Fund.

Duerksen, S. (January 10, 1993). Getting a grip on jargon of a national health plan. *San Diego Union Tribune,* B-3.

Dunham-Taylor, J., Marquette, P., & Pinczuk, J. Z. (1996). Surviving capitation: How to minimize your risk and maximize your opportunities as the eclipse of fee-for-service pricing continues. *American Journal of Nursing, 96*(3), 26–29.

Every, N. R., Fihn, S. D., Maynard, C., Martin, J. S., & Weaver, D. (1995). Resource utilization in treatment of acute myocardial infarction: Staff-model health maintenance organization versus fee-for-service hospitals. *Journal of the American College of Cardiology, 26,* 401–406.

Feldstein, P. J. (1993). *Health care economics* (4th ed.). Albany, NY: Delmar.

Gale, B. J., & Steffl, B. M. (1992). The long-term care dilemma: What nurses need to know about Medicare. *Nursing & Health Care, 13,* 34–41.

Harris, M. (1996). Medicare as secondary payer. *Home Healthcare Nurse, 14*(1), 51–53.

Hart, S. (1995). *Managed care curriculum for baccalaureate nursing programs.* Washington, DC: American Nurses Foundation of the American Nurses Association.

Hosek, J., & Levine, R. (1996). An introduction to the issues. In J. Hosek & R. Levine (Eds.), *The new fiscal federalism and the social safety net* (pp. 1–17). RAND.

Jordan, S. (1994, October). Special interests pay high premium for no health care reform. *The Nation's Health,* 4.

Karpatkin, R. H., & Shearer, G. E. (1995). A short-term consumer agenda for health care reform. *American Journal of Public Health, 85,* 1352–1355.

Kerr, C. E. (1996). The case for managed care. In E. D. Baer, C. M. Fagin, & S. Gordon (Eds.), *Abandonment of the patient: The impact of profit-driven health care on the public* (pp. 57–64). New York: Springer.

Kletke, P. R., Emmons, D. W., & Gillis, K. D. (1996). Current trends in physicians' practice arrangements. *JAMA, 276,* 555–560.

Lamm, R. R. (1990). The 10 commandments of health care. In P. R. Lee & C. L. Estes (Eds.), *The nation's health* (3rd ed.) (pp. 124–133). Boston: Jones and Bartlett.

Leibowitz, A., & DuPlessis, H. (1996). Restructuring the Medicaid program. In J. Hosek & R. Levine (Eds.), *The new fiscal federalism and the social safety net* (pp. 101–126). RAND.

Longest, B. B., Jr. (1994). *Health policy making in the United States.* Ann Arbor, MI: AUPHA Press.

Ludlam, D. (1992, Spring). Curing what ails our health-care system. *USD Magazine,* 8–13.

MacLaren, E. (June 2, 1994). Basics of managed care. *NURSEweek,* 10–11.

Melillo, K. D. (1996). Medicare and Medicaid: Similarities and differences. *Journal of Gerontological Nursing, 22*(7), 12–21.

Miller, D. F. (1995). *Dimensions of community health* (4th ed.). Dubuque, IA: W. C. Brown.

Mundinger, M. O. (1994). Health care reform: Will nursing respond? *Nursing & Health Care, 15,* 28–33.

National Center for Injury Prevention and Control. (1994). Medical-care spending—United States. *MMWR, 43,* 581–586.

National Immunization Program. (1994). Implementation of the Medicare influenza vaccination benefit—United States, 1993. *MMWR, 43,* 771–773.

National League for Nursing. (1993, April). The financing of health care reform. *NLN's Health Care Update,* 1–2.

Newell, M. (1996). *Using nursing case management to improve health outcomes.* Gaithersburg, MD: Aspen.

Nichols, L. (1996, January). *Nonphysician health care providers: Use of ambulatory services, expenditures, and sources of payment.* Washington, DC: U.S. Department of Health and Human Services.

NURSEweek. (1994, April). NPs stymied in battle over Medicaid reimbursement. 4.

O'Grady, T. P. (1994). Building partnerships in health care: Creating whole systems change. *Nursing & Health Care, 15,* 34–38.

Perkins, C. B., & Perkins, K. C. (1992). Uncompensated care: The millstone around the neck of U.S. health care. *Nursing & Health Care, 13,* 20–23.

Powell, S. K. (1996). *Nursing case management: A practical guide to success in managed care.* Philadelphia: Lippincott-Raven.

Raymond, A. G. (1994). *HMO health care companion: A consumer's guide to managed care networks.* New York: Harper Perennial.

Regan, M. (1994). Medicaid reimbursement: Can we save money by paying doctors more? *American Journal of Public Health, 84,* 548–549.

Riley, G. F., Potosky, A. L., Lubitz, J. D., & Brown, M. L. (1994). Stage of cancer at diagnosis for Medicare HMO and fee-for-service enrollees. *American Journal of Public Health, 84,* 1598–1604.

Rooney, E. (1990). Corporate attitudes and responses to rising health care costs. *AAOHN Journal, 38,* 304–311.

Rowland, S., & Salganicoff, A. (1994). Lessons from Medicaid: Improving access to office-based physician care for the low-income population. *American Journal of Public Health, 84,* 548–549.

Salmon, M. E. (1995). Public health policy: Creating a healthy future for the American public. *Family and community health, 18*(1), 1–11.

U.S. Department of Commerce. (1993). *Statistical Abstract of the United States, 1993* (113th ed.). Washington, DC: Government Printing Office.

U.S. Department of Commerce. (1996). *Statistical Abstract of the United States, 1996* (116th ed.). Washington, DC: Government Printing Office.

U.S. Department of Health and Human Services. (1996). *HCFA Statistics.* Washington, DC: U.S. Department of Health and Human Services.

U.S. Preventive Health Services Task Force. (1995). *Guide to clinical preventive services* (2nd ed.). Baltimore: Williams & Wilkins.

Vladek, B. (1996). The corporatization of American health care and why it is happening. In E. D. Baer, C. M. Fagin, & S. Gordon (Eds.), *Abandonment of the patient: The impact of profit-driven health care on the public* (pp. 9–19). New York: Springer.

Ware, J. E., Bayliss, M. S., Rogers, W. H., Kosinski, M., & Tarlov, A. R. (1996). Differences in 4-year health outcomes for elderly and poor, chronically ill patients treated in HMO and fee-for-service systems. *JAMA, 276,* 1039–1047.

White House Domestic Policy Council. (1993). *Health security: The President's report to the American people.* Washington, DC: Government Printing Office.

Young, Q. D. (1993). Health care reform: A new public health movement. *American Journal of Public Health, 83,* 945–946.

RESOURCES FOR HEALTH CARE FINANCING

Committee for National Health Insurance
1757 N Street, NW
Washington, DC 20036
(202) 223–9685

Health Economics Research, Inc.
300 Fifth Avenue, 6th Floor
Waltham, MA 02154
(617) 487–0200

International Health Policy and Management Institute
c/o Paul Detrick
Christian Health Service Development Corporation
10133 Dunn Road, Ste. 400
St. Louis, MO 63136
(314) 355–0009

Nurses for National Health Care
PO Box 441021
Somerville, MA 02144
(617) 623–3001

Physicians for a National Health Program
332 S Michigan Avenue, Ste. 500
Chicago, IL 60604–4302
(312) 554–0382

U. S. Department of Health & Human Services
Health Care Financing Administration
200 Independence Avenue, SW
Washington, DC 20201
(202) 690–6726

U.S. Department of Health & Human Services
Social Security Administration
6401 Security Bldg.
Baltimore, MD 21235
(301) 594–3120

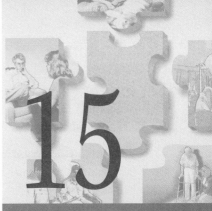

ETHICAL INFLUENCES ON COMMUNITY HEALTH

The goal of community health nurses is to enhance the health of the public. But what happens when enhancing the health of one segment of the population harms others? Or, what happens when enhancing the health of a single individual harms that individual in some other way?

Community health nurses are concerned with such ethical questions. Medical ethics deals with values, choices, and personal moral behavior as they pertain to interactions with individual clients. Community health ethics, on the other hand, relates to those same values, choices, and social morality as applied to the health of population groups. Although both types of ethics are important to community health nurses, the ethics of providing health care for individuals and their families is addressed in other books. This chapter focuses on the ethics of providing health care to population groups.

To answer ethical questions, community health nurses need a working knowledge of ethical theory. That knowledge assists the community health nurse first, to recognize ethical issues. Second, it is the basis for discussing and understanding moral issues. Finally, it creates an openness to alternative interpretations of correct behavior in a given situation (Zucker, Borchert, & Stewart, 1992). When community health nurses develop insight into the values underlying their own perspectives of an ethical situation, they are better able to appreciate the perspectives of others. This chapter presents an overview of several perspectives on ethical decision making.

▶ ## Chapter Objectives

After reading this chapter, you should be able to:

- Describe the relationship between ethics and values.
- Distinguish between consequentialist and nonconsequentialist ethical perspectives.
- Describe at least five perspectives on ethical decision making.
- Identify at least two sources of ethical dilemmas in health care.
- Describe at least four ethical dilemmas encountered in community health practice.
- Identify two levels of nursing diagnosis related to an ethical dilemma.
- Describe two tasks in planning to resolve an ethical dilemma.

▶ ## ETHICS AND VALUES

Ethics is defined as a "philosophic analysis of morality, the systematic endeavor to understand moral concepts and justify moral principles and theories" (Pojman, 1992). Principles provide general guides to action (Husted & Husted, 1991). Rules, on the other hand, are somewhat more specific and delineate what must be done, must not be done, or may be done, morally speaking, in a given situation.

Relationship of Values to Ethical Decision Making

An *ethical dilemma* is a conflict between two or more possible courses of action in a given situation. The conflict arises when strongly held values that underlie the potential choices are incompatible with each other. For example, as nurses we value self-determination for clients. We also value the client's safety. What course of action do we take, then, when an elderly client at high risk for falls persists in getting out of bed alone? If we restrain the client, we are violating his or her right to self-determination. If we do not, we jeopardize his or her safety. Both outcomes, safety and self-determination, are equally desirable, but only one can be achieved, leading to an ethical dilemma or a need to choose the best or "right" course of action.

When faced with an ethical dilemma, we engage in moral reasoning to choose the best course of action. *Moral reasoning* is the thought processes used to differentiate among possible courses of action and to select a moral or "right" alternative. The actions selected constitute ethical nursing practice, or the actions taken by nurses in ethical situations.

Perspectives on Ethical Decision Making

Values conflicts give rise to ethical dilemmas. Values also underlie the perspectives from which we attempt to resolve these dilemmas. Over the years, philosophers and ethicists have developed a variety of perspectives on ethical decision making. Some early or traditional perspectives have been supplanted by or refined in more contemporary perspectives. Each of these perspectives is based on one or more values that are given priority and that guide action in ethical situations. Several of these traditional and contemporary perspectives and their underlying values are listed in Table 15–1.

From the perspective of *altruism,* love of others is the determining principle or value. Doing what is best for others, even at the risk of one's own harm, becomes the guiding rule in ethical decisions. Related ethical perspectives are found in virtue ethics, stoicism, and the ethics of care. The decision maker with a *virtue ethics* perspective chooses a course of action that exemplifies heroism and virtues valued in society.

Stoicism is an ethical perspective that values virtues of another kind, those dealing with personal fortitude rather than interactions with others. The emphasis in the *ethics of caring* is on care for others who are in need. This is a particularly relevant perspective for caring professions such as nursing. Potential for conflict arises between the perspectives of stoicism and caring when the stoic in need of care refuses it. Another difficulty with the caring perspective is that it does not provide guidelines for deciding between two individuals or groups who need care when care can only be provided to one (Bandman & Bandman, 1995).

Rational paternalism is another ethical perspective that focuses on a caring attitude toward others. From this perspective, however, the decision maker is assumed to know what is best for the beneficiary of action. The paternalistic perspective is in direct opposition to those perspectives that value self-determination (Husted & Husted, 1992).

Collectivism focuses on the good of the larger society and equality in the distribution of goods and services. Collectivism is the underlying principle that gave rise to communism. The concept of societal benefit is also the underlying principle of the utilitarian perspective. *Utilitarianism* is an ethical approach in which decisions are based on perceptions of the greatest good or happiness (or the least harm) for the greatest number of people (Ashley & O'Rourke, 1994). The overriding ethical principle in this perspective is *beneficence,* the doing of good for the client.

The principle of beneficence requires that the community health nurse or other health care provider

TABLE 15–1. SOME TRADITIONAL AND CONTEMPORARY ETHICAL PERSPECTIVES AND THEIR UNDERLYING VALUES

Traditional		Contemporary	
Perspective	**Values**	**Perspective**	**Values**
Altruism	Love of others	Altruism	Love of others
		Collectivism	Group good, equality, social change
Duty-based	Free will, equality, promise keeping, truth telling	Duty-based	Obligations and responsibilities
Egoism	Personal good		
Epicureanism	Pleasure		
		Ethics of caring	Care for others
Eudaimonism	Happiness, high-mindedness, generosity, friendship, liberality, confidence, self-realization		
Existentialism	Authenticity, good faith	Existentialism	Individual decision making, responsibility
Individualism	Self-regard	Libertarianism	Self-determination, individual liberty
		Justice-based	Equality, fairness
Relativism	Determined by individual or group	Relativism and subjectivism	Determined by culture
Rational paternalism	Love, wisdom, well-being, knowledge, courage, temperance, piety		
		Rights-based	Self-determination
Stoicism	Endurance, resignation, self-denial	Stoicism	Endurance, resignation, self-denial
Utilitarianism (classic)	Greatest good	Utilitarianism (contemporary)	Majority good
		Virtue ethics	Courage, honesty, wisdom, prudence, responsibility, temperance

(Source: Bandman and Bandman, 1995.)

take positive steps to help clients. These steps may involve preventing harm to the client (sometimes referred to as nonmaleficence or nonmalfesance [Nelson, 1997]), removing harm, or actively promoting the client's good (Smith, 1995).

The perspective of individualism is in direct opposition to those of collectivism and utilitarianism. The overriding principles of *individualism* are those of personal liberty, self-determination, self-reliance, initiative, and self-realization. Individualistic principles underlie capitalism and are strongly valued in U.S. society. *Existentialism* is one form of individualism in which individuals are to be held responsible for their actions because they have freedom of choice with respect to those actions. Collectivism, on the other hand, absolves individuals and places responsibility for action with society as a whole (Bandman & Bandman, 1995).

Libertarianism is another ethical perspective related to individualism. In *libertarianism,* the overriding value to be considered in an ethical dilemma is individual liberty. From this perspective, no action should be taken that violates freedom of choice even if that action would bring benefit to the persons constrained. A closely related perspective is *rights-based ethics,* in which the right to self-determination is one of several rights attributed to people by virtue of their humanness. Belief in innate rights to life, liberty, and the pursuit of happiness provided the philosophical justification for the American Revolution. One hotly

debated issue in this area is the notion of a right to health care.

A perceived right to a share of society's goods is the source of the related justice-based ethical perspective. The principle of *justice,* or equity, involves the fair distribution of benefits and burdens among members of society (Drane, 1994). Under the principle of justice, all things being equal, all groups of people should be treated equally. There are several ways of viewing justice. The first is in terms of the *egalitarian principle*—that all individuals are entitled to an equal share of available goods and services. The second view is that goods and services should first be provided to those most in need. In this view, distribution of goods and services should benefit those who are the least advantaged in society.

From the perspective of *duty-based ethics,* one acts on the basis of duties and responsibilities that arise out of an assumed position, a contractual arrangement, or duty to God as expressed in commandments. Other terms used for this perspective are *deontology* (Ashley & O'Rourke, 1994) and *contractarianism.*

The last three ethical perspectives to be addressed are those that benefit the person making the ethical decision. *Egoism* is an ethical perspective in which ethical decisions are based on what is best for the decision maker. The community health nurse, or other policy maker, who acts from an egoist perspective makes decisions based on self-interest.

From the perspective of *epicureanism,* action should be based on what brings the greatest pleasure for oneself. Like egoism and epicureanism, *eudaimonism* is based on self-interest, but the good sought is happiness as a result of self-realization (Bandman & Bandman, 1995).

Many ethicists classify the perspectives presented here as either consequentialist or nonconsequentialist. *Consequentialist perspectives* are those in which ethical decisions are based on the consequences (intended or actual) of an action rather than on the action itself. Other terms used for consequentialist perspectives are *situational ethics* and *teleological ethics* (Ashley & O'Rourke, 1994). Examples of consequentialist perspectives include individualism, egoism, utilitarianism, and libertarianism. From the consequentialist perspective, the morality of a particular act is judged on whether or not it results in a good outcome.

Nonconsequentialist perspectives are those in which ethical decisions are based not on the outcome of an action, but on the rightness or wrongness of the action itself (Drane, 1994). According to these perspectives, certain rules or duties are unchanging and apply to all situations. Professional codes of ethics such as the American Nurses Association Code of Ethics and the International Council of Nurses Code for Nurses are based on notions of duty and are derived from nonconsequentialist perspectives. Examples of nonconsequentialist perspectives include duty-based ethics, altruism, and virtue ethics.

Each of the ethical decision-making perspectives presented here may be brought to bear on ethical dilemmas encountered in community health nursing. Next we turn to some of the sources of ethical dilemmas and the types of dilemmas faced by community health nurses.

Sources of Ethical Dilemmas in Health Care

Ethical dilemmas in health care arise from societal factors that place values in conflict. One source of ethical dilemmas in health care is society's choice of some goals over others. When society chooses to work toward certain goals, values implicit in those goals are emphasized, and the values implicit in other goals are minimized. For example, because the U.S. health care system has emphasized curative care, the value of preventive care has been minimized. Conversely, a focus on prevention would minimize the values inherent in the care of people with existing health problems. In a society that does not have the resources to provide the needed level of care in both areas, the need to choose one focus over the other create an ethical dilemma.

Another source of ethical dilemmas in health care is the choice of target groups that will benefit from health care programs. The choice of one segment of the population as beneficiaries discriminates against other groups constrained by limited resources. For instance, health care programs that assist the poor, such as Medicaid, discriminate against those with moderate incomes who are not eligible for services but who must pay for them through taxes.

A third source of ethical dilemmas is the means chosen to achieve some common public health care goal. Approaches that seem to benefit the majority of the population might infringe on the right of certain other individuals. Prohibiting smoking in public buildings, for example, infringes on the rights of smokers.

Finally, ethical dilemmas in health care can arise as consequences of social change. For example, a declining economy and reduced tax base might force policy makers to curtail some health care services. The choice of what services to curtail could constitute an ethical dilemma because any reduction in services will affect some group of consumers adversely.

Ethical Dilemmas in Community Health

Health care providers, including community health nurses, are faced with a variety of ethical dilemmas that affect the health status of population groups. These include determining whether responsibility for health lies with the individual or with the society; deciding on the preeminence of one individual's rights over another's; individual or societal good; allocating scarce resources; and dealing with issues related to quality versus quantity of life.

Personal or Societal Responsibility for Health

Ethical questions related to responsibility for health can be of two types. The first deals with a person's right to make health-related decisions; the second deals with the extent to which society is responsible for providing health care for its citizens.

Personal freedom is one of the hallmarks of American society. But freedom can have its limits. Should one be free to make one's own decisions regarding health matters, or is this an area in which government regulation is appropriate?

The ethical dilemma here often takes the form of controversies over whether individuals should be compelled to engage in behaviors that are for their own good. Examples of such dilemmas include controversies over compulsory helmet laws for motorcyclists or compulsory tests of thyroid function for all newborns. For cases in which the activity of one person is obviously harmful to another, it is easier to decide that the freedom of one individual should not be construed as liberty to harm others; however, when it can be argued that one's behavior (eg, not wearing a seat belt or riding a motorcycle without a helmet) does not directly harm others, should one be allowed to make one's own decisions? An affirmative answer to this question would be based on the value of self-determination, whereas arguments that people need to be prevented from engaging in unhealthful behaviors would be based on a duty to safeguard one's health. A related question is that of client noncompliance, an area found to be of concern to community health nurses in one study (Turner, Marquis, & Burman, 1996).

Should one who chooses to act in an unhealthful manner be held responsible for the consequences of that choice, or does society have a responsibility for the health of these people? Should the smoker who develops lung cancer, for example, be held responsible for the costs of expensive therapy needed to treat his or her disease? Or does society have some responsibility to assist the individual to deal with the consequences of his or her actions?

Questions of individual versus societal responsibility repeatedly arise in health care. Who should pay for the lifetime expenses of the quadriplegic injured in a motorcycle accident? Should the person injured pay the costs for care if he or she was not wearing a helmet? Should society assume these costs if the motorcyclist took appropriate precautions, but injury occurred anyway? Some authors point out that assigning responsibility for one's behavior assumes that the specific consequences of that behavior for health are known (eg, supported by research findings) and understood by the individual involved. They caution that this perspective may result in *blaming the victim* or assigning total responsibility for health to the actions of the individual without acknowledging the influence of social and environmental factors.

The second aspect of the question of personal versus societal responsibility for health is the extent of society's responsibility to provide health care services. The answer lies in the way in which society defines health (Reinhardt, 1990). If health is defined as a *social good*, one that benefits all of society, health care should be financed by the society at large. If health and health care are perceived as *private consumption goods*, goods that benefit the individual and can be obtained if one can afford them, like a car or a swimming pool, health care should be financed by the individual recipient. Unfortunately, this question has not yet been adequately resolved in American society.

Individual Versus Individual

A second type of ethical dilemma arises in community health when the rights of one individual are incompatible with the rights or another. One example of this type of dilemma lies in the decision to prosecute women who continue their pregnancies after known fetal drug exposure. The values in conflict are the safety of the fetus and the women's right of self-determination (Weiss & Hansell, 1992). A similar conflict of values occurs in questions of abortion. If the sanctity of life is the paramount value, abortion is unethical. If one's right to self-determination is the more important value, abortion is an ethical choice. This choice is difficult in view of nurses' respect for the worth and dignity of each individual.

Another conflict between the rights of individuals lies in decisions by health care providers to refuse care to certain clients when that care may threaten their own health or safety. Arguments in support of providers' right to refuse to care for someone with HIV infection, for example, are based on libertarian values of self-determination, whereas counterarguments are supported by duty-based or justice perspectives. Nursing has attempted to address the question of refusal to care for a client based on potential harm to the nurse. According to the American Nurses Association Committee on Ethics, nurses must care for clients except when the risk to the nurse outweighs the benefit to the client (Thomasma & Marshall, 1994). Denial of service would occur before the community health nurse or other provider has assumed responsibility for care of the client. Client *abandonment*, on the other hand, is defined as the severing of a nurse–client relationship for which the nurse has accepted responsibility without providing for another source of needed care (Claar-Rice, 1993).

A related conflict of individual rights arises from the converse situation in which a health care provider is infected with HIV virus (Thomasma & Marshall, 1994). Does the provider have an obligation to inform clients and give them the opportunity to find another provider? The values in conflict here are the client's safety and the health care provider's rights to privacy, self-determination, and a source of livelihood.

Individual Versus Societal Good

An ethical dilemma closely related to the previous discussion is the relative merit of individual rights or good versus those of the society at large, when the two are in conflict. Does a person with a communicable disease, for instance, have a right to refuse treatment if he or she is likely to infect others? Or does society have a right to impose some restrictions on individual freedoms to protect the health of the majority?

Perhaps the most compelling ethical conflict of this sort today is the need to protect the identity of individuals who test positive for HIV, the virus that causes AIDS, versus the need to protect others from becoming infected. Control of AIDS is hampered in many jurisdictions because of privacy laws that expressly prohibit notifying contacts that they have been exposed to HIV. In this instance, the right of the individual to privacy has been given primacy over the rights of others to know of possible infection and over the rights of still others to be protected from exposure to a fatal disease. In view of concerns for both confidentiality and protection from harm, several criteria have been proposed for determining the appropriateness of mandatory screening and reporting of HIV test results (Gostin & Curran, 1987). These criteria include expectations that:

1. The target population has an identified reservoir of infection.
2. The environment of the population poses a significant risk of spreading the disease.
3. Knowledge of test results would enable authorities to take preventive measures.
4. The consequences of testing would not outweigh the benefits.
5. There are no other alternatives that would be as effective in meeting health objectives.

In some states confidentiality statutes have been relaxed to allow notification of contacts to persons with HIV-positive tests. Contacts can then engage in measures to prevent the spread of the disease to others; however, many HIV-infected persons fail to notify sexual partners of their exposure (Bayer & Toomey, 1992). In one California case, the court ruled that health care providers have an obligation to protect third parties from harm even if doing so means violating client confidentiality (Kleinman, 1987). Although the legal status of the issue may have been addressed, the ethical question remains whether the individual right to confidentiality outweighs the right of others to know of their possible exposure. Another aspect of harm that must be considered in contact notification is the potential for violent abuse of HIV-infected individuals by their sexual partners (Rothenberg & Paskey, 1995).

Some ethicists have asserted that any situation in which societal rights clearly take precedence must be necessarily related to the common good. In many instances, however, it is difficult to make that distinction, and health care providers must use their own ethical principles to resolve the ethical dilemma.

Others have made the point that an emphasis on populationwide benefits may distort decisions with respect to individual clients. It may be that, in the interests of enhancing the overall health status of society, individuals are being subtly coerced to more healthful behaviors. A case in point is the tremendous pressure brought to bear on people to quit smoking. The ethical conflict lies in the individual's freedom to determine his or her own behavior versus society's right to decrease the societal costs of such conditions as heart disease and cancer.

Resource Allocation

Another ethical dilemma that faces today's public health policy makers is the allocation of scarce health care resources (Zucker, Borchert, & Stewart, 1992). Modern medical technology makes possible many previously undreamed of health benefits. Unfortunately, because of limited economic resources, not all of this medical technology can be made available to everyone.

Allocation decisions take place at two levels. *Macroallocation* involves decisions about the distribution of health care resources among groups of people. *Microallocation,* on the other hand, is allocation of resources to individuals within the groups selected at the macroallocation level. Examples of macroallocation decisions would be choosing to allocate a larger portion of health care resources to children than to the elderly or to wellness-oriented rather than illness-oriented services. A microallocation decision might be to provide a kidney transplant for child A rather than child B. Both types of allocation decisions are, essentially, forms of rationing although this term is rarely used (Kelly, 1994). Without a clear national direction for health care policies related to resource use, allocation decisions are made in a fragmented and ineffective way. In fact, the United States has been described as having a "nonsystem of rationing" (Berkowitz, cited in Gray, 1995).

Quality Versus Quantity of Life

Ethical dilemmas related to the quality of life versus the length or quantity of life abound in today's society. Does a person have the right to refuse extraordinary treatment to prolong life? Does one have the right to terminate his or her life? Does one have the right to decide the manner in which he or she dies when death is imminent? Some of the approaches taken to resolve these dilemmas are examined here.

Extraordinary Treatment Measures. Most of the ethical perspectives discussed earlier, except perhaps stoicism, would recognize an individual's right to refuse extraordinary treatment measures to prolong life when death is imminent. American society has legalized this moral right through the mechanism of advance directives. *Advance directives* are legal statements, made by a mentally competent client before the need for extraordinary measures arises, delineating their wishes in this area.

Advance directives usually take one of two forms, instructional documents or proxy documents (Clark, 1994). The most common type of instructional document is a *living will*, a document drawn up and signed by an individual stating that the signer chooses not to be subjected to certain extraordinary lifesaving measures should the time arise when he or she is unable to make choices regarding care.

Because a client's wishes may change with circumstances and because a living will cannot specify every conceivable circumstance, many people have chosen to execute proxy documents, the most common of which is a durable power of attorney, instead of a living will. A *durable power of attorney* is a legal document giving a designated person the authority to make health care decisions for the client in the event he or she becomes mentally incapacitated and incapable of making such decisions (Clark, 1994).

The use of advance directives was further institutionalized in American society by the passage of the federal Patient Determination Act which took effect in 1991. Under this legislation, all health care institutions that receive reimbursement under Medicare and Medicaid are required to inform clients of their rights to refuse treatment and to execute advance directives. Paradoxically, some ethicists have suggested that informing clients of this right may subtly pressure them to execute advance directives when they do not wish to do so, violating the value of self-determination while attempting to protect it.

Clients' desires may change, and advanced directives may provide some leeway in the kind of decisions that can be made. For this reason, the community health nurse may want to explore with competent clients who have executed advance directives how closely they wish their advance directives followed. Community health nurses should also determine whether or not clients' primary providers are aware of the existence of advanced directives. Some studies have shown that providers may not be aware of advance directives for their clients (Connors, et al., 1995; Morrison, Olson, Mertz, & Meier, 1995). When advanced directives are brought to providers' attention, however, they tend to influence treatment decisions (Morrison, et al., 1995).

Another consideration related to use of specific treatment measures is medical futility. Occasionally, it is not the client, but the provider, who makes the decision that a specific treatment, or indeed any treatment, may be inappropriate in a given situation. *Medical futility* is the determination that a particular therapy is of no value and should not be given. Decisions of medical futility are usually made on the basis of four considerations. Is the treatment physiologically capable of achieving the desired effect? For example, antibiotics cannot cure cancer and so would not be used for this purpose. Would the treatment benefit the client or cause disproportionate harm? For example, removal of a stomach tumor would be of little benefit if the cancer has metastasized to multiple organs, or surgery might cause additional pain without providing any marked benefit. A third consideration is whether the treatment is likely to achieve the desired result in view of the overall client situation. Finally, a therapeutic approach may be futile if there is minimal research to support the probability of the desired effect despite its theoretical plausibility (Miles, 1994).

Euthanasia.   Advance directives and medical futility are related to the issue of withholding extraordinary measure to prolong life. A related issue not addressed by these responses is euthanasia. *Euthanasia is* the practice of providing a merciful death for those who are hopelessly sick or injured. Euthanasia can be voluntary, involuntary, or nonvoluntary, active or passive (Perrett, 1996). In voluntary euthanasia, life is terminated with the consent of the person involved. In involuntary euthanasia, the person's consent has not been obtained even though he or she is capable of consenting; whereas in nonvoluntary euthanasia, the person is incapable of consent or dissent. Legally, both involuntary and nonvoluntary euthanasia are equivalent to murder. Passive euthanasia involves failure to use measures that would prolong life and is addressed by advance directives.

Active euthanasia involves the use of interventions that bring about death sooner than would otherwise be the case. Active euthanasia, or "mercy killing," is currently illegal in all states. Another concept related to active voluntary euthanasia is *assisted suicide*. In assisted suicide, health care personnel provide clients with the means or information to facilitate death. In euthanasia, on the other hand, the provider engages in actions that directly cause death (Devine, 1996). Legislative efforts to legalize the practice are aimed at eliminating criminal prosecution for health care providers and loved ones who assist terminally ill individuals to commit suicide.

Arguments supporting legislation permitting active voluntary euthanasia often advance the claim that current laws force physicians to keep clients alive in violation of clients' wishes, force clients to endure pain and loss of dignity, and abrogate clients' absolute rights to control their own health care decisions. Opponents of such legislation argue that individuals can choose to refuse treatment and die in the normal course of events. Further, it is argued that although terminally ill patients may suffer pain and other consequences of disease, termination of life is an inappropriate approach to symptom control (Kowalski, 1993). Rather, efforts should be directed at providing symptom relief and restoring the dignity of the terminally ill.

Finally, opponents of legislation permitting active voluntary euthanasia argue that the right to self-determination may not be exercised to the harm of others. Such legislation might be interpreted as a mandate requiring health care providers to assist clients in active euthanasia, possibly forcing providers to violate their own ethical principles. Harm might also occur to clients and society if such legislation is interpreted as condoning involuntary euthanasia, as has occurred in The Netherlands. In such an event, persons felt to be a drain on society might be eliminated with or without their consent. To prevent the potential for such harm to individuals, to health care providers, and to society, many ethicists believe continued prohibition of active euthanasia is warranted (Carlson, 1997).

▶ THE DIMENSIONS MODEL AND ETHICAL DILEMMAS

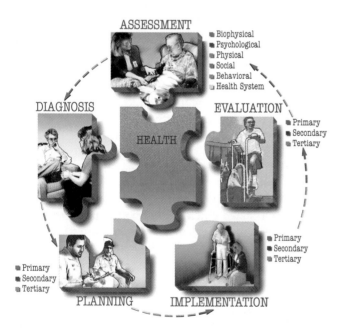

The ethical dilemmas discussed here have implications for the behavior of community health nurses at both individual and aggregate client levels. At the individual level, the community health nurse would function as a client advocate, ensuring that the health care provided to clients and their families is based on sound ethical principles. Community health nurses do not usually make unilateral ethical decisions at the aggregate level, but they have a responsibility to ensure that health policy is consistent with ethical principles.

To promote ethical action at both the individual and aggregate client levels, community health nurses must examine their own ethical values and use an approach to ethical decision making consistent with those values. Ethical decision making should be a deliberative process engaged in by nurses and others involved in an ethical dilemma. Deliberation in an ethical dilemma can be guided by the use of the Dimensions Model. Using the model in an ethical dilemma, the community health nurse would not only facilitate assessment and diagnosis of the ethical situation but also participate in planning, implementing, and evaluating actions to be taken to resolve the dilemma.

Critical Dimensions of Nursing in an Ethical Dilemma

The most important elements of nursing in an ethical dilemma lie in the skills and interpersonal dimensions. In the skills dimension, the community health nurse uses the intellectual skills of diagnosis and analysis to identify the factors creating the ethical dilemma and influencing its resolution. The ability to prioritize values, another intellectual skill, will assist the community health nurse to determine an appropriate course of action in an ethical dilemma. In the interpersonal dimension, communication skills will aid the nurse in communicating the ethical dilemma, as well as the clients' perspective of the situation, to other members of the health care team.

Elements of other dimensions of community health nursing are also important. In the cognitive dimension, the nurse must have a sound knowledge of the client's condition and the likely effects of various forms of therapy. Knowledge of cultural beliefs and values will also allow the nurse to intervene more effectively in ethical situations. Finally, the process dimension elements of leadership, change, and group dynamics may also assist the nurse to promote more effective ethical decision making.

 Assessing the Dimensions of the Ethical Dilemma

The community health nurse and others involved in ethical decision making assess both factors that contribute to an ethical dilemma and those that influence decisions on an appropriate course of action. Some ethicists refer to this as the expository phase of ethical decision making (Devine, 1996; Drane, 1994). This assessment can be conducted from a health dimensions perspective.

The Biophysical Dimension

Human biological factors can influence both an ethical dilemma and decisions regarding its resolution. For example, the ages of persons involved might be an influencing factor. The decision to perform a hysterectomy would be easier if the woman is past childbearing age than if she is younger and wants to have children. On the one hand, the younger woman may want to be cured of her uterine cancer; on the other hand, she may also desire to have a child. The decision becomes even more complicated if the physiologic factor of pregnancy is added. Should the woman have the hysterectomy, or should she carry the pregnancy to term?

Another example of age as an influencing factor might arise in resource allocation decisions related to the use of expensive medical technology. If the recipients of organ transplants are primarily young children, policy makers may decide that this is a more worthwhile expenditure of available health care funds than if most recipients are elderly. The reasoning here is that children who are saved through transplants have their entire lives ahead of them and can become productive members of society, whereas older persons have already lived most of their lives and would have a limited number of productive years left even with the transplant.

As noted earlier with respect to pregnancy, physiologic factors may also affect ethical dilemmas and decisions related to them. For example, in a situation of limited resources, policy makers might choose to provide care to those who are in relatively good health, judging that their chances of survival are greater than those who have other debilitating life-threatening conditions.

The Psychological Dimension

Ethical issues are usually emotionally charged, and the psychological dimension can greatly influence decisions. For example, the fear of contracting AIDS has led some health care providers to refuse care to people with AIDS. Similarly, feelings about crime and criminals influence decisions about the provision of health care in correctional settings.

The Social Dimension

Social dimension factors can also influence ethical dilemmas. Fear of malpractice suits may influence providers in decisions to terminate or continue life support services. The cost of health care and lack of access to care also contribute to ethical dilemmas. For example, should parents be held responsible for their child's death from pertussis because they failed to obtain immunizations they could not afford?

Cultural beliefs about human dignity, self-determination, and the worth of human life also contribute to ethical dilemmas. In the United States, for example, where personal liberty is a predominant value, health care policies that curtail individual freedom in favor of the common good are frequently resisted. In making such decisions, policy makers have to take into account the relative merits of personal liberty versus the benefit to society of curtailing certain liberties.

Similarly, beliefs about the worth of individuals often influence situations in which policy makers must decide between allocating resources to care for those with existing illness and preventing illness in the larger population. With a cultural value of individual worth, it is difficult to decide that society will not pay for a liver transplant for a sick child because the money is needed to keep other children healthy. Beliefs about human dignity and the value of life can also influence policy decisions related to living wills, hospice care, and euthanasia.

Predominant values may differ widely from one cultural group to another. For this reason, the community health nurse involved in an ethical dilemma not only must consider the values held by a particular group, but must also ascertain the degree to which a given clients' acculturation has altered those values. Religious background also plays a significant part in determining values.

The Behavioral Dimension

Behavioral factors play a part in the development or resolution of ethical dilemmas. Sometimes the dilemma itself arises out of behaviors related to lifestyle. For example, should society accept the burden of care for someone who is injured while hang gliding? Should the motorcyclist who refuses to wear a helmet or the person who drinks and drives be eligible for public assistance in overcoming the effects of a serious accident?

Other ethical dilemmas arise out of Americans' commitment to personal freedom and independence. To what extent should society be allowed to compel healthful behaviors such as the use of seat belts and the avoidance of smoking? In what circumstances does the protection of society supersede individual rights?

ASSESSMENT TIPS: Ethical Dilemmas

Biophysical Dimension

What are the ages of persons involved in the ethical dilemma?

Is age likely to make a difference in the outcome of the ethical dilemma?

What is the physiologic status of persons involved in the ethical dilemma?

What is the prognosis in the ethical dilemma?

Are there other physiologic conditions (eg, pregnancy) that may influence ethical decision making?

Psychological Dimension

What are the emotional responses of those involved in the ethical dilemma?

What are the potential psychological effects of alternative courses of action in the ethical situation?

Social Dimension

What beliefs and values are held by persons involved in the ethical dilemma? How are these values prioritized?

Is fear of legal action a factor in the ethical dilemma?

What are the economic implications of alternative courses of action in the ethical dilemma?

What cultural or religious values or practices are relevant to the situation?

Do persons involved in the ethical dilemma hold different beliefs on the value of human life?

Behavioral Dimension

What influence will consumption patterns (eg, substance abuse) have on the ethical decision, if any?

To what extent do alternative courses of action restrict the behavior or rights of others?

Health System Dimension

Do the rights and needs of health care providers conflict with those of the client?

Do the values held by health care providers conflict with those held by clients?

The Health System Dimension

Health care system factors give rise to ethical dilemmas when the rights and needs of health care providers conflict with other societal values. For example, do providers have a right to charge fees that afford them a reasonable income despite the inability of some clients to pay those fees? Should providers be expected to be on call 24 hours a day, 7 days a week? Should government have the right to dictate how health care providers practice their professions? What happens when the moral beliefs and values of a provider conflict with the desires of clients, or the policies of an employer or society at large? Must providers jeopardize their own safety in the care of clients who have potentially communicable diseases or who are violent? Should employers be required to protect health care personnel from hazardous conditions? Should they, for example, be required to provide expensive immunizations against hepatitis B?

 Diagnostic Reasoning and Ethical Dilemmas

Based on factors identified in assessing the ethical situation, the community health nurse derives nursing diagnoses at two levels. The first level relates to the existence of an ethical dilemma, whereas second-level diagnoses address the values and value conflicts involved in the dilemma.

Diagnosing the Existence of an Ethical Dilemma

The first level of nursing diagnosis involves confirming that an ethical dilemma does, in fact, exist. The nurse supports this diagnosis with a description of both the problem and the disadvantages posed by all of the potential alternatives to its solution that constitute an ethical dilemma. When there is an alternative without ethical disadvantages, there is no ethical

Critical Thinking in Research

Morrison and associates (1995) examined the availability of clients' advanced directives to health care providers and the extent to which those directives were honored. Advanced directives were available for only 26% of clients during hospitalization for acute illness. Advanced directives were similarly available for only 26% of those judged incompetent to make medical decisions. In 86% of cases in which advanced directives were available, the directives influenced treatment decisions. The authors concluded that advanced directives are not readily accessible to providers when needed, but that providers tend to adhere to them when they are aware of their existence.

1. What nursing interventions could make advanced directives more available to clients' health care providers?
2. How might you test the effectiveness of these interventions in resolving the problem of inaccessibility of advanced directives?
3. Is there a potential role for case managers in making providers aware of clients' advanced directives? How would you determine case managers' attitudes to the incorporation of this responsibility into their role?

dilemma to be solved. An example of a nursing diagnosis at this level is the community's "need for an ethical decision on what programs will be eliminated due to reduced funds."

Diagnosing Conflicting Values

The second level of nursing diagnosis involves identifying the values and value conflicts inherent in the ethical situation. The community health nurse would specify the values operating in the situation and identify the individuals holding those values. For example, in the case of mandatory use of motorcycle helmets, cyclists who oppose such a law may value freedom of choice, convenience, and lack of constraints on vision encountered in helmet use. Health care providers supporting legislation for mandatory helmet use value protection of life and health, whereas lawmakers may value personal freedom, protection of life and health, and protection of society from the economic burden of caring for individuals injured because of failure to use helmets. A nursing diagnosis in this situation might be "conflict between the values of personal freedom and protection of life and health." Another nursing diagnosis might reflect the conflict between the values of personal freedom and protection of society from the costs of accidental injuries.

 Planning to Resolve an Ethical Dilemma

In the Dimensions Model, planning to resolve an ethical dilemma involves three tasks. The first task is to give priority to the values involved in the dilemma, the second task is to evaluate alternative courses of action, and the third task is to select the alternative that best fits the paramount values operating in the situation.

Giving Priority to Values Involved in the Dilemma

The first consideration in planning to resolve ethical dilemmas is assessing the priority of the values involved. Values would be given priority on the basis of the ethical perspective selected by community health nurses as most in keeping with their personal and professional values. Suppose, for example, a group of community health nurses are trying to decide whether to support proposed legislation for mandatory helmet use by motorcyclists.

An egoistic perspective on the part of the nurses might result in no action being taken by the group in regard to the proposed legislation. If the nurses perceive that they will neither gain nor lose as a result of the decision, they may ignore the issue altogether. If, however, the nurses perceive the costs of medical care for motorcycle injuries as the cause of increases in their taxes, they will probably decide to support the legislation. If, on the other hand, the costs of enforcing the legislation were perceived as likely to increase their taxes, they would probably take collective action to oppose the legislation.

If a duty-based perspective is being used by the nurses, top priority will be given to values that conform to notions of duty and obligation. For example, the nurses might believe that individuals have a duty to protect their own health and that the legislature has a duty to protect society. In this situation, the nurses would give protection of health and protection of society greater priority than personal freedom, and would support mandatory helmet use.

Viewing the dilemma from a utilitarian perspective, the nurses would see the good of society as the primary deciding factor. For this reason, they would probably assign first priority to the value of protecting society from economic burdens and again support the legislation.

The libertarian perspective used in this situation would result in personal freedom being considered the most important value. For nurses using this perspective, the right to choose for oneself always supersedes all other rights and values. Given the priority of this value over the values of protecting individuals and society from harm, the nurses would decide not to support the legislation.

Evaluating and Selecting a Course of Action

Once the values operating in a given ethical situation have been assigned priority, it is possible to evaluate alternative courses of action in terms of their conformity to the values given highest priority. Then the course of action that best supports those values would be selected. Using the previous example, if the highest priority is protection of society, legislation mandating helmet use would be supported. If the value of personal freedom is given greater priority, nurses would vigorously oppose proposed legislation.

Implementing an Ethical Decision

Once a course of action in keeping with the ethical principles of the decision makers has been selected, steps are taken to implement the decision. In the example above, if the community health nurses have decided to support the proposed legislation for mandatory helmet use, they will employ some of the political strategies described in Chapter 13 to influence legislators to support their position. They would use these same strategies to implement the decision to oppose the legislation.

Evaluating an Ethical Decision

Two aspects are involved in evaluating decision making in an ethical dilemma. The first is evaluating the outcome of actions taken. Did the selected course of action result in an outcome consistent with important values? In the case of laws mandating helmet use, for example, one might evaluate whether helmet laws decreased the severity of motorcycle injuries and thereby reduced the economic burden on society.

The second aspect of evaluation deals with the decision-making process used. Were the nurses involved in the ethical decision unsure of the ethical theory to which they subscribed? Were they unclear on what values were really most important to them? If the answer to these and similar questions is yes, there is a need for individual or group clarification of the moral principles and values that are espoused before dealing with another ethical dilemma.

Ethical dilemmas can pose difficult situations for community health nurses. A broad knowledge of ethical theory and the process of ethical decision making is required. Some of the agencies and organizations included in the Resource List at the end of this chapter can assist the community health nurse to develop this knowledge base.

Critical Thinking in Practice: A Case in Point

A community health nurse is helping with casualties resulting from collapse of her apartment building after a major earthquake. Many severely injured persons need immediate care. At present, the nurse is the only health care provider available, and decisions must be made as to who should receive care first. One of the victims who will probably not survive unless she receives immediate attention is the 88-year-old mother of the community health nurse. This older woman has had a heart attack. Other victims include an 8-year-old who has a head injury and a woman with a sprained wrist who is hysterical because her toddler is trapped in the building. A neighbor who was trying to help others trapped in the rubble has suffered a severe laceration on his thigh and needs to have the would cleaned and dressed. All of these people require help from the community health nurse. Who should she care for first?

1. What biophysical, psychological, physical, social, behavioral, and health system factors will influence the community health nurse's decision?
2. What values are operating in this situation?
3. How would the egoist resolve this situation? The duty-based ethicist? The utilitarian? The altruist? The libertarian?
4. How would you resolve the dilemma? Why would you take this approach?

TESTING YOUR UNDERSTANDING

1. Distinguish between consequentialist and nonconsequentialist theories of ethical decision making. (p. 306)
2. Describe the basis for ethical decisions in each of four perspectives on ethical decision making. (pp. 304–306)
3. Identify at least two sources of ethical dilemmas. Give an example of an ethical dilemma related to community health that might arise from each. (p. 306)
4. Describe at least four types of ethical dilemmas encountered in community health practice. Give an example of each. (pp. 306–310)
5. What are the two levels at which nursing diagnoses are made in an ethical dilemma? (p. 312)
6. What are the tasks in planning to resolve an ethical dilemma? (pp. 313–314)

WHAT DO YOU THINK?
Questions for Critical Thinking

1. How should health care resources be allocated among different age groups in the population? Why?
2. Do you think health care funds should be used primarily for preventive health care or curative care? Why?
3. Should all taxpayers have access to health services funded by taxes? If so, why do you think so? If not, who should be eligible for those services?
4. Should health care providers assist terminally ill clients to end their lives if they request help?
5. What perspective do you use in making ethical decisions? Do you use the same perspective in all ethical situations? If not, under what circumstances do you use particular perspectives and why?

REFERENCES

Ashley, B. M., & O'Rourke, K. D. (1994). *Ethics of health care* (2nd ed.). Washington, DC: Georgetown University Press.

Bandman, E. L., & Bandman, B. (1995). *Nursing ethics through the life span* (3rd ed.). Norwalk, CT: Appleton & Lange.

Bayer, R., & Toomey, K. E. (1992). HIV prevention and the two faces of partner notification. *American Journal of Public Health, 82,* 1158–1163.

Carlson, E. (1997). An ethicist's view of "suicide." *AARP Bulletin, 38*(2), 2, 7.

Claar-Rice, U. (1993). BRN adopts policy on patient abandonment. *The BRN Report, 8*(2), 5.

Clark, D. B. (1994). The patient self-determination act. In J. Monagle & D. C. Thomasma (Eds.), *Health care ethics: Critical issues* (pp. 93–108). Gaithersburg, MD: Aspen.

Connors, A. F., Dawson, N. V., Desbians, N. A., et al. (1995). A controlled trial to improve care for seriously ill hospitalized patients. *JAMA, 274,* 1591–1598.

Devine, R. J. (1996). *Good care, painful choices: Medical ethics for ordinary people.* Mahwah, NJ: Paulist Press.

Drane, J. F. (1994). *Clinical bioethics: Theory and practice in medical decision-making.* Kansas City, MO: Sheed & Ward.

Gostin, L., & Curran, W. J. (1987). AIDS screening, confidentiality, and the duty to warn. *American Journal of Public Health, 77,* 361–366.

Gray, B. B. (1995). Nurses face ethics of rationing as healthcare industry evolves. *NURSEweek, 8*(8), 1.

Husted, G. L. & Husted, J. H. (1991). *Ethical decision making in nursing.* St. Louis: Mosby.

Kelly, K. (1994). *Health care rationing: Dilemma and paradox.* St. Louis: Mosby.

Kleinman, I. (1987). Transmission of human immunodeficiency virus: Ethical considerations and practical recommendations. *Canadian Medical Association Journal, 137,* 597–599.

Kowalski, S. (1993). Assisted suicide: Where do nurses draw the line? *Nursing and Health Care, 14,* 70–76.

Miles, S. H. (1994). Medical futility. In J. E. Monagle & D. C. Thomasma (Eds.), *Health care ethics: Critical issues* (pp. 233–240). Gaithersburg, MD: Aspen.

Morrison, R. S., Olson, E., Mertz, K. R., Meier, D. E. (1995). The inaccessibility of advance directives on transfer from ambulatory to acute care settings. *JAMA, 274,* 478–482.

Nelson, J. N. (1997). Ethical, legal, and economic foundations of the education process. In S. B. Bastable (Ed.), *Nurse as educator: Principles of teaching and learning* (pp. 16–30). Boston: Jones and Bartlett.

Perrett, R. W. (1996). Buddhism, euthanasia, and the sanctity of life. *Journal of Medical Ethics, 22,* 309–313.

Pojman, L. P. (1992). *Life and death: Grappling with the moral dilemmas of our times.* Boston: Jones and Bartlett.

Reinhardt, U. E. (1990). Rationing health-care surplus: An American tragedy. In P. R. Lee & C. L. Estes (Eds.), *The nation's health* (3rd ed.) (pp. 104–111). Boston: Jones & Bartlett.

Rothenberg, K. H., & Paskey, S. J. (1995). The risk of domestic violence and women with HIV infection: Implications for partner notification, public policy and the law. *American Journal of Public Health, 85,* 1569–1576.

Smith, D. (1995). Doubts, dilemmas, and conundrums. *Inside Case Management, 2*(7), 7.

Thomasma, D. C., & Marshall, P. (1994). Ethical pitfalls and benefits of disclosure of HIV positive status. In J. E. Monagle & D. C. Thomasma (Eds.), *Health care ethics: Critical issues* (pp. 188–198). Gaithersburg, MD: Aspen.

Turner, L. N., Marquis, J. D., Burman, M. E. (1996). Rural nurse practitioners: Perceptions of ethical dilemmas. *Journal of the American Academy of Nurse Practitioners, 8,* 269–274.

Weiss, J., & Hansell, M. J. (1992). Substance abuse during pregnancy: Legal and health policy issues. *Nursing & Health Care, 12,* 472–479.

Zucker, A., Borchert, D., & Stewart, D. (Eds.). (1992). *Medical ethics: A reader.* Englewood Cliffs, NJ: Prentice-Hall.

RESOURCES FOR NURSES DEALING WITH ETHICAL ISSUES

American Nurses Association
Center for Ethics and Human Rights
600 Maryland Avenue, SW, Ste. 100W
Washington, DC 20024-2571
(202) 651–7000

American Society of Law and Medicine
765 Commonwealth Avenue
Boston, MA 02215
(617) 262–4990

Association for Practical and Professional Ethics
410 Park Avenue
Bloomington, IN 47405
(812) 855–6470

Hastings Center
Institute of Society, Ethics, and the Life Sciences
255 Elm Road
Briarcliff Manor, NY 10510
(914) 762–8500

Kennedy Institute of Ethics
Georgetown University
Washington, DC 20057
(202) 687–3885
(800) MED–ETHX

Park Ridge Center
211 E Ontario, Ste. 800
Chicago, IL 60611–3215
(312) 266–2222

Society for Health and Human Values
6728 Old McLean Village Drive
McLean, VA 22101
(703) 556–9222

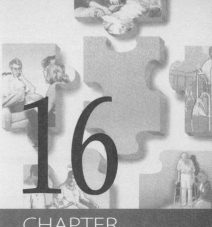

CULTURAL INFLUENCES ON COMMUNITY HEALTH

The health status of individuals, families, and communities is the product of interaction between the client and environment. One significant component of the environment that has considerable influence on clients' health is culture. Culture is a pervasive social phenomenon that colors attitudes, values, and beliefs about the world, and guides interactions with that world. Culture directs most human behavior, including health-related behavior. For this reason, it is particularly important for community health nurses to consider their clients' cultural backgrounds in formulating care to meet health needs.

▶ KEY TERMS

acculturation
cultural
   accommodation
cultural blindness
cultural conflict
cultural imposition
cultural pluralism
cultural relativism
cultural sensitivity
cultural shock
cultural universals
culture
culturebound
   syndromes
culture brokering
discrimination
ethnic culture
ethnic identity
ethnicity
ethnocentrism
prejudice
race
racism
stereotyping

▶ Chapter Objectives

After reading this chapter, you should be able to:

- Differentiate among culture, race, and ethnicity.
- Identify six characteristics common to all cultures.
- Describe at least four potential negative responses of nurses to people from another culture.
- Describe at least three positive responses by nurses to people of another culture.
- Apply four principles of cultural assessment to individuals, families, and groups.
- Use the dimensions of health to identify cultural factors influencing health.
- Describe at least three similarities and four differences between folk and scientific health care systems.
- Describe at least four considerations in assessing the influence of folk health care systems.

In the United States, society is characterized by *cultural pluralism,* the simultaneous existence of many cultures within the larger society. Almost from its beginnings, the United States has been a nation of people from multiple ethnic heritages. Early colonization of what is now the United States was accomplished by such diverse groups as the English and the Spaniards. Later, other European and Chinese immigrants and African slaves supplied the labor force for continued expansion. More recently, refugees from Asia and South America have come to change the complexion of the population even more. Each of these groups brought with them cultural beliefs and practices, sometimes similar and sometimes different, that influenced their interaction with each other and also influenced their health. *Acculturation,* the process of adapting to facets of the dominant culture, has resulted in modification of some of these beliefs and behaviors, but many remain intact to influence everyday activities including those related to health.

▶ **THE NEED FOR CULTURALLY RELEVANT CARE**

Community health nurses, like the clients they serve, come from a wide variety of cultural backgrounds. Without knowledge of culture and its influences on daily life and health, cultural differences experienced by community health nurses and their clients can lead to ineffective nursing care. Cultural relevance, on the other hand, can enhance the effectiveness of community health nursing care.

There are several reasons why culturally relevant care is essential to effective community health nursing. Respect for oneself and acceptance as a worthwhile individual are universal desires. Respect and acceptance must encompass differences in cultural beliefs, values, and behaviors as well as other features of the person that make him or her unique. Respect and acceptance facilitate the rapport required by the level of intimacy between nurse and client that is characteristic of community health nursing.

Rapport between client and nurse sets the stage for effective nursing care, but culturally relevant care has other, more practical, implications for interactions between nurses and clients. Knowledge of cultural factors on the part of the nurse can facilitate communication and minimize miscommunication. For example, in many German American households, visitors are always offered substantial refreshment. A community health nurse who does not understand this may inadvertently insult a client by refusing the offer of coffee and cake. Similarly, knowledge of the client's culture will allow the nurse to more accurately identify potential health problems. For example, if an African American client says she has "high blood," the knowledgeable nurse would understand this to mean an excess of blood and would explore the use of folk remedies commonly used to treat "high blood" that may contribute to uncontrolled hypertension.

Knowledge of cultural beliefs and practices will also allow the nurse to tailor the intervention plan to the client's lifestyle. This enhances the potential for compliance with health care recommendations. For example, a Mexican American client may be more likely to comply with a diabetic diet that incorporates traditional foods than one based on a typical European American diet.

Culturally relevant care is particularly important for some ethnic minority groups who experience more health problems than the general population. Community health nurses need to be cognizant of the increased incidence and prevalence of specific conditions in minority populations and actively work to reduce the burden of illness in these groups. For example, many persons of Mediterranean descent are at increased risk of thalassemia, whereas African Americans are at high risk for hypertension and obesity (Office of Surveillance and Analysis, 1994) and have elevated mortality rates for heart disease, cerebrovascular disease, cancer, homicide, and HIV infection (U.S. Department of Health and Human Services, 1996). Common health problems among Native Americans include infant mortality (Blane, 1995), fetal alcohol syndrome (Division of Birth Defects and Developmental Disabilities, 1995), obesity, hypertension, heart disease, and diabetes (Huttlinger, 1995; Maynard, 1996). Tuberculosis and heart disease are serious problems among Asians, particularly Southeast Asians (Ginsberg, Gage, Martin, Gerstin, & Acuff, 1994; Klatsky, Tekawa, Armstrong, & Sidney, 1994). Other common problems include respiratory infections and cancer, as well as parasitic infestations, hepatitis, malaria, goiter, hypertension, diabetes, arthritis, and hearing and vision problems (Chen & Hawks, 1995). For Latinos, common health problems include tuberculosis (Chavez & Torres, 1994), cardiovascular disease (Juarbe, 1996), injury, homicide, liver disease, and diabetes (Ginsberg, et al., 1994). These differences in illness and mortality were the impetus for developing more than a hundred national health objectives for the year 2000 specifically targeted to these four ethnic groups (U.S. Department of Health and Human Services, 1991). Some of these objectives are presented in Appendix A.

At the aggregate level, culturally relevant care by community health nurses has implications that go beyond health. Planning and implementing culturally relevant health care programs conveys respect for and acceptance of multiple cultural groups and sets the stage for greater cohesion and cooperation in society at large.

▶ RACE, CULTURE, AND ETHNICITY

Three terms that are frequently, and inaccurately, used synonymously in discussions of client groups are *race, culture,* and *ethnicity.* **Race** is an attribute that allows classification of human beings on the basis of certain biological characteristics, such as color of skin, eyes, or hair; hair texture; and shape of eyes, nose, and lips (Randall-David, 1989). Such distinctions, however, are unreliable as scientific classifications. A case in point is the racial admixture found among Latinos, whose forebears may have included whites, Native Americans, African Americans, and Asians. Racial distinctions are useful primarily as risk markers for health problems caused by social, rather than biological, factors (Centers for Disease Control, 1993).

Definitions of culture abound in the literature. Culture, according to one observer, is "the unique achievement of a human group that distinguishes it from other groups" (Banks, 1991). For others, culture is learned systems of patterns of beliefs, behaviors, values, and meanings shared by a group of people (Galanti, 1991; Kavanaugh & Kennedy, 1992). For the purposes of this chapter, *culture* is the collection of beliefs, values, and behaviors that permit a group of people to interact effectively with their environment.

A group's culture is unique. The beliefs and behaviors that constitute a particular culture arise from the unique constraints faced by a given group of people in dealing with problems common to humanity. These unique situational constraints are the source of cultural variation among groups of people. For example, exposure to periodic drought and famine in India may have resulted in the Hindu prohibition on killing cattle (Harris, 1989). Because the cow was a source of milk and assistance in plowing the farmer's fields, killing and eating the family's only cow in a time of deprivation would decrease the family's chances of long-term survival and also jeopardize the survival of the society. Reinforcing this supposition is the observation that, in areas where droughts and famine were not experienced on a regular basis, the need to protect cattle did not arise. In this instance, the environmental constraints imposed on Hindu society led to the development of a specific cultural practice that ensured society's survival in times of drought or famine.

Ethnicity is the designation by self or others as being a member of a distinct population group with an historical origin and a shared heritage as well as a sense of peoplehood and interdependence (Banks, 1991). Research has suggested three dimensions of ethnicity: ethnic culture, ethnic group membership, and ethnic identity (Keefe, 1992). *Ethnic culture* is a pattern of beliefs and behaviors unique to the group. Ethnic group membership reflects an affiliative network including other persons belonging to a particular ethnic group. Finally, *ethnic identity* consists of one's perceptions of affiliation with the group and the degree of one's emotional attachment to the group and its heritage. From this perspective, culture may contribute to ethnic distinctions, but is not equivalent to ethnicity.

In this chapter we explore some of the cultural differences that contribute to ethnic diversity and influence the health status of specific population groups in the United States. In addition to identifying cultural differences, we investigate their implications for planning, implementing, and evaluating health care activities in the community health setting.

▶ CHARACTERISTICS OF CULTURE

Although cultures vary among groups, certain identifiable characteristics are common to all cultures. Culture is a universal experience. All people engage in culturally prescribed behavior patterns. Examples of *cultural universals*—areas addressed by all cultures—are family, marriage, parenting roles, education, health, work, and modes of communication. Curiously, though, the influence of culture on an individual occurs largely subconsciously. Culture encompasses and directs most aspects of life; however, the influence of culture is rarely consciously noted, unless one purposefully undertakes a study of one's own culturally determined behavior. As aptly noted by one author, "Culturally learned assumptions control our lives, with or without our permission" (Pedersen, 1995). Moreover, the culture of any particular group is unique. Although several cultures may exhibit certain commonalities, no two cultures, like no two individuals, are exactly alike.

Another characteristic of culture is its stability. Cultural characteristics tend to endure across generations. Culture, however, is neither static nor immutably fixed; it is subject to change (Schrefer, 1994). Although the superficial aspects of culture can change relatively easily, basic cultural values and beliefs change slowly and may provide the basis for strong resistance to change.

Finally, the degree to which an individual adheres to cultural beliefs, values, and customs is affected by many factors. Among these are an individual's education level, social status, facility with the dominant language, length of exposure to the culture of the larger society, and residence in an urban or rural setting in the country of origin. Often, a person's education level is associated with greater use of the dominant language. It cannot always be assumed, however, that use of the dominant language is indicative of an individual's identification with the culture of the larger society or that an individual adheres less to subcultural norms.

▶ RESPONSES TO CLIENTS FROM ANOTHER CULTURE

Community health nurses frequently encounter clients whose cultures differ from their own. The response of nurses to these differences may be either positive or negative. Negative attitudes that may be displayed by community health nurses in crosscultural situations include ethnocentrism, cultural blindness, cultural shock, cultural conflict, and stereotyping. Other negative responses include racism, prejudice, discrimination, and cultural imposition.

Ethnocentrism is a conviction that one's own way of life, values, beliefs, and customs are superior to those of others (Galanti, 1991). *Cultural blindness* involves ignoring or denying cultural differences between nurse and client, behaving as if these differences do not exist. *Cultural shock* occurs when the

▶ CHARACTERISTICS OF CULTURE

Universality
    Culture is a pervasive phenomenon that involves all human populations.
Subliminality
    Expression of cultural meanings through behaviors and symbols often occurs without conscious awareness.
Uniqueness
    All cultures are unique and, although similarities may exist among cultural groups, no two cultures are exactly alike.
Stability
    Culture is lasting and endures through generations.
Changeability
    Culture changes over time. Superficial aspects of culture change more readily than deeply held beliefs and values.
Variability
    The degree of adherence to cultural beliefs, values, and behaviors varies with individual members of the culture and depends on a variety of factors.

nurse is only too aware of cultural differences and is stunned and immobilized by the "shocking" aspects of the alien culture (Leininger & Reynolds, 1993). Cultural shock is most likely to occur in response to behaviors approved in one culture that are disapproved in another. The stronger the taboos against the behavior in the disapproving culture, the greater the shock when that behavior is accepted, or even encouraged, in the other. Clients, as well as nurses, experience cultural shock. In fact, clients from other cultural groups may experience two levels of culture shock, one in response to exposure to the dominant U.S. culture and the other in response to exposure to the health care culture which may be quite alien to them (Dreher, 1996; McGee, 1992).

In *cultural conflict,* the nurse is aware of cultural differences and is threatened by them. This threat arises when recognition of cultural differences causes the nurse to doubt the validity of personal beliefs and values, threatening self-esteem. In response to this perceived threat, the nurse may actively seek to support personal beliefs and behaviors by denigrating those of others. *Stereotyping* is attributing a cultural pattern to all members of a group on the basis of prior opinions, attitudes, and interactions (Samovar & Porter, 1991). Stereotypes may have their basis in fact or fiction. But, even when the stereotypical notion conforms to an actual cultural norm, expecting that all members of the group accept that norm can be as detrimental to nurse–client interactions as ignoring cultural differences. Stereotyping must be distinguished from generalization. Generalizations are expectations based on knowledge of behaviors and beliefs common to a particular cultural group. A *stereotype*, on the other hand, is an assumption that a member of a particular group will always act in accord with the cultural expectation (Galanti, 1991). The difference lies not so much in the content of the generalization or stereotype, which may be very similar, but in their use. For example, many European Americans use tea and toast to settle an upset stomach. Assuming that a particular client does so is a stereotype. The nurse operating from a generalization, on the other hand, recognizes that a European American client may practice this health measure and asks the client if such is the case.

The negative attitudes discussed thus far can lead to other negative responses by nurses and others caring for members of another cultural group. *Racism* is the belief that people can be classified on the basis of biophysical traits into groups that differ in terms of mental, physical, and ethical capabilities, with some groups being intrinsically superior or inferior to other groups. *Prejudice* is a set of attitudes unfavorable to a given group of people based on preconceptions rather than fact. Both racism and prejudice may lead to discrimination. *Discrimination* is differential treatment of an individual or group based on unfavorable attitudes toward the group (Banks, 1991).

Cultural imposition is another potential course of action in response to negative attitudes toward another culture. *Cultural imposition* refers to the nurse's expectation that everyone should conform to the nurse's cultural practices, whatever their own personal beliefs (Leininger & Reynolds, 1993). This response to cultural differences is an extension of ethnocentrism in that the nurse not only believes that other practices are inferior, but expects them to be abandoned and those of the nurse's culture assumed. For example, an Asian American nurse might be appalled when a European American adolescent challenges his parent's opinion and expect the parent to chastise the son.

Positive attitudes toward members of another culture include cultural sensitivity, cultural relativism, cultural accommodation, and culture brokering. *Cultural sensitivity* is an acknowledgement by the nurse of the significance of cultural factors in health and illness characterized by respect for people as individuals and for their culture and acceptance of culturally prescribed health beliefs and practices. *Cultural relativism* is the ability to view beliefs and behaviors within the contest of the culture in which they originated (Luna, 1994; Pedersen, 1995). Cultural accommodation is the behavioral response to sensitivity and relativism. *Cultural accommodation* is the modification of health care services in keeping with the client's cultural background (Leininger & Reynolds, 1993; Luna, 1994). This may involve incorporating cultural health practices whenever possible. Another positive response by nurses is *culture brokering,* the act of mediating between groups or individuals from different cultures to reduce conflict or foster change. Positive and negative responses to clients from another culture are summarized in Table 16–1.

TABLE 16–1. **RESPONSES TO CLIENTS WITH DIFFERENT CULTURAL BELIEFS/PRACTICES**

Positive Responses	Negative Responses
Cultural sensitivity: recognition of significance of cultural factors in health	*Ethnocentrism:* belief that one's own culture is superior to that of others
Cultural relativism: ability to view beliefs and behaviors in the context of the culture in which they originated	*Cultural blindness:* failure to recognize cultural differences
Cultural accommodation: modification of health care delivery in light of cultural factors	*Cultural shock:* immobilization due to perceptions of overwhelming cultural differences
Culture brokering: mediation between individuals or groups from different cultures	*Cultural conflict:* ridicule of cultural beliefs and practices of others because of perceived threats to one's beliefs
	Stereotyping: belief that all members of a cultural group conform to a set of real or perceived beliefs and behaviors
	Racism: belief that people can be classified by biophysical traits that indicate innate superiority or inferiority
	Prejudice: unfavorable attitudes toward an individual or group based on preconceptions rather than fact
	Discrimination: differential treatment of an individual or group based on unfavorable attitudes to the group
	Cultural imposition: belief that everyone should conform to the dominant culture

▶ RELATIONSHIPS BETWEEN CULTURE AND HEALTH

Culture has both direct and indirect effects on health. Direct effects stem from specific culturally prescribed practices related to diet and food or to health and illness. For example, all cultures have prescribed practices intended to promote health and prevent illness or to restore health when illness occurs. Similarly, all cultures have particular dietary practices that contribute to the nutritional status and, thereby, to the health status of their members.

Culture also affects health indirectly. These indirect effects result from cultural definitions of health and illness, acceptability of health care programs and providers, and cultural influences on compliance with suggested health or illness regimens. Cultural definitions of health and illness determine what kinds of health problems are considered worthy of attention and what conditions are likely to be disregarded. If, for example, certain behaviors that are perceived as evidence of mental illness by the larger society are considered normal in the client's culture, then the client is unlikely to take any action to deal with those behaviors. Similarly, minor illnesses may be ignored if health is defined in terms of one's ability to work or to perform other social roles. In general, people are likely to disregard any type of condition that is not defined as illness in their own culture. This cultural propensity can lead to serious health consequences.

Cultural factors may also determine the acceptability of both health programs and health providers. For example, cultures that eschew scientific medicine in favor of healing based on faith in God may view immunization programs as inimical to their beliefs. In other cultures, health care providers may be considered lower-class persons not to be associated with, effectively preventing people from taking advantage of many health opportunities. For example, nursing is considered a lower-class occupation in India, and nurses have little opportunity to influence the health of their clients for the better because of their low social status.

Finally, cultural factors often determine whether clients will comply with recommendations when they do seek professional help. If the recommendations of health care providers are too far removed from normal cultural practices in a given situation, the client is unlikely to comply with those recommendations. For example, a community health nurse may suggest reducing the caloric intake of an infant who is overweight. If the mother's culturally derived perception is that a fat baby is a healthy baby, she is unlikely to follow the nurse's suggestions.

▶ THE DIMENSIONS MODEL AND CULTURALLY RELEVANT CARE

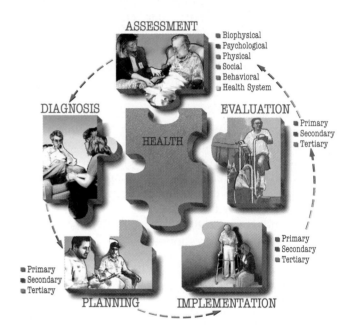

The Dimensions Model can be used as a framework for exploring other cultures as well as for organizing care for clients from specific cultural groups. Using the model, the community health nurse examines racial, ethnic, and cultural factors that influence clients' health. The nurse then uses the model to design culturally sensitive interventions to meet the needs of specific clients.

Critical Dimensions of Nursing in Culturally Relevant Care

Elements of each of the six dimensions of community health nursing come into play in designing culturally relevant care for all segments of the U.S. population. In the cognitive dimension, community health nurses must have a clear understanding of the influence of culture on health and knowledge of their own culture and other cultural groups whose members they are likely to encounter in practice. In particular, the nurse needs to arrive at an understanding of the origin, intent, and meaning of beliefs and behaviors within a culture. In addition to having accurate knowledge of the beliefs and practices of a given culture, the nurse will also need to know how members of that cultural group perceive the individual nurse and nursing as a profession (Pedersen, 1995).

Several elements of the interpersonal dimension are critical to effective intervention with clients from another culture. Probably the most important element in this dimension is the nurse's attitude toward members of other cultural groups and their beliefs, values, and behaviors. Both positive and negative attitudes on the part of the nurse were addressed earlier in this chapter. Development of positive attitudes is fostered when nurses explore their own cultures and the influence of culture on their lives.

Communication skills are another important element of the interpersonal dimension. The nurse working with clients from another culture must be aware of cultural proscriptions and prescriptions within the culture. The nurse muse also consider the effect that his or her culturally prescribed modes of communications have on the client. Communication within and between cultures will be addressed in more detail later in this chapter.

In the ethical dimension, the nurse may be called upon to act as an advocate for clients from another culture to assure that they receive culturally competent and sensitive health care. The nurse may need to express for clients needs they cannot express for themselves because of language barriers, perceptions of powerlessness, lack of understanding of the health care culture, or other cultural factors. Nurses function as advocates when they interpret to other team members the sociodynamics influencing the client. They may provide information on cultural beliefs and practices to others caring for the client. They also fulfill an advocacy role in considering cultural influences on target groups for specific health care programs. Other avenues of cultural advocacy include fostering recognition of cultural differences among nurses and nursing students and recruiting members of other cultural groups into nursing.

Ethical dilemmas related to culture may arise when clients' cultural health practices are harmful to themselves or others. In this instance, the nurse is faced with the dilemma of respecting and maintaining the client's culture while attempting to modify harmful cultural practices (Kikuchi, 1996).

Skills needed by nurses working with clients from other cultures include intellectual abilities to identify cultural barriers to effective intervention or cultural practices that are adversely affecting health. Creativity in health care planning may also be required to incorporate cultural beliefs and practices whenever possible and appropriate. Health assessment skills will need to be adapted to biophysical differences among some cultural groups. For example, assessment of the skin for jaundice is somewhat more difficult in African American clients than in Anglo-European populations.

Elements of the change, leadership, group, and political processes may be used by community health nurses working with clients from other cultures to help assure the availability of culturally competent health care services. Community health nurses may be very effective in organizing members of cultural groups to advocate for their own needs. Other elements of the process dimension that may be employed by the community health nurse are the home visit and health education processes which may need to be modified to reflect cultural expectations for interactions in clients' homes. For example, while a visiting nurse might not ordinarily accept a gift offered by a client, it would be extremely important to do so in working with clients from certain cultural groups.

All three of the elements of the reflective dimension of nursing are relevant to culturally competent health care. In providing such care, the nurse may employ transcultural nursing theory developed by such theorists as Madeleine Leininger and others (Leininger, 1994; Leininger & Reynolds, 1993). Leininger's theory incorporates three modes of decision and action by nurses working in transcultural situations (Luna, 1994): (1) activities designed to preserve and maintain the client's culture; (2) activities designed to adapt nursing intervention to cultural expectations; and (3) activities designed to eliminate or modify cultural practices that may be harmful in nature. Research, a second element of the reflective dimension, can assist nurses to become conversant with different cultures and their health effects. Finally, evaluation can assist the nurse to identify the most effective means of providing culturally competent health care to members of another cultural group.

Assessing the Dimensions of Health in a Cultural Context

The first task in working with clients from another culture is obtaining information about the culture. Community health nurses can use the dimensions perspective to collect, organize, and analyze information about cultures frequently encountered in their practice. Prior to examining some of the biophysical, psychological, physical, social, behavioral, and health system factors arising from culture, several general principles involved in the study of another culture are explored.

Principles of Cultural Assessment

Four basic principles should guide nurses engaged in the study of another culture. First, view all cultures in the context in which they developed. As noted earlier, cultural practices arise out of a need to meet common human problems in a particular human setting. That setting must be considered in exploring another culture.

Second, examine the underlying premise of culturally determined behavior. What was the intended purpose for the behavior when it originated? Does the behavior still fulfill this purpose? When one knows the underlying reason for behaviors that seem strange, the behaviors may not seem quite so strange after all. The nurse should also examine the meaning of the behavior in the cultural context. The meaning of certain behaviors from the perspective of the nurse's culture may be very different from the behavior's meaning in the context of the client's culture. For example, resistance to having one's head shaved for a cranial surgical procedure may be interpreted as vanity from a European American nurse's perspective. When the nurse understands that some clients view the head as the home of the soul, however, such resistance is more understandable.

Finally, recognize the existence of intracultural variation. Not every member of any given cultural group displays all of the typical cultural behaviors. There may be several subgroups within one cultural group with different behavior patterns. Or, individual clients may be more or less acculturated to the dominant U.S. culture. The nurse who expects to find intracultural variation tends to avoid stereotyping and responding to clients as if they were typical representatives of their cultural group. Principles of cultural assessment are summarized below:

- View all cultures in the context in which they developed.
- Examine underlying premises for culturally determined beliefs and behaviors.
- Interpret the meaning and purpose of behavior in the context of the specific culture.
- Recognize the potential for intracultural variation.

Obtaining Information About Another Culture

How does one become knowledgeable about another culture? Perhaps the best way to begin is to become conversant with one's own culture, recognizing the influences of culture on one's life and behavior. Personal insights regarding culture will enable the nurse to accept cultural beliefs and behaviors that may differ from his or her own. Once familiar with his or her own cultural heritage, the nurse can begin to read literature related to other cultures of interest. In reading, the community health nurse should examine the qualifications of the authors writing. Was the book or article written by a member of the culture? Is it based on empirical data derived from research, on personal experience with a particular culture, or on stereotypes?

A second means of acquainting oneself with another culture is to interview colleagues who are members of that culture. Explore with them their concepts of health and illness and attitudes and practices affecting health. Discover how these may differ from those held by previous generations or other members of their family. Health care professionals, by virtue of their knowledge of health matters, are likely to have achieved a greater degree of acculturation and conformity with the dominant U.S. culture with respect to health practices than nonprofessionals from the same group; however, these individuals remain a valid source of information regarding cultural health beliefs and practices.

One of the best ways to become familiar with a particular culture is to spend time living within it. This approach, however, is not always feasible. Alternatives include home visits to families within the group to observe daily living in the cultural context and questioning clients and families regarding health-related beliefs and practices. Another possible approach is observing activities and interactions at health facilities and community or religious functions.

When assessing another culture directly, the community health nurse should follow a few general guidelines. First, look and listen before asking questions or taking action. Observation aids in asking pertinent and timely questions and forestalls actions that may be inappropriate. Second, explore how the group feels about being studied. Explain that your reasons for studying the culture are practical and do not arise out of idle curiosity. Third, discover any special protocols. Should one speak to a local leader before beginning to observe a group? Is there a council or leadership group who should grant permission for participation in group activities? Fourth, foster human relations, putting them before the need to obtain information. Information will not assist the nurse to provide care if he or she alienates members of the group. Social amenities are very important in many cultures and should be attended to before the "business" of information gathering begins in earnest. In fact, information about social amenities is part of the data needed by the nurse.

Many people, in exploring another culture, look for differences from their own culture. The nurse, however, should also look for cultural similarities to use as a foundation in aiding clients to accept and use health care services. Cultural differences should be accepted as normal.

Locate group leaders and respected residents, those considered wise, "ordinary" group members, and clients who can converse knowledgeably about another culture. Critics of the traditional aspects of the

► MODES OF CULTURAL EXPLORATION

Become conversant with your own culture and its influences on your life.

Review the existing literature on beliefs, values, and behaviors of specific cultural groups.

Interview colleagues who are members of the cultural group in question.

Immerse oneself in the culture to be studied.

Observe members of specific cultural groups.

Interview members of cultural groups, particularly group leaders.

Interview other persons who are conversant with the culture.

culture may also be interviewed to provide a balanced picture.

Participate as well as observe. The nurse must assess each situation as it occurs to determine whether participation or observation is the more appropriate activity. Participation conveys an openness to cultural differences and a willingness to engage in culturally prescribed activities rather than ridicule them. Some activities, however, are closed to outsiders, and the community health nurse's participation would not be welcomed.

When exploring another culture, the nurse should also consider the feelings of group members about questions asked. The nurse should ascertain what types of questions are acceptable or offensive in a particular culture. For example, Americans in India find it difficult to adjust to frequent questions about their salary or how much their clothes cost. Such questions are perfectly acceptable in India, but considered impolite or "nosy" in the United States.

A little forethought as to the phrasing and timing of questions can prevent serious mistakes. Ask questions positively without implying value judgments. For example, "I notice you put garlic on a string around the baby's neck; can you tell me what it's used for?" is far more acceptable than "Why in the world do you hang garlic around the baby's neck?"

Nurses might ask the same questions of themselves and gauge their own emotional reaction to the questions. A nurse can also try out questions on colleagues who are members of the culture being explored. Suggestions for modes of cultural exploration are listed above.

The Biophysical Dimension

Biophysical variations have usually arisen in adaptive response to environmental conditions to ensure survival (Young, 1994). It is important to keep in mind that a thorough assessment of persons from other ethnic and cultural groups should not focus exclusively on social factors or culturally determined behaviors. Differences related to age, genetic inheritance, and physiologic function must be considered as well.

Age.   Age is relevant to cultural assessment in two respects. First community health nurses should be aware of cultural attitudes to age in the cultural groups with which they work. In many cultural groups, older persons tend to be highly respected and influential. Children are highly valued, although boy children may be more highly valued than girls by some groups (eg, some Asian and Arab populations). In most cultural groups, children are expected to be quiet and respectful of their elders and do not participate in family decisions. This is not the case in many Native American tribes where children are expected to make decisions for themselves and physical punishment is infrequent (Hanley, 1991).

The nurse also considers the age composition of the cultural group because this information will help to identify potential age-related health concerns. Statistical data on group composition by age is available from census figures for Native Americans, African Americans, Asian Americans, and Latinos, but is not readily available for other cultural groups. Many ethnic groups have a higher proportion of children under 5 years of age than the general population. They also frequently have larger adolescent populations and fewer elderly than the general population (U.S. Department of Commerce, 1996). These facts suggest that some cultural groups have higher proportions of young people subject to a variety health problems common among the young than the general population and help to guide health care planning at the aggregate level.

Genetics.   Physical differences deriving from genetic inheritance have implications for nursing. For example, African American youngsters tend to exceed standard heights and weights at all ages except at birth (Cherry, 1991), whereas Asian Americans are usually smaller (Schrefer, 1994). Groups also differ in rates of maturation, with African and Asian Americans reaching puberty earlier than whites. The dry ear wax normal in Asian or Native American clients is best dealt with using irrigation techniques, whereas the wet wax common in African Americans and whites is more appropriately removed with a curette.

Epicanthic folds are commonly seen among Asian Americans, and lumbar lordosis is a common finding in African American children. The size, number, and shape of teeth also differ among ethnic groups. Differences in skin pigmentation of some groups can hinder assessment of changes in skin coloration unless one recognizes variations in normal coloration for a particular group. In some groups, palpation may be a more effective means of identifying erythema or bruises than inspection (Spector, 1996). Hair texture differences, food intolerances, and differences in drug metabolism may necessitate changes in approaches to physical care and require knowledge of such variations on the part of the nurse. For example, milk is not always considered a suitable source of protein for African Americans, Latinos, Native Americans, and some Asians owing to the relatively high incidence of lactose intolerance in these groups (Hanley, 1991; Schrefer, 1994). Community health nurses working with these clients would suggest other sources of protein in place of milk. Differences exist in normal laboratory values among different cultural groups. For example, normal hematocrit levels are slightly lower for African American clients than for whites.

Genetic inheritance may also play a part in the types of health problems commonly seen in members of some ethnic and cultural groups. For example, diabetes is a common problem among Latinos and many Native American tribes (Hanley, 1991; Kuipers, 1991), whereas sickle cell disease is a genetically transmitted disease particularly prevalent among African Americans. Among Chinese Americans, thalassemia and glucose-6-phosphate dehydrogenase disorders occur more frequently than in the general population (Shrefer, 1994). Research has also indicated that genetically determined pathways for alcohol metabolism leading to rapid rise in and slow clearance of blood acetaldehyde levels may explain differences in physiologic responses to alcohol among Native and Asian Americans. Tay-Sacks disease and several other genetic disorders occur more frequently among Jewish groups than in other populations (Schrefer, 1994).

Physiologic Function. Physiologic function is the second aspect of human biology considered in the study of another culture. Two categories of physiologic considerations need to be addressed. These include attitudes toward body parts and physiologic functions as well as folk designations of physical illness commonly encountered in the particular group.

ATTITUDES TOWARD BODY PARTS AND PHYSIOLOGIC FUNCTIONS. The physical differences described previously may lead to different cultural attitudes and approaches to physiologic function in different cultures. Care of one's body and attention to basic physiologic functions differ from one group to another. One area the nurse should explore is approaches to hygiene. The nurse may ask how and when group members bathe and how hair, skin, and teeth are cared for.

Special significance may be attached to certain body parts in a particular culture. For instance, in some cultures, the head is considered sacred and is to be treated with respect. In these cultures, bumping someone's head is considered an insult. Among many Vietnamese and Hmong, for example, touching the head is thought to cause loss of the soul or vital force (Geissler, 1994).

In many cultures, certain body parts are believed to be responsible for functions and conditions that are not in accordance with scientific knowledge of physiology. In many Asian folk medicine systems, for example, the heart is thought to be responsible for insomnia, dreams, forgetfulness, insanity, and delirium. The kidneys, on the other hand, are believed to control water, birth, development, reproduction, and maturation (Cargill, 1994). Beliefs and attitudes toward body parts and physiologic function may influence acceptance of such scientific medical procedures as transfusions, venipuncture, transplantation, and autopsy.

Exposure of certain body parts is appropriate in some cultures and not in others. In some regions of the world, neither men nor women cover their breasts, yet for the U.S. female, exposing the breasts is generally unacceptable. In India, uncovering the shoulders and upper arms is considered indecent.

Differences also exist between cultures in terms of what body parts may appropriately be touched and who may touch them. Touching members of the opposite sex or members of the same sex may be restricted. For example, it would be unusual for adult members of the same sex to hold hands or to kiss in public in the United States. In other cultures, same-sex touching or kissing may be perfectly acceptable, whereas similar behavior toward members of the opposite sex is thought to be inappropriate (Geissler, 1994).

Another consideration to be addressed relative to physiologic function is privacy. Cultures differ in terms of what physiologic functions may be performed in public and those for which privacy is required. Latinos and other cultural groups, for instance, exhibit a great deal of modesty regarding urination and defecation as well as bathing and dressing. Similarly, people from other cultural groups may have difficulty accepting the presence of the husband or father during delivery. In some cultures, children are allowed or even encouraged to observe a delivery; in the U.S. health care culture, however, children are excluded from the birth setting.

In exploring cultural attitudes toward physiologic function, the nurse may also need to determine whether there are periods during which individuals are considered ritually unclean. In many cultures, for example, postpartum or menstruating women are considered unclean, and their activities and interactions with others are restricted. A final consideration with respect to physiologic function is the culturally appropriate response to the physiologic experience of pain. Asian clients, for example, tend to be stoic and uncomplaining; whereas pain expression among Arabs is particularly vocal and demanding of immediate relief as evidence of care and concern (Geissler, 1994).

RECOGNIZED FOLK ILLNESSES.   Health is an area of concern to most people, and there are few cultural groups that do not have some systematized way of dealing with illness. Many folk cultures have a unique method of classifying illnesses that aids in their identification and their treatment within the culture. A term frequently used to describe these illnesses unique to specific cultures is *culturebound syndromes* (Frye, 1995).

African American and Appalachian folk medicine systems recognize a number of similar conditions related to the character of the blood. Among these are high blood, low blood, thin blood, bad blood, and poison blood. Some of the recognized folk illnesses among Latino cultural groups include *susto, empacho, caida de mollera, mal de ojo* (evil eye), *mal puesta, serena,*

and *coraje.* Belief in the "evil eye" as a cause of illness is fairly widespread and may be encountered among people of Jewish, Italian, German, Greek, Arab, Asian, and Filipino origin among others (Geissler, 1994; Luna, 1994; Spector, 1996). Culturebound syndromes can be found among some Asian groups as well. *Toa* is a culturebound syndrome experienced by Khmer women after childbirth and is a condition of extreme cold that causes physical collapse and death if not treated. *Koucharang, latah, koro,* and *amok* are other Asian culturebound syndromes that result in psychiatric rather than physical symptoms (Frye, 1995). These and other culturebound syndromes are described in Table 16–2.

The Psychological Dimension

Areas to be considered in assessing the psychological dimension include attitudes and beliefs regarding mental illness and the prevalence of mental illness in the cultural group, the importance of individual versus group goals, modes of authority and decision making, attitudes toward change, and the character of relationships with the larger society. The importance of culture in relation to mental health is highlighted by findings that treatment programs specifically de-

TABLE 16–2. SELECTED EXAMPLES OF CULTUREBOUND SYNDROMES

Condition	Cultural Groups	Description
High blood	African American, Appalachian	An excess of blood in the body (not related to hypertension)
Low blood	African American, Appalachian	Too little blood (comparable to anemia)
Thin blood	African American, Appalachian	Increased susceptibility to illness
Bad blood	African American, Appalachian	Sexually transmitted disease acquired through sexual promiscuity (not necessarily related to bacterial or viral infection)
Poison blood	African American, Appalachian	Septicemia or illness due to witchcraft
Susto	Latino	Magical fright resulting in soul loss
Empacho	Latino	Adherence of a bolus of food to the walls of stomach or intestine
Caida de mollera	Latino	A depressed fontanel resulting from an infant being bounced too vigorously or having a nipple suddenly or forcefully withdrawn from the mouth
Mal de ojo (evil eye)	Latino, Arab, Asian, Italian, Greek, Scottish, German, Jewish, Filipino	Disease caused by someone with the evil eye looking at, admiring, or envying the victim (may not be intentional)
Mal puesta	Latino	Unusual behavior caused by magic
Serena	Latino	Upper respiratory symptoms caused by dampness, draft, or evil spirits
Coraje (rage)	Latino	Hyperactivity, screaming, or crying due to an extreme emotional reaction
Espanto	Latino	Severe fright caused by witnessing supernatural beings or events
Pujos	Latino	Umbilical protrusion and grunting in an infant exposed to a menstruating woman
Pasmo	Puerto Rican	Paralysis due to an imbalance of hot and cold forces
Ataque	Puerto Rican	Hyperkinetic activity, aggression, or stupor due to tension, stress, or grief
Toa	Khmer	Extreme cold after childbirth leading to physical collapse
Koucharang	Cambodian	Preoccupation with distressing thoughts and memories due to "thinking too much"
Latah, koro, amok	Cambodian	Conditions characterized by tic-like movements, withdrawal or panic, and aggressive behavior

signed for certain ethnic groups have better compliance rates than generalized programs (Takeuchi, Sue, & Yeh, 1995).

Attitudes Toward Mental Illness. Many cultures fail to make a distinction between mental and physical illness. Emotional distress may be somatized and experienced as physical symptoms or an inability to perform one's usual social roles (D'Avanzo, Frye, & Froman, 1994). Several cultural groups, however, do have some concept of disease caused by psychological factors. African Americans, for example, view stress as a source of illness. Stress is believed to arise from negative emotions such as envy, guilt, and ineffective interpersonal relationships. Similarly, Laotians may believe that worry results in illness. For Cambodian refugees, stress-related disorders may arise from *koucharang,* thinking too much about past traumatic events (Frye, 1995; Geissler, 1994).

Many Latinos also distinguish between physical and emotional illness. The client with a mental illness is seen as a victim of circumstances with no responsibility for his or her condition. The client's condition may be the result of a blow to the head, fright, or anxiety, or may be due to the malign effects of witchcraft. Another example of emotional illness is seen as the result of moral weakness on the part of the client and might be manifested as excessive emotion, as in the case of *coraje;* weakness of character, as in alcoholism; or a propensity for engaging in vice, such as drug abuse. Puerto Ricans perceive mental illness as caused by evil spirits; however, their definition of abnormal behavior may differ from that of the dominant culture. For example, seeing visions and hearing voices are not aberrant, but are to be accepted.

A diagnosis of mental illness may be perceived by members of many cultural groups as shameful. Chinese clients, for example, might try to hide mental illness in a family member, keeping the person at home as long as possible. Typical Western approaches to psychotherapy are frequently ineffective with members of non-Western cultures because assertiveness and independence, expression of feelings, and confrontation are culturally prohibited behaviors frequently encouraged in psychotherapy.

Vietnamese clients may differentiate between mental health problems of an organic nature, caused by damage to the brain and nerves, and bizarre behavior caused by sin, disobedience, or possession (Stauffer, 1991). Vietnamese believe that sorrow and grief are "natural." Vietnamese clients seek professional help for a mental health problem only when psychosomatic symptoms present.

Appalachian clients may exhibit a dichotomous approach to unusual behavior. Being thought "crazy"

may carry social stigma, (Lewis, Messner, & McDowell, 1985) or may warrant punishment through the criminal justice system (Small, 1991). On the other hand, it is not considered abnormal to have "bad nerves" (emotional problems) or be "odd turned" (exhibit neurotic behavior) (Lewis, Messner, & McDowell, 1985).

Cultural groups differ with respect to the types of behavior considered abnormal and when intervention is required. A behavioral classification schema of four categories has been suggested to explore these differences among cultures (Helman, 1994). The first type of behavior is normal controlled behavior, that which any typical person displays on a daily basis. Abnormal, but controlled, behavior is unusual but expected in certain culturally acceptable circumstances. Examples include religious visions and trance states, many of the culturebound syndromes discussed earlier, or the excesses of Mardi Gras season. A third category of behavior is considered normal but uncontrolled. In this category, the individual engages in "bad" behavior by choice and is aware of doing so. In the final category of abnormal and uncontrolled behavior, the person is unaware of the behavior and might be considered "mad" rather than bad. It is this last category of behavior that is most likely to result in attempts at intervention. What specific behaviors fit into each of the four categories is culturally defined and will color people's responses to a given behavior.

In addition to identifying cultural attitudes to mental illness and definitions of aberrant behavior, the community health nurse will also assess the extent of mental illness in the cultural group and the ways in which mental illness is manifested. For example, mental health problems may be highly somatized by some cultural groups because of the associated stigma. Common somatic symptoms include fatigue, dizziness, weight loss, nausea, headache, chest pain, or insomnia. High rates of homicide or suicide are also indicators of psychological stress within the group.

Individual Versus Group Goals. The nurse exploring the norms of another culture would assess the relative importance of individual versus group goals. Western medicine (and nursing in particular) emphasizes the worth of each individual. In many other cultures, however, the needs of the family, work group, or larger society may take precedence over the needs or desires of the individual.

Among Native Americans, the individual is considered an independent agent. This orientation is particularly true of the Navajo, among whom even small children are encouraged to voice their opinion (Hanley, 1991). Individualism is also characteristic of the values of many European Americans, but does not extend to young children who are generally expected to conform to parental directives.

Commitment to family and to tribe is also strong among Native Americans, but does not take precedence over individual development or freedom of choice. Family goals tend to hold less sway among European Americans.

In contrast, the Asian client's individuality is subordinated to the family. In traditional Chinese society, for example, the family or clan and some other community associations fulfilled the social needs of the individual. As families were separated after coming to America, the newly arrived family groups and benevolent associations took on the responsibility of meeting the social welfare needs of immigrant Chinese. The relationship of the individual Chinese to the group remains very strong, and the individual is expected to direct his or her energies to the benefit of the group. Group ties are also strong in many Arab and Latino cultural groups.

Authority and Decision Making. Cultural patterns of authority and decision making often correspond to individual versus group goal orientations. Groups that emphasize family or community goals frequently vest authority and decision-making power in elders rather than individuals.

Respect for authority is another feature of culture that influences the psychological environment and its effects on health. Seeming agreement and compliance of the part of some clients may only reflect an attitude of respect for the health care provider rather than genuine motivation toward healthy behavior. Respect for authority can enhance or detract from a therapeutic regimen. When a client's respect for authority leads to compliance with medication orders and other recommendations, for example, it enhances the therapeutic effect of health care. A client's respect for authority can also hinder health care providers' efforts. For example, a client's respect for authority may detract from the effectiveness of a community health nurse's efforts to enhance the client's reliance on his or her own abilities to resolve health problems.

Decision-making processes within a cultural group are indicative of its attitude toward authority. The community health nurse should assess how decisions are made. Are they arrived at in a democratic fashion where all concerned have equal input? Or, are they made by a central authority figure or group? The traditional, Asian or Latino family identifies the husband/father as the primary decision maker. More recent research indicates that many decisions are made jointly by husband and wife, particularly in those families where the woman is employed (Geissler, 1994; Kanellos, 1993; Zinn, 1994). In some Native

American tribes, on the other hand, all family members (including children) help make decisions. In other tribes, decisions are made by the female head of the family. Grandparents' opinions are of particular importance.

Attitudes Toward Change. Group attitudes toward change also influence the psychological environment and health care for group members. In assessing a particular cultural group, the nurse explores what changes are taking place within the culture itself as well as how open or resistant to change the group is. Closely allied to group attitudes toward change are culturally based attitudes of resignation and acceptance. In many areas of the world, notably underdeveloped countries, people have little access to the means to change the circumstances of their lives. Over many generations, people in such cultures often become resigned to their condition. Widespread resignation within a cultural group can frustrate health care professionals who see ways in which people could better their situation if they were only motivated to act. In fact, an attitude of resignation is often misinterpreted as a lack of motivation on the part of clients from other cultures.

Relations with the Larger Society. Another cultural feature that may significantly influence the effects of the psychological environment on health is the quality of a cultural group's relationships with the larger society. Relationships between subcultures and the larger cultural group can be complementary, "colonial," competitive, or conflictive. Complementary relationships exist when interaction between groups is mutually supportive. To a large extent, complementary relationships exist between Americans and Canadians. Colonial relationships occur when one group is exploited by another. This type of relationship is frequently seen in the United States in interactions between Latino migrant farm workers and the larger society and occurred historically with the Chinese brought to the United States to build the railroads and the black Africans brought as slaves to the southern states.

Competitive relationships occur when cultural groups compete for the same resources on an essentially equal basis. This type of interaction was typical between Irish and Italian immigrants during the industrial development of the northeastern United States. Finally, a conflictive relationship exists when one cultural group attempts to dominate the other and the second group resists attempts at domination. Attempts by the white population to continue to dominate African Americans have been actively resisted since the advent of the civil rights movement in the

United States, creating conflictive relationships in many parts of the country.

In assessing a subculture's relationships with the larger society, the community health nurse considers how the subculture views itself with respect to the larger society. Do group members tend to assume a subservient posture or one of superiority in their interactions with the larger group? Do they view themselves as the equals of other members of the society? How do members of the larger society view the subculture? Are the views of members of the subculture respected by the larger society? Is their participation in society sought or rejected?

The Physical Dimension

The geographic isolation created by some physical environments may contribute to the development and continuation of cultural variations. For example, the isolation of many Appalachian mountain communities led to the development of a unique culture that has withstood many incursions by the dominant U.S. society. The insularity created by geographic or social isolation also contributes to lack of change within a culture over time (Hansen & Resnick, 1990).

Cultural groups differ in their view of the relationship between human beings and their environment. These differences can be referred to as the "man–nature" orientation of a culture (Kluckhohn & Strodtbeck, 1961). This orientation may reflect a view of people as subject to, in harmony with, or having mastery over the environment. African American, Latino, and Appalachian clients tend to perceive human beings as subject to the environment and as having little control over their own destiny. Many Arab Americans are believers in *Islam* which translated from Arabic means submission to the will of Allah (Luna, 1994) also suggesting a certain fatalistic attitude. Asian and many Native American cultures tend more toward the view of people acting in harmony with nature, whereas European American culture emphasizes society's mastery of nature.

The type of man–nature orientation typically exhibited by members of a cultural group has implications for health-related action. For example, people who see themselves as subject to the environment may see little use in attempts to change environmental factors impinging on their health.

In addition, cultural groups found in rural areas, such as migrant Latino and Haitian farm workers, may experience environmental conditions that increase their risk of exposure to hazardous substances (Delgado, Metzger & Falcon, 1995) or decrease the availability of health care. Distances to health care providers and facilities, poor roads that flood, and

bridges that wash out with heavy rains may limit access to health care. Lack of indoor plumbing and outdoor privies in rural areas present potential sources of water contamination and subsequent communicable diseases. In addition, wells, a major source of potable water in rural areas, periodically go dry, leaving families without a source of safe drinking water. Similar problems might be encountered among rural Native Americans and African Americans.

The Social Dimension

The social dimension within a specific culture also influences health and health practices. Each culture has norms that govern the social interaction of its members. Areas for consideration in assessment include interpersonal relationships, communication, beliefs and values, and the place of religion and magic in the culture. The nurse also explores the effects of the larger society on the subculture.

Interpersonal Relationships. The types of interpersonal relationships that are important in a particular culture and the rules governing those relationships can profoundly influence the health of members of the cultural group and their relationships with health care providers.

One of the primary concerns in cultural assessment is determining the place of the family within the culture and the role of the family with respect to health and illness. The community health nurse should be aware of the influence that the family exerts on its members in a particular culture. To what extent do family beliefs and values influence individuals' behavior?

The structure of family life also merits exploration, including the family's typical organizational structure and patterns of residence. Do families tend do be nuclear or extended in structure? Who lives with whom? For example, although a multigenerational extended family structure is traditional in many Asian cultures, the exigencies of relocation have changed this norm for many refugee families (Frye, 1995). Economic forces are also causing movement away from extended family structures in cultures of origin such as China and Taiwan (Chao, 1997). Another area for consideration is that of descent. Is descent determined matrilineally (through the mother, as in the case of some Native American tribes) or patrilineally (through the father)?

Another consideration is family roles. What tasks do family members typically assume? Are these tasks interchangeable, as is often the case in African American families? Who assigns tasks? Are family tasks gender specific, with males taking on certain functions and females responsible for others? The development of gender roles in ethnic groups is influenced by several conditions in the larger society. These conditions include position of the cultural group vis-à-vis other groups in the larger society, presence of an identifiable ethnic community, and degree to which group members self-identify with the cultural group. The greater the identification with the group, the greater the identifiability of an ethnic community, and the less the interaction with the larger society, the more likely it is that gender roles follow traditional cultural patterns. In exploring any particular cultural group, the community health nurse identifies typical gender roles and patterns and how they are exhibited within families.

The role and status of individual family members are major considerations with implications for health care. In some cultures, children are central figures in the family. In others, life centers around the older members. Who in the family makes decisions regarding health and illness? In some instances, individuals decide for themselves when and where to seek health care. In others, those decisions are made by the authority figures within the family. Arab women, for example, may have considerable decision power within the family, but their husbands interact with the outside world (Geissler, 1994).

What roles are assumed by family members with respect to illness? There may be specific family members whose task it is to care for the sick. Or, the entire family may expect to participate in the care of ill members (Wing, Crow, & Thompson, 1995).

Appropriate Demeanor. Another aspect of interpersonal relationships within a specific culture that is of particular concern to community health nurses is the demeanor or behavior expected in one's interactions with others. In every culture certain behaviors are acceptable and others are not. If community health nurses are to work effectively with clients from other cultures, they must engage in acceptable behaviors and avoid behaviors that might give offense.

Behaviors acceptable in one culture are not necessarily acceptable in another. For example, it is not unusual in some cultures for men to embrace or for women to hold hands while walking down the street. In the United States, however, such behavior might be interpreted as homosexuality. Members of the opposite sex, however, holding hands in public is acceptable in the United States and unacceptable in other parts of the world. Community health nurses need to consider how their behavior is perceived by clients as well as how clients' behavior should be interpreted. Interpretation of the meaning of a given behavior is

based on four assumptions of attribution theory (Gropper, 1996):

- Behavior has meaning.
- The meaning of behavior can be derived from observation alone, without validation of the interpretation.
- The meaning of a behavior is assigned on the basis of past experience.
- Different cultural groups may attribute different meanings to the same behavior.

Community health nurses need to be aware of and validate their interpretations of client behavior. They must also recognize that clients are using a similar attribution process to assign meaning to the behavior of the nurse. Therefore, it is important to understand the usual meaning of a given behavior in the client's culture to avoid misunderstanding or giving offense. Table 16–3 presents examples of acceptable and unacceptable behaviors for several cultural groups.

Communication. Communication is another important consideration in assessing social dimension factors in culture. Both verbal and nonverbal forms of communication should be explored.

Language is the major means of transmitting culture. As such, it is an important consideration in cultural assessment. In the United States, 32 million people speak a language other than English as their primary language (Spector, 1996). For a large segment of this population, Spanish is their primary language (Gonzales, 1997). The community nurse should determine the language with which the client is most comfortable. Whenever possible, the client's native language (and dialect, if relevant) is employed. This is particularly important when there is a need to discuss intimate topics. Such areas are even more difficult to discuss in a second language than in one's mother tongue.

As far as possible, the community health nurse should strive to become familiar with the spoken language of a cultural group. Some languages include both formal and informal modes of address, and the nurse should become familiar with the circumstances in which each mode of address is used. For example, one would usually use an informal mode when speaking to a family member, a close friend, or a child. Formal modes of address are usually used when conversing with strangers and casual acquaintances, people in positions of authority, and older persons. In Korean culture, for example, it is considered disrespectful to address elders in the informal mode; only children are addressed by name (Rowles & Johansson, 1993).

It is wise to remember that the nurse with a poor

TABLE 16–3. SELECTED EXAMPLES OF CULTURALLY UNACCEPTABLE BEHAVIOR

Unacceptable Behavior	Recommended Approach
Disrespect for elders and others in authority, especially men (Asian, African American, Latino Appalachian, Native American, Gypsy, Arab)	Show respect for elders and those in authority, incorporate into treatment decisions
	Give things to elders with both hands (Hmong)
Using informal forms of address inappropriately (Asian, Latino, African American, European American)	Use appropriate forms of address (eg, using formal mode of speech with older persons); ask about preferred form of address
	Use last name with Mexican American clients
	Use first name only with close African American friend
Using titles of "Miss" or "Mrs." for women (dominant U.S.)	Use title "Ms."
Direct eye contact (Native American, Latino, Appalachian, Arab—sexual overture between sexes, Navajo—may cause soul loss, Asian—implies equality)	Look at the ground or to the side when speaking to others
Not maintaining eye contact (European American)	Maintain eye contact when speaking to others
Assuming authority over others (Appalachian)	Avoid conflict
	Mind your own business
Arguing with authority figures (Asian, Latino, Appalachian)	Show respect and acceptance
	Avoid conflict
Competing with others (Native American, Appalachian)	Cooperate with others
Causing others to "lose face" (Asian)	Prevent others from losing face
Strong hand clasp (Native American)	Moderate grasp when shaking hands
	Lightly touch hand (Native American)
Weak hand clasp (European American)	Firm handshake
Writing a "life story" (Native American)	Display modesty and respect for privacy
Self-disclosure (Native American, Asian, Latino, Appalachian, Gypsy, Arab)	Use tact in obtaining health history
	Use trusted interpreters from family
	Provide for physical privacy
Overt discussion of sexuality (Asian, Latino, Arab, Hmong)	Discuss sexual matters without members of opposite sex present; ensure availability of same-sex health provider
Aggressiveness or self-assertion (Native American, Latino, Asian, Appalachian)	Display humility and self-effacement
Lack of motivation or initiative (European American)	Display initiative in task accomplishment
Drawing attention to oneself (Native American, Asian)	Display humility and self-effacement
Expressing personal opinions (Asian)	
Ridiculing others, teasing (Asian, Appalachian)	Direct humor at self (especially with Appalachian clients)
Dependence on others, being a burden (Asian, Appalachian, European American)	Display self-reliance
Complaining (Asian)	Accept without complaining
Displaying emotion (Asian, Native American, Appalachian)	Control emotions
Accepting things when first offered (Asian)	Repeat offers of food, pain medication
Giving negative information or disagreeing (Asian, Arab)	Give a polite response (whether or not true)
Giving misinformation (European American)	Tell the truth however hurtful
Putting personal needs before family needs (Asian, Latino, Appalachian, Vietnamese)	Try to incorporate personal needs into family goals
Physical contact by opposite sex (Asian, Appalachian, Latino)	Avoid physical contact when possible
Physical contact with same sex (dominant U.S.)	" "
Touching the head (Hmong, Vietnamese)	Avoid touching the head if possible
Pointing at others, especially with feet (Vietnamese, Indian, Native American)	Avoid pointing objects at others
Being more successful than one's husband (Navajo, Arab)	Help with role conflict
Interrupting, chattering (Native American)	Maintain silence, do not interrupt
	Allow time to formulate answers
Failure to understand others (Asian—causes loss of face for teacher)	Validate understanding of client
Getting right down to business (Asian, Latino, Native American, Appalachian)	Observe social amenities before business
Wasting time (European American)	Come to the point immediately
Saying no, refusing a request (Asian)	Graciously accept requests
Refusing hospitality (Asian, Appalachian, Arab, European American)	Graciously accept hospitality
Being late for an appointment or social event (European American)	Arrive on time

command of a foreign language is at the same disadvantage as a client with little facility in English. In this situation, an interpreter is in order, preferably one with a cultural background similar to that of the client and conversant with the larger society as well. An interpreter who is not familiar with the larger culture may not be able to translate a concept he or she does not understand. For example, the interpreter may not be able to translate a question about the use of contraceptives unless that individual understands the meaning of contraception. Other considerations in the use of interpreters include gender and age differences between client and interpreter, membership in opposing groups or different socioeconomic classes, and the potential for an interpreter to inject his or her personal bias into the conversation (Schrefer, 1994).

Knowledge of a client's language also allows community health nurses to obtain or create health-related literature in the client's native tongue for clients who are literate. Unfortunately, many foreign-language materials related to health are literal translations of materials written in English and may not be comprehensible to the client. Translated educational materials should make use of native idioms whenever possible.

The words used are only one aspect of communication. Another aspect is the context in which the message is conveyed (Hall, 1976). In a "low-context" culture such as that of the United States, the essence of a message is conveyed in the *words* used. In a "high-context" culture, on the other hand, much of the message is communicated by the *context* in which the message is relayed rather than in the words used. Suppose, for example, that the nurse asks a mother when she plans to follow up on an immunization referral. In some cultures, it is polite to respond with the answer that one believes is expected, and the client might reply that she plans to get the immunizations that week. When the nurse visits the following week and finds that the mother has not yet had the child immunized, the nurse may interpret the client's previous statement as a lie. Yet, in the context of the client's culture, she was giving the appropriate response. If the nurse is aware of this cultural context, he or she is more likely to interpret correctly the mother's response as meaning that she will get the immunizations in the not too distant future.

Conflict can occur between individuals from high-context and low-context cultures primarily as a result of misinterpretation of communications. Those from the high-context culture may be reading into the message contextual considerations that might not exist. At the same time, the low-context person may be missing a large portion of the content of the message through neglect of contextual considerations.

Contextual considerations might include the need to observe certain social amenities before directing the conversation to the area of interest. For example, Puerto Ricans, as well as members of other cultures, might expect to learn something about the nurse as a person before getting down to the business at hand.

Culturally prescribed reticence, courtesy titles, epithets, and gestures are other culturally determined aspects of communication. Culturally prescribed reticence refers to the relative openness about personal matters expected in casual encounters with others. Asians, for example, display a high degree of reticence. They traditionally consider it impolite to ask personal questions and are uncomfortable discussing personal matters with casual acquaintances, including health care professionals. Native Americans are also socialized to little self-disclosure. Reticence may be particularly problematic in group therapy situations where participants are expected to share intimate information with virtual strangers (Wing, Crow, & Thompson, 1995).

Latinos are also frequently reluctant to discuss personal matters with strangers (Zuniga, 1997). In a similar vein, Latinos tend to provide responses that they believe are expected by health care professionals and often keep their true feelings to themselves (Medina, 1987).

Gestures are another important contextual factor. Gestures, like words, can convey totally different meanings in different cultures. In the dominant U.S. society, for example, one apologizes for accidentally bumping into someone else, but thinks nothing of pointing the sole of one's shoe at another. Clients from India would be highly insulted to have the soles of one's shoes directed toward them or, worse yet, to be touched by someone's shoe. Footwear is considered dirty and contaminated in India, and the implications of intentionally touching someone with your shoe would be comparable to spitting in someone's face in the United States. For Iranians, the typical American "thumbs up" and "V for victory" signs would be offensive (Geissler, 1994).

Other gestures, even if not insulting, may convey different meanings in different cultures. For instance, in the dominant U.S. culture, one indicates agreement by nodding the head, whereas in India one says yes by tilting the head toward the shoulder. In Vietnamese culture it is unacceptable to crook one's finger to beckon another person, as that is how Vietnamese call dogs.

Cultures also differ with respect to their use of first or last names and courtesy titles. As with any client, it is wise to ask how a client from another culture wishes to be addressed. Often the use of a first name is restricted to close friends or children. Adults may be referred to by last name with or without the appropriate title (eg, "Gordon" vs. "Mrs. Gordon"). In Korean culture, family members are addressed in terms of their relationship to the youngest child in the family (eg "Sung's grandmother"). As other children are born into the family constellation, the individual's relationship changes and forms of address change. For this reason, many elderly Koreans may not remember their given name after being addressed in terms of multiple relationships for years (Sich, 1988). Vietnamese prefer to be called by their given first name.

Some epithets are considered insulting in different cultures. An epithet is a word or phrase used in place of the correct designation and may or may not be derogatory in nature. When cultural differences intervene, generally innocent words may take on the character of insults. Most nurses are sensitive enough to refrain from calling an African American male "boy." Some Mexican Americans may or may not be offended by being referred to as *chicano* depending on what part of the United States they are from and their level of acculturation. Again, ask the individual client the preferred form of address.

Beliefs and Values. Cultural beliefs and values also influence health-related behavior. A culture's value orientations should be investigated as part of cultural assessment, as should the values attached to material goods, success, and competition.

All cultures develop value orientations related to questions common to all groups of people (Kluckhohn & Strodtbeck, 1961). These value orientations address the character of human nature (the human nature orientation), the relation of human beings to their natural environment (the man–nature orientation), the temporal focus of life (time orientation), the modality of human activity (the activity orientation), and the relation of human beings to each other (the relational orientation).

Variations in these five value orientations are believed by some researchers to result in the major differences that occur between cultures. Many cultural groups differ markedly from the value orientations typical of the dominant U.S. culture. Understanding these variations in value orientations helps the community health nurse understand differences in behaviors that arise out of beliefs and values. Such an understanding also aids the nurse in planning culturally consonant interventions.

Earlier in this chapter, the man–nature orientation was described as the way in which members of a specific cultural group view their interaction with the physical environment. The human nature orientation

refers to the cultural view of human beings as inherently evil, inherently good, or any of several combinations of good and evil. Native American and Asian cultural groups tend to see humanity as fairly neutral, neither good or evil. Traditional Appalachian, African American, and Latino cultures, on the other hand, view human beings as sinful, but redeemable.

All cultures deal, to some extent, with the three aspects of time orientation: past, present, and future. Differences between cultures lie in the emphasis placed on each aspect. For example, Native Americans, African Americans, Latinos, and Appalachians tend to be oriented to the present, whereas Asian clients may be oriented to the past and to tradition or may view time in a cyclic fashion. Middle Eastern clients may also be present oriented and Muslin Arabs may regard planning for the future as defying the will of Allah (Geissler, 1994). American society in general is oriented to the future.

Another aspect of time orientation is that of scheduling. Members of European American cultures tend to order much of their lives in relation to the clock. Crosscultural conflicts can arise as a result of different orientations to time. For example, Puerto Rican and Egyptian clients are oriented in the present and value completing a current activity, particularly a social interaction, rather than interrupting it to keep an appointment (Geissler, 1994). Clients from other cultural groups are also less concerned with specific schedules than health care professionals are likely to be and may, in fact, have the perspective that an activity will start when they arrive (Cherry, 1991).

Another consideration in cultural orientations to time relates to the timing of home visits. As noted in Chapter 10, community health nurses should cultivate knowledge of the daily habits of all clients and plan home visits (or clinic appointments) at times that are least disruptive to family life. A home visit at an inappropriate time is likely to be unproductive and may even be destructive of the rapport between client and nurse. As a general rule, times to be avoided include rest periods, periods when intensive work is performed, times of religious ceremonies and rituals, and bathing times. Mealtimes should also be avoided unless the nurse has a specific purpose in visiting at that time. For instance, visiting during lunch is one way of validating a client's compliance with a special diet. Because the times at which certain activities are routinely performed may vary from culture to culture, the community health nurse should become familiar with daily patterns typical of specific cultural groups.

One of the most frustrating manifestations of different cultural orientations to time for health care providers is late or broken appointments. Because some cultural groups are not as time conscious as the typical health care provider, clients may tend to arrive at a time convenient to them, not at their appointed time. Latino clients, for example, do not adhere rigidly to schedules, and in some Asian cultures it is considered polite to arrive late for an appointment. Appalachians also have a different orientation to time, which may give rise to difficulties with formal work schedules and in keeping appointments. Other groups, such as the Japanese, value punctuality in general, and still others, like Laotians, value punctuality for important events (Geissler, 1994).

A variety of approaches can be employed to deal with the problem of differing cultural orientations to time. Appointments can be made for a specific day rather than a specific hour, with clients seen on a first-come, first-served basis. Another possibility is to schedule several clients at the same hour in the hope that at least one will be there on time. A third approach is to do away with scheduling altogether or schedule people 2 to 3 hours before you actually expect them to appear. Clinics can also be scheduled at more convenient times (eg, evenings or weekends, or during slow periods for seasonal workers). None of these approaches may prove successful, however, and community health nurses might need to learn to cultivate patience to cope with their feelings of frustration.

The activity orientation refers to the purpose of human activity. "Being" is emphasized in Latino, African American, and Native American cultures. In these cultures the emphasis is on spontaneous self-expression. In the "being-in-becoming orientation," the purpose of human activity is developing all aspects of the self as an integrated whole. This is the typical emphasis among Asian cultures. A "doing orientation," on the other hand, characterizes European American cultural groups and U.S. society in general. This orientation emphasizes activities that lead to visible accomplishments such as career success and wealth.

A culture's relationship orientation describes the value that members of the group place on specific categories of relationships. In some cultures the most important relationships are those that occur between generations within the family. This is typical of Asian clients, who function within a group identified primarily by direct lineal descent from father to son.

Collaterally oriented cultures place more emphasis on relationships with others on one's own level (eg, among one's siblings and cousins). The extended families of African American and Native Americans are examples of this type of relationship. Arab, Appalachian, and Latino cultures, however, tend to emphasize both lineal and collateral relationships. In contrast, European American cultures and U.S. society as a whole tend to place greater emphasis on individualistic relationships in which relationships with those outside the family are often more highly valued than those with family members. Individualistic relationships are characterized by impersonality, whereas more intimate personal relationships are characteristic of lineal and collateral orientations.

Cultural values related to material goods, success, and competition are also explored in relation to the particular culture studied. Do members of the cultural group value economic success as measured by material goods and wealth? Is career success valued? Formal education, work, and achievement are valued in African American, Asian, and Latino cultures, but attitudes toward material measures of success are viewed somewhat differently from what is typically the case in U.S. society as a whole. For example, achievement is valued by the Asian client because it reflects on family honor and status. Among many Native Americans, formal education is valued because it enhances prosperity. Although prosperity is valued, generosity commands the respect of others, and acquisition of material goods can lead to social ostracism.

Another important value involves the emphasis placed on competition. Competition and personal achievement have been highly valued by the European American cultural groups that influenced the dominant U.S. culture. In other cultures, however, emphasis is placed on cooperation, and competition is considered rude and inappropriate.

Religion and Magic. Religion and belief in magic are other important considerations in cultural exploration. Religion is an organized system of beliefs regarding the origin, nature, and purpose of the universe. Individual and group experiences related to religion differ along five dimensions: the experiential, ritualistic, ideologic, intellectual, and consequential dimensions (Andrews & Hanson, 1990). The experiential dimension reflects the emotional aspects of religion. For example, religious beliefs and practices may bring feelings of comfort, joy and elation, and remorse for different people or different groups. Religions also have a ritualistic dimension. Members of most religious groups are expected to engage in certain prescribed behaviors or practices. These may include lighting candles, chanting specific prayers, participating in special ceremonies like a Mass or worship service, handling snakes, and using hallucinogenic substances. The ideologic dimension of religion consists of the spiritual beliefs held by members of the religious group. For example, Christians believe that Christ is the Son of God sent to save the world. For members of other religious groups, Christ is one of several prophets. The intellectual dimension of a religion reflects members' knowledge of these beliefs and their familiarity with the sacred writings of the group. Finally, the consequential dimension of religion consists of the standards of conduct expected of group members. The five dimensions of religion are summarized below:

- *Experiential dimension:* emotional effects of participation in religion and religious observances
- *Ritualistic dimension:* expectations regarding participation by group members in specific rituals and practices
- *Ideologic dimension:* beliefs held by the members of the group
- *Intellectual dimension:* knowledge of religious beliefs and sacred writings and how these are conveyed to group members
- *Consequential dimension:* expectations regarding standards of conduct based on religious beliefs

Religion can be a contributing factor in the phenomenon of resignation noted earlier. "Who can challenge the will of God?" may be the fatalistic response to efforts toward change in Appalachian, Asian, and Latino cultures. African American culture is more amenable to change, whereas belief in destiny and the will of Allah is strong in many Arab cultures and among black Muslims (Geissler, 1994; Spector, 1996).

Religion can affect health in ways other than contributing to fatalistic attitudes. The nurse exploring another culture may encounter religious practices that enhance or detract from health. Most people are familiar with the prohibition against blood transfusions among some religious sects and the stand of the Roman Catholic Church against artificial forms of birth control. Either of these practices can be detrimental to health in situations where a transfusion is indicated or where pregnancy is medically contraindicated. On the other hand, Jewish and Muslim proscriptions against pork probably originated as a measure designed to promote health by preventing infestation with trichinosis (Harris, 1989).

A community health nurse needs to assess several features of a culture's relationships to religion to determine the importance of religions in the health of a community. First, one would explore the extent to which religion is involved in health care. Are there specific religious beliefs regarding the cause of illness or appropriate treatments? Do members of religious groups play a role in the diagnosis and treatment of illness? For example, belief in faith healing is strong in Appalachia and among African Americans (Galanti, 1991). Here, religion takes on a direct curative aspect in the treatment of illness. The healer is believed to have been "called by God" and exercises healing powers through divine intervention.

Second, one should explore the influences of religion on the health of a cultural group's members and on the health care system. Are certain religious practices detrimental to health? Examples of potentially dangerous religious practices are snake handling in some parts of Appalachia (Covington, 1995) and the use of peyote and other hallucinogens in some Native American religious ceremonies (Huttlinger & Tanner, 1994). Another related area of inquiry is determining the degree to which religious and health care systems either conflict with or complement each other.

A third aspect of the impact of religion on health is the effect of religious sponsorship on the use of health services. Does this sponsorship enhance or detract from the acceptability of health programs? For example, if the only hospital in the community is a Roman Catholic hospital, are Protestant Appalachian clients reluctant to obtain services there? The fourth consideration is the relationship of religious leaders and healers to health care personnel. Is this a cooperative relationship? Or are they in competition with each other?

Religion and magic are closely intertwined in many cultures. Distinctions between the two are based on the agent of action. Religion is viewed as supplicative; the person typically conciliates personified supernatural powers, requesting specific action on their part. For example, a particular client may make an offering to gods or spirits or pray for a cure for his or her illness or relief from suffering. Magic on the other hand is considered manipulative. In using magic, an individual manipulates impersonal powers to achieve a desired result (Murphree, 1968). Magic is based on the principle of sympathy. Sympathetic magic arises from an assumed connection between everything in the universe and the belief that an understanding of the connection provides the power of manipulation (Cherry, 1991).

Magical practices are divided into two categories: contagious magic and imitative magic. Contagious magic is based on the assumption that things that have been connected remain connected even though physically separated from each other. Whatever one does to the part influences the whole. This is why fingernail parings or locks of hair are frequent ingredients of magical rituals. It is believed that damage done to these things formerly connected to an individual will cause damage to the individual (Cherry, 1991).

In imitative magic, the operating principle is "like follows like" in which similar objects have similar properties and react in similar ways. Pins inserted into a doll made to look like an enemy, for example, will cause the enemy pain and injury. By the same token, a knife placed under the bed of a woman in labor is believed to "cut the pain" of contractions.

Knowledge of beliefs regarding the influence of magic on health and health practices is useful to community health nurses. If a nurse determines that the client or family attributes illness to witchcraft, he or she can encourage consultation with a practitioner of folk medicine *in addition* to compliance with a medically prescribed regimen. An understanding and acceptance of such beliefs also enable the nurse to contribute to the client's emotional health by promoting expression of fears and anxieties.

Economic Status.   Assessment of a cultural group also includes consideration of the economic status of group members relative to the larger society. Members of many ethnic subcultures tend to be economically and educationally disadvantaged as a result of a number of factors, including language barriers and limited job opportunities. Community health nurses should assess the economic and educational status of members of the cultural group and of the effects of these factors on the health of group members.

The Behavioral Dimension

The lifestyle typical of a particular cultural group can also have significant effects on the health status of its members. Aspects of the behavioral dimension to be assessed by the community health nurse include dietary practices, practices related to specific life events, sexual practices, and other health-related behaviors.

Dietary Practices.   Generally, cultural groups classify foods in five types of systems: food versus nonfood items, sacred versus profane foods, parallel foods, social foods, and foods used as medicine (Helman, 1994). What is considered food may vary considerably among cultural groups. For example, dogs and snails are considered delicacies by members of some cultures, but are repulsive to others. Sacred foods are those used for religious purposes (eg, corn for many Native Americans or bread and wine for Christians). Profane foods are unclean and forbidden. For example, pork and pork products are forbidden to Jews and Muslims. Many cultures classify foods (and other substances such as medications) in a parallel system of "hot" and "cold," although cultures differ significantly in what is considered hot or cold. Social foods are those that signify relationships, gender, occupation, or group identity. A great deal of symbolism is attached to food in every culture. Food can function as a focus of emotional association, a channel for interpersonal relationships, or as a means of communicating love, disapproval, or discrimination. What parent has not shown love of a child by providing a favorite food or indicated disapproval by sending a child to bed without dessert?

In most cultures, the sharing of food indicates acceptance and intimacy. When new neighbors move in, for example, one might invite them over for coffee to get acquainted. Food practices also convey many associations with family sentiment. In many households, it is not Christmas without a special cookie, dessert, or meal. Many cultural traditions revolve around food. For many generations, eating fish on Fridays symbolized sacrifice on the part of Roman Catholics. Fasting still has this connotation in many cultures. Muslim Arabs fast for 30 days during the feast of Ramadan and are permitted to eat only after sundown during this period.

Within everyday family life, certain meals have more or less symbolism than others. In many cultures, the evening meal is the specific gathering time of the family. Morning and noon meals have less significance in these cultures. In rural America, however, the noon meal may still be the most important meal of the day.

Food items can also be used for preventive and therapeutic purposes by members of cultural groups. For example, many cultures use a variety of herbal teas to prevent or cure illness. Some of the therapeutic uses of specific foods are presented later in this chapter.

Methods of preparation can affect the nutritional status of many foods. For example, the rapid cooking of vegetables by many Asians helps to retain the vegetables' vitamin content, whereas overcooking by other groups causes loss of nutrients. Frying foods in animal fats, a common practice among many southern blacks, increases their cholesterol consumption and dietary fat content.

Other areas for consideration in nutritional assessment include the frequency of meals eaten away from home and the degree of regularity of consumption patterns. For example, African Americans tend to eat larger, more elaborate meals on weekends than during the week. For this reason, a 3-day diet history, a frequent method of assessing dietary patterns, may not provide an accurate picture of an African American client's nutrition or food consumption patterns. Even the times at which specific meals are eaten can vary among cultural groups. For instance, in warmer climates, the evening meal is often eaten quite late to provide a cooler, more relaxed atmosphere in which to dine.

As is the case with other culturally determined behavior, dietary practices vary with the extent to which an individual client has adopted the culture of the larger society. Pressures to change food practices arise from two sources: the environment and demands for acculturation. The environment causes changes in dietary practices when usual food sources or ingredients are not available or when changes in one's living environment make certain foods or practices inappropriate. For example, movement from a nomadic hunter society to a sedentary existence has caused the fat consumption of some Native American groups to become inappropriate and has resulted in widespread obesity.

Demands for acculturation, or a desire not to be "different," can lead to either positive or negative changes in eating habits. For instance, the desire to fit Western cultural norms has led to decreased breast-feeding among Southeast Asian women, a negative result of acculturation.

Other Consumption Patterns. Another consideration in investigating behavioral dimension factors in another culture is that of consumption patterns other than dietary practices. These include the use of tobacco, alcohol, and other abused substances. Alcoholism is a serious problem among Native Americans and has contributed to rising mortality rates due to alcohol-related motor vehicle accidents. In addition, alcohol is involved in five of the ten leading causes of death among Native Americans (May & Moran, 1995). Alcohol abuse among Native Americans also accounts for the high prevalence of fetal alcohol syndrome in this population. Native Americans also have higher self-reported rates for use of other drugs than other population groups. For example, approximately, 20% of Native American youths use some form of drugs and 71% use alcohol (Beauvais, 1996). In addition, almost 40% of Native American men, 29% of women, and 78% of young people smoke (Office of Surveillance and Analysis, 1994; Young, 1994), compared to less than 20% of Asian men and 10% of Asian women (Office of Surveillance and Analysis, 1994).

Use of alcohol is disapproved by many Appalachian families, although brewing alcoholic beverages for sale to outsiders is a lucrative enterprise in some parts of Appalachia. Asians have a relatively low incidence of alcoholism, which many believe is due to early introduction of children to moderate use of alcoholic beverages such as fruit wines and saki and to the high value placed on self-control. Among African Americans and Latinos, use of alcohol is considered part of the male adult image. Alcohol is proscribed among Muslim Arabs, but in one study as many as one third of the participants admitted to occasionally drinking alcohol (Haddad & Lummis, 1987).

Life Events. A great deal of variation exists among cultural groups in the attitudes and behaviors expected in relation to certain life events such as conception, birth, and death.

CONCEPTION AND CONTRACEPTION. Beliefs and practices related to conception and contraception vary from culture to culture. In very traditional Latino families, the wife may expect to become pregnant shortly after marriage. Should conception not occur, certain herbs may be used to "heat the womb" and promote conception. Korean women traditionally define their self-identity in terms of the mother role and their duty to produce an heir, so conception shortly after marriage is valued (Sich, 1988). For Arab clients, contraception is apt to be perceived as challenging Allah's will (The Crib Sheet, 1993). Family planning information is likely to be unwanted by women who adhere to such traditional beliefs about childbearing.

African and Native Americans tend to view contraception as an individual decision or one made for the good of the family. Latinos, on the other hand, may not be open to artificial forms of contraception such as birth control pills and intrauterine devices (IUDs) because of religious doctrines of the Roman Catholic Church, the primary religion of many Latinos. In addition, use of condoms may be strongly resisted by Latino women because "only prostitutes need to use condoms" (Organista & Organista, 1997). Filipinos often resist contraception on similar religious grounds. Asian women might be reluctant to seek family planning services if they believe that they will be examined by male health care providers; feminine modesty is highly valued in Asian culture.

BIRTH. Birth is a life event surrounded by many cultural beliefs and practices. Many folk health beliefs and practices are related to conception, pregnancy, labor and delivery, and postpartum care. The Navajo, for example, may hold special ceremonies just before or after birth. The Owl Way Ceremony is one used to safeguard both mother and child (Bell, 1994).

Among Asians, childbirth is not considered an illness, but is a period of danger for both mother and infant. Special foods and herbs such as ginseng are used to safeguard the pregnant woman. Iron in the prenatal period is thought to harden the bones and make delivery more difficult. Therefore, many Asian women will resist taking vitamin preparations containing iron. To facilitate delivery, a pregnant Vietnamese woman is encouraged from the seventh month of pregnancy to sit in a squatting position as much as possible.

Many Asians, including Vietnamese, Cambodians, and Chinese, believe that body heat is lost during labor and delivery (Geissler, 1994). The Vietnamese use hot coals beneath the bed to counteract this, and both Vietnamese and Chinese use "hot" foods to replenish body heat. Hot foods include rice, chicken soup, peanuts, vinegar, and ginger. Cold foods such as most fruits and vegetables are avoided.

Practices related to birth itself vary from one group to another. Among the Hmong, for example, the placenta is buried after delivery with the place of burial specifically defined for male and female infants. The placenta is to be buried near the center pole of the house after the birth of a male child and under the parents' bed for a girl. It is believed that the place where the placenta is buried is the person's "true home" and burial in the wrong place will lead to misfortune (Lee, 1986).

Some Mexican American women view colostrum as "bad milk" and may refuse to begin breastfeeding until several days after delivery. This belief is common in several cultures, and a variety of substances may be given to satisfy the baby until breast milk production begins. For example, Latinos may give milk, juice, herb teas, or sugar water. Herbal teas and waters may also be given in some African American and Arab cultures (Mennella, 1996).

Traditional Appalachian practices used in the postpartum period include bed rest, a dose of castor oil or paregoric to purge impurities from the mother, and avoidance of fresh fruit. In both Appalachian and African American cultures, catnip tea may be given to the newborn to cleanse the liver and bring out impurities. Arab infants may be tightly swaddled or have a band called a *zunaad* wrapped around the abdomen to prevent illness from cold entering the body. Another practice is to place *ko'hl* on the umbicial stump. Since ko'hl may have a high lead content, this last practice may be hazardous to the infant's health (Luna, 1994). Selected cultural beliefs and behaviors related to childbearing are presented in Table 16–4.

DEATH AND DYING.   The last life event to be considered in a cultural assessment is death. All cultural groups have beliefs and practices related to death and drying, and culture influences attitudes to death and dying in a number of ways. One area of influence is the need for comfort experienced by the dying client. In those cultures where death is seen as a normal part of life, there may be less need to comfort the dying and his or her family; conversely, in cultures where death is feared, comfort may be needed and appreciated.

The community health nurse should assess whether those he or she is dealing with have a cultural belief in an afterlife. Some non-Western religions, including Hinduism, believe in reincarnation until the soul has achieved perfection and passes to Nirvana. Do religious beliefs regarding death and afterlife offer a source of comfort to clients and families or do they engender fear and anxiety?

Attitudes toward death within a cultural group can also vary depending on the nature of the death. Violent deaths may be more difficult to accept as a normal part of life. Among African Americans, violent deaths provoke more emotional outbursts, anger, and rage than do natural deaths, and the Lao people see violent death as punishment for misdeeds (Westermeyer, 1988). For the Cheyenne, violent death is believed to lead to a disturbance in spiritual balance and eternal wandering of the departed soul.

Cultural responses to suicide differ from cultural responses to death from natural causes. For example, Latinos are more likely to conceal a suicide than members of other groups. This may be a result of past refusal by the Catholic Church to bury suicide victims in hallowed ground. Among Filipinos, suicide is considered shameful, whereas ritual suicide may restore family honor in other Asian cultural groups.

Culture also influences the selection and perception of health care providers when death is imminent. People from some cultures believe that death should occur at home and are, therefore, unlikely to seek medical care for a dying client for fear that he or she will be removed from the home and placed in a hospital to die. For many people, going to the hospital means that death is inevitable. For example, Asian, Native American, African American, and Appalachian clients may equate hospitalization with imminent death.

Care of the body following death and funeral and burial practices are also influenced by culture, as are expectations regarding grief and mourning and practices to be observed during this period. Mourning is a cultural expression of grief following death, and mourning practices may vary from group to group.

Finally, culture influences communication regarding death, particularly with respect to children and their knowledge of and participation in the rites that accompany a death. For example, Appalachians are usually quite open in their communication about death, and Native American and Latino children help with the care of the dying family member and participate in funeral and grieving practices. Despite this participation, members of many cultural groups may resist telling the client or others regarding imminent death. This resistance may stem from three causes, reluctance to eliminate hope and beliefs that discussing an event will either cause it to happen or prevent it from happening (Gropper, 1996). Because of these beliefs, some clients may actually resist signing advance directives (Blackhall, Murphy, Frank, Michel, & Azen, 1995; Koenig & Gates-Williams, 1995).

Other questions relate to who should attend the

TABLE 16–4. SELECTED BELIEFS AND BEHAVIORS REGARDING CHILDBEARING

Focus	Belief or Behavior
General	• The uterus is the center of female energy. (Hmong) • Menstrual cramping can be alleviated by avoiding hot spicy food. (Appalachian, Latino) • Menstruation is a "hot" condition, so "cold" foods should be eaten. (Appalachian) • Childbirth is a natural event. (Appalachian)[a] • A pregnant woman is considered ill or weak. (Latino) • Pregnancy is a time of danger for mother and child, but is not an illness. (Asian) • Children are a sign of a man's virility. (Latino) • Wives should become pregnant as soon as possible after marriage. (Latino, Korean) • Sexuality should not be discussed between men and women. (Asian, Latino, Arab)
Contraception	• Herbal preparations can be used to prevent pregnancy. They may be given as teas, suppositories, or douches, or applied topically, or inhaled. (Latino) • Pregnancy should be prevented by abstinence. (Chinese, Filipino, Latino, Roman Catholic) • Oral contraceptives cause birth defects and ill health for the mother. (Appalachian) • Abortion can be caused by drinking ginger root tea, jumping from a height, or stepping over a rail fence. (Appalachian) • A wife who asks her husband to use a condom marks herself as a prostitute. (Latino) • Nine drops of turpentine taken 9 days after intercourse will prevent conception. (Appalachian) • Charms and ceremonies may prevent conception. (Native American) • Contraception challenges the will of God. (Latino, Arab)
Conception	• Herbs can be used to "heat" the womb to promote conception. (Latino) • The fertile period for a woman is a few hours of a "heat cycle" midway between menstrual periods. (Appalachian) • The child's sex is determined by the side the mother turns to after intercourse. (Appalachian) • The right ovary produces "girl seeds;" the left produces "boy seeds." (Appalachian)
Pregnancy	• Pregnant women should eat a balanced diet and avoid sweets and snacks. (Appalachian)[a] • Pregnancy is a "hot" condition so meat should be avoided and sodium intake increased. (African American)[b] • "Hot" foods including protein foods should be avoided in pregnancy. (Latino)[b] • Red meat should be avoided during pregnancy to prevent "high blood." (African American, Appalachian)[b] • Iron in the prenatal diet causes hardening of the bones and a difficult labor. (Asian)[b] • Milk during pregnancy may result in a large baby and a hard labor. (Latino)[b] • Soy sauce and shellfish should be avoided during pregnancy. (Asian) • Unclean foods should be avoided during pregnancy. (Asian) • Cravings should be satisfied to prevent a defect related to the food craved. (Appalachian, Latino) • Ginseng tea will strengthen the pregnant woman. (Asian) • Strong emotions during pregnancy will leave a mark on the baby. (Appalachian, Latino) • Fright or surprise during pregnancy can injure the baby. (Latino, Appalachian) • A pregnant woman's workload should be reduced. (Native American) • Pregnant women should avoid raising their arms or hanging laundry to prevent knots in the umbilical cord. (Latino) • Sitting cross-legged will cause knots in the umbilical cord. (Latino) • Bathing should be encouraged during pregnancy. (Latino)[a] • Pregnant women should sleep on their backs. (Latino) • Pregnant women should keep active. (Latino)[a] • Nausea and vomiting can be treated with a mixture of flour and water, lemon and water, or chamomile tea. (Latino) • Violent purging herbs can be used for constipation in pregnancy. (Latino)[b] • Prenatal care and delivery by a woman is preferred. (Appalachian, Asian) • Pregnant women should be accompanied to the doctor by husbands or female family members. (Latino) • Periodic massage during pregnancy can help fix the uterus in the correct position for delivery. (Latino) • Baby showers should be held close to the time of delivery to prevent envy and the "evil eye." (Latino) • Planning for the baby prior to delivery defies God's will. (Arab) • Sexual activity should be continued throughout pregnancy to keep the birth canal lubricated. (Latino)
Delivery	• There is a correlation between the hour of conception and time of delivery. (Appalachian) • Labor can be stimulated by the use of herbal preparations. (Latino) • Tea made of winter fat leaves and roots will enhance contractions. (Hopi) • Wrapping warm cloths around the mother's ankles will speed delivery. (Appalachian) • The presence of the father or an article of his clothing will speed delivery. (Appalachian) • The father or one of his relatives should deliver the child. (Hmong) • Husbands should not be present during labor and delivery. (other Asian, Latino, Arab) • Husbands should be present during delivery. (dominant U.S.) • Children should be excluded from delivery. (dominant U.S.) • Physical exertion will initiate labor in women who go over term. (European American) • The pregnant woman's mother-in-law should attend her during delivery. (Chinese) • Birth attendants should be female. (Native American)

TABLE 16–4. SELECTED BELIEFS AND BEHAVIORS REGARDING CHILDBEARING (Continued)

Focus	Belief or Behavior
Delivery (continued)	• The person who delivers and "breathes life into" the baby has a special bond with the baby. (Native American)
	• It is inappropriate to exhibit pain during labor. (Asian, many European Americans)
	• Emotional expression is expected during labor. (Arab, Italian)
	• Labor pains can be "cut" by placing a sharp implement under the bed. (Appalachian)
	• Aspirin given for pain will thin the blood and cause increased bleeding. (Appalachian)[a]
	• Recitation of certain biblical passages will stop hemorrhage. (Appalachian)
	• Delivery should take place in a squatting position. (Asian)
	• Delivery causes a loss of body heat that must be replaced. (Asian)
	• Delivery is a "hot" condition, so no pork (a hot food) should be eaten afterward, also no penicillin, which is a hot medicine. (Latino)
	• Delivery is a "cold" experience that may allow spirits to leave the body. (Hmong)
	• Spinal anesthesia/epidural is dangerous. (Arab)
Postparum	• Castor oil or paregoric should be given to the woman after delivery. (Appalacian)[b]
	• Boiled cedar tea should be drunk to cleanse the mother after delivery. (Native American)
	• Cleansing rituals including washing, incense, or burning sage may be used after delivery. (Native American)
	• Fresh fruit and other "cold" foods should not be eaten after delivery. (Appalachian, Asian, Hmong, Mexican)
	• Incompatible "hot" and "cold" foods should be avoided during hospitalization after delivery. (Arab)
	• A postpartum diet should include chicken, soup, nonsticky rice, and special herbs to "wash out" the uterus. (Hmong)
	• Warm or hot fluids should be drunk after delivery. (Hmong)
	• Ginseng tea should be drunk after delivery to build the blood. (Chinese)
	• Salads and sour foods cause postpartum incontinence. (Asian)
	• Postpartum fluid intake should be decreased to prevent stretching the stomach. (Asian)[b]
	• Beef and seafood cause itching at the episiotomy site. (Asian)
	• Alcohol in rice wine causes bleeding. (Asian)
	• Prolonged bed rest and avoidance of strenuous activity prevent complications after delivery. (Appalachian, Asian, Hmong)[b]
	• Bathing should be avoided after delivery. (Mexican)
	• Outside visitors should be discouraged after delivery. (Korean)
	• Strangers after delivery may steal the mother's milk. (Hmong)
	• Postpartum pain can be relieved by whiskey or by hanging the husband's pants over the bedpost. (Appalachian)
	• Herbal preparations can relieve afterpains. (Latino)
	• Burning or burying the placenta will prevent harm to mother and child. (Appalachian, Hmong)
	• The placenta should be disposed of in the Rio Grande with a prayer ceremony. (southwestern Native American)
	• Drinking cold water should be avoided after delivery. (Asian)
	• No water should be drunk for 4 months after delivery; then water from the Rio Grande should be drunk. (Native American)
	• Intercourse should be avoided 2 to 3 months after delivery to prevent disease. (Asian)
Infant	• Infants should not be fussed over or cuddled or evil spirits may steal them. (Vietnamese)
	• A beautiful baby may provoke envy and the evil eye so praise should be given to the mother for her performance in delivery rather than to the baby. (Arab)
	• Wearing of amulets and not mentioning the number 5 will protect against the evil eye. (Arab)
	• Massage of the newborn by the mother promotes bonding. (Native American)[a]
	• The infant should not be named until it is brought home. (Vietnamese)
	• An Indian name may be given at a traditonal naming ceremony and a saint's name at baptism. (Native American)
	• An infant's name may be given by an older relative or tribal leader. (Native American)
	• An infant's name may be selected on the basis of his or her horoscope or personal characteristics. (Asian)
	• Colostrum is "bad milk" and may make the infant ill; breastfeeding should not start until actual milk comes in. (Latino)
	• Castor oil will seal the umbilical stump. (Appalachian)
	• Ko'hl should be put on the umbilica stump. (Arab)[b]
	• A raisin on the umbilical stump will prevent air from entering the infant's body. (Latino)[b]
	• A belly band on the infant will prevent umbilical hernia or protruberant umbilicus. (Latino)
	• Infants should be given a purge or tonic (may contain lead). (Asian, African American)[b]
	• A second stillbirth can be prevented by placing a dead infant face down in the coffin. (Appalachian)
	• Exposure to a menstruating woman may cause an umbilical hernia. (African American, Latino)
	• Infants should be kept wrapped on a cradle board provided by the father. (Native American)[a]
	• Infants should be warmly clothed and wrapped. (European American)
	• Infants should not be cuddled too much to avoid spoiling them. (European American)
	• The child should be kept physically close to the mother for the first year. (Mexican)
	• Breastfeeding may continue for several years. (Asian)
	• Males do not do child care. (Middle Eastern)

[a]Beliefs or practices consistent with scientific health care.
[b]Potentially harmful beliefs or practices

dying client. The eldest son of a Chinese client should be present with his dying parent, whereas in some Native American tribes, the maternal aunt is the more important figure. Members of other tribes believe that the spirit cannot leave the body until family members are present.

Nurses should be familiar with the death rites of specific cultural groups so they can assist the family through their time of grief. Should the nurse wash and prepare the body or is a family member responsible for this? Should personal belongings be left with the body or given to the family? The nurse should learn the answers to such questions when working with clients from other cultures.

Generally speaking, there is no belief in an afterlife among traditional Native American tribes. Nurses who use this approach to comfort clients with terminal disease will find it ineffective. Nurses may be confused and frustrated by the lack of response by some clients to such efforts unless an understanding of the cultural beliefs involved has been achieved.

Another area for consideration is preparation of the body. Members of many Native American tribes see the body as a "seed to be planted" and believe that the body must be disposed of in its entirety. Thus, family members may request amputated limbs to be kept until death and disposal of the body. They may also resist having an autopsy performed. In a similar view, some Native Americans may request the return of hair or nail clippings from hospitalized clients to prevent their use by witches. Disposal of the body can vary among tribes. For example, cremation is traditionally practiced by the Tlingit and Quechan tribes, whereas the Sioux place the dead on elevated platforms, and members of Pueblo tribes bury their dead. Among many tribes, such as the Navajo, the body is dressed in fine clothes and jewelry and wrapped in new blankets. The Tlingit fear to touch a dead body, so the client may be dressed in funeral clothes several days before death.

Mourning can be very emotional in some cultural groups and may last for varying periods of time. For instance, following 4 days of mourning, the Cheyenne and Quechan cease grieving, as do members of some other tribes. In some tribes, the name of the deceased is never spoken again and memory of the deceased is actively suppressed.

Clothing assumes special meanings when it comes to dying. The clothing of a deceased Chinese person is believed to contain evil spirits. Family members of hospitalized clients should be encouraged to take clothing home until the client is discharged. If the client should die, the family may be reluctant to accept the deceased's personal effects. Clothing is also used to symbolize mourning, and mourning garments are worn for varying lengths of time in different cultures. The color of mourning can also vary. For example, black is the color of mourning for many cultures, but among the Hmong and Vietnamese, white signifies mourning and black is worn for weddings and other celebrations.

In traditional African American culture, death is perceived as a passage from one realm of life to another. Funerals are generally occasions for celebration despite the grief of family members left behind. Some African Americans also practice passing a child over the dead body to carry away any illness the child may have. As is true in the larger society, funerals and wakes are seen as a psychosocial mechanism that facilitates grieving. Funerals for many Latinos are evidence of their deep religious belief in an afterlife.

As we have seen, beliefs and behaviors regarding death and dying vary among different cultures. Table 16–5 presents selected cultural behaviors related to death and dying.

Sexual Practices. Another element of the behavioral dimension that is influenced by culture is sexual behavior. Behavior related to contraceptive use has already been addressed, but other aspects of sexuality should be considered by the community health nurse. Homosexuality is one of these areas. Homosexuality may be defined differently in some cultures than in the dominant U.S. culture. For example, Latino, Middle Eastern, and Greek men who have sex with other men are only considered homosexual if they assume a receptor role; whereas for Haitians, intercourse with other men is not homosexual if it is done for money (Gropper, 1996; Organista & Organista, 1997). Among Khmer women, lesbianism is generally disregarded rather than ostracized (Thompson, 1991).

Attitudes regarding heterosexual activity are another area for consideration. Some Arab Muslims believe any sexual activity makes one unclean and must be followed by purification rituals (Luna, 1989). Adultery is regarded with extreme disapproval and may result in death in some traditional Muslim countries (Haddad & Lummis, 1987). Among Latinos, extramarital sexual activity is accepted for men, but not women (Peragallo, 1996). "Good" women are not sexually experienced or knowledgeable and may not be willing to discuss sexual issues with their partners for fear of being thought prostitutes (Hubbell, Chavez, Mishra, & Valdez, 1996; Organista & Organista, 1997). These cultural attitudes place Latinos at risk for sexually transmitted diseases and cervical cancer since sexual beliefs have been found to influence willingness to obtain Pap smears.

One area of increasing concern related to sexuality is female genital mutilation (FGM). This practice is

TABLE 16–5. SELECTED CULTURAL BELIEFS AND BEHAVIORS REGARDING DEATH

Focus	Belief or Behavior
General	• Death is a normal part of life. (Native American, Asian) • Death is passage from one realm of life to a better one. (African American, Appalachian) • Death is passage into the next life. (Asian) • No belief in an afterlife. (Native American) • Flowers should not be given to the living because they are reserved for the dead. (Vietnamese) • Visitation by a clergy member may be perceived as indicating imminent death. (Vietnamese)
Violent death	• Violent death provokes stronger emotional outbursts than does a normal death. (African American) • Violent death is punishment for misdeeds. (Lao) • Violent death creates a ghost to wander forever. (Navajo, Cheyenne)
Suicide	• Suicide should be concealed because of its shameful nature. (Latino, Filipino) • Suicide may be used to restore family honor. (other Asian)
Time and place of death	• Hospitalization means death is imminent. (African American, Asian, Native American, Appalachian) • Death should occur at home. (Hmong, Vietnamese) • Removal of life support should be postponed until an "auspicious" time. (Asian)
Preparation and disposal of body	• Touching a dead body may bring misfortune. (Navajo, Tlingit) • Touching an animal struck by lightning can bring misfortune. (Navajo) • Passing an ill child over a dead body may cure illness. (African American) • Entire body must be disposed of together. Autopsy may be resisted. (Native American, Vietnamese) • Bodies should be cremated. (Tlingit, Quechan) • Bodies should be buried. (Pueblo tribes) • Bodies should be exposed to air on a funeral platform. (Sioux) • The dying person should be dressed in funeral clothes before death. (Tlingit) • Family members should prepare the body for disposal. (Sioux) • Bodies are prepared for burial by commercial mortuary. (Latino, European American) • Bodies should be richly dressed and wrapped in new blankets. (Navajo) • Clothing of a dead person may contain evil spirits. (Chinese) • The hair of the dead person should be unraveled. (Navajo) • The home of a dead person may contain evil spirits and should be sealed to prevent its future use. (Navajo) • Touching articles belonging to a dead person may bring misfortune. (Navajo) • The dead should be buried in family graveyards when possible. (Appalachian) • Graveyards should be placed on hilltops to prevent the graves from being covered by water. (Appalachian) • If a body is exhumed and reburied, the person will not go to heaven. (Appalachian) • The body should be buried facing Mecca. (Arab) • Organ donation is prohibited. (Arab)
Grief and mourning	• Emotional grieving lasts 4 days, after which the name of the dead is never spoken. (Cheyenne, Quechan, Navajo) • White should be worn during the mourning period. (Hmong) • Black should be worn during the mourning period. (Latino, European American) • Social activities should be restricted during the mourning period. (Latino) • The dead should be included in rituals commemorating ancestors. (Vietnamese) • Homage paid to ancestral spirits will prevent illness. (Hmong, Vietnamese) • The funeral and wake are a time to rejoice for the dead and comfort the living. (African American) • Funeral Mass is preceded by saying the Rosary. (Latino) • The first Monday after death begins 9 days of evening prayer for the dead. (Latino) • Funerals should be followed by food. (European American) • Condolences should be offered with a handshake and special phrases of consolation. (Arab)
Participation and knowledge	• Dying clients should be protected from knowledge of impending death. (Latino, Chinese, Japanese, Arab, African American) • Bad news should be mixed with an element of hope. (Hmong) • Children should participate in the care of dying family members, funerals, and mourning. (Native American, Latino) • The eldest son should be present at the death of a parent. (Chinese) • Family members must be present for the spirit to leave the body. (Native American)

frequently associated with the Muslim religion, but it is also practiced by some non-Islamic groups (including some Christians, Animists, and the Fallasha Jews of Ethiopia). Not all Muslim cultural groups practice FGM and it is not supported by the Qur'an. Cultural groups that practice FGM, however, are found in Africa, the Middle East, Latin America, India and the Far East, North America, and Europe (Wright, 1996). Community health nurses should be alert to the possible practice of FGM in client populations with whom they work because of the serious physical and psychological health effects including infection and difficulties with fertility, pregnancy, and delivery.

The Health System Dimension

Areas of cultural assessment related to the health care system include the folk health system within the culture, as well as group members' use of the scientific system. Components of the folk health system to be addressed include cultural perceptions of health and illness and disease causation, folk health practitioners, and culturally prescribed health practices.

Perceptions of Health and Illness and Disease Causation. All cultures have concepts of health and illness and theories of disease causation, although these may differ widely from group to group. It has been suggested that each culture has an "explanatory model" that defines the nature of illness, its treatment, and the type of relationships that should occur between client and health care provider. European Americans, for example, often view exposure to cold weather as a contributing factor in illness. Other cultural groups have similar explanations of the cause of disease. Nurses who wish to understand clients' conceptions of health and illness must investigate the explanatory models found in each client's culture.

Among Native Americans, for example, health is viewed in terms of the life cycle, which encompasses birth, life, and death. Health is the result of harmony and order between man and universe, congruence with other people, the environment, and supernatural forces. The Navajo term for this state of harmony is *hozhoni* (Huttlinger & Tanner, 1994).

The Asian concept of health involves achieving a state of *Qi* (pronounced "chee"), which is a balance of Yin and Yang (Spector, 1996). An imbalance between Yin and Yang results in disharmony or illness. Most Asian cultures believe that all components of the universe, including humans, are composed of a Yin and a Yang (Cargill, 1994). The Yin is the negative female force, characterized by darkness, cold, and emptiness. The Yang is the positive male force producing light, warmth, and fullness. An overabundance of either Yin

or Yang is thought to trigger illness. Other recognized causes of illness in some Asian cultures include soul loss or theft, spirit possession, breach of taboo, and object intrusion in which a magical foreign object enters the body. Similar causes of disease are also noted among some Native American tribes.

African Americans tend to classify illnesses as natural or unnatural, and they place them in three etiologic categories: environmental hazards, divine punishment, and impaired social relationships that may result in worry or the incursion of spells and witchcraft (Cherry, 1991). In traditional African American culture, all illnesses are thought to be curable, and the concept of chronic disease is difficult to accept (Gropper, 1996). The belief in a cure for every illness is derived from the principle that for everything, including disease, there exists its opposite. African Americans tend not to separate mental and physical illness.

In some Latino subgroups, illness is viewed as more than a mere biological occurrence and is seen in terms of its spiritual and social ramifications. Latino clients also differentiate between natural and unnatural illnesses. Natural illnesses are thought to occur as the result of a personal violation of the balance among human beings, nature, and God (Schrefer, 1994). Unnatural or supernatural illness is secondary to satanic forces. Illness can also be a result of imbalance in "hot" and "cold" humors, concepts similar to the hot-and-cold balance seen in Asian cultures (Autotte, 1995).

In some Latino subgroups, chronic illness is seen as punishment for evil. The traditional Latino attitude toward health and illness can be fatalistic. It is believed that health is a matter of chance and little can be done to maintain or enhance it. Health is perceived as a gift from God (Spector, 1996) and is defined in terms of three criteria: freedom from pain, a well-fleshed body, and a high level of physical activity. Health is equated with strength, and illness is equated with weakness. Selected cultural beliefs regarding disease causation are presented in Table 16–6.

Folk Health Practitioners. Every culture has its own folk health practitioners. The most important attributes of folk practitioners were well captured in this description:

> The folk practitioner uses a combination of rational, irrational, and psychological techniques in curing; his diagnosis is minimal; he has folk medical theories based on such things as a simplified notion of the body, religion, astrology, and plant lore; he treats more commonplace or chronic conditions than he does acute ailments or infectious diseases; he is charismatic and a good showman; and he reinforces the value system of his clients (Green, 1978).

TABLE 16–6. SELECTED CULTURAL BELIEFS REGARDING DISEASE CAUSATION

Focus	Belief
General	• Illness can result from either natural or supernatural causes. (Native American, Asian, Appalachian, African American, Latino, Vietnamese)
Natural illness	• Illness can result from violation of a natural law. (Native American)
	• Natural phenomena such as storms, lightning, and other disturbances may cause disease. (Native American)
	• Germs may cause disease. (Appalachian, Vietnamese, dominant U.S.)
	• Environmental hazards (eg, bad air, water) may result in illness. (African American, Vietnamese, Mexican)
	• Imbalance among person, nature, and God may cause illness. (Latino)
	• Imbalance between "hot" and "cold" forces may cause illness. (Arab, Appalachian, Vietnamese, Puerto Rican, Mexican, Hmong, Chinese)
	• Natural illnesses may result from insect bites, bruises, or injuries that cause fractures. (Zuni)
	• Bad blood may cause disease. (African American, Hmong)
	• Illness may be due to inharmonious relationships or inappropriate behavior by client, relatives, and/or neighbors. (Southeast Asian, Chinese, Native American, Mexican, African American)
	• Natural diseases occur when one confronts the forces of nature without adequate protection. (African American)
	• Poor health habits and bad hygiene may cause disease. (African American, Appalachian)
	• Irregular bowel habits might bring on illness. (African American, Appalachian, European American)
	• "Nerves" can cause illnesses such as depression, gastrointestinal upset, weight loss, and headache. (Appalachian)
	• Disease may result from dislocation of a body part. (Latino)
	• Being deprived of certain foods may cause illness. (Saudi)
	• Cutting one's hair may result in weakness or illness. (Native American)
	• Fright may cause soul loss and illness. (Latino, Hmong)
	• Exposure to cold weather may cause illness. (European American)
Supernatural illness	• "Bad" illnesses are caused by the evil action of people or spirits. (Otomi)
	• "Airs" or wandering ghosts of those who met violent ends may cause illness. (Otomi)
	• Disease may result from spirit intrusion or object intrusion. (Otomi, Zuni, other Native American, Asian)
	• Breach of taboo may result in disease. (Zuni, Asian)
	• Germs must be activated by a sorcerer before they can cause disease. (Thai)
	• Evil spirits cause disease. (Hmong, African American, Latino, Zuni, Navajo)
	• Illness may be punishment for sins or a test of faith. (African American, Appalachian, Latino, Vietnamese)
	• Soul loss may cause disease. (Hmong, Lao, Native American, Latino)
	• Illness may be due to witchcraft. (African American, Latino, Asian, Appalachian, Vietnamese, Native American)
	• Disease may result from exposure to an "evil eye." (Scot, Latino, Asian, Jewish, Italian, Iranian, Indian, Greek, Central American, Mediterranean, Middle Eastern, African American, Filipino)
	• Illness may be the will of God. (Latino, Filipino, Muslim, African American, Appalachian, European American)
	• Having blood drawn may cause disease. (Hmong)

Folk practitioners may come to their calling in several ways including inheritance, family position, birth portents, revelation, apprenticeship, and self-study (Helman, 1994). Healing skills are sometimes believed to be passed down in families from generation to generation, or one's position within the family may suggest special abilities (eg, the seventh son of a seventh son). Unusual occurrences during pregnancy or at birth, such as being born with a "caul" or amniotic sac over the face, may also herald healing skills. Other practitioners may be called in dream or vision or after recovering from a life-threatening illness themselves. Others show an aptitude for healing and may be apprenticed to an experienced healer. Finally, some practitioners learn their calling on their own due to personal interest.

There is wide variation in the types of folk healers found in different cultural groups, from the family member or friend with expertise in dealing with illness to the specialist practitioner. Most of us have family members who have a repertoire of home remedies used for illness. For example, your mother may recommend peppermint tea for an upset stomach or honey and lemon for a sore throat. Generally speaking, most people first seek advice on health from these knowledgeable family members or friends before seeking more professional assistance. That professional assistance, however, may be sought from a variety of different practitioners depending on one's cultural background. There is also a growing tendency among the general public to seek health care from providers of other cultural groups. Many clients with AIDS, for example, are seeking relief of symptoms through acupuncture, and the use of chiropractic services for back pain is also increasing. In fact, some health insurance plans are even beginning to cover some more traditional folk healing practices, and there is a growing body of scientific research attesting to the efficacy of many traditional forms of healing.

Some cultural groups include a wide array of health providers, many of them highly specialized. Zuni healers, for example, are divided into twelve highly secret medicine societies, each of which specializes in the treatment of specific conditions (Hultkrantz, 1992). Navajo healers or singers may also specialize in the kinds of sings they are qualified to perform (Bell, 1994). Asian practitioners are often divided into the categories recognized in Chinese medicine including acupuncturists and herbalists. Herbalists are also found among African American, Latino, and Appalachian cultural groups.

Religious healers, faith healers, or spiritualists are found among many cultural groups, including Asians, Latinos, African Americans, and Appalachians. Religion as a source of healing is common, and prayer and other religious rituals may accompany more scientific forms of healing for many of us. The charismatic healing tradition of the Roman Catholic Church is another example of the use of religious practices in healing. Other cultural groups embrace the practice of psychic healers (Cavender, 1996) thought to possess healing energy that can be transmitted to others, usually by some form of touch. Belief in this transfer of energy underlies the practice of therapeutic touch as a nursing intervention.

Practitioners of healing magic may also be found in a number of cultural groups. For example, the *abolarios* in the Latino folk health tradition of *curanderismo* specialize in the treatment of illness due to witchcraft (Weaver, 1994). The voodoo priest or priestess found among some African American groups is another example of magic used in healing. Another group of health practitioners found in many cultures specializes in massage and is exemplified by the *sabador* in some Latino cultures. Finally, many cultural groups include midwives as recognized health practitioners. In fact, midwifery as a specialized practice is a growing phenomenon in nursing that is gaining in popularity throughout the United States.

In assessing any cultural group, the nurse explores several areas related to folk health practitioners. Among these are the types of practitioners recognized by the group, the health-related services provided, and the methods employed. Who and where are the practitioners? Is there a recognized hierarchy among practitioners? Does referral or cooperation exist between folk and professional practitioners? Who uses the folk practitioner and what is the prevailing attitude of community members toward folk practitioners? Finally, the nurse explores the expectations involved in the client–practitioner relationship.

Folk Health Practices. Members of all cultural groups engage in certain culturally prescribed health practices. It is wise for the community health nurse exploring the health practices employed by a cultural group to recognize that these practices are designed to meet specific needs and have meaning and importance to group members.

Traditional health practices can be categorized into those related to primary and secondary prevention. Childbirth practices, a special category of primary preventive measures, were discussed earlier in this chapter.

PRIMARY PREVENTIVE PRACTICES. Health promotion and illness prevention are important aspects of a folk health system. Table 16–7 presents some cultural beliefs and behaviors related to health promotion and illness prevention. Although health-promotive and illness-preventive measures vary considerably from one culture to another, there are several common types of primary prevention measures found in many cultures. One such common practice is the use of diet to promote health and prevent illness. For example, ginseng preparations as well as other special foods may be given to pregnant Asian women to provide strength and prevent complications. African Americans, on the other hand, may avoid red meat to prevent "high blood." Among both Latinos and Asians, maintenance of a balance between "hot" and "cold" foods is used to prevent illness, whereas a traditional Appalachian client may eat raw onions or take baking soda to prevent influenza (Green, 1978).

The use of herbal and other medicinal preparations is another common preventive strategy in a number of cultures. For example, many European Americans take large doses of vitamins C or E to prevent illness. Herbal teas are widely used among Native Americans and Asians as well as other cultural groups, although the herbs used may vary from one group to another.

Many cultural groups also use religious or magical amulets or charms to prevent disease or misfortune. For example, many European American and Latino Catholics wear medals of patron saints or the Virgin Mary. Similarly, Arab Americans may use amulets to ward off evil spirits or the evil eye. Amulets may include verses from the Qur'an, turquoise, or a five-fingered hand (Geissler, 1994). Among some Native American tribes, a medicine bundle, or *gist*, is carried to ensure blessing. A most powerful charm used by the Lao is made from the fat of a person who has met a violent death (Westermeyer, 1988), and charms and amulets are common among other Asian cultural groups as well.

Cleansing is another health promotion strategy

TABLE 16–7. SELECTED CULTURAL BELIEFS AND BEHAVIORS RELATED TO HEALTH PROMOTION AND ILLNESS PREVENTION

Focus	Belief or Behavior
General	• Moving in a clockwise direction in the home maintains balance with the environment. (Navajo) • A variety of herbal preparations can be used to promote health and prevent illness. (Asian, Latino, African American, Native American, Appalachian, European American) • Periodic purges keep the system open and prevent disease. (African American) • Silver or copper bracelets worn by young girls warn of impending illness by turning the surrounding skin black. (African American) • A *limpia* or cleansing ceremony may be used as a general preventive measure. (Otomi) • Herbal remedies must be gathered at appropriate times to be effective. (Chinese, Appalachian) • Avoid water after engaging in a "hot" activity. (Mexican) • Sulfur and molasses rubbed on the back provides a spring tonic. (African American) • Hanging garlic or onions in the home can prevent illness. (Native American) • Burning refuse will prevent disease. (Native American)[a] • Dressing warmly can prevent illness. (European American)
Diet	• Children, pregnant women, convalescents, and the elderly should avoid red meat to prevent "high blood." (African American, Appalachian)[b] • Pork, cabbage, instant coffee, "store tea," fish with scales, round-hoofed animals, oysters, potatoes, plums, grapefruit, cherries, cranberries, graham crackers, salt, and saccharin lead to waste buildup and illness and should be avoided. (Appalachian) • A balance of "hot" and "cold" foods should be eaten. (Asian, Latino, Appalachian, Arab) • "Hot" foods include beef, pork, potatoes, and whiskey. "Cold" foods include chicken, fish, fruit, and beer. (Pakistani) • Eating three meals, including breakfast, promotes health. (African American, dominant U.S.) • Eating a 1000-year-old egg can prevent illness. (Chinese)
Lifestyle	• Excess in food, drink, and activity should be avoided. (African American) • Keeping the body clean inside and out will prevent illness. (African American) • Rest promotes health. (African American) • Staying active promotes health. (Appalachian)
Prayer and magic	• Carrying a printed prayer on one's person will prevent mishap. (African American, Appalachian) • Prayer and veneration of the relics of saints can prevent illness. (Latino and other Roman Catholic) • Blessing throats on St. Blaise's feastday (Feb. 3) can prevent choking. (Latino and other Roman Catholic) • Wearing garlic on one's person wards off evil spirits. (African American) • Charms made of the fat of a person who died a violent death can scare away evil spirits. (Lao) • Amulets, chains, and tattoos prevent spirit invasion. (Khmer) • A string on the wrist or neck protects the infant from evil spirits. (Hmong) • Charms and fetishes will ward off evil. (Native American) • Wearing religious medals or displaying religious statues in the home can prevent misfortune. (Latino and other Roman Catholic) • Carrying or wearing a medicine bundle can prevent illness. (Native American) • Placing a red ribbon on a child can prevent illness. (Mexican) • Prevent evil spirits by wearing amulets in the hair or in a red bag pinned to clothing or hanging them over doors, on walls, or on curtains. (Chinese) • Jade charms bring health. If the charm dulls or is broken, misfortune follows. (Chinese) • Tying a string on an arm, leg, or around the neck controls spirits. (Vietnamese) • A gold ring on a red ribbon around the neck will prevent anxiety. (Latino) • Keeping a black animal will prevent witchcraft. (Mexican) • Wearing coral around the neck or wrist will prevent depression and "evil eye." (Latino) • Touching a child while admiring him or her will prevent evil eye. (Mexican) • Moistening a finger with saliva and tracing a cross in a child's forehead can prevent evil eye. (Filipino) • Charms can prevent the evil eye. (Mediterranean) • Wearing copper or silver bracelets, necklaces, or anklets prevents soul loss by locking the soul into the body. (Hmong)
Specific prevention	• Eating onions or baking soda will prevent "flu." (Appalachian)[b] • Avoiding tomatoes will prevent cancer. (Appalachian) • Immunization prevents smallpox. (ancient Chinese)[a] • *Asafetida*, or rotten flesh, worn in a bag around the neck prevents communicable disease. (African American) • Avoiding cutting infants' fingernails will prevent heart disease. (Asian) • Nosebleeds can be prevented by not becoming overheated. (Latino, dominant U.S.) • Prevent chills by not eating or drinking cold things when hot. (Latino) • Not cutting one's hair will prevent loss of strength. (Native American) • Avoid writing one's story to prevent loss of life spirit. (Native American) • Isolation will prevent the spread of communicable diseases. (Native American)[a] • Isolating ill persons will prevent their condition from becoming worse. (Native American)[a] • Not going barefoot will prevent tonsillitis. (Latino) • Chachayotel, a seed, tied around the waist will prevent arthritis. (Mexican) • Cod liver oil prevents colds. (African American) • Avoid sitting under a mango tree when hot to prevent kidney infection and back problems. (Puerto Rican) • Avoid baby formula for infants because it causes rashes. (Puerto Rican) • Avoid going into the coffee fields when hot to prevent respiratory illness. (Puerto Rican) • Avoid drinking cold water when hot to prevent colds. (Puerto Rican)

[a]Belief or practice consistent with scientific health care.
[b]Potentially harmful belief or practice.

that may be employed either figuratively or literally. Sweat baths are used by several Native American tribes to remove impurities. Among the Otomi, the *limpia,* or cleansing ceremony, may be used on a regular basis both as a preventive and curative measure (Dow, 1986). Ritual cleansing is also employed by Muslim Arabs. African Americans and Appalachians, on the other hand, may engage in internal cleansing of impurities through the use of laxatives to purge the body.

Some cultural groups also engage in measures designed to limit the transmission of communicable diseases. Interestingly, African American slaves practiced smallpox inoculation well before the acceptance of this practice in the larger society (Spector, 1996). Similarly, some Native American tribes developed a number of precautions for communicable diseases without benefit of knowledge of pathogenic organisms. Some of these practices included isolation, burning or washing of contaminated articles, and burning of refuse. Meditation and massage are other primary prevention practices used in some cultural groups.

SECONDARY PREVENTIVE PRACTICES.   When illness occurs, members of a cultural group turn to practices designed to diagnose and treat illness. Many similarities exist between cultures in such practices. Table 16–8 includes selected cultural beliefs and practices related to diagnosis and treatment of illness.

Several diagnostic techniques are used in different cultures. For example, some Native American and Asian cultural groups use dreams as diagnostic tools. Seers or prophets within some Native American tribes may be responsible for interpreting dreams. Other types of Native American diagnosticians include the "hand trembler" and "crystal" or "star gazers" who identify the locale and cause of disease.

Asian medicine employs four diagnostic techniques: glossoscopy, osphretics, anamnesis, and sphygmopalpation (Spector, 1996). *Glossoscopy* involves primarily inspection of the tongue; *osphretics* assesses sounds and odors. *Anamnesis,* or questioning, addresses many of the same areas covered in a routine health history. In *sphygmopalpation,* the practitioner examines several pulses (Cargill, 1994), the abdomen and chest, the back, and the meridians that carry the *Qi* (pronounced "chee") or life force. One other diagnostic approach that may be used by some practitioners is iridology, or examination of various parts of the iris that reflect the condition of specific body parts (Yetiv, 1988). Some African Americans and traditional Appalachians may consult the signs of the zodiac. Specific signs of the zodiac may be associated with particular body parts. Aries, for example, is the "head" sign, so persons under this sign are particularly susceptible to head colds (Green, 1978).

Treatment modalities also vary among cultural groups, but certain categories of treatments are found among several groups. These include diet and herbal remedies, prayer and magical interventions, massage and other treatment techniques involving the skin, and sophisticated treatment systems such as acupuncture, acupressure, and reflexology. Many of these treatments are based on the homeopathic principle that "like cures like" (Davidson & Gaylord, 1995).

Special foods are often used to treat illness. For example, chicken soup is used as a restorative in many cultures and JELL-O water is often given to people with diarrhea. In many cultural groups, dietary interventions are used to restore the balance of "hot" and "cold" or Yin and Yang. "Hot" foods should be taken to treat "cold" illnesses and vice versa. What is considered hot or cold, however, may vary considerably from culture to culture. For example, fruits and vegetables are considered cold foods in some cultures, while many meats are considered hot foods.

A variety of herbal preparations and other medicinals are also used. For example, goldenrod tea is used for colds, sore throat, and cough among the Zuni, and sassafras for lung fever, ulcers, and gout among Appalachians. Ginseng is widely used among Asian cultural groups. Cooked prickly pear cactus may be used by Latinos to treat diabetes. This preparation has a mild lowering effect on blood glucose and should be used with care in clients taking hypoglycemic medications (Smith, 1988).

Some medicinal preparations may have adverse health effects. For example, the relatively common practice in the dominant U.S. culture of taking baking soda for gastric upset may lead to electrolyte imbalance or mask the symptoms of myocardial infarction. Other folk remedies contain poisonous substances. Use of Jin Bu Huan, a Chinese herbal remedy for pain and insomnia, for example, has been implicated in cases of drug-induced hepatitis and alkaloid poisoning (*NURSEweek,* 1994; National Center for Infectious Diseases, 1993). Other hazardous remedies may result in lead poisoning. These include the Southeast Asian preparation *paylooah,* Asian Indian *surma,* and an unnamed Tibetan ayurvedic substance, as well as *greta* and *azarcon,* two Latino folk remedies widely used for treating *empacho* (Flattery, et al., 1993). Another Latino folk health practice that may have harmful effects is the use of rattlesnake capsules, an old remedy used to treat a variety of chronic illnesses. The capsules, made of pulverized rattlesnake, often contain *Salmonella arizona,* a pathogenic bacterium that causes diarrheal disease (Waterman, Juarez, Carr, & Kilman, 1990).

TABLE 16–8. SELECTED CULTURAL BELIEFS AND PRACTICES RELATED TO DIAGNOSIS AND TREATMENT OF ILLNESS

Focus	Belief or Behavior
Diagnosis	• Diagnosis is by means of dreams, "hand tremblers," "star gazers," or "crystal gazers." (Native American) • Diagnosis is made using techniques of inspection, listening, questioning, and palpation. (Chinese) • Diagnosis of women should be made on the basis of pulses only. (Asian) • Women may point to areas on an alabaster figure to indicate areas of complaint. (Chinese) • Diagnosis is made by iridology, the condition of the iris. (Asian) • Susceptibility to certain illnesses is determined by signs of the zodiac. (Appalachian)
General treatment	• Exercise may be suggested as a remedy for illness. (Asian)[a] • Herbal preparations are used to treat illness. (Asian, Native American, Latino, African American, Appalachian) • Sweat baths may be used to treat illness. (Native American, Lao, Khmer) • Massage may be used to treat illness. (Zuni, Otomi, Lao, Hmong, Chinese) • Onions placed on the wall of a sickroom will absorb illness. (Appalachian) • Signs of the zodiac should be consulted when planning surgery. (African American) • Pressure on specific points on the foot (reflexology) may relieve illness. (Japanese) • Medication should be discontinued when symptoms disappear. (Lao, other Asian, African American) • Wounds should be covered to keep them clean. (Lao)[a] • Medicines are usually prepared by boiling herbs in a prescribed amount of water and taking all of the preparation. (Chinese, other Asian)[b] • Scientific medicines are considered "hot" and may not be taken for a "cold" illness. (Otomi, Asian)[b] • Scientific medicines are considered very strong so clients may take only half the prescribed dose. (Vietnamese) • Everything has an opposite; every disease has a cure. (African American)
Diet	• "Hot" foods should be taken to treat "cold" illnesses and "cold" foods taken to treat "hot" illnesses. (Asian, Latino, Appalachian) • Treat "cold" illnesses like diarrhea and fever with "hot" foods like sweets, candies, and spices. Treat "hot" illnesses like pimples, boils, and skin problems with "cold" foods like vegetables, fruits, and water. (Vietnamese) • "Cold" foods used to treat "hot" illnesses include tropical fruit, dairy products, goat, fish, chicken, honey, cod, raisins, bottled milk, and barley water. "Hot" foods used to treat "cold" illnesses include chocolate, cheese, temperate-zone fruits, eggs, peas, onions, aromatic beverages, oils, beef, waterfowl, mutton, goat's milk, cereals, and chili peppers. (Mexican) • Eating snake flesh improves vision. (Chinese) • Use green vegetables and onions to treat respiratory disease. (Otomi) • Use cooked onions to gain weight, raw onions to lose weight. (Otomi) • Avoid spices, salt, and garlic when ill and eat plain food and soup. (Hmong) • Treat constipation with vegetables, tea, honey, or prunes. (Chinese)[b] • Karo syrup added to the bottle will help constipation in an infant. (dominant U.S.)[b] • Chicken soup stimulates recovery from illness. (Jewish, dominant U.S.) • JELL-O water or flat soft drinks should be given to persons with diarrhea. (dominant U.S.)
Prayer and magic	• Prayer may bring about cure of illness. (Latino, Native American, Filipino) • Promises, visiting shrines, offering medals or candles, and prayer may help cure illness. (Mexican) • Gather bark from the east side of a tree to appease the Gods (Native American) or for greater potency. (Appalachian) • Use cornmeal in healing rituals. (Native American) • *Gist,* or medicine bundles, are used in healing rituals. (Native American) • Like cures like. (African American, Appalachian) • Use invocations to spirits accompanied by rattle or drum in healing rituals. (Native American) • Prayers and laying-on-of-hands may cure illness. (African American, Appalachian) • Songs or chants amplify the forces of good in their battle with evil. (Otomi, other Native American) • A *limpia,* or cleansing of evil, may be accomplished by passing an object over the body to pick up evil spirits. (Otomi, Latino) • Recital of the Twenty-third Psalm, reading Scripture, prayer, and positive reminiscences may cure illness caused by a hex. (African American) • A *baci* ceremony may be used to placate spirits causing illness. (Lao)
Herbal treatments	• "Hot" herbs or medicines used for "cold" illnesses include ginger, garlic, cinnamon, anise, penicillin, tobacco, vitamins, iron, cod liver oil, castor oil, and aspirin. "Cold" herbs or medicines include orange flower water, linden, sage, milk of magnesia, and sodium bicarbonate. (Mexican) • Herbal teas may be used for fatigue, cold, sore throat, cough, chest ailments, and other conditions. (Appalachian) • Sassafras is used for agues, lung fever, ulcers, stomach problems, skin conditions, sore eyes, catarrh, gout, dropsy, syphilis, and anemia (Appalachian) or for colds. (African American) • Use goldenseal (an herb) for weak stomach, liver, or intestinal problems, hemorrhages, poor circulation, and "nerves." (Appalachian) • Use ginseng for stomach and female problems, aging, sore eyes, asthma, poor appetite, rheumatism, longevity, and luck (Appalachian) or for anemia, colic, depression, indigestion, impotence, rheumatism, or as a sedative (cannot be prepared in any metal container). (Chinese) • Any plant root or plant with a yellow cast can be used to treat jaundice. (Appalachian) • A hot, moist tea bag held in the mouth relieves canker sores. (European American) • Oil of clove is good for a toothache. (European American) • Whiskey rubbed on the gums will sooth a teething baby. (European American)[b]

(continued)

TABLE 16–8. SELECTED CULTURAL BELIEFS AND PRACTICES RELATED TO DIAGNOSIS AND TREATMENT OF ILLNESS (Continued)

Focus	Belief or Behavior
Herbal treatments (continued)	• Honey and lemon are effective for sore throat. (dominant U.S.) • Vicks Vaporub is useful for chest congestion and cough or stuffy nose. (dominant U.S.)[b] • Use yellow root tea for sore throat, stomach upset, high blood pressure, canker sores, or tonic. (Appalachian) • Treat diarrhea with boiled green persimmons. (Appalachian) • Treat indigestion with chrysanthemum, crystal, ginseng, or other teas. (Chinese) • Smoke jimson weed for asthma. (Appalachian) • Use ginger to strengthen the heart and treat nausea and dyspepsia. (Asian) • Grind up guava and put in the mouth to treat sores. (Otomi) • Boiled banana peel or stems will stop heavy or prolonged menstrual bleeding. (Otomi) • A tamarind bath can be used for the chronically fatigued child. (Otomi) • Chopped garlic, onion, parsley, and water can be used as a expectorant. (African American) • Onions applied to the feet wrapped in warm blankets will cure fever. (African American) • Goldenrod tea is used for colds, sore throat, and cough. (Zuni) • Thistle concoctions can be used for fever, gastrointestinal problems, or genitourinary infections (Zuni) or to treat worms. (Hopi) • Blanket flower can be used to treat painful urintation. (Hopi) • A tea made from painted cup can be used for menstrual pain. (Hopi) • Witch hazel or sweet flag is used for colds. (Oneida) • Elderberry flowers can be used for diarrhea. (Oneida) • Dried raspberry leaves can be used for mouth sores. (Oneida) • Mustard plant can be used to treat headache or sunburn. (Zuni) • Use sage to treat burns. (Zuni) Or on boils. (Hopi) • Tansy and sage can be used to treat headache. (Oneida) • Use a sunflower water bath for spider bites. (Hopi) • Chew the root of a bladder pod plant and put it on a snake bite. (Hopi) • Fleabane can be bound to the head or used in a tea for headache. (Hopi) • Yucca stem can be used as a laxative. • Raw potato soaked in vinegar may be placed on the forehead to treat headache. (Latino) • Treat skin conditions with grated potato or tomato. (Latino) • Oregano tea may be used for cough. (Latino) • Earache is treated with a preparation of rue on cotton placed in the ear. (Latino) • Hot tea or a dock (weedy plant) or saline gargle can be used to treat sore throat (Latino) or use comfrey. (Oneida) • Fever may be treated with an enema of "malva leaves." (Latino) • Chamomile tea (Latino) or garlic (Vietnamese) is good for high blood pressure. • High blood pressure may be treated by eating pears, being tranquil, and eating garlic (to prevent stroke). (Latino) • Put globe mallow on cuts and wounds. Chew the root for broken bones. (Hopi) • Use cliff rose to wash wounds. (Hopi)
External treatments	• Coining is used to treat pain, colds, vomiting, and headache (Khmer), heat stroke, indigestion, and colic (Chinese), colds, flu, and wind entering the body. (Vietnamese) • Pinching is used for headache and sore throat. (Vietnamese) • Cupping is used to treat headache by removing noxious elements (Khmer), to treat arthritis, abdominal pain, abscess, and stroke paralysis (Chinese), to treat joint or muscle pain. (Vietnamese, also some Europeans) • Moxibustion is used to treat mumps, convulsions, and nosebleed, and during labor and delivery. (Chinese) • Balms and medicated plasters can be applied to the skin for bone and muscle problems. (Vietnamese) • Treat pain with acupuncture, acupressure, blowing in the ear, painting with a purple spot, pinching, cupping, or coining. (Asian) • Acupuncture may also be used to treat any "hot" illness. (Chinese) • Sweatbaths are useful for childbirth, opium withdrawal, mental disorder, and psychosomatic illness. (Lao) • Warts can be removed with water from the rotted stump of a chestnut tree. (Appalachian)
Other treatments	• Deer antler strengthens bones, improves potency, and eliminates nightmares. (Chinese) • Rhino horn can be used for pus boils and snakebite. (Chinese) • Turtle shell can be used to stimulate the kidneys and cure gallstones. (Chinese) • Seahorses can be used to treat gout. (Chinese) • Use quicksilver (mercury) to treat venereal disease. (Chinese)[b] • Treat object intrusion with massage to draw the object up; then suck over the area. (Otomi, other Native American) • Dissolve certain tree insects in the mouth to treat sores or drink the juice of the insect. (Otomi) • Poultices may be used to treat heart pain (Otomi), inflammation. (African American) • Take sugar and turpentine by mouth to treat worms. (African American) • Purgatives should be used for "poison." (Otomi)

TABLE 16–8. SELECTED CULTURAL BELIEFS AND PRACTICES RELATED TO DIAGNOSIS AND TREATMENT OF ILLNESS (Continued)

Focus	Belief or Behavior
Other treatments (continued)	• Drink sugar and turpentine for worms; rub it for backache. (African American) • Use "bluestone" powder in open wounds or for poison ivy. (African American) • Use stale bread or sour milk or salt pork on lacerations. (African American) • Clay in a dark leaf can be wrapped around a sprained ankle. (African American) • Use the skin from inside the shell of a raw egg for boils. (African American) • For stiff neck, place crossed pieces of silverware over the area. (African American) • Fluid intake should be decreased with fever. (Khmer)[b] • Pinon sap is used to treat ulcers. (Zuni) • Pinon gum may be used as an antiseptic and to keep air from wounds. (Zuni, Hopi, Navajo) • Anemia may be treated with blood pudding. (Latino) • Tape treated with camphor balm can be placed over the temples to treat headache. (Lao) • Greta or azarcon can be used to treat *empacho* (both have high lead content. (Latino)[b] • Rattlesnake capsules may be used for a variety of chronic conditions. (Latino)[b] • Use warmth to treat fever. (Japanese, other Asian, Latino, African American)

[a]Belief or practice consistent with scientific health care.
[b]Potentially harmful belief or practice.

Community health nurses should be aware that many cultural groups have different orientations to medication use. Many European Americans, for example, believe that there is a pill to cure every ill, others prefer not to take medications at all if they can possibly avoid doing so. Chinese clients may believe that one dose of an herbal preparation should cure the condition and are confused by multiple-dose therapies. Laotians, on the other hand, may take several doses of medication in the belief that if one is good, more is better.

Religious or magical rituals are frequently used in many cultures to treat illness. Among the Navajo, for example, "sings" are major healing rituals performed by a medicine man or singer (Hultkrantz, 1992). Different chants or songs are used for different types of health problems. Religious treatment rituals are also used by many Roman Catholics as well as Protestants and Muslims, and magical treatments may be employed in several cultural groups. Among some African Americans, for example, remedies used for diseases caused by evil spirits include reading Scripture, recitation of the Twenty-third Psalm, and prayer (Flaskerud & Rush, 1989).

A number of external treatments may also be employed. These may include techniques such as massage, cupping, pinching, coining, moxibustion, and the use of poultices or rubs. Massage is widely used in Asian cultures and may be combined with medicinal preparations to improve its effectiveness. For example, among some Appalachians, a combination of "white lightning" and snake oil is used as a rub for sore muscles (Green, 1978).

Cupping involves burning an alcohol swab in a cup and placing the heated cup over a painful area to draw out noxious elements (Stauffer, 1991). Pinching, believed to bring out wind (Frye, 1995), produces bruises or welts and is commonly done on the neck and over the bridge of the nose. Coining or rubbing is performed on lubricated skin with the edge of a coin or spoon and leaves ecchymotic strips in symmetrical rows. Moxibustion consists of the application of pulverized and heated wormwood or moxa plant over specific meridians or areas that indicate points of entry to channels leading into the body and may produce characteristic burn marks on the skin (Cargill, 1994). Each of these treatments modalities is widely used in many Asian cultural groups and the resulting skin lesions are often mistaken for evidence of child abuse. The community health nurse working with Asian populations should be aware of these practices and their beneficial intent and should not view them as abuse.

Poultices are another externally applied treatment measure and may be used for a variety of conditions in different cultures. The Zuni, for example, use poultices of juniper ash to reduce edema due to injury, and tape treated with camphor balm is used by the Lao for headache (Westermeyer, 1988). Poultices of raw potato slices soaked in vinegar may be used for headache or grated potato and tomato for skin condition in some Latino cultures (Gonzales-Swafford & Gutierrez, 1983). Cucumber poultices have been used in many cultures for removing freckles.

Acupuncture makes use of small needles inserted into specific points that control the flow of *Qi* along the body's meridians. Acupressure, a related Japanese technique, makes use of pressure rather than needles to stimulate the flow of *Qi* (Phillips & Gill, 1995). Both acupressure and acupuncture have demonstrated effectiveness in treating a variety of conditions (Baischer, 1995; Phillips & Gill, 1995). Reflexology is another related technique in which certain points on the hand, foot, and ear are stimulated with pressure to achieve specific therapeutic effects in related parts of the body (Oleson & Flocco, 1993). Jin Shin Acutouch also employs touch to certain meridians to effect cure or pain relief. Areas of particular emphasis in this therapy are the fingers (Arguin, 1993).

Folk Versus Professional Health Care. When the health practices followed by individual members of a culture are not successful and illness results, there is a need to seek assistance from a health care provider. Given the relative inaccessibility of professional health care, coupled with a distrust of professional providers in some groups, it is not surprising that members of many cultures turn to folk healers for assistance.

In many cultures, illnesses tend to be divided into two major categories: those amenable to folk medicine and those amenable to scientific medicine. Illnesses considered amenable to folk medicine tend to be chronic, nonincapacitating maladies and those believed to be caused by supernatural agents. Critical, incapacitating conditions, on the other hand, tend to require scientific medicine.

Several similarities can be observed in both folk and scientific health care systems (Gomez & Gomez, 1985). Both employ similar diagnostic skills such as listening and observation and both make use of verbal and nonverbal communication skills. Both systems engage in psychological and somatic techniques of naming illnesses, creating positive expectations, suggestion, interpretation, emotional support, and manipulating the environment. In addition, both systems use medicinal substances and engage in some forms of laying on of hands or massage. Finally, both the folk and scientific systems are based on an unequal relationship in which one party is an expert and one is a layperson.

Additional similarities between folk and scientific health systems include provision of a rationale for treatment, and explanation of illness, and a rationale for social and moral norms. For example, both traditional African American culture and the scientific health care system explain the cause of AIDS in terms of lifestyle behaviors related to sexual behavior and drug use. They also provide rationale for selective sexual activity and refraining from drug abuse as a means of preventing AIDS (Flaskerud & Rush, 1989). The reasoning process used to reach these conclusions, however, is different in each system.

Differences between the two systems are also evident. Traditional folk medicine takes into account the religious and moral implications of disease, the scientific system does not. Scientific medicine makes a definite distinction between mental and physical illness, whereas many folk health systems do not. Folk medicine is community-oriented, whereas scientific medicine is more oriented to the individual client. Folk medicine also tends to take place in familiar surroundings, whereas care in the scientific system is frequently provided in a distinctly foreign environment (Gomez & Gomez, 1985).

Other differences have also been noted between folk and professional health care systems. Folk health care is primarily humanistic, whereas scientific care is impersonal. Emphasis is placed on familiar, practical, and concrete facts in the folk system and on unfamiliar and more abstract concepts in the scientific system. The folk system is holistic in its orientation; the scientific system tends to be more fragmented. Generally speaking, the focus is on *caring* in the folk system and on *curing* in the scientific system. The folk system stresses prevention of illness; the scientific system emphasizes diagnosis and treatment.

Cost of services is another significant difference between the two systems, with moderate costs for folk health care and high costs for scientific care. There is also less emphasis on cultural support systems in the scientific system than in the folk system. Similarities and differences between folk and scientific health care systems are summarized in Table 16–9.

The choice of one system over the other is influenced by a variety of factors. Reasons for choosing folk health practices over scientific medicine include the following:

1. Underestimating the severity of disease
2. Inability to afford scientific medicine
3. Religious beliefs and practices
4. Inability to communicate because of language barriers
5. Distrust of health care professionals owing to impersonality of service, long waits, and so on
6. Pride and modesty
7. Fear of unfamiliar practices and hospitalization
8. Desire for a quick, easy cure with a minimum of pain and frustration
9. A wealth of misinformation regarding health (Cornacchia, 1992)

TABLE 16–9. SIMILARITIES AND DIFFERENCES BETWEEN FOLK AND SCIENTIFIC HEALTH CARE SYSTEMS

Similarities

• Employ similar diagnostic techniques including observation and listening	• Use medicinal substances and employ some form of laying on of hands in the care of the sick
• Use verbal and nonverbal communication	• Based on asymmetric relationships between experts and laypersons
• Engage in naming of illnesses and creation of positive expectations	• Provide an explanation of disease, a rationale for treatment, and a rationale for social and moral norms
• Employ suggestion, interpretation, emotional support, and manipulation of the environment as therapeutic modalities	

Differences

The Folk Health System	*The Scientific Health System*
• Takes into account the religious and social implications of disease	• Focuses primarily on the personal implications of disease
• Does not make a definite distinction between mental and physical illness	• Makes a definite distinction between mental and physical illness
• Oriented to the community	• Oriented to the individual
• Takes place in familiar surroundings	• Takes place in unfamiliar surroundings
• Emphasizes humanistic care	• Emphasizes impersonal care
• Emphasizes familiar, practical, and concrete facts	• Emphasizes abstract concepts
• Provides holistic care	• Provides fragmented care
• Emphasizes caring	• Emphasizes curing
• Stresses prevention	• Stresses diagnosis and treatment
• Emphasizes cultural support	• Does not emphasize cultural support
• Is of moderate cost	• Is of high cost

Two additional phenomena that support continued use of folk health practices and practitioners are spontaneous remission and the placebo effect. The client improves in both cases and attributes improvement to the folk healer or remedy used. Yetiv (1988) noted that approximately 80% of the effects of all medical practice may be due to placebo and that nontraditional healers are "able to offer the caring touch, the confidence in their healing powers" and are able to "concentrate more effectively on the placebo aspects of their contact with the patient."

Members of many cultural groups may seek services from both folk and scientific health care systems. For example, in one study 20% of Latino parents had taken their children to traditional healers (Risser & Mazur, 1995). In others, as many as 74% had used some form of traditional healing practice for asthma (Pachter, Cloutier, & Bernstein, 1995) and 71% of people had used some type of herbal remedy (National Center for Environmental Health, 1995). Integration of folk and scientific health care systems has implications for community health nurses assessing cultural influences on health. Areas for consideration include the potential for adverse interactions between therapies, unhealthful therapies, and client expectations of providers. Adverse interactions between therapies may occur when traditional and scientific treatments counteract each other. For example, use of

brine to treat "high blood" among African Americans counteracts the effects of antihypertensives. In other instances, treatments may potentiate each other. For example, ginseng has an antihypertensive effect that, combined with antihypertensive medication, may result in severe hypotension. As noted earlier, some traditional remedies and practices (and some scientific ones) may actually be harmful. Tonics high in lead may result in lead poisoning; overuse of antibiotics by Western physicians, on the other hand, has contributed to antibiotic resistance in some bacteria.

A client's culture may influence expectations of providers. Arabs, Asians, and Latinos, for example, may prefer (or insist on) a provider of the same sex. Similarly, many cultural groups expect preliminary social amenities from providers. Some European Americans, Arabs, and Asians will expect to receive a prescription, whatever their complaint. Members of some cultural groups, particularly Asians, will expect to be told what to do by an authoritative provider, while others will expect to be given several options among which to choose.

Knowledge of these differences is important for community health nurses and other providers to interact effectively with clients from another culture. As noted by some authors, "Traditional and contemporary ways of healing are not in conflict with each

ASSESSMENT TIPS: Assessing Cultural Influences on Health

Biophysical Dimension

Age

What is the age composition of the cultural group?

What attitudes toward age and aging are prevalent in the culture?

At what age are members of the culture considered adults?

Are there cultural rituals associated with coming of age?

Genetic Inheritance

Do members of the cultural group display genetically determined physical features or physiologic differences?

Do group members display differences in normal physiologic values (eg, hematocrit, height)?

What genetically determined illnesses, if any, are prevalent in the cultural group?

Physiologic Function

What are the cultural attitudes to body parts and physiologic functions?

Are there specific culturebound syndromes recognized by the group? If so, what are they?

What scientific medical diagnoses are prevalent in the group?

Psychological Dimension

What are the cultural attitudes toward mental health and illness?

What behaviors are considered aberrant in the culture?

Are individual or group goals more salient among members of the cultural group?

How are authority and decision making exercised in the group? By whom? What are group members' attitudes toward authority?

What is the cultural group's attitude toward change?

What is the quality of interaction between the cultural group and the dominant society?

Physical Dimension

Have members of the cultural group been physically isolated from the dominant society?

What are the attitudes of members of the group toward the environment?

Do environmental hazards hold particular risk for members of the cultural group (eg, potential for pesticide exposure)?

Social Dimension

Interpersonal Relationships

What is the typical family organizational structure within the culture?

What roles are typically performed by family members? How interchangeable are these roles? How congruent are family roles with those of the dominant culture?

What are the attitudes of group members toward children?

What childrearing practices are typical of the cultural group?

Communication

What is the primary language spoken by members of the culture?

How important is context to communication?

Are there formal and informal modes of address within the cultural group? In what circumstances is each used?

Is a certain degree of personal reticence expected by group members?

What courtesy titles are used and for whom?

What gestures are considered appropriate or inappropriate?

Demeanor

What behaviors are expected in interactions with others?

What behaviors are considered unacceptable by members of the cultural group?

Beliefs and Values

Where does the group lie in terms of the basic cultural values orientations?

Does the group value health? Material gain? Punctuality? Education? Individualism?

What is the relative priority given to different values within the culture?

Religion and Magic

What is the typical religious affiliation of group members?

Does religion influence health? If so, in what way is this influence exerted?

Are religious leaders or groups involved in health care? If so, how?

What is the effect of religious sponsorship on use of health services?

Are religious beliefs and practices incorporated in health care? If so, how?

ASSESSMENT TIPS: Assessing Cultural Influences on Health (cont.)

Do members of the group express belief in magical causes or treatments for illness?

Economic Status

What is the economic status of group members?

What occupations are typical of group members?

Behavioral Dimension

Dietary Patterns

What are the usual food preferences and consumption patterns in the culture?

How are foods usually prepared?

Do certain foods have special symbolism in the culture? If so, what foods and in what circumstances?

Are certain foods used as primary or secondary prevention measures within the culture?

Are there specific nutrients typically lacking in the diets of group members?

Other Consumption Patterns

What are the attitudes of group members toward the use of alcohol, tobacco, and other drugs?

To what extent do group members use these substances?

What is the extent of caffeine consumption by group members?

Life Events

Conception and Contraception

What are the attitudes of members of the cultural group toward conception and contraception?

Is conception expected early in marriage?

Are there special cultural practices to promote or prevent conception? If so, what are they?

Are there certain behaviors expected during pregnancy? If so, what are they?

Are there behaviors or circumstances that should be avoided during pregnancy? If so, what are they?

What is the attitude of group members toward prenatal care?

Birth

Are there special cultural practices related to labor and delivery? If so what are they?

Who should be present during labor and delivery?

Where should labor and delivery occur?

Are there special practices related to disposal of the placenta?

What behaviors are expected of the mother during the postpartum period?

What does cultural care of the newborn entail? Who provides this care?

What are the cultural attitudes toward breastfeeding?

Death and Dying

What are the attitudes of the cultural group toward death?

Do group members wish to be informed of terminal illness?

Do group members believe in an afterlife?

Where should death occur?

Who should be present at the time of a family member's death?

Who should be involved in preparation of the body after death?

What is the typical mode of disposal of the body after death?

Are there special practices related to grief and mourning in the culture? If so, what are they?

Who should participate in rituals and practices related to death?

Sexual Practices

What are the attitudes of members of the cultural group toward homosexual activity?

What are group members' attitudes toward heterosexual activity?

Do group members engage in any specific sexual practices?

Do group members practice female genital mutilation?

Health System Dimension

How do members of the cultural group define health and illness?

Do group members hold specific theories of disease causation? If so, what are they?

Are there recognized folk health practitioners within the culture? If so, who are they? How do they learn their craft? What health-promotive, diagnostic, and treatment measures do they employ?

To what extent do members of the group use the services of folk health providers?

What primary preventive measures are typical within the culture? What secondary preventive measures are used?

Are any folk health practices used by group members potentially harmful?

What is the relationship of folk and scientific health care systems within the cultural group?

To what extent do group members use both systems?

other, not antagonistic; rather they can be complimentary" (Perrone, Stockel, & Krueger, 1989). Research has indicated that culture-specific health programs are effective in meeting the needs of group members, and scientific providers are becoming more willing to integrate alternative approaches to care. In one study, for example, more than 60% of physicians actually made referrals to alternative providers (Borkan, Neher, Anson, & Smoker, 1995). Some providers are also integrating alternative therapies into their conventional practice.

Assessing Individual Clients

Up to now we have examined beliefs, attitudes, and behaviors typical of groups of people. It is important for community health nurses to recognize that the degree of a particular client's participation in folk health practices will vary. Social class and the concomitant degree of acculturation to the prevailing U.S. culture are two of the factors that mediate the influence of folk health practices. Generally speaking, members of lower socioeconomic groups tend to adhere more closely to belief in and use of traditional health practices. Members of a cultural group who are part of the American middle class may continue to use the folk health system while expressing disbelief in its efficacy. Scientific medicine is also widely used by middle-class individuals. The upper class tends to use scientific medicine as a mark of prestige and may scoff at folk health practices.

Acculturation, a complex phenomenon, is associated with a number of factors in addition to social class. These include the amount of exposure to the dominant culture, the closeness of kinship ties, the extent of family use of traditional practices, and the degree of familiarity with the English language (Galanti, 1991). Nurses working with clients from another culture must ascertain for each client the extent to which he or she adheres to traditional health practices. The assessment tips suggested for assessing cultural groups can also be used to assess individual clients.

Diagnostic Reasoning and Culture

Once client-specific data on cultural affiliation have been obtained, the nurse makes note of areas in which the client conforms to the typical patterns and areas in which the client does not. This information can be useful in identifying underlying factors in a variety of

client health problems identified as nursing diagnoses. For example, the nurse might make a diagnosis of "inadequate nutritional intake due to nonavailability of usual dietary components." Having made such a diagnosis, the nurse can then assist the client to incorporate foods as close as possible to the traditional diet to create a healthy diet.

Nursing diagnoses made at the aggregate level can also be related to cultural factors. For example, the nurse might diagnose a "widespread lack of prenatal care due to failure to provide prenatal services acceptable to Asian clients." Or the nurse might find that clients receive prenatal care from traditional midwives within the cultural group. Efforts might then be directed toward incorporating these midwives into prenatal services provided in the scientific health care system.

Planning and Implementing Culturally Relevant Care

As is the case with most clients in community health nursing, clients from another culture will be largely responsible for implementing health care activities suggested by the community health nurse. The nurse will enhance client compliance with these suggestions by encouraging both clients and their families to participate in planning health care.

The nurse should discuss the client's perceptions of problems, the usual plan of care, and any anticipated difficulties with the suggested plan. It is important that the nurse and client engage in mutual goal setting, because nursing and family goals may not be perfectly congruent. The plan of care can be adapted as much as possible to incorporate traditional health care practices and to avoid introducing drastic changes in the client's lifestyle (Leininger, 1994).

One aspect of a client's ability to act on advice is the question of who must give permission for such action. Sometimes a client cannot act on his or her own initiative because of cultural proscriptions. In such instances, nurses must identify the person responsible for health care decisions and incorporate that person in planning health care.

Community health nurses endeavor to integrate new health behaviors into the client's existing lifestyle as much as possible. This can be accomplished in several ways. The nurse can plan special diets around usual food preferences or tailor care to the client's normal routine. Other practices that may be revised in light of cultural practices are bathing and exercise. Incorporating family members whose role includes health care into the intervention plan is another way of providing culturally sensitive health care.

Another means of integrating new ideas into existing cultural patterns is the incorporation of folk health practices into the plan of care whenever they are not harmful to the client. Allowing the client to wear an amulet or drink herbal tea will not usually hurt and may actually benefit the client. The client's faith in the efficacy of folk remedies may go a long way to accomplish healing. When folk remedies are harmful, the nurse can explain the potential harm and assist clients to identify other actions that will meet the cultural need without harm (Wing, Crow, & Thompson, 1995).

Nurses may also incorporate folk healers into the plan of care, encouraging the *curandero*, medicine man, or elderly female practitioner to attend the client at home or in the health care facility. A nurse may choose to participate in healing rituals if comfortable with this role and if the client has grown to accept and trust the nurse. When appropriate, the nurse may make referrals to a folk healer in place of or in conjunction with the usual plan of care. This may be warranted particularly when the client considers his or her condition to be the result of magical intervention. Resources for nurses working to incorporate cultural variables into their care of clients can be found at the end of this chapter.

Evaluating Culturally Relevant Care

Evaluation of care provided to clients from another cultural group should focus on both the outcomes of care and the delivery processes employed. In terms of outcomes, nurses should examine indicators for health status for individual clients and for subcultural groups. For example, has the nurse been able to improve the client's nutritional status without changing the client's cultural dietary pattern? Has a woman from another cultural group had a successful pregnancy outcome? Have parents ceased giving potentially harmful tonics to their children?

The nurse should also evaluate the outcomes of health care for subcultural groups within the population. One avenue for evaluation at this level is assessment of the level of accomplishment of national health objectives targeted to racial and ethnic minorities. As of 1995, more than half (53%) of the objectives for minority health were moving toward established targets, 27% were actually moving away from the target, and 3% showed no change. No tracking data were available for the remaining 17% of minority-related objectives. Movement away from targeted objectives was most evident for African Americans, for whom data indicate worsening conditions related to 35% of relevant objectives. For Native Americans, 31% of objectives were moving in the wrong direction, compared to 14% for Latinos and 11% for Asian Americans (U.S. Department of Health and Human Services, 1995).

Attention should also be given to evaluating the way in which care is provided. Are health programs designed with cultural sensitivity as a central focus? Is the care provided to the individual client indicative of cultural sensitivity on the part of the particular community health nurse? Answers to these and similar questions are the focus of evaluation of the care provided to individuals from cultural groups other than that of the nurse.

TESTING YOUR UNDERSTANDING

1. How does culture differ from race and ethnicity? (p. 319)
2. What are the six characteristics common to all cultures? Give an example of each characteristic. (pp. 319–320)
3. Describe at least four potential negative responses of nurses to people from another culture and give an example of each type of response. (pp. 320–321)

Critical Thinking in Practice: A Case in Point

In 2 weeks, the Ramirez family expect their fourth child. Mr. Ramirez works in an avocado grove for minimum wage. Because the family cannot afford to pay a physician or hospital, Mrs. Ramirez is not receiving prenatal care. Although the Ramirez family seems pleased about the pregnancy, they have made no plans for the new baby and seem to have no interest in family planning after delivery.

Mr. Ramirez makes all the decisions for the family. The Ramirez family believe that good health and illness are gifts of God and there is very little that they can do to promote their health. All of their relatives are still in Mexico and they rarely communicate with any of them. They believe that the people around them are out to take their money if possible and have not made any friends in the rural neighborhood where they live.

Neither parent attended school. The oldest child is in second grade, but is frequently absent when Mr. Ramirez needs his help in the groves. The public health nurse has talked with Mrs. Ramirez several times regarding the need for immunizations for the younger children, family planning, and prenatal care. Mrs. Ramirez has not attended any of the clinics even though she and her husband own an old truck and come to town regularly on Saturday to buy groceries.

1. Are the family roles depicted in this situation typical or atypical of the traditional Latino family?
2. What are the family's apparent values as evidenced by data in the case study?
3. How do the family's values conflict or coincide with those of the dominant U.S. society?
4. What might the nurse do to provide culturally relevant health care for this family?

---

4. Describe at least three positive responses to clients from another culture. Give an example of each. (p. 321)
5. Describe four principles of cultural assessment. Give an example in which each principle has been violated. (pp. 323–324)
6. Describe three considerations in assessing the biophysical dimension of a culture. Given an example of each. (pp. 325–327)
7. Identify at least five aspects of the psychological and social dimensions to be considered in a cultural assessment. (pp. 327–337)
8. Describe at least three life events to be considered in a cultural assessment. Give an example of the effects of culture related to each life event. (pp. 338–342)
9. Describe three similarities and four differences between the folk and scientific health care systems. Give an example of each. (pp. 352–356)
10. Describe four considerations in assessing the influence of folk health care systems. (pp. 352–355)

WHAT DO YOU THINK?
Questions for Critical Thinking

1. How has your own culture influenced your health-related behavior? Have these influences been positive or negative?

2. What are some aspects of the culture of professional nursing? How might nursing's professional culture interfere with effective interaction with clients?
3. Why is it important to assess the degree to which a particular client conforms to the norms of his or her cultural group?
4. What effect, if any, do you think cultural differences have on racial conflict?
5. Using the references cited in this chapter and the suggested readings at the end of the book as a starting place, explore a culture with which you are not familiar. Do a similar cultural assessment of your own culture. How are the two cultures similar? How do they differ? How might those differences and similarities affect your care if you were the client and your nurse was from the other culture?

REFERENCES

Andrews, M. M., & Hanson, P. A. (1990). Religious beliefs: Implications for nursing practice. In J. S. Boyle & M. M. Andrews (Eds.), *Transcultural concepts in nursing* (pp. 119–166). Philadelphia: Lippincott.

Arguin, S. S. (1993). *Jin Shin Acutouch: Self-help.* Encinitas, CA: North County Healing Arts Center.

Autotte, P. A. (1995). Folk medicine. *Archives of Pediatric and Adolescent Medicine, 149,* 949–950.

Baischer, M. D. (1995). Acupuncture in migraine: Long-term outcome and predicting factors. *Headache, 35,* 472–474.

Banks, J. A. (1991). *Teaching strategies for ethnic studies.* Needham Heights, MA: Allyn and Bacon.

Beauvais, F. (1996). Trends in drug use among American Indian students and dropouts, 1975–1994. *American Journal of Public Health, 86,* 1594–1598.

Bell, R. (1994). Prominence of women in Navajo healing beliefs and values. *Nursing & Health Care, 15,* 232–240.

Blackhall, L. J., Murphy, S. T., Frank, G., Michel, V., & Azen, S. (1995). Ethnicity and attitudes toward patient autonomy. *JAMA, 274,* 820–825.

Blane, D. (1995). Social determinants of health—Socioeconomic status, status, and ethnicity. *American Journal of Public Health, 85,* 903–904.

Borkan, J., Neher, J. O., Anson, O., & Smoker, B. (1995). Referrals for alternative therapies. *Journal of Family Practice, 39,* 545–550.

Cargill, M. (1994). *Acupuncture: A viable medical alternative.* Westport, CT: Praeger.

Cavender, A. (1996). Local unorthodox healers of cancer in the Appalachian south. *Journal of Community Health, 21,* 359–373.

Centers for Disease Control. (1993). Use of race and ethnicity in public health surveillance. Summary of the CDC/ATSDR workshop. *MMWR, 42*(RR–10), 1–17.

Chao, S. (1997). *The experience of Taiwanese women caregiving for parents-in-law.* Unpublished doctoral dissertation, University of San Diego, California.

Chavez, L. R., & Torres, V. M. (1994). The political economy of Latino health. In T. Weaver (Ed.), *Handbook of Hispanic cultures in the United States: Anthropology* (pp. 226–243). Houston: Arte Publico Press.

Chen, M. S., & Hawks, B. L. (1995). A debunking of the myth of healthy Asian Americans and Pacific Islanders. *American Journal of Health Promotion, 9,* 261–268.

Cherry, B. (1991). Black Americans. In J. N. Giger & R. E. Davidhizar (Eds.), *Transcultural nursing: Assessment and intervention* (pp. 147–182). St. Louis: Mosby Year Book.

Cornacchia, H. J. (1992). *Consumer health: A guide to intelligent decisions* (5th ed.). St. Louis: Mosby Year Book.

Covington, D. (1995). *Salvation on Sand Mountain.* Reading, MA: Addison-Wesley.

The Crib Sheet. (1993). The Arab American patient, 7(1), 2, 4.

Davidson, J., & Gaylord, S. (1995). Meeting of minds in psychiatry and homeopathy: An example in social phobia. *Alternative Therapies, 1*(3), 36–43.

D'Avanzo, C. E., Frye, B., & Froman, B. (1994). Stress in Cambodian refugee families. *Image, 26,* 101–105.

Delgado, J. L., Metzger, J. P., & Falcon, D. M. (1995). Meeting the health promotion needs of Hispanic communities. *American Journal of Health Promotion, 9,* 300–311.

Division of Birth Defects and Developmental Disabilities. (1995). Use of International Classification of Diseases coding to identify fetal alcohol syndrome—Indian Health Service facilities, 1981–1992. *MMWR, 44,* 253–255, 261.

Dow, J. (1986). *The Shaman's touch: Otomi Indian symbolic healing.* Salt Lake City: University of Utah.

Dreher, M. (1996). Nursing: A cultural phenomenon. *Reflections, fourth quarter,* 4.

Flaskerud, J. H., & Rush, C. E. (1989). AIDS and traditional health beliefs and practices of black women. *Nursing Research, 38,* 210–215.

Flattery, J., Gambatese, R., Schlag, R., et al. (1993). Lead poisoning associated with use of traditional ethnic remedies. *MMWR, 42,* 521–524.

Frye, B. A. (1995). Use of cultural themes in promoting health among Southeast Asian refugees. *American Journal of Health Promotion, 9,* 269–280.

Galanti, G. (1991). *Caring for patients from different cultures: Case studies from American hospitals.* Philadelphia: University of Pennsylvania Press.

Geissler, E. M. (1994). *Pocket guide: Cultural assessment.* St. Louis: C. V. Mosby.

Ginsberg, C., Gage, L., Martin, V., Gerstin, S., & Acuff, K. (1994). *America's urban safety net hospitals: Meeting the needs of our most vulnerable populations.* Washington, DC: National Association of Public Hospitals.

Gomez, G. E., & Gomez, E. A. (1985). Folk healing among Hispanic Americans. *Public Health Nursing, 2,* 245–249.

Gonzales, G. M. (1997). The emergence of Chicanos in the twenty-first century: Implications for counseling, research, and policy. *Journal of Multicultural Counseling and Development, 25,* 94–106.

Gonzales-Swafford, M. J., & Gutierrez, M. G. (1983). Ethnomedical beliefs and practices of Mexican-Americans. *Nurse Practitioner, 8*(10), 29–34.

Green, E. C. (1978, Autumn). A modern Appalachian folk healer. *Appalachian Journal, 2,* 15.

Gropper, R. C. (1996). *Culture and the clinical encounter: An intercultural sensitizer for the health professions.* Yarmouth, ME: Intercultural Press.

Haddad, Y. Y., & Lummis, A. T. (1987). *Islamic values in the United States: A comparative study.* New York: Oxford University Press.

Hall, E. T. (1976, July). How cultures collide. *Psychology Today, 10,* 66–74.

Hanley, C. E. (1991). Navajo Indians. In J. N. Giger & R. E. Davidhizar (Eds.), *Transcultural nursing: Assessment and intervention* (pp. 215–238). St. Louis: Mosby Year Book.

Hansen, M. M., & Resnick, L. K. (1990). Health beliefs, health care, and rural Appalachian subcultures from an ethnographic perspective. *Family and Community Health, 13*(1), 1–10.

Harris, M. (1989). *Cows, pigs, wars and witches: The riddles of culture.* New York: Random.

Helman, C. G. (1994). *Culture, health, and illness* (3rd ed.). Oxford: Butterworth-Heinemann.

Hubbell, F. A., Chavez, L. R., Mishra, S., & Valdez, R. B. (1996). Beliefs about sexual behavior and other predictors of Papanicolaou smear screening among Latinos and Anglo women. *Archives of Internal Medicine, 156,* 2353–2358.

Hultkrantz, A. (1992). *Shamanic healing and ritual drama: Health and medicine in native North American religious traditions.* New York: Crossroad.

Huttlinger, K. W. (1995). A Navajo perspective of diabetes. *Family and Community Health, 18*(2), 9–16.

Huttlinger, K. W., & Tanner, D. (1994). The peyote way: Implications for culture care theory. *Journal of Transcultural Nursing, 5*(2), 5–11.

Juarbe, T. C. (1996). The state of Hispanic health: Cardiovascular disease and health. In S. Torres (Ed.), *Hispanic voices: Hispanic health educators speak out.* New York: National League for Nursing Press.

Kanellos, N. (1993). *The Hispanic-American almanac: A reference work on Hispanics in the United States.* Detroit: Gale Research.

Kavanaugh, K. H., & Kennedy, P. H. (1992). *Promoting cultural diversity: Strategies for health care professionals.* Newbury Park, CA: Sage.

Keefe, S. E. (1992). Ethnic identity: The domain of perceptions of and attachment to ethnic groups. *Human Organization, 51*(1), 35–43.

Kikuchi, J. F. (1996). Multicultural ethics in nursing education: A potential threat to responsible practice. *Journal of Professional Nursing, 12,* 159–165.

Klatsky, A. L., Tekawa, I., Armstrong, M. A., & Sidney, S. (1994). The risk of hospitalization for ischemic heart disease among Asian Americans in Northern California. *American Journal of Public Health, 84,* 1672–1675.

Kluchohn, F. R., & Strodtbeck, F. L. (1961). *Variations in value orientations.* Evanston, IL: Peterson.

Koenig, B. A., & Gates-Williams, J. (1995). Understanding cultural differences in caring for dying patients. *Western Journal of Medicine, 163,* 244–249.

Kuipers, J. (1991). Mexican Americans. In J. N. Giger & R. E. Davidhizar (Eds.), *Transcultural nursing: Assessment and intervention* (pp. 184–212). St. Louis: Mosby Year Book.

Lee, P. A. (1986). Traditional medicine: Dilemmas in nursing practice. *Nursing Administration Quarterly, 10*(3), 14–20.

Leininger, M., & Reynolds, C. L. (1993). *Cultural care diversity and universality theory.* Newbury Park, CA: Sage.

Leininger, M. (1994). *Transcultural nursing: Concepts, theories, and practice.* Columbus, OH: Greyden Press.

Lewis, S., Messner, R., & McDowell, W. A. (1985). An un-

changing culture. *Journal of Gerontological Nursing, 11*(8), 21–24, 26.

Luna, L. (1994). Care and cultural context of Lebanese Muslim immigrants: Using Leininger's theory. *Journal of Transcultural Nursing, 5*(2), 12–20.

Luna, L. J. (1989). Care and cultural context of Lebanese Muslims in an urban U.S. community: An ethnographic and ethnonursing study conceptualized within Leininger's theory. *Doctoral Abstracts International.* (University Microfilms No. 9022423).

May, P. A., & Moran, J. R. (1995). Prevention of alcohol misuse: A review of health promotion efforts among American Indians. *American Journal of Health Promotion, 9,* 288–299.

Maynard, M. (1996). Promoting older ethnic minorities health behaviors: Primary and secondary prevention considerations. *The Journal of Primary Prevention, 17,* 219–229.

McGee, P. (1992). *Teaching transcultural nursing: A guide for teachers of nursing and health care.* London: Chapman and Hall.

Medina, C. (1987). Latino culture and sex education. *SIECUS Report, 15*(3), 1–4.

Mennella, J. A. (1996, summer). The flavor world of infants: A cross-cultural perspective. *Pediatric Basics,* 2–8.

Murphree, A. H. (1968). A functional analysis of southern folk beliefs concerning birth. *American Journal of Obstetrics and Gynecology, 103,* 125–134.

National Center for Environmental Health. (1995). Self-treatment with herbal and other plant-derived remedies—Rural Mississippi, 1993. *MMWR, 44,* 204–207.

National Center for Infectious Diseases. (1993). Jin Bu Huan toxicity in children—Colorado, 1993. *MMWR, 42,* 633–635.

NURSEweek. (1994, April). Illegally sold Chinese herbal tablets may cause hepatitis, poisoning, 8.

Office of Surveillance and Analysis, National Center for Chronic Disease Prevention and Health Promotion. (1994). Prevalence of selected risk factors for chronic disease by educational level in racial/ethnic populations—United States, 1991–1992. *MMWR, 43,* 894–899.

Oleson, T., & Flocco, W. (1993). Randomized controlled study of premenstrual symptoms treated with ear, hand, and foot reflexology. *Obstetrics & Gynecology, 82,* 906–911.

Organista, P. B., & Organista, K. C. (1997). Culture and gender sensitive AIDS prevention with Mexican migrant laborers: A primer for counselors. *Journal of Multicultural Counseling and Development, 25,* 121–129.

Pachter, L. M., Cloutier, M. M., & Bernstein, B. A. (1995). Ethnomedical (folk) remedies for childhood asthma in a mainland Puerto Rican community. *Archives of Pediatric and Adolescent Medicine, 149,* 982–988.

Pedersen, P. B. (1995). Culture-centered counseling skills as a preventive strategy for college health services. *Journal of American College Health, 44,* 20–25.

Peragallo, N. (1996). Latino women and AIDS risk. *Public Health Nursing, 13,* 217–222.

Perrone, B., Stockel, H. H., & Krueger, V. (1989). *Medicine women, curanderas, and women doctors.* Norman, OK: University of Oklahoma Press.

Phillips, K., & Gill, L. (1995). The use of simple acupressure bands reduces post-operative nausea. *Complementary Therapies in Medicine, 2,* 158–160.

Randal-David, E. (1989). *Strategies for working with culturally diverse communities and clients.* Bethesda, MD: Association for the Care of Children's Health.

Risser, A. L., & Mazur, L. J. (1995). Use of folk remedies in a Hispanic population. *Archives of Pediatric and Adolescent Medicine, 149,* 978–981.

Rowles, G. D., & Johansson, H. K. (1993). Persistent elderly poverty in rural Appalachia. *Journal of Applied Gerontology, 12,* 349–367.

Samovar, L. A., & Porter, R. E. (1991). *Communication between cultures.* Belmont, CA: Wadsworth.

Schrefer, S. (Ed.). (1994). *A quick reference to cultural assessment.* St. Louis: Mosby-Year Book.

Sich, D. (1988). Childbearing in Korea. *Social Science and Medicine, 27,* 497–504.

Small, C. S. (1991). Appalachians. In J. N. Giger & R. E. Davidhizar (Eds.), *Transcultural nursing: Assessment and intervention* (pp. 240–259). St. Louis: Mosby Year Book.

Smith, L. S. (1988). Ethnic differences in knowledge of sexually transmitted diseases in North American black and Mexican-American migrant farmworkers. *Research in Nursing and Health, 11*(1), 51–58.

Spector, R. E. (1996). *Cultural diversity in health and illness* (4th ed.). Norwalk, CT: Appleton & Lange.

Stauffer, R. Y. (1991). Vietnamese Americans. In J. N. Giger & R. E. Davidhizar (Eds.), *Transcultural nursing: Assessment and intervention* (pp. 403–428). St. Louis: Mosby-Year Book.

Takeuchi, D. T., Sue, S., & Yeh, M. (1995). Return rates and outcomes from ethnicity-specific mental health programs in Los Angeles. *American Journal of Public Health, 85,* 638–643.

Thompson, J. L. (1991). Exploring gender and culture with Khmer refugee women: Reflections on participatory feminist research. *Advanced Nursing Science, 13*(3), 30–48.

U.S. Department of Commerce. (1996). *Statistical abstract of the United States, 1996.* Washington, DC: U.S. Government Printing Office.

U.S. Department of Health and Human Services. (1991). *Healthy people 2000: National health promotion and illness prevention objectives.* Washington, DC: U.S. Government Printing Office.

U.S. Department of Health and Human Services. (1995). *Healthy people 2000: Midcourse review and 1995 revisions.* Washington, DC: U.S. Government Printing Office.

U.S. Department of Health and Human Services. (1996). *Health United States, 1995.* Hyattsville, MD: U.S. Public Health Service.

Waterman, S. H., Juarez, G., Carr, S. J., & Kilman, L. (1990). *Salmonella arizona* infections in Latinos associated with rattlesnake folk medicine. *American Journal of Public Health, 80,* 286–289.

Weaver, T. (1994). The culture of Latinos in the United States. In T. Weaver (Ed.), *Handbook of Hispanic cultures in the United States: Anthropology* (pp. 15–38). Houston: Arte Publico Press.

Westermeyer, J. (1988). Folk medicine in Laos: A comparison between two ethnic groups. *Social Science and Medicine, 27,* 768–778.

Wing, D. M., Crow, S. S., & Thompson, T. (1995). An ethnonursing study of Muscogee (Creek) Indians and effective health care practices for treating alcohol abuse. *Family and Community Health, 18*(2), 52–64.

Wright, J. (1996). Female genital mutilation: An overview. *Journal of Advanced Nursing, 24,* 251–259.

Yetiv, J. Z. (1988). *Popular nutritional practices: A scientific approach.* New York: Dell.

Young, T. K. (1994). *The health of Native Americans: Toward a biocultural epidemiology.* New York: Oxford University Press.

Zinn, M. B. (1994). Mexican-heritage families in the United States. In F. M. Padilla (Ed.), *Handbook of Hispanic cultures in the United States: Sociology.* Houston: Arte Publico Press.

Zuniga, M. E. (1997). Counseling Mexican American seniors: An overview. *Journal of Multicultural Counseling and Development, 25,* 142–155.

RESOURCES FOR NURSES WORKING WITH CLIENTS FROM OTHER CULTURES

Ethnic Groups

Administration for Native Americans
370 L'Enfant Promenade, SW
Washington, DC 20447
(202) 690–7776

Black, Indian, Hispanic, and Asian Women in Action
122 West Franklin Avenue, Ste. 306
Minneapolis, MN 55404
(612) 870–1193

Indian Health Service
5600 Fisher's Lane
Rockville, MD 20857
(301) 443–3593

National Coalition of Hispanic Health and Human
   Service Organizations
1501 16th Street, NW
Washington, DC 20036
(202) 387–5000

National Indian Health Board
1385 South Colorado Blvd., Ste. A-708
Denver, CO 80222
(303) 759–3075

U.S. Senate Select Committee on Indian Affairs
SH-838 Hart Senate Office Bldg.
Washington, DC 20510
(202) 224–2251

Healers and Healing

Acupuncture Research Institute
313 W Andrix Street
Monterey Park, CA 91754
(213) 722–7353

American Acupuncture Association
4262 Kissena Blvd.
Flushing, NY 11355
(718) 886–4431

American Association for Acupuncture
   & Oriental Medicine
433 Front Street
Catasauqua, PA 18032–2506
(610) 266–1433

American Center for Chinese Medical Sciences
c/o Yng-Shiuh Sheu
4623 Rosedale Avenue
Bethesda, MD 20814

American Herbalist's Guild
Box 1683
Soquel, CA 95073

Center for Attitudinal Healing
23 Buchanan Drive
Sausalito, CA 94964
(415) 331–6161

Council of Colleges of Acupuncture
   and Oriental Medicine
1010 Wayne Avenue, Ste. 1270
Silver Spring, MD 20901
(301) 608–9175

G-Jo Institute
4950 Southwest 70th Avenue
Davie, FL 33314
(305) 791–1562

International Foundation for Homeopathy
PO Box 7
Edmunds, WA 98020
(206) 776–4147

Ohashi Institute
12 W 27th Street, 9th Floor
New York, NY 10001
(212) 684–4190

Psychic Science International
Special Interest Group
7514 Belleplain Drive
Huber Heights, OH 45424
(513) 236–0361

Nursing

American Holistic Nurses Association
4104 Lake Boone Trail, Ste. 201
Raleigh, NC 27607
(919) 787–5181

National Association of Hispanic Nurses
1501 16th Street, NW
Washington, DC 20036
(202) 387–2477

National Black Nurses Association
1511 K Street, NW, Ste. 415
Washington, DC 20005
(202) 393–6870

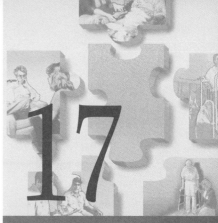

ENVIRONMENTAL INFLUENCES ON COMMUNITY HEALTH

During much of history, human beings have been subjected to the effects of the natural environment. Earthquakes, famines, floods, droughts, and other environmental calamities created upheavals in human society. Human progress has, to a certain extent, been measured in terms of capabilities for controlling the environment. Environmental factors, however, continue to exert an impact on human health and welfare. Air, water, noise, radiation, and waste present a variety of hazards to human health.

Community health nurses are concerned with the effects of environmental factors on the health of individuals, families, and communities. Interventions related to environmental concerns may occur at any of these levels. For example, a community health nurse may teach a family how to reduce the indoor air pollution in the home, or work for legislation to promote safe disposal of hazardous wastes. To engage in effective action at all levels, community health nurses must have an understanding of environmental influences on health.

▶ Chapter Objectives

After reading this chapter, you should be able to:

- Identify three physical health hazards arising from the environment.
- Describe three biological health hazards that may be present in the environment.
- Identify three chemical or gaseous hazards to human health arising from environmental conditions.
- Describe at least two health effects of environmental conditions in each of six human target organs or body systems.
- Identify two levels of nursing diagnoses related to environmental influences on health.
- Describe at least five primary prevention measures for health problems related to environmental conditions.
- Describe at least three secondary preventive measures for health problems related to environmental conditions.
- Describe at least three tertiary preventive measures for health problems related to environmental conditions.

▶ **ENVIRONMENT, HEALTH, AND NURSING**

It is estimated that as much as 15% of the world's population are affected by environmentally caused diseases (Kime, 1992). Among health care providers, community health nurses are some of those most likely to become aware of environmental health problems, yet they are often unprepared to recognize and deal with these problems. The Institute of Medicine has recommended that environmental health should be given new emphasis in nursing education, practice, and research and that nurses become actively involved in environmental protection efforts at both the individual and aggregate levels (Pope, Snyder, & Mood, 1995). Protection of the environment is one of the core functions of public health, and community health nurse participation in this function is essential (Josten, Clarke, Ostwald, Stoskopf, & Shannon, 1995).

Public Health and Ecological Perspectives

Environmental health and protection is defined as the "art and science of protecting against environmental factors that may adversely impact human health or adversely impact the ecological balances essential to long-term human health and environmental quality" (Gordon, 1997). As this definition indicates, there are both public health and ecological perspectives relevant to environmental concerns. The public health

perspective concerns itself with the effects of the environment on human health, for example, the effects of lead exposure on child growth and development. The ecological perspective is one of concern for the preservation of the environment, for example, preventing species extinction. In the past, nursing in general has subscribed to an egocentric perspective in which the needs of the individual are paramount. Community health nursing, on the other hand, has focused on the public health perspective which is homocentric in nature. In a homocentric perspective, the emphasis is on the good of the group, but still exclusively focused on concern for humanity. More recently, nursing has become more attuned to the ecological, or ecocentric, perspective in which the concern is with the cosmos, the total environment (Kleffel, 1996). This ecological perspective has been described as a concern for "environmental security" which is viewed as any ecological development that influences societal welfare (Soroos, 1995) including a variety of global changes that may not be directly related to human health (Kotchian, 1995). Another way to express the ecological perspective is the concept of "stewardship." Stewardship is a middle ground view between the poles of seeing the earth as a machine to be used for human pleasure and as a living organism in itself. The concept of stewardship acknowledges humanity as preeminent among species, but with a caretaking responsibility for the rest of the cosmos (Artson, 1995).

Ecological Issues

Issues from the ecological perspective that are of concern include a variety of global changes that are affecting the balance of the environment and its ability to maintain itself. Some of these issues include deforestation, desertification, loss of biodiversity, global warming, ozone depletion, planetary toxification, and overpopulation.

Deforestation, Desertification, and Loss of Biodiversity

Deforestation, desertification, and loss of biodiversity are interrelated issues that are affecting the face of the earth more intensely each year. *Deforestation* refers to the clearing of forests to create crop lands. Deforestation may involve cutting trees, but is more efficiently accomplished by burning. In addition to eliminating natural habitats for many plant and animal species, deforestation contributes to soil erosion and changes in climatic and hydrologic cycles, and the method of burning forest lands also contributes vast quantities of pollutants to the air. *Desertification* is the conversion of fertile land into desert. In part, desertification occurs as a result of deforestation and the subsequent climate changes achieved by altering the rain cycle. Desertification also results from poor land management, overgrowth of crops that deplete essential nutrients from soil, and climatic changes due to global warming (Kime, 1992). *Loss of biodiversity* refers to the extinction of certain species of plants and animals which may result from loss of natural habitat as well as desertification, overhunting, and reproductive changes related to other environmental changes.

Global Warming

Global warming is an overall increase in temperature throughout the world. Whether or not such an increase is actually taking place is a matter of some controversy in environmental circles (Gordon, 1997). One suggested contributing factor to global warming is the *greenhouse effect* in which gases resulting in large part from the use of fossil fuels collect in the atmosphere and reflect heat back to the earth rather than letting it dissipate (Kime, 1992; Soroos, 1995). Whether the suggested climatic changes are a long-term trend or not, they do have other effects on the environment and on health. Increasing warmth has been associated with increased worldwide incidence of infectious diseases such as malaria and dengue fever (*The Nation's Health,* 1995). Other health effects linked to increasing temperature and humidity include heat-related mortality (National Center for Environmental Health, 1997) and premature labor (Lajinian, Hudson, Applewhite, Feldman, & Minkoff, 1997).

Ozone Depletion

The protective stratospheric layer of ozone is gradually being destroyed. This destruction is a result of chemical interactions between air pollutants, primarily chlorofluorocarbons (CFCs), and ozone. As we will see later, ozone is itself an air pollutant in ambient air. In the stratosphere, however, the ozone layer performs a filtering function that reduces the extent of ultraviolet radiation that reaches the earth. Without the ozone layer, it is estimated that skin cancer incidence rates would increase 60% and 20,000 more fatalities would occur each year in the United States.

Planetary Toxification

Planetary toxification refers to the accumulation of a variety of wastes on the planet with their consequent environmental effects. Some of those effects, such as air and water pollution and acid rain, will be addressed later in this chapter. Other aspects of planetary toxification include the accumulation of both solid and hazardous wastes. In the United States alone, 160 to 200 million tons of solid waste materials are generated annually. Each American household generates approximately 87 gallons of solid waste a week, 30 to 40% of which is packaging materials for products used. Just one element of this household waste is 216 million pounds of plastic grocery bags discarded each year. The annual amount of solid waste generated increased 80% between 1960 and 1992 (Kime, 1992).

In addition, the United States produces 250 million tons of toxic wastes a year, an estimated 50% of which is dumped illegally (Kime, 1992). In 1995, there were 700 million tons of toxic wastes deposited in some 30,000 to 40,000 sites in the United States. Over 500 of these sites are considered health hazards (Cordasco & Zenz, 1995), and an estimated 40 million people live within 4 miles of waste sites deemed health threats by the Environmental Protection Agency (Pope, Snyder, & Mood, 1995). Solid and toxic wastes contribute to a variety of health problems including cancers, heavy metal poisoning, and infectious diseases.

Overpopulation

Overpopulation is another area of environmental concern from an ecological perspective. Despite efforts in many parts of the world, most notably China, to achieve zero population growth, the world's population continues to increase rapidly. For the United States alone, total population is expected to increase by more than 27% from 1995 to 2025 (U.S. Department of Commerce, 1996), and most of this growth will be due to births rather than immigration. Population growth, combined with economic and environmental factors, is expected to result in food shortages in many parts of the world. These shortages will be the result of actual insufficiency rather than maldistribution of food because of the diminishing technologic ability to increase food yields commensurate with population growth (Brown, 1995). Water will also be in short supply if population growth continues unabated. Not only are there more people who require water, but per capita water consumption has increased dramatically. In fact, per capita use is expected to double between 1980 and 2000 (Kime, 1992).

▶ ENVIRONMENTAL PUBLIC HEALTH ISSUES

In recent years, greater attention has been given to the health risks posed by environmental conditions. This attention is evident in the number of national health objectives for the year 2000 that focus on environmental health issues. Sixteen objectives related to environmental health were included in the objectives for the year 2000 (U.S. Department of Health and Human

Services, 1991). Some of these objectives are summarized in Appendix A.

Another indicator of the increased importance of environmental health problems throughout the world is the existence of ecological refuges. *Ecological refugees* are people who have chosen or who have been forced to leave certain areas because of environmental deterioration. It is estimated that worldwide more than 15 million people have been made ecological refugees by desertification of arable land, toxic chemical contaminations, nuclear disasters, and retreat from coastal areas as sea levels rise with the melting of the polar ice caps (Zuk & White, 1990).

Many environmental forces influence human health. Microorganisms such as bacteria, viruses, and fungi, for example, cause communicable diseases, and animals contribute to the spread of these diseases.

Plants may contribute to accidental poisoning or to allergic reactions. Industry, vehicles, and buildings add to air and water pollution and excess noise. Climate and terrain contribute to natural disasters, which are discussed in Chapter 29. In addition, climate and terrain add to air and water pollution that have long-term effects on health. All of these facets of the environment give rise to environmental hazards that affect human health. Some of the environmental components that produce health hazards are presented in Figure 17–1. Health hazards arising from environmental conditions fall into five categories: physical hazards, biological hazards, chemical and gaseous hazards, mechanical hazards, and psychosocial hazards (Pope, Snyder, & Mood, 1995). Mechanical and psychosocial hazards are addressed elsewhere in this book and are not dealt with here except as they influence the other categories.

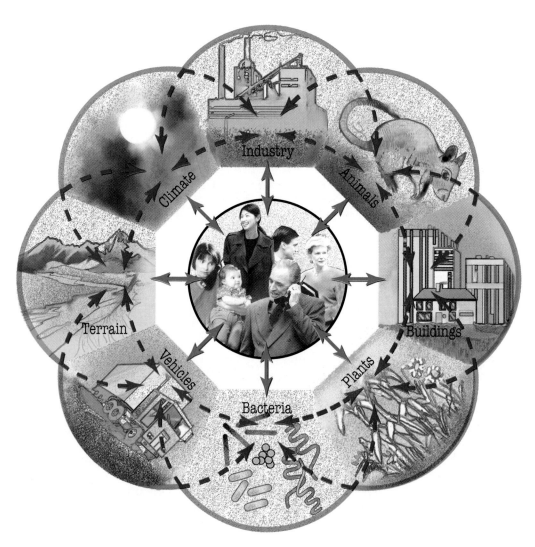

Figure 17–1. Selected environmental components that produce health hazards.

Physical Hazards

Physical hazards to health arising from environmental conditions are those related to the physical objects and conditions that surround human beings. Physical hazards to be addressed here include radiation, lead and other heavy metals, and noise.

Radiation

Radiation is energy in motion that occurs in the form of waves or particles. Two forms of radiation can be health hazards: ionizing radiation and nonionizing radiation.

Ionizing radiation is the transfer of energy through electromagnetic waves or subatomic particles that cause ionization. *Ionization* is a process in which atoms gain or lose electrons to become electrically charged (Diehl, 1995). When ionizing radiation passes through human tissue, atoms are ionized, creating a variety of health effects. Ionizing radiation is created when radioactive elements break up. Ionizing radiation occurs naturally in the soil and rock, and humans are exposed to this form of radiation daily. In fact, more than 80% of human exposure to ionizing radiation arises from natural sources (MacIntyre & Saha, 1995). Exposure to natural ionizing radiation is greater in some parts of the country than in others depending on the extent of radioactive elements found. Exposure to artificial ionizing radiation may occur as a result of some forms of technology. X-ray procedures, for example, are a form of ionizing radiation. Ionizing radiation also results from a variety of industrial processes and processes used to create nuclear power.

The percentage of ionizing radiation typically received from natural and artificial sources is presented in Table 17–1. Radon accounts for 55% of human exposure to ionizing radiation. Radon is a radioactive gas created by the breakdown of radium occurring naturally in the soil and in many building materials, particularly pumice stone and granite. Radon is also found in some well water and may be expelled into household air through seepage from cracks in foundations or during showers and baths. Radon gas can be inhaled in free form or attached to dust particles. After inhalation, the radioactive gas continues to decompose, releasing alpha particles that damage lung tissue and may result in lung cancer. Radon exposure has been indicated as a significant contributing factor in cancer incidence (Pershagen, et al., 1994). In fact, after smoking, radon is the second most common cause of lung cancer (Environmental Protection Agency, 1993).

Cosmic radiation comes from outer space, whereas terrestrial radiation arises from radioactive

TABLE 17–1. DISTRIBUTION OF HUMAN EXPOSURE TO IONIZING RADIATION AMONG NATURAL AND ARTIFICIAL SOURCES

Type and Source of Radiation	Percentage of Total Exposure
Natural radiation	88
Radon	55
Cosmic radiation	8
Terrestrial radiation	8
Internal radiation	11
Artificial radiation	18
Medical x-rays	11
Nuclear medicine	4
Consumer products	3
Other	<1
Occupational exposure	0.3
Fallout	<0.3
Nuclear fuel cycle	0.1
Miscellaneous	0.1

(Source: Moeller, 1992.)

substances found in the earth. Internal radiation sources include radioactive substances ingested or inhaled and deposited in body tissues. Dietary potassium isotopes, for example, emit small amounts of ionizing radiation. Radium is also found in some well water and in Brazil nuts (Moeller, 1992).

Medical and dental x-ray procedures are the source of approximately 11% of human exposure to ionizing radiation, and nuclear medicine treatments account for another 4% (MacIntyre & Saha, 1995). There is some question of the health effects of medical irradiation. Some studies have found no relationship between diagnostic x-rays and diseases such as leukemia and non-Hodgkin's lymphoma, whereas others have found relationships with multiple myeloma and breast cancer. The uncertainty in this area underscores the need for keeping medical exposures to ionizing radiation to a minimum.

Some consumer products such as smoke detectors using americium, some tinted glasses, and glazes on some dentures and "fiesta-ware" china are also sources of ionizing radiation. Tobacco is another consumer product commonly containing radioactive material (MacIntyre & Saha, 1995).

The health hazards of nuclear power were demonstrated by the effects of the bombing of Japanese cities that occurred at the close of World War II. These effects were demonstrated more recently in the morbidity and mortality that occurred as the result of the nuclear accident at Chernobyl, in the former Soviet Union. In this type of acute radiation exposure over a short period, adverse health effects can be expected to begin at exposures of 25 rem or 0.25 Sievert (Sv). (A rem is a measure of the biological damage produced in human tissue by radiation, and a mrem is one-thousandth of a rem. The Sievert, a more recent measurement term, equals 100 rem.) When acute exposures reach 300 to 600 rem (3–6 Sv), there is a 50% fatality rate within weeks of exposure. Death may occur within hours at exposures of 5000 rem (50 Sv) or greater (Moeller, 1992). Barring nuclear accidents, however, nuclear fallout and power sources generally account for less than 0.4% of ionizing radiation exposures; occupational exposures account for another 0.3% (MacIntyre & Saha, 1995).

The vast majority of people are not exposed to high levels of ionizing radiation. Evidence, however, reveals that long-term exposure to low levels of ionizing radiation may have cumulative health effects. In one study, the risk of death due to cancer increased by nearly 5% for every rem of cumulative radiation exposure incurred by employees of nuclear power plants. The findings of this study reinforce those of earlier studies (Gibbons, 1991).

Because little can be done about most natural sources of ionizing radiation, minimizing human exposure to radiation focuses primarily on control of exposure to artificial radiation. For this reason, the International Commission on Radiological Protection (ICRP) in 1990 recommended cumulative exposure limits for artificial ionizing radiation of less than 1 mSv or 100 mrem per year over a 5-year period for the general public and 20 mSv per year for occupational exposures (Moeller, 1992).

Nonionizing radiation passes through matter without any transfer of energy and does not result in ionization. Forms of nonionizing radiation include electromagnetic fields, ultraviolet radiation, visible light, infrared radiation, and microwaves. Electromagnetic fields (EMFs) are created in the generation of electricity, and occur around power lines, electrical wiring, and electrical equipment and appliances (NIOSH Fact Sheet, 1996). Video display terminals (VDTs) also create electromagnetic fields (March of Dimes, 1992).

The health effects of this type of radiation are not yet fully known, but there is some evidence that chronic exposure to microwave radiation may contribute to fatigue, headaches, blood dyscrasias, cataracts, memory loss, arrhythmias, decreased fertility, and genetic defects. Video display terminals have been suggested as sources of headache, eyestrain, visual disturbances, cataracts, and genetic defects. In several studies, however, no relationship was found between exposure to VDTs during pregnancy and risk of spontaneous abortion (March of Dimes, 1992; Schnorr, Grawjewski, Hornung, & Thun, 1991). Some evidence suggests that the health effects of using VDTs are due not to the radiation produced,

but to glare from the screen and other aspects of the work.

Ultraviolet radiation consists of waves of light energy beyond the capability of the human eye to see. Ultraviolet radiation occurs naturally in sunlight and is created by fluorescent lights and sunlamps. Ultraviolet radiation has several positive uses including destroying pathogenic microbes and producing light that is less harsh and uses less energy than incandescent lighting. Ultraviolet light is also involved in producing vitamin D when human skin is exposed to sunlight. Unfortunately, ultraviolet light also results in sunburn, and exposure contributes to the incidence of basal and squamous cell carcinomas and malignant melanomas. More than 500,000 cases of skin cancer are diagnosed each year and account for 2000 deaths annually in the United States. The potential for skin cancer due to exposure to ultraviolet radiation is increased by the destruction of the protective stratospheric layer of ozone discussed earlier.

Visible light radiation includes not only sunlight and artificial light, but also laser beams. Potential health effects of visible light include retinal burns from looking directly at the sun, eyestrain from inadequate or excessive light, and laser burns to the retina or skin.

Infrared radiation is produced by the sun and by heating devices such as stoves and molten metals. Infrared energy is basically heat energy. Health effects may include burns to the skin, cataracts, heat exhaustion, and heat stroke.

In addition to creating electrical and magnetic fields in microwave ovens, microwaves are emitted by radar, radio, and television transmitters, as well as satellite communication systems. Health effects of microwave radiation tend to localize to the testes, causing temporary sterility, and the eyes, causing cataracts. Microwaves may also produce thermal burns (Moeller, 1992).

Lead and Other Heavy Metals

Other physical hazards to health arise from the presence of lead and other heavy metals in the environment. Eliminating elevated blood lead levels in young children is one of three priority environmental objectives included in *Healthy People 2000* (Lum, 1995). Lead may be present in soil, in water, and in the air, as well as in dust or paint chips in older dwellings painted with lead-based paint. Sources of lead in the air include vehicle emissions, stationary source fuel combustion (eg, burning coal to generate electrical power), industrial processes, and decomposition of solid wastes. Lead in vehicle emissions was significantly reduced with the introduction of unleaded gasoline. From 1979 to 1988, for example, the amount of lead expelled into the air each year declined 89% (Moeller, 1992).

Use of lead-based paint in residential units was prohibited in 1977 (Tesman & Hills, 1994). These efforts have resulted in lower blood lead levels in children and the absence of overt signs of lead toxicity in most pediatric practices (Schoen, 1993). Seventy-four percent of private homes built prior to 1980 contain some lead-based paint (Tesman & Hills, 1994), however, and an estimated 4.4% of all children in the United States under age 5 have blood lead levels high enough to cause declining intelligence and retarded development. This latter figure doubles for children in poverty (Division of Health Examination Statistics, 1997). Another source of lead for some children is traditional folk remedies (California Department of Health Services, 1996; Goldman, 1996). Some traditional remedies with high lead content are included in Table 17–2. Prenatal lead exposure may also occur and result in premature delivery (Amaya & Ackall, 1996).

Young children are particularly at risk for lead poisoning because of their propensity to place objects that may be contaminated with lead-bearing dust in their mouths. Children may also ingest paint chips from peeling walls in deteriorating buildings. Painting over old surfaces with nonlead-based paint does not help, because as later coats of paint flake off, the older lead-contaminated layers peel as well. In addition, children absorb and retain higher levels of lead than adults due to their higher rate of mineral turnover in the bones (Committee on Advances in Assessing Human Exposure to Airborne Pollutants, 1991). Infants may also develop high lead levels through formula mixed with lead-contaminated water as well as congenital exposure to elevated maternal lead levels (Shannon & Graef, 1992).

Abatement procedures to remove lead-based paint in older homes traditionally consist of open-flame burning or sanding techniques with minimal clean up of the resulting dust. This dust is heavily contaminated with lead and may present subsequent exposure risks. Research has indicated that neither traditional abatement methods nor modified methods incorporating better clean up procedures are effective in reducing lead levels in house dust on a long-term basis (Farfel & Chisholm, 1990), so community health nurses working in older residential areas may still encounter clients with lead poisoning. In fact, some abatement efforts have resulted in increased blood lead levels in children living in affected homes (Tesman & Hills, 1994).

Exposure to lead and other heavy metals can also occur through drinking water. These metals enter water as it passes through soils containing lead, nickel, mercury, arsenic, cadmium, and other metals. This process is facilitated if water is acidified as a result of acid rain caused by chemical air pollution. Metals are also leached into the water system from improper solid waste disposal. Finally, lead and copper may be leached from lead and copper pipes in older homes. Again, acidification of water due to acid rain enhances leaching of metals from pipes.

Lead interferes with red blood cell production and may cause damage to the brain, liver, and other vital organs. Typical symptoms of lead poisoning include headache, irritability, weakness, abdominal pain, vomiting, and constipation. In later stages, victims may exhibit convulsions, coma, and paralysis. Low-level exposure to lead in children can result in mental retardation as well as behavior problems (Tesman & Hills, 1994). Mildly elevated blood lead levels have also been associated with a 2- to 3-point decline in IQ for every 10 μg/dL increase in blood lead (Lanphear, et al., 1996). Elevated blood lead levels may also contribute to learning disability and school dropouts (Lee & Moore, 1990). Treatment for lead exposure involves correcting dehydration and electrolyte imbalances and using chelating agents to facilitate urinary excretion of lead.

Mercury poisoning manifests initially as listlessness and irritability. Recurrent rashes, photophobia, and a pinkish coloration of fingertips, toes, nose, hands, and feet are characteristic of the disease. Severe perspiration, pruritus, desquamation of hands and feet, and a burning sensation of hands and feet are also typical. Neurologic symptoms include neuritis, mental apathy, and loss of deep tendon reflexes. Chelating agents and maintenance of nutrition and fluid and electrolyte balances are the key to therapy. Prior to 1991, mercury could be found in some interior and exterior paints. Mercury may also be sprinkled

TABLE 17–2. **FOLK REMEDIES WITH HIGH LEAD CONTENT**

Culture Group	Remedy	Typical Use
Latino	Greta	Empacho (intestinal illness)
	Azarcon (Alarcon, Coral, Liga, Maria Luisa, Rueda)	Empacho
Hmong	Pay-loo-ah	Rash or fever
Asian Indian	Ghasard	Digestive aid
	Bala Goli	Stomachache
	Kandu	Stomachache
Arab	Ko'hl (Alkohl)	Umbilical stump, skin infection, cosmetics

(Source: California Department of Health Services, 1996.)

around the home ceremonially by some religious and ethnic groups (Environmental Protection Agency, 1994).

Arsenic is used in both pesticides and herbicides and is found in water contaminated by runoff in agricultural areas. Arsenic is also found in the home in over-the-counter ant poisons and may be a source of accidental poisoning. Symptoms of acute arsenic poisoning include nausea, vomiting, diarrhea, severe burning of the mouth and throat, and acute abdominal pain. Chronic poisoning may manifest as weakness, prostration, muscle aches, desquamation and hyperpigmentation of the trunk and extremities, and linear pigmentation of fingernails.

Cadmium poisoning can occur when acidic foods are prepared in cadmium-lined containers (eg, mixing lemonade in metal cans) or from contaminated drinking water. Another source of cadmium contamination of water supplies is decomposition of rechargable batteries in landfills. Cadmium filters through into groundwater (Koren, 1991b). Symptoms of cadmium poisoning include nausea, vomiting, diarrhea, and prostration within 10 minutes of ingestion. Cadmium fumes can also be produced by some industrial processes and, when inhaled, cause a severe pneumonitis.

Noise

In addition to the physiologic effect of noise on hearing, evidence suggests that prolonged exposure to noise contributes to increased anxiety and emotional stress that may manifest as nausea, headaches, and sexual impotence. Other effects include insomnia, skin problems, swollen ankles, increase in the incidence of minor accidents, heart trouble and hypertension, cardiac dysrhythmias, and drug use. The psychological effects of noise can include irritability, depression, and diminished work productivity (Kime, 1992).

Hearing loss due to noise exposure is a serious problem in industry. Exposure to noise outside the work environment is also a problem. Approximately 8 million people are exposed to hazardous noise levels in the United States, and 1.5 million experience detectable hearing loss (Kime, 1992). Examples of noise sources that exceed the hearing impairment threshold include buses, trucks, motorcycles, garbage trucks, trains, subways, recreational and off-road vehicles such as snowmobiles, motor boats, and airplanes, and loud music. The health effects of noise are a function of both the intensity of sound (decibels) and the duration of exposure. For example, one could tolerate a sound level of 90 decibels for 8 hours a day without hearing loss, but just over an hour a day at 105 decibels would cause hearing impairment (Auerbach, 1985).

Biological Hazards

Biological hazards are those caused by living organisms in the environment. Biological hazards of concern to community health nurses include infectious agents, insects and animals, and plants.

Infectious Agents

Many infectious agents are transmitted by means of contact with an infected person. Others are transmitted by environmental means. Water is a primary means for environmental transmission of infectious agents. It is estimated that 80% of communicable diseases throughout the world are water-related. Approximately 70% of people worldwide do not have access to safe water (Kime, 1992). In the United States, sanitation and water treatment have limited the extent of waterborne infectious diseases, but transmission via contaminated water still occurs. In fact, there has been an increase in waterborne disease outbreaks in the United States since 1955. During 1991 and 1992, 34 waterborne disease outbreaks occurred in 17 states, resulting in more than 17,000 illness episodes (Moore, Herwaldt, Craun, Calderon, Highsmith, & Juranek, 1993).

In large part, contamination of drinking water supplies occurs via improper sewage treatment and improper solid waste disposal. Septic tanks may have leach lines that are too short to permit adequate filtration of water contaminated with human wastes before it enters the groundwater supply. Approximately 30% of the population use septic tanks to dispose of wastes, and 3.5 billion gallons of human waste are introduced into the soil and portions of it into groundwater each day. Sewer systems prevent this sort of occurrence, but because of population expansion in many parts of the country, sewage treatment plants are inadequate to meet the demand for services. In some areas, untreated sewage contaminates water supplies. In San Diego, for example, untreated sewage from neighboring Tijuana, Mexico, contaminates both ground and surface water supplies, thus creating a biological health hazard.

Biological contamination of water supplies also occurs when solid wastes are improperly handled and rain water is contaminated as it flows through waste disposal sites that breed bacteria, viruses, and other disease-producing microorganisms (Koren, 1991b). There is also potential for contamination of both drinking water and food supplies through the use of reclaimed water. Increased demands for water have led to an upsurge in wastewater recycling. This is particularly true in some parts of the country such as Southern California where wastewater reclamation programs are being developed or are already in operation in many communities. Most of this water is used for crop irrigation, a use that not only provides needed water, but recharges groundwater basins and provides a nitrogen-rich fertilizer for crops. Because of its high nitrogen content, however, recycled wastewater could contaminate drinking water supplies. Use of wastewater to irrigate food crops must be closely monitored to prevent contamination of fruits and vegetables with organic wastes.

Chlorination assists in reducing the hazards of bacterial contamination of water, but water systems are occasionally recontaminated after chlorination due to surface water leaking into faulty pipes. Chlorination can produce its own hazards, though, because the chlorine can react with organic compounds that may be present in water to create carcinogenic compounds (Doyle, et al., 1997). Currently, however, chlorination remains the most efficient and cost-effective mode of water treatment available.

Biological hazards also occur with improper disposal of medical wastes such as needles, syringes, and other objects contaminated with human blood or other secretions and excretions. Although disposal of biological hazards from medical facilities is supposed to be strictly controlled, medical wastes have been found on beaches, apparently washed ashore from ocean dumping. Contaminated medical wastes have also surfaced among ordinary solid wastes where they pose risks to waste industry workers as well as contribute to the potential for biological contamination of water through solid waste disposal sites.

Finally, infectious agents can be transmitted through the air. This transmission is enhanced by technology when improperly cleaned air-conditioning units and heating systems provide breeding grounds for disease-causing microorganisms. For example, contaminated heating, cooling, and water systems have been implicated in the spread of Legionnaires disease (Benenson, 1995; National Center for Infectious Diseases, 1997c).

Insects and Animals

As noted in Chapter 8, insects and animals serve as reservoirs and vectors for a variety of communicable diseases that affect human beings. Insects such as flies, cockroaches, and mosquitoes and animals such as rats transmit communicable diseases. Again, improper solid waste disposal can provide a breeding ground for these and other insect and animal vectors.

The presence of large numbers of wild animals such as skunks, foxes, bats, coyotes, bobcats, and raccoons increases the potential for transmission of rabies to humans. Large numbers of unimmunized domestic animals such as dogs and cats also present a

biological health hazard for the human population. In addition, animal feces provide breeding grounds for flies and other insects that transmit disease.

Plants

Plants can pose biological health hazards in two ways. First, many plants are poisonous and present the opportunity for accidental poisoning among small children. A variety of plants commonly found in homes and yards are potential poisons. Several of these common plants are listed here:

Arrowhead vine	Mistletoe
Asparagus fern	Mountain-ash
Azalea	Oak
Begonia	Oleander
Chrysanthemum	Oregon grape
Climbing nightshade	Philodendron
Dumbcane	Poinsettia
"Fiesta" pepper	Poison ivy
Firethorn	Pokeweed
Flame violet	Rhododendron
Holly	Rubber plant
Honeysuckle	Schefflera
Jade plant	Spider plant
Jerusalem cherry	Weeping fig tree
Medicine aloe	

Plants also pose a biological hazard to those individuals who are allergic to pollen. Allergic responses to plant pollens may include mild to severe hay fever symptoms or asthma. Other plants such as poison ivy and poison oak produce severe dermatologic symptoms.

Chemical and Gaseous Hazards

The environment also provides opportunities for human contact with a variety of *chemical and gaseous hazards.* These hazards are created by the effect of certain chemicals and gases on human tissue, and can involve poisons and air and water pollution.

Poisons

Chemical poisons include insecticides, herbicides, fungicides, and rodenticides as well as a variety of household and industrial chemicals. The use of pesticides has been a primary factor in the increased agricultural production experienced in the United States, but it has also contributed to the occurrence of a number of health-related effects. Pesticide poisoning occurs through massive exposures such as when several thousand people died as a result or exposure to methyl isocyanate resulting from a leak at a chemical plant in Bhopal, India, in 1984. Poisoning also occurs with cumulative exposures among people over a period of time. Herbicide use has been associated with increased incidence of sarcomas, lymphomas, chloracne, multiple myelomas, and respiratory and prostate cancers (Committee to Review the Health Effects in Vietnam Veterans of Exposure to Herbicides, 1994). Home pesticide use has also been implicated in some childhood cancers (Leiss & Savitz, 1995).

Pesticides are used in large volume, and numerous exposures are reported to poison control centers every year. From 1970 to 1989, production of synthetic organic pesticides increased from 469 million kilograms to 572 million kilograms (U.S. Department of Commerce, 1993). Pesticide exposures can occur as a result of working with the chemicals or servicing and repairing equipment used to apply them. Indirect exposure occurs through contamination of food and water that are then ingested by humans and by animal sources of human food. In particular, DDT is absorbed in body fat and is found in animals who consume treated vegetation. These animals, in turn, serve as a food source for humans, who are thus exposed to the stored DDT. Although DDT use has been banned in the United States, it may still be present in foods imported from other countries.

Chemical poisoning can also result from several household and industrial products and medications. Generally, such poisoning occurs in young children who ingest chemical compounds or medications improperly stored in the home. In 1993, the rate of accidental poisoning due to drugs and medicines among all age groups was almost 3 per 100,000 persons (U.S. Department of Commerce, 1996). Accidental poisoning is addressed in more detail in Chapters 20 and 31.

Air Pollution

Chemicals and gaseous materials add to air pollution, thus presenting additional hazards to human health. Both volatile chemicals and particulate matter contribute to the problem, and air pollution occurs in both indoor and outdoor, or "ambient," air. Pollution of the ambient air is measured in terms of the Pollutant Standards Index (PSI). PSI ratings between 100 and 200 are considered "unhealthful," ratings from 200 to 300 "very unhealthful," and levels over 300 "hazardous" to health. Specific pollutants that are routinely monitored include carbon monoxide, ozone, sulfur oxides, volatile organic compounds, nitrogen oxides, lead, and particulates (U.S. Department of Commerce, 1996).

Some progress has been made in controlling pollutants in the ambient air. From 1988 to 1994, the amount of particulate matter in ambient air declined by 25%, and the level of sulfur dioxide decreased by 28%. Declines were noted for carbon monoxide and nitrogen oxides as well (28 and 10%, respectively) (U.S. Department of Commerce, 1996).

Air pollution is more evident in some parts of the country than in others. For example, in 1994, Los Angeles had nearly five times as many days during which carbon monoxide levels exceeded the Environmental Protection Agency (EPA) standards as any other metropolitan area. Similarly, Los Angeles experienced 88 days when ozone levels exceeded standards, compared with 32 days for the San Joaquin Valley, also in California, which had the next highest number of days in excess of ozone standards in the nation (U.S. Department of Commerce, 1996).

Social factors such as widespread automobile use contribute to air pollution. Unfortunately, although vehicles produced today emit fewer hazardous and polluting substances than in the past, the number of autos on U.S. roads has doubled from that of 20 years ago. Each vehicle also travels more miles than ever before and spends more time idling in traffic. Automotive engineering appears to have made the greatest contribution to clean air possible without a complete revolution in the type of engine built.

Sources of ambient air pollution include technological processes used to manufacture consumer goods required to maintain the U.S. standard of living. The level of emissions permissible by large industries is controlled under Clean Air Act standards, but contributions to air pollution are made by numerous small businesses such as dry cleaning and other processes and the use of nail polish remover, paints, aerosols, and other household products that are not controlled. In fact, individuals rather than industry are the most significant contributors to air pollution (Kime, 1992).

Pollutant emissions have a cumulative effect compounded by geographic features in some parts of the country. For example, in Los Angeles a persistent inversion layer, or increase in air temperature with increasing altitude, results in decreased dispersion of pollutants that would normally occur with air movements. The effect of the inversion layer is further compounded by the barrier to air movement presented by nearby mountains. In addition, sunlight interacts with particulate and gaseous matter to produce a photochemical smog (Godish, 1990).

Ambient air pollution is normally dispersed by wind, but wind speed is slowed by the physical features of the earth's surface. The buildings of major urban areas reduce wind speed and thus hinder the dispersion of air pollutants (Godish, 1990).

Health effects of air pollution include respiratory symptoms, eye irritation, fatigue, and headache. Occasionally, air pollution causes death. From 1880 to 1966, for example, there were 12 major air pollution episodes worldwide. Deaths per episode ranged from 20 to the more than 4700 fatalities that occurred during a 3-week period in London in 1952. Air pollution-related mortality generally occurs in the elderly and those with chronic respiratory diseases. Air pollution can also result in increased nonfatal respiratory illness, particularly in children (Buchdahl, Parker, Stebbings, & Babiker, 1996; Dockery, et al., 1993). Air pollution levels have also been associated with increased incidence of cardiovascular and cerebrovascular disease (Ponka & Virtanen, 1996).

Air pollution causes acid rain, which contributes to chemical pollution of both groundwater and surface water supplies. As noted earlier, acid rain enhances leaching of a variety of compounds from soil and solid waste disposal sites and from lead and copper pipes. Air pollution also produces a chemical reaction that depletes the stratospheric ozone layer and reduces the extent of atmospheric filtering, contributing to the adverse health effects of ultraviolet radiation.

Indoor air pollution is also a cause for concern to community health nurses. Pollutants commonly found in household air include formaldehyde, carbon monoxide, carbon dioxide, nitrogen oxides, benzo(*a*) pyrene, asbestos, and other household chemicals (Koren, 1991a). Indoor air pollution tends to be most severe in newer buildings that have been designed, for reasons of energy conservation, to reduce air exchange with the outdoors.

Sources of indoor air pollution include contaminants such as formaldehyde, asbestos, organic dust, and fibrous glass particles released by structural components of buildings or by furnishings. Other sources of pollution indoors include smoking, cooking, heating, cleaning with a variety of household products, and the use of personal hygiene products such as aerosol deodorants (Rogers & Guidotti, 1995). The high cost of energy has also resulted in a shift to new forms of home heating that increase the number and types of pollutants present in dwellings. For example, the use of wood stoves or kerosene heaters, particularly in poorly ventilated areas, leads to the build up of combustion products in the air.

Indoor air pollution is particularly serious since most people spend more than 90% of their time indoors. Those at particular risk for health effects of this type of pollution (children, the elderly, and the infirm) spend an even greater portion of their day inside. Health effects of indoor air pollution range from nose, throat, and eye irritation to respiratory impairment, heart disease, central nervous system damage, and a variety of cancers (Environmental Protection Agency, 1994).

Water Pollution

Only 3% of the earth's water is fresh water and two thirds of that amount comprises glaciers and polar ice caps, leaving less than 1% of the earth's water for human consumption. Because of increased world population, water consumption increases each year. Per capita withdrawal in the United States, for example, has risen from 1000 gallons per day in 1940 to 1600 gallons per day in 1990 (U.S. Department of Commerce, 1996). Daily personal water use typically includes 15 to 20 gallons for bathing, 2 quarts for cooking and drinking, and 15 to 25 gallons for flushing toilets. It takes approximately 250 gallons of water to carry 1 pound of fecal material through a sewer system. An additional 140 billion gallons are used each day for irrigation purposes (Moeller, 1992). Given this level of water use and the limited availability of water, it is not surprising that water pollution is of serious concern.

As noted earlier, acid rain is one source of water pollution, but other sources exist as well. Some 17 chemical carcinogens have been identified in drinking water across the nation, and 33 hazardous chemicals have been identified in groundwater in Pennsylvania, New York, New Jersey, Maine, Connecticut, Massachusetts, Hawaii, California, Arizona, and Delaware. Chemical contamination of groundwater is a particularly serious concern because groundwater constitutes 70% of all fresh water in the United States (Moeller, 1992) and is the source of drinking water for half of the American population.

Manufacturing industries are major sources of chemical pollution of the water, but pollution also arises from mining operations, underground storage of chemicals, septic tanks, and the use of salt and deicing chemicals on highways. Another source of contamination is the 7 million tons of sewage sludge containing both organic and inorganic chemicals produced in the United States each year. By the year 2000, this figure is expected to rise to 14 million tons per year (Koren, 1991b). In 1995, 35% of U.S. rivers and streams violated fecal coliform bacteria standards (U.S. Department of Commerce, 1996). Pesticides and fertilizers also find their way into the water supply to create chemical pollution. Health effects of chemical water pollution include bladder and colorectal cancers, central nervous system effects, skin irritation, alopecia, peripheral neuropathies, seizures, hepatitis and cirrhosis, infertility, congenital anomalies, developmental disabilities, anemia, renal failure, esophagitis, gastritis, stomach cancer, and heart disease.

▶ THE DIMENSIONS MODEL AND ENVIRONMENTAL INFLUENCES ON HEALTH

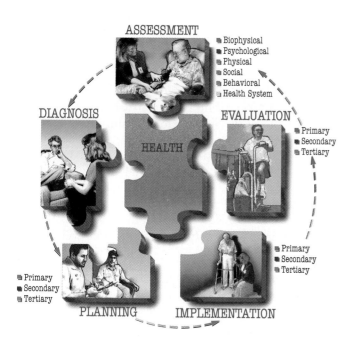

The Dimensions Model can be used by community health nurses to assess the existence of environmental health hazards and their effects on health and to plan, implement, and evaluate primary, secondary, and tertiary preventive measures to address these hazards. The model can be used with individuals, families, and population groups as the focus of care.

Critical Dimensions of Nursing and Environmental Influences on Health

Elements of several dimensions of nursing are relevant to the control of environmental influences on community health. In the cognitive dimension, community health nurses require knowledge of a variety of environmental health hazards, exposure pathways, health effects, and interventions for preventing or mitigating those effects. In order to recognize the health effects of environmental hazards, nurses must also have knowledge of their symptomatology.

Interpersonal dimension capabilities needed by nurses dealing with environmental issues include personal attitudes that promote protection of the envi-

ronment. These attitudes reflect the ecocentric perspective discussed earlier. Communication and collaboration skills are also needed. Nurses will not usually be able to resolve environmental problems with unilateral action. Environmental health problems are collaborative problems and require the interaction of nursing and other disciplines for their resolution. Community health nurses must be able to communicate with policy makers regarding the existence of environmental health problems and to collaborate with members of other disciplines and the general public regarding their resolution.

In the ethical dimension, nurses must consider the ethical implications of environmental health problems, particularly when approaches to problem resolution infringe on the rights of individuals. For example, legislation prohibiting smoking in public places provides for a healthier environment but infringes on the right of individuals to smoke. Community health nurses must also serve as advocates for the public in promoting attention to environmental issues.

Process dimension skills needed to resolve environmental health problems include expertise in the change and leadership processes as well as the political process. The community health nurse will also need to employ the health education process to educate individual clients and the public regarding environmental issues.

 Assessing the Dimensions of Health

The first step in ameliorating environmental health problems is an assessment of the factors contributing to them and their effects on human health. This assessment can be conducted from the perspective of the Dimensions Model considering elements in each of the dimensions of health. Considerations in the biophysical dimension include the interactions of age and genetic make-up with environmental factors and the physiologic effects of environmental conditions. Other existing physiologic conditions may also influence the effects of environmental factors on health. Generally speaking, young children and the elderly are more susceptible to the effects of many environmental hazards than people of other ages. Children's higher metabolic rate increases the rate of absorption of toxins, and very young children are closer to the floor, where air pollutants, in particular, accumulate. In addition, the rapid rate of growth and cell differentiation in children fosters genetic alteration and carcinogenesis. Finally, the hand-to-mouth activity of many young children places them at higher risk for ingestion of toxins from the environment (Pope, Snyder, & Mood, 1995). Older adults, because of changes in cardiovascular, renal, pulmonary, and immune systems, are less able to detoxify environmental toxins placing them at increased risk of adverse health effects. Skin changes in the elderly also increase the rate of absorption of environmental toxins (Pope, Snyder, & Mood, 1995).

Existing genetic and physiologic conditions may also increase the potential for health effects of environmental factors. For example, levels of environmental toxins that might not harm an adult may be harmful to the fetus in a pregnant woman. There is also evidence that preexisting tuberculosis may increase the risk of lung cancer by 50% (Vena, 1995) exacerbating the effects of environmental conditions. The effects of some environmental conditions are influenced by genetic susceptibility. For example, exposure to the herbicide *agent orange,* has been associated with porphyrian cutanea tarda, a disfiguring skin condition, in Vietnam veterans with genetic predisposition to the disease (Committee to Review the Health Effects in Vietnam Veterans of Exposure to Herbicides, 1994).

Another assessment consideration in the biophysical dimension is the physiologic effect of environmental factors. Environmental factors have been implicated in several diseases. For example, environmental factors cause an estimated 11% of cancers in some populations (Zenz, Velasco, Demeter, & Cordasco, 1995), and approximately 60% of the world's population develop sensitization to environmental allergens (O'Rourke & Lebowitz, 1995). The physical, biological, chemical, and gaseous environmental hazards discussed earlier affect a number of target organs in the body. Target organs and systems include the central nervous, respiratory, cardiovascular, gastrointestinal, genitourinary, reproductive, integumentary, hematopoietic, lymphatic, metabolic/endocrine, and musculoskeletal systems, as well as the eyes and ears.

Air pollution, for example, affects the respiratory system primarily, but may also produce cardiovascular, central nervous system, or hematopoietic effects. Air pollution also irritates the eyes and mucous membranes of the respiratory system. Water pollution can affect the gastrointestinal system, skin, liver, and reproductive, hematopoietic, lymphatic, cardiovascular, and genitourinary systems. Pesticides can adversely affect the central nervous system and produce kidney damage, a variety of cancers, and chromosomal changes. Radiation can cause skin cancer, visual impairment, cataracts, and genetic mutations, as well

as lung and other cancers. Lead poisoning damages the central nervous system as well as the gastrointestinal system and can impair growth and development. Other metals and hazardous chemicals may cause cancers or central nervous system, gastrointestinal, and metabolic damage. Finally, high levels of noise not only compromise human hearing, but can contribute to gastrointestinal, dermatologic, central nervous system, cardiovascular, and psychological problems. Some of the effects of these environmental hazards are presented in Figure 17–2.

In the psychological dimension, environmental factors such as pollution and noise decrease the aesthetic aspects of the environment and contribute to stress. The environmental factors discussed earlier, such as air pollution, solid wastes, radiation, and so on, are elements of the physical dimension that affect health. There may also be interaction between elements in the physical dimension that worsen environmental health problems. For example, the chemical reactions that contribute to air pollution are enhanced by heat during warm weather.

The primary social dimension factor relating to environmental health problems is occupation. Occupational settings give rise to multiple opportunities for exposure to environmental hazards. For example, mushroom growers may develop hypersensitivity pneumonitis from exposure to fungal spores and grain workers may develop organic dust toxic syndrome (Musgrave & McCawley, 1995). Miners, on the other hand, may be exposed to high levels of radon, and sawmill workers are at higher risk for lymphomas (Hertzman, et al., 1997). Other social factors, such as socioeconomic status, may influence exposure to environmental hazards. For example, children in families with lower income levels are at higher risk for lead poisoning (Lee & Moore, 1990).

Aspects of the behavioral dimension interact with elements of the physical environment to cause or exacerbate health problems. Smoking, for example, increases lead absorption levels for both smokers and their children, and similar findings have been noted for cocaine users. In addition, inadequate calcium and iron intake in either smokers or cocaine users may further enhance lead absorption (Neuspiel, Markowitz, & Drucker, 1994). Recreational activities may also contribute to environmental exposures. For example, ice skaters have been found to be at particularly high risk for carbon monoxide (CO) poisoning due both to CO accumulation in indoor rinks and to strenuous activity that increases oxygen consumption (National Center for Environmental Health, 1996). "Adventure tourism" is another recreational activity that increases the potential for exposure to environmental hazards,

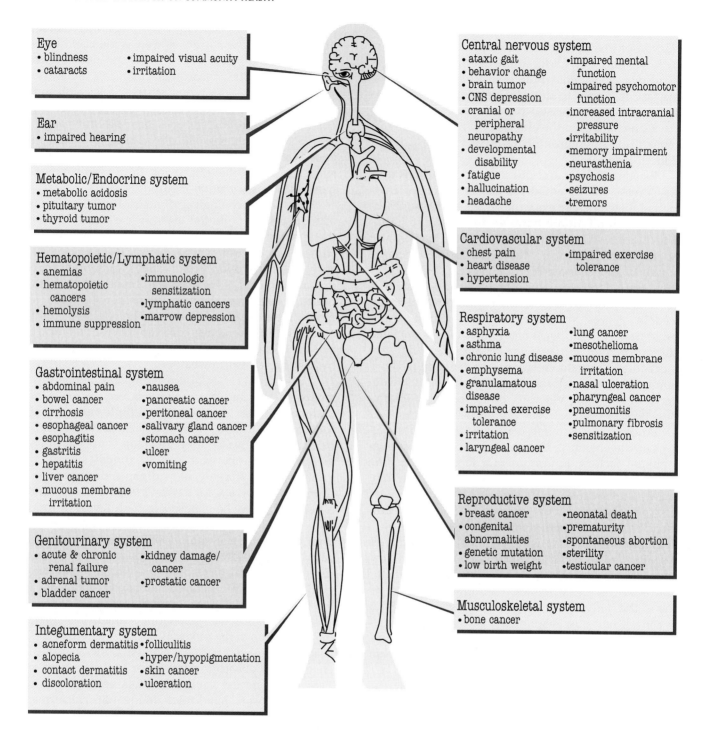

Eye
- blindness
- cataracts
- impaired visual acuity
- irritation

Ear
- impaired hearing

Metabolic/Endocrine system
- metabolic acidosis
- pituitary tumor
- thyroid tumor

Hematopoietic/Lymphatic system
- anemias
- hematopoietic cancers
- hemolysis
- immune suppression
- immunologic sensitization
- lymphatic cancers
- marrow depression

Gastrointestinal system
- abdominal pain
- bowel cancer
- cirrhosis
- esophageal cancer
- esophagitis
- gastritis
- hepatitis
- liver cancer
- mucous membrane irritation
- nausea
- pancreatic cancer
- peritoneal cancer
- salivary gland cancer
- stomach cancer
- ulcer
- vomiting

Genitourinary system
- acute & chronic renal failure
- adrenal tumor
- bladder cancer
- kidney damage/cancer
- prostatic cancer

Integumentary system
- acneform dermatitis
- alopecia
- contact dermatitis
- discoloration
- folliculitis
- hyper/hypopigmentation
- skin cancer
- ulceration

Central nervous system
- ataxic gait
- behavior change
- brain tumor
- CNS depression
- cranial or peripheral neuropathy
- developmental disability
- fatigue
- hallucination
- headache
- impaired mental function
- impaired psychomotor function
- increased intracranial pressure
- irritability
- memory impairment
- neurasthenia
- psychosis
- seizures
- tremors

Cardiovascular system
- chest pain
- heart disease
- hypertension
- impaired exercise tolerance

Respiratory system
- asphyxia
- asthma
- chronic lung disease
- emphysema
- granulamatous disease
- impaired exercise tolerance
- irritation
- laryngeal cancer
- lung cancer
- mesothelioma
- mucous membrane irritation
- nasal ulceration
- pharyngeal cancer
- pneumonitis
- pulmonary fibrosis
- sensitization

Reproductive system
- breast cancer
- congenital abnormalities
- genetic mutation
- low birth weight
- neonatal death
- prematurity
- spontaneous abortion
- sterility
- testicular cancer

Musculoskeletal system
- bone cancer

Figure 17–2. Human health effects of environmental hazards.

particularly biological agents (National Center for Infectious Diseases, 1997a; 1997b).

Finally, factors in the health system dimension may contribute to environmental health problems. In some instances, the health system may be a direct contributing factor in environmentally caused disease.

For example, hospital environments are a frequent site for Legionnaires disease outbreaks. In fact, from 1980 to 1989, 23% of the cases of Legionnaires disease were nosocomially acquired (National Center for Infectious Diseases, 1997c). Failure of health care providers to attend to environmental concerns is another contribut-

ASSESSMENT TIPS: Environmental Influences on Health

Biophysical Dimension

Will environmental conditions have differential effects on different age groups in the population? If so, what will those effects be?

How do environmental conditions affect existing physiologic conditions present in the population?

Do environmental conditions interact with genetic predispositions present in the population? If so, in what way?

What are the physiologic effects of environmental conditions? How do those effects manifest themselves?

Psychological Dimension

What effect do environmental conditions have on the aesthetic quality of the environment?

To what extent do environmental conditions contribute to stress (eg, via noise)?

Physical Dimension

Do other physical dimension factors (eg, weather) interact with environmental conditions to affect health?

Social Dimension

What attitudes do members of the population hold toward environmental conditions?

Do occupational factors contribute to exposure to environmental conditions? If so, how?

Does economic status influence exposure to environmental conditions? If so, how?

Behavioral Dimension

Does smoking interact with environmental conditions to exacerbate their effects?

Do dietary patterns influence the effects of environmental conditions?

Do recreational activities influence exposure to environmental conditions?

Health System Dimension

Do health care environments contribute to adverse effects on health? If so, how?

Are health care providers alert to evidence of illness caused by environmental conditions?

---

ing factor. Despite recommendations for routine lead screening for all children, only 12% of physicians in one survey were testing blood lead levels in their pediatric patients (Tesman & Hills, 1994).

Community health nurses assess the dimensions of health to identify environmental hazards present in the community, the factors contributing to them, and the health effects that result. They then use this information to develop nursing diagnoses and plan interventions to control environmental health problems.

Diagnostic Reasoning and Environmental Influences on Health

The environmental assessment conducted by the community health nurse gives rise to two levels of nursing diagnoses. The first level reflects the presence of health hazards within the client's environment. For example, the nurse may make a diagnosis of "increased potential for lead poisoning due to lead-based paint in deteriorating older housing." Such a diagnosis would signal environmental risks for individuals who live in the area affected as well as for the community at large. In another instance, the nursing diagnosis may relate to risks experienced by a particular family, rather than the entire community. For example, the nurse might make a diagnosis of an "increased potential for poisoning due to the presence of young children and improper storage of household chemicals in the home."

The second level of nursing diagnosis reflects the presence of existing health problems related to environmental conditions. For example, the nurse might derive a diagnosis of "possible lead poisoning due to eating paint chips" in a young child. Or, the nurse might diagnose an "increased incidence of respiratory illnesses due to inadequate cleaning of air-conditioning and heating units" in an energy-efficient office building.

As can be seen in the examples given, both levels of diagnoses may be made in relation to individuals, families, and groups or communities. For an individual or a family, diagnoses can reflect an increased risk of health problems due to specific environmental conditions or the identification of existing health problems related to those conditions. The same is true for diagnoses related to groups of people. The nurse may diagnose environmental conditions that pose risks for the entire community or existing health problems due to environmental factors.

Planning the Dimensions of Environmental Health Care

Based on the findings of the nursing assessment and the nursing diagnoses derived from that assessment, the community health nurse plans interventions to control environmental influences on health. These interventions can occur at the primary, secondary, or tertiary level of prevention.

Primary Prevention

Primary preventive measures are directed toward modifying or eliminating environmental hazards or reducing the potential for exposure to them. Primary prevention can occur with individuals and their families or with groups of people. For instance, the community health nurse might discourage the use of industrial paints that may still contain lead for painting surfaces in a family's home. Or, the nurse may suggest that the family run the tap for a while before getting water for drinking or cooking and to use only cold water. The effects of acidified water in leaching lead and copper from pipes in older homes are enhanced by heat, so warm water or water that has been standing in sun-heated pipes for some time contains higher levels of lead than cold water that has been allowed to run. Another primary preventive measure directed toward the health of individuals and families would be education on the safe storage of medications and household chemicals to prevent accidental poisonings.

At the group level, community health nurses can engage in political efforts to minimize environmental hazards. For example, a nurse might campaign for a local ordinance that requires landlords to engage in safe and effective lead abatement procedures in older dwellings or a law that prevents improper disposal of hazardous wastes. Community health nurses can also educate the public regarding preventive measures. For example, a nurse might be involved in developing a campaign to educate people on the appropriate disposal of hazardous household chemicals. Other primary preventive measures for individuals, families, and communities are listed in Table 17–3.

Secondary Prevention

Secondary prevention with individuals and their families would be geared to identifying and resolving existing health problems caused by environmental conditions. For example, community health nurses might be involved in screening for elevated lead levels or hearing loss. They might also make referrals for testing of water supplies for clients who are concerned about potential contamination. When possible environmentally caused health conditions are identified, community health nurses might make referrals for medical diagnosis and treatment as needed. They might also make referrals for assistance with eliminating environmental hazards. For example, the nurse might be aware of lead-based paint in dwellings in some parts of town. He or she can screen young children in the area for elevated blood lead levels and make referrals for treatment for children with positive test results. The nurse might also make a referral for assistance in removing lead-based paint from the homes of affected children. Finally, the nurse might monitor children's responses to therapy and potential for continued exposure to lead.

Political activity might again be used as a secondary preventive measure at the aggregate level. For example, a nurse might influence health care policy makers to provide adequate access to diagnostic and treatment facilities for people with health problems caused by environmental conditions. Or, a nurse might campaign for stricter standards for pollutant emissions in air and water. Potential secondary preventive measures for individuals, families, and communities are listed in Table 17–4.

Tertiary Prevention

Community health nurses may need to work with individuals or families to prevent recurrence or complications of environmentally caused health problems. For example, a community health nurse might assist a family to find housing where exposure to lead is not a problem. Or, the nurse might provide parents with referrals for assistance in coping with the mental effects of longstanding lead poisoning in their children. Another tertiary preventive measure might involve suggestions for decreasing noise levels in the home to prevent further impairment of hearing.

TABLE 17–3. PRIMARY PREVENTIVE MEASURES FOR SELECTED ENVIRONMENTAL HAZARDS FOR INDIVIDUALS, FAMILIES, AND COMMUNITIES

Environmental Hazard	Individual/Family	Community
Radiation	• Refer for assistance with testing and sealing a home against radon leaks	• Educate the public on the hazards of radon exposure and preventive measures
	• Encourage spending most of one's time in higher levels of the home	• Engage in political activity to promote building standards that safeguard occupants in areas with high levels of natural radiation
	• Discourage overuse of diagnostic x-rays	• Educate public about the hazards of overuse of diagnostic x-rays
	• Encourage adequate cleaning of door seals on microwave ovens and maintenance of safe distance while microwave is in operation	• Engage in political activity to promote and enforce safety standards for nuclear reactors
	• Discourage sunbathing	• Educate the public about the hazards of exposure to ultraviolet radiation
	• Encourage use of sunscreen and protective clothing when outdoors	
Lead and heavy metals	• Encourage families to remove lead-based paint from older homes	• Encourage communities to remove lead-based paint form older homes
	• Encourage families to wash small children's hands as well as toys to remove lead-contaminated dust	
	• Encourage close supervision of small children	
	• Encourage families to use cold water to drink and cook with and to allow the tap to run for a few minutes	• Promote legislation to ban air pollution and acid rain to prevent pollution of water with heavy metals
		• Encourage policy makers to set and enforce standards for solid waste sites to prevent metal contamination in waters
Noise	• Encourage families to limit noise in the home	• Promote noise abatement ordinances
	• Encourage use of ear protection in high-noise areas	
Infectious agents	• Promote routine immunization for all ages	• Educate the public on need for immunizations
		• Encourage policy makers to provide low-cost immunization services
	• Encourage good hygiene	
	• Encourage washing fruits and vegetables before eating	
	• Encourage adequate refrigeration of food	• Encourage enforcement of regulations for food processing and food handlers
	• Encourage susceptible individuals to boil water for cooking and drinking in areas with unsafe water	• Promote adequate sanitation, waste disposal, and water treatment
Insects and animals	• Encourage immunization of family pets	• Encourage development and enforcement of immunization and leash laws
	• Refer for assistance in eliminating insects, rats, and other pests from the home	• Promote ordinances controlling insect breeding areas
	• Encourage use of insect repellent and protective clothing when outdoors	
Plants	• Eliminate poisonous house plants	• Eliminate poisonous plants from recreational areas
	• Eliminate poisonous plants from the yard	
	• Eliminate other hazardous plants (eg, poison ivy, plant allergens) from home environment	
	• Encourage close supervision of small children	
Poisons	• Educate families on proper use and storage of household chemicals and medications	• Educate public on hazards of household chemicals and medication
	• Encourage close supervision of children	• Promote legislation to limit use of hazardous chemicals in home and industry
Air pollution	• Encourage limiting physical activity on days with high air-pollutant levels	• Promote legislation to prevent air pollution
	• Encourage car pooling	
	• Discourage use of space heaters in poorly ventilated areas	• Promote legislation to develop safety standards for home heating devices
	• Encourage frequent cleaning of heater and air-conditioning filters	• Promote building standards that ensure adequate ventilation
	• Encourage opening doors and windows to permit air exchange	
	• Encourage replacing asbestos insulation as needed	
Water pollution	• Encourage use of bottled water by high-risk persons in areas with heavily polluted water	• Promote legislation to prevent water pollution

Tertiary prevention might also be needed to deal with environmental problems at the aggregate or group level. An example of tertiary control measures at this level might include political activity to mandate standards that prevent the recurrence of a leak at a nuclear power plant or to pass a bond issue to renovate a water treatment plant and prevent recontamination of drinking water with sewage. Other possible tertiary preventive interventions by community health nurses are presented in Table 17–5.

TABLE 17–4. SECONDARY PREVENTIVE MEASURES FOR SELECTED ENVIRONMENTAL HAZARDS FOR INDIVIDUALS, FAMILIES, AND COMMUNITIES

Environmental Hazard	Individual/Family	Community
Radiation	• Look for signs of health problems among clients and members of their families that may be caused by radiation • Refer for diagnosis and treatment as needed • Monitor effectiveness of treatment	• Monitor incidence of health problems caused by radiation • Promote accessibility of diagnostic and treatment facilities • Monitor longevity to determine effects of treatment in groups of people
Lead and heavy metals	• Screen for elevated blood levels of heavy metals in persons at risk • Observe for signs of heavy metal poisoning • Refer for diagnosis and treatment as needed • Monitor effects of treatment	• Promote accessibility of screening services • Monitor incidence of heavy metal poisoning • Educate the public on the signs and symptoms of heavy metal poisoning • Promote accessibility of diagnostic and treatment facilities • Monitor prevalence of complications due to heavy metal poisoning
Noise	• Screen for hearing loss in persons at risk • Refer for diagnosis and treatment as needed • Monitor effects of treatment	• Promote accessibility of screening services • Promote accessibility of diagnostic and treatment services
Infectious agents	• Screen for selected communicable diseases in high-risk persons • Observe for signs of communicable diseases	• Promote accessibility of screening services • Monitor incidence of communicable diseases
Insects and animals	• Educate families about first aid for insect and animal bites • Observe for signs and symptoms of diseases caused by insects or animals • Refer for medical assistance as needed	• Promote accessibility of treatment facilities for animals bites • Monitor the incidence of diseases caused by insects or animals • Promote accessibility of diagnostic and treatment services for diseases caused by insects or animals
Plants	• Inform families of poison control center activities • Refer families for poison control center services as needed • Refer for treatment of allergies and other conditions caused by plants	• Educate the public about poison control center activities • Promote community support of poison control centers
Poisons	• Educate families about first aid for poisoning • Observe for signs and symptoms of poisoning • Refer families for poison control services as needed	• Educate the public about first aid for poisoning • Monitor the incidence of accidental poisoning • Promote access to poison control center services
Air pollution	• Observe for signs and symptoms of diseases caused by air pollution • Refer for diagnosis and treatment as needed	• Promote legislation to reduce pollutant emissions • Promote access to diagnostic and treatment services
Water pollution	• Observe for signs and symptoms of water-related diseases • Refer for diagnosis and treatment of water-related diseases	• Promote legislation to control water pollution • Promote availability of diagnostic and treatment services for water-related diseases

Implementing Environmental Measures

Implementing environmental control measures can involve both creating support for action to be taken and reducing resistance to action. The community health nurse may need to make individuals and families aware of the risks presented by environmental hazards. For example, the avid runner may not realize that vigorous exercise actually enhances the adverse effects of air pollution on lung tissue and may be unwilling to limit the amount of physical exertion on smoggy days. Or, a family may not be aware of the need to wash children's toys frequently when there is potential for lead exposure.

In addition, the nurse may need to take steps to decrease resistance to action designed to modify environmental hazards. Resistance can arise from perceived barriers to action. The runner, for example, may be unwilling to reduce his or her exercise on days with elevated levels of air pollutants. Or, a landlord

may be unwilling to replace lead or copper pipes with synthetics that minimize the potential for heavy metal poisoning. In the first instance, the nurse might suggest alternative exercises that the runner can perform

Critical Thinking in Research

Because environmental factors surround us on a daily basis, we often grow accustomed to them and fail to recognize their significance for health. How might you go about conducting an environmental assessment in your community? What kinds of data collection strategies would you use? How would you get data about the attitudes of community members toward environmental health issues? Whose attitudes would you examine?

1. What implications would the findings described above have for community health nursing practice in your community?
2. Do you think people's attitudes toward environmental issues would vary among cultural groups in the community? If so, in what way would they differ? How would you find out?

TABLE 17–5. TERTIARY PREVENTIVE MEASURES FOR SELECTED ENVIRONMENTAL HEALTH HAZARDS FOR INDIVIDUALS, FAMILIES, AND COMMUNITIES

Environmental Hazard	Individual/Family	Community
Radiation	• Remove or seal off radiation sources in homes to prevent further exposure • Assist clients to deal with effects of diseases caused by radiation	• Advocate steps to prevent recurrence of radiation exposures in the community • Promote community long-term treatment services for diseases caused by radiation
Lead and heavy metals	• Refer families for help in removing lead-based paint and lead-bearing dust from homes • Encourage families to replace lead and copper pipes if possible • Encourage use of bottled water if needed to prevent subsequent exposure to waterborne metals • Provide assistance in dealing with long-term effects of heavy metal poisoning	• Advocate lead-abatement programs in older residential areas • Educate the public on the hazards of lead and copper pipes • Advocate legislation to promote reductions in water pollutants • Promote access to services needed to deal with effects of heavy metal poisoning
Noise	• Monitor for subsequent hearing loss • Assist client/family to adjust to hearing loss	• Advocate noise abatement legislation • Promote community programs for the hearing impaired
Infectious agents	• Encourage immunization • Encourage hygiene to prevent the spread of communicable diseases to other family members • Monitor for complications of communicable diseases • Maintain overall health status to prevent relapse	• Advocate access to immunization services • Educate the public to prevent the spread of communicable diseases in the community • Promote access to long-term care for effects of communicable diseases
Insects and animals	• Assist clients to adjust to effects of diseases caused by insects and animals	• Promote access to long-term care as needed • Advocate eradication of insect and animal vectors to prevent the spread of disease
Plants	• Assist clients to live with long-term effects of plant poisoning or allergy	• Promote access to long-term care as needed
Poisons	• Assist clients to deal with effects of poisons • Encourage removing potential poisons from the home and proper storage of poisonous substances • Encourage better supervision of young children	• Promote access to long-term care for victims as needed • Advocate removal of potential poisons from the environment
Air pollution	• Assist clients to adjust to effects of diseases caused by pollution • Encourage activity limitation when air pollution is severe	• Promote access to long-term care services as needed • Advocate measures to prevent pollutant emissions
Water pollution	• Assist client to deal with long-term effects of diseases due to water pollution • Encourage use of bottled water by those at risk for recurrence of diseases due to water pollution	• Advocate measures to eliminate existing water pollution and prevent further pollution

indoors. In the second example, the nurse might need to advocate for the family, encouraging the landlord to take the needed action. Or, the nurse might assist the family to move to safer housing. If the family owns its own home, the nurse might refer members to agencies that will help with the cost of removing hazardous materials from the home. For example, some power companies assist homeowners with the cost of installing nonasbestos insulation.

Implementation of environmental controls at the aggregate level also requires developing support and measures to decrease or circumvent resistance to action. The community health nurse may use some of the political strategies described in Chapter 13 to create public support for legislation related to environmental measures. Community health nurses may also be involved in educating the public regarding the risks posed by environmental hazards and in motivating people to take collective action to reduce those risks.

Evaluating Environmental Measures

Community health nurses are also involved in evaluating the effectiveness of environmental control measures. Evaluation would focus on the effectiveness of primary, secondary, and tertiary preventive measures related to individuals, families, and population groups. For example, the nurse might monitor blood lead levels of children in housing with lead-based paint to determine whether primary preventive measures have prevented initial elevation. For those children who already have elevated blood lead levels, evaluation would focus on the effects of chelating agents in reducing blood levels and the prevention of symptoms of lead poisoning. Evaluation of tertiary measures would be aimed at the effectiveness of

TABLE 17–6. SAMPLE QUESTIONS FOR EVALUATING PRIMARY, SECONDARY, AND TERTIARY PREVENTION OF ENVIRONMENTAL HAZARDS

Environmental Hazard	Primary Prevention	Secondary Prevention	Tertiary Prevention
Radiation	Have exposures to radiation been eliminated or reduced? Has the incidence of radiation-related illness been reduced?	Have those with radiation-related diseases received adequate treatment? Have the effects of radiation exposure been minimized?	Have reexposures to radiation been reduced or prevented altogether?
Lead and heavy metals	Have environmental sources of exposure to heavy metals been eliminated? Has the incidence of heavy metal poisoning decreased?	Have blood levels for heavy metals decreased after treatment? Have long-term sequelae of heavy metal poisoning been prevented?	Has reexposure to heavy metals been prevented? Have lowered blood levels for heavy metals been maintained after treatment?
Noise	Have noise levels been reduced to prevent hearing loss? Has the incidence of hearing loss been reduced?	Have persons with hearing impairment received needed services? Has hearing been restored by means of hearing aids or other devices?	Has further deterioration of hearing been prevented?
Infectious agents	Has the incidence of communicable diseases declined? Has the proportion of persons immunized against immunizable communicable diseases increased?	Have individuals with communicable diseases been adequately treated?	Have recurrent cases of communicable diseases been prevented?
Insects and animals	Has the incidence of diseases spread by insects and animals decreased? Have insect and animal vectors been eliminated?	Have individuals with diseases spread by insects and animals been adequately treated?	Have recurrent episodes of diseases caused by insects and animals been prevented?
Plants	Have poisonous plants been removed from the environment? Has the number of cases of plant-related poisoning declined?	Has mortality due to plant poisoning been reduced?	Have recurrent plant poisonings been prevented?
Poisons	Has the incidence of poisoning decreased? Are hazardous substances disposed of appropriately?	Has poisoning mortality declined?	Have recurrent episodes of poisoning been prevented?
Air pollution	Has the level of pollutants in ambient or indoor air been reduced? Has the incidence of diseases due to air pollution declined?	Have individuals with diseases due to air pollution received adequate diagnostic and treatment services?	Has further contamination of ambient or indoor air been prevented?
Water pollution	Has the number of exposures to polluted water been reduced? Has the incidence of diseases due to water pollution declined?	Have individuals with diseases due to water pollution been adequately treated?	Have recurrent episodes of diseases due to water pollution been prevented? Has recontamination of water by pollutants been prevented?

abatement procedures in preventing blood lead levels from rising again after treatment. Similar approaches to evaluation of primary, secondary, and tertiary preventive interventions could be used for each of the environmental health problems addressed in this chapter. Evaluation at the aggregate level would focus on the extent to which national objectives for environmental health have been achieved. Possible foci for evaluating primary, secondary, and tertiary preventive measures for other environmental hazards are listed in Table 17–6.

An examination of the status of the national objectives for environmental health revealed that of the 17 related objectives, 3 have been met, 11 are progressing toward the targeted goal, and 4 are moving away from the goal (U.S. Department of Health and Human Services, 1997). The most significant progress has been made with respect to decreasing

the number of persons with blood lead levels above 15 μg/dL, reducing the number of waterborne disease outbreaks, and increasing the number of states requiring disclosure of lead prior to the sale of homes. This last objective was achieved by federal legislation in 1996 for all homes built prior to 1978. Movement away from projected targets has occurred for objectives related to the number of waterborne disease outbreaks, solid waste generation, the proportion of people with access to safe drinking water, and contamination of surface water. Pollution of lake waters, for example, has worsened by 142%, and the amount of solid waste generated per person per day has increased by approximately 80% rather than decreasing (U.S. Department of Health and Human Services, 1995). Progress toward meeting national objectives related to environmental health is summarized in Table 17–7.

TABLE 17–7. STATUS OF SELECTED NATIONAL HEALTH OBJECTIVES FOR ENVIRONMENTAL HEALTH

	Objective	Base	Most Recent	Target
11.1	Reduce asthma hospitalizations (per 100,000 population)	188 (1987)	194 (1995)	160
11.2	Reduce mental retardation (per 1,000 school-age children)	3.1 (1987)	4 (1992)	2
11.3	Reduce waterborne disease outbreaks	16 (1988)	11 (1994)	11
11.4	Reduce blood lead levels exceeding			
	a. 15 µg/dL	3 million (1984)	274,000 (1992)	300,000
	b. 25 µg/dL	234,000	NDA[a]	0
11.5	Increase proportion of people living in counties meeting air pollution control standards	49.7% (1988)	67.1% (1995)	85%
11.6	Increase number of homes tested for radon	<5% (1989)	11% (1994)	40%
11.7	Reduce release of toxic agents on Department of Health and Human Services' list of carcinogens (billion pounds)	0.32 (1988)	0.17 (1994)	0.12
11.8	Reduce solid waste production (lbs/person/day)	4 (1988)	3.4 (1994)	3.2
11.9	Increase safe community water systems	74% (1988)	73% (1995)	85%
11.10	Reduce percentage of contaminated surface water	25% (1988)	Increased (1994)	15%
11.11	Increase percentage of homes tested for lead-based paint	<5% (1991)	9% (1993)	50%
11.12	Increase number of states with construction standards to minimize radon	1 (1989)	3 (1993)	35
11.13	Increase number of states requiring disclosure prior to home sales			
	a. Lead	2 (1989)	50 (1996)	30
	b. Radon	1 (1989)	25 (1995)	30
11.14	Eliminate immediate and significant health threats from hazardous waste sites	NDA	90% (1995)	100%
11.15	Increase percentage of population with recycling programs	26% (1991)	46% (1995)	50%
11.16	Increase number of states that track environmental events	NDA	27 (1996)	35
11.17	Decrease percentage of children exposed to tobacco smoke at home	39% (1986)	27% (1994)	20%

[a]NDA, no data available.

(Source: U.S. Department of Health and Human Services, 1991, 1997.)

Critical Thinking in Practice: A Case in Point

Janice Wu, a community health nurse, is visiting a new client in a nursing home in an inner-city area in Los Angeles. As she enters the nursing home, she notices that several of the residents are doing calisthenics in the yard. Some of the residents are sitting on the sidelines and appear quite short of breath. When Janice checks to be sure they are all right, they tell her that they usually have a hard time breathing when they exercise on smoggy days like today. The residents say that they usually try to continue their exercises because it is one of the few activities that gets them out of the building. They also enjoy the social aspects of the exercise sessions. Many of them state that they have always been active and want to maintain their strength and mobility as long as possible. They express fears of being bedridden and unable to care for themselves.

After Janice is sure that all of the residents will be all right, she goes on to see her client. When she enters the building, she notices that it is quite hot inside, even though all of the windows and doors are open. Although it is only 10 A.M., it promises to be one of L.A.'s scorching summer days. After seeing her client, Janice talks to the director about the heat in the building. The director tells her that the building is always hot and that the air conditioning has never worked properly. The last time the repairmen came to fix the air-conditioning unit, they said it could not be repaired and would have to be replaced. The nursing home is run by a large national corporation, and the director says she has been told that they will have to wait until the next budget year (October) before money will be available for a new air conditioner. Fortunately, the heating system is separate, so there will be heat when the colder weather starts. The director says that staff members have been particularly careful about maintaining hydration in the residents during the hot weather, but many of the residents seem fatigued and listless with the heat.

1. What environmental hazards are present in this situation? What health effects, if any, are these hazards causing?
2. What biophysical, psychological, social, behavioral, and health system factors are interacting with hazards in the physical dimension to contribute to problems?
3. What level(s) of prevention is(are) warranted in this situation? What might Janice do to intervene?

TESTING YOUR UNDERSTANDING

1. Discuss the need for both public health and ecological perspectives on environmental concerns. (p. 364)
2. Summarize at least five of the national health objectives for the year 2000 related to environmental health. (p. 383)
3. What are three physical hazards to health arising from the environment? Give an example of the effects of each on human health. (pp. 367–370)
4. Describe three types of biological hazards to health that may be present in the environment. Discuss how each might adversely affect health. (pp. 370–371)
5. What three types of hazards to human health are posed by chemical or gaseous materials? Give an example of the effect of each type of hazard. (pp. 371–374)
6. Describe at least two health effects of environmental conditions on each of six human target organs or body systems. (pp. 374–377)
7. What are the two levels at which nursing diagnoses may be made with respect to environmental influences on health? Give an example of a nursing diagnosis at each level. (pp. 377–378)
8. Describe at least five primary preventive measures for health problems related to environmental conditions. (p. 378)
9. Describe at least three secondary preventive measures for health problems related to environmental conditions. (p. 378)
10. Describe at least three tertiary preventive measures for health problems related to environmental conditions. (pp. 378–379)

WHAT DO YOU THINK?
Questions for Critical Thinking

1. What type of hazardous wastes do you generate? How could you cut down on the amount of hazardous waste generated?
2. To what extent does your educational institution recycle materials? What interventions by nursing students might promote recycling?
3. What are the relative risks and benefits of medical irradiation?
4. What health hazards are present in your campus environment? What actions could be taken to minimize the health risks of environmental hazards on campus?

REFERENCES

Amaya, M., & Ackall, G. (1996, 3rd quarter). Perinatal lead exposure. *Reflections,* 18–19.

Artson, B. S. (1995). Humanity's relationship to earth. *National Forum, 75*(1), 10–12.

Auerbach, L. (1985). The Occupational Health and Safety Act. In D. S. Blumenthal (Ed.), *Introduction to environmental health* (pp. 169–178). New York: Springer.

Benenson, A. S. (1995). *Control of communicable diseases in man* (16th ed.). Washington, DC: American Public Health Association.

Brown, L. R. (1995). The world food prospect: Entering a new era. *National Forum, 75*(1), 16–19.

Buchdahl, R., Parker, A., Stebbings, T., Babiker, A. (1996). Association between air pollution and acute childhood wheezy episodes: Prospective observational study. *British Medical Journal, 312,* 661–665.

California Department of Health Services. (1996). *Lead in home remedies.* Sacramento, CA: California Department of Health Services.

Committee on Advances in Assessing Human Exposure to Airborne Pollutants. (1991). *Human exposure assessment for airborne pollutants: Advances and opportunities.* Washington, DC: National Academy of Science.

Committee to Review the Health Effects in Vietnam Veterans of Exposure to Herbicides. (1994). *Veterans and agent orange.* Washington, DC: National Academy Press.

Cordasco, E. M., & Zenz, C. (1995). The relationship of occupational to environmental respiratory diseases. In E. M. Cordasco, S. L. Demeter, & C. Zenz (Eds.), *Environmental respiratory diseases* (pp. 141–157). New York: Van Nostrand Reinhold.

Diehl, J. F. (1995). *Safety or irradiated foods* (2nd ed.). New York: Marcel Dekker.

Division of Health Examination Statistics. (1997). Update: Blood lead levels—United States, 1991–1994. *MMWR, 46,* 141–146.

Dockery, D. W., Pope, C. A., Xu, X., et al. (1993). An association between air pollution and mortality in six U.S. cities. *New England Journal of Medicine, 329,* 1753–1759.

Doyle, T. J., Zheng, W., Cerhan, J. R., et al. (1997). The association of drinking water source and chlorination by-products with cancer incidence among postmenopausal women in Iowa: A prospective cohort study. *American Journal of Public Health, 87,* 1168–1176.

Environmental Protection Agency. (1993). *Radon: The health threat with a simple solution.* Washington, DC: Environmental Protection Agency.

Environmental Protection Agency. (1994). *Indoor air pollution: An introduction for health professionals.* Washington, DC: Environmental Protection Agency.

Farfel, M. R., & Chisolm, J. J., Jr. (1990). Health and environmental outcomes of traditional and modified practices for abatement of residential lead-based paint. *American Journal of Public Health, 80,* 1240–1245.

Gibbons, W. (1991). Low level radiation: Higher long-term risk? *Science News, 139,* 181.

Godish, T. (1990). *Air quality* (2nd ed.). Chelsea, MI: Lewis.

Goldman, R. R. (1996). *Public health nursing in a multi-cultural society: Lead poisoning from non-traditional sources.* Los Angeles: Los Angeles County Department of Health Services.

Gordon, L. J. (1997). Environmental health and protection. In F. D. Scutchfield & C. W. Keck (Eds.), *Principles of public health practice* (pp. 300–317). Albany, NY: Delmar.

Hertzman, C., Teschke, K., Ostry, A., et al. (1997). Mortality and cancer incidence among sawmill workers exposed to chlorophenate wood preservatives. *American Journal of Public Health, 87,* 71–79.

Josten, L., Clarke, P. N., Ostwald, S., Stoskopf, C., & Shannon, M. D. (1995). Public health nursing education: Back to the future for public health sciences. *Family and Community Health, 18*(1), 36–48.

Kime, R. E. (1992). *Environment and health.* Guilford, CT: Dushkin.

Kleffel, D. (1996). Environmental paradigms: Moving toward an ecocentric perspective. *Advances in Nursing Science, 18*(4), 1–10.

Koren, H. (1991a). *Handbook of environmental health: Principles and practices* (Vol. 1) (2nd ed.). Chelsea, MI: Lewis.

Koren, H. (1991b). *Handbook of environmental health: Principles and practices* (Vol. 2) (2nd ed.). Chelsea, MI: Lewis.

Kotchian, S. B. (1995). Environmental health services are prerequisites to health care. *Family and Community Health, 18*(3), 45–53.

Lajinian, S., Hudson, S., Applewhite, L., Feldman, J., & Minkoff, H. L. (1997). An association between the heat-humidity index and preterm labor and delivery: A preliminary analysis. *American Journal of Public Health, 87,* 1205–1207.

Lanphear, B. P., Weitzman, M., & Winter, N. L., et al., (1996). Lead-contaminated house dust and urban children's blood lead levels. *American Journal of Public Health, 86,* 1416–1421.

Lee, W. R., & Moore, M. R. (1990). Low level exposure to lead. *British Medical Journal, 301,* 504–506.

Leiss, J. K., & Savitz, D. A. (1995). Home pesticide use and childhood cancer: A case-control study. *American Journal of Public Health, 85,* 249–252.

Lum, M. R. (1995). Environmental public health: Future direction, future skills. *Family and Community Health, 18*(1), 24–35.

MacIntyre, W. J., & Saha, G. B. (1995). Sources of ionizing radiation and their effects on humans. In E. M. Cordasco, S. L. Demeter, & C. Zenz (Eds.), *Environmental respiratory diseases* (pp. 337–348). New York: Van Nostrand Reinhold.

March of Dimes Birth Defects Foundation. (1992). *Public health education information sheet.* White Plains, NY: March of Dimes.

Moeller, D. W. (1992). *Environmental health.* Cambridge, MA: Harvard University Press.

Moore, A. C., Herwaldt, B. L., Craun, G. F., Calderon, R. L., Highsmith, A. K., & Juranek, D. D. (1993). Surveillance for waterborne disease outbreaks—United States, 1991–1992. *MMWR, 42* (SS-5), 1–22.

Musgrave, K. J., & McCawley, M. A. (1995). Respiratory health risks in agriculture. In E. M. Cordasco, S. L. Demeter, & C. Zenz (Eds.), *Environmental respiratory diseases* (pp. 363–394). New York: Van Nostrand Reinhold.

National Center for Environmental Health. (1996). Carbon monoxide poisoning at an indoor ice arena and bingo hall—Seattle, 1996. *MMWR, 45,* 265–267.

National Center for Environmental Health. (1997). Heat-related deaths—Dallas, Wichita, and Cooke Counties, Texas, and United States, 1996. *MMWR, 46,* 528–531.

National Center for Infectious Diseases. (1997a). Malaria in an immigrant and travelers—Georgia, Vermont, and Tennessee, 1996. *MMWR, 46,* 536–539.

National Center for Infectious Diseases. (1997b). Outbreak of leptospirosis among white-water rafters—Costa Rica, 1996. *MMWR, 46,* 577–579.

National Center for Infectious Diseases. (1997c). Sustained transmission of nosocomial Legionnaires disease—Arizona and Ohio. *MMWR, 46,* 416–421.

The Nation's Health. (1995, March). Global warming, infectious disease spread linked, 2.

NIOSH Fact Sheet. EMFs in the workplace. (1996). Washington, DC: U.S. Department of Health and Human Services.

Neuspiel, D. R., Markowitz, M., & Drucker, E. (1994). Intrauterine cocaine, lead, and nicotine exposure and fetal growth. *American Journal of Public Health, 84,* 1492–1494.

O'Rourke, M. K., & Lebowitz, M. D. (1995). Environmental allergens and the development of chronic and allergic obstructive lung diseases. In E. M. Cordasco, S. L. Demeter, & C. Zenz (Eds.), *Environmental respiratory diseases* (pp. 295–335). New York: Van Nostrand Reinhold.

Pershagen, G., Akerblom, G., Axelson, O., et al. (1994). Residential radon exposure and lung cancer in Sweden. *New England Journal of Medicine, 330,* 159–164.

Ponka, A., & Virtanen, M. (1996). Low-level air pollution and hospital admissions for cardiac and cerebrovascular diseases in Helsinki. *American Journal of Public Health, 86,* 1273–1280.

Pope, A. M., Snyder, M. A., & Mood, L. H. (Eds.). (1995). *Nursing, health, and environment: Strengthening the relationship to improve the public's health.* Washington, DC: National Academy Press.

Rogers, R. E., & Guidotti, T. L. (1995). Indoor air quality and building associated outbreaks. In E. M. Cordasco, S. L. Demeter, & C. Zenz (Eds.), *Environmental respiratory diseases* (pp. 179–207). New York: Van Nostrand Reinhold.

Schnorr, T. M., Grawjewski, P. A. Hornung, P. A., & Thun, M. D. (1991). Video display terminals and the risk of spontaneous abortion. *New England Journal of Medicine, 324,* 727–733.

Schoen, E. J. (1993). Childhood lead poisoning: Definitions and priorities. *Pediatrics, 91,* 504–505.

Shannon, M. W., & Graef, J. W. (1992). Lead intoxication in infancy. *Pediatrics, 89,* 87–90.

Soroos, M. S. (1995). Environmental security: Choices for the twenty-first century. *National Forum, 75*(1), 20–24.

Tesman, J. R., & Hills, A. (1994). Developmental effects of lead exposure in children. *Social Policy Report, VIII*(3), 1–16.

U.S. Department of Commerce. (1993). *Statistical abstract of the United States, 1993* (113th ed.). Washington, DC: Government Printing Office.

U.S. Department of Commerce. (1996). *Statistical abstract of the United States, 1993* (116th ed.). Washington, DC: Government Printing Office.

U.S. Department of Health and Human Services. (1991). *Healthy people 2000: National health promotion and illness prevention objectives.* Washington, DC: Government Printing Office.

U.S. Department of Health and Human Services. (1995). *Healthy people 2000: Midcourse review and 1995 revisions.* Washington, DC: Government Printing Office.

U.S. Department of Health and Human Services. (1997). *Healthy people 2000: Progress review—Environmental Health.* Washington, DC: Government Printing Office.

Vena, J. E. (1995). Environmental lung cancer. In E. M. Cordasco, S. L. Demeter, & C. Zenz (Eds.), *Environmental respiratory diseases* (pp. 417–443). New York: Van Nostrand Reinhold.

Zenz, C., Velasco, J. A. V., Demeter, S. L., & Cordasco, E. M. (1995). From workplace to the general environment. In E. M. Cordasco, S. L. Demeter, & C. Zenz (Eds.), *Environmental respiratory diseases* (pp. 1–19). New York: Van Nostrand Reinhold.

Zuk, G., & White, S. (1990). Six pressing environmental problems: An interview with Lester Brown. *National Forum, 70*(1), 8–11.

RESOURCES FOR PROMOTING ENVIRONMENTAL HEALTH

Agency for Toxic Substances and Disease Registry
1600 Clifton Road, NE
Mail Stop E-28
Atlanta, GA 30333
(404) 639–0501

Center for Atomic Radiation Studies
PO Box 2082
Acton, MA 01720–6082
(508) 263–2065

Centers for Disease Control
Center for Environmental Health and Injury Control
4470 Buford Highway, Room 1218
Chamblee, GA 30341
(404) 488–4111

Consumer Product Safety Commission
East West Towers
4340 East West Highway
Bethesda, MD 20814
(301) 540–0580

Environmental Action Foundation
6930 Carroll Avenue, 6th Floor
Takoma Park, MD 20912
(301) 891–1100

Environmental Protection Agency
401 M Street, SW
Washington, DC 20460
(202) 260–2090

Ministry of Concern for Public Health
PO Box 1487
Williamsville, NY 14231

National Council on Radiation Protection
   and Measurements
7910 Woodmont Avenue, Ste. 800
Bethesda, MD 20814
(301) 657–2652

National Environmental Health Association
720 S Colorado Boulevard, Ste. 970, S Tower
Denver, CO 80222
(301) 756–9090

Nuclear Regulatory Commission
1717 H Street, NW
Washington, DC 20555
(301) 492–7000

Office of Lead-based Paint Abatement
  and Poisoning Prevention
Department of Housing and Urban Development
451 7th Street, SW
Washington, DC 20401
(202) 708–1422

Pesticide Education Center
PO Box 420870
San Francisco, CA 94142–0870
(415) 391–8511

Sierra Club
730 Polk Street
San Francisco, CA 94109
(415) 776–2211

U.S. Department of Agriculture
Agricultural Marketing Service
PO Box 96456
Washington, DC 20250
(202) 720–8999

U.S. House of Representatives
Committee on Energy & Commerce
Subcommittee on Health & the Environment
2415 Rayburn House Office Bldg.
Washington, DC 20515
(202) 225–0130

Water Environment Federation
601 Wythe Street
Alexandria, VA 22314–1994
(703) 684–2400

World Watch Institute
1776 Massachusetts Avenue, NW
Washington, DC 20036
(202) 452–1999

WIDOW

Alma Brown
sits alone
one alone
where yesterday
there were two
Alma and Jesse.
Two alone
passing the years
in a boarding house basement
with flowers on the bookcase
and clocks for Jesse to fix.

"Sometimes he'd drink
and then we'd fight
but come the next morning
I'd always go lean over
his chair and ask him
if he still loved me.
The answer was yes
I could tell by his eyes.

"He died easy
I'm glad for that.
I didn't even believe
he was dead, his toes
stayed warm so long.
He woke up in the night
and started coughing up blood
didn't struggle or nothing
just held my hand tight
like he did the night
we met the first time
drinking beers at the Derby Bar.

Then he lay back
and closed his eyes
and that was it."

"I come in and look
at the empty bed.
I say to myself, well
he must've got up.
Then I look at the chair

and he's not there …
Oh, it's alright
I haven't broke down yet."

She sits straight
on a straight-back chair
feet planted firm on the floor
hands on her knees
head erect on broad shoulders.

"The ambulance came first.
They were nice but they said
it was no use taking
a dead man. The police
came next. They called
the doctor and helped me
phone the undertaker.
The undertaker said
not to worry, just leave it
all in his hands.
The only thing I'd need to do
is pay him on Monday
so they can start
digging the grave.

I don't know if I can stay
in this place alone
or not. Jesse wants me to
but I don't know …
We lived here twenty years."

"The ambulance left
and then the police.
The undertaker sent his helper
out to the car, then he
took me out to the kitchen
and when I came back
Jesse was gone."

Excerpted with permission from V. Masson (1993). just who. *Washington, DC: Crossroads Health Ministry.*

CARE OF CLIENTS

The essence of community health nursing is the care that is provided to clients to enhance their health. Clients are men, women, children, families, groups, and communities. They include all racial, ethnic, and cultural groups, both rich and poor. In Unit IV, the Dimensions Model is applied to the care of diverse clients with differing health needs.

Nursing care for an individual differs, of course, from that for families and groups. The unique health care needs of families and the community or target group are discussed in Chapters 18 and 19. Assessment is described as well as considerations in planning, implementing, and evaluating care.

The age and sex of clients (Chapters 20 to 23) influence community health nursing services. If children are taught to engage in healthy behaviors, their lifetime health status may be influenced. Health promotion and prevention for this age group can make a tremendous impact on the overall future health of a population. Chapter 20 addresses some of the health concerns that confront our children, including drug and alcohol exposure, chronic illness, AIDS, and psychological problems.

Men and women experience unique health care needs, in part due to sexual differences in susceptibility to specific health problems, but also due to social conditions that are amenable to change. The unique needs of men and women and how to address them are the focus of Chapters 21 and 22.

Much can also be done by community health nurses to enhance the health status of the elderly population, improve their quality of their life, and decrease the health care costs that are associated with the needs of this population (Chapter 23).

As noted in Chapter 14, economic resources have great impact on the health and well-being of clients. The homeless population is particularly influenced by the economics of a community. Community health nurses should be in the forefront of efforts to meet the health needs of homeless individuals and families, whose numbers continue to grow (Chapter 24).

Each type of client discussed in this unit has unique health care needs for which community health nurses can intervene. By adapting the Dimensions Model, clients' needs may be identified, and interventions planned, implemented, and evaluated. The health of the client and ultimately the overall health status of the population is thereby enhanced.

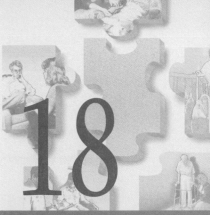

18

CARE OF THE FAMILY CLIENT

Patricia Caudle

The family, although changeable and as unique as its individual members, is the oldest and most enduring social institution. The family has been the basis for procreation, socialization, and continuation of cultures since the beginning of human history. As social norms have evolved over the centuries, many have predicted that the family would cease to exist as a social institution. This prediction, however, has not been realized. Despite periodic experimentation with communal living and other forms of social organization, the family unit is still the social unit most prevalent in society. Consequently, the family as a unit of service is an important consideration for community health nurses. Community health nurses contribute to the growth and health of the community and society through the assistance given to family groups. Knowledge of family health care principles also prepares community health nurses to minister to individual family members, a topic examined in later chapters in this unit.

▶ KEY TERMS

binuclear family
cohabiting family
communal family
crisis
ecomap
extended family
family
formal roles
foster families
genogram
homosexual family
informal roles
maturational crisis
nuclear conjugal
    family
nuclear dyads
role conflict
role overload
roles
single-parent family
situational crisis
skip-generation families
stepfamily
stress

▶ ## Chapter Objectives

After reading this chapter, you should be able to:

- Describe at least five family types and their characteristic features.
- Identify at least three characteristics of families.
- Identify at least four considerations to be addressed in assessing family communication patterns.
- Differentiate between formal and informal family roles.
- Differentiate between situational and maturational crises.
- Describe the structure of a crisis event.
- Identify at least four principles of crisis intervention.

▶ ## FAMILIES

The family is the basic social unit of American society. Defining family is difficult, however, because families can assume so many different forms. For the purposes of community health nursing, a *family* is a social system composed of two or more people living together who may be related by blood, marriage, or adoption, or who stay together by mutual agreement. Family members usually share living arrangements, obligations, goals, the continuity of generations, and a sense of belonging and affection (Murray & Zentner, 1997). This broad definition of family suggests that the principles of community health nursing applied to family clients must be flexible enough to meet the needs of many different family forms.

Types of Families

Nuclear Conjugal Families

The *nuclear conjugal family,* or, more simply, the nuclear family, is composed of husband, wife, and children. Husband and wife are joined by marriage and their children are either biological offspring or adopted. The nuclear family is found in all ethnic and socioeconomic groups and is sanctioned by all religions. In the past, this type of family has been accepted as a social institution necessary to raise children properly and is sometimes referred to as an "intact" family (Janosik & Green, 1992). Today the high rate of divorce, increased sexual freedom, women's liberation, and the decreased social stigma attached to illegitimacy and alternative sexual lifestyles have contributed to changes in the form of the family. The nuclear conjugal family is becoming less common in response to societal changes. In fact, it is

expected that by the year 2000 only 34% of American families will consist of a married couple with children. Almost half (43%) of families will be *nuclear dyads,* married couples without children (Hanson & Boyd, 1996). Nuclear dyads occur by choice, because of infertility, or because children are grown and away from home (Ross & Cobb, 1990).

Extended Families

The *extended family* consists of the family kin network such as grandparents, aunts, uncles, and cousins (Grove, 1996). Like the nuclear family, the extended family has been affected by societal change. In the past, members of extended families often lived in close proximity to the nuclear family. But owing to increased mobility and the enticement of better jobs in other areas, families are more likely to live away from their extended kin network. Thus, the extended family is now more likely to be a long-distance unit with whom the nuclear family corresponds and visits. This phenomenon has limited the social, economic, and emotional support formerly available to members of a nuclear family from older and more experienced relatives.

As time passes and circumstances change, the nuclear family may take extended family members into the home. This typically occurs as a consequence of early marriage of children where the newlyweds must live with parents or when adult children return home following a divorce, an economic setback, or some other life crisis. Some adult children are remaining in the home due to economic constraints and older age at marriage. Approximately 30% of people aged 25 to 29 years, for example, still live with their parents (Hanson & Boyd, 1996). New living arrangements to incorporate extended family members into the nuclear family can also occur when aging parents can no longer live alone. The parent of a grown child may present adjustment problems for the nuclear family that has been separated from the parent for some time.

Single-parent Families

The most common family unit to be encountered by community health nurses is the *single-parent family.* Single-parent families consist of an adult woman or man and children. Single-parent families result from divorce, out-of-wedlock pregnancies, absence or death of a spouse, or adoption by a single person. From 1970 to 1990, births to single women increased from 11% to 27% of all births, and the proportion of single-parent households more than doubled. Most (86%) of single-parent families are headed by women (Hanson & Boyd, 1996). The number of single-parent families is expected to continue to increase. Single-parent families headed by men are expected to increase at a faster rate than those headed by women through the year 2000 (Person, 1993).

Stepfamilies

Stepfamilies are increasingly evident in American society. A *stepfamily* is composed of two adults, at least one of whom has remarried following divorce or death of a spouse. Stepfamilies can include children from either adult's previous marriage, as well as offspring from the new marriage. Approximately 50% to 60% of marriages end in divorce, and two thirds of divorces involve children. Seventy-five percent of divorced adults eventually remarry (Hanson & Boyd, 1996) contributing to the formation of more than 250,000 new stepfamilies each year (Ross & Cobb, 1990). Other terms used for stepfamilies include "blended," "remarried," or "reconstituted" families (Ballard, 1996; Grove, 1996; Ross & Cobb, 1990). The extended kin network of a stepfamily can include stepgrandparents, stepaunts, stepuncles, and stepcousins, as well as an ex-spouse who is the biological parent of some of the children, but no longer a part of the household. Closely similar is the *binuclear family,* which exists when a child is a member of two nuclear households as a result of a joint-custody arrangement following the divorce of the child's parents (Grove, 1996).

Cohabiting Families

A *cohabiting family* consists of a man and a woman living together without being married. Individuals who choose cohabitation range in age from teens to retired elderly persons. The reasons cited for preferring this arrangement include the desire for a "trial marriage," the increased safety of living with another, and financial necessity. Cohabitation is becoming more prevalent in the United States. The number of unmarried couples increased from nearly 2 million in 1985 to 3.3 million in 1992 (U.S. Department of Commerce, 1993).

Homosexual Families

The *homosexual family* is a form of cohabitation in which a couple of the same sex live together and share a sexual relationship. Homosexual couples constitute 2% of U.S. households (Hanson & Boyd, 1996). The homosexual family might include children and might resemble the traditional nuclear family in terms of the mutual support and sexual and economic interdependence of the couple involved. It may be difficult, however, for the homosexual family to stay together over time because of the lack of social sanction and support for their lifestyle (Janosik & Green, 1992).

Communal Families

A *communal family* is made up of several adults and children living together, usually because of a common religious or ideological bond or financial necessity. Communal families typically resemble traditional extended families in qualities of affection and interdependence, rituals, migration, and influence or control. Communal living can be more stressful than the typical nuclear family; this is because of crowding, more people and roles to deal with, and a general lack of privacy for couples and children to resolve differences. Communal families may exhibit monogamous or polygamous sexual relationships (Ross & Cobb, 1990).

Other family forms that are being seen with increasing regularity by community health nurses are foster families and skip-generation families (Hanson & Boyd, 1996). *Foster families* consist of at least one adult and one or more foster children placed by the court system. Foster families may also include the adults' own biological or adopted children. Foster family composition may change frequently and exemplifies what has been called a *permeable family structure* which encompasses many different kinship arrangements (Elkind, 1995). *Skip-generation families* are those in which grandparents are raising their grandchildren. Skip-generation families may occur because of working parents, drug or alcohol abuse, or child abandonment. Approximately 5% of U.S. children are being raised by grandparents (Hanson & Boyd, 1996). The family types presented here are summarized in Table 18–1.

TABLE 18–1. **TYPES OF FAMILIES AND THEIR CHARACTERISTICS FEATURES**

Family Type	Characteristic Features
Nuclear conjugal family	Mother and father who are married with one or more biological or adopted children
Extended family	Kin network of the adult male and female of a nuclear family (eg, grandparents, aunts, uncles, cousins)
Single-parent family	One adult male or female with biological or adopted children
Stepfamily	Reconstituted or blended family created by a second marriage in which one or both spouses have children from a previous marriage and possibly children of the new union
Binuclear family	A child (or children) who is part of two nuclear households as a result of divorce and joint custody
Cohabiting couple	A male and a female living together without marriage, with or without children
Homosexual family	A cohabiting couple of the same sex, with or without children
Communal family	Multiple adults and children in one household
Foster family	One or more adults and one or more court-designated foster children, with or without other biological or adopted children
Skip-generation family	One or both grandparents raising one or more grandchildren

Community health nurses may record information regarding family composition and relationships among family members in the form of genograms or ecomaps. A *genogram* is a diagram of a family tree incorporating information regarding family members and their relationships over at least three generations. Information that may be included in a genogram includes dates of births, deaths, marriages, separations, and divorces; health status; ethnicity; occupation or unemployment; retirement; and significant family problems such as trouble with the law, family violence, or incest (Hanson, 1996). A sample genogram is included in Figure 18–1.

By convention, certain symbols have certain meanings in a genogram. For example, females are represented by circles and males by squares. Squares and circles marked with an "X" indicate deceased family members. A double circle or square indicates the *index person* or identified client. The lines connecting persons in the diagram indicate the character of relationships between them. Broader lines indicate stronger relationships, broken lines reflect distant or tenuous ones, and cross-hatched lines indicate conflictual relationships (Roth, 1996).

An *ecomap* is a visual representation of relationships both within and outside of the family (Hanson, 1996). An ecomap can be used to depict the relationships of family members with each other and with outside forces such as health care providers, employers, and extended family members. The segment of the

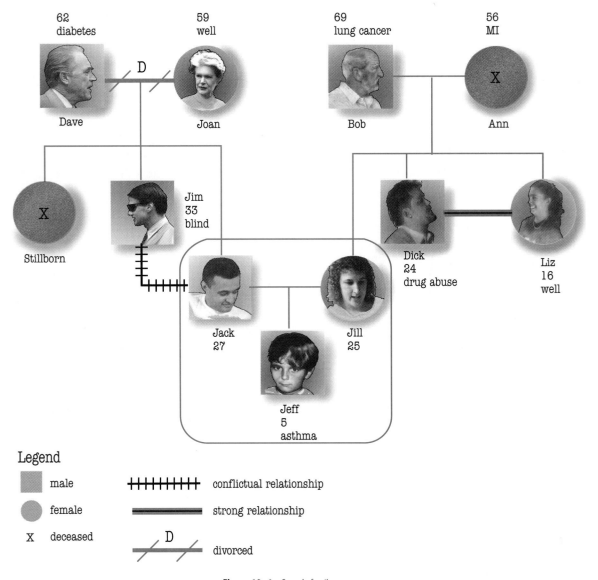

Figure 18–1. Sample family genogram.

genogram including the household of interest may be contained within the larger central circle of the ecomap. Outside forces are represented by smaller circles on the periphery. Again, relationships are represented by the types of lines connecting the circles in the diagram. Figure 18–2 presents a sample ecomap in which there are strong supportive relationships between the wife and the community health nurse and between the son and his teacher and conflictual relationships between the husband and his employer and between the family and the next door neighbor. There is also a tenuous relationship with the extended family.

Characteristics of Families

Despite the outward variations in family form, all families share certain characteristics. Every family is a social system that has its own cultural values, specific functions, and structure, and that moves through recognizable developmental stages.

Family as a Social System

The family is a basic social system. A *social system* is a group of people who share common characteristics and who are mutually dependent on one another. Be-

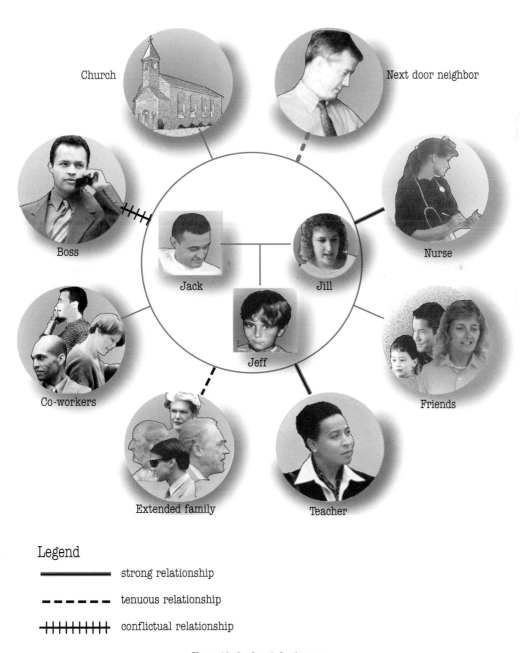

Legend

———————— strong relationship

- - - - - - tenuous relationship

+++++++++ conflictual relationship

Figure 18–2. Sample family ecomap.

cause of this mutual dependence, community health nurses work with the family unit, not just the individual. What affects one member affects the entire family and vice versa.

Families have certain features that differ from those of other social systems. First, families last longer than many other social groups. Second, families are intergenerational social systems with kin networks consisting of three or possibly even four generations. Third, family systems include both biological and *affinal* relationships. Affinal relationships are those created by law or interest. For example, marriage and adoption create legal relationships, while cohabitation and homosexual unions are created out of interest. Finally, the biological aspects of family relationships create links to a larger kin group that are not found in other social systems (Klein & White, 1996).

Family Cultural Values

A family's cultural values can greatly influence the way a family views health and the health care system (Friedman & Ferguson-Marshalleck, 1996). A family's culturally mediated values and behaviors can either facilitate or impede a community health nurse's efforts to promote health and prevent disease. This subject was explored in detail in Chapter 16.

Structure and Function

Family structure is the organized pattern or hierarchy of members that determines how family members interact. In other words, it is the way family members or subgroups are arranged to form a complete, interacting family unit. Components of a family's structure include the roles of each family member and how they complement each other and the family's value system, communication patterns, and power hierarchy. The power hierarchy typically places parents in charge of decision making for the family. A family's structure affects how a family functions.

Family functions are those activities a family performs to meet the needs of its members. Members must be fed, clothed, housed, and given emotional support and guidance. Children must be socialized to societal and family cultural values and expectations. Members need economic security and mutual support as they adapt to changes in the environment and within the family. Many of these traditional family functions have, in part, been delegated to other social institutions such as schools and churches or synagogues. Additional newer family functions have arisen including a relationship function of providing opportunities to love and be loved and a health function of meeting health care needs of family members (Hanson & Boyd, 1996). All families, regardless of type, have in common these basic needs that require the family to function in ways that ensure family survival over time.

Family Development

Movement through developmental stages is characteristic of all families, regardless of the type. As the family expands and contracts, new role behaviors and communication skills are needed to cope with developmental crises and change. It has been suggested that each family passes through eight developmental stages beginning with family formation and continuing to the dissolution of the family (Duvall & Miller, 1990). During each stage, which is demarcated by acquisition of members and by the age of the oldest child, the family has certain patterns of expected changes in family interactions that must be accomplished (Klein & White, 1996). Achievement of each change is necessary for successful movement through subsequent stages.

Single-parent, divorced, and reconstituted families experience developmental stages much like those of two-parent families. Single parents may not establish or maintain a marriage. Their family adjustments are limited to dealing with added roles, socializing the children, encouraging education and separation of children from the family constellation, providing a healthful environment, and adjusting to the independence and eventful departure of the children to form families of their own.

Single parenthood that is precipitated by divorce or the death of a partner causes a pile-up of stressor events that can lead to crisis for many families. The single parent must assume roles that were once fulfilled by the missing partner while continuing to perform his or her own roles.

Binuclear and stepfamilies, created by remarriage of single parents, also experience predictable life cycle stages (Danielson, Hamel-Bissell, & Winstead-Fry, 1993). Their experience, however, is much more complex. There are many more adjustments to be made because more people are involved in the transition. The central focus of family development is still the children, but at the same time the adults in the family are trying to adjust to each other. To sustain such families over a long period takes considerable compromise.

It is important to remember that, in addition to contributing to the accomplishment of the developmental tasks of the family unit, each family member is involved in accomplishing personal developmental tasks. These tasks can either parallel family tasks or conflict with them. The family must meet both individual and family developmental tasks to function as an effective unit. Thus, there may be conflict or stress when the accomplishment of a family task is in direct opposition to task achievement by the individual. The healthy family develops effective mechanisms for dealing with this type of conflict when it arises. Stages of individual and family development and the developmental tasks to be accomplished in each were presented in Chapter 6.

▶ THE DIMENSIONS MODEL AND CARE OF THE FAMILY

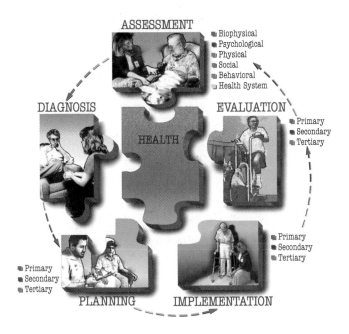

When working with families, the community health nurse's goal is to promote optimal health for each family member and for the family as a unit. The community health nurse can achieve this goal by using the Dimensions Model to facilitate care to family clients.

Critical Dimensions of Nursing in the Care of Families

In the early days of their practice, community health nurses saw families primarily as a source of care for sick members (Capuzzi, 1996). It was not long, however, before community health nurses began to see families as an important unit of service. In providing care to families as a unit, community health nurses employ many of the elements of the dimensions of nursing. In the cognitive dimension, the nurse must have knowledge of family dynamics and healthy family interaction. Knowledge related to specific problems encountered by families, and particularly of family crisis intervention strategies, will also be required. In the interpersonal dimension, the nurse must de-

velop a trusting relationship with the family, one that is nonjudgmental and accepting of family beliefs and values. Community health nurses working with families may discover that they require a high level of emotional investment on the part of the nurse as well as excellent communication and collaboration skills. In addition to using good communications skills themselves, community health nurses often need to teach and model effective communication with family members.

Interpersonal skills often interact with elements of the ethical dimension in the care of families. Nursing intervention with families may necessitate functioning as an advocate for the family unit or for individual family members. This is particularly true when family relationships include violence directed at one or more members. This responsibility for advocacy may create ethical dilemmas for the community health nurse when an abused family member does not wish legal action to be taken or when the nurse must weigh the benefits of removing an abused child from the home against the effects of disrupting the family system. The presence of violence in the family may make it difficult for the nurse to set aside personal attitudes and values and to work effectively with all family members, abuser and abused alike. A nonjudgmental attitude is particularly important in such cases and requires particular strength to sustain. The nurse may also need to deal with suspicion and hostility on the part of the abuser which will require even more interpersonal skill on the nurse's part.

In the skills dimension, the community health nurse working with families will engage in the intellectual skills of assessment and analysis of problems, diagnostic reasoning, and planning for intervention. Intervention may also require the use of manipulative skills to provide direct care to family members or to teach family members to care for each other. The nurse may employ the health education process to teach these skills as well as to provide other health education needed for the family to engage in healthful behavior. Other process dimension elements that may come into play in the care of families are the case management and home visit processes and the change and leadership processes. The case management process is particularly important in assisting families with multiple health and social problems. At the aggregate level, the political process may be needed to assure adequate social and health care support for families. Finally, in the reflective dimension, nursing research will provide the knowledge base for effective care of families as well as for the development of family theory as it relates to nursing practice. Evaluation, another aspect of the reflective dimension, is also important in assessing the care given to individual families as well as the effectiveness of health care programs designed to serve families.

Assessing Family Dimensions of Health

The Biophysical Dimension

When the community health nurse first encounters a family, assessment begins by gathering data to identify the physical needs of family members. It is important to note that the physical status of each family member should be weighed as part of the family assessment. The physical health status of each member affects how the family functions and how members relate to each other. For example, if a child has a chronic disease, the entire family must make adjustments to accommodate the youngster's special needs. The parents have to adjust their schedules to care for the child and ensure that the child is seen by appropriate health care providers. Siblings can assume household chores and provide some measure of care for their ill brother or sister. Other family members can assist with care and offer emotional support for the parents and children.

Knowledge of the sex, age, and race of family members, as well as information related to genetic inheritance, can guide the nurse in identifying problems and planning family care. For example, knowing that there are several young children in the home, the nurse may emphasize safety precautions when interacting with the family. An elderly family is more likely to have members with chronic, debilitating illnesses and may need closer scrutiny for evidence of these problems. The presence of older family members may contribute to *filial crises* in which they and their adult children are faced with acknowledging their mortality and accommodating role reversals. Multiple generations in the household may also result in the *sandwich generation* phenomenon in which younger adult members are caught between meeting the needs of their children and their aging parents (Richards, 1996). Or, a family's race may increase its members' risks for certain diseases such as sickle cell disease among African Americans and those of Eastern Mediterranean descent.

The Psychological Dimension

Communication Patterns. Communication patterns are an indicator of functioning in the psychological dimension. Both verbal and nonverbal modes of family communication should be considered, as should the listening ability of family members. How do members communicate values and ideas? When one family member talks, do others listen? Do they show anger or boredom while listening?

Mealtime is a good time to assess family interaction. It is here that the nurse can determine whether meals are a time of light conversation or heated argument, whether all family members eat together, and whether mealtimes contribute to family solidarity.

It is also important to assess the content of communications. Are they superficial or does the family engage in values clarification discussions? The type of statements made or questions asked tell the nurse a great deal about family interactions. For example "You are wrong about that" and "Tell me more about your feelings" indicate different attitudes about interactions among family members. The latter, open-ended response facilitates communication, whereas the previous accusatory statement impedes it.

The feeling tone expressed in communication is another indicator of the psychological environment. Family communications may be "incendiary," contributing to interpersonal difficulties, or "affirming," facilitating cohesion and problem resolution (McCubbin & Van Riper, 1996). Sarcastic and resentful statements could block further communication between family members. For example, "When are you ever going to use your head?" does not facilitate communication. Other types of one-way communication include repeated complaints, manipulation through covert requests, insulting remarks, lack of validation, and inability to focus on one issue (Friedman, 1998).

The nurse should ascertain what areas of communication are taboo (off limits) for family members. Typical areas include feelings, sexual issues, and religion. If certain topics are found to be taboo, the nurse may need to alter his or her approach to data gathering. For example, if one of the areas closed to discussion involves feelings, the nurse might try engaging in self-disclosure, thus acting as a role model. Another way to alter the approach is to gather data by examining areas related to the taboo issue. This may also help the nurse to identify the reason for resistance to communication about a specific area.

Communication patterns can influence the effectiveness of parenting, particularly in the area of discipline. Praise enhances the development of self-worth in the child, whereas negative or condescending communications restrict its development. More about communications and child discipline can be found in Chapter 20.

The nurse should be aware of several dysfunctional communication patterns that may be employed within families. For instance, messages may be passed from one family member to another in a chainlike fashion that does not allow for reciprocal discussion.

Or, communication may isolate a family member, as when the mother and children exclude the father from their discussions. Another problematic pattern is the wheel in which a central person directs what communication will be passed between family members. By way of comparison, a successful pattern of communication is the "switchboard" in which there is reciprocal communication among all family members. Figure 18–3 illustrates these patterns of communication.

A final consideration is the degree of communication between the family and the suprasystem. Is the family open to new ideas and opinions from people outside the family? Are outsiders invited to participate in family discussions or are they expected to "mind their own business"?

Family Developmental Stages. As noted in Chapter 6, each family passes through developmental stages that have specific developmental tasks for the family to attain. The community health nurse should assess each family to determine the developmental stage the family is currently experiencing and whether or not developmental tasks of that and previous stages have been accomplished. For example, the Da Costa family is expecting the arrival of their second child. Their first child is 4 years old and has begun preschool this fall. The family developmental stage is that of the preschool family (stage III) and the tasks to be accomplished are (1) to integrate the second child into the family; (2) to separate from the oldest child to a greater degree as he or she goes off to school; and (3) to socialize the children. The degree to which the Da Costas have achieved the tasks

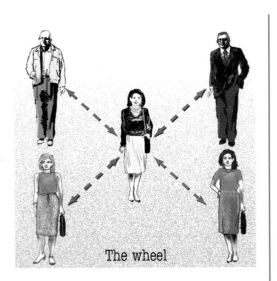

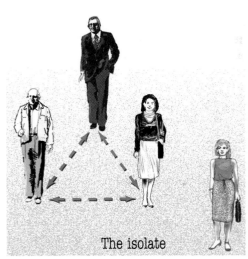

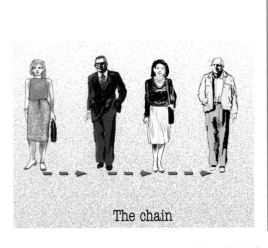

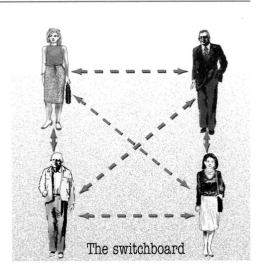

Figure 18–3. Family communication patterns.

of the beginning family (stage I) and early childbearing (stage II) will affect their ability to meet the tasks of stage III. For example, if the couple had been unable to establish a satisfying marriage, a task of stage I, the second pregnancy may cause stress that will lead to the dissolution of the marriage.

Assessing the family's developmental stage assists the community health nurse to provide anticipatory guidance that helps the family incorporate new members, adjust to the addition, and avert maturational crisis. Family maturational crisis is addressed in some detail later in this chapter.

Family Relationships and Family Dynamics. Family relationships and family dynamics are areas of concern in the community health nurse's assessment of the family's psychological environment. *Family relationships* are those bonds between family members that create identifiable patterns, such as subgroups and isolated members. *Family dynamics* describes the hierarchical patterns within the family. Power and leadership are the central focus for this area of assessment.

How does one assess relationships within the family? Initially, information regarding subgroups is compiled. For example, the nurse may notice that a mother–daughter subgroup has excluded the father from the decision-making process.

Communication within and between subgroups is then assessed in terms of both content (what is said) and process (who says it and how it is said). This is followed by identification of the relationship as supportive or close, demanding, maternal, and so on. Subgroups are described in terms of how they relate. For example, one may describe the sibling group as one that shares feelings and actions, or they may be described as alienated from each other.

Family dynamics is assessed by observing family leadership patterns. Who are the primary decision makers? Who controls conversations? Is there a leader in the family? What leadership style does the leader employ? (See Chapter 12 for a discussion of leadership styles.) Do family members respect the leader? Do they respect each other? Respect requires that children view parents as individuals as well as parents. Likewise, parents need to learn to respect their children as individuals.

Family Emotional Strengths. A family's emotional strengths become evident as the nurse observes interactions and communicates with family members over time. The nurse should look for evidence of family cohesion and the degree of sensitivity to others displayed by each family member. For example, the nurse might observe whether a mother anticipates the child's needs or whether there is a general feeling of warmth and car-

ing. The nurse should also estimate the degree to which family members support and praise each other. The results of these observations help the nurse to estimate how well the family is meeting the emotional and psychological needs of its members.

A positive self-image on the part of a family member is the result of daily family interactions that bolster the individual's feelings of self-worth. A child who is criticized too often may develop a poor self-image. The nurse can assess the self-esteem of each family member by observing nonverbal behavior as well as their communication patterns with others.

Coping Strategies. Identifying a family's coping strategies and defense mechanisms enables the nurse to assist families to deal realistically with stress and crisis. *Coping strategies* are behaviors that help a family to adapt to stress or change and are characterized by positive problem-solving methods that prevent or resolve crisis situations. Coping involves specific actions taken to manage demands on the family and to bring resources to bear on family problems (McCubbin & McCubbin, 1993). Coping strategies may be internal or external (Friedman & Ferguson-Marshalleck, 1996). Internal coping strategies rely on resources contained within the family. Role flexibility, joint problem solving, and controlling the meaning of stressful conditions are examples of internal strategies. In external strategies, the family links to outside resources to enhance their ability to meet demands. Examples of external coping strategies are seeking information, maintaining community linkages, and seeking spiritual or social support.

Defense mechanisms are tactics for avoiding recognition of problems. They may be used when the family cannot immediately determine how to solve a problem. Defense mechanisms are not considered problematic unless they interfere with coping and may actually be helpful in allowing time to marshal resources before facing a problem. Examples of defense mechanisms include denial, rationalization, selective inattention, isolation, intellectualization, and projection.

The use of coping strategies or defense mechanisms is seen most often when the family is faced with change. The community health nurse can assess how the family deals with change by observing behavior during life change events or by obtaining information on how the family has dealt with a major move, job change, or loss of a family member in the past. Working with a family in crisis is discussed more fully later in this chapter.

Child-rearing and Discipline Practices. Another consideration is assessing the psychological dimension of family

► COMMONLY USED DEFENSE MECHANISMS

Denial
　Ignoring threat-provoking aspects of a situation or changing the meaning of the situation to make it less threatening

Rationalization
　Giving a "good" or rational excuse, but not the real reason for responding to a situation with a particular behavior

Selective Inattention
　Attending to only those aspects of the situation that do not cause distress or pain

Isolation
　Separating emotion from content in a situation so one can deal objectively with otherwise threatening or emotionally overwhelming conditions

Intellectualization
　Focusing on abstract, technical, or logical aspects of a threatening situation to insulate oneself from painful emotions generated

Projection
　Attributing one's own motivation to other people

health is that of child-rearing and discipline practices. Such practices have the potential either for causing psychological problems among family members or for strengthening a sense of right and wrong in each child.

The nurse should determine the type of discipline used, who administers it, and behavior that elicits disciplinary action. The nurse should also determine whether parents and other adults in the family support each other's decisions in matters of discipline. For example, if the child is punished by the mother, does the child attempt to avoid punishment by manipulating the father? If so, are the adults able to discuss and support a joint decision? Ultimately, parents need to teach self-discipline, so it is important to assess whether they provide adequate role models for the child. For a more detailed discussion of discipline, see Chapter 20.

Family Goals.　Family goals are an element of the psychological environment that may be difficult to assess because families often are not consciously aware of them. The nurse, however, can be aware of and observe for evidence of family goals; these include producing children and ensuring their survival, ex-changing love and affective support, and providing economic survival or affluence.

Family goals are a function of family values and reflect a family's cultural background. Family goals also vary with a family's developmental stage, economic status, and physical health of family members. Problems arise when there is disagreement on family goals. For example, the O'Reilly family worked hard to send their son to college (a family goal). Before his sophomore year, the son refused to return to school, preferring instead to work as a plumber's apprentice.

The Physical Dimension

The community health nurse's observational and interpretive skills are especially needed to assess the home environment. Within this setting, the family develops either functional or dysfunctional relationships. A chaotic, crowded, unsanitary, or unsafe home can contribute to physical and psychological health problems among family members.

To begin the assessment it is important to describe the home and its condition. Information such as the address, whether the family owns or rents the home, whether the home is big enough for the family, the presence of safety hazards, and family plans for fire or other disasters are all pertinent to the nurse's plan of care for the family. The nurse should consider several potential hazards in assessing a family's physical environment:

- Absence of fire alarms in the home
- Peeling paint (especially lead-based paint in older homes)
- Broken furniture
- Loose throw rugs
- Broken stair railings (inside or outside the home)
- Broken stairs
- Broken porch floor boards or railings
- Hazardous materials within children's reach
- Plumbing that does not allow for sanitary disposal of human wastes
- Toys in walkways
- Overcrowding
- Lack of a fire plan
- Lack of an earthquake, tornado, or other disaster plan
- Lack of a poison control plan (posted telephone numbers)
- Numerous house pets such as cats, chickens, or dogs
- Close proximity to a heavily traveled highway
- Lack of a fenced-in yard for small children

For example, note the following concise description of a home environment:

> Mrs. Turner, age 35, lives with her husband and 6 children in a run-down, single-family home. The home, consisting of 8 rooms (3 bedrooms), is well furnished and adequately heated. Health and safety hazards are presented by broken stairs and railings to the upstairs, peeling paint, and the lack of running water for the last 2 days. The owner has been notified of these conditions.

Information about the neighborhood should also be obtained. Physical characteristics include the types of homes in the area, degree of industrialization, crime rate, and level of sanitation. Other important considerations include population density, common occupations of neighbors, availability of transportation, shopping facilities, health services, churches, schools, and recreational facilities. Each of these areas is assessed in relation to the specific needs of individual family members and of the family as a whole.

The community health nurse should note if there are any air, water, or noise pollution problems in the area that would increase the family's risks of disability and illness. It is important to determine what the sources of pollution are and the effects of pollution on the family.

After making this assessment, the community health nurse may want to question family members about perceptions of their environment. Does the family feel safe in this neighborhood? What are the hazards they perceive? Do they have an emergency plan if their safety should be jeopardized? Is the family aware of any existing pollutants in their neighborhood?

The Social Dimension

The social dimension of family health shares some of the influences of the psychological environment. For instance, relationships outside the family are the basis for a portion of personality development. Leadership ability of individual family members is developed in school and in cultural, social, and political organizations where family members have the opportunity to interact with others and to contribute to community endeavors. Family discussions of social, cultural, and political issues help to develop social awareness as children grow and encourage the children to become involved in community, county, state, and national politics or social movements. Areas for consideration in assessing the family's social dimension include family members' roles, religion, culture, social class and economic status, employment and occupational factors, and external resources.

▶ INFORMAL FAMILY ROLES

Encourager
Praises others and is able to draw others out and make them feel that their ideas are important

Harmonizer
Mediates differences by use of humor and smoothing over

Blocker
Tends to be negative to all ideas

Follower
Passively goes along with the group

Martyr
Wants nothing for self but sacrifices for the sake of others

Scapegoat
Identified problem member, serves as a safety valve, relieving family tensions

Pioneer
Moves the family into unknown territory and new experiences

Go-between
Transmits and monitors communications among family members (often the mother)

Blamer
Fault finder and dictator

Roles.   One of the most interesting aspects of the social dimension is role enactment within families. *Roles* are socially expected behavior patterns that are determined by a person's position or status within a family. Each person in a family occupies several roles by virtue of his or her position. For example, the adult woman in a family typically has the roles of wife, mother, cook, and confidante. Roles can take two forms: formal and informal. *Formal roles* are expected sets of behaviors associated with family positions such as husband, wife, mother, father, and child. Examples of formal roles are those of breadwinner, homemaker, house repairman, chauffeur, child caretaker, financial manager, and cook. *Informal roles* are those expected behaviors not associated with a particular position. Informal roles influence the social dimension within the family by determining whether, how, and by whom emotional needs are met. Informal roles that may be present within any family group include the encourager, the harmonizer, the follower, the martyr, the scapegoat, the pioneer, the go-between, and the blamer. The nurse identifies the presence or absence of these and similar informal roles and examines their effects on family function and cohesiveness.

Next, the nurse may want to assess for evidence of role conflict. *Role conflict* occurs when the demands of a single role are contradictory or when the demands attending several roles contradict or compete with each other (Anderson, 1996). For example, a mother who works will experience role conflict when a business meeting she is expected to attend conflicts with her child's school play. Role conflict can also occur when one individual's definition of a role does not correspond with someone else's definition of the same role (Janosik & Green, 1992). For example, a husband may expect his wife to be responsible for all the cooking for the family, but the wife may work late and expect the husband to prepare an evening meal.

Role overload is another phenomenon that occurs in families when members assume multiple roles. *Role overload* occurs when an individual is confronted with too many role expectations at one time, even though these expectations do not contradict each other (Ballard, 1996). For example, a mother with four children who returns to school and also has a part-time job may experience role overload in trying to meet the demands of housekeeping, cooking family meals, performing well on the job, and making straight A's.

Flexibility of family roles and mutual respect for individuality are also considered in the assessment of the social dimension of family health. Family roles often change when a family member is absent, ill, or incapacitated and cannot fulfill his or her usual roles. It is important to assess the ability of family members to take on these unfilled roles and make the necessary role adjustments. When the ill or absent member is ready to resume roles, a readjustment may again be necessary. For example, when Frank had his heart attack, Beth had to go to work and assume the breadwinner role. Now Frank is recovered and can return to work. Beth likes her job and does not want to quit. Assistance in adjusting to changes in roles can alleviate conflict and stress in this and in similar situations.

Role adjustments may also be required as the family progresses through its various developmental stages. For example, the parental role should be enacted differently with an adolescent child than with a preschooler. The nurse can assess the family's ability to adjust roles to the changing needs of its members and can also provide anticipatory guidance about adjustments that will be needed.

Religion. The influence of religious beliefs and practices on the health of the family can be assessed by asking specific questions about the importance of religion in family interactions and decision making and the role of religion for the family as a whole. For example, strong religious beliefs may prohibit the use of contraceptives, or health teaching may need to be modified in keeping with the family's religious convictions. Close affiliation with an organized church may also provide a source of emotional and/or material support for family members in time of need.

Culture. Family cultural information is an invaluable aid in building relationships and designing family interventions that will not conflict with cultural values. Does the family engage in cultural practices related to health? If so, are these practices helpful or harmful? What cultural factors will affect attempts to resolve family health problems? The nurse can compare the family's culture with that of the community in which they live and determine if there are differences present that may create problems for the family or the children of the family. Principles of cultural assessment, discussed in Chapter 16, are applicable to assessment of the social dimension of families.

Social Class and Economic Status. Social class delineations involve cultural groupings of people based on financial status, race, occupation, education, lifestyle, and language. In America, the lower social class consists of people with less money, less education, and less access to resources such as health care.

The family's social class is important to the extent that it affects lifestyle, interactions with the external environment, and the structural and functional characteristics of the family. Economic status is closely tied to social class and education level. For instance, many single parents are members of lower socioeconomic groups, and most single-parent households are poor. For example, children of single mothers are four times more likely than other children to be poor (Allen, 1994). In 1994, 44% of female-headed households had incomes below the poverty level (U.S. Department of Health and Human Services, 1996). The single female parent in many of these families either works outside the home or accepts welfare for economic support of her family. Often the jobs available to such women are minimum-wage, menial jobs that allow some flexibility so they can care for their children. The single female parent often has no other adult to share in family decision making and must call on her children to carry out functions within the family that might have been her own if a male parent were present.

The social class and economic status of a family can profoundly affect its health. Lack of financial resources can mean that the family does not have enough nutritious food, adequate shelter, or access to health care. The community health nurse can assess the family's social class and economic status and begin to make plans to assist the family through referral to community resources that will increase their access to food, better shelter, and health care.

Employment or Occupational Factors.   Job-related factors that influence family health may present in three forms. First, the job might produce stress for the adult that results in illness. Second, the adult might be exposed to hazards that he or she brings home to other family members. Third, job-related problems and time constraints might interfere with family commitments.

Occupational or workplace stress can lead to a number of stress-related illnesses. Safety hazards within the work setting may cause injury and disability to the family breadwinner(s). The financial burden and stress an occupation-related illness can cause have led to divorce and the dissolution of families, among other problems.

Sometimes substances to which a working parent is exposed not only threaten the parent, but may also inadvertently be brought home to other family members. For example, nurses and other health care workers need to be aware that some infectious diseases may be transmitted to young children via clothing and shoes. Working with lead or other hazardous substances may also result in exposure of family members through contaminated clothing and other articles worn on the job.

Job-related family problems also might arise if a family member's work commitment conflicts with family commitments. For example, Dad may have to work late on the night the family was to attend a play, or a new job may interfere with family vacation plans. The nurse can assist family members to establish priorities and to plan quality time together.

External Resources.   To assist families in dealing with social environmental stressors, the community health nurse needs to identify external resources available to the family. External resources include those materials or sources of assistance available to the family from the community. The nurse's assessment of the family's external resources may suggest ways of dealing with identified health problems. Questions that elicit this information are those related to neighborhood sources of financial assistance, transportation, housing, health care, and education. The nurse should also investigate relational support systems such as kin networks, friends, and neighbors. Usually each community has service agencies that can assist families in need.

The Behavioral Dimension

The fifth component in the assessment phase of the Dimensions Model is family behavior. Areas of focus here include family consumption patterns, rest and sleep patterns, and exercise and leisure activities.

Family Consumption Patterns.   A family's nutritional status can be assessed through physical assessment of each member and by observing the way in which the family selects, purchases, and prepares food. If any family members are nutritionally impaired, the nurse will need to determine the underlying causes. Is it lack of money to buy food? Does the person who prepares food lack information that would ensure good family nutrition? How is food prepared? Are cultural patterns evident in food selection, preparation, and consumption? For example, the excessive use of fried or high-fat foods sometimes seen among Latinos or families in the southern United States contributes to the increased incidence of atherosclerosis, heart disease, and stroke among members of these populations.

Other consumption patterns of interest to the nurse include the use of alcohol, drugs, medications, tobacco, and caffeine. Is the use of any of these substances causing a family member to be unable to carry out his or her role and functions within the family? Does the mother's smoking, for instance, aggravate a child's respiratory condition? Are prescription drugs being used as prescribed? Are any side effects evident from the use of prescription drugs? Are over-the-counter (OTC) products used appropriately? The answers to these and similar questions assist the nurse to identify problems arising from family consumption patterns.

Rest and Sleep.   Family rest and sleep patterns may be a source of problems. For example, a new baby may sleep during the day and cry at night. This will adversely affect parents' rest and their subsequent performance the next day.

Another problem frequently encountered with respect to family sleep patterns is that of differing work schedules. If, for example, one parent works days and the other works nights, this situation may limit their opportunities to interact with each other and with their children. A parent's typical rest and sleep schedule may also require children to play at a neighbor's house during the day or find quiet pastimes at home. The nurse can assist the family in making decisions about how to deal with these and similar problems.

Exercise and Leisure. Regular exercise is necessary for good health. The earlier children are included in activities, the more likely they are to build lifetime habits of exercise. Exercise and leisure activities that include the entire family promote cohesion. Assessment in this area includes consideration of the type and frequency of exercise engaged in by family members. At times it is also helpful to plan leisure activities that are unique to certain members of the family. This allows for individuality among family members and promotes a balance between family togetherness and separateness that is needed for individual development. The nurse should explore whether there are exercise or leisure activities that include only the adults or only the children.

The nurse can also help the family to identify potential health risks involved in leisure activities. For example, are safety helmets worn by all family members on bike trips? What are the safety rules when the family goes swimming? Is a backyard pool fenced in and covered when not in use to prevent a child from going in alone or falling in accidentally?

High costs and low income may limit the activities that families can do together, but should not eliminate them. The nurse can help the family plan low-cost activities that enhance family cohesion. For example, the family could take part in a picnic in the park followed by a game of ball or horseshoes.

Household and Other Safety Practices. Safety practices such as use of seat belts, infant safety seats, cribs with safe spacing between rails and proper mattress width, proper disposal of hazardous substances, and safety education for children are important considerations in family assessment. Are these behavioral safety factors evident in the household? Who is the person most attentive to family safety issues? What family behaviors contribute to health risks for members? In assessing the behavioral dimension of family health, several safety practices should be considered:

- Consistent seat belt use
- Use of safety equipment such as eye and ear protection
- Use of infant safety seats
- Cribs with safe spacing between rails and proper mattress width
- Proper disposal of hazardous substances
- Safety education of children regarding not talking to or going with strangers, crossing the street safely, and using seat belts and safety equipment such as helmets, goggles, and ear protection
- Safe use of appliances and craft equipment such as saws, glues, and drills

The Health System Dimension

Family Response to Illness. Assessing the biophysical, psychological, physical, social, and behavioral dimensions of health within the family should give the nurse a general idea of the health of the family and of the strategies family members use to remain healthy. But how do family members deal with illness? Part of learning about this aspect of family life is determining who in the family decides when an ill family member should stay home from work or school and whether an ill member should receive health care. For example, in some families the mother decides who is ill and consults the father when she believes that the illness is severe enough to require the services of a health care provider.

In some families, folk remedies or cultural health practices are used before consulting a health care provider. The community health nurse needs to assess whether these practices are harmful to the sick family member and whether to encourage the family to seek professional assistance. Chapter 16 provides more information on how the nurse can determine which cultural health practices may be harmful and how to help the family member choose other modes of care.

Use of Health Care Services. Accessibility, availability, and use of health care services by family members need to be assessed by the nurse. The community health nurse should explore how the family deals with health problems. Family functions with respect to illness vary with the type of illness. For example, family functions in the case of acute illness include providing or obtaining health care, reassigning roles, and supporting the sick person. Additional functions in dealing with chronic illness include avoiding or coping with medical crises, preserving the family's quality of life, and arranging treatment modes and mechanisms. In the face of terminal illness, family functions also include dealing with shock and fear and minimizing pain and discomfort (Janosik & Green, 1992).

Do family members have a source of health care? Often there may be providers available for the mother and children because of federal and state programs. The father and other young adults, however, are often excluded from these programs. The nurse may be asked to help the family find health care for excluded family members who become ill.

It is important to learn where family members go for health care and whether their choice provides any preventive health services or dental care. Many private medical doctors provide only sickness care,

ASSESSMENT TIPS: Assessing the Family Client

Biophysical Dimension

Age

What are the ages of family members?

What is the developmental level of each family member?

Have family members successfully completed age-appropriate development tasks?

Do individual family members' developmental stages create stress in the family?

How knowledgeable are family members about normal development in individuals?

Genetic Inheritance

Is there a family history of genetic predisposition to disease? If so, to what diseases?

Physiologic Function

Do any family members have existing physical health problems? If so, what are they?

What are the effects of existing physical health problems on the family?

Is any member of the family pregnant? If so, what is the family's response to the pregnancy?

Psychological Dimension

Communication Patterns

What are the typical modes of communication in the family?

Does family communication address values?

What is the feeling tone of typical family communications?

What are the purposes of communication in the family (eg, give direction, provide support)?

What areas are taboo in family communication?

Is communication a two-way process?

Do family members engage in dysfunctional communication patterns? If so, what are they?

What is the extent and quality of communication between the family and the outside world?

Family Development

What is the family's stage of development?

Has the family adequately completed the tasks of prior stages of development?

Is the family achieving the tasks of the present developmental stage?

Family Relationships and Dynamics

How cohesive is the family? Do family members exhibit close supportive relationships?

How are decisions made in the family? By whom? Which family members have input into decisions?

Who is responsible for carrying out family decisions?

Who is the leader in the family? What leadership style does the leader use? Is it appropriate to the age and abilities of other family members?

Do family members express respect for each other?

Is there evidence of violence within the family?

Emotional Strengths and Coping Abilities

What emotional strengths does the family exhibit?

How does the family deal with change?

What coping strategies does the family use? How effective are these strategies?

How well does the family deal with crisis?

Child Rearing and Discipline

Who in the family is responsible for socialization of children?

What forms of discipline are used in the family? Is the discipline used appropriate?

Are expectations of family members realistic?

Family Goals

What are the family's goals?

Do individual goals conflict or complement family goals?

What values are reflected in the family's goals?

Physical Dimension

Where does the family live (eg, house, apartment, shelter)?

What is the physical condition of the home? Is it in good repair?

Are there physical hazards in the home (eg, peeling paint, broken stairs)?

How are hazardous items (eg, paint, medications, knives) stored?

Is plumbing adequate?

Is the amount of space available adequate for the number of persons in the family?

Are safety features in the home appropriate to the ages and development of family members?

Does the family have an emergency plan (eg, fire evacuation)?

Are there environmental hazards in the neighborhood? If so, what are they?

How safe is the neighborhood?

Does the family have access to necessary goods and services (eg, grocery stores)?

ASSESSMENT TIPS: Assessing the Family Client (cont.)

Social Dimension

Family Structure

What is the family structure (eg, nuclear, extended)
Who lives in the home?
What is their relationship to each other?

Roles

What formal and informal roles are typically performed by each family member?
How flexible and interchangeable are these roles?
How congruent are family roles with those of the dominant culture?
Is there evidence of role conflict in the family? If so, what form does that conflict take?
Do family members exhibit role overload?
How adequate were family role models?
Are essential family roles being adequately performed? If not, why not?
How are family roles assigned? Is role assignment appropriate? Do assigned roles meet family members' needs?
Are there expected changes in family roles (eg, with the advent of a new baby)? How will the family adapt to these changes?

Religion

Do family members have any particular religious affiliation? If so, what is it?
How important is religion to the family?
What influence, if any, do religious beliefs and practices have on family health?
Is there a religious group that serves as a social support for the family?

Culture

What language(s) do family members speak? Does language pose a barrier to health care services?
Does the family engage in cultural practices related to health? If so, what are these practices?
Are cultural health practices helpful or harmful?
How congruent is the family's culture with that of the dominant society? Does lack of congruence create problems for the family?

Social Class and Economic Status

What is the family's socioeconomic status?
What is the family's income? Is income sufficient to meet the family's needs?
How effectively does the family budget their income?

Employment and Occupation

Are family members employed?
What are the occupations of family members?
Do family members' occupations pose any health hazards for themselves or for other family members?
Do occupational roles conflict with family roles? If so, how? What is the effect of this conflict?

Behavioral Dimension

Dietary Patterns

What are the usual food preferences and consumption patterns of the family?
How are foods usually prepared? Who prepares food for the family?

Other Consumption Patterns

Do family members smoke? What precautions, if any, are taken to avoid exposing other family members to second-hand smoke?
Do family members use alcohol? If so, what is the extent of alcohol consumption?
What medications are used by family members? Is medication use appropriate? Are medications stored safely?
Is there evidence of substance abuse by family members? If so, what is the effect on the family?

Rest, Exercise, and Leisure

Do family members get adequate rest?
Are family sleeping arrangements appropriate to family members' needs?
What are the family's usual sleep patterns?
What is the extent of family members' exercise? Is it adequate to maintain health?
What kinds of leisure activities do family members engage in? Do leisure activities pose any health hazards?

Other Health-related Behaviors

Do family members use appropriate safety precautions (eg, seat belts, childproof cabinet latches)?
Who in the family engages in sexual activity? Is there a need for contraceptives?
What is the attitude of family members to sexual activity? Are these attitudes appropriate to family members' ages and developmental levels?
What is the level of sexual satisfaction of adult family members?

(continued)

ASSESSMENT TIPS: Assessing the Family Client (cont.)

Health System Dimension

How do family members deal with illness?

Who makes health-related decisions in the family? Who carries out those decisions?

To what extent do family members engage in health promotion?

Who in the family is responsible for care of the sick?

Do family members engage in any folk health practices or use home remedies? If so, what?

What is the family's usual source of health care?

Is the family's use of health care services appropriate?

Does the family have health insurance? If so, are all family members covered? What services are covered?

---

and the family needs information about where to go for preventive services such as immunizations, health teaching, and dental care.

Health care may be limited because of a lack of funds, language barriers, distance of the health care facility from the family and transportation limitations, and many other problems. The nurse needs to determine these deterrents to access and find resources within the community to help the family obtain health care.

Occasionally, even when a family has health insurance, members are not able to take full advantage of this resource because they do not understand what services are covered (or not covered). The nurse can help them understand their insurance benefits or refer the family to resources in the community who can explain insurance benefits and how to use them.

Appendix H is a tool to assist in gathering family assessment data.

 Diagnostic Reasoning and the Family as Client

The data obtained during the assessment phase of the Dimensions Model enable the nurse to make informed decisions about how to intervene with families who need assistance. The best way to demonstrate how diagnostic reasoning progresses using the model is to present an example. The accompanying case study serves as the basis for discussion of the use of the Dimensions Model with a family. Diagnostic reasoning, and planning, implementing, and evaluating health care for the Smith family are discussed in the following sections. Refer to the Family Nursing Case Study on page 409.

Mrs. Smith is pregnant and has hypertension. These are physical conditions that affect her ability

to fulfill her roles as wife and mother. Mrs. Jones, the community health nurse, must assist Mr. and Mrs. Smith to choose health care services that provide affordable care. The question of affordability depends on whether the couple have health insurance. If they do not, Mrs. Jones can help them apply for assistance.

The psychological dimension within the family is strained because of impaired communication between Mr. and Mrs. Smith and because of frequent quarrels between Mr. Smith and his son, Brian. Communication in the family may not have been effective before the pregnancy or may have deteriorated because of the unplanned pregnancy. Further evaluation of the communication pattern between father and son is needed to determine the best mode of intervention.

There is also a behavioral risk factor evident in Mr. Smith's employment pattern. Holding down two jobs over an extended period can cause extreme fatigue and stress. Fatigue and tension can contribute to decreased safety precautions and increased risk of accidents. In addition, Mr. Smith is increasing his risk for stress-related illnesses such as hypertension. The following sample nursing diagnoses for the Smith family are based on the data contained in the case:

1. Need for changes in family nutritional patterns due to mother's pregnancy and hypertension
2. Increased stress and anxiety due to poor communication patterns and frequent arguments
3. Inability to meet financial demands due to forthcoming birth of fourth child
4. Need for contraception to prevent subsequent pregnancies
5. Need for changes in family roles to accommodate addition of another family member

FAMILY NURSING CASE STUDY

Arlene Jones, RN, a community health nurse, has been visiting the Smith family for a month. Mrs. Smith, age 30, is pregnant with her fourth child. The other children are ages 12, 10, and 6. This pregnancy was unplanned.

Mrs. Smith has been quite depressed and experiences frequent episodes of crying. She also has hypertension. Mrs. Smith has talked with the nurse about difficulties she is having with her husband and 12-year-old son, Brian. Mr. Smith is seldom home because he needs to hold two jobs to meet the family's financial needs. When he is home, his presence is characterized by frequent arguments with Brian. Brian is experiencing problems at school and is often truant. Mrs. Smith thinks her son's problems are due to his strained relationship with his father.

Mr. Smith has expressed concern about being able to provide for a fourth child. Perhaps for this reason, his relationship with his wife has deteriorated and there is little communication between them. Mrs. Smith is close to her neighbors and active in her church.

  ## Planning and Implementing Health Care for the Family

From the nursing diagnoses and the assessment database, Mrs. Jones can compile a health status summary for the Smith family. Together, Mrs. Jones and the Smith family can give priority to identified health care needs. Collaboration with the family is important. Without an agreement or contract with the family dealing with the needs most important to them, members may not enter into any of the planned interventions that involve their active participation.

The health status summary for the Smith family might include the following needs and concerns:

1. Income inadequate to meet needs
2. Ineffective communication among family members
3. Anticipated role changes with the birth of a fourth child
4. Mrs. Smith's depression and hypertension
5. School truancy by the 12-year-old son
6. Mr. Smith's potential for stress-related accidents or diseases

Nursing interventions that may take place at primary, secondary, or tertiary levels of prevention must be designed for each health care need. Goals and objectives for each need should be stated in measurable terms. The objectives should also state a date for attainment of expected outcomes. For example, Mrs. Jones has made a diagnosis related to the ineffective communication between husband and wife. The goal of intervention is to facilitate open communication and strengthen the marital bond. One objective that may promote goal achievement might be: "The Smiths will plan a weekend together without the children within the next month."

There may be several alternative solutions for each of the Smith family's identified problems. In an attempt to choose the most appropriate course of action, Mrs. Jones would discuss these alternatives with the Smiths. Together, they would evaluate the advantages and disadvantages of each alternative and select the most appropriate solution to each problem.

Not all of Mrs. Jones's goals need to be shared with the Smiths. It is appropriate for some goals to remain in the mind of the nurse (Wright & Leahy, 1993). For example, Mrs. Jones may feel that Mr. Smith is using an authoritarian approach with his son that is blocking communication between the two. She would not share the goal of changing Mr. Smith's approach because doing so might destroy the trust she has developed with the Smiths. Instead, she will work with the family to establish a communication pattern that is supportive of each member's needs, thereby changing the father's approach to his son without labeling the interaction "authoritarian."

Primary Prevention

Planning primary preventive strategies for the Smith family requires that the nurse consider the data in the assessment. For example, based on the fact that the Smiths will soon be having their fourth child, the nurse can help them plan ahead for immunizations and other well-child services for the new baby.

The psychological environmental assessment revealed that the Smiths are in stage IV of family development, the family with school-age children. As they are also expecting a new baby, one of the tasks of stage III will need to be repeated. The developmental tasks with which the Smiths may need assistance include integrating a fourth child into the family, fostering education and socialization of the school-age children, and maintaining the marriage. For the Smiths, the community health nurse focuses on anticipated role changes for each family member that will occur with the arrival of the new baby. For example, she will plan to discuss with Mr. and Mrs. Smith such topics as who will get up with the baby at night, who will assist with household tasks, and the possibility of sibling rivalry.

Anticipatory guidance to develop new communication channels will be important to avert developmental crises as the son Brian enters adolescence. Allowing Brian to accept more responsibility and to have more freedom, while maintaining discipline, will set the pattern for the way his brothers and sisters will progress through adolescence.

Referrals for financial assistance (depending on the family's eligibility) may decrease some of Mr. Smith's burden as sole breadwinner. Relieving the stress he is experiencing may prevent development of stress-related health problems.

Secondary Prevention

Secondary prevention is employed when Mrs. Jones plans meetings to give family members opportunities for mediated communication that will assist them to become more supportive of each other. With increased and enhanced communications, the family's power structure can be more equally divided and the changes in roles that will occur with the new baby can be planned.

With the resolution of the spousal communication problem and economic assistance, Mrs. Jones can look for a decrease in Mrs. Smith's depression. When this has occurred, Mrs. Jones will initiate dietary teaching related to Mrs. Smith's hypertension, an important secondary preventive measure.

Intervention to resolve the conflict within the father–son subsystem cannot begin until Mrs. Jones has gathered more data; however, because a behavioral problem and truancy have been identified, a referral can be made to the school counselor. The Smiths can meet with the counselor to determine how their son's problems can be resolved. After gathering more data about the communications block between father and son, Mrs. Jones will facilitate communication between them by acting as a mediator to permit open communication. She can also help Mr. Smith become more accepting of the changes in his son and his son's developmental need to interact with his peers.

Tertiary Prevention

Work with the Smiths to improve communications can also be considered a tertiary preventive measure. From this perspective, improved communications will prevent complications of family discord such as divorce. It will also prevent the recurrence of many of the family problems that have stemmed from poor communication between husband and wife. Another tertiary preventive measure might be a referral for contraceptive services to prevent another unplanned pregnancy.

Evaluating Health Care for the Family

Evaluation begins as the nurse examines the adequacy of the assessment database and continues as he or she evaluates alternative approaches to meeting the family's health care needs. The primary focus for postintervention evaluation is the objectives of care. If these objectives were adequately developed, they are measurable and provide criteria for evaluating the outcome of the intervention. For example, Mrs. Jones set the following objectives for her intervention with Mr. Smith and Brian:

1. Mr. Smith will praise his son at least once a day.
2. Mr. Smith will agree to listen to his son for at least 5 minutes a day.

Mrs. Jones must then determine the means for collecting data to compare outcomes with the stated objectives. In this instance, she could ask Mrs. Smith whether the desired communication pattern has been achieved. If the objectives are not met, an alternative solution can be attempted.

Evaluation is a continuous process throughout the nurse's relationship with the family. If evaluation is not planned at the same time as nursing intervention, it may be impossible to obtain the data needed to evaluate outcomes.

When Mrs. Jones finds that all goals and objectives have been achieved, she will terminate her relationship with the Smiths. Termination, like evaluation, should be planned and discussed early in the relationship. Termination is necessary because the goal of nursing intervention is to help the family become independent.

Both the Smiths and Mrs. Jones may experience some degree of grief during the termination process. Resolution of that grief is necessary and, when achieved, indicates growth. Mrs. Jones should leave the phone number and address of the health unit in case of a future need for services. If necessary, Mrs. Jones can refer the family to other agencies that may be of assistance.

▶ THE DIMENSIONS MODEL AND CRISIS INTERVENTION

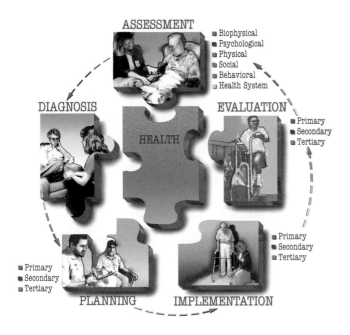

Family Stress

Stressful life events and change are inevitable for families. Some families experience more stressful life events than do others and some are less able to cope with stress. Community health nurses can contribute much to families experiencing varying degrees of stress. In addition, community health nurses can offer anticipatory guidance based on an understanding of family development and stress theory that will assist families to prepare themselves for change and thus minimize stress.

Understanding stress theory enables the community health nurse to identify signs and symptoms of stress within families. It also helps the nurse to assist families experiencing stress whose methods of coping are inadequate to the situation. Stress theory is a scientific explanation for the physiologic and psychological effects of change on individuals or groups of people. Stress theory, in effect, states that any change, emotion, or activity that an individual or family experiences will cause stress. *Stress* is a nonspecific response to any demand that includes both physiologic and psychological components (Selye, 1978). This response is triggered by *stressors* or changes in the internal or external environment. When an individual or a family experiences stress, it may disrupt *homeostasis*, or balance. When this occurs, the individual or family attempts to adapt. *Adaptation* is a process of adjustment to change. Stress may be either positive or negative. Negative stress creates unpleasant effects

and is called *distress*. If distress is extreme, the result may be disease in an individual or family dysfunction and disruption (Selye, 1978).

An example of family stress is the disruption of family homeostasis that occurs when a mother of four returns to work. This change has both positive and negative effects and necessitates other changes within the family. For example, the father may have to act as chauffeur for the children, cook occasional evening meals, or assist with other household chores. Another problem might be difficulty in obtaining adequate child care. The community health nurse can assess how the family is coping with the stress engendered by the mother's return to work and make suggestions to facilitate adaptation.

The experience of stress and successful adaptation to stressful events can be a growth-producing experience for the family. Families who learn together how to solve problems and adjust to stressors increase their resistance to the detrimental effects of future stress. Families who do not adapt well or ignore signs of distress are more likely to experience crisis.

Definition of Crisis

A family can view any situation as a crisis. What is a crisis for one family may not be a crisis for another. Moreover, some families function and thrive on daily crises and would deteriorate if crisis situations were eliminated from their lives. Assessment and intervention, then, must be based on the family's perception of a crisis event.

A *crisis* occurs when a family faces a problem that is seemingly unsolvable. None of their methods of problem solving work. The problem becomes psychologically overwhelming, and anxiety and tension increase until the family becomes disorganized and unable to cope (McCubbin & McCubbin, 1993). A crisis state is unlikely to be sustained for more than 6 weeks because it is difficult to endure the high stress and tension associated with crisis without breakdown or change. The result of a crisis can be either resolution, resulting in a healthier, more positive state of being, or loss of well-being and a higher potential for recurrent crisis. Temporary relief can be gained from the use of defense mechanisms, environmental action, or both. Resolution and more permanent relief and growth require appropriate coping mechanisms (McCubbin & McCubbin, 1993).

During periods of crisis, families are more susceptible to change and are usually more open to help when it is offered. This receptiveness affords the nurse the opportunity to produce change with very little intervention.

Types of Crises

There are two types of crises: maturational and situational. A *maturational crisis* is viewed as "normal" transition point where old patterns of communication and old roles must be exchanged for new patterns and roles (Murray & Zentner, 1997). Every family experiences maturational crisis points, whether or not a crisis is actually experienced. Examples of transitional periods when maturational crises may occur are adolescence, marriage, parenthood, and one's first job. Such periods in life are usually predictable, so families can be prepared to use coping mechanisms that assist them through each transition period.

All the transitional periods experienced by families have in common a change in roles or the addition of new roles, and crises occur when a family is unable or unwilling to accept new roles. There may be a history of poor role modeling from parents that leaves children unprepared for new roles and unable to leave home successfully. There may be family members who are unable or unwilling to view one member in a new role. For example, it is sometimes difficult for parents to acknowledge that their teenage children need to make decisions for themselves.

A *situational crisis* can occur when the family experiences an event that is sudden, unexpected, and unpredictable. Such events threaten either biological, psychological, or social integrity leading to disorganization, tension, and severe anxiety. Examples include illness, accidents, death, and natural disasters.

Some crises may arise that contain elements of both situational and maturational crisis events. For example, a female may be going through the maturational transition of adolescence and encounter the situational crisis of an unwanted pregnancy. The multiplicity of crisis events further impairs the family's ability to cope.

Factors That Increase Susceptibility to Crisis

Why do some families go into crisis while others do not? Four categories of factors seem to play a part in determining whether or not a crisis will occur. These factors relate to the stressor itself and the family's perceptions of the stressor, other stressors impinging on the family, family coping ability, and the extent of family resources. Factors related to the stressor and how it is perceived by the family include the extent of the impact of the stressor on the family and the severity of that impact, the duration of the stressor and whether its onset was sudden or gradual, and the degree of perceived control the family has over the stressor. A stressor that is perceived as manageable is less likely to cause a crisis situation than one that is seen as

uncontrollable. The cause and predictability of the stressor may also influence the occurrence of crisis. Stressors with unknown causes or unpredictable effects create greater anxiety and greater potential for crisis. A final factor related to the stressor and how it is perceived is the degree of stigma that may be attached to the stressor (Danielson, Hamel-Bissell, & Winstead-Fry, 1993).

The family's perception of the stressor may be distorted by previous experience with crises that were not growth producing. For example, there are crisis-prone families who have a chronic inability to perceive or solve existing problems. Their inability to cope with problems results in an exaggerated response to new changes, and crises occur for them that would be averted by other families.

The extent of other concurrent stressors affecting the family may also be a determining factor in the development of a crisis. Multiple stressors may have additive effects that precipitate crises (McCubbin & McCubbin, 1993). As noted earlier, maturational and situational crises may occur simultaneously stretching family coping abilities beyond their limits. Existing family problems such as illness, unemployment, and marital strife, may make a seemingly minor stressor a precipitating factor in a crisis. Situational demands created by the stressor may also increase the potential for crisis. Unfortunately, situational demands created by the health care system may enhance the potential for crisis. For example, the illness of a child is a stressor; if taking the child to the clinic necessitates losing work time and money, this creates an additional burden for the family.

The family's coping mechanisms represent internal family resources important to crisis resolution. Among these resources are cohesion or closeness among family members, open communications, use of humor, control of the meaning of the problem, and role flexibility. The family's ability to cope lessens the impact of any crisis event. It is important to assess what degree of success has been achieved using these mechanisms in the past and whether the family is aware of the mechanisms used.

Situational support arises from external resources such as the extended family, community agencies, churches, neighbors, and friends of the family. The degree of security felt by family members in relationships with these support systems may be sufficient to avert crises.

Structure of a Crisis Event

In every crisis there are contributing factors that culminate in the crisis event. A hazardous incident or stressor of some sort triggers the sequence of events

(Bomar & Cooper, 1996). Hazardous situations can arise from human biology as a result of aging, genetic factors, or illness; from the physical, psychological, or social dimensions; as a result of behavior patterns such as drug or alcohol use; or from health care system problems such as lack of affordable medical care.

The hazardous situation is stressful and causes anxiety. The family experiences a reaction to the event characterized by depression or anger. Family members may use defense mechanisms, such as denial, to ease their discomfort before beginning to use coping mechanisms that help them deal constructively with the situation.

A precipitating event might occur that throws the family into acute anxiety and crisis. This event may be seemingly minor, but serves to tip the scales toward crisis. It overtakes coping mechanisms already stretched to the limits. For example, father's unemployment is a hazardous event that makes the family vulnerable to crisis. Because of the mother's job and other supports, members are not yet in crisis. Then the car breaks down! This last event is perceived by the family as overwhelming and pushes members beyond their ability to cope. A crisis has occurred.

When coping mechanisms fail, the family resorts to different strategies. One person may laugh or cry a great deal; another might withdraw. Finally, the family is in full crisis, evidenced by inappropriate behavior and painful, stressful feelings. During this time they are unable to focus or concentrate and need clear, direct, precise direction. Figure 18–4 depicts the structure of a crisis event.

Crisis Intervention

 ## Assessing the Crisis Situation

Interviewing during a crisis requires empathy, a calm demeanor, and a sensitivity to feeling tones that may not be readily apparent to others. Nondirective techniques are used. Inquiries and instructions need to be precise, concrete, and simple; a family in crisis is unable to focus and narrow the field to what must be done. Open-ended statements are used to encourage family members to speak spontaneously.

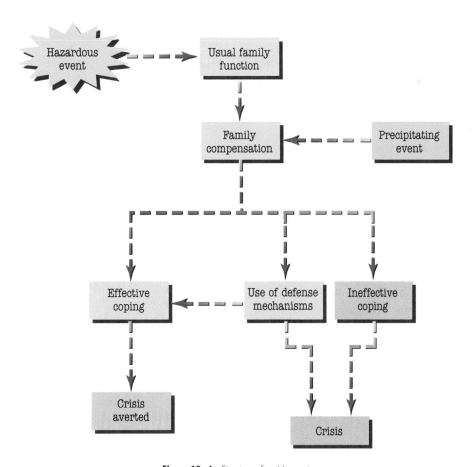

Figure 18–4. Structure of a crisis event.

The Biophysical Dimension

Human biological factors such as aging, genetic factors, and illness can contribute to the crisis. For example, Mr. Simon is 74 years old and has to move into a nursing home because he can no longer buy his own groceries and cook for himself. He becomes very agitated and cannot make decisions.

The Psychological Dimension

The initial step in assessing a crisis situation is to review the events leading to the crisis. This gives family members a chance to discuss their perceptions of the event and affords the nurse an opportunity to assess perceptions, defense mechanisms, and coping strategies. A detailed history is not necessary. Just let the family members talk.

The nurse should determine if the family has ever experienced a similar event and how the family has reacted in the past. Past successful coping can be used to reassure members that they can cope with the current problem as well. Or, discussion of past events can be used to identify patterns that were not successful, and plans can be made to use alternative coping mechanisms.

A major concern during a crisis is the potential for physical danger that may be present within the family. Individual family members must be assessed for suicidal or homicidal tendencies. If there are indications that a family member is contemplating violence to oneself or to others, immediate referral for psychiatric help is warranted.

The Social Dimension

When family members have had an opportunity to discuss the situation and are emotionally open to exploring solutions, an assessment can be made of external resources arising from the social environment. Find out if there are extended family members nearby, agencies that have been helpful for the family in the past, clergy, church members, or friends that the family want near them now.

Sometimes social dimension factors such as unemployment, racial discrimination, and poverty can contribute to a crisis. For example, Mr. Lloyd's son needs surgery so he can walk. Arrangements were made but had to be canceled when Mr. Lloyd lost his job and his health insurance benefits. In this case, the community health nurse may want to determine whether an agency is available that can help the family to obtain the care their son needs.

The Behavioral Dimension

Behavioral dimension factors such as alcohol or drug use can constitute the hazardous event, be a precipi-

tating event, or act as a defense mechanism for a family experiencing crisis. Alcohol and drug abuse can also impair a family's response to maturational and situational crises. The nurse must be alert to any evidence of alcohol or drug abuse and assist the family in seeking and obtaining counseling.

The Health System Dimension

Assessment in this area includes determining whether the family has insurance coverage for counseling, emergency care, or hospitalization should these be required to deal with the crisis. Counseling and medical services for potentially suicidal family members, accident victims, or members with drug and alcohol problems often must be sought for families that do not have any insurance or money. Identifying local, county, and state resources for families in need is an important responsibility for the community health nurse.

Diagnostic Reasoning and Crisis Intervention

Often diagnostic reasoning and planning for crisis intervention occur at the same time. Working with a family in crisis requires expertise in quickly determining the family's needs, knowledge of resources available that can be used spontaneously or with very little delay, and ability to teach problem solving. The fam-

Critical Thinking in Research

Zerwekh (1992) analyzed anecdotal stories of 30 expert public health nurses making home visits to families to determine the competencies required for effective family caregiving and development of family self-help skills. The competencies identified included locating highly mobile families, building trust between nurse and family, and building family strengths which included helping families develop faith in their own capabilities.

1. Do you think these findings would be more applicable to some groups of families than others? If so, what kinds of families might they characterize?

2. What specific nursing interventions do you think might assist families to develop self-help capabilities?

3. How would you design a study to determine if these interventions do, indeed, make a difference?

ily crisis case study is used to illustrate how Mr. James, a community health nurse, assisted the Robbins family during a crisis. Refer to Family Crisis Case Study on this page.

From these data, Mr. James derives some nursing diagnoses. First, this is a situational crisis precipitated by son Bob's drinking and his argument with his father. Elements of a maturational crisis are also present because Mr. Robbins seems reluctant to accept Bob's new role as a young adult. Second, the family does not know how to deal with a teenage son who has a drinking problem. Third, son John is being left out of the discussions at a time when he is old enough to be a contributing member. Mr. James also surmises that the family seems to have drawn together to help each other survive this crisis.

Intervention in a crisis situation is guided by several general principles. First, the nurse should listen actively and with concern to family members' perceptions of and feelings about the event. Second, the nurse should encourage open expression of feelings and help the family gain an understanding of the crisis event. The nurse should also help the client accept reality and explore new ways of coping with problems presented by the crisis situation. The nurse may also need to link family members with a social network that can assist them to deal with the crisis. The community health nurse also engages in problem solving with the family and reinforces new coping strategies. Finally, the nurse needs to follow up with the family after the crisis has been resolved to engage in primary prevention for future crisis events.

Intervention with the Robbins family focuses on secondary prevention and is directed toward helping members to discuss and define the problem and to express their feelings concerning Bob. The nurse is an active listener and participates attentively, but the family must do the work. The emphasis is on bringing feelings out into the open. Mr. James must be truthful, honest, and forthright. He does not give false reassurance about son Bob or his whereabouts.

It is important at this stage not to let the anxiety become contagious. If Mr. James begins to experience anxiety, he should step out and perhaps make a phone call to maintain perspective.

Exploration of coping mechanisms already used enables the nurse to help the family examine ways to cope. Mr. James's involvement includes helping the family to explore other options for dealing with the situation. The pros and cons of each of these alternatives should be discussed with the family.

Mr. James would discourage Mr. Robbins from blaming himself or others for the problem. Suggestions are made about how to find Bob and what to do once he is found. Mr. James recommends the alcohol

FAMILY CRISIS CASE STUDY

The Robbins family includes five members: Dad, 46, Mom, 43, and three children, Bob, 18, John, 16, and Debbie, 6 months. Bob will finish high school this year. He and his father seem to argue all the time about Bob's friends, Bob's drinking, and the way he drives. Last evening Bob and his father had a heated argument and Bob left the house in a rage. He drove away, squealing tires and swerving at the corner. When the community health nurse, Mr. James, visits the next morning, the family is agitated. Bob did not come home. Dad has not gone to work and the family cannot seem to decide what to do to find Bob. They are worried that he may have had an accident.

During his assessment, Mr. James discovers that part of the reason Mr. Robbins is so upset is his past experience with a similar crisis event. Mr. Robbins' brother died in an alcohol-related automobile accident 20 years ago, after an argument with his brother. It is obvious that Bob's leaving has had a tremendous impact on Mr. Robbins. Mrs. Robbins is trying to console her husband, but she too is very upset about Bob and the danger he may be in. John is sitting nearby pounding the arm of the chair because his parents will not listen to what he has to say about why Bob left. Debbie is sleeping.

and drug rehabilitation center nearby. In addition, he refers the family for counseling with an experienced counselor.

Implementing Primary Prevention to Avert Crisis

Primary crisis prevention techniques are widely used by community health nurses because all families experience crises. Primary prevention includes providing anticipatory guidance related to common crises of family life and assisting families to develop effective coping strategies to combat the stress of situational crises.

It is impossible, and sometimes undesirable, to prevent a crisis situation from occurring; however, the nurse can assist the family to prepare for and cope with the event. For example, the birth of a child or change of employment may be a very desirable event. Such an event requires changes in lifestyle and family adaptation that might precipitate a crisis. The nurse can assist the family to explore areas in which change will be required, avenues for accomplishing these changes, and strategies for dealing with the anxiety related to change. Through primary prevention implemented via anticipatory guidance, a potential crisis may be averted even though the stressful event takes place.

Evaluating Crisis Intervention

The evaluation process in crisis intervention is continuous as the nurse assesses the family's progress through the crisis event. More formal evaluation may also be conducted to review the entire process of intervention with the family. This includes systematic review of the crisis, the coping mechanisms used (old and new), and the result achieved. The emphasis is on reinforcing learning and strengthening the family for future crises.

TESTING YOUR UNDERSTANDING

1. List at least five different types of families. What are the characteristic features of each type? (pp. 392–394)
2. Identify at least three characteristics of families. Give an example of each characteristic. (pp. 395–397)
3. Describe four considerations to be addressed in assessing family communication patterns. Give an example of each consideration. (pp. 398–399)
4. What are the two central themes in assessing patterns of family dynamics? Give an example of the influence of each. (p. 400)
5. How do formal family roles differ from informal roles? Give an example of each type of role. (pp. 402–403)

Critical Thinking in Practice: A Case in Point

You are a community health nurse, and you have received a request to visit the Miller family. On arriving at their home, you find that the family recently moved to your district from Georgia and that they have been married only 18 months.

Sandy, age 26, is 3 months pregnant and does not have a source of prenatal care. She is an experienced elementary school teacher but needs a state credential to teach in this district.

Jim, age 30, is an engineer. This is his second marriage; Jane, age 13, is his daughter from his previous marriage. Jane resents Jim's marriage to Sandy. Jim does not understand why Jane and Sandy argue so much. Many of the couple's disagreements occur over discipline for Jane. Jane is particularly hard to handle after a weekend spent with her own mother. Jane refuses to obey Sandy or to help around the house.

During your visit, Jane arrived home from school. Sandy asked her to go to her room and change clothes. Instead, Jane flopped down on the floor to watch television. At this point, Sandy yelled, "Wait 'til your father comes home, young lady!" You and Sandy moved into the kitchen so you could talk away from the noise of the TV.

Sandy tells you that Jim is not happy about the pregnancy. He is worried about the effect of another child on an already stretched budget. Sandy is pleased about the baby, even though at present she is experiencing a lot of nausea and backaches. She has not mentioned this to Jim because she does not want him to think she complains a lot. When asked, Sandy tells you that she has not obtained prenatal care because of the cost. She also tells you that she and Jim have not discussed her need for care or made any plans for the new baby.

To add to Sandy's current problems, Jim has never assisted with housework. He feels that this is "woman's work." Sandy has been doing her best to keep up the house, but she resents Jim's attitude, especially since she has not been feeling well. She also resents Jim making the decision that she will not work until the baby starts first grade when she has not even been consulted.

1. What biophysical, psychological, social, behavioral, and health system factors are operating in this situation?
2. What nursing diagnoses might you derive from the data included in the case description?
3. What primary prevention measures would be appropriate with this family? Why?
4. What secondary intervention strategies would you employ to deal with existing health problems? What tertiary prevention might be warranted in this situation?
5. What client care objectives would you set for dealing with this family? How will you go about evaluating the achievement of those objectives?

6. Define stress, distress, homeostasis, and adaptation. Give an example of each. (p. 411)
7. Give two examples of family stressors. (p. 411)
8. Differentiate between maturational and situational crises. Give an example of each type. (p. 412)
9. Describe the structure of a crisis event. Identify points at which nursing intervention could occur. (pp. 412–413)
10. Identify at least four principles of crisis intervention. (p. 415)

WHAT DO YOU THINK?
Questions for Critical Thinking

1. How would you intervene to help a family adjust to the stress of a young wife's return to work with three young children at home? How might your interventions differ if the stress was due to the children leaving home?
2. How do you cope with stress in your life? Are your coping mechanisms compatible with those used by other family members?
3. Why should community health nurses intervene to resolve families' socioeconomic problems as well as health problems?
4. What resources are available to families in your community? Are they adequate to meet the needs of families living in the community?

REFERENCES

Allen, C. E. (1994). Families in poverty. *Nursing Clinics of North America, 29,* 377–393.

Anderson, E. (1996). Family roles. In P. Bomar (Ed.), *Nurses and family health assessment: Concepts, assessment, and intervention* (2nd ed.) (pp. 70–82). Philadelphia: W. B. Saunders.

Ballard, N. (1996). Family structure, function, and process. In S. M. H. Hanson & S. T. Boyd (Eds.), *Family health care nursing: Theory, practice, and research* (pp. 57–78). Philadelphia: F. A. Davis.

Bomar, P., & Cooper, S. (1996). Family stress. In P. Bomar (Ed.), *Nurses and family health assessment: Concepts, assessment, and intervention* (2nd ed.) (pp. 121–138). Philadelphia: W. B. Saunders.

Capuzzi, C. (1996). Families and community health nursing. In S. M. H. Hanson & S. T. Boyd (Eds.), *Family health care nursing: Theory, practice, and research* (pp. 351–368). Philadelphia: F. A. Davis.

Danielson, C. B., Hamel-Bissell, B., & Winstead-Fry, P. (1993). *Family health and illness: Perspectives on coping and intervention,* St. Louis: Mosby Year Book.

Duvall, E., & Miller, B. (1990). *Marriage and family development* (6th ed.). New York: Harper College.

Elkind, D. (1995). The family in the postmodern world. *National Forum, 75*(3), 24–28.

Friedman, M. (1998). *Family nursing: Research, theory, and practice* (4th ed.). Stamford, CT: Appleton & Lange.

Friedman, M. M., & Ferguson-Marshalleck, E. G. (1996). Sociocultural influences on family health. In S. M. H. Hanson & S. T. Boyd (Eds.), *Family health care nursing: Theory, practice, and research* (pp. 81–98). Philadelphia: F. A. Davis.

Grove, K. A. (1996). The American family: History and development. In P. Bomar (Ed.), *Nurses and family health assessment: Concepts, assessment, and intervention* (2nd ed.) (pp. 36–45). Philadelphia: W. B. Saunders.

Hanson, S. M. H. (1996). Family assessment and intervention. In S. M. H. Hanson & S. T. Boyd (Eds.), *Family health care nursing: Theory, practice, and research* (pp. 147–172). Philadelphia: F. A. Davis.

Hanson, S. M. H. & Boyd, S. T. (1996). Family nursing: An overview. In S. M. H. Hanson & S. T. Boyd (Eds.), *Family health care nursing: Theory, practice, and research* (pp. 5–37). Philadelphia: F. A. Davis.

Janosik, E., & Green, E. (1992). *Family life: Process and practice.* Boston: Jones and Bartlett.

Klein, D. M., & White, J. M. (1996). *Family theories: An introduction.* Thousand Oaks, CA: Sage.

McCubbin, M. A., & McCubbin, H. I. (1993). Family coping and illness: The resiliency model of family stress, adjustment, and adaptation. In C. B. Danielson, B. Hamel-Bissell, & P. Winstead-Fry, *Family health and illness: Perspectives on coping and intervention* (pp. 21–63). St. Louis: Mosby Year Book.

McCubbin, M., & Van Riper, M. (1996). Factors influencing family functioning and the health of family members. In S. M. H. Hanson & S. T. Boyd (Eds.), *Family health care nursing: Theory, practice, and research* (pp. 101–121). Philadelphia: F. A. Davis.

Murray, R., & Zentner, J. (1997). *Health assessment and promotion strategies through the life span* (6th ed.). Stamford, CT: Appleton & Lange.

Person, J. (Ed.). (1993). *Statistical forecasts of the United States.* Detroit: Gale Research.

Richards, B. S. (1996). Gerontological family nursing. In S. M. H. Hanson & S. T. Boyd (Eds.), *Family health care nursing: Theory, practice, and research* (pp. 329–348). Philadelphia: F. A. Davis.

Ross, B., & Cobb, K. L. (1990). *Family nursing: A nursing process approach.* Redwood City, CA: Addison-Wesley.

Roth, P. (1996). Family social support. In P. Bomar (Ed.), *Nurses and family health assessment: Concepts, assess-*

ment, and intervention (2nd ed.) (pp. 107–120). Philadelphia: W. B. Saunders.

Selye, H. (1978). *The stress of life* (2nd ed.). New York: McGraw-Hill.

U.S. Department of Commerce. (1993). *Statistical abstract of the United States 1993* (113th ed.). Washington, DC: Government Printing Office.

U.S. Department of Health and Human Services. (1996). *Health United States, 1995.* Hyattsville, MD: U.S. Public Health Service.

Wright, L., & Leahy, M. (1993). *Nurses and families: A guide to family assessment and intervention* (2nd ed.). Philadelphia: F. A. Davis.

Zerwekh, J. V. (1992). Laying the groundwork for family self-help: Locating families, building trust, and building strength. *Public Health Nursing, 9,* 15–21.

RESOURCES FOR NURSES WORKING WITH FAMILIES

Emotional Support

Emotions Anonymous
PO Box 4245
St. Paul, MN 55104–0245
(612) 647–9712

Family Service America
11700 West Lake Park Drive
Milwaukee, WI 53224
(414) 359–1040

National Mental Health Association
1021 Prince Street
Alexandria, VA 22314–2971
(703) 684–7722

Family Counseling Services of the Court System
Local, county, parish, or state offices

Catholic Community Services
Department of Family Services, local office

Families Anonymous
PO Box 3475
Culver City, CA 90231–3475
(310) 313–5800

Nutrition

U.S. Department of Agriculture
Food & Nutrition Service
Supplemental Food Program Division
Special Supplemental Food Program for Women, Infants, & Children
3101 Park Center Drive
Alexandria, VA 22302
(703) 305–2062

RESOURCES FOR NURSES WORKING WITH FAMILIES IN CRISIS

National

National Council on Child Abuse & Family Violence
1155 Connecticut Avenue, NW, Ste. 300
Washington, DC 20036
(202) 429–6695

National Council of Community Mental Health Centers
12300 Twinbrook Parkway, No. 320
Rockville, MD 20852
(301) 984–6200

American Cancer Society
National Office
1599 Clifton Road, NE
Atlanta, GA 30329
(404) 320–3333

Local

County or parish mental health services

Office of counselor of mental health

Superior court

Rape crisis centers

Family crisis centers

Police

Social services

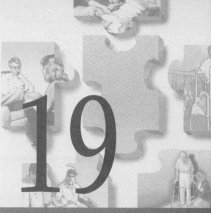

CARE OF THE COMMUNITY OR TARGET GROUP

▶ KEY TERMS

age-specific death rate
Area Resource File (ARF)
cause-specific death
  rates
community activation
community assessment
crude death rate
forecasting
health index
key informants
normative planning
participant observation
planning
rate under treatment
screening
sensitivity
specificity
strategic planning
tactical planning
target group

When a community health nurse provides care to aggregates, the recipient of care—the client—may be an entire community or a subgroup within the community (Kuehnert, 1995), called a target group. A *target group* can be either a particularly vulnerable subgroup within the population, such as the elderly, or a group with known health needs, such as people with AIDS. In either case, the nurse would apply the Dimensions Model to the care of the group rather than to specific individuals within the group. This chapter examines the application of the model to communities and target groups. The process used with both is the same, but information gathered differs with the group addressed.

Chapter Objectives

After reading this chapter, you should be able to:

- Identify at least three purposes for assessing a community or target group.
- Describe at least three factors that influence the scope of a community or target group assessment.
- Describe at least two factors in each of the six dimensions of health to be considered in assessing a target group or a community.
- Describe two levels of community nursing diagnoses related to the health status of a community or target group.
- Identify interventions at the primary, secondary, and tertiary levels of prevention that will influence the health of communities or target groups.
- Describe at least three considerations in planning screening programs for communities and target groups.
- Identify at least six tasks in planning health programs to meet the needs of communities or target groups.
- Describe three levels of acceptance of a health care program.
- Describe three types of considerations in evaluating a health care program.

► THE DIMENSIONS MODEL AND CARE OF COMMUNITIES AND TARGET GROUPS

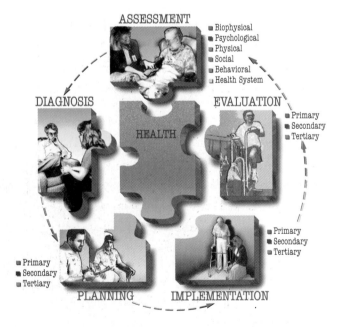

Community health nurses working with communities or target groups as clients use the Dimensions Model

to identify client needs and to direct action to meet those needs. The process employs the six dimensions of nursing, begins by assessing group needs, and proceeds to a diagnosis of health problems. These steps are followed by the planning and implementation of health programs to meet the health needs of the group. The process concludes with an evaluation of the adequacy of those programs.

Critical Dimensions of Nursing in the Care of Communities and Target Groups

Although elements of each of the six dimensions of nursing are needed, aspects of the interpersonal and process dimensions are apt to be the most useful to the community health nurse caring for communities and target groups. The nurse certainly will require cognitive knowledge of communities and community organization and specific knowledge of the communities and groups with which he or she works. In order to use that knowledge to enhance the health of population groups, however, the nurse will have to be adept at communicating and collaborating with the myriad other disciplines that must act together to promote public health (Flynn, Rider, & Bailey, 1992). Negotiation skills will also be needed in the interpersonal dimension (Dees & Garcia, 1995). Similarly, the intellectual skills of analysis and organization in the skills dimension can best be brought to bear on community health problems through the exercise of the group, change, leadership, and political processes embodied in the process dimension of community health nursing. Elements of the reflective dimension, such as research, theory development, and program evaluation provide the knowledge base that permits effective use of these processes. Within the ethical dimension, the nurse must function as a community advocate, while simultaneously guarding the rights of individuals within the community and achieving a balance between individual freedoms and public good. Care of communities or population groups provides the most complex arena for use of any of the dimensions of nursing and forms the crux of community health nursing practice.

 Assessing the Dimensions of Health in Communities and Target Groups

Community assessment has been identified as one of the primary tasks of community health nurses. *Community assessment* is the process by which data are compiled regarding a community's health status and from which nursing diagnoses are derived. Another term used is a "needs assessment" (Soriano, 1995). Such assessment consists of the collection of two types of data: (1) data specific to the community or target group itself and (2) general information about particular problems of interest such as adolescent pregnancy, incidence of AIDS, and motor vehicle fatalities. General information is used to make comparisons between the community or target group and larger segments of society that aid in identifying strengths and weaknesses. General information collected might include state and national data on the extent of particular problems as well as information on factors contributing to those problems.

An accurate assessment is the basis of any community health endeavor and is essential to planning any program designed to meet health-related needs. Community or target group assessment provides a *health index,* a summary of a population's health status, which serves as a basis for planning to meet health care needs. Without a clear picture of the health needs of the community or target group, health care providers have no way of determining whether current programs meet health needs or how to plan programs that will.

Preparing to Assess the Health of a Community or Target Group

Prior to beginning an assessment of the health status of a community or target group, the community health nurse should determine the purpose and scope of the assessment, types of data to be collected, sources of data, and methods for data collection, organization, and analysis.

Determining the Purpose and Scope of the Assessment. The purpose for assessing a target group or community determines the types of data to be collected as well as the scope of the assessment. Community or group needs assessment may be conducted for a variety of reasons. For example, one may demonstrate the need for a specific kind of program to justify program funding, or a needs assessment may fulfill a legal mandate to identify the health care needs of a community. Needs assessments may also be used as a basis for resource allocation decisions or to identify the needs of certain underserved segments of the population, such as the elderly or persons with AIDS (Soriano, 1995). Community health nurses and others use the data derived from a community needs assessment to develop diagnoses and to plan, implement, and evaluate programs designed to promote health and resolve existing health problems.

The scope, or depth and complexity, of a community or target group assessment depends on a number of factors. First, if the purpose of the assessment is to determine the group's health status, the assessment needs to be much more extensive than if the purpose is to obtain additional data about a known problem. Second, the size of the population also affects the assessment. A small target group can be assessed in greater depth than can a community at large for the same expenditure of money and effort. Third, the time available for the assessment may limit its scope. If information is required within a specified period, the nurse may be limited in the depth of assessment possible. Fourth, a limiting factor may be the degree of expertise of those conducting the assessment (Barton, Smith, Brown, & Supples, 1993). Fifth, the relationship between the cost and the perceived benefits of an in-depth assessment may also contribute to limitations on the scope of the assessment undertaken. Finally, the political environment within the community may affect the comprehensiveness of any assessment. If policy makers or group members do not place a high priority on health, they are unlikely to support an extensive assessment of health needs.

Selecting Data Collection Methods and Sources. When the scope of an assessment is limited, the community health nurse needs to decide what categories of data are already available and what additional data are needed to accomplish the purpose of the assessment (Witkin & Altschuld, 1995). In this chapter the focus is on categories of data that would be collected in a comprehensive assessment of a community or a target group. In an assessment of lesser scope, the community health nurse must determine what categories of data are essential to accomplish the purpose of the assessment and what information may safely be left out.

Usually, a variety of methods are used to collect the data. Both quantitative and qualitative approaches should be used to assess the health status of communities or target groups. *Quantitative* approaches involve the collection of numbers of events. *Qualitative* approaches focus on examination of perceptions of health, attitudes, and health concerns as voiced by members of the population. For example, in obtaining information on the use of health care services by group members, quantitative methods would be used to gather data on the numbers of people who received care at various facilities; group members' perceptions of health care services and their reasons for using or not using them would be more easily obtained using qualitative methods of data collection.

Quantitative data may be obtained by reviewing statistics compiled by health care agencies and other sources at the local, state, and national levels. For example, the nurse might obtain information on the racial composition of a community from published census figures, or on the incidence of child abuse from records kept by child protection agencies or law enforcement officials. Newspaper reports are a source of quantitative data about injuries, crime, and residential fires. It has been noted that news stories often contain more detailed information about such incidents than official reports (Rainey & Runyan, 1992). The community health nurse might also obtain quantitative data by conducting surveys and compiling figures on the frequency of certain responses. For example, the nurse might ask a sample of elderly persons how often they see a physician.

The nurse might also obtain quantitative data through observation. For example, one way the adequacy of protective services in a community could be assessed is to determine the location of fire stations. The nurse might drive through the community, note each fire station on a map, and then calculate the maximum distance of any point in the community from a fire station.

Surveys and observations can also provide qualitative data about a community or target group. Community or group members can be asked about their attitudes toward health and health care services or about their perceptions of community health needs. Qualitative data can also reflect community leadership and the readiness of a community for change. Because people's opinions and perceptions vary greatly, a diversity of community members should be approached for information. Such diversity is particularly evident in comparing opinions of residents in a community and those of health care providers in the area.

Community health nurses might also interview members of the community and "key informants." *Key informants* are people who, because of their position in the community, possess information and insights about the community. Examples of key informants include public officials, school and health care personnel, prominent business people, and local clergy. Again, it is important not to restrict interviews to these sources, but also to interview typical residents of the community because of the possible differences in perceptions of the community's health needs.

Participant observation is another means of gathering qualitative data. In *participant observation,* the community health nurse participates in the life of the community or target group, making observations about health and health needs in the course of that participation. For example, the nurse might look for housing in the community and, in the search, observe housing conditions and determine rents typical of different areas of the community. Or, a nurse assessing

the needs of the alcoholic population might attend meetings of an Alcoholics Anonymous (AA) group or visit a detoxification center.

Different methods of data collection are appropriate to different types of information. Appropriate methods for gathering specific data needed to assess the health of communities or target groups are addressed later in this chapter.

Where does one find the information needed for a community or target group assessment? Before beginning an assessment, the community health nurse should identify several potential sources. Additional sources are usually uncovered during the course of the assessment, but the nurse needs an identified starting point for data collection.

A community or target group is assessed using data from many sources. Usually the local chamber of commerce can supply information regarding community size, history, industry, and facilities for transportation, communication, and recreation. Information about many population characteristics such as age, sex, race and language, income and education levels, employment, and marital status can be obtained from the most recent census figures, as can some statistics related to housing. Similar information related to a particular target group may be less easy to find unless the group is one that is of interest to government officials or other agencies that gather statistics. For example, the nurse might be able to get information about people with certain types of cancer from a local cancer registry, or about older persons from the local office on aging.

Basic data from the most recent census may be found in public and university libraries. More detailed census information is available from libraries designated as government document repositories. Libraries of large universities and large metropolitan areas are usually so designated. If no repository of government documents is nearby, information can be obtained directly from the Bureau of Census located in Atlanta, Georgia. This office also has recently collected data on microfiche.

Local school systems are good sources of information regarding the availability of education facilities and immunization levels. Various religious groups in the community can be identified in the yellow pages of the telephone directory; further information on religious affiliation can be sought from local houses of worship.

The yellow pages also lists health care services and resources, transportation, and formal communication networks. In some communities, local agencies compile lists of referral resources for a variety of health-related services. A local Headstart program, for example, is required by federal standards to provide this type of information to parents of children enrolled.

Information about protective services can be obtained from the local government or police and fire departments. Statements of the adequacy of services can be validated in interviews with members of the community or target group or with insurance company representatives. The local health department can provide statistics related to births, deaths, and morbidity, as well as data on the availability and use of health resources and services. Information on water supply and waste disposal can also usually be obtained from health department sources.

Local government officials can provide information on the priority given to health care programs in the budget. Many industries provide some forms of health care services and would also have records of expenditures of this nature, as would insurance companies. Local voluntary and official health care agencies can also be sources of information on health care financing.

Area maps define the size of a community and the presence or absence of recreational facilities. Maps also show thoroughfares that link the community with other areas.

Other possible sources of organized data include the local hospital association, local chapters of professional and business organizations, and voluntary agencies, such as the American Diabetes Association. Key persons in the community, both official and unofficial, can provide information as well. Specific sources of information are addressed later in this chapter in relation to the categories of data that constitute a community or target group assessment. General sources of qualitative and quantitative assessment data are listed in Table 19–1.

For some types of information, however, no records are available. Such information must be obtained by the nurse through personal observation and through contact with members of the community or target group. Community attitudes toward health are one example of this type of data. Figures on the use of health care services can provide a partial and indirect indication of attitudes, but nonuse may reflect the effects of cost or other barriers rather than a low priority given to health. The perceptive community health nurse derives information about attitudes based on the feeling tone of contacts with group members. For example, the nurse would note whether community members are receptive to suggestions regarding health practices and whether they would expend energy or resources to resolve an identified health problem.

Selecting Methods for Organizing and Analyzing Data. In addition to determining appropriate data collection methods,

TABLE 19–1. SOURCES OF COMMUNITY ASSESSMENT DATA

Type of Data	Source	Example
Quantitative	Census figures	• Age composition of population
		• Racial composition of population
	Local agencies	• Child abuse incidence figures from child protective services
		• Diabetes admissions from hospitals
	Community surveys	• Frequency of health services use
		• Common health problems
	Observation	• Number and types of educational institutions
		• Number and types of recreational opportunities
	Newspaper reports	• Incidence of homicide
		• Incidence of motor vehicle fatalities
	Telephone book	• Number and types of health care providers
		• Number and types of churches
Qualitative	Community surveys	• Attitudes toward health
		• Attitudes toward specific health issues
	Key informant interviews	• Perceptions of community health needs
	Resident interviews	• Perceptions of health needs
	Observation	• Quality of housing
	Participation observation	• Barriers to health care for handicapped individuals

the nurse preparing to assess a community explores methods for organizing and analyzing the data. Data organization may be facilitated by the use of a computerized database management system (DBMS) (Hettinger & Brazile, 1992). In designing such a system, a nurse would first identify the data entry categories needed, for example, age, race, and sex composition of a population and morbidity and mortality data. Information obtained through qualitative methods might also be codified and entered in the database. For example, data entry categories might be created for community health problems identified in interviews with key informants. Not all community assessment data can be computerized. The community health nurse should, therefore, explore other methods of data organization and analysis such as thematic analysis of interview data. When modes of data organization and analysis are identified as much as possible prior to data collection, interpretation of the masses of information obtained becomes much easier.

Dimensions of a Community Assessment

Community health nurses can use a dimensions of health perspective to guide the assessment of a total population or community. Biophysical, psychological, physical, social, behavioral, and health system factors influencing community health are examined.

The Biophysical Dimension. Human biological factors influencing community health reflect specific physical attributes of community members. The first of these attributes is age. Others reflect the genetic inheritance and physiologic function of community members.

AGE. The age composition of the population is an important indicator of probable health needs. Typically, there is an increased need for health services in areas with large numbers of the very young and the very old (Ellencweig, 1992). Large numbers of women of childbearing age increase needs for prenatal and family planning services. Accident prevention is a major consideration in communities with large numbers of school-age and younger children. Information on the age composition of the population can be obtained from census figures for the census tracts that make up the community.

Another community factor related to age composition is the annual birth rate, which provides information on the growth of the younger segments of the population. The annual birth rate is calculated on the basis of the number of live births during the year in relation to the total population of the community. As is true of several of the other rates discussed in Chapter 8, the proportion of live births to the population is multiplied by 1000 to give the rate of births per 1000 persons. Birth statistics are usually compiled by local and state health agencies and can be obtained from these sources.

Age-specific death rates also provide valuable information regarding the health status of the community (Rohrer, 1996). An *age-specific death rate* is the number of deaths in a particular age group compared with the population within that group. Because of the relatively small number of deaths in some age groups, the multiplier used in calculating age-specific death rates is 100,000. Excess deaths (deaths over the number that would be expected for that age group in the general population) for any age group in the community would indicate the presence of health problems. Mortality statistics are available from state and local health agencies.

The average age at death also provides an indication of overall community health. If people in the community typically die at a relatively young age, this suggests the existence of health problems that are contributing to these early deaths. Native Americans, for example, have shorter expected life spans than the rest of the population because of the high incidence of such health problems as chronic disease and alcoholism and high rates of homicide. A large proportion of the Native American population die in middle age compared with an average life expectancy of 75 years for the general public (U.S. Department of Commerce,

1996). Information on age at death may be compiled by local health agencies, but may also be obtained by a review of death certificates or examination of obituaries published in local newspapers.

Some typical community assessment data related to age composition are included in Table 19–2. It is often helpful to include comparison data to identify trends over time. The community represented in Table 19–2, for example, has experienced a slight increase in the older adult population and a decline in the number of youngsters.

GENETIC INHERITANCE. One feature of the genetic inheritance of the population is its distribution by gender. Many health problems such as obesity, hypertension, and various forms of cancer are more prevalent in one sex than in the other. Knowing the sex distribution in the community sharpens the index of suspicion with regard to these problems. Knowing the composition of the population with respect to gender assists the nurse to identify health needs and plan programs to meet them. For example, the knowledge that women constitute 79% of a community's population might suggest the need for easily accessible detection programs for cancer of the cervix and breast.

The racial composition of a community is another important factor in assessment. Knowledge of

TABLE 19–2. **SAMPLE COMMUNITY ASSESSMENT DATA RELATED TO AGE**

		1995		1985	
		N	Percent	N	Percent
AGE COMPOSITION	Birth–1 year	5,827	6	6,380	7
	1–5 years	7,932	9	7,863	9
	6–12 years	9,347	10	8,476	10
	13–20 years	12,701	14	9,340	11
	21–30 years	10,838	12	11,795	13
	31–50 years	12,397	14	14,832	17
	51–65 years	10,492	11	9,508	11
	66–80 years	15,438	17	13,802	16
	Over 80 years	6,739	7	5,127	6

		1995	1985
AGE SPECIFIC DEATH RATE PER 100,000 POPULATION	Birth–1 year	27	35
	1–5 years	58	40
	6–12 years	110	80
	13–20 years	154	175
	21–30 years	75	77
	31–50 years	90	87
	51–65 years	169	185
	66–80 years	203	213
	Over 80 years	254	267

Average annual birth rate for last 10 years: 268 per 100,000 population
Average age at death: 72 years

the ethnicity and racial origin of the population helps to pinpoint health problems known to be prevalent in certain groups, such as sickle cell disease in African Americans and diabetes in some Native American tribes. Data on both the sex and racial composition of the community population are available in census figures as well as from state and local agencies. Sample assessment data reflecting a community's genetic inheritance are included in Table 19–3.

PHYSIOLOGIC FUNCTION.   Information about physiologic function in a community is derived from morbidity and mortality data as well as other health status indicators such as immunization levels. Mortality rates of concern to the community health nurse include the crude death rate, cause-specific death rates, and death rates among specific segments of the population, such as the elderly, minority groups, and homeless.

The *crude death rate* reflects all deaths in the population regardless of age or cause of death and is calculated using the formula presented in Chapter 8. The crude death rate presents a picture of the overall health status of the community, but it does not suggest the presence of specific health problems that may be contributing to deaths.

Cause-specific death rates, on the other hand, provide information about a community's specific health problems. Cause-specific death rates are the number of deaths in the population attributable to specific conditions such as diabetes, heart disease, and suicide. They are calculated in proportion to the total population using a multiplier of 100,000. When death rates due to specific causes are higher than those of populations with a comparable age composition, health care programs may be needed to deal with these causes of death. Mortality statistics are compiled by state and local health departments. Information on mortality may also be available from other sources. For example, insurance companies or trauma centers

might be able to provide information on motor vehicle fatalities, and homicide figures may be available from local law enforcement agencies.

The majority of health problems are nonfatal, and many existing health problems in the community are not brought to light by examining mortality statistics alone. For this reason, the nurse must consider morbidity as well as mortality rates. Morbidity rates reflect the extent of illness present in the community. The two morbidity statistics of greatest significance in community assessment are prevalence and incidence rates. Prevalence rates indicate the *total* number of cases of a particular condition at any given time. Incidence rates indicate the number of *new* cases of the condition identified over a period. For example, eight new cases of tuberculosis may have been diagnosed in Buffalo County last month (incidence), but 39 people in the county are currently under treatment for active tuberculosis (prevalence).

Local and state health departments compile statistics on the incidence and prevalence of certain reportable health conditions. These conditions include many communicable diseases, but may also include other conditions for which special surveillance programs are in place. For example, in some areas information is compiled on newly diagnosed cases of hypertension. Another indicator of community morbidity is the *rate under treatment* or the number of people seeking assistance for specific health problems (Witkin & Altschuld, 1995). For example, the number of people being treated for depression says a great deal about the mental health of the population and may be obtained from local treatment facilities. For other conditions, the nurse may need to seek other sources of data. Cancer registries, may be a source of information about the incidence and prevalence of certain forms of cancer, and local health care facilities and providers may have figures related to the incidence of other conditions. The local hospital may have data on the number of clients hospitalized for diabetes, myocardial infarction, and other conditions.

Immunization levels within the community also provide information on the physiologic function of community members. Information on immunization levels is usually extrapolated from immunization figures derived from school records. In areas where a large number of school-age children are not immunized, there are probably also large numbers of unimmunized younger children, and overall immunization levels in the general population are also likely to be low. School immunization records, however, are not always an accurate indicator of high immunization levels. Because immunization is required for school entry in most places, school-age children may be immunized, while younger children remain unimmu-

TABLE 19–3. **SAMPLE COMMUNITY ASSESSMENT DATA RELATED TO GENETIC INHERITANCE**

Race/Ethnic Group	Male		Female		Total	
	N	*Percent*	*N*	*Percent*	*N*	*Percent*
White non-Hispanic	19,003	56	33,511	58	52,514	57
Hispanic	6,787	20	8,667	15	15,454	17
Asian/Pacific Islander	3,733	11	8,089	14	11,822	13
African American	3,393	10	6,355	11	9,748	11
Native American	1,017	3	1,156	2	2,173	2
Total	33,933	100	57,778	100	91,711	100

nized. For additional data on immunization levels, the nurse might want to examine the records of public immunization clinics as well as those of private physicians who provide immunization services.

Comparison figures on morbidity and mortality at state and national levels can be obtained from state health departments and from various federal publications, respectively. One publication that contains a great deal of information on morbidity and mortality statistics is the *Morbidity and Mortality Weekly Report* published by the Centers for Disease Control. National morbidity and mortality data can also be obtained from health and life insurance companies as well as specialty agencies concerned with specific health problems, such as the American Cancer Society and the American Heart Association. Sample data reflecting a community's physiologic status are presented in Table 19–4. Again, comparison data indicate changes in community health problems over time.

The Psychological Dimension. The psychological environment within the community influences the health of community members by increasing or mediating their exposure to stress and affects the ability of the community to function effectively. In addition, elements of the psychological dimension may enhance or impede community action to resolve identified health problems. Some of the areas to be considered in assessing the psychological environment include the future prospects of the community, significant events in community history and the community's response to those events, communication networks existing within the community, and the adequacy of protective services. Other considerations in this area include evidence of psychological problems such as suicide and homicide rates and identifiable sources of stress within the community.

Learning about a community's prospects helps the nurse gain a clearer picture of the psychological

climate within the community. If a community is growing and productive, for example, apathy regarding community problems is less likely than might be the case if the community is economically depressed and faltering. A community that is in decline or has multiple problems is also more likely to have multiple sources of stress that affect the health of its residents.

Similarly, information about a community's history can provide insight into previous and current health problems and how the community has dealt with them. Historical information may also provide some clue as to how the community will deal with subsequent problems and where community strengths lie. For example, historical information on the cohesive response of community members to a past crisis suggests a strength that will enable the community to face future crises.

The psychological environment created by relationships between subgroups within the community should also be explored. Harmonious relations between groups indicate a psychological climate that is conducive to concerted community action to resolve identified problems. Tension and distrust between groups, on the other hand, may make resolution of community health problems more difficult. The community health nurse should be alert to unrest and conflict between groups within the community and the implications of such psychological tensions for the health of the community and its members.

The adequacy of protective services provided by law enforcement, fire, and other emergency personnel can profoundly influence the psychological climate of an area. Adequate protective services help to create a psychological environment that enhances feelings of personal safety and security. Where these services are inadequate to meet residents' needs, stress and insecurity are created and can negatively influence the health of the population. The nurse assessing the health of a community would obtain information about the availability and quality of police and fire services, as well as information on the availability and adequacy of legal services, services for victims of abuse, and consumer protection services.

Communication is an important contributing factor in the psychological climate of a community, therefore, the nurse should explore the communication network. Communication may be formal or informal. Formal channels include media such as radio, television, and newspapers, as well as the form that public announcements may take. Informal communications take place outside of these channels and may also influence the health of the community. For example, rumors about a particular religious or ethnic group may serve to exacerbate intergroup tension and strife. The degree of trust placed in official formal

TABLE 19–4. SAMPLE COMMUNITY ASSESSMENT DATA RELATED TO PHYSIOLOGIC FUNCTION

Data Element	1995	1985
MORTALITY		
• Cardiovascular death rate (per 100,000 population)	568 deaths	793 deaths
• AIDS death rate (per 100,000 population)	207 deaths	150 deaths
• Cancer death rate (per 100,000 population)	350 deaths	317 deaths
MORBIDITY		
• Measles incidence (per 100,000 population)	35 cases	30 cases
• Hypertension incidence (per 100,000 population)	2,130 cases	2,353 cases
• Hypertension prevalence (per 100,000 population)	8,875 cases	8,038 cases
• Immunization level among school-age children	92%	85%

communications is another element of the psychological dimension that may enhance or detract from community health.

Other indicators of the psychological environment in a community include annual incidence rates for homicide and suicide. Rates for specific subgroups within the community should also be examined, for there is usually considerable variation among different racial and ethnic groups. For example, both suicide and homicide rates are frequently higher for minority group members than for the general population in most communities. Examination of these figures and their distribution in the population may help the nurse to identify factors contributing to poor psychological health in certain subgroups or in the population in general.

Finally, the nurse would want to identify common sources of stress within the environment. Widespread unemployment, lack of available housing, and crowded living conditions are sources of stress in a community. These and other sources of stress serve to create a psychological environment that is not conducive to health.

Information on the psychological dimension of community health is obtained primarily through observations by the community health nurse and through interviews with area residents. Again, it is important to get a broad representation of community membership among the people interviewed. Data about the psychological environment of a rural community with severe problems might include:

- Community population has declined by 15% in the last 5 years
- 25% of the town was destroyed in a tornado and flood 7 years ago; only 20% of the buildings destroyed have been replaced
- 10% of local businesses have gone bankrupt in the last 3 years
- The only local newspaper closed 2 years ago
- There are no radio or television stations in town
- The volunteer fire department is able to respond to fire calls within an average of 15 minutes
- All medical emergency calls receive a response within an average of 20 minutes
- Suicide incidence is 50 per 100,000 population

The Physical Dimension. Physical environmental factors affecting a community include its location, its type (eg, rural, urban, or suburban) and size, topographical features, and climate. Other physical factors to be assessed include the type and adequacy of housing in the community and considerations related to water supply, nuisance factors, and potential for disaster.

The location, climate, and physical geography or topography of the community provide indications of some health problems likely to be identified in the course of the nurse's assessment. An area that is heavily wooded, for example, might increase the index of suspicion for problems such as Rocky Mountain spotted fever and Lyme disease. On the other hand, a dry, arid desert area would be more conducive to problems of heat exhaustion and dehydration.

Size and population density, as well as the type of community, are other factors that influence the types of health problems encountered. Certain health problems are more prevalent in urban areas than in rural ones and vice versa. Statistics indicate that suicide is more prevalent in urban communities, whereas one would expect a problem like rabies to occur more often in a rural area where wild animals are likely to be infected. Urban dwellers are less likely to encounter rabid animals because of regulations regarding vaccination of pets.

Housing is another important physical environmental factor. Inadequate, unsafe, or unsanitary housing conditions contribute to a variety of health problems including communicable diseases spread by poor sanitation, lead poisoning due to lead-based paint in older homes in poor repair, and unintentional injuries resulting from safety hazards. Overcrowding has been found to increase the incidence of a number of health concerns. Communicable diseases are spread more rapidly in crowded conditions, but the prevalence of stress-related conditions such as alcohol abuse, suicide, and other forms of violence increases with crowding as well.

The source of a community's water supply is another important physical environmental consideration. Are most residents supplied by local water systems or do they have independent wells? The nurse should investigate the *potability,* or drinkability, of the community's water. Is the community's water supply safe for drinking, or does it pose biological or chemical hazards to health? Moreover, the nurse should explore the presence or absence of fluoride in the water supply as an indicator of dental health.

Disposal of wastes is another area of consideration in assessing the physical environment of a community. The nurse should ascertain disposal methods for various types of materials. Of particular concern is the disposal of hazardous wastes. Do disposal methods ensure adequate safeguards for the health of the public, or is there potential for environmental pollution as a result of waste disposal? Concerns about hazardous waste disposal were addressed in Chapter 17.

The nurse may also need to assess whether physical factors within the community contribute to accidental injuries. For example, particularly dangerous intersections may be the sites of frequent motor vehicle accidents, or large numbers of swimming pools in the area may contribute to the incidence of drownings.

Nuisance factors such as insects, noxious plants, and other substances may provide physical health hazards or prove offensive to the senses, thereby decreasing the quality of life in the community. Nearby dairy farms, for example, might provide insect breeding grounds that contribute to the incidence of insect-borne diseases. Or there might be an airport that presents a noise hazard. Another consideration in terms of nuisances is the presence of various pollutants in the environment. The effects of pollution and the community health nurse's responsibility with regard to pollution were discussed in Chapter 17. In doing a community assessment, the nurse would obtain information related to the presence of environmental pollutants in the community being served.

Finally, within the community's physical environment there may be the potential for either natural or manmade disasters. Is the community located on a major fault line and subject to earthquakes? Is a chemical manufacturing plant close by that presents a potential hazard? Assessment of the potential for disaster and the community health nurse's role in planning for disaster response are addressed in more detail in Chapter 29.

For the most part, the physical environmental characteristics of a community can be observed. For example, the nurse might drive through the community assessing its geographic features, nuisance factors, and the general adequacy of housing. Information about pollution, water supply, and waste disposal might be obtained from local government bureaus or the nearby public health agency. Data on population size and density are available from census figures or from local government agencies. This information, as well as information on the typical climate and geographic features, may also be available in local publications or from the chamber of commerce. Sample assessment data reflecting features of a rural community's physical environment include:

- 50% of residential units contain lead-based paint
- Annual temperature ranges from 33° to 109° F
- Rabies incidence is 53 per 1000 wild skunks and raccoons
- 13% of local wells are contaminated with pesticides
- Poor maintenance of local roads and wandering livestock pose safety hazards
- 30% of surrounding land is forested; 70% is used for dairy farming
- River running through town floods approximately every 5 years

The Social Dimension. From the previous discussion it is clear that social and psychological dimensions are closely interrelated. Social dimension factors influence the psychological environment and have other effects on health as well. Considerations in assessing the social dimension include information about community government and leadership, language, income and education levels, employment levels and occupations, marital status and family composition, and religion. Other areas to be addressed include transportation and the availability of goods and services needed by residents.

A community's government and power structure are important considerations in terms of planning and implementing programs designed to solve community health problems. Who holds the purse strings? How are decisions made? Who are the decision makers in the community? The community health nurse should discover who are the formal and informal community leaders. In one isolated community, for example, no program was successful unless it first received approval from one elderly matriarch. It was she who controlled the community despite the presence of elected officials.

Information on the community's official leadership can be obtained from the mayor's office or from other local government agencies. Informal leaders may be more difficult to identify, but the nurse can ask key informants in the community (eg, school principals, clergy, and official leaders) who the informal leaders are. Other health care providers and business leaders might also provide information on informal leadership within the community.

Language is another important social factor affecting the health of community members. The nurse should assess the degree to which language presents a barrier to health education or to the provision of other health care services. Again, key informants in the community can provide the nurse with information about languages spoken. School teachers and principals, for example, are knowledgeable about languages spoken by their students. The nurse may also derive this information from personal observation in the community. For example, the nurse may spend time observing stores where large segments of the population shop or check for newspapers and radio and television broadcasts in languages other than English. Another aspect of language to be assessed is the use of colloquialisms by local residents. Are there unique ways in which community members express themselves? Unfortunately, much of this information is gleaned by trial-and-error on the part of the nurse; however, the nurse can ask key informants about the use of colloquialisms and about their meaning.

Closely related to language are the cultural affiliations of community members. The nurse needs to assess the host of cultural factors within the community that affect its health status (see Chapter 16). Information on cultural groups in the community can be obtained from key informants and through observation.

The average income of community residents also has bearing on a community's health status. It has been noted, for example, that there is a near linear relationship between the economic status of the population and certain critical indicators of health (Blane, 1995; Ellencweig, 1992). Economic status influences the ability of residents to provide for basic necessities and to gain access to health care services. In addition, the income of residents influences the tax base of the community and the types of services the community is able to provide its citizens. For example, when many residents are unemployed or have low incomes, they have less money to spend. Businesses take in less money and community revenues from sales and other taxes are decreased. Consequently, the community is less able to provide essential services for its citizens.

Income is closely related to education level. Less well-educated people may have lower paying jobs. They also tend to have less health-related knowledge, and, consequently, lower levels of health. Both income and education levels are indicators of a community's standard of living and, indirectly, of its health status. The prevalence of several acute and chronic conditions in the population (eg, tuberculosis, pneumonia, and heart disease) tends to decline as income and education levels rise. Information on income and education levels can be obtained from census figures. This information may also be available from local government agencies or school districts.

In addition to determining the education level of the population, the nurse assesses the community's education resources. This information enables the nurse to make diagnoses regarding the adequacy of community resources for meeting identified health needs. The telephone directory is a good starting place for obtaining information on education facilities in the area. The nurse can then interview administrators of those facilities or review their brochures and other publications to determine the types of education programs offered. Local school personnel can also provide information on education opportunities in the community.

Because large numbers of people within a community are usually employed, it is important to assess the types of occupations and health hazards involved. Persons in some occupational groups are at higher risk for certain health problems than those in other groups. For example, histoplasmosis is a frequent occurrence among people who work with birds (eg, poultry farmers), and black lung (pneumoconiosis) is prevalent among coal miners. Information about community businesses and industries is available from the local chamber of commerce. The numbers of people employed in specific occupations can be obtained from major employers in the area.

Questions should be asked about other health hazards presented by jobs in the community. Address the potential for exposure to hazardous substances (eg, asbestos and chlorine gas), radiation, noise, or vibration, as well as the potential for injury due to falls or use of hazardous equipment. In addition to determining the potential for occupational injury or illness, the nurse would obtain figures on the extent to which such conditions occur. This type of information may be obtained from the illness and accident records of major employers or may be available from the state occupational health agency.

In addition to information about employment, the level of unemployment in the community provides an indication of possible health problems. Unemployment contributes to stress and to decreased income levels that affect access to health care as well as other necessary goods and services. Unemployment figures can be obtained from state or local employment offices. Occupational data derived from a community assessment might include:

- 10% of the local workforce is unemployed
- 75% of working adults are employed in textile manufacture; 25% are in service occupations
- Local health care workers are at increased risk of HIV exposure because of the high rate of HIV seropositivity in the community
- There is a moderate to severe risk of chemical exposures in the manufacture of synthetic textiles
- 15% of textile workers report significant hearing loss

Religious affiliations within a community can either foster or impede health practices. The nurse should be aware of religious beliefs that may affect health or may influence the acceptability of health programs to community members. For example, some religious groups may be averse to the idea of providing on-site health care services in high schools because of the fear that contraceptive services will be provided (see Chapter 16 for more information on the influence of religion on health). Again, the telephone directory can provide a picture of the religious groups represented in the community, and the membership rosters of specific houses of worship can provide information on the number of people affiliated with each religious group.

Marital status and family composition are social environmental factors that might influence the health of communities. The nurse determines the number of single-parent families and older persons living alone. Generally, married individuals have lower death and illness rates than those who are unmarried; therefore information about marital status in the community can provide clues to overall health status. Information on marriage and family composition is available from census data for the community.

Accessibility of transportation is an important factor related to the use of health services and is, therefore, a necessary component of the nurse's community assessment. Transportation difficulties compound health problems where large numbers of people are poor or elderly, chronically ill or disabled, mothers with small children, and persons who are poorly motivated with respect to health. The nurse can obtain information on the number of families with cars from community census data. Information on other forms of transportation can be gleaned from the telephone directory and by contacting bus and taxi companies to determine routes and fares.

In addition, the community health nurse obtains data on the types and adequacy of goods and services available to community members including recreational programs, local shopping facilities, prices for goods and services, and the social service programs for community members. Much of this information can be obtained through participant observation. For example, the nurse might shop in local stores or look for recreational pursuits. Information about the number and types of stores and services is also available in the telephone directory. Newspaper advertisements provide information on local prices. Finally, the nurse can contact personnel at local social service agencies to obtain information about the services offered. Data related to a community's social environment might include the following information:

- Elected community officials represent the white segment of the population; all have been in office a minimum of 15 years.
- A large influx of Spanish-speaking migrant workers (5000 to 6000 people) occurs every spring.
- The average annual family income of year-round residents is $28,000; the average annual income for migrant families is $12,000.
- The average number of years of school completed by the resident population is 12; for migrant workers, the average is 3.
- 90% of adult residents are married; 60% of the migrant population consists of males without families in the area.

- The town contains 3 elementary schools, 1 junior high school, and 1 high school.
- 90% of the resident population is Protestant (major denominations: Methodist and Lutheran); 80% of the migrant population is Roman Catholic.
- 75% of the residents and 25% of the migrant workers own cars; there is no public transportation available in town.

The Behavioral Dimension. Behavioral factors influence the health status of a community and its members. Areas to be addressed in this portion of the assessment include community consumption patterns, leisure pursuits, and other health-related behaviors.

CONSUMPTION PATTERNS. Consumption patterns play a major part in the development of health or illness. In assessing consumption patterns in the community, the nurse would examine dietary patterns and the use of potentially harmful substances.

Information is needed on the general nutritional level of community members and on specific dietary patterns. For example, the nurse might want to know the prevalence of overweight individuals in the population or the incidence of anemia in school-age children. Another area for consideration is any ethnic nutritional patterns that might influence health either positively or negatively. For example, movement away from traditional tribal foods to typical American dietary practices has contributed to obesity and a variety of chronic diseases among many Native Americans. Information on dietary patterns may be obtained by interviews and surveys of community residents as well as by observation of foods purchased in grocery stores.

The use of harmful substances is another area to explore. The nurse should determine the level of alcohol consumption within the community, both for the community at large and for specific target groups. The extent of both legal and illegal drug use may also merit investigation: the types of substances abused and the typical sources of abused substances. Finally, the nurse would determine the number of residents who smoke and whether that number is increasing or decreasing. Indirect indicators of use of alcohol, drugs, and tobacco include the extent of sales of these items in the community. This information can be obtained from interviews with personnel in stores that sell these items or from information about the related taxes collected. Information on substance abuse may be reflected in law enforcement agencies' records regarding arrests or accidents related to drugs and alcohol. Information can also be obtained on the number of admissions to drug and alcohol treatment facilities. Community self-help groups, such as a local chapter of Alcoholics Anonymous, may also provide information on the extent of substance abuse problems. Data reflecting a community's consumption patterns might include:

- Local diets are typically high in saturated fats due to frying foods; diets are also low in calcium, iron, and vitamin C
- The incidence of moderate to severe anemia is 150 per 1000 children
- Annual per capital alcohol consumption is 3.64 gallons
- 10% of the adult population smoke
- The annual rate of arrests for illicit drug use is 15 per 1000 population
- The annual rate of arrests for driving under the influence of drugs or alcohol is 30 per 1000 population
- The annual death rate for motor vehicle accidents involving alcohol is 202 per 100,000 population
- 35% of all motor vehicle accidents in town are alcohol-related

LEISURE PURSUITS. Information about leisure activities prevalent in the community can also indicate the potential for certain kinds of health problems. For example, boating, waterskiing, and related recreational activities increase the risk of drowning and similar accidents. On the other hand, if watching television is the primary form of recreation, there may be increased potential for heart disease and other conditions associated with a sedentary lifestyle. The presence or absence of recreational opportunities in the community may also affect the psychological environment and the ability of community members to deal with stress effectively. Information on leisure-related exercise is usually obtained by means of interviews and surveys. To determine the extent of community interest in various forms of exercise, the nurse might also contact groups that offer exercise-related classes or sell related equipment. In addition, the nurse can observe for joggers or other exercise enthusiasts as he or she moves about the community. Information on recreational opportunities can be obtained from the telephone directory, from direct observation, and from events publicized in the newspaper or other means of communication employed in the community.

OTHER BEHAVIORS. The community health nurse also assesses the prevalence of other health-related behaviors by community members. For example, the nurse would obtain information on the extent of seat belt use in passenger vehicles or the use of safety devices in certain occupational settings. The nurse would also be interested in such behaviors as the extent of hetero-

sexual and homosexual activity and use of condoms and other forms of protection against conception and sexually transmitted diseases. Two negative indicators of contraceptive use are the proportion of births that are illegitimate and the local abortion rate. In areas with a high prevalence of intravenous drug use, the nurse would also try to obtain information on the extent of needle sharing and other practices that contribute to the spread of diseases such as AIDS and hepatitis. Much of this information is available to the community health nurse only through observation and through interviews of key informants in the community.

The Health System Dimension. Health system factors can profoundly affect the health of a community. Needs assessment in this dimension involves identifying existing services, assessing their level of performance, and identifying areas in which services are lacking (Timmreck, 1995). In assessing the community's well-being, community health nurses would obtain information on the type of health services available to residents. What types of primary, secondary, and tertiary preventive services are available? How adequate are these services to meet the needs of the people? The nurse would examine the availability and accessibility of specific types of services and how effectively they are used. For example, one might inquire as to the percentage of pregnant women who receive prenatal care and at what point in the pregnancy care usually begins. The nurse might also investigate the availability of services provided by emergency medical personnel and by emergency rooms or trauma centers. Other questions relate to the availability and accessibility of certain types of health care providers. For example, there may be several physicians in town, but none of them provide prenatal services because of malpractice concerns.

Information on health care services available in the community may be obtained from the telephone directory and from personal observation. Referral services provided by professional organizations or agencies such as local senior citizens groups can also supply information on health care providers and facilities in the community. Health care institutions are also a source of information on services provided and fees involved. Another source is the *Area Resource File (ARF),* a computerized, county-based data system containing information on available health care professionals, facilities, and education as well as other information. The ARF is maintained by the Office of Data Analysis and Management of the federal Health Resources and Services Administration.

The nurse would also determine to what extent available services are overused or underused. What factors contribute to overuse and to underuse? For example, emergency room services might be overused because many community members cannot afford a regular source of health care and seek care only in crisis situations. Conversely, the services of clinics and physicians might be underused because they are offered at inconvenient times or places or because people have no means of transportation to such services. Or, residents may simply not be aware of the need for or availability of certain services. Utilization figures can be obtained from health care facilities and providers in the community.

Another area for consideration is the financing of community health care. Questions to be addressed include who pays for health care services, adequacy of funding sources for meeting community health needs, priority given to health-related concerns in planning community budgetary allocations, extent of health insurance coverage among community members, and availability of funds to pay for care for the indigent (see Chapter 14). Information on health insurance may be available from insurance agencies or major health care facilities in the area. Health care facility records may also contain data on the percentage of the population without health insurance. Information about recipients of Medicaid and Medicare benefits is available from the agencies that administer these programs.

Financing of health care can also provide an indirect indication of prevailing community attitudes toward health. For example, adequate health care budgeting indicates that health is considered a public priority. Budgetary information can be solicited from public officials. Other considerations related to the health care system include community definitions of health and illness and the use of culturally prescribed health practices and practitioners. Community assessment data related to the health care system might include:

- 10% of the local government's budget is allocated to health services
- Local insurance coverage is as follows:
  Eligible for military health care services—15%
  Covered by Medicare/Medicaid—30%
  Covered by private insurance—43%
  Uninsured—12%
- Only 3% of private health care providers accept Medicaid
- 70% of Medicaid-reimbursable services are provided in emergency departments
- Civilian health care providers in town include:
  Family practice physicians—3
  Internist—1

  Pediatricians—2
  Dermatologist—1
  Cardiologist—1
  Neurosurgeon—1
  Orthopedist—1
  Obstetrician/gynecologist—1
  Osteopath—1
  Advanced practice nurses—5 (1 nurse midwife, 2 pediatric nurse practitioners, 2 family nurse practitioners)
- There is one hospital in town; its utilization rate is 85% of capacity
- The local emergency medical service receives an average of 3440 calls per month

A tool for assessing the health status of a community from the perspective of biophysical, psychological, physical, social, behavioral, and health system dimensions is included in Appendix I, Health Intervention Planning Guide—Community Client.

Dimensions of a Target Group Assessment

Similar factors are considered in assessing the health of a target group. Biophysical, psychological, physical, social, behavioral, and health system elements influence the health of subgroups in the population as well as the total population.

The Biophysical Dimension.   In examining human biological factors, the nurse would obtain information on the age, race, and sex composition of the target group. Other necessary information in this category relates to the incidence and prevalence of specific health conditions among group members. For example, the incidence of alcohol abuse is particularly high among Native Americans, whereas tuberculosis is prevalent among Asian refugee groups.

Mortality data related to the group, such as the crude death rate, cause-specific death rates, and age-specific death rates, are also important. For example, the infant mortality rate for African Americans in 1993 was more than twice that of white infants (U.S. Department of Commerce, 1996). Similarly, homicide death rates are seven times as high for African American males as white males (U.S. Department of Health and Human Services, 1996).

The Psychological, Physical, and Social Dimensions.   Assessment of a target group would entail identification of special concerns in the physical, psychological, and social dimensions that influence the health of the group. For example, if preschool children are the target group, special attention would be given to home safety factors. Similar considerations would be appropriate to

ASSESSMENT TIPS: Assessing the Community or Target Group

Biophysical Dimension

Age

What is the age composition of the population?

What is the community's annual birth rate?

What are the age-specific death rates in the community?

What is the average age at death of community members?

Genetic Inheritance

What is the racial composition of the population?

What is the relative proportion of men and women in the community? In specific age groups?

What genetically determined illnesses, if any, are prevalent in the community?

Physiologic Function

What are the cause-specific mortality rates for the community?

What physiologic conditions are prevalent in the community?

What is the extent of disability within the community?

What is the overall immunization level in the community?

How does the community compare with state and national morbidity and mortality figures?

Psychological Dimension

What stressors are present in the community?

How does the community deal with crisis?

What significant events have occurred in the history of the community? What was the community's response to those events?

What are the community's prospects for the future?

How cohesive is the community? Is there evidence of tension between groups in the community?

How adequate are protective services in the community?

What are the formal communication channels in the community? The informal channels?

What are the prevalence rates for mental illnesses in the community?

What is the community homicide rate? Suicide rate?

What are the rates of crime in the community? What types of crimes are prevalent?

Physical Dimension

What type of community is this (eg, rural, urban)?

Where is the community located? How large is the community? How densely populated?

What topographical features could influence the health of community members?

What is the local climate like? How might climate affect health in the community?

What is the quality of housing in the community? Is affordable housing available? Are dwellings in good repair?

What is the community's source of water?

Is the community water supply adequate to meet community needs? Is it safe for consumption?

How does the community handle waste disposal? Does waste disposal pose health hazards?

What plants and animals are common in the area? Do they pose health hazards for community members?

Is there evidence of environmental pollution that may affect health?

Are there nuisance factors present in the community? If so, what are they? How do they affect health?

Is there potential for disaster in the community? If so, what kind of disasters are likely? What is the extent of community disaster preparation?

Social Dimension

Governance and Leadership

How are community decisions made? Who makes them?

Who holds power in the community? How is that power exercised?

What is the community's governance structure? How effective is community governance?

Who are the formal and informal leaders in the community?

Culture and Religion

What cultural groups are represented in the community?

What languages are spoken by community members?

What cultural beliefs and behaviors are prevalent in the community?

What is the character of relationships between members of different cultural groups in the community?

What religious affiliations are represented in the community? What effect do they have on community life and health?

Socioeconomic Status

What is the education level of community members?

What education resources and facilities are present in the community?

What is the income level and distribution within the community?

(continued)

ASSESSMENT TIPS: Assessing the Community or Target Group (cont.)

What is the rate of unemployment in the community?

Who are the major employers in the community?

What kinds of occupations are represented within the community?

What occupational health hazards are present in the community?

Other Factors

How accessible is transportation in the community?

What is the marital status of community members?

What is the typical family structure in the community?

How accessible are goods and services to community members?

Behavioral Dimension

Consumption Patterns

What are the usual food preferences and consumption patterns in the community?

What is the nutritional level in the community? What percentage of the population is overweight? Underweight?

What is the extent of drug abuse in community? What drugs are abused? How easy is it to obtain drugs?

What is the extent of alcohol and tobacco sales in the community?

What is the prevalence of arrests related to alcohol and other drugs?

What is the extent of smoking in the community?

What is the rate of hospital admissions for health problems related to alcohol, drug, and tobacco use?

Exercise and Leisure

What exercise opportunities are available to community members? To what extent are they utilized?

What opportunities for leisure activity are present in the community?

Do typical community leisure activities pose any health or safety hazards?

Sexual Practices

What is the attitude of the community to sexual activity? To homosexuality?

What is the extent of homosexuality in the community?

What is the prevalence of unsafe sexual practices in the community?

What is the extent of contraceptive use in the community?

Other Behaviors

To what extent do community members engage in safety practices (eg, seat belt use)?

Health System Dimension

What types of primary, secondary, and tertiary preventive services are available in the community? How accessible are these services to community members?

Are the types of services available adequate to meet community health needs?

Are available services culturally relevant to members of the population?

To what extent are available health care services utilized? What barriers to service utilization exist in the community?

Are there folk health services available in the community? To what extent do members of the community use folk health services?

What is the level and quality of interaction between folk and scientific health care systems in the community?

How are health care services financed? What proportion of the population has health insurance?

What level of priority is given to health care services in budgeting local funds?

What are community attitudes toward health care services and providers?

the assessment of the physical environment for a group of elderly clients.

In addition to concerns with the psychological environment discussed earlier, the nurse assessing a target group would examine the effects of attitudes toward group members on their health. For example, society's attitude toward drug abusers creates a psychological environment that makes resolution of the problem difficult. Because of the stigma attached to drug abuse and the potential for incarceration, drug abusers may not seek help for their problem. Nor are they likely to seek screening services for HIV infection despite their increased risk of infection via needle sharing and other practices. Social dimension concerns are similar to those considered in the assessment of a community.

The Behavioral Dimension. Specific behavioral factors may also need to be considered in the assessment of a target group. For example, cultural factors might greatly influence the dietary patterns of some target groups such as Latinos. As noted earlier, were the target group drug abusers, the nurse would want to assess behaviors such as needle sharing that put this group at higher risk for specific diseases such as AIDS and hepatitis. Similarly, sexual activity would be a more pressing concern were the target group adolescents rather than a group of preschoolers.

The Health System Dimension. Specific health system factors can influence the health of some target groups more than others. For example, the unwillingness of many health care providers to work in rural areas creates an influence on health not found in urban populations. Similarly, fear and anxiety on the part of some health care providers may lead to their refusal to care for clients with AIDS, thereby further decreasing this population's access to necessary health care services.

In assessing a target group, the nurse often obtains data similar to those needed to assess the health of a community. Depending on the particular target group, however, some of the data that would be obtained regarding a community may not be relevant. For example, information on employment and education levels is not relevant to an infant target group. Likewise, there may be information specific to the target group that one would not necessarily obtain in assessing a community, as was the case with the information about needle sharing among a group of drug users. A general tool that can be used to assess the health status of a target group is provided in Appendix J, the Health Intervention Planning Guide—Target Group. The tool can be adapted to fit the needs of a particular target group to provide the information needed for the community health nurse to derive nursing diagnoses and to plan interventions to meet group health needs.

Diagnostic Reasoning and Group Health Status

The collection of data on factors influencing the health status of a community or a target group is the first step in identifying group health needs. To be of any value, the data must be interpreted and analyzed to derive nursing diagnoses. In other words, assessment data are used to identify health-related needs that are amenable to nursing action. Needs are deficits between a desired state of affairs and the actual situa-

tions (Loos, 1996). Community nursing diagnoses reflect discrepancies between needs and the community's ability to meet those needs. Community or group nursing diagnoses should reflect existing, emerging, and potential threats to public health, as well as community and group strengths or competencies.

Diagnostic reasoning in the care of communities involves comparing community needs assessment data to identified standards to uncover community or group health problems. One type of standard that may be used in data analysis is the general health status of the state or the nation. For example, the community health nurse can compare data for the community or target group with data for the state or the nation as a whole. In doing so, the nurse might ask the following questions: How does this group stand in relation to the larger population on a variety of measures of health status? Is the local birth rate higher or lower than that of the state or the nation? How do death rates compare? For example, the southern region of Georgia is considered the "stroke belt" because the death rate for cerebrovascular accidents far exceeds that of the rest of the nation. Do morbidity rates for various illnesses exceed national and state rates? How do income and education levels compare?

Another standard with which to compare present data is found in the history of the community or target group. How do current rates compare with those of a year ago? Five years ago?

Members' perceptions of areas of need are a third type of standard with which to compare the data gathered. What health problems are mentioned in interviews with group members? What problems are perceived by other health care professionals and community or target group leaders? What are the expectations of the community or target group regarding these problems?

Diagnostic reasoning gives rise to statements of health needs or risk in the population. A second stage of community diagnosis involves a comparison of the health care needs identified and the resources available to meet those needs. This may be referred to as a diagnosis of "need–service match" or mismatch (Porter, 1987). Data for this level of nursing diagnosis would be found in the nurse's assessment of the health care system. If the community health nurse found community health care resources inadequate to meet the needs posed by the increased risk of suicide in a vulnerable population, he or she would make a diagnosis of "need–service mismatch due to inadequate (or inaccessible) suicide prevention services."

The nurse might also make positive diagnoses related to the health status of a community or target group. For example, a preliminary diagnosis might indicate a vulnerable population group (eg, children) at risk for certain health problems (such as communicable diseases). Examination of assessment data, however, might indicate that there are few problems with immunizable childhood diseases because of easy accessibility of immunization services and high immunization levels in the population. In this situation, the nurse's diagnosis might be a "need–service match due to accessibility and use of immunization services."

Planning the Dimensions of Health Care for Groups and Communities

Whenever a diagnosis of need–service mismatch is made, planning to meet the unmet need is warranted, and the community health nurse should become involved in planning health care delivery programs to meet the identified needs of the population. The importance of systematic planning for health care services was succinctly put in the comment "Failing to plan is like planning to fail" (Terry, 1992). Systematic planning is essential to effective health care programming. The importance of community health nurses' involvement in planning was noted by the Secretary of the U.S. Department of Health and Human Services Commission on Nursing (1988). Community health nurses, in particular, are aware of community health needs and of the kinds of programs that will be acceptable to members of target populations. The process used in planning health programs is similar to that used to plan care for other types of clients but is somewhat more involved. Considerations in planning at the group level include setting priorities, determining the level of prevention involved in meeting identified health needs, and developing health care programs to meet those needs.

Setting Priorities

Once nursing diagnoses have been derived, they must be assigned priority for intervention. The community health nurse, along with other health care providers, must be able to set priorities that allow for the best use of available resources. This is even more important when the client is a community or a target group than in the care of individuals or families, because care of communities and target groups usually necessitates a greater expenditure of resources than care of an individual. This frequently means that only the highest-priority needs will be addressed because of limited resources available.

Prioritization has been described as a process of superimposing the values and expectations of the community on the findings of the needs assessment (Timmreck, 1995). This means that priorities may need to be based as much on local value systems as on the concerns of health care providers (Rohrer, 1996). The criteria used to prioritize community or target group needs are essentially the same as those used in working with individuals and families: (1) severity of the threat to the community's health, (2) degree of the community's concern about the need, and (3) extent to which meeting one need depends on meeting other needs.

It is likely that the priorities of the community or target group involve needs that are easily perceived. Community health nurses may find that they must deal first with a need they consider relatively minor, but which is of concern to the community, before tackling other more major problems. In other words, the nurse must establish credibility with the community before he or she can expect community support for subsequent efforts.

The process of assigning priority to the health needs identified in a community assessment involves the development of criteria for decision making, establishing standards for minimally acceptable levels of the criteria, and assigning weights to the criteria (Loos, 1996). For example, a high priority problem will usually meet criteria of severity, significant community concern, and high cost to society. A standard for severity might be that a minimum of 20% of the population be affected by the problem; whereas significant community concern would be evident if 10% of community members surveyed mentioned a particular problem as needing attention. Possible standards for cost to society might be the number of days of lost school or work attendance or the actual monetary cost for medical treatment for the problem. Each of these three criteria (and others developed) would be given a weight reflecting its relative importance in decisions about priorities. For example, high societal cost might be given greater value than the level of community concern about a given problem. All of the problems identified in the community needs assessment would be evaluated in terms of the weighted criteria, and those with higher priority scores would be addressed first in efforts to resolve community health problems.

Determining the Level of Prevention

Programs for meeting the health needs of communities or target groups may be needed at any of the three levels of prevention.

Primary Prevention Programs.   Primary prevention programs are designed to promote the health of the population and prevent specific illnesses. An exercise program for senior citizens is an example of a health promotion program aimed at a target group. Community education programs on water safety or prevention of accidents in the home are primary preventive measures for a community. Primary prevention involves education programs of any kind designed to promote the public's overall health. For example, parenting classes for expectant couples could help prevent child abuse, and sex education in the school system could minimize problems of adolescent pregnancy and sexually transmitted diseases. Immunization programs are another example of primary prevention for a community or target group.

Secondary Prevention Programs.   Secondary prevention involves identifying and resolving existing health problems in members of the community or target group. Specific secondary interventions may focus on screening programs or control programs for community health problems.

SCREENING PROGRAMS.   One major area of program planning related to secondary prevention for communities and target groups is the development of screening programs. *Screening* is the preliminary examination or testing of a person to determine whether or not he or she might have a particular condition and whether further diagnostic testing is indicated. Screening procedures are not diagnostic. Instead, they serve to indicate the possibility that a particular disease or condition is present. Positive screening test results are always an indication of the need for further diagnostic procedures. Screening is frequently used with large population groups because it is considerably less expensive than conducting a battery of diagnostic tests when the majority of people can be expected to have negative results. Screening procedures are available and recommended for breast and cervical cancer, testicular cancer, colorectal cancer, skin cancer, hypertension, and diabetes. Screening may also be done for several sexually transmitted diseases such as syphilis and gonorrhea and for the human immunodeficiency virus (HIV) that causes AIDS. Screening for tuberculosis is also available. Another form of screening is the periodic health examination in which the person is examined for signs and symptoms of several common diseases.

Several factors need to be considered in decisions to implement large-scale screening programs. These factors can be divided into three groups: (1) considerations regarding the condition that is being screened, (2) considerations regarding the test itself, and (3) considerations related to the target group for the program. Any condition for which screening is warranted should have several characteristics. First, the condition should affect a sufficient number of people to make screening cost-effective. Second, the condition should be a relatively serious condition. For example, although it would be cost-effective to screen for the common cold because of the number of people affected, the effects of colds are usually minor and thus do not justify screening. The third consideration is the availability of an acceptable treatment. It is not realistic, generally speaking, to screen for a disease for which there is no treatment. (A significant exception to this criterion is screening for HIV infection. In this case, knowledge of being HIV-positive allows the infected individual to take precautions that can help limit the spread of the disease and minimize its effects.) Fourth, there should be a significant preclinical period between the time of exposure and the development of clinical symptoms to allow for treatment before the person becomes symptomatic. Finally, early diagnosis and treatment need to make a difference. If the outcome is the same whether the condition is treated early or late in its course, there is no point in screening. If, on the other hand, earlier treatment increases the chances of being cured, as is the case in breast cancer, then screening is appropriate.

The second group of factors influencing decisions for mass screening relates to the screening test itself. These factors are the sensitivity and specificity of the screening test as well as the cost, ease of administration, and acceptability of the procedure. *Sensitivity* refers to the ability of the test to identify accurately those persons with the disease (Harkness, 1995). A sensitive screening test would be able to detect the presence of a condition even when very little of the indicator that the test reacts to is present. For example, if a screening test relies on the presence of a particular substance in the blood, a sensitive test would give a positive result even when a small amount of that substance is present. The *specificity* of a screening test reflects the extent to which it excludes those who do not have the disease (Harkness, 1995). A positive result on a highly specific test would indicate the potential presence of only one condition, rather than two or three possible conditions.

Other considerations with respect to the screening test itself are cost, ease of administration, and acceptability. Screening tests should be relatively inexpensive compared with specific diagnostic tests. They should also be easy to administer to large groups of people and not require expensive or sophisticated equipment to conduct the test. Finally, the test should be acceptable to those who are intended to participate in the screening. This means that the test should not be overly painful, embarrassing, or anxiety-provok-

► DISEASE, TEST, AND TARGET GROUP
CONSIDERATIONS IN SCREENING

Disease Considerations

The disease affects a sufficient number of people to make
screening cost-effective.

The disease is relatively serious.

An effective treatment is available for the disease.

The preclinical period is sufficient to allow treatment before
symptoms occur.

Early diagnosis and treatment make a difference in terms of
outcome.

Test Considerations

The screening test is sensitive enough to detect most cases of
the disease.

The screening test is specific enough to exclude most other
causes of positive results.

The screening test costs little, is easy to administer, and has
minimal side effects.

Target Group Considerations

The target group is identifiable.

The target group is accessible.

ing. The test should not have objectionable side effects. It would be unwarranted to screen people using
a test whose potential side effects are worse than the
symptoms of the disease in question.

Another consideration in deciding for or against
mass screening projects is the population to be
screened. The target group must be identifiable and
accessible to screeners. If the target group for screening is not easily identifiable, screening programs may
not reach those most in need. Adult women, for example, have been identified as being vulnerable to breast
and cervical cancer, and this population can easily be
screened for these conditions during the course of
routine check-ups for all adult women. If the appropriate target group is less easily identified or unlikely
to come forward (eg, intravenous drug users or homosexuals), screening programs are less likely to be successful.

When conditions related to the illness, the
screening test, and the target population are met,
large-scale screening programs can prove worthwhile.
When these conditions are not met, screening is unlikely to be effective in improving the health of communities. Disease, test, and target group considerations in planning large-scale screening programs are
summarized above.

CONTROL PROGRAMS.   Some of the same programs described as primary preventive measures may also be
employed in secondary prevention designed to alleviate existing health problems. When a community or
target group is already experiencing a high rate of sexually transmitted diseases (STDs), education on the
transmission and prevention of STDs would be a secondary preventive measure. The intent of the program is to control an existing problem (high rate of
STD), rather than prevent a problem from occurring.

The kind of secondary prevention programs
planned for a given community or target group varies
with the types of problems identified in the assessment. For example, if child abuse is prevalent in the
community, parenting classes for abusive parents
would be an appropriate secondary preventive measure. Similarly, if there is a high rate of hypertension
among group members, clinics could be established to
screen for, diagnose, and treat this problem. In another community, a program to enforce seat belt legislation could be used as a secondary preventive measure for a high rate of motor vehicle accident fatalities.

Tertiary Prevention Programs.   Tertiary prevention programs
for communities or target groups are designed to prevent complications of identified problems or prevent
the recurrence of a problem. For example, if a community is experiencing an epidemic of measles, mass immunization programs to control the epidemic would
be used as a secondary preventive measure. When the
epidemic is under control, a program designed to
maintain immunity levels among community members would be a tertiary preventive measure designed
to thwart future epidemics.

Tertiary prevention is also designed to prevent
consequences of existing problems. For example,
when an earthquake occurs and safe water supplies
are limited, programs to conserve or to purify water
help to limit additional health effects of the earthquake that may arise from drinking contaminated
water.

Planning the Health Program

Planning is a collaborative and systematic process
used to attain a goal. Planning is collaborative in the
sense that persons who will be affected by the
planned program need to be involved in its planning.
It is systematic in that change is consciously and deliberately brought about.

Some authors differentiate among several levels
of planning including normative planning, strategic
planning, and tactical or operational planning. *Normative planning* deals with the level of policy planning and focuses on the general directions that health

care planning should take (Dever, 1991). Normative planning is long range and comprehensive. *Strategic planning* focuses on action that can be taken to achieve desired goals and is somewhat more specific than normative planning. Expected outcomes of strategic planning include clarification of future directions, development of resource allocation priorities, examination of alternative courses of action, development of a sound basis for decisions, and rapid adjustment to changing conditions (Lantz, Fullerton, & Dowling, 1993). *Tactical planning* brings planning to the program operation level in terms of how specific health care services will be provided (Dever, 1991). This last level is the main focus of planning in the remainder of this chapter.

Reasons for Planning.   Until fairly recently, health care programs were designed and implemented with little regard for principles of planning. Why the recent concern with planned efforts in terms of health care? For one thing, those in the health care professions are coming to realize that limited resources are available. Grass roots popular movements have done a great deal to curb government spending and have brought this realization home quite forcefully. Adequate planning helps to ensure that limited resources are used most effectively with the least waste possible.

A second concern is that consumers are demanding organized planning efforts into which they have some input. Gone are the days when taxpayers provided money on request. They now require adequate justification for the expenditure of tax dollars. Another consideration in the push for organized planning efforts is the psychological impact of planning. Systematic planning allows people to feel that they are in control. In an age when much of daily life seems dictated by circumstances beyond one's control, concerted efforts at program planning allow some degree of say over one's destiny. Finally, planning encourages health care professionals and community members to take positive steps to ensure health rather than wait for events to dictate the future state of the community's health.

General Principles of Program Planning.   Several general principles of program planning have been identified in the literature. Program planning should be population-based. In other words, health programs planned should be appropriate to the population to be served and based on an understanding of the community's circumstances and the health problems experienced.

Also very important is that the community, as well as health care professionals, should be actively involved in developing solutions to health problems. Eliciting community participation in planning may in-

▶ GENERAL PRINCIPLES
OF PROGRAM PLANNING
··

- Planning must be population-based and include broad community participation.
- The community must share responsibility for health problems and their solution.
- Planning should be based on epidemiologic and scientific data.
- Multiple interventions are needed to deal with the multiple causes of most community health problems.
- Planning should focus on both long-term and short-term change.
- Planning should balance needs and resources.
- Planning should be based on a recognition of the interactive nature of influences on health.
- Planning should be flexible.

volve *community activation*, a process of coordinating various segments of the community to increase awareness of health problems and to mobilize resources for dealing with them (Wickizer, et al., 1993). Community activation begins with a feeling of dissatisfaction with present circumstances, an awareness of the need for change, and a desire for change to occur. This is followed by a group decision to take action and concerted and collaborative planning of the action that is to be taken. The activation process concludes with action taken and a sense of satisfaction with its outcome. Community health nurses may need to actively promote the process of community activation to facilitate community participation in health care planning.

Programs should be based on epidemiologic and scientific data. Epidemiologic data suggest factors contributing to health problems that might be amenable to intervention. Research findings from the social sciences should also be used to plan programs that are acceptable to community residents.

Multiple approaches are often needed to address health problems arising from multiple causes. For this reason, planning should focus on both long-term and short-term outcomes that address the multiple contributing factors involved. Planning should also balance community needs and resources, and should make the best use of those resources to resolve identified health problems.

Planning should be based on a recognition of the interaction of multiple factors influencing health. This suggests that interventions encompassing the health care sector alone may not be comprehensive enough to resolve health care problems. For this reason a wide variety of societal segments should be involved in health problem resolution. This means that intersectoral components of the community must work collaboratively rather than in isolation.

Broad community participation in health program planning has several advantages. Extensive participation promotes multiple points of view and may generate a wider array of potential solutions to community problems. Broad participation also leads to better refinement of programs and greater acceptance within the community. With multiple agencies and segments of society involved, there is also less chance for duplication of existing programs and more effective use of community resources. Finally, broad community participation enhances community abilities for self-advocacy via the community activation process (Loos, 1996).

Finally, health care planning should be flexible enough to accommodate changes in community circumstances. This necessitates the development of broad strategies that can be implemented in a variety of ways. Flexibility may also require the interchangeability of some health care personnel within a plan, for example, using both physicians and nurse practitioners to provide primary care services to underserved populations.

The Planning Process.   The process of planning health care programs for groups of people involves several discrete activities. These include selecting the planning group, developing planning competence, formulating a philosophy, establishing program goals, developing alternative solutions, evaluating alternatives and selecting a solution, and developing program objectives. Other planning activities are identifying resources, delineating actions required to accomplish objectives, evaluating the plan, and planning evaluation. These activities may or may not occur in the sequence in which they are presented here, but may occur simultaneously or in a slightly different order. What is important is that each one does occur at some point in the process.

SELECTING THE PLANNING GROUP.   Those involved in planning should include key community or target group members expected to benefit from the program (Dees & Garcia, 1995). Potential beneficiaries of the program need to feel a sense of "ownership" of the program. For example, if the health need is one arising from adolescent sexuality (eg, high incidence rates for STDs among teenagers), adolescents should be encouraged to provide input into planning a viable program to meet the need. They are the best judges of what will be acceptable to themselves and to their peers.

Other categories of persons to be included in the planning group depend, to a certain extent, on the type of problem to be solved; however, some general guidelines may prove helpful. It is wise to involve diverse segments of the community whenever possible to provide a widespread base of support for the resulting program. Individuals who have the authority to deal with the problem should certainly be included in the planning group. Those in a position to promote acceptance of the program such as media representatives, key community leaders, and influential citizens should also be invited to participate.

Another group that should be involved are those who are going to implement whatever program is planned. For example, if the program involves some type of educational campaign, local educators should be included in the planning process. Experts knowledgeable about the problem should also be included. These individuals can contribute to the group's understanding of the problem and provide knowledge of possible alternative solutions.

Both implementer and expert categories may involve health care professionals. The need to involve health care professionals in planning health care programs may seem obvious, but there are some additional, not so obvious, advantages to their inclusion in the planning group. In addition to providing technical input into the plan, health care professionals, especially community health nurses, have insights into local health care practices that affect problem resolution either positively or negatively. Furthermore, they can help legitimize the program and foster its acceptance in the community. Finally, health care professionals may be able to make the structural changes in the community's health care system that will be required for a successful program.

The last category of persons who should be involved in planning are individuals or groups who are likely to resist the program. This is one effective way of reducing opposition. Once these people have contributed to a plan that is acceptable to them, they are usually committed to the program and will work toward its acceptance by others.

DEVELOPING PLANNING COMPETENCE.   Once the planning group is assembled, the first step in program planning is developing necessary planning competence. Few health care professionals or consumers have any educational background or experience in program planning. For this reason, the community health nurse may find it necessary to educate members of the planning group in regard to planning processes and activities. It may also be necessary to prevent the group from engaging in activities for which an adequate foundation has yet to be provided. In doing so, the community health nurse needs to exercise well-developed skills in leadership and group dynamics addressed in Chapter 12.

FORMULATING A PHILOSOPHY. The next step, formulating a philosophy, is not often carried out as a conscious activity, but is an assumption on the part of group members. For example, there must be some type of commitment to adequate health care for prison inmates before a group would even consider planning a program to meet prisoners' needs. It is, however, important that the philosophies of various members of the planning group be compatible. Therefore, group members should be encouraged to verbalize their philosophies and to identify and deal with areas of conflict between philosophies.

ESTABLISHING PROGRAM GOALS. Goals flow from the group's philosophy and describe the overall intent of the group with respect to the problem to be solved. Again, goals must be developed by the group as a whole to ensure consistency. Goals are usually stated in general terms as a desired ultimate outcome. In the prison example, a possible goal might be "to provide adequate health care services for inmates." This goal, stated very generally, gives no indication of possible means of achieving the desired outcome. Objectives, on the other hand, are stated as specific expected outcomes that contribute in some way to realizing the goal. Objectives are discussed more thoroughly later in this chapter.

DEVELOPING ALTERNATIVE SOLUTIONS. The next step in the program planning process is developing alternative solutions to the identified health need. Here the planning group should be encouraged to exercise creativity in attempts to develop alternatives. A suggestion that appears absurd on first presentation may be found to be quite feasible on investigation. In appropriate alternatives will eventually be eliminated during the next step of the planning process—evaluation of alternatives in terms of critical criteria for problem resolution.

EVALUATING ALTERNATIVES AND SELECTING A SOLUTION. As noted in Chapter 7, one of the components in the planning stage of the nursing process is the development of critical criteria against which any solution to a particular problem must be weighed. Critical criteria for solutions are also required when the client is a community or target group rather than an individual or a family. Examples of critical criteria for solutions to community problems might be that such solutions fit within available budgetary resources or that they be acceptable to ethnic or religious groups within the community.

Potential solutions to community problems should always be evaluated in terms of cost, feasibility, acceptability, availability of necessary resources, efficiency, equity, political advantage, and identifiability of the target group. Generally speaking, an alternative that costs less will be viewed more favorably, other factors being equal, than one that costs more. Or, one alternative may be selected over another because its implementation is more feasible. For example, it is considerably easier to install a traffic light at an accident-prone intersection than to build a bridge to route one intersecting road over the other.

Potential solutions should also be evaluated in terms of their acceptability to policy makers, implementers, and the community. Policy makers are unlikely to approve an alternative that diminishes their power or authority, and implementers are certainly unlikely to accept a potential solution that requires them to work overtime or without pay if another alternative is available. Similarly, community members affected by the proposed program may find one alternative more acceptable than another for a variety of reasons.

Alternative solutions may also differ in terms of the resources needed to implement them. Generally speaking, an alternative that requires fewer resources or for which resources are already available is more likely to be endorsed than one that requires extensive or scarce resources. For example, a group seeking to improve the nutritional status of schoolchildren may select an alternative that makes use of existing facilities used to prepare meals for senior citizens rather than one that necessitates providing kitchen facilities in each school. Efficiency is a related criterion on which alternative solutions to a particular problem can be evaluated. An efficient alternative makes better use of available resources and is usually viewed more favorably in making planning decisions than an inefficient one.

Questions of equity also arise in evaluating alternative solutions to a problem. Alternatives that unfairly discriminate against one segment of the population are usually rejected. For example, one alternative to the problem of dealing with teen pregnancy might be to provide contraceptive services in the larger high schools. If, however, these schools tend to serve the upper-middle-class segment of the community while lower-class students attend smaller schools, this alternative would discriminate against a segment of the community also needing service.

Political consequences also need to be considered in evaluating the alternative solutions to specific problems. For instance, an alternative plan that provides services to a highly vocal voting bloc might be viewed more favorably by politicians than one that serves a less politically involved minority group. Evaluation of alternatives may also involve forecasting regarding the effects of other possible events on the problem or its solution. For example, if a vaccine for HIV infection is likely to be available in the near future, the community may not want to put a lot of resources into a condom promotion program.

Finally, alternative solutions should be evaluated in terms of the identifiability of the target group. One potential solution for preventing the spread of AIDS might be to screen all prostitutes in the community for HIV infection. It is somewhat difficult, however, to identify this group of people, as prostitution is an illegal activity in most places. It might be easier to screen everyone who requests services for STDs because this group is sexually active and is also identifiable.

The community health nurse should assist the planning group to determine the relative weight to be given to each of these considerations in evaluating alternative solutions. Those considerations that are weighted most heavily become the critical criteria against which all potential solutions are evaluated. The remaining considerations are those that are nice if they can be met, but not absolutely necessary. For example, if there is an unlimited source of funding for dealing with certain types of problems, cost might not be a critical criterion for selecting a solution to the problem in question. Or, it may be that criteria of cost, feasibility, and acceptability are considered critical and others are viewed as less important. Once the criteria have been established, the group can proceed to evaluate all of the potential solutions generated and select the one most appropriate to the situation.

Consideration of possible sources of opposition also contributes to selection of the most appropriate alternative. If it is known that members of the community PTA would vigorously oppose a "sex fair" as a means of educating adolescents on sexual issues, another less threatening alternative would be more appropriate.

There are two basic types of opposition to proposed programs: rational and irrational. Rational opposition is based on sound reasoning and should be seriously considered, as it may prove beneficial to the planning effort. Rational opposition does pose problems to the extent that it lends support to irrational opposition and also tends to sway individuals who are undecided as to the merits of the planned program.

Irrational opposition can arise from several sources. It may result from a general attitude of conservatism in which only proven interventions are held to be acceptable. As a rule, conservatives usually discount innovative ideas as possible solutions and prefer to remain with more traditional approaches.

The second type of irrational opposition arises out of cultural patterns and social reactions to change in general. For example, agricultural change programs initiated by Peace Corps volunteers in India were considerably less successful than programs fostering small industries. The farmers were responding to centuries of culturally ingrained patterns of farming, whereas the small businessmen were engaged in pursuits that held no strong cultural connotations.

Opposition may also arise from perceptions that a particular course of action poses a threat to the power, prestige, or economic security of certain members in or outside of a group or community. For example, starting a clinic staffed by nurse practitioners to improve the accessibility of health care may be seen by local physicians as a threat to their economic security.

Another source of irrational opposition is usually unconscious in nature and results from feelings of overall vulnerability. This type of opposition is usually found in the same group of people, whatever the issue addressed. Because of their own personal insecurity, change of any type may be threatening to these individuals.

Additional sources of resistance to health care programs include reluctance to spend money on health care, legal obstacles across jurisdictions, and unreasoning self-reliance. Reluctance to spend money can often be overcome by accurate documentation of the costs of the problem and the cost-effectiveness of problem resolution. For example, a county sheriff's department got council approval for a nursing clinic in the county jail by documenting the decrease in the cost of health care for prisoners when a nurse was available.

Jurisdictional obstacles can be overcome by including in the planning body persons with authority and prestige in the problem area. Pride or unreasoning self-reliance can also be an obstacle to utilization of health programs. For this reason, any alternative selected must be acceptable to the group for which it is designed. One method of accomplishing this is including members of the target group in the planning body.

DEVELOPING PROGRAM OBJECTIVES.   Once alternative solutions have been evaluated in light of critical criteria and a solution selected, the process of planning a specific program based on that alternative begins. At this point, the planning group sets specific program objectives. Objectives are statements of specific outcomes expected to result from the program that contribute to the realization of the overall goal.

For objectives to be useful, they should meet several criteria (Timmreck, 1995). Perhaps the most essential of these is that the objective be clearly stated and measurable. A well-stated objective includes some means of measuring the outcome expected and evaluating the effectiveness of the effort. For example, if the overall goal is to improve children's nutritional status, one program objective might relate to hematocrit levels. It is not, however, sufficient to state that hematocrit levels will improve as no measure of the degree of improvement expected has been stated. A measurable objective could be that "75% of school-age children in the community (or target group) will have hematocrit levels within normal limits." A more precise objective would include a definition of normal hematocrit levels: "75% of school-age children in Evanston will have hematocrit levels of 35% or greater." In this objective, a measure of the expected hematocrit level is specified as is a measure of the number of children expected to achieve it. This objective is measurable and precise.

Another criterion of good program objectives is the inclusion of a specific time frame within which the outcome is expected to occur. A time frame can easily be added to the previous objective to state that "a hematocrit reading of 35% or greater will be achieved in 75% of the school-age children in Evanston within 6 months of initiating a food supplement program in the schools." As stated, this objective also meets several other criteria for program objectives. It is reasonable and practical to expect a significant increase in hematocrit levels after 6 months of an iron-rich diet. To expect it in 2 weeks would not be reasonable. It would also be unreasonable to expect that all of the children would achieve normal hematocrit levels as a result of the program. Seventy-five percent is reasonable.

The objective also meets the criterion of being within the competence of the planning group to accomplish. This would not be true, however, were the planners a group of electrical engineers. It is also legal, provided one has the permission of parents to provide nourishment to children in need of it and to obtain hematocrit levels. It fits the moral and value framework of the community and carries minimum unpleasant side effects. The latter would not be true, however, if the alternative chosen called for injectable iron preparations that are painful to administer. Finally, the objective, as stated, will probably be acceptable to those implementing the program, and it is hoped that it will fit within the budgetary limitations of the school system.

Program planners usually develop two types of program objectives: outcome objectives and process objectives. The examples of objectives provided above

> ## ▶ CRITERIA FOR EFFECTIVE PROGRAM OBJECTIVES
>
> *Measurability*
> The objective is measurable so as to determine whether it has been achieved.
>
> *Precision*
> The expected outcome is clear and precisely stated.
>
> *Time Specificity*
> The objective includes a statement of the time within which it is expected to be accomplished.
>
> *Reasonability or Practicability*
> The objective is practical and able to be met with a reasonable amount of effort.
>
> *Within Group Competencies*
> The objective is within the competence of the planning group to accomplish, given members' expertise and authority.
>
> *Legality*
> The objective is legal.
>
> *Congruence with Community Morals and Values*
> The objective is consistent with the values and morals of implementers and members of the community or target group.
>
> *Carries Minimal Side Effects*
> The objective has minimal side effects, and these effects are acceptable to program beneficiaries.
>
> *Fits Budgetary Limitations*
> The objective fits the community's budgetary limitations.

are outcome objectives and specify the expected results of the program in terms of changes in clients' health status or behavior. Process objectives specify the means to achieve outcome objectives. A process objective related to the problem of childhood anemia, for example, might be "provision of 75% of the recommended dietary allowance for iron in a school meal program." The inclusion of iron-rich foods in a school meal program is the means by which normal hematocrit levels among school-age children are expected to be achieved. Process objectives are later broken down in the planning process into specific activities necessary for their achievement.

IDENTIFYING RESOURCES.   Once objectives have been established, the planning group can proceed to identify resources needed to implement the program. Resources include personnel, money, materials, and time. To continue with the previous example of improving the nutritional status of children, if the alternative selected was an iron-rich school meal program, a variety of resources are required to institute such a program. Personnel needed include people to develop menus incorporating iron-rich foods palatable to school-age children and people to purchase, prepare, and serve the food as well as to wash dishes. Funds to purchase food and the equipment with which to prepare and serve it are also needed. Material resources needed include the dishes, silverware, pots and pans, and cooking facilities. Other needs include the equipment and health care personnel who will check hematocrit levels. Not only must the planning group decide what resources are required but they must also specify how these resources can be obtained. Will the PTA have a fund-raising drive? Will a grant proposal for federal assistance be submitted? The final consideration with respect to resources is that of time. The time needed to put the program into operation must be determined.

DELINEATING ACTIONS TO ACCOMPLISH OBJECTIVES. The next step in the planning process is delineating specific actions required to carry out the program. This is usually considered the "nitty-gritty" of planning, and many planning groups mistakenly jump immediately to this phase of activity. For planning to be effective, however, this step must be preceded by those discussed earlier.

In this phase of planning, the step-by-step details of the plan are developed. Using the example of the school meal program, some of the actions needed include presenting the problem and the proposed solution to the PTA, planning fund-raising projects, and purchasing equipment and supplies. In addition, the health department nutritionist would plan adequate menus. Advertisements for cooks and enlistment of parent volunteers to help prepare and serve food would be initiated, and so on, down to the last detail. Other areas that may need to be addressed include legal issues, development of program policies and procedures, ways of informing families of the program, and forms and recording processes (Timmreck, 1995).

EVALUATING THE PLAN. When the detailed plan has been constructed and specific activities delineated, the plan itself should be evaluated. Is the plan based on identified needs of the target group or is it unrelated to those needs? Is the plan flexible enough to adapt to changing circumstances in the foreseeable future? How efficient will the planned program be? Could program efficiency be improved by modification of the plan? Finally, how adequate is the plan? Have all constraints and contingencies been addressed? Answers to these and similar questions enable the plan-

> ### STEPS IN THE PLANNING PROCESS
>
> - Selecting the planning group
> - Developing planning competence
> - Formulating a philosophy
> - Establishing program goals
> - Developing alternative solutions
> - Evaluating alternatives and selecting a solution
> - Developing program objectives
> - Identifying resources
> - Delineating action to accomplish objectives
> - Evaluating the plan
> - Planning evaluation

ning group to evaluate the plan and to identify the need for any modifications before implementation.

PLANNING EVALUATION. The final component to be considered in program planning is planning evaluation of program effectiveness. This may seem a bit premature because the program has not even started; however, it is essential. Unless planning for program evaluation is incorporated at this stage, the data needed for evaluating program outcomes will not be available when the time arrives for actual evaluation.

Planning evaluation involves four considerations. The first of these is determining criteria on which the program should be evaluated. The second consideration is the types of data to be collected and the means used to collect the data. Determining the resources needed to carry out the evaluation is the third consideration in planning evaluation. Finally, the planning group should determine who will evaluate the program. All of these considerations are addressed in greater detail under the heading "Evaluating the Program." At this juncture it is sufficient to reemphasize the point that planning evaluation begins during program planning, not after the program has been implemented.

Effective health program planning involves all of the steps discussed up to now. When steps are ignored or bypassed, the program planned is likely to be less effective and its implementation may prove more difficult.

Implementing the Plan

It is not enough for the planning group to plan for a health care program to meet identified health care needs. The group must also ensure that the plan is implemented. Implementing a health program involves several considerations. These include getting the plan accepted, performing the tasks involved in implementing the program, and using strategies that foster implementation of the program as planned.

Plan Acceptance

Acceptance of the planned program occurs at three levels. The first level is acceptance by community policy makers. If policy makers have been represented on the planning group, this level of acceptance should already have been achieved.

The second level of acceptance involves convincing those who are to implement the plan to implement it for everyday operation. Again, if program implementers have been adequately represented in the planning effort, this level is already partially achieved. It only remains for the implementers to convert the plan into an operational program.

Acceptance and participation in the planned program by members of the target group is the third level of acceptance. If, for example, the planned program involves providing contraceptive services to sexually active adolescents, the third level of acceptance involves adolescents' participation in the program. Acceptance at this third level may require marketing the program to the intended target population.

Tasks of Implementation

Three basic tasks are involved in program implementation: activity delineation and sequencing, task allocation, and task performance. Necessary activities have been broadly outlined in plan development. Now they must be specified and subactivities identified. This involves identifying needed categories of action and the skills required for their performance. At this point, implementers would determine the appropriate sequencing of activities and might establish a time frame for their accomplishment.

Task allocation involves identifying the expertise of program implementers relative to the skills needed for effective implementation of the plan. Also at this point, responsibility is assigned for various activities delineated. Such assignments must be communicated to those involved, and they must be provided with whatever education or training is required for implementing the plan. Finally, the activities themselves are carried out and the planned program is put into operation.

Strategies for Implementation

Program implementation can be enhanced if several specific implementation strategies are employed. The first of these strategies is to assign responsibility for coordination of the total effort to one person. Identifying preparatory steps to each activity and listing them in sequence also fosters implementation of the program as planned.

Another strategy that enhances program implementation is periodic consultation with those implementing the program to address any difficulties that arise. Finally, the chances of implementing the program as planned are enhanced when everyone involved is clearly informed of expectations and the time frame for meeting expectations.

Using the school meal program as an example, implementing the plan might involve designating the school nurse as the program coordinator, staging a PTA bazaar to raise funds after delineating all of the activities involved in doing so, hiring and training personnel, and developing menus. Other implementation activities would include purchasing food, supplies, and equipment and preparing and serving the meals.

 Evaluating the Program

Evaluating the effects of health care programs is an essential feature of the epidemiologic prevention process model as applied to the care of communities and target groups. Program evaluation is needed for many of the same reasons that a systematic process is used in program planning. Health care providers recognize the limitation of available resources and must be accountable to the community members who use the program and, particularly, to the community members who pay for the program. They must be able to justify the program's existence and continuation. This can be done only by documenting the effectiveness of the program in solving the problem at hand.

Evaluation of a particular program may be undertaken for a variety of reasons. Some of these include justifying program continuation or expansion, improving the quality of service provided, determining future courses of action, and determining the impact of the program (Fink, 1993). Other reasons for evaluation might be to call attention to the program, to assess personnel performance, or to assuage political expectations. Evaluation is frequently conducted because it is required by a funding agency.

Considerations in Program Evaluation

Purpose Considerations.   The purpose of the evaluation influences all other aspects of the process. For example, if the purpose of the evaluation is to justify continuing a program, the evaluation will focus on determining whether the program has a beneficial effect on the health of the population group for which it is designed. On the other hand, if the purpose is to decide whether programs are under- or overused, evaluation will focus on the number of persons served. In other words, the purpose of the evaluation influences the types of data collected and how they are used.

Evaluator Considerations. The second area for consideration is who should conduct the evaluation. A number of choices are possible. The program can be evaluated by those who implement it or who benefit from it. Evaluation by people who are involved in the program has some disadvantages in that there is a certain amount of bias on the part of those with a vested interest in retaining the program. The advantages of an inside evaluator are familiarity with the program and knowledge of sources of data that will be needed.

Another possibility is to employ someone from outside the program to conduct the evaluation. This person is likely to be relatively objective in his or her approach to evaluation, but faces the disadvantages of not being well acquainted with the program and, possibly, of being unable to identify appropriate sources of data. This alternative is also rather expensive.

The third option is the use of an academician to evaluate the program. Faculty members who have expertise in the program area are likely to be familiar with the general operation of the program but also remain relatively unbiased. Because college faculty are usually open to opportunities for research, it may also be possible to acquire their services for a lower fee.

Ethical Considerations. Ethical conflicts must be anticipated in program evaluation. Participation in the evaluation should be voluntary for staff and clients alike. This poses some problems in that staff members are sometimes unwilling to reveal information that reflects poorly on them or on the program that employs them. To circumvent this reluctance, the evaluator needs to have a variety of sources of data that provide an overall picture of the program and its effects.

Confidentiality is another issue. Persons who provide data need to be assured that their individual responses will not be identifiable. There is also the question of who will have access to the findings of the evaluation. Should findings be shared only with those involved in the program? With their supervisors? With funding agencies or regulatory bodies? The use to which findings can be put is also of concern. Can the evaluator publish the information? Will it be used to fire personnel?

Finally, the evaluator must consider the risks and benefits accruing from the evaluation. Is there potential for harm to the participants, either clients or staff? Do the anticipated benefits of the evaluation outweigh any possible risks?

Type of Evaluation. The last major consideration in evaluating a health care program is the type of evaluation to be conducted. There are two basic types of evaluation, outcome and process evaluation, each of which can be broken down into subtypes or approaches.

OUTCOME EVALUATION. *Outcome evaluation* focuses on the extent to which program goals and objectives have been met, irrespective of how well organized or how efficient the program was. Outcome evaluation documents the effects of the program and justifies decisions to continue, modify, or eliminate it. The two subtypes of outcome evaluation are evaluation of *effect* and assessment of *impact*.

A program's effect is the degree to which specific outcome objectives were met. Using the previous example of the school lunch program, the effect of the program is evaluated when one determines whether 75% of the school-age children have a hematocrit level of 35% or greater within 6 months of the start of the program. If they do, the program can be considered effective. If not, the evaluator must determine to what degree the objective has been met and whether continuation of the program is warranted. For example, if the objective was achieved with 60% of the participating children, extending the program would probably be considered. If, on the other hand, only 20% of the children achieved normal hematocrit levels, alternative solutions to the problem may need to be considered.

The impact of a program is how well it serves to attain overall goals. If the goal was improving the nutritional status of school-age children, for example, the achievement of improved hematocrit levels does contribute to goal achievement. If, however, the goal was to improve the children's learning ability through adequate nutrition, increasing hematocrit levels may or may not contribute to its achievement. In this case, one would need to know not only the hematocrit levels but also the amount of learning that has taken place to state that the program has had an impact on meeting the overall goal. One may find that hematocrit levels did indeed rise, but no improvement in learning ability occurred. In this instance, the program was effective in accomplishing its objective, but accomplishing the objective did not lead to achievement of the overall goal.

Health programs can have a number of outcomes. Often the outcomes arise out of the program's stated objectives as in the examples above. Other outcomes may also be of interest. Usually, however, it is not feasible or even possible to examine all of a program's possible outcomes, so the program evaluator will need to decide which outcomes will be the focus of program evaluation. Several criteria have been suggested for making this decision. First, the outcomes studied should be valued by persons involved in the program, the recipients, the implementers, or the funders. Second, a multidimensional array of outcomes should be examined to provide information about the overall worth of the program. Outcomes should be selected for which objective and measurable data can be obtained. Fourth, the outcomes selected should be logically connected to the program and should be effects that can be attributed to the program rather than to other factors. Finally, both long-term and short-term outcomes of the program should be assessed whenever possible (Schalock, 1995).

PROCESS EVALUATION. The second type of evaluation is *process evaluation.* Here one is concerned with the operation of the program vis-à-vis established standards of performance (Des Harnais & McLaughlin, 1994). Process-evaluation examines program performance and may take the perspective of quality assurance or quality improvement. The focus in quality assurance is on making sure that the processes by which care is provided meet certain established standards (Speake, Mason, Broadway, Sylvester, & Morrison, 1995). If the standard has been met, no action is warranted and program operation continues unmodified. Quality improvement, on the other hand, is designed to produce "a continuous stream of improvements in order to provide health care that meets or exceeds consumer expectations" (McLaughlin & Kaluzny, 1994). The philosophy behind quality improvement, also referred to as continuous quality improvement (CQI) or total quality management (TQM), is that client's needs and expectations change over time and that an effective health care program is continually changing to better meet those needs. This can only be achieved if the processes of care are being continually examined and improved as needed. Quality improvement focuses on enhancing the processes of care to create more effective outcomes. General areas to be examined include the effectiveness of services in meeting client needs, the accessibility and acceptability of services to the client population, optimization of resource

---

Critical Thinking in Research

Community assessment should form the basis for health program planning. How would you conduct a study to determine if this is, indeed, occurring? What health programs would you examine? How would you obtain information on any needs assessments that were conducted prior to planning the programs? What criteria would you use to evaluate the adequacy of needs assessments done? How could you determine the extent of community health nurse participation in the needs assessments?

---

use, and needs for improvement in care processes (Speake, et al., 1995).

The types and aspects of program evaluation presented here are summarized below:

Outcome Evaluation
- *Effect:* evaluation of achievement of outcome objectives
- *Impact:* evaluation of the program's influence on meeting overall goals

Process Evaluation
- *Quality assurance:* evaluation of care processes based on identified standards
- *Quality improvement:* continuous improvement in care processes to better meet or exceed client expectations

In designing a program evaluation, the community health nurse needs to decide which of the types of evaluation are appropriate. A particular program can be evaluated with respect to any one aspect or a combination of several. The aspects selected depend on the purposes of the evaluation and the time and other resources available. Most health program evaluations will incorporate aspects of both outcome and process evaluation.

The Evaluation Process

Like any other systematic process, evaluation takes place in a series of specific steps. Some of these steps, such as planning the evaluation, have already been completed as part of the total planning process. Other steps include collecting data, interpreting data, and using evaluative findings.

Planning Evaluation. Goals for the evaluation, evaluative criteria, types of data needed, and appropriate methods of data collection were established as part of the planning process. Evaluative criteria and type of evaluation are based on the purpose of the evaluation. If the intent of the evaluation is to determine the extent to which outcome objectives are met, evaluative criteria will be derived from those objectives. In the school meal program example, evaluative criteria related to outcome objectives would be hematocrit levels of children participating in the program. If the intent is to assess the efficiency of the program, evaluative criteria would include the amount of food wasted and the number of hours spent implementing the program.

Data needed to conduct the evaluation are determined and data collection procedures established. Planning evaluation also involves determining the necessary equipment and supplies. Items needed to evaluate accomplishment of the school meal program's outcome objectives would include parental consent forms for hematocrit testing, capillary tubes, lancets, and a microcentrifuge. Other equipment and supplies would be needed to evaluate other aspects of the program.

Collecting Data.   The evaluative criteria chosen influence the types of data collected and the manner in which they are collected. For the hematocrit criterion, data include participating children's hematocrit levels, which need to be collected by testing blood samples at periodic intervals before and during the program. There needs to be a baseline level for each child before the program to determine whether hematocrit levels have increased, so data collection related to evaluation must begin before the program itself starts. Data collection related to food wasted might include review of purchase orders and periodic observation of the amount of food discarded at the end of the day.

Interpreting Data.   The next step in the evaluation process is interpreting the data collected. In this step, data are compared with the evaluative criteria. In evaluating the achievement of the outcome objectives of the school meal program, the nurse would compare the children's hematocrit levels after starting the program with those obtained before the program. If an increase is noted in most children, the program has been somewhat effective. The nurse would also determine how many of the children had now achieved a normal hematocrit level. If 75% or more of the children now have normal levels, the program has met its objective.

In examining data related to the efficient use of supplies, the nurse would look at what percentage of food purchased is actually consumed and what percentage is wasted. If the criterion derived from process objectives specified that less than 5% of food and supplies purchased is wasted and the nurse finds that closer to 10% is actually wasted, program processes are not operating as efficiently as planned.

Using Evaluative Findings.   The findings of the evaluation are then used to make decisions about the program. Basically, three decisions can be made based on evaluative findings: to continue, to modify, or to discontinue the program. If the nurse finds that the program's objectives are being achieved, he or she may decide to continue the program. If the nurse finds that only a few children are participating in the program, the nurse may decide either to stop the program or take steps to increase participation. For example, perhaps the menu needs to be changed to include nutritious foods that are more acceptable to the target group. Looking at program efficiency, if the nurse finds that 10% of the food purchased is being wasted, various waste control practices may need to be instituted. The use of evaluative findings and the other steps in program evaluation are summarized below:

Critical Thinking in Practice: A Case in Point

You are the community health nurse assigned to Copper City, a small town in New Mexico with a population of 3000. You have just arrived in town and have been given the task of assessing the health needs of the community and developing a plan to meet those needs.

During your assessment, you obtain the following information: Copper City is a small town run by a city council and a mayor. Most of these officials are administrators of the local copper mines or owners of large chicken farms in the area. The town is in a largely rural area, and lies 50 miles from Tucumcari. The surrounding countryside is hot and arid.

The ethnic composition of the town is 80% Caucasian of European ancestry and 20% Latino, primarily of Mexican descent. Fifty percent of the town's population is under 8 years of age. There are very few elderly persons in the community, because Copper City is a relatively new town that grew up around copper mines discovered in the last 20 years. The birth rate is 30 per 1000 population. Approximately 10% of all births are premature, and the neonatal death rate is 50 per 1000 live births. Only about 10% of the women receive prenatal care during their pregnancies.

The major industries in the area are copper mines and chicken farms, which employ approximately 85% of the adult men and 50% of the women. The majority of the Latino population works on the chicken farms. The remaining 15% of the adult men and another 20% of the adult women are employed in offices and shops in the town. The unemployment level is 0.5%, far lower than that of the state and the nation.

The average annual family income is $8000, and 75% of the population is below the poverty level. Nearly one third of those below the poverty level receive some form of aid such as Medicaid or AFDC.

The predominant religion among the Caucasian population is Methodist, and among the Latino group it is Roman Catholic. These are two Methodist churches in town, one Catholic church, and a small Southern Baptist congregation.

Many of the Latino group subscribe to folk health practices. They frequently seek health care from a local *yerbero* (herbalist). They may also drive to a nearby town to solicit the services of a *curandera* (faith healer). Close to one third of the Latino population speaks only Spanish.

The average education level for the community is tenth grade. For the Spanish-speaking group, however, it is only third grade. Education facilities in the town include a grade school and a high school. The high school also offers adult education classes at night. There is a Head Start program that enrolls 50 children, but no other child care facilities are available.

There is a high incidence of tuberculosis in the community, and anemia and pinworms are common problems among the school-age children. Several of the men have been disabled as a result of accidents in the mines.

The only transportation to Tucumcari is by car or by train, which comes through town morning and evening. About half of the families in town own cars.

There is one general practice physician and one dentist in the town. The nearest hospital is in Tucumcari, and the funeral home hearse is used as an ambulance for emergency transportation to the hospital. The driver and one attendant have had basic first aid training. The county health department provides family planning, prenatal, well-child, and immunization services one day a week in the basement of the larger of the two Methodist churches. In addition to yourself, the staff consists of a physician, one licensed practical nurse, a masters-prepared family nurse practitioner, and a nutritionist. The well-child and immunization services are heavily used, and immunization levels in the community are high among both preschoolers and school-age youngsters.

1. What are the biophysical, psychological, physical, social, behavioral, and health system factors influencing the health of this community?
2. What community nursing diagnoses might you derive from these data?
3. What health problems are evident in the case study? Which are the three most important problems for this community? Why have you given these problems priority over others?
4. Select one of the three top-priority problems and design a health program to resolve it. Be sure to address the following:
    a. Level of prevention involved
    b. Who should be involved in the planning group and why
    c. Additional information you would need, if any, and where you would obtain that information
    d. Goals and objectives for the program
    e. Resources needed to implement the program
5. How would you gain acceptance of your program?
6. How would you go about implementing the program?
7. How would you conduct outcome and process evaluation of the program?

1. Planning Evaluation
    a. Setting evaluation goals
    b. Developing evaluative criteria
    c. Determining the data needed
    d. Establishing data collection procedures
    e. Determining resources needed
2. Collecting data
3. Interpreting data
4. Using evaluative findings to make decisions regarding
    a. Continuing the program
    b. Modifying the program
    c. Discontinuing the program

TESTING YOUR UNDERSTANDING

1. Describe at least three purposes for assessing a community or a target group. (p. 421)
2. Identify at least three factors that influence the scope of a community or target group assessment. Give an example of the influence of each factor. (p. 421)
3. List at least four considerations related to the biophysical dimension to be addressed in a community or target group assessment. Explain how each could affect the health of a community. (pp. 424–426)
4. Describe at least six factors in the psychological, physical, and social dimensions to be considered in assessing a target group or a community. Give an example of the influence of each factor on the health of a community. (pp. 426–430)
5. Describe at least four ways in which behavioral factors can influence the health status of a community or a target group. (pp. 430–431)
6. What are three considerations in assessing the impact of the health system on the health of a community or target group? (pp. 431–432)
7. Describe two levels of nursing diagnoses related to the health status of a community or a target group. Give an example of a diagnosis at each level. (pp. 436–438)
8. Describe at least three considerations in planning screening programs for communities or target groups. (pp. 437–438)
9. Identify at least six tasks in planning a health program to meet the needs of communities or target groups. (pp. 440–444)
10. What are three levels of acceptance of a health care program? (p. 445)
11. Describe three types of considerations in evaluating a health care program. (pp. 445–447)

WHAT DO YOU THINK?
Questions for Critical Thinking

1. Should sex education be a required topic in public junior and senior high schools? How would you go about getting such a program accepted by the community?
2. What are the top three environmental hazards in your community?
3. How can nurses influence public financial support for health programs in your community?
4. Why have nurses not been very active or visible in health program planning efforts in the past? What could be done to promote their involvement in program planning?

REFERENCES

Barton, J. A., Smith, M. C., Brown, N. J., & Supplies, J. S. (1993). Methodological issues in a team approach to community health needs assessment. *Nursing Outlook, 41,* 253–261.

Blane, D. (1995). Editorial: Social determinants of health—Socioeconomic status, social class, and ethnicity. *American Journal of Public Health, 85,* 903–905.

Dees, J. P., & Garcia, M. A. (1995). Program planning: A total quality approach. *AAOHN Journal, 43,* 239–244.

Des Harnais, S., & McLaughlin, C. P. (1994). The outcome model of quality. In C. P. McLaughlin & A. D. Kaluzny (Eds.), *Continuous quality improvement in health care: Theory, implementation, and applications* (pp. 47–69). Gaithersburg, MD: Aspen.

Dever, G. E. A. (1991). *Community health analysis: Global awareness at the local level.* Gaithersburg, MD: Aspen.

Ellencweig, A. Y. (1992). *Analyzing health systems: A modular approach.* Oxford: Oxford University Press.

Fink, A. (1993). *Evaluation fundamentals: Guiding health programs, research, and policy.* Newbury Park, CA: Sage.

Flynn, B. C., Rider, M. S., & Bailey, W. W. (1992). Developing community leadership in healthy cities: The Indiana model. *Nursing Outlook, 40,* 121–126.

Harkness, G. A. (1995). *Epidemiology in nursing practice.* St. Louis: Mosby.

Hettinger, B. J., & Brazile, R. P. (1992). A database design for community health data. *Computers in Nursing, 10,* 109–115.

Kuehnert, P. L. (1995). The interactive and organizational model of community as client: A model for public health nursing practice. *Public Health Nursing, 12*(1), 9–17.

Lantz, J., Fullerton, J. T., & Dowling, W. (1993). A community strategic planning process for elder services. *Journal of Nursing Administration, 23*(1), 47–52.

Loos, G. P. (1996). *Field guide for international health project planners and managers.* London: Janus.

McLaughlin, C. P., & Kalunzy, A. D. (1994). Defining total quality management/continuous quality improvement. In C. P. McLaughlin & A. D. Kaluzny (Eds.), *Continuous quality improvement in health care: Theory, implementation, and applications* (pp. 3–10). Gaithersburg, MD: Aspen.

Porter, E. J. (1987). Administrative diagnosis: Implications for the public's health. *Public Health Nursing,* 4, 247–256.

Rainey, D. Y., & Runyan, C. W. (1992). Newspapers: A source for injury surveillance. *American Journal of Public Health, 82,* 745–746.

Rohrer, J. E. (1996). *Planning for community-oriented health systems.* Washington, DC: American Public Health Association.

Schalock, R. L. (1995). *Outcome-based evaluation.* New York: Plenum Press.

Secretary's Commission on Nursing. (1988). *Final report,* (Vol. 1). Washington DC: U.S. Department of Health and Human Services.

Soriano, F. I. (1995). *Conducting needs assessments: A multi-disciplinary approach.* Thousand Oaks, CA: Sage.

Speake, D. L., Mason, K. P., Broadway, T. M., Sylvester, M., & Morrison, S. P. (1995). Integrating indicators into a public health quality improvement system. *American Journal of Public Health, 85,* 1448–1449.

Terry, P. E. (1992). Health education. In A. E. Barnett & G. G. Mayer (Eds.), *Ambulatory care management and practice* (pp. 209–231). Gaithersburg, MD: Aspen.

Timmreck, T. C. (1995). *Planning, program development, and evaluation: A handbook for health promotion, aging, and health services.* Boston: Jones and Bartlett.

U.S. Department of Commerce. (1996). *Statistical abstract of the United States, 1996* (116th ed.). Washington, DC: Government Printing Office.

U.S. Department of Health and Human Services. (1996). *Health United States, 1995.* Washington, DC: Government Printing Office.

Wickizer, T. M., et al. (1993). Activating communities for health promotion: A process evaluation method. *American Journal of Public Health, 83,* 561–567.

Witkin, B. R., & Altschuld, J. W. (1995). *Planning and conducting needs assessments: A practical guide.* Thousand Oaks, CA: Sage.

RESOURCES FOR NURSES INVOLVED IN HEALTH PROGRAM PLANNING

American Health Planning Association
7245 Arlington Blvd, Ste. 300
Falls Church, VA 22042
(202) 371–1515

American Public Health Association
Community Health Planning and Policy
    Development Section
1015 15th Street, NW
Washington, DC 20005
(202) 789–5600

Forum for Health Care Planning
1101 Connecticut Avenue, NW, Ste. 700
Washington, DC 20036
(202) 857–1162

CARE OF CHILDREN

One of the most effective ways to improve the health status of a community is to maintain and enhance the health of its children. In 1991, children under 15 years of age constituted 22% of the U.S. population (U.S. Department of Commerce, 1996). Children who receive effective health care services, particularly health-promotive and illness-preventive services, are less likely to develop a variety of acute and chronic health problems. When working with children with physical, mental, or emotional health problems, community health nurses also endeavor to promote the child's ability to reach his or her fullest potential.

Goals for primary prevention for children include promoting normal growth and development, developing positive parent–child relationships, preventing health problems, and developing strengths and resources. When children are ill or have a health problem, the community health nurse also works toward goals related to secondary and tertiary prevention. Goals of secondary prevention reflect efforts to accurately diagnose and treat health problems. Tertiary prevention goals in the care of children include restoring function and preventing problem recurrence, preventing complications, adapting to long-term effects of illness, and minimizing the effects of health problems on the child and family.

Community health nurses encounter children in a variety of settings. The focus of this chapter is community health nursing activities with children seen in the home or in the clinic or office setting. Pediatric care in acute care settings is addressed in detail in many pediatric nursing textbooks, and care of the child in the school setting is addressed in Chapter 25.

▶ Chapter Objectives

After reading this chapter, you should be able to:

- Identify at least five problems of particular concern to community health nurses working with children.
- Differentiate between growth and development and describe how one would assess each.
- Identify at least three safety considerations in assessing infants, toddlers and preschool children, and school-age children.
- Describe at least five areas to be addressed in assessing the psychological dimension of children's health.
- Identify at least three behavioral dimension considerations in assessing the health status of a child.
- Describe at least five primary prevention measures appropriate to all children.
- Identify at least three approaches to providing secondary preventive care for children.
- Describe three tertiary preventive considerations in the care of children.

▶ HEALTH PROBLEMS OF CONCERN IN THE CARE OF CHILDREN

In addition to concerns for health promotion and illness prevention, several specific health problems are of concern to community health nurses caring for children. Some of these problems are infant mortality and low birth weight, congenital anomalies, HIV infection, unintentional injury, handicapping and chronic conditions, fetal drug and alcohol exposure, and child abuse.

The importance of community health efforts to improve the health of the nation's children is seen in the fact that 49 of the national health objectives for the year 2000 directly address the health needs of children, and another 37 objectives address those needs indirectly (U.S. Department of Health and Human Services, 1991). These objectives are summarized in Appendix A.

Infant Mortality

In 1996, the United States ranked sixteenth in the world in terms of infant mortality rates, far higher than many other developed and even underdeveloped areas. The infant mortality rate in the United States was 6.7 deaths for every 1000 live births. Infant mortality is even higher for some segments of the population. More than twice as many infants in minority groups die before they are a year old (U.S. De-

partment of Commerce, 1996), and infant mortality is 60% higher among babies born to poor women than the nonpoor (Infant and Child Studies Bureau, 1995). Although current infant mortality rates are the lowest in history in this country, the rate of decline has slowed considerably in the last decade. Primary causes of death are congenital anomalies, respiratory distress syndrome and other consequences of prematurity, sudden infant death syndrome, and effects of maternal complications during pregnancy (U.S. Department of Commerce, 1996).

Low Birth Weight

Low birth weight among those infants who survive also presents problems. *Low birth weight* is a weight less than 2500 grams at birth (O'Campo, Xue, Wang, & Caughy, 1997), and *very low birth weight* is a birth weight less than 1500 grams (Alberman, 1994). Approximately 7% of all babies born in the United States are of low birth weight (Ginsberg, Gage, Martin, Gerstein, & Acuff, 1994) and an estimated 742 low birth weight babies are born each day (Berg, Bryant, & Bach, 1994). Again, figures are worse for certain segments of the population. For example, more than twice as many African American babies have low birth weight as white babies, and babies born to women with lower education levels are more likely to have lower birth weights (U.S. Department of Health and Human Services, 1996b).

Low birth weight is associated with younger and older maternal age, poor maternal weight gain, multiparity, lack of prenatal care, and substance abuse. Other factors associated with low birth weight include low income and maternal smoking and alcohol and drug use (Alberman, 1994). Low birth weight has also been associated with public assistance, fatalism (Shiono, Rauh, Park, Lederman, & Zuskar, 1997), increased altitude (Jensen & Moore, 1997), and maternal hypertension, diabetes, or urinary tract infection during pregnancy (DeBaun, Rowley, Province, Stockbauer, & Cole, 1994).

Low birth weight infants are more likely to die in the first year of life than infants with normal birth weights (Alberman, 1994). Effects of low birth weight include lower IQ, cerebral palsy, seizure disorders, and blindness. Approximately one fourth of very low birth weight babies exhibit moderate to severe disabilities, whereas 2 to 4% of low birth weight babies are affected (U.S. Department of Health and Human Services, 1991). In addition, low birth weight children have been found to have sensory, learning, and behavior disorders; respiratory problems; cerebral palsy; visual and hearing defects; growth retardation; hyperactivity; and scarring due to invasive procedures (Alberman, 1994). Very low birth weight babies are even

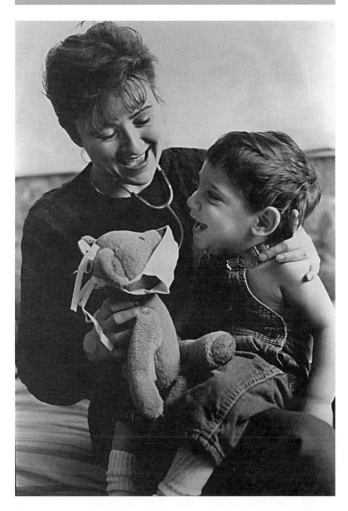

One of the most effective ways to improve the health status of a community is to enhance and maintain the health of its children.
Photo courtesy of Visiting Nurses Society of New York.

more likely to exhibit many of these problems (Becker, Grunwald, Moorman, & Stuhr, 1993).

Congenital Anomalies

In 1993, infant mortality due to congenital anomalies was 1.8 per 1000 live births (U.S. Department of Commerce, 1996). Although many children with congenital anomalies die in utero or during infancy, modern medical technology has increased the number of children with anomalies who survive. In recent years, there has been an increasing prevalence of several congenital abnormalities in newborns. These abnormalities include anomalies of the central nervous system (hydrocephalus, encephalocele); eye (congenital cataract); cardiovascular system (ventricular and atrial

septal defects, tetralogy of Fallot, pulmonary and aortic valvular stenosis, patent ductus arteriosus); gastrointestinal system (intestinal atresia, tracheoesophageal anomalies); genitourinary system (renal agenesis and hypoplasia); and musculoskeletal system (club foot), as well as cleft lip and palate and chromosomal abnormalities (Down syndrome, trisomy 13, trisomy 18). The societal cost of care for these children is staggering. In 1992 alone, the cost due to 18 congenital conditions was $8 billion. The cost per case for some conditions can be over $500,000 (Waitzman, Romano, Scheffler, & Harris, 1995). In addition to physical effects and societal costs, congenital anomalies also lead to parental reactions of guilt, revulsion, anxiety, hopelessness, and isolation (Evans, Le Mar, Pitzen & Thompson, 1997).

HIV Infection and AIDS

Other areas of concern are HIV infection and the growing number of AIDS cases in children. As of September 1996, more than 7000 cases of AIDS had been diagnosed in youngsters under 13 years of age. Of these cases, 90% are attributable to perinatal transmission from infected mothers. Approximately 6000 to 7000 babies are born each year to infected mothers (Division of HIV/AIDS Prevention, 1996).

A large proportion of infants born to HIV-infected mothers are themselves infected. Vertical transmission of HIV infection occurs in 15 to 30% of babies born to HIV-infected mothers (Davis, Byers, Lindegren, Caldwell, Karon, & Gwinn, 1995). *Vertical transmission,* transmission from mother to baby, may occur in utero, during delivery, or, less commonly, via breastfeeding. In addition to newborn infection, vertical transmission of HIV is thought to be related to fetal demise and miscarriage (Langston, et al., 1995). With the increasing incidence of HIV infection among women of childbearing age, there will be continued increases in the number of children with HIV infection and with symptomatic AIDS.

Unintentional Injury

Unintentional injuries are a frequent occurrence among children, resulting in extensive morbidity as well as mortality. In fact, approximately one in every four children in the United States experiences an accidental injury requiring treatment each year (Scheidt, Harel, Trumble, Jones, Overpeck, & Bijur, 1995). Injuries account for 40% of mortality in children aged 1 to 4 years and 70% of mortality in the 15- to 19-year-old group. Specific causes of injury mortality differ with age, with infants more likely to die of choking and toddlers and preschool children of burns, poison, and drownings. Motor vehicle accidents are a frequent cause of death for all children (Rivara, 1994).

Unintentional injuries among children also result in significant morbidity. For example, in 1990, there were 729 nonfatal poisonings for every 100,000 children under the age of 4 in the United States. Head trauma is also a frequent cause of injury, accounting for 464,000 emergency room visits in 1991. Forty percent of these injuries in children and adolescents occur during sports and recreational activities, and three fourths of recreational injuries are related to playground equipment (Baker, Fowler, Li, Warner, & Dannenberg, 1994). In one study of children's playgrounds, more than half of all climbing equipment was situated over nonresilient surfaces, creating a potential for serious injuries due to falls. Only 5% of the playgrounds studied had no identifiable hazards, and a mean of 16 hazards each was noted at the other 95% of playgrounds. The study further noted that making playground directors aware of safety hazards did not result in their elimination (Sacks, Brantley, Holmgreen, & Rochat, 1992).

Firearms injuries are a serious concern in the health of children. In 1992, for example, accidental mortality due to firearms ranged from 0.1 per 100,000 children among white children under 5 years of age to 2 per 100,000 among black male children aged 10 to 14 years (U.S. Department of Commerce, 1996). It is estimated that for every fatality related to firearms, there are 105 nonfatal injuries, suggesting the magnitude of the problem in the United States. Most of these injuries occur in the home and involve improperly stored weapons. It is estimated that modification of guns with childproof safety devices and loading indicators could prevent almost one fourth of unintentional firearms fatalities.

Handicapping and Chronic Conditions

The health of children in the United States is also influenced by a variety of chronic or handicapping conditions. In fact, according to a national survey, in 1991 and 1992 more than 9% of U.S. children under age 18 had some form of disability (National Center for Chronic Disease Prevention and Health Promotion, 1995). The percentage of disability caused by selected conditions is reflected in Table 20–1. Roughly 15% of school-age children experience some form of disability that requires assistance, and 4.3 million children receive educational services related to one or more handicap (Berkson, 1993).

Chronic and handicapping conditions in children fall into several categories: sensory impairments; motor handicaps; mental retardation; pervasive developmental disorders; learning disabilities; speech and

TABLE 20–1. PERCENTAGE OF DISABILITY DUE TO SELECTED CONDITIONS IN CHILDREN UNDER 18 YEARS OF AGE

Condition	Percentage of Disability
Learning disability	29.5%
Speech problems	13.1%
Mental retardation	6.8%
Asthma	6.4%
Mental illness	6.3%
Blindness or vision problem	3.0%
Seizure disorder	2.6%
Deafness/hearing impairment	2.4%
Heart problems	0.9%
Cancer	0.5%
Diabetes	0.3%
Other	28%

(Source: National Center for Chronic Disease Control and Health Promotion, 1995.)

language disorders; emotional, behavioral, and conduct disorders; and chronic diseases. The prevalence of sensory impairments related to hearing or vision is approximately 260 per 100,000 schoolchildren (Berkson, 1993). Fortunately, most of these impairments are relatively mild, but the community health nurse must be aware of the potential for impairment and alert to the need for correction of vision or hearing problems.

Motor handicaps include such conditions as developmental delays, cerebral palsy, motor paralyses, problems with coordination, and bone malformations or injuries that may arise from a variety of causes. These types of conditions affect approximately 140 of every 100,000 school-age children (Berkson, 1993). Cerebral palsy, for example, occurs in 2 per 1000 children (Kennel & Seibold, 1997), and Down syndrome in 1 per 800 (Ross, 1997). Mental retardation, on the other hand, occurs in 2.5% of the population (Seibold & Kennel, 1997). *Mental retardation* is defined as a low Intelligence Quotient (IQ) that poses adaptive problems for the individual involved (Berkson, 1993). Many individuals can cope with the demands of adult life, but have difficulty adapting to the requirements of the school setting.

Pervasive developmental disorders include such conditions as autism and childhood schizophrenia. Autism affects approximately 5 to 15 of every 10,000 children born in the United States (Hellerman, 1997); schizophrenia is found in 130 of every 100,000 youngsters. Far more children are affected by learning disabilities, the next category of disabling condition. A *learning disability* is defined as being 2 or more years behind agemates in one academic area. Three to five percent of school children experience dyslexia, and as many as 9% of boys and somewhat fewer girls are affected by attention deficit disorder with or without hyperactivity (Berkson, 1993).

Speech and language difficulties are experienced by roughly 3% of school-age children and most often involve stuttering. Emotional disorders are characterized by fears, shyness, and anxiety; behavioral disorders may take one of two forms: undercontrolled behavior and overcontrolled behavior. Undercontrolled behavior may manifest as hyperactivity, delinquency, or aggression, whereas overcontrolled behavior may result in displays of anxiety, depression, obsessive–compulsive behavior, or somatic complaints (Berkson, 1993).

Young children also experience a variety of chronic physical health problems such as asthma, diabetes, cancer, sickle cell disease, and obesity. Approximately 5.5% of schoolchildren in the United States experience these and similar problems (Berkson, 1993). For example, according to National Health Interview Survey (NHIS) data, the prevalence of asthma is 42.5 cases per 1000 children under 18 years of age. In 1991, asthma resulted in an average of nearly 5 days of school absence per child per year (Newacheck & Taylor, 1992).

Each year, more than 6500 children under age 15 are diagnosed as having cancer. More than 50% of these children survive to live with cancer as a chronic health threat. The most common childhood cancers are leukemia (30% of all cancers in youngsters), lymphomas (5%), neuroblastomas (50% of cancers occurring in infancy), Wilms tumor (5–6%), sarcomas (5–8%), and bone tumors (Diamond, 1994). Childhood risk factors for malignant neoplasms include environmental exposures to carcinogens, viral exposures (eg, the Epstein–Barr virus that causes infectious mononucleosis), genetic characteristics, and other existing conditions such as some congenital anomalies, immunodeficiency states, and chromosomal anomalies.

Insulin-dependent diabetes mellitus (IDDM) occurs in one of every 600 school-age children (Kirchgessner, 1997). More than 35% of children with diabetes in the NHIS had been hospitalized in the year prior to the study, and children with IDDM reported an average of 3 days of school absence per year due to their disease. Diabetes also caused 30% of children affected to experience activity limitations (Newacheck & Taylor, 1992).

Approximately 15 of every 1000 children under 18 years of age are affected by some form of heart disease, with boys more often affected than girls and white children more often affected than their African American counterparts. According to the NHIS, more than 15% of these children used medications and nearly 8% had been hospitalized in the last year (Newacheck & Taylor, 1992). Hypertension, a risk fac-

tor for heart disease, may be associated with childhood obesity, but it is more likely due to an underlying medical condition such as coarctation of the aorta, renal artery stenosis, drug and toxin ingestion, and chronic pyelonephritis and glomerulonephritis (Kenney, 1997). Routine blood pressure measurements starting at 3 years of age are recommended to identify youngsters with hypertension.

Juvenile arthritis is a collection of syndromes that have in common chronic arthritis beginning in childhood. Although precise incidence and prevalence are unknown, it is estimated that approximately 4 to 5 of every 1000 American children may be affected. This amounts to about 290,000 youngsters in the United States (Newacheck & Taylor, 1992). Arthritis in children can affect single or multiple joints, and virtually any joint may be involved. Anywhere from 10% to more than 50% of children with various forms of juvenile arthritis will have severe joint involvement during their lifetime.

Approximately 2 to 5% of children experience at least one seizure sometime during their childhood (Berg, 1994). Most seizures experienced by children are a manifestation of underlying acute systemic or central nervous system diseases such as meningitis and encephalitis, metabolic disturbances such as hypoglycemia and hypocalcemia, or intoxications. Some children, however, experience recurrent seizures that constitute a seizure disorder or epilepsy. Prevalence rates for epilepsy and seizures in the NHIS was 2 to 4 per 1000 children or 151,000 cases in the U.S. child population (Newacheck & Taylor, 1992). Most of these children obtain good seizure control with antiepileptic drug therapy, but the disease is still a frightening one for both parents and children.

The presence of these and other chronic illnesses in children creates special needs for community health nursing care. These illnesses may also necessitate creative approaches to general health promotion and illness prevention in these youngsters.

Attention Deficit Hyperactivity Disorder

As noted earlier, attention deficit hyperactivity disorder (ADHD) affects as many as 6 to 7% of school-age children (Safer, Zito, & Fine, 1996), with boys more likely to be affected than girls (U.S. Department of Health and Human Services, 1996a). As many as one quarter to one half of these children have associated learning disabilities (Gabby, 1994). *Attention deficit hyperactivity disorder* is characterized by poor attention span, impulsive behavior, and hyperactivity. Hyperactive children frequently have difficulties with school performance, peer interactions, and unacceptable behavior. Attention deficit with associated hyperactivity is frustrating for the children affected and for everyone who interacts with them. A relatively large number of school-age children receive psychostimulants as treatment for ADHD, yet only about three fourths of these children show improvement of problematic behaviors, and their effects on academic performance are unclear (Gabby, 1994). Behavior modification has been shown to be effective with some children. Children with ADHD are at increased risk for conduct and anxiety disorders, depression, and personality and substance abuse disorders (U.S. Department of Health and Human Services, 1996a).

Fetal Alcohol and Drug Exposure

It is estimated that 1 in every 10 babies born in the United States has been exposed to alcohol or illicit drugs in utero. In a 1994 National Institute on Drug Abuse survey, 20% of pregnant women smoked, 19% drank alcohol, 5.5% used other illicit drugs, 0.9% used crack cocaine, and 10% used some form of psychotherapeutic medication (Stratton, Howe, & Battaglia, 1996). Community health nurses are often involved in assisting either biological or foster parents to care for these children. *Fetal alcohol syndrome* (FAS) is a condition resulting from maternal alcohol consumption during pregnancy and is characterized by growth retardation, facial malformations, and central nervous system dysfunctions that may include mental retardation. In 1993, 6.7 babies of every 10,000 live births exhibited evidence of FAS. This is six times the FAS incidence rate of 1979 (Birth Defects and Genetic Disease Bureau, 1995). Incidence of FAS is even higher in some segments of the population. For example, FAS incidence rates for Native American infants are four times higher than for the general population (Centers for Disease Control, 1996a). Long-term effects of FAS include inability to hold down a job, impulsivity, social withdrawal, poor judgment, and mental retardation.

Even those infants exposed to moderate amounts of alcohol during pregnancy may have long-term effects (Larroque, Kaminski, Dehaene, Subtil, Delfosse, & Querleu, 1995). It is estimated that three to ten times as many infants have fetal alcohol effects as have FAS (Ginsberg, et al., 1994). In 1995, 16% of pregnant women participating in the Behavioral Risk Factor Surveillance Survey (BRFSS) continued to drink throughout their pregnancies (National Center for Chronic Disease Prevention and Health Promotion, 1997), increasing the potential for fetal alcohol effects in their offspring.

Fetal drug exposure also has adverse effects on children. Use of cocaine during pregnancy, for example, increases the incidence of stillbirth, low birth weight, and congenital malformations (Bateman, Ng,

Hansen, & Haggarty, 1993; Division of Reproductive Health, 1996). Fetal drug exposure has also been shown to result in neurological abnormalities and developmental delays and increased risk of sudden infant death syndrome (SIDS).

Child Abuse

Child abuse is an area of serious concern to community health nurses. Increasing incidence of all forms of child abuse has been noted since 1980, and in 1993, an estimated 2.8 million children experienced some form of abuse or neglect. Less than half of these cases were reported to child protective services, and only 28% of those reported were actually investigated (HHS survey, 1996). These figures do not include the thousands of "thrown away children" (those forced to leave home or who are not sought when they run away) (Christoffel, 1994) or "boarder babies" left in hospitals. Child abuse is addressed in detail in the section on family violence included in Chapter 34.

Evidence of all of the problems discussed above highlights the need for community health nursing services to children. Such services can help to prevent the occurrence of these and other problems affecting children and to minimize their effects on both the child and the child's family.

▶ THE DIMENSIONS MODEL AND CARE OF CHILDREN

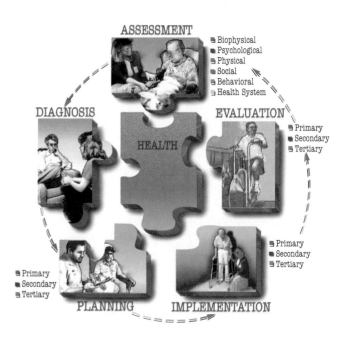

The Dimensions Model provides a framework for community health nursing efforts to accomplish the goals of primary, secondary, and tertiary prevention in the care of children.

Critical Dimensions of Nursing in the Care of Children

Community health nurses caring for children will use elements of each of the six dimensions of nursing. In the cognitive dimension the nurse will need knowledge of normal child growth and development as well as knowledge about common child health problems and interventions appropriate to those problems. Interpersonal dimensions skills of communication and collaboration remain critical to effective care of children as well as other client groups. The nurse will need to be able to communicate and collaborate effectively with the child, the family, other health care providers, teachers, and others working with children.

Advocacy, an element of the ethical dimension, may be needed at the level of the individual child and at the aggregate level. The most frequent need for individual advocacy occurs in the case of child abuse or neglect, but the nurse may also need to advocate with overprotective parents of handicapped children or with the teachers of a child with ADHD. At the aggregate level, advocacy may take the form of political activity to assure safe environmental conditions or access to health care for all children.

Both intellectual and manipulative skills may be required in the care of children. Intellectual skills of diagnosis, analysis, and planning will be based on information derived, in part, from physical assessment skills. Other manipulative skills may also be needed. For example, the nurse may need to demonstrate to parents how to suction a tracheostomy, instill eye drops, or bathe a newborn. Nursing care of children is, of course, grounded in the nursing process, but other elements of the process dimension may also be needed. Health education is a process commonly employed in the care of children as the community health nurse educates parents and children for health promotion, illness prevention, and care of existing health problems. Case management, leadership, change, and home visiting processes may also be employed. As noted earlier, the political process may be used in advocacy at the aggregate level. Finally, reflective dimension elements of theory development, research, and evaluation are needed to create a sound knowledge and theory base for community health nursing intervention with children.

 Assessing the Dimensions of Child Health

As always, the use of the model begins with assessing the client's health status to identify the need for nursing intervention. Assessment of children should be thorough, but it is not necessary to obtain all of the assessment data in the first encounter with the child. Data collected during a first encounter depend on the child and the situation. If the child is basically well, more data may be collected than if the child is ill at the time of the initial encounter. With an ill child, one would obtain data related to current problems and defer gathering additional data until a later time. Over time, however, the nurse elicits information on factors in each of the six dimensions of health.

The Biophysical Dimension

Human biological factors that may influence a child's health include age and maturation levels, genetic inheritance, and physiologic function.

Age and Maturation

ASSESSING GROWTH.   *Growth* is an increase in body size or change in the structure, function, and complexity of body cells until a point of maturity. Growth parameters considered in the nurse's assessment of the child include weight, height, and head and chest circumferences. With respect to height and weight, the nurse assesses the child in relation to normal values for the child's age and in comparison to the child's own previous growth pattern. Height and weight should be plotted on a graph at periodic intervals to establish the child's growth pattern. Plotting facilitates comparisons with age norms. Height and weight are also examined in relation to each other and to other growth parameters. Plotting a child's height in relation to his or her weight is demonstrated in Figure 20–1. Marked deviations from normal values for the child's age,

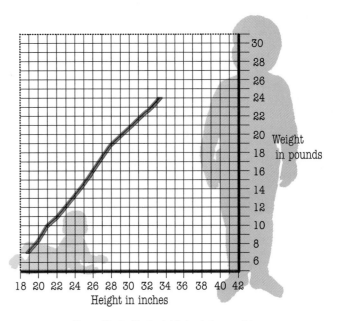

Figure 20–1. Plotting height in relation to weight.

changes in previous growth patterns, and marked incongruence among growth parameters are indications of a need for further evaluation.

Head circumference is another indicator of growth that is usually measured and plotted on a graph until 1 to 2 years of age. Head circumference is measured at the largest diameter of the head, with the tape measure circling the forehead and the occipital bulge as indicated in Figure 20–2. Head circumference is always evaluated in conjunction with chest circumference measured at the nipple line as indicated in Figure 20–2. The ratio between head and chest circumference changes dramatically in the first year of life. At birth, head circumference is approximately three fourths of an inch greater than chest circumference. By 1 year of age, the two measurements are approximately equal. Beyond 1 year of age, chest circumference should exceed head circumference, and the difference in the two measurements will continue to increase with age until adult proportions are reached.

A marked departure from the expected ratio between head and chest circumference may indicate neurological, cardiovascular, or respiratory problems. For example, an overly large head might indicate hydrocephaly, whereas a small head may be related to microcephaly or poor bone growth of the skull. A large chest might be due to respiratory difficulties or cardiac enlargement. A small chest, on the other hand, could reflect malnutrition or other causes of poor bone growth.

The nurse assesses the child in terms of these growth parameters, noting deviations from age norms or changes in the child's own growth pattern. Such deviations or changes are examined to determine whether they indicate the presence of health problems. For example, deviation from age norms may be related to metabolic or hormonal disorders, poor feeding, overfeeding, neglect, or familial characteristics, to name a few underlying factors. Unexpected changes in the child's previous growth patterns may result from either physical or emotional causes. General guidelines for assessing growth patterns in children are presented in Table 20–2.

ASSESSING DEVELOPMENT. *Development* is a process of patterned, orderly, and lifelong change in structure, thought, or behavior that occurs as a result of physical or emotional maturation. The community health nurse assesses the child's development in terms of *developmental milestones,* which are critical behaviors expected at specific ages. Developmental assessment may be approached in a number of ways. The most widely used tool for assessing the development of children from birth to age 6 is the Denver Developmental Screening Test (DDST). This test provides a gross measure of the child's fine motor and gross motor development, personal–social development, and language development. Although the test is easy to administer and can indicate problem areas related to the child's development, it is *not* a diagnostic tool and does not indicate the possible causes of developmental delays. The DDST is also useful as an aid in providing parents with anticipatory guidance regarding their child's behavior. (Test kits, score sheets, and directions for performing a DDST can be purchased from DDM, Inc., PO Box 6919, Denver, CO 80203–0911.)

TABLE 20–2. GENERAL PARAMETERS FOR ASSESSING GROWTH IN CHILDREN OF SELECTED AGES

Age Group	Assessment Parameter
Neonate (birth–30 days)	• Median weight of a full-term infant: 7 to 7¼ lbs. • Loss of several ounces in first few days • Return to birth weight by 10 to 14 days of age • Median length at birth: 19¾ to 20 in.
Infant (1–12 months)	• Doubles birth weight by 4 to 5 months of age • Triples birth weight by 1 year of age • Gains 10 in. in length by 1 year of age • Head circumference increases by about 4¾ in. (12 cm) by 1 year of age
Toddler and preschool child (2–5 years)	• Quadruples birth weight in the second year of life • Gains 5 in. height in the second year of life • Gains 3 to 5 lbs. per year from age 2 to age 5 • Grows 2 in. per year from age 2 to age 5 • Head circumference increases by 1 in. in the second year
School-age child (6–12 years)	• Gains 3 to 5 lbs. per year through age 10 • Grows 1½ to 2½ in. per year through age 10 • Boy: Gains 15 to 20 lbs. per year through age 12; grows 4½ to 5 in. per year through age 12 • Girl: Gains 20 to 25 lbs. per year through age 12; grows 5 to 6 in. per year through age 12

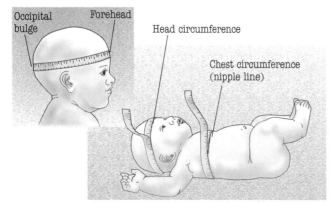

Figure 20–2. Measuring head circumference and chest circumference.

An abnormal DDST should be repeated in 2 to 3 weeks. If results on the retest are similar, a more in-depth developmental assessment is warranted. In addition to retesting, the nurse would also explore factors that may be contributing to delayed development. For example, if the child is not given the opportunity to engage in certain activities, a developmental delay may occur. Mothers who will not let their children feed themselves because of the "mess" may be contributing to a delay in personal–social development on the part of the individual child. Similarly, if the child always gets what he or she wants by pointing, language development may be delayed. Other potential reasons for developmental delay include neurological deficits, mental retardation, and neglect.

The DDST is a useful tool for assessing the development of children from birth through age 6. The development of older children should also be assessed. A few assessment tools are available for use with older children, but these are less widely used and less well known than the DDST. For children over age 6, a general assessment in terms of accomplishment of specific milestones for their age is probably sufficient. Major developmental milestones for children of various ages were presented in Chapter 6.

Genetic Inheritance. Two intrinsic genetic factors that influence the health of the child are the child's sex and racial background. Male and female children and children of different racial groups tend to experience different types of health problems. For example, the nurse would want to direct more attention to a review of systems related to the urinary tract in school-age girls than boys because urinary tract infections occur more frequently in girls than in boys in this age group (Gray & Johnson, 1997). Similarly, screening tests for sickle cell anemia would be routinely conducted on an African American child, but not a child of European descent (U.S. Preventive Health Services Task Force, 1995).

Other information about genetic inheritance is obtained from the family history. Information obtained in the family history should include the age and health status of family members as well as any history of illnesses that may have a genetic component. If family members are deceased, the cause and age at time of death should be recorded, if known. The community health nurse should ask specifically about the presence of such conditions as cancer, heart disease, allergies, diabetes, kidney disease, hypertension, seizure disorders, emotional problems, and other chronic conditions in family members. Notations about conditions identified in the family history should include the family member or members affected. Notations should also be made of the absence of specific diseases within family configuration. Family information can be described in a narrative format or diagrammed in a "genogram" as described in Chapter 18.

Physiologic Function. Information on various aspects of the child's physiologic functioning can be obtained from the history of present and past health problems, review of systems, physical examination, results of routine screening tests, and review of the child's immunization status. The review of systems is tailored to the age of the child. For example, the nurse would not need to ask questions related to sexual activity when the client is an infant. Similarly, questions about urinary tract function for an infant would center around the number of wet diapers and any strong odor to the child's urine.

Physical examination of a child is also somewhat different from that of an adult. Differences are found in both the way the examination is conducted and in the findings. Most examiners adopt a head-to-toe approach when systematically examining an adult. This is not particularly appropriate with young children. With children, the nurse starts the examination with noninvasive techniques and leaves invasive procedures, such as the examination of ears and throat, until last. Similarly, different techniques may need to be adopted to examine the ears of a child or the abdomen of a ticklish child. The examination also takes place at a slower rate because of the need for extensive explanation and reassurance for the child.

There are also differences in what is considered normal and abnormal in the findings of a pediatric physical. For example, normal values for vital signs vary considerably in young children compared with those for adults. Also, some findings that would be considered definitely abnormal in an adult are perfectly normal in children of certain ages. One such finding is a positive Babinski reflex in an infant. This is an expected response, and a negative Babinski reflex at this age would be an abnormal finding. It is beyond the scope of this book to describe all of the differences in physical findings between children and adults. Community health nurses working with youngsters should, however, become familiar with these differences so they can accurately assess children's health status.

Assessing physiologic function also involves obtaining information about current and past conditions experienced by the child. Of particular concern are the types of conditions discussed at the beginning of this chapter. The nurse should ask about the presence of these conditions or any other diagnosed health problem. In addition, the nurse would also be alert to the signs and symptoms of a variety of problems that commonly occur in children. Some of these common problems are listed in Table 20–3.

Information about the child's physiologic function may also be obtained by means of several routine screening tests performed at periodic intervals. The following are indications for the use of several routine screening measures (U.S. Preventive Health Services Task Force, 1995). Screening measures for other age groups are included in Appendix K.

Age	Screening Test
Birth	Phenylketonuria (PKU), T_4
6 months	Hematocrit or hemoglobin, lead
9 months	Tuberculin skin test (PPD)
1 year	Hematocrit or hemoglobin, sickle cell (for African American), lead
2 years	Hematocrit or hemoglobin
3–4 years	Hematocrit or hemoglobin, lead, blood pressure, hearing, vision, dental
5–6 years	Hematocrit or hemoglobin, lead, blood pressure, hearing, vision, dental, urinalysis (for girls)
7–8 years	Hematocrit or hemoglobin, lead, blood pressure, hearing, vision, dental
9–10 years	Hematocrit or hemoglobin, lead, blood pressure, hearing, vision, scoliosis, dental
11–12 years	Hematocrit or hemoglobin, lead, blood pressure, hearing, vision, scoliosis, dental

TABLE 20–3. COMMON PHYSICAL HEALTH PROBLEMS IN CHILDREN AND ORGAN SYSTEMS AFFECTED

Organ System	Commonly Encountered Problem
General	Anemia, communicable diseases, fever, failure to thrive, physical abuse
Cardiovascular system	Murmurs
Gastrointestinal system	Abdominal pain/appendicitis, colic, constipation, diarrhea, food allergy, spitting up, vomiting
Integumentary system	Abrasions, bruises, burns, diaper rash, eczema, impetigo, lice and scabies, monilial infection, other rashes, swollen lymph nodes
Musculoskeletal system	Congenital hip displasia (CHD), fractures, scoliosis, sprains and other muscle injuries
Neurological system	Headache, hearing loss, visual problems, speech problems, developmental delay
Respiratory system	Allergic rhinitis, asthma, bronchitis, bronchiolitis, croup, otitis media, pharyngitis, pneumonia, upper respiratory infection
Urinary system	Bedwetting, urinary tract infection

In many states, screening for PKU and thyroid dysfunction (T_4) occurs at birth. Early intervention in these two conditions can prevent lasting consequences such as mental retardation, so early diagnosis is important and warrants routine screening of all newborns. Other screening tests are performed at intervals throughout childhood. Hematocrit or hemoglobin levels are usually tested at 6 months, 1 year, and yearly thereafter. Another blood test routinely performed on children in high-risk groups is that for sickle cell disease. Sickle cell screening is recommended for African American children at birth. Routine screening for tuberculosis (TB) is conducted in areas with a high incidence of this disease. The Mantoux intradermal test is recommended and is usually given before 1 year of age and periodically thereafter depending on the incidence of TB in the community. Formal testing of vision and hearing can begin at 3 to 4 years of age, when children are old enough to understand and to cooperate in testing. Prior to that time, gross assessment of hearing and vision is performed as part of the physical examination. Blood pressure measurement is also recommended yearly, starting at age 3, because of the number of children who are found to be hypertensive. The final routine screening procedure for children is a urinalysis for little girls at age 4 or 5 (U.S. Preventive Health Services Task Force, 1995).

The nurse should also assess the child's immunization status. Has the child received immunizations appropriate to his or her age? Guidelines for childhood immunizations are summarized in Table 20–4. For the very young infant, the nurse would also explore the mother's immune status, as immunity in the newborn is derived from transplacental transfer of maternal antibodies. If the mother has had chickenpox, for example, the child will probably have some protection against this disease. This is also true for diseases against which the mother has been immunized.

TABLE 20–4. ROUTINE PEDIATRIC IMMUNIZATION SCHEDULE

Age	HBV	DTP	Hb	IPV	OPV	MMR	Td	Var
Birth	#1							
2 months	#2	#1	#1	#1				
4 months		#2	#2	#2				
6 months	#3	#3	#3					
12 months		#4	#4		#3	#1		#1
4–6 years		Booster			#4	Booster		
11–12 years, then every 10 years							Booster	

(Sources: Centers for Disease Control, 1996b; 1997.)

The Psychological Dimension

There are large numbers of seriously emotionally disturbed children in the United States, many of whom go unrecognized and untreated. The estimated prevalence of mental health problems among U.S. children is 17 to 20%. Child mental health problems may manifest as emotional or internalizing disorders characterized by internal feelings of anxiety or depression, or as behavioral or externalizing disorders characterized by disruptive behavior (Anderson & Werry, 1994). Community health nurses should routinely assess children for evidence of emotional problems and should explore factors in the psychological environment that may contribute to those problems. The child's psychological environment is a product of forces within and outside the child. Areas for consideration related to the psychological environment include the child's reactivity patterns, parental expectations and discipline, parental coping abilities and mental health status, parent–child interaction, and the child's self-image. The nurse should also consider the potential for child abuse within the family or child care environment.

Reactivity Patterns. Children react differently to their environment based on their individual temperament. These differences in response are the child's reactivity patterns (Pilletteri, 1987). *Reactivity patterns* are a set of typical responses to environmental stimuli displayed by a particular child. These patterns are part of the child's internal psychological environment. Reactivity patterns may persist throughout life and may influence the way others react to the child, thereby affecting the child's self-image and ability to interact meaningfully with others.

There are nine areas in which children's reactivity patterns may differ: activity level, rhythmicity, approach to new situations, adaptability, intensity of reaction, distractibility, attention span, threshold of response, and mood. The characteristic features of differences in these reactivity patterns and their implications for the child's interactions with others are presented in Table 20–5.

The nurse can determine the child's reactivity patterns or typical patterns of response to his or her environment by means of the client interview and by observation. In the interview, either the child or caretaker—in the case of a young child—can be asked how the child responds in each of the areas addressed. The nurse will be able to determine reactivity patterns by also observing the child. For example, perseverance can be seen in the child who repeatedly returns to an activity when told "no" or when a hand has been slapped. Similarly, response to new situations can be gauged on the basis of the child's response to the nurse as a stranger or to the environment of the clinic or office.

Knowledge of a child's reactivity patterns can suggest some potential problems that the child may encounter in his or her interactions with the outside world. Such knowledge also aids the nurse in designing interventions to assist families to adapt to their youngster's reactivity patterns or to aid children in adapting patterns to better fit the world around them.

Parental Expectations. Many of the difficulties in relationships between parents and children, and between the father and mother regarding their children, stem from unrealistic beliefs about things that children should and should not do. Community health nurses can help prevent such difficulties by assisting parents to develop realistic expectations of children's behavior. For example, it is unrealistic to expect a 3-year-old not to wet the bed occasionally. The community health nurse can explain to parents that the depth of a child's sleep at this age is such that urges to empty one's bladder are not sufficient to wake the child and so accidents occur. Similarly, the negativism of a 2-year-old is normal behavior, not evidence of deliberate disobedience. The nurse should explore with parents their expectations of children's behavior to determine whether these expectations are realistic in light of the child's age and developmental level, as well as his or her physical status.

Discipline. Discipline is frequently an area of concern for parents and children alike. Many parents need assistance in knowing when and how to discipline children appropriately. The nurse should assess parental approaches to discipline and the appropriateness of disciplinary measures used. The nurse should also determine the extent to which parents adhere to the principles that should guide discipline. These principles and related assessment questions are presented in Table 20–6.

Discipline can take any of several forms, and the community health nurse should ascertain the approach taken to discipline and the effectiveness of that approach. Verbal discipline is very effective with some children. When verbal discipline is used, the nurse should make sure that parents are focusing on the child's behavior and not the child. The idea should be conveyed that it is the *behavior* that is unacceptable, not the child. Physical punishment, such as spanking, may be used, but the nurse should ascertain that it is used with caution. Children should not be hit with anything other than the hand and then only where no damage can occur (eg, on the buttocks). The nurse

TABLE 20–5. CHARACTERISTIC FEATURES AND IMPLICATIONS OF DIFFERENCES IN REACTIVITY PATTERNS AMONG CHILDREN

Reactivity Pattern	Characteristic Feature	Implications
ACTIVITY LEVEL		
Active	• Curious and motivated to learn new things • Always into something • Doesn't always consider consequences of action • Gets dirty frequently	• Responds rapidly to new ideas or directions • Needs close supervision • Needs to channel energy productively • Delay dressing for important occasions until the last minute
Placid	• Slow to react • Frequently late • Needs more time to complete activities	• Need to encourage interaction with environment • May need to be awakened early to get to school on time • Need to allow extra time for activities • Need to allow time for child to respond
RHYTHMICITY		
Regular	• Tends to eat, sleep, and defecate at the same time each day • Responds poorly to schedule changes • Schedule may not coincide with that of family members	• Predictable behavior allows planning • Need to maintain a regular schedule • Easier to toilet-train • Need to adjust family schedules to accommodate child • Need to accept fussiness related to schedule changes
Irregular	• Eating, sleeping, and other habits unpredictable • Responds well to schedule changes	• Unable to plan daily schedule • More difficult to train • Need to maintain flexibility in family schedules • May need relief of caretaker to carry out other duties
APPROACH TO NEW SITUATIONS		
Adventurous	• Accepts new ideas and people easily • Willing to try new things • Frequently unaware of danger	• Need to caution on talking to strangers • Needs close supervision • Need to discuss consequences of action • Need to provide safe "adventures"
Shy	• Slow and cautious in new situations • May have difficulty meeting new people • May have difficulty adjusting to new situations	• Less likely to engage in dangerous activities • Needs advance warning of changes • Needs extra time to adjust to change • Need to reinforce similarities to previously encountered situations • Need to implement changes slowly
ADAPTABILITY		
Adaptable	• Adjusts easily to changes in situation	
Rigid	• Adjusts poorly to changes in situation	• Need to assist child to adjust to changes • Need to accept and deal with child's feelings of anger and frustration • Need to introduce changes slowly if possible
INTENSITY OF REACTION		
Intense reaction	• Reacts strenuously to stimuli • Cries with little stimulus • Emotionally wearing for caretakers • Difficult to know when there is cause for concern	• Need to accept and legitimize child's expression of feelings • Need to arrange respite for primary caretaker • Need to help child express emotion in appropriate ways • Need not to ignore in case of serious injury
Moderate	• Slow to anger • Easy to soothe and comfort	• Need to be aware of subtle signs of distress • Need to encourage child to express feelings
DISTRACTIBILITY		
Easily distracted	• Easily distracted from current activity	• Use distraction to halt unacceptable behavior • Need to promote task accomplishment by removing distractions or refocusing attention • Needs frequent reminders • Provide extra time for task completion • Acknowledge small accomplishments
Persevering	• Perseveres in current activity despite distractions	• May need to remove child from temptation • May need help in recognizing futility of efforts • May need help in dealing with failure

TABLE 20–5. **CHARACTERISTIC FEATURES AND IMPLICATIONS OF DIFFERENCES IN REACTIVITY PATTERNS AMONG CHILDREN (Continued)**

Reactivity Pattern	Characteristic Feature	Implications
ATTENTION SPAN		
Long	• Can work at the same activity for extended periods • May bore others with continued attention to a "dead" topic	• May need to be made to stop one activity to move on to others • May need to set time limits on activities • Need to help child understand others may not have same level of interest
Short	• Easily bored with an activity	• Needs to be kept busy to avoid mischief • Need to refocus attention on task accomplishment
THRESHOLD OF RESPONSE		
High	• Requires extensive stimulus to react	• Need to be aware of subtle signs of distress • Need to watch for extreme reaction when threshold is reached
Low	• Requires minimal stimulus to react • Emotionally wearing for caretakers	• May need to help child channel reaction in productive ways • Need to arrange respite for primary caretaker
MOOD		
Happy	• Basically happy with life	• May need to be sure child is not taken advantage of
Unhappy	• Unhappy with most of life • Frequently critical of others or situation • Emotionally wearing for caretakers	• Need to accept feelings of discontent • Need to help child be less critical of others or express criticism in socially acceptable ways • Need to arrange respite for primary caretaker

should also be sure that parents refrain from using too much force even in spanking.

Removal of privileges is another effective means of discipline. When parents use this approach to discipline, the nurse should determine that the "punishment fits the crime" whenever possible and that the child is helped to see the connection between his or her behavior and the restriction imposed. For example, if a young child has purposefully broken another child's toy, he or she can be made to give up a similar toy for a certain period of time. Another effective method of discipline is "time-out." Time-out effectively stops the behavior and affords the child an opportunity to contemplate its consequences. Whatever the form of discipline used, the nurse should ensure that it is employed in a way that leads to the accomplishment of its purposes.

Parental Coping Skills and Mental Health. The ability of a child's parents to cope with the stresses and frustrations of parenthood and everyday life is another factor that influences the child's psychological environment. Parents who are unable to cope with their own frustrations are likely to take some of their frustration out on the child. Even when this is not so, children are sensitive to the atmosphere around them and may feel insecure and uncertain in a situation in which parents are under obvious stress.

Three basic approaches can be taken to cope with the stresses of parenthood. The first of these is to change the situation that is creating stress. If a child's behavior is creating stress, the parent can attempt to alter the child's behavior. Or the parent can temporarily remove oneself from the situation by hiring a babysitter and leaving the home for a few hours.

The second approach is to change one's attitude toward the situation. Parents may stop to consider that they will only have their children at home for a few more years or that their own children could be twice as bad (like the neighbor's child) and so decide that the situation is not as bad as it first seemed. Finally, parents can change their response to the situation. This may occur when the parents channel their frustrations into a floor-scrubbing spree or other activity, or decide that the situation is not worth worrying about.

Community health nurses should assess whether parents use any of these three methods of coping and the effectiveness of their use. In addition, community health nurses can identify ineffective parental coping mechanisms that may contribute to a psychological environment that is not conducive to the child's physical or emotional health. Parents can be asked what stressors they perceive in their lives and how they deal with stress.

In addition to parental coping skills, the presence of parental psychopathology can influence the health of children in the home. For example, parental depression may contribute to child neglect when one or both parents do not have the psychic energy to meet children's physical or emotional needs. Antiso-

TABLE 20–6. PRINCIPLES OF EFFECTIVE DISCIPLINE AND RELATED ASSESSMENT QUESTIONS

Principle	Assessment Question
1. Determine what is important.	• Have parents determined what behaviors are never acceptable? • Is there good rationale for this determination? • Do parents say "No" automatically?
2. Be consistent.	• Are parents consistent in what is considered unacceptable behavior? • Do parents allow children to wear them down until they let unacceptable behavior pass? • Do parents agree on what behavior is unacceptable, or can children manipulate parents? • Have parents determined situations in which certain behaviors, otherwise allowed, are not acceptable? • Have parents explained to children the reason for the difference in what is allowable at some times and not at others?
3. Never act in anger.	• Do parents control their anger before disciplining children? • Do parents use a "cooling off" period when needed? • Have parents explained the reason for the cooling off period so children will learn appropriate ways of dealing with anger?
4. Allow time for compliance.	• Do parents allow time for children to comply with directions, or do they expect instant obedience? • Do parents respect children's need to complete a task in which they are engaged before complying with parental instructions?
5. Set limits ahead of time.	• Do parents establish rules of behavior prior to disciplining certain behaviors on the part of the child? • Do parents use knowledge of child growth and development to anticipate children's behavior? • When children engage in unacceptable behavior that is not addressed in previously established rules, do parents give a warning before instituting punishment?
6. Be sure the child understands the rules.	• Are parents clear on what behavior is expected of the child and what behavior is unacceptable?
7. Prevent rather than punish unacceptable behavior.	• Do parents take steps to prevent unacceptable behavior before it occurs, rather than punishing it afterward? • Do parents remove sources of temptation for young children? • Do parents provide adequate supervision for children?
8. Be sure that discipline is warranted.	• Do parents ascertain the facts of a situation before punishing children? • Are parental expectations warranted given the developmental level of the child? • Have rules been clearly established and made clear to the child? • Do parents attempt to determine the reason for the child's behavior and explain what is wrong when the child's intentions were good?
9. Be sure that discipline is meaningful.	• Do parents make sure that the child understands the reason for punishment? • Do parents explain how the child can correct his or her behavior? • What form of discipline do parents use? • Is the form of discipline used effective in modifying the child's behavior?

cial behavior by young women has been correlated with later hyperactivity, depression, peer conflict, social withdrawal, immaturity, and dependency in their children (Martin & Burchinal, 1992). Similarly, parental psychopathology (eg, anxiety, affective, and substance abuse disorders) has been associated with attention deficit hyperactivity disorder (ADHD), conduct disorders, and emotional disorders among children. History of parental hyperactivity also seems to be a risk factor for similar problems in male offspring (Schachar & Wachsmuth, 1990).

Parent–Child Interaction. The quality of interaction between parent and child is another important factor in the child's psychological environment. In assessing this area, the nurse would observe the pattern of interaction between parent and child in the nurse's presence. Do parents relate well to the child, or do they scream and yell over minor misbehavior? Do parents

convey a sense of concern for the child and his or her welfare, or do they ignore the child unless the behavior impinges on the parents' level of comfort? Answers to these and similar questions provide the nurse with a picture of typical interactions between parent and child.

In the child with a chronic illness or disability, the quality of parent–child interactions may be profoundly influenced by the parents' response to the child's condition. These children tend to have higher incidence rates for emotional problems than do healthy children. The community health nurse can assess the parental response to the child's condition and identify any problem areas that may adversely affect the child's emotional status.

Parental responses to chronic illness or disability in their children usually occur in four stages: disbelief, anger, demystification, and conditional acceptance (Austin, 1990). The community health nurse should assess the stage of parental response and the effects of that response on interactions with the child.

In the stage of disbelief, the parent denies the condition. If prolonged, this denial could result in unrealistic expectations of the child and frustration for the child who is unable to meet those expectations.

In the second stage, anger, the parent begins to understand the implications of the child's condition for the parent and for other family members. The parent is faced with additional duties and responses that he or she may not be willing to assume. Feelings of anger related to the disruption of life caused by the child's condition may be turned against the child and may be exhibited in emotional or physical abuse. Other feelings that may be experienced in this stage are guilt, anxiety, and depression. These feelings may also interfere with healthy parent–child interactions. Guilt, for example, can lead to attempts to "make up to the child for his or her condition" that interfere with appropriate discipline for the child or encourage the child to manipulate parental behavior by playing on that guilt. Anxiety may contribute to an attitude of overprotectiveness on the part of the parent, and the child may not be allowed opportunities for development appropriate to his or her age and health status. Depression can result in parental immobilization and consequent neglect of the child.

In the demystification stage, parents actively seek information about the child's condition. In addition, they begin to cope with the problem through a mechanism called "downward comparison" (Austin, 1990). *Downward comparison* is a coping strategy in which one compares one's own situation with those of others whose circumstances are worse. In this stage, parents also begin to develop a sense of control over the situation, which they can communicate to the child, thus decreasing the child's level of fear and anxiety and improving the child's self-image.

The final stage is conditional acceptance, when parents incorporate the child's condition into their view of reality. Parents and child accommodate to the condition and normalize family life as much as possible. Parents also exhibit control of the problem by developing contingency plans to deal with potential problems. In addition, family members may come to see positive effects of the child's condition such as drawing the family closer together. Parents who have accepted the child's condition foster the child's ability to develop as normally as possible. Acceptance does not mean that the child's condition is no longer stressful for the parents. Parents of chronically ill children have identified triggers that increase their uncertainty and stress. Some of these triggers include routine medical appointments, bodily changes in the child, changes in therapy, negative outcomes of treatment,

and new developmental demands (Cohen, 1995). Other sources of stress for these parents include inadaptibility on the part of the child, high caregiving demands, lack of response from the child or support from others, and the parents' own health status (Holaday, 1997).

Each of the stages of parental response presented here are normal. When parents fail to proceed to later stages, however, their response may have adverse effects on interactions with the child and on the child's psychological environment. The community health nurse should identify any problems resulting from parental response to chronic illness or disability in the child.

Self-image. Another area to be addressed in relation to the child's psychological environment is the child's self-image. The nurse can determine the child's self-perceptions by asking the child to "Tell me about yourself." A similar approach would be to ask the child to describe things that he or she does well. A child who has difficulty answering this question may not have a very strong self-image. For younger children who cannot easily articulate their feelings about themselves, nurses might watch for self-punishing behavior (eg, slapping oneself or saying "I'm dumb") or ask them to draw and explain pictures of themselves.

Child Abuse. Inability to cope with life's stresses is one of the primary contributors to child abuse, a growing area of concern for community health nurses. The community health nurse should be alert to evidence of actual or potential child abuse. Although child abuse has both physical and psychological effects on children, it is factors in the psychological environment that place families at risk for the occurrence of abuse. Guidelines for child abuse assessment include considerations of parent characteristics and role expectations, child characteristics and behavior, and environmental stressors. Parental characteristics that increase the potential for child abuse include a history of abuse or parental abandonment when they themselves were children, feelings of hostility to or alienation from their own parents, and physical or emotional health problems experienced by the child's parents. Unrealistic parental expectations of the child, verbalizations of hostility or disappointment in the child, parental expectations that the child will always understand the parents' feelings, and a belief that the child does not love the parents enough are also parental indicators of potential for abuse.

Characteristics of the child may also signal potential for abuse. Such characteristics include prematurity, early separation from parents, developmental disability, obvious differences from siblings, difficulty concentrating, and inappropriate ways of expressing needs. The nurse should also be aware of environmental stressors such as financial pressures, social isolation, alcoholism or drug abuse, spousal abuse, and poor school performance that may indicate a potential for abuse.

Community health nurses should also be alert to signs of actual abuse or neglect. Some of these include evidence of obvious injury; torn, stained, or bloody underwear; an enlarged anal opening; signs of malnutrition and poor hygiene; and failure to thrive. Nurses should also be suspicious of stories that are inconsistent with injuries presented or with the child's stage of development and of inappropriate behavior on the part of adults in the situation (eg, belligerence, being overly concerned, or refusing to allow diagnostic tests). Children may also display unusual behavior such as being excessively withdrawn or extremely passive. Abused children may cling to parents with unusual force or be remarkably detached from them.

The nurse should be alert to families at risk for child abuse and work to help them develop positive parenting skills as described in this chapter. The development of such skills may help to prevent abuse or to eliminate it in families where it already exists. The problem of child abuse and potential nursing interventions are addressed in more detail in Chapter 34.

The Physical Dimension

Safety hazards are a major factor in the physical dimension that influence the health of children of all ages. Safety concerns are related to the child's physical surroundings and the child's ability to gain access to dangerous substances. The nurse should assess both the presence of hazardous conditions in the child's environment and the child's knowledge of safety-related behaviors.

The community health nurse also assesses the knowledge of and adherence to safety practices among parents and other caretakers. Areas for consideration relative to caretaker practices include the amount of supervision provided for the child and parental use of safety devices. Child safety practices in both the home and the child care environment should be considered if they are different.

Considerations in assessing child safety factors vary with the age of the child. Specific questions related to safety assessment for infants, toddlers and preschool children, and school-age children are presented in Table 20–7.

For the infant, the nurse assesses parental safety practices, sleeping arrangements, and toys. The nurse should determine whether parents are aware of the potential for falls and the danger in leaving an infant unattended on an elevated surface. The use of safety belts in high chairs, swings, strollers, and infant seats should also be explored. The safety of sleeping arrangements should be addressed as well. Areas to be considered are the spacing between crib slats, use of plastic film to cover mattresses, and use of nontoxic paint on crib surfaces. The nurse should also make sure that no cords are dangling from drapes near the crib in which the child could become entangled and thus strangle. Toys should be soft with no sharp edges and should not have small parts that can be detached and swallowed. Care should also be taken that toys with small parts belonging to older siblings are kept out of the infant's reach.

Safety concerns for the toddler or preschool child include supervision of play activities, use of safety equipment, safety education, the extent to which the home or child care center has been "child-proofed," toy safety, and playground safety.

Considerations in childproofing include covering electrical outlets, eliminating dangling electrical cords, and storing sharp objects or hazardous substances appropriately. Sharp objects should be locked away as should any poisonous substances. Placing these items up high is not a sufficient precaution, as children rapidly learn to climb and can devise ingenious methods of obtaining objects placed out of reach. Locks or childproof latches should be used on drawers or cabinets where hazardous substances are kept, and children should be closely supervised at all times.

Access to medications and other potentially poisonous items should be prevented. Most poisonings occur in the home. Potential poisons include medications, cleaning agents, paints, and paint removal substances. The Poison Prevention Packaging Act of 1970 requires child-resistant containers for 15 categories of products. Ever since the implementation of this legislation, poisonings from products in these categories have declined. Poisonings related to unregulated products, however, have increased. Possible causes for the still overwhelming numbers of unintentional child poisonings include failure to use child-resistant packages correctly, improper storage of potential poisons, ignorance of first aid measures for poisoning, and failure of some pharmacies to use child-resistant packaging.

Toys are another safety concern for children in this age group. Many toy-related injuries result from physical impact with or ingestion of the toy. The primary factors involved in toy-related injuries are selection of toys inappropriate to the child's age and improper use of the toy. In conjunction with the U.S. Consumer Product Safety Commission, the Toy Manufacturers of America has developed guidelines for the selection and use of toys that the community

TABLE 20–7. QUESTIONS FOR ASSESSING ENVIRONMENTAL SAFETY FOR CHILDREN OF SELECTED AGES

Age Group	Assessment Questions
Infant (birth–1 year)	• Is the child left unattended on elevated surfaces? • Is an approved car seat restraint used consistently? • Do parents routinely fasten safety straps in high chairs, strollers, swings, and infant seats? • Do parents use flame-retardant sleepwear? • Does the infant have his or her own crib? • Is plastic film that might suffocate the child left on or in the crib? • Are there dangling drapery or other cords near the crib in which the child could strangle? • Are slats on the crib sufficiently close together that the child cannot get his or her head stuck? • Has nontoxic paint been used on crib surfaces? • Are bumper pads used to prevent injury? • Are soft pillows removed from the bed? • Do mobiles or toys have sharp surfaces or small parts that can be swallowed? • Are toys free of strings that could choke the child? • Are siblings' toys with small parts kept out of the infant's reach? • Do parents refrain from giving a bottle in bed or propping a bottle?

Toddler (2–3 years)	• Are car seats used consistently?
	• Is the child adequately supervised during waking hours?
	• Do parents check the child periodically during naps?
	• Has the environment been child-proofed so that:
	  —Electrical outlets are covered?
	  —Sharp objects and poisonous substances are locked away, not just placed out of reach?
	  —Medications and other hazardous substances are kept in appropriate containers?
	  —Safety latches or locks are on cabinets used to store hazardous items?
	  —Child-resistant containers are used correctly?
	  —Dangling electrical cords have been eliminated?
	  —Stairs are gated?
	  —Bathroom doors are kept closed to prevent the child from falling in the toilet?
	• Have parents inspected play equipment for hazards?
	• Is the surface below playground equipment padded in some way?
	• Are toys appropriate to the child's age and ability?
	• Do parents leave the child unattended in the tub?
	• If the family has a pool, is it adequately fenced?

Preschool child (3–6 years)	• Has the home been child-proofed as above?
	• Are pot handles turned away from the edge of the stove?
	• Are car seats or seat belts used consistently?
	• Is play equipment safe?
	• Are toys used appropriately, with adult supervision as needed?
	• Is the child adequately supervised at all times?
	• Has the child been given safety education regarding:
	  —Talking to or going with strangers?
	  —Crossing the street?
	  —Fire safety?
	  —Water safety?

School-age child (6–12 years)	• Is play equipment safe?
	• Are sports and play activities well supervised?
	• Are sports activities age appropriate?
	• Are seat belts used consistently?
	• Has the child been given safety education regarding:
	  —Sports?
	  —Bicycling?
	  —Water safety?
	  —Opening the door to strangers or letting others know one is home alone?
	  —Correct use of medications?
	• Does the child know how to swim?
	• Is a helmet used consistently for bike riding and other activities as appropriate?
	• Are firearms kept in the home? If so, are they locked up? Is ammunition kept locked in a separate place from guns?

health nurse can pass on to parents to enable them to make their child's environment a little safer:

- Select toys appropriate to the child's age, ability, and interest.
- Establish ground rules for playing with the toy.
- Select toys with clear instructions for parents and child on use of the toy.
- Select toys that are sturdily constructed.
- Avoid toys with small parts for young children.
- Avoid toys that propel or shoot objects.
- Supervise use of toys with electrical heating elements (use recommended for children over 8 years of age only).
- Consider the environment in which toys are used.

Playground safety is another area of concern. In 1991, more than 43,000 head injuries were associated with playground equipment (Baker, et al., 1994). The nurse should assess the safety of any playground equipment in the home or day care environment. Some considerations include the ground surface on which equipment is placed and the state of repair of equipment. Energy-absorbing mats, wood chips, and sand under equipment reduce the likelihood of injuries due to falls. Concrete, asphalt, and packed earth, however, are very dangerous. The nurse should also determine whether equipment is properly anchored and free of obstructions. Equipment should also be in good repair and children should be supervised in its use.

Safety assessment for school-age children should include considerations of playground safety described above and the correct and appropriate use of toys. Other considerations include supervision of sports activities and seeing that such activities are appropriate to the age and development of the child. Elementary school children, for example, should not engage in contact sports such as football. Youngsters of this age should be taught safety rules for sports and bicycling, including the use of helmets and other protective equipment. Seat belt use and the ability to swim are other important areas for assessment.

A major concern with this age group is exposure to firearms. The nurse should explore whether firearms are present in the home, or in the homes of friends, and how access to firearms is controlled. Guns should be kept away from all children, and youngsters in early adolescence should be taught how to handle them correctly for supervised sporting use.

The Social Dimension

Factors in the child's social environment that contribute to health or illness should also be assessed. In younger children, the nurse might observe interactions with others in the environment, including the nurse. Parents can be asked about the child's interaction with siblings and with peers. The nurse should determine whether such interactions are normal for the child's age. For example, parallel play (play alongside of, rather than with, other children) is to be expected of toddlers; sharing and interactive play would not be expected to occur until preschool years. Competitive games and activities with rules are normal interactive behaviors for school-age children.

Older youngsters can also be asked about their friends and what kinds of things they do together. In addition, parents may offer their perspective on how the child interacts with agemates at school and in other settings.

Another area for assessment related to the child's social environment is exploration of family culture and its effects on children's health. Other social factors within the family environment may also influence the health of the child. For example, a parent's unemployment may mean a lack of available health care for children or, in some cases, lack of money for adequate nutrition, housing, and other necessities. In 1994, more than 14 million children (over 21%) lived in families with incomes below poverty level. For minority children, figures are even more alarming. For example, over 43% of black children and 41% of Hispanic children live at poverty level or below (U.S. Department of Commerce, 1996). Low income is a significant factor in homelessness among children; children currently make up more than one third of the homeless population in some areas (Reimer, Van Cleve, & Galbraith, 1995). Health concerns of the homeless are addressed in more detail in Chapter 23.

Prejudice in the social environment may also affect children. For instance, they may be subjected to ridicule by other children at school because of their dress, physical appearance, family culture, or religion. Family religious affiliation may also lead to potential health problems. For example, during early 1994, persons in religious groups that do not permit immunization accounted for half of all reported measles cases (National Immunization Program, 1994b).

The Behavioral Dimension

Behavioral factors can be important contributors to health or illness in children. Areas of primary concern include nutrition, rest and exercise, child care, school performance, and use of hazardous substances.

Nutrition. Childhood growth and appropriate development are facilitated by adequate nutrition. Both malnutrition and obesity contribute to childhood morbidity and mortality (Cohn & Deckelbaum, 1993; Pelletier, Frongillo, & Habicht, 1993). A review of several recent studies, for example, indicated a strong association between declining weight for age and increased mortality. Forty-five percent of malnutrition deaths in these studies were attributable to mild to moderate, rather than severe, malnutrition, indicating the potential for health effects of even slight undernourishment (Pelletier, et al., 1993).

Much of the malnutrition found among children in this country is due to inadequate knowledge of nutrition on the part of parents. The community health nurse should assess parental knowledge of child nutritional needs as well as nutritional practices related to children. Nutritional status should be assessed in relation to the child's age and nutritional needs. Specific questions related to assessment for children of different ages are included in Table 20–8.

Rest and Exercise. Another area for consideration with respect to lifestyle factors and their influence on child health is the ratio of rest to exercise. With infants, the nurse would assess sleeping patterns and the length of periods of sleep and periods of wakefulness. One problem that may become evident at this point is the child whose schedule does not coincide with that of the rest of the family, so the nurse should be sure to ask when sleep periods occur. The nurse would also note whether the child appears to be sleeping more or less than would be expected at that age.

Activity level should also be assessed. Is the child normally active or listless and apathetic? Lethargy may be a sign of a variety of physical health problems including acute illness, hypothyroidism, and anemia. Hyperactivity should also be noted. Hyperactivity in young infants is a frequent aftereffect of drug exposure during pregnancy.

TABLE 20–8. QUESTIONS FOR ASSESSING THE NUTRITIONAL STATUS OF CHILDREN OF SELECTED AGES

Age Group	Assessment Question
Infant (birth–1 year)	• Is the child breast- or bottlefed?
	• If breastfed,
	—How often does the child nurse?
	—How long does the child nurse?
	—Does mother alternate breasts?
	—Is mother's nutritional intake adequate?
	—Does the child seem satisfied?
	• If bottlefed,
	—How often does the baby eat?
	—How much formula is consumed in 24 hours?
	—What type of formula is used? Is it iron-fortified?
	—Do parents prepare formula correctly?
	—Do parents use appropriate feeding techniques (eg, not propping the bottle)?
	—Does the infant tolerate the formula well?
	• Is the infant gaining weight?
	• At what point did parents introduce solids? (Recommendations are for cereal at 6 months, followed by vegetables, fruits, and meat.)
	• How much solid food does the baby eat?
	• Do parents use individual foods rather than less nutritious combination foods (like vegetable and beef combinations)?
	• Is one new food introduced at a time? Over several days?
	• Has the child started eating table food? (This usually occurs at about 9 months of age.)
	• Is the child weaned from the bottle by 1 year?
Toddler and preschool child (2–5 years)	• What foods is the child eating?
	• How much food is the child eating?
	• Is the child's diet well balanced?
	• Are finger foods and variety encouraged?
	• Are nutritious snacks provided?
	• Is the child given small portions initially and allowed to ask for more to enhance independence?
	• Is the child's growth pattern normal for his or her age?
School-age child (6–12 years)	• Is the child's diet well balanced?
	• Is junk food avoided?
	• Are snacks nutritious?
	• How much does the child eat?
	• Is the child overweight or underweight?
	• Is the child's height within normal limits for his or her age?

Lack of exercise among children is a factor contributing to the increasing prevalence of childhood obesity. For many children, television and video games have largely replaced outdoor play. The community health nurse should assess the extent of regular exercise obtained as well as the type of activity performed.

Recreational activities may also pose health hazards, and potential for injury or other health effects should be assessed. Do children use appropriate safety equipment during sports activities? Are helmets consistently used for bicycling, skate boarding, roller blading, and skiing? Do hazardous substances used in children's or parents' hobbies pose potential health hazards? These and other similar areas should be considered by the nurse in his or her assessment of child health.

Child Care.   Child care is a factor in the health of a child that coincides with a family's dual wage-earner lifestyle or with a single-parent lifestyle when the parent works. The nurse assessing factors influencing the child's health should ask the following questions about child care arrangements:

- Who cares for the child?
- Where does child care take place?
- Are child caretakers qualified to care for children?
- Have parents requested references from private child caretakers other than family members?
- Is there more than one adult in the child care setting?
- Have parents inspected the child care premises for potential safety hazards?
- Do parents "drop in" to witness the quality of care provided to children in the child care setting and the extent of supervision of children's activities?
- Do parents investigate unusual stories reported by children?
- Have parents made contingency plans for care of the child when he or she is ill or when the child caretaker is unavailable?
- Are child care facilities licensed, if appropriate?

Child care for children of working parents tends to occur in one of four arrangements (Berg, et al., 1994), the most common of which is nonresidential care in a recognized child care center. Other possibilities are family day care, in which the caretaker supervises several children in his or her home, care by relatives, or in-home care by a nonrelative. Each arrangement has both advantages and disadvantages that should be considered by working parents. In addition to those children involved in specific child care arrangements, there are 7 million "latchkey" children in the United States, children aged 5 to 13 years who are left to care for themselves for several hours each day (Berg, et al., 1994).

School Performance.   Another area for consideration with respect to lifestyle relates to school-age children. The nurse obtains information on the child's response to the school environment and on performance in school. Children can be asked how they like school. Information on performance can be obtained from both children and parents. Areas of academic and interpersonal strength and weakness should be identified, and the nurse should also try to gain some insight into family attitudes toward education because these will influence the child's performance. Do parents assist the child with learning tasks? What are parental expectations with regard to school performance? Are they too high or too low? What efforts, if any, are being made to assist the child with problems related to school performance? The child's ability to interact with peers and any school behavior problems should also be determined.

Exposure to Hazardous Substances.   The effects of fetal drug and alcohol exposure were discussed earlier in this chapter. Unfortunately, infants are not the only members of the pediatric population exposed to drugs and alcohol, not to mention tobacco. Both passive and active exposure to tobacco occurs among children. Maternal smoking, for example, is a contributing factor in 19% of annual expenditures for childhood respiratory conditions (Stoddard & Gray, 1997). Breastfeeding infants are exposed to tobacco by-products not only through smoke inhalation, but also via breast milk (Stepans & Wilkerson, 1993). Other children may experience passive smoking, which has been linked to increased incidence of respiratory infections, otitis media, asthma, poor school performance, ADHD, and behavior problems (Weitzman, Gortmacher, & Sobol, 1992). Older children may actively experiment with tobacco or use alcohol and drugs. For example, in 1994, 10% of 12 to 17 year olds had smoked cigarettes in the last month, 16% had used alcohol, 7% marijuana, and 0.4% had used cocaine (U.S. Department of Health and Human Services, 1996b). Family substance use and abuse should also be explored. For instance, an estimated 7 million children have parents who abuse alcohol (Palfrey, 1994), and abuse of other drugs is common as well.

The Health System Dimension

Assessment of the health system dimension includes consideration of the attitudes of the child and the family toward health and health care, the usual source of

ASSESSMENT TIPS: Assessing Children's Health

Biophysical Dimension

Age and Development

What is the child's age? Is the child's developmental level commensurate with his or her age?

How do the child's height, weight, and head circumference compare to age standards?

Are there impediments to normal development in the child's circumstances?

Do parental behaviors foster child development?

Genetic Inheritance

Is the child a boy or girl? Is the child's sex congruent with parental desires?

Is there a family history of genetic predisposition to disease? If so, to what disease(s)?

Physiologic Function

Does the child have any existing physical health problems?

Are there any problems with physiologic function (eg, constipation, spitting up)?

Does the child have a history of frequent illnesses?

What is the status of routine screening of the child?

Are the child's immunizations up-to-date for his or her age?

Psychological Dimension

Does the child exhibit evidence of psychological health problems?

What is the attitude of family members toward the child?

What are the child's reactivity patterns? Do the child's reactivity patterns create conflict within the family?

Are parental expectations of the child realistic?

How is the child disciplined? Is discipline appropriate to the child's age and abilities? Is discipline warranted?

How adequate are parental coping skills? Do parents exhibit evidence of mental illness?

What is the quality of parent–child interaction?

How adequate is the child's self-concept?

Is there evidence of child abuse in the family?

Physical Dimension

Are there safety hazards present in the home environment? Is the home effectively child-proofed?

Do parents use age-appropriate safety measures?

Are the child's toys safe and age-appropriate? Is play equipment safe and in good repair?

Does the neighborhood present any health or safety hazards for the child?

What are the sleeping arrangements for the child? Are these arrangements safe?

Social Dimension

Does the child interact effectively with others?

What roles does the child play in the family? Are these roles age-appropriate?

What are the effects of family culture on the child's health?

Are there factors in the family's social environment that may affect health (eg, unemployment)?

What is the family's economic level? Is family income adequate to meet the child's needs?

Are parents employed outside the home?

Behavioral Dimension

Consumption Patterns

What is the child's usual diet? Is it adequate for growth?

Is there evidence of substance abuse in the family?

Is the child exposed to tobacco smoke?

Doe the child use alcohol, tobacco, or other drugs?

Rest and Exercise

What is the child's usual sleep pattern? Is it appropriate to the child's age?

What is the child's activity level? Is it age-appropriate?

What is the extent of the child's exercise? Is the amount of exercise obtained adequate?

Is the child involved in sports activities? If so, does the child use appropriate safety equipment?

What recreational activities is the child involved in? Do these activities pose any health or safety hazards?

Child Care/School

Who provides care for the child? Is the child involved in child care outside the home?

Are child care arrangements safe and appropriate to the child's age and developmental level?

Is the child care setting free of health and safety hazards?

Do parents have plans for contingency care if the child is ill?

(continued)

health care, and use of health care services. Particular consideration should be given to the use of primary preventive services related to immunization and dental care.

Another area for consideration is how health care services are financed by the family. Children under 18 years of age constitute more than one fourth of the uninsured population in the United States (Berg, et al., 1994). Homeless children are particularly unlikely to be insured. Not surprisingly, as family incomes decline, the percentage of uninsured children increases. These figures indicate that those least able to afford out-of-pocket health care costs are those least likely to have health insurance coverage. The end result is lack of access to health care. Other health system factors may also influence the health of children. In one study, for example, early newborn discharge (within 48 hours) was associated with 50% more hospital readmissions and 70% more emergency department use than later discharge (Kinsella, 1996).

The nurse should also explore parental knowledge of the care of minor illness in the home. Do parents know not to give aspirin to children? Does the caretaker know how to take a child's temperature? Are parents aware of when to take a child for medical care? What illness care practices are employed by the family? Are any of these practices potentially harmful? Appendix L is a tool that may be used by the community health nurse to assess the health needs of children.

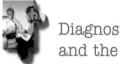

Diagnostic Reasoning and the Care of Children

Based on the data gathered in assessment of the child, the community health nurse derives diagnoses or statements of the child's health status and health care needs. Both positive and problem-focused nursing diagnoses should be made based on the child's situation. Diagnoses may reflect the need for primary, secondary, or tertiary preventive measures. For example, a positive nursing diagnosis related to primary prevention is "immunizations up-to-date due to high parental motivation and access to health care services." On the other hand, a problem-focused nursing diagnosis related to immunizations is "lack of appropriate immunizations for age due to lack of transportation to immunization clinic." Another problem-focused nursing diagnosis related to primary prevention is "potential for child abuse due to unrealistic parental expectations of child, parental stress, and poor parental coping abilities."

Nursing diagnoses related to secondary prevention are necessarily problem-focused because secondary prevention is warranted when actual health problems exist. Examples of nursing diagnoses at this level include "need for medical evaluation and treatment due to possible otitis media" and "need for referral to child protective services due to probable child abuse." Nursing diagnoses at this level might reflect physical, psychological, or social problems affecting the child's overall health status.

At the level of tertiary prevention, nursing diagnoses focus on the need to prevent complications of existing problems or to prevent the recurrence of problems. For example, the nurse might derive a nursing diagnosis of "need for education on proper infant feeding techniques due to practice of propping bottle" to prevent recurrent middle ear infections. Or the nurse might diagnose a "need for emotional support due to imminent death of child" for a child with AIDS. The intent in this latter diagnosis is to direct nursing care to preventing family complications of a terminal illness. Community health nurses may also derive nursing diagnoses related to the health needs of groups of children. An example of a diagnosis at this level might be "potential for measles epidemic among preschool children due to low immunization rates."

Planning the Dimensions of Health Care for Children

As in the care of any client, planning nursing care for children involves prioritizing needs, developing criteria for approaches to meeting those needs, evaluating alternatives, and selecting a course of action. Objectives for care must be developed and specific interventions related to needs for primary, secondary, and tertiary prevention planned.

Client participation in planning is desirable. Most often this participation includes the child's parents or other caretakers; however, it is important for the nurse to remember that participation by the child in planning for his or her own care is also important. Even young children can be involved in some of the decisions about their care, particularly when problems can be addressed by relatively simple interventions. For example, if the school-age child is anemic, he or she may be given a choice of iron-rich foods to be included in the diet. Similarly, if the problem is related to behavior, the child may have some ideas of strategies that will help to alter that behavior.

The interventions selected should be appropriate to the problems identified as well as to the age and developmental level of the child. For example, toys designed to enhance motor development should be challenging but not beyond the child's capability to use. If such strategies are not capable of implementation by the child, frustration will result. As another example, it may be appropriate to make a preadolescent responsible for soaking a sprained ankle periodically, but this would not be appropriate for a first-grader.

Nursing intervention for the health problems of children include primary, secondary, and tertiary preventive measures. In dealing with the well child, emphasis is placed on primary prevention—health promotion and prevention of illness. Initial intervention for the acutely ill child is geared to secondary prevention for the illness, with later attention to primary and tertiary prevention. For the child with a chronic illness, the initial focus of care may be either secondary or tertiary prevention, depending on the child's status. Primary prevention with this child, however, would not be neglected.

One general measure that cuts across all three levels of prevention is the provision of access to health care services for health-promotive, illness-preventive, restorative, and rehabilitative care. The community health nurse may be instrumental in referring children and their parents to appropriate sources of health care. The nurse may also need to refer families for financial assistance with health care needs.

Primary Prevention

Primary preventive activities are designed to promote the health of the child and to prevent illness. Major considerations in primary prevention include promoting growth and development, nutrition, safety, immunization, dental care, and support for parenting.

Promoting Growth and Development. To develop properly, the child needs an environment conducive to growth and development. Community health nurses can assist parents in creating such an environment. One of the ways in which this assistance may be provided is in the form of anticipatory guidance. *Anticipatory guidance* is the act of providing information to parents regarding behavioral expectations of children at a specific age before the child reaches that age.

Such information allows parents to engage in activities that promote development and to cope with some of the more negative aspects of that development. For example, the community health nurse might warn parents who have a child about to turn 2 of the negative behavior typical of this age group. Parents need to know that this negativism is an attempt on the child's part to become autonomous and is normal behavior. They should be assisted to deal with this behavior in such a way that autonomy is fostered while the child's safety is ensured and discipline is maintained. The community health nurse can also reinforce the consistent use of the principles of discipline presented earlier.

Most parents are concerned about their child's development and ability to accomplish developmental milestones. Parents can be told when to expect the child to perform various activities, but should also be informed that children develop at different rates. Toilet training is a common parental concern. Many parents attempt toilet training before the child is physically ready. The nurse can inform parents that toilet

GOALS OF PRIMARY PREVENTION

- Promote normal growth and development
- Develop positive parent–child relationships
- Prevent the occurrence of health problems
- Develop strengths and resources

training is not appropriate until the child is walking. It is not until this time that sufficient sphincter muscle development has occurred to permit the child to control defecation. Parents can be encouraged to look for signs that a child is ready to begin toilet training, such as squatting behaviors, hiding behind furniture, or pulling at their clothing when they feel the urge to defecate. Children may also demonstrate readiness by displaying curiosity about parents' eliminative behavior.

When the child has begun to demonstrate some of the signs of readiness for toilet training, parents should determine patterns of defecation and urination and should time trips to the bathroom to coincide with these patterns. If the child normally defecates after a meal, then meals should finish with a trip to the toilet. Children should not be left unattended in the bathroom and should not be encouraged to play during this time. Two to three minutes on a "potty seat" is sufficient. If the child is successful in defecating or urinating on the potty seat, he or she should be praised. Accidents, however, should be ignored. Parents should also be aware that early in the training process, children have very limited sphincter control. When a child indicates a need to go to the bathroom, they mean "now!" Parents who tell the child to "wait" are inviting trouble, and accidents that occur in these situations are not the child's fault, but the parents'.

Teething is another developmental concern for parents. Children are frequently irritable when cutting their first teeth. Parents can be encouraged to provide safe teething objects for the child. Teething objects that can be placed in the freezer are comforting. Parents can even place an ice cube inside a washcloth to make a cold, hard surface for children to teeth on. The nurse should discourage the use of commercial teething preparations as these may irritate the gums.

Promoting growth and development in children with chronic illnesses or disabilities should also be a concern for the community health nurse. Parents may need to be encouraged to allow their youngster to engage in behaviors that facilitate the child's development. For example, the nurse may need to remind parents of a blind child that the child can use other senses to compensate for lack of vision and that they should encourage the child to engage in activities appropriate to his or her age, rather than overprotect the child. Parents may also need to learn about specialized activities they can do to facilitate the child's development. Information on these types of activities can be obtained from a variety of agencies and organizations that address the needs of children with specific conditions or special needs. Some of these agencies are listed at the end of this chapter.

Providing Adequate Nutrition. Childhood growth and appropriate development are facilitated by adequate nutrition. Here again, the primary function of the community health nurse is educating parents to provide adequate nutrition for their children. The nurse may also provide referrals to assistance programs as needed.

Much of the malnutrition found among children in this country is due to inadequate knowledge of nutrition on the part of parents. The community health nurse can help to alleviate such problems by educating parents on the nutritional needs of children at various ages. Parents should be told that children under 6 months of age should be maintained on breast milk or formula alone, because early introduction of solid foods contributes to food allergies and overweight in later life. The community health nurse may want to encourage prospective parents in decisions to breastfeed rather than bottlefeed their infants because of the number of advantages posed by breastfeeding. These advantages include facilitating maternal–child bonding, improved developmental outcomes, fewer infections, reduced allergy potential, convenience, faster return to a prepregnancy weight, and reduced fertility. This last holds true at the aggregate level, not necessarily for the individual, therefore breastfeeding should not be suggested as a mode of contraception. The nurse should also be alert to factors that may impede breastfeeding success: lack of peer and professional support for breastfeeding, the need to return to work and inability to effectively pump one's breasts, and commonly experienced problems such as sore nipples. Parents planning to breastfeed need relevant education prior to delivery (Ajl & Senft, 1993).

Some parents, for a variety of reasons, prefer to bottlefeed their infants and should be supported in this decision by the community health nurse. These parents may also need information prior to delivery to ensure that they use an appropriate and nutritious formula, prepare formula properly, adequately refrigerate formula and clean bottles and nipples, and provide nurturance during feeding using correct feeding techniques. Both the nurse and parents of breast- or bottlefed infants should be aware that growth patterns differ somewhat between the two groups. Breastfed infants, for example, can be expected to taper off in their weight gain after the first 2 or 3 months, whereas bottlefed infants continue to gain at a relatively constant rate for several months (Ajl & Senft, 1993).

When solid foods are introduced, parents need to be aware that they should introduce new foods slowly to allow for identification of food allergies. They should give a new food for several days without introducing any other new substance to allow time for the development of allergic symptoms. Juices can be introduced between 4 and 5 months of age with the exception of orange juice, which may cause some allergies. Parents should be cautioned against using adult apple juice as it has not been pasteurized and may contain bacteria that can cause severe diarrhea in infants. Solid foods should be introduced at about 6 months of age, beginning with easily digestible cereals such as rice cereal.

Once the baby has been able to tolerate several different types of cereal, parents can begin to introduce an array of vegetables, beginning with yellow vegetables and progressing to green. Vegetables should be introduced before fruits to avoid the development of a preference for the sweeter fruits and later resistance to eating vegetables. After the child is eating a variety of cereals and vegetables, fruits can be introduced followed by meats. Again, parents should start with the more easily digested meats such as lamb.

Parents can either prepare pureed foods themselves or purchase commercially available baby foods. If using commercially processed foods, parents should be taught to evaluate food products for their nutritive value. They should be made aware that they should buy plain items rather than combinations of foods. For example, they should purchase vegetable and meat separately and mix them if desired, rather than buy the vegetable and meat combination. This is both more economical and more nutritious for the baby. Plain fruits should be purchased over the baby desserts as these merely add unneeded calories and expense.

Parents also need to understand the eating habits of children. The nurse should encourage parents to provide nutritious meals and snacks for youngsters of all ages and to avoid offering junk food. Parents should also avoid food fads such as the use of raw milk and other "natural" foods that may actually be harmful to children (examples of potentially harmful foods are raw eggs and unpasteurized honey).

Many children begin eating finger foods at 8 to 9 months of age. Parents should see that children are carefully supervised to prevent choking on small pieces of food. Table foods may also be started at about this age, and children may begin drinking from a cup at mealtime (retaining the bottle at nap- or bedtime). Parents can try any table food to see how a child responds. They should, however, be sure that their children are getting a well-balanced diet and that they are carefully supervised to prevent choking. If small vegetables such as peas and lima beans are provided, parents might want to mash them, as children have been known to put such small objects into any bodily orifice, including the ears, nose, and vagina.

Many parents become concerned about their toddler's apparent loss of appetite. Community health nurses need to reassure parents that this is a normal phenomenon resulting from the slower rate of growth that occurs at this age. Again, the primary concern should be the quality of what is eaten rather than the amount. Parents may want to arrange several small meals and nutritious snacks throughout the day rather than the usual three meals. Toddlers and preschoolers also react well to foods that can be eaten "on the go" because they are much more interested in playing than eating. Small portions and colorful meals also tempt a flagging appetite.

School-age children should receive well-balanced diets that provide them with sufficient energy to engage in all of their activities in and out of school. At this age, children tend to be very strongly influenced by what their peers are doing and eating, and parents may need to insist on nutritious foods without making the child feel too different from his or her peers.

Besides providing parents with information on nutritional needs and eating habits of children at various ages, the community health nurse may be called on to provide assistance in budgeting for adequate nutrition. In this area the nurse can assist parents in the development of lower-cost menus that provide adequate nutrition. Nurses may also be involved in referring parents to sources of financial assistance with nutrition.

Special attention may be needed in meeting the nutritional needs of children with chronic conditions or disabilities. For example, the parents of a young child with diabetes may need to adapt family dietary patterns to accommodate the child's diabetic diet. Or the parents of a child with a cleft lip and palate may need assistance in learning feeding techniques to prevent aspiration of food. Based on an assessment of parents' (and children's) knowledge of special dietary needs, the nurse may educate parents or help them develop the skills needed to meet the nutritional needs of their children.

Promoting Safety.   Adequate supervision is the major primary preventive measure for promoting the safety of children of all ages. The community health nurse can educate parents regarding safety hazards and measures to keep children safe. Infants and young children should never be left unsupervised, even for short periods, unless they are sleeping soundly in a crib or are otherwise confined, as in a playpen. Even then, frequent checks by parents are indicated.

Children, even when securely restrained, can somehow manage to climb out of high chairs or strollers. Even small children can tip over swings and infant seats. For these reasons, as well, children should not be left unattended. Parents should also be

Critical Thinking in Research

Luepker and colleagues (1996) studied the effects of food service modifications, revised physical education curricula, and classroom health education on serum cholesterol levels, eating patterns, physical activity, and several physiologic measures among third grade students in four states. In experimental schools, the fat content of school lunches declined compared to control schools, and fat intake of individual students was significantly less in the experimental schools. Intervention students also had more physical activity, but did not differ from control students in terms of blood pressure, body size, or cholesterol levels.

1. How might you gather information on the long-term effects of these interventions on the children's health?
2. What would be the implications of your findings if the intervention children continued to get more exercise and ate less fat than the control students, but continued to show no differences in blood pressure, body size, or cholesterol levels as adults?
3. What might be some possible explanations for the lack of differences noted in body size, cholesterol levels, and blood pressure between experimental and control groups in this study?
4. What factors do you think might contribute to high fat content in school lunches? How could you determine whether or not your suppositions are correct?

taught not to leave infants alone on elevated surfaces from which they might fall. Care should also be taken that young children are not left unsupervised, even for a few minutes, in the bath.

Another primary preventive measure is instructing parents on the need for consistent use of safety devices such as seat belts and restraints in cars, strollers, high chairs, infant seats, and swings. Parents can also be encouraged to insist on the use of safety helmets for any child over 6 months of age in any form of wheeled conveyance. Helmets are particularly important for older children riding bicycles or skateboards or roller blading or skiing. Community health nurses may also need to be involved in advocacy programs to make safety equipment, such as car seats, available to children in low income families (Louis & Lewis, 1997).

The community health nurse should also instruct parents about age-appropriate toys and the need to examine toys frequently for sharp edges, damage, or other conditions that might present safety hazards. Parents can also be encouraged to establish rules for the appropriate use of toys and for toys that are not to be used without adult supervision.

Parents may also need assistance in providing safety education for their children. The community health nurse can inform parents of safety issues to be addressed with children of specific ages and assist parents with ways of presenting this information to their children. Areas that should be addressed include watching for cars, crossing streets, talking to strangers, answering the phone or the door, playing with fire, and poisonous substances. Children should also be taught safety rules for sports and bike riding, water safety, and safety with firearms.

Childproofing the home is another area of primary prevention for the young child. This involves placing hazardous objects where children cannot access them and eliminating other safety hazards from the environment. Safety instruction for parents should be geared toward the age and developmental level of the child. Before the child begins creeping, parents need to think of covering electrical outlets and keeping small objects out of the reach of young children. Stairways should be inaccessible, as should sharp objects and medications of all kinds. Because children learn at a surprisingly early age to climb to reach an objective, sharp objects and poisons should be kept in areas with sturdy locks or latches that the child cannot open, rather than placed out of reach.

Parents should also be discouraged from putting toxic substances in unlabeled or usually innocuous containers. The child who sees liquid in a soda bottle may drink it, even if it tastes as bad as bleach or gasoline. Special attention should be given to supervising the activities of young children when visiting friends or relatives whose homes may not be child-proofed.

Dealing with firearms is an important safety consideration for school-age children. Parents should be encouraged to eliminate firearms or to make them inaccessible to children, never to leave a gun loaded, and to store ammunition apart from weapons. As noted earlier, preadolescent youngsters should be taught the principles of gun safety, and all children should be discouraged from pointing even toy guns at other people.

Immunization. Immunization is a particular concern of the community health nurse working with children and their families. Immunization not only protects the individual who is immunized, but maintaining high immunization levels in the community leads to smaller numbers of susceptible persons and less risk of exposure for those who are not immunized. Unless contraindicated, a child's immunizations should begin at 6 to 10 weeks of age. All infants should be immunized against diphtheria, tetanus, and pertussis, (DTP); polio (IPV followed by OPV); measles, mumps, and rubella (MMR); *Hemophilus influenza* b (Hb); hepatitis B (HBV), and varicella (chickenpox). A rotavirus vaccine may also soon be available to pre-

STANDARDS FOR PEDIATRIC IMMUNIZATION SERVICES

- Readily available services
- Absence of barriers or unnecessary prerequisites to services
- Free or low-cost services
- Utilization of all pediatric clinical encounters to assess and update immunization status
- Parental education on the importance of immunizations
- Parental education on side effects and potential adverse effects of immunizations
- Postponement of immunizations only for true contraindications
- Simultaneous administration of all vaccines for which the child is eligible
- Complete and accurate recording
- Incorporation of immunizations into appointments for other child health services
- Prompt reporting of adverse effects by providers
- Use of immunization tracking systems
- Use of correct procedures for vaccine management
- Semiannual record audits to determine immunization coverage in the client population
- Use of up-to-date immunization protocols
- Use of both patient-oriented and community-based approaches
- Administration of immunizations by trained personnel
- Ongoing provider education

vent gastroenteritis which causes 100 deaths and 70,000 hospitalizations each year in the United States (Rennels, et al., 1996). The routine schedule for these immunizations was presented in Table 20–4. Older children should also be immunized with DTP, OPV, HBV, and MMR vaccines. A single dose of the recently approved chickenpox vaccine is recommended for children under age 13. Health care providers and family members in households with immunocompromised clients should also receive varicella vaccine if they do not have antibody titers suggesting they have had the disease (U.S. Department of Health and Human Services, 1997). Adolescents and adults are generally given two doses of varicella vaccine (Stutman, 1996).

Because a recent decline in childhood immunization had led to periodic outbreaks of communicable disease, the National Vaccine Advisory Committee has established a set of standards for pediatric immunization services (National Vaccine Advisory Committee, 1993).

The community health nurse is able to inform parents regarding the schedule for immunizations and refer them to an appropriate provider. In addition, the nurse should inform parents of the expected side effects of immunizations and interventions to minimize them. Parents should also be informed about the signs and symptoms of unusual reactions.

Immunization is of particular concern for children with immunodeficiency problems. For example, live virus vaccines such as oral polio vaccine (OPV) are usually contraindicated for children with AIDS. Inactivated polio vaccine (IPV) should be given both to the child with AIDS and to his or her siblings. Measles immunization may be considered in children with AIDS, as measles in individuals who have AIDS can be extremely serious, and the benefits of immunization outweigh its risks. Immunization for pneumococcal pneumonia and annual influenza immunization should be provided for children with chronic illnesses or disabilities, including those with AIDS (Immunization Practices Advisory Committee, 1992).

Community health nurses may also need to educate other health care providers regarding valid contraindications for immunization to avoid missed opportunities for immunizing children. In a series of studies, for example, immunization opportunities were overlooked in 64 to 82% of children (National Immunization Program, 1994a), and 61% of providers reported basing immunization decisions on invalid contraindications (National Immunization Program, 1996).

Dental Care. Dental health is another area of concern in primary prevention with children. Dental hygiene should begin as soon as the first tooth erupts. At this time parents can be encouraged to rub teeth briskly with a dry washcloth. Later, parents can begin to brush the child's teeth with a soft toothbrush. Older children can be taught to brush and floss their own teeth with adult supervision. Use of a fluoridated toothpaste should be encouraged in areas with unfluoridated water; parents can give fluoride-containing vitamins to infants in such areas.

Community health nurses can instruct parents to wean infants from the bottle before a year of age to prevent bottle-mouth syndrome. The use of sugarless snacks and rinsing the mouth after eating—when brushing is not possible—can also be encouraged. Finally, community health nurses should encourage parents to obtain regular dental check-ups for children and to get prompt attention for dental problems. Financial assistance may be needed for such services for low-income families. In such cases, the community health nurse should make a referral for Medicaid in those areas where dental care is covered.

Support for Parenting.   Another major consideration in primary preventive activities for child health is that of support for parenting. As noted earlier, unrealistic parental expectations of children, excessive parental stress, and poor parental coping skills may contribute to child abuse. These conditions also create a psychological environment that is not conducive to health for either parents or children. Such conditions can be modified by community health nursing support in the parenting role. Parents can be assisted to develop realistic expectations of child behavior through anticipatory guidance and help with skills related to communications and discipline. The community health nurse can also help parents to identify children's reactivity patterns and develop approaches to dealing with children that minimize some of the negative aspects of specific patterns. Some of these approaches were discussed earlier in this chapter.

In addition, community health nurses can engage in activities that minimize parental stress. This may involve referral for financial assistance, arrangement of respite care, assistance with finding work or adequate housing, or whatever is required to meet family needs. At the same time, the nurse can assist parents to identify coping strategies that work for them. Parents may also need assistance in problem-solving skills to decrease their own stress levels.

Support for parenting is particularly needed by parents of children with chronic or terminal illnesses or disabilities. Parents may need assistance or referral in dealing with feelings of guilt and anxiety engendered by the child's condition. In addition, the community health nurse may provide assistance in developing new child care skills necessitated by the child's condition. Referral to groups of parents with children who have similar problems may provide parents with avenues of emotional, social, and material support.

Another area in which the community health nurse may be able to support parents of children with serious health problems is respite care. Parents need to be able to maintain their own lives and care for other children, in addition to meeting the needs of the ill child. The nurse may need to encourage parents to take some time for themselves. Frequently, this entails assisting parents to obtain respite care so they can be sure the child's needs are adequately being met while they are away.

Parents and other family members also need to be encouraged to maintain a family life that is as normal as possible. The ill or disabled child should be incorporated into family activities whenever possible, and family members should be encouraged not to let the child's condition become the focus of family life. Family members should be assisted to discuss problems posed by the child's condition and to engage in active problem solving to resolve those concerns. Other avenues for providing support to parents of chronically ill or disabled children include giving information about the child's condition and its treatment, providing emotional support, focusing on positive aspects of the situation, encouraging use of existing support networks, and helping families to expand sources of support (Austin, 1990).

Families of terminally ill children need additional support in coming to terms with the eventuality of death. The nurse can determine the family's stage in the grief process and design interventions that help them successfully pass through these stages. The stages of grief are similar to those described earlier in parental response to a chronic illness. Referrals for counseling or for hospice services may also be helpful in working with families of terminally ill children.

Other Primary Preventive Activities.   Additional primary preventive measures may be warranted for children with specific illnesses. For example, parents of children with AIDS and other immunosuppression conditions should be taught how to minimize exposure to opportunistic infections. Special intervention may also be warranted to create a healthy self-image in children with chronic conditions or disabilities. For example, the physically handicapped child can be helped to develop skills such as artistic ability that contribute to a positive self-image. Primary preventive interventions employed by community health nurses in caring for children are summarized in Table 20–9.

Secondary Prevention

Secondary prevention is geared toward resolution of health problems currently experienced by the child. Activities are directed toward screening for conditions, care of minor illness, referral for diagnostic and treatment services, and dealing with illness and treatment regimens.

Additional Screening Procedures.   Although many screening tests are routinely conducted as part of the assessment of a child's health status, assessment data may indicate a need for additional screening tests. As part of secondary prevention aimed at detecting existing health problems, the nurse can either conduct or make referrals for these additional tests. For example, lead screening may be indicated for children who live in areas with high lead levels in ambient air or who reside in areas where lead-based paint was used. Blood lead levels would also be obtained for children who exhibit signs of lead poisoning (see Chapter 17).

Other screening tests may be warranted by assessment data. Children who are at risk for HIV infec-

TABLE 20–9. PRIMARY PREVENTIVE INTERVENTIONS IN THE CARE OF CHILDREN

Promoting growth and development	• Provide anticipatory guidance to parents. • Assist with accomplishment of developmental tasks. • Provide assistance with developmental concerns.
Promoting adequate nutrition	• Educate parents regarding children's nutritional needs. • Provide assistance in meeting nutritional needs.
Promoting safety	• Encourage parents to provide adequate supervision of children. • Educate parents regarding safety concerns appropriate to the child's age. • Eliminate hazardous conditions from the environment. • Assist parents to provide safety education appropriate to child's age and health status.
Immunization	• Educate parents regarding the need for immunization and immunization schedules. • Refer parents to immunization services. • Educate parents about side effects of immunizations. • Modify immunization practices or provide additional immunizations for children with special needs.
Dental care	• Encourage adequate dental hygiene. • Encourage regular dental check-ups.
Support for parenting	• Assist parents to develop realistic expectations of children. • Take action to minimize parental stress. • Assist parents to develop effective coping strategies and learn child care skills. • Assist parents to deal with the special needs of children with chronic illnesses or disabilities. • Assist parents to deal with feelings of guilt, anger, and frustration engendered by a chronic or terminal condition in a child. • Arrange respite care as needed for parents of children with chronic conditions or disabilities.

tion should be referred for screening. Children at risk include those born to mothers who are intravenous drug users or partners of intravenous drug users or of bisexual males. Children who exhibit signs of immunodeficiency or opportunistic infections associated with AIDS (see Chapter 30) should also be referred for screening. Similarly, screening for hepatitis B antibodies may be conducted for children who have been exposed to the disease.

Care of Minor Illness.   Many of the health problems experienced by children can be treated by parents at home; however, many parents are quite inexperienced in dealing with minor childhood ailments. They may require help in determining when illness can be dealt with at home and when the assistance of health care professionals is required. The community health nurse can educate parents on the signs of illness in children, appropriate measures to be taken at home, and when to seek medical intervention. Common areas of concern that the nurse addresses are teething, fever, diarrhea and constipation, vomiting, and rashes. Parents should be acquainted with what is normal and what is abnormal, as well as what home remedies are appropriate and what might be harmful.

Besides providing such information, the community health nurse frequently is called on to assess a child's health status and recommend appropriate interventions or make a referral for medical assistance. Potential interventions for minor problems in children and indications for referral for medical assistance are addressed in Appendix M, Nursing Interventions for Common Health Problems in Children.

Referral.   Community health nurses frequently encounter health problems in children that require further diagnostic evaluation and treatment. Unless the nurse is also a nurse practitioner, he or she will most probably refer the family to another source of diagnostic and treatment services. Referrals made should be appropriate to the condition suspected and to the circumstances of the situation. Considerations in making referrals and the referral process were addressed in Chapter 11.

In addition to making referrals for diagnosis and treatment services, the nurse may also educate parents and children about probable diagnostic and treatment procedures. For example, if the nurse suspects that a child may have hepatitis, he or she will explain the need for diagnostic blood tests to the parent (and to the child, if the child is old enough to understand) and will describe the typical treatment for hepatitis.

Referrals may be made for assistance with physical, psychological, or social health problems. In the

GOALS OF SECONDARY PREVENTION

- Promote accurate diagnosis of health problems
- Facilitate treatment for health problems
- Eliminate existing health problems

case of child abuse, for example, the nurse might make a referral for evaluation and treatment of the physical effects of abuse on the child. At the same time, the nurse may refer both the perpetrator and the victim of abuse (or other family members) for psychological counseling. Finally, the nurse may refer for assistance those families whose social factors create stress and contribute to the potential for abusive behavior.

Dealing with Illness and Treatment Regimens.   When an illness requiring medical intervention has been diagnosed, the community health nurse may engage in several secondary preventive interventions related to the diagnosis and its treatment. These interventions include educating parents and children about the condition and its treatment. For example, parents of a child with a newly diagnosed case of diabetes may need information on diet, exercise, and the effects of infection on insulin needs, as well as instruction on how to give insulin. Or parents of a child with otitis media may need directions on the use of the antibiotic prescribed. Parents and children should also be given information on the side effects of medications or treatments. For example, parents should be warned about the potential side effects of radiation therapy for cancer and educated on ways to minimize these consequences as much as possible.

Secondary prevention may also entail informing parents and children about what to expect regarding a chronic disease and its treatment. For example, they should be informed that diabetes or essential hypertension can usually be controlled with therapy, but will not be cured, and that the child will probably need to take medication for the rest of his or her life. On the other hand, parents should be informed that symptoms of an ear infection should abate within a day or so of starting antibiotic therapy, but that medication should be completed.

The community health nurse may also be responsible for monitoring the effect of treatment and the child's health status between visits to a physician or nurse practitioner. In addition, the nurse will observe the child for evidence of medication side effects or other adverse effects of therapy. For example, the nurse may observe a child with ADHD to determine whether medication results in diminished hyperactivity or whether the child exhibits any medication side effects.

Monitoring compliance with a treatment regimen is another secondary preventive measure in the care of children with acute and chronic conditions. The community health nurse periodically needs to assess the child's or family's compliance with medication or other treatments. If noncompliance occurs, the nurse needs to determine factors contributing to noncompliance and plan interventions that enhance compliance. For example, if parents have not been giving their child prescribed antiepileptics because they cannot afford them, the nurse may make a referral for financial assistance or help the family budget their income more effectively. If, on the other hand, parents stopped giving antibiotics prescribed for the child's otitis media because the child got better, the nurse will educate them on the need to finish the prescribed medication.

Secondary prevention for children with conditions like arthritis, cancer, or other illnesses that cause pain include interventions for pain control (Muller, Harris, Wattley, & Taylor, 1996). Parents and children may need to be encouraged to use pain medications before pain becomes uncontrollable, or they may need suggestions for dealing with side effects related to pain medication.

Tertiary Prevention

As is the case with secondary prevention, tertiary prevention is geared toward the particular health problems experienced by the child. Generally, there are three aspects to tertiary prevention with children: preventing recurrence of problems, preventing further consequences, and, in the case of chronic illness or disability, promoting adjustment.

Preventing Problem Recurrence.   Community health nurses may educate parents and children to prevent the recurrence of many health problems experienced by children. For example, the parent may need information on the relationship of bottle propping to otitis media to prevent subsequent infections. Similarly, education about the need to change diapers frequently, to wash the skin with each diaper change, and to refrain from using harsh soaps to wash diapers may help prevent continued diaper rash.

Preventing Consequences.   Tertiary prevention related to preventing further consequences of health problems is most often employed with children with chronic conditions. For example, the child with diabetes requires attention to diet, exercise, and medication to control the diabetes and prevent physical consequences of the

 GOALS OF TERTIARY PREVENTION
- Restore function and prevent problem recurrence
- Prevent complications of existing conditions
- Promote adjustment to chronic conditions

disease itself. At the same time, attention must be given to promoting the child's adjustment to the condition and normalizing his or her life as much as possible. Nursing interventions would be geared toward convincing the child to stick to one's diet and promoting the child's social interactions with peers.

The nurse might also need to intervene to prevent or minimize the consequences of the child's condition for the rest of the family. For example, the nurse might need to point out to parents that in their concern for the child with a chronic heart condition, they are neglecting the needs of siblings. Or tertiary prevention for an infant with AIDS may entail educating parents on the disposal of bodily fluids and excreta to prevent infection of other family members. Tertiary prevention may also extend to helping the child and his or her family deal with death if the child's condition is terminal.

Tertiary prevention may entail a wide variety of activities on the part of the nurse, from education on how to deal with a specific condition to referral for assistance with major medical expenses. Nurses may also need to act as advocates for children with chronic conditions. The example that most readily comes to mind is the need for advocacy for children with AIDS who are still well enough to attend school.

Emotional support by the nurse is a very important part of tertiary prevention for children with chronic conditions. Parents' and children's feelings about the condition need to be acknowledged and addressed. The nurse can also reinforce positive activities on the part of parent or child. Again, this support may need to be extended as families go through the grieving process. Grieving will probably occur with most chronic illnesses, even those that are not terminal, and the nurse should be prepared to reassure families that their feelings of grief are normal and to support them through this process.

Promoting Adjustment. The community health nurse may also engage in activities that are designed to return the child and family to a relatively normal state of existence. For children with chronic illnesses or disabilities, this means restoring function as much as possible, preventing further loss of function, and assisting the child and his or her family to progress through the stages of family response to chronic illness discussed earlier in this chapter. The community health nurse might accomplish this by encouraging the family to discuss problems posed by the child's condition and to view the condition in the most positive light possible. The nurse should also encourage the family to normalize family life as much as possible. For example, if the Little League activities of a sibling have been curtailed because of an exacerbation of the

child's illness, parents should make an attempt to re-institute those activities as soon as the youngster's condition is stable. Or the family can be encouraged to call on members of their support network to take the sibling to baseball practice and games.

 ## Implementing Nursing Care for Children

Planned nursing interventions may be implemented by the nurse, by family members or others responsible for the child, or by the child. The nurse should be certain that the child or family members are motivated and capable of carrying out planned care activities. This might necessitate interventions by the nurse to improve motivation or to help the child or family members develop the skills needed to implement the plan. The processes involved in motivating and educating people to take action were addressed in Chapters 9 and 12.

During the implementation phase of nursing intervention, the nurse should check frequently with the child and the family to determine that the plan is indeed being implemented. If it is not, the nurse would assess reasons for noncompliance and plan interventions to facilitate implementation. The nurse should also determine whether the family is experiencing any problems with implementation. Perhaps the nurse has arranged for physical therapy for a handicapped child, but visits by the therapist are interfering with the mother's work schedule. In this case, the nurse might explore the options for providing therapy in the school or in a day care setting instead of the home.

 ## Evaluating Nursing Care for Children

The effectiveness of nursing interventions for the child is assessed in the same manner that care of any individual client is evaluated. Has intervention fostered the child's growth and development? Is the child's nutrition adequate for normal needs? Is the child up-to-date on his or her immunizations? Are physical or psychological hazards present in the child's environment? Is the child receiving health care as needed? Have acute health care problems been resolved?

The community health nurse would also examine the extent to which care has contributed to the adjustment of the child and family to existing chronic disease or disability. Are parents comfortable and adequately prepared to parent a child with special needs? Do they

TABLE 20–10. STATUS OF SELECTED NATIONAL HEALTH OBJECTIVES FOR CHILDREN

	Objective	Base	Most Recent Status	Target
2.4	Reduced growth retardation	11% (1988)	met (1995)	10%
2.10	Reduce iron deficiency (children 1–2 years)	9% (1980)	NDA[a]	3%
3.8	Reduce tobacco smoke exposure of children	39% (1986)	27% (1993)	20%
6.3	Reduce prevalence of mental disorders	20% (1992)	NDA	10%
7.4	Reduce incidence of child abuse (per 1000 children)	22.6 (1986)	NDA	<22.6
9.3a	Reduce motor vehicle accident deaths (per 100,000)	6.2 (1987)	5.3 (1993)	5.5
9.12	Increase seat belt use	48% (1988)	NDA	85%
11.4	Reduce blood lead levels exceeding 15 µg/dL	3 mil (1984)	274,000 (1992)	300,000
	Reduce blood lead levels exceeding 25 µg/dL	234,000 (1984)	NDA	0
14.1	Reduce infant mortality (per 1000 live births)	10.1 (1987)	6.7 (1996)	7
17.8	Reduce prevalence of mental retardation (per 1000 children)	2.7 (1988)	NDA	2
20.11	Increase immunization levels in children under 2	54–64% (1985)	75% (1995)	90%

[a]NDA, no data available.

(Sources: U.S. Department of Health and Human Services, 1993; 1995; 1996c; 1996d.)

perform this role adequately? Have complications of the child's condition been prevented?

The community health nurse would identify criteria that provide the answers to these and similar questions. Data would then be collected relative to the criteria to determine whether nursing intervention has resulted in improved health status for the child and whether specific client care objectives have been met. If, for example, the child is anemic, the criteria used to evaluate nursing interventions related to this problem might include hemoglobin or hematocrit levels and the number and type of iron-rich foods in the child's diet. Evaluative data would be used to modify the plan of care or to determine the appropriateness of terminating services.

The community health nurse may also be involved in evaluating the effects of interventions at the aggregate level. Evaluative data regarding the status of national health objectives related to children's health are summarized in Table 20–10.

Critical Thinking in Practice: A Case in Point

You have received a referral to visit Mrs. Kwon, a 24-year-old mother with a newborn baby. There is also another child in the family, Mandy, who is 3. Mother's pregnancy and delivery were uneventful, and mother and baby were discharged after 2 days in the hospital. When you make your home visit, Mrs. Kwon tells you that the baby is spitting up an ounce or so of formula after each feeding but had gained almost a pound at her 2-week visit to the pediatrician yesterday. Otherwise the baby is doing well.

When you first arrive in the home, Mandy is sitting with her back to you watching cartoons on television. The TV is rather loud and she does not seem to be aware that a visitor has arrived. While you are talking to Mrs. Kwon, Mandy turns around and sees you. She picks up her rag doll and comes to lean against her mother's knee with her thumb in her mouth. She seems to be rather pale compared with her mother's coloring.

Mandy pulls at her mother's sleeve to get her attention. When Mrs. Kwon continues to tell you about the baby spitting up, Mandy hits the infant with her doll. Mrs. Kwon scolds her and then tells you that Mandy used to be a very good girl, but ever since they brought the new baby home, she has been throwing tantrums and sucking her thumb.

1. What biophysical, psychological, social, behavioral, and health system factors are influencing the health of these two children?
2. What screening tests and immunizations should these two children have had?
3. Based on the data presented above, what are your nursing diagnoses?
4. How could you involve members of the family in planning to resolve the problems identified?
5. What primary, secondary, and/or tertiary preventive measures might you employ with this family?
6. How would you go about evaluating the effectiveness of your nursing interventions?

TESTING YOUR UNDERSTANDING

1. Describe at least five problems of concern to community health nurses working with children. (pp. 454–458)
2. Differentiate between growth and development. How would you go about assessing each? (pp. 459–462)
3. What are three safety considerations in assessing the physical environment of infants? Toddlers and preschool children? School-age children? (pp. 468–470)
4. List at least five areas to be addressed in relation to the child's psychological environment. Describe how factors in each of these areas might affect the child's health. (pp. 463–468)
5. Identify at least three behavioral considerations in assessing the health status of a child. Give an example of the influence of each on a child's health. (pp. 470–472)
6. What are five primary preventive measures appropriate to all children? What modifications might be needed in these measures when caring for a child with a chronic or terminal illness or a disability? (pp. 475–480)
7. Describe at least three approaches in providing secondary preventive services to a child with existing health problems. Give an example of the use of each. (pp. 480–482)
8. What are the three considerations in tertiary preventive measures for children with existing health problems? Give an example of each consideration. (pp. 482–483)

WHAT DO YOU THINK?
Questions for Critical Thinking

1. Why are community health nurses better prepared than some other providers to promote health and prevent illness in children?
2. How does the information that you would collect in assessing a child differ from assessment information for an adult?
3. How can we assure that all children are adequately immunized?
4. Should dying children be told about their prognosis? Why or why not? Should some children be told and not others?

REFERENCES

Ajl, S., & Senft, C. (1993). Infant feeding practices. In R. J. Karp (Ed.), *Malnourished children in the United States: Caught in the cycle of poverty* (pp. 47–58). New York: Springer.

Alberman, E. (1994). Low birthweight and prematurity. In I. B. Pless (Ed.), *The epidemiology of childhood disorders* (pp. 49–65). New York: Oxford University Press.

Anderson, J., & Werry, J. S. (1994). Emotional and behavioral problems. In I. B. Pless (Ed.), *The epidemiology of childhood disorders* (pp. 304–338). New York: Oxford University Press.

Austin, J. K. (1990). Assessment of coping mechanisms used by parents and children with chronic illness. *MCN, 15,* 98–102.

Baker, S. P., Fowler, C., Li, G., Warner, M., & Dannenberg, A. L. (1994). Head injuries incurred by children and young adults during informal recreation. *American Journal of Public Health, 84,* 649–652.

Bateman, D. A., Ng, S. M., Hansen, C. M., & Haggarty, M. C. (1993). The effects of intrauterine cocaine exposure in newborns. *American Journal of Public Health, 83,* 190–193.

Becker, P. A., Grunwald, P. C., Moorman, J., Stuhr, S. (1993). Effects of developmental care on behavioral organization in very-low-birthweight infants. *Nursing Research, 42,* 214–219.

Berg, B. O. (1994). The nervous system. In A. M. Rudolph & R. K. Kamei (Eds.), *Rudolph's fundamentals of pediatrics* (pp. 617–647). Norwalk, CT: Appleton & Lange.

Berg, C. N., Bryant, N. A., & Bach, M. L. (1994). *America's children: Triumph or tragedy.* Washington, DC: American Public Health Association.

Berkson, G. (1993). *Children with handicaps: A review of behavioral research.* Hillsdale, NJ: Erlbaum.

Birth Defects and Genetic Diseases Bureau. (1995). Update: Trends in fetal alcohol syndrome—United States, 1979–1993. *MMWR, 44,* 249–251.

Centers for Disease Control. (1996a). Alcohol and other drug-related birth defects awareness week, May 12–18, 1996. *MMWR, 45,* 378–379.

Centers for Disease Control. (1996b). Recommended childhood immunization schedule—United States, July–December, 1996. *MMWR, 45,* 635–638.

Centers for Disease Control. (1997). Poliomyelitis prevention in the United States: Introduction of a sequential vaccination schedule of inactivated poliovirus vaccine followed by oral poliovirus vaccine. *MMWR, 46*(RR-3), 1–25.

Christoffel, K. K. (1994). Intentional injuries: Homicide and violence. In I. B. Pless (Ed.), *The epidemiology of childhood disorders* (pp. 392–411). New York: Oxford University Press.

Cohen, M. (1995). The triggers of heightened parental uncertainty in chronic, life-threatening childhood illness. *Qualitative Health Research, 5*(1), 63–77.

Cohn, L., & Deckelbaum, R. J. (1993, Fall). Early childhood nutrition: Eating today for tomorrow's health. *Pediatric Basics, 66,* 7, 10–15.

Davis, S. F., Byers, R. H., Lindegren, M. L., Caldwell, B., Karon, J. M., Gwinn, M. (1995). Prevalence and incidence of vertically acquired HIV infection in the United States. *JAMA, 274,* 952–955.

DeBaun, M., Rowley, D., Province, M., Stockbauer, J. W., & Cole, F. S. (1994). Selected antepartum medical complications and very-low-birthweight infants among black and white women. *American Journal of Public Health, 84,* 1495–1497.

Diamond, C. (1994). Oncology. In A. M. Rudolph & R. K. Kamei (Eds.), *Rudolph's fundamentals of pediatrics* (pp. 439–457). Norwalk, CT: Appleton & Lange.

Division of HIV/AIDS Prevention. (1996). AIDS among children—United States, 1996. *MMWR, 45,* 1005–1010.

Division of Reproductive Health. (1996). Population-based prevalence of perinatal exposure to cocaine—Georgia, 1994. *MMWR, 45,* 887–891.

Evans, J. C., Le Mar, K. L., Pitzen, K. R., & Thompson, D. (1997). Newborn assessment. In J. A. Fox (Ed.), *Primary health care of children* (pp. 109–143). St. Louis: Mosby-Year Book.

Gabby, T. (1994). Behavioral pediatrics. In A. M. Rudolph & R. K. Kamei (Eds.), *Rudolph's fundamentals of pediatrics* (pp. 617–647). Norwalk, CT: Appleton & Lange.

Ginsberg, C., Gage, L., Martin, V., Gerstein, S., & Acuff, K. (1994). *America's urban safety net hospitals: Meeting the needs of our most vulnerable populations.* Washington, DC: National Association of Public Hospitals.

Gray, M., & Johnson, V. Y. (1997). Urinary system. In J. A. Fox (Ed.), *Primary health care of children* (pp. 540–567). St. Louis: Mosby-Year Book.

Hellerman, S. P. (1997). Autism. In J. A. Fox (Ed.), *Primary health care of children* (pp. 900–913). St. Louis: Mosby-Year Book.

HHS survey. (1996, October). *The Nation's Health,* p. 5.

Holaday, B. (1997). What causes stress in mothers of chronically ill children? *Reflections, 26*(1), 24.

Immunization Practices Advisory Committee. (1992). Prevention and control of influenza: Recommendations of the Immunization Practices Advisory Committee (ACIP). *MMWR, 41*(RR-9), 1–17.

Infant and Child Health Studies Bureau. (1995). Poverty and infant mortality—United States, 1988. *MMWR, 44,* 922–927.

Jensen, G. M., & Moore, L. G. (1997). The effect of high altitude and other risk factors on birthweight: Independent or interactive effects. *American Journal of Public Health, 87,* 1003–1007.

Kennel, S., & Seibold, E. (1997). Cerebral palsy. In J. A. Fox (Ed.), *Primary health care of children* (pp. 913–919). St. Louis: Mosby-Year Book.

Kenney, K. (1997). Hypertension. In J. A. Fox (Ed.), *Primary health care of children* (pp. 452–454). St. Louis: Mosby-Year Book.

Kinsella, J. L. (1996, Fall). Perinatal discharge: How soon is too soon? *Perinatal Care Matters,* 102.

Kirchgessner, J. (1997). Diabetes mellitus. In J. A. Fox (Ed.), *Primary health care of children* (pp. 858–867). St. Louis: Mosby-Year Book.

Langston, C., Lewis, D. E., Hammill, H. A., et al. (1995). Excess intrauterine fetal demise associated with maternal human immunodeficiency virus infection. *Journal of Infectious Diseases, 172,* 1451–1460.

Larroque, B., Kaminski, M., Dehaene, P., Subtil, D., Delfosse, M., & Querleu, D. (1995). Moderate prenatal alcohol exposure and psychomotor development at preschool age. *American Journal of Public Health, 85,* 1654–1661.

Luepker, R. V., Perry, C. L., McKinlay, S. M., et al. (1996). Outcomes of a field trial to improve children's dietary patterns and physical activity. *JAMA, 275,* 768–776.

Louis, B., & Lewis, M. (1997). Increasing car seat use for toddlers from inner-city families. *American Journal of Public Health, 87,* 1044–1045.

Martin, S. L., & Burchinal, M. R. (1992). Young women's antisocial behavior and the later emotional and behavioral health of their children. *American Journal of Public Health, 82,* 1005–1010.

Muller, D. J., Harris, P. J., Wattley, L. A., & Taylor, J. (1996). *Nursing children: Psychology, research, and practice* (2nd ed.). London: Chapman & Hall.

National Center for Chronic Disease Prevention and Health Promotion. (1995). Disabilities among children aged <17 years—United States, 1991–1992. *MMWR, 44,* 609–613.

National Center for Chronic Disease Prevention and Health Promotion. (1997). Alcohol consumption among pregnant and childbearing-aged women—United States, 1991 and 1995. *MMWR, 46,* 345–350.

National Immunization Program. (1994a). Impact of missed opportunities to vaccinate preschool-aged children on vaccination coverage levels—Selected U.S. sites, 1991–1992. *MMWR, 43,* 709–711, 717–718.

National Immunization Program. (1994b). Outbreak of measles among Christian Science students—Missouri and Illinois, 1994. *MMWR, 43,* 463–465.

National Immunization Program. (1996). Use of a data-based approach by a health maintenance organization to identify and address physician barriers to pediatric vaccination—California, 1995. *MMWR, 45,* 188–193.

National Vaccine Advisory Committee. (1993). Standards for pediatric immunization practices. *MMWR, 42*(RR-5), 1–13.

Newacheck, P. W., & Taylor, W. R. (1992). Childhood

chronic illness: Prevalence, severity, and impact. *American Journal of Public Health, 82,* 364–371.

O'Campo, P., Xue, X., Wang, M., Caughy, M. O. (1997). Neighborhood risk factors for low birthweight in Baltimore: A multilevel analysis. *American Journal of Public Health, 87,* 1113–1118.

Palfrey, J. S. (1994). *Community child health: An action plan for today.* Westport, CT: Praeger.

Pelletier, D. L., Frongillo, E. A., & Habicht, J. (1993). Epidemiologic evidence for a potentiating effect of malnutrition on child mortality. *American Journal of Public Health, 83,* 1130–1133.

Pilletteri, A. (1987). *Child health nursing: Care of the growing family* (3rd ed.). Boston: Little, Brown.

Rennels, M. B., Glass, R. I., & Dennehy, P. H., et al. (1996). Safety and efficacy of high-dose Rhesus–human reassortant rotavirus vaccines—Report of the national multicenter trial. *Pediatrics, 97,* 7–13.

Reimer, J. G., Van Cleve, L., & Galbraith, M. (1995). Barriers to well child care for homeless children under age 13. *Public Health Nursing, 12,* 61–66.

Rivara, F. P. (1994). Unintentional injuries. In I. B. Pless (Ed.), *The epidemiology of childhood disorders* (pp. 369–391). New York: Oxford University Press.

Ross, L. J. (1997). Down syndrome. In J. A. Fox (Ed.), *Primary health care of children* (pp. 919–926). St. Louis: Mosby-Year Book.

Sacks, J. J., Brantley, M. D., Holmgreen, P., & Rochat, R. W. (1992). Evaluation of an intervention to reduce playground hazards in Atlanta child-care centers. *American Journal of Public Health, 84,* 649–652.

Safer, D. J., Zito, J. M., & Fine, E. M. (1996). Increased methylphenidate usage for attention deficit disorder in the 1990s. *Pediatrics, 98,* 1084–1088.

Schachar, R., & Wachsmuth, R. (1990). Hyperactivity and parental psychopathology. *Journal of Child Psychology and Psychiatry, 31,* 381–392.

Scheidt, P. C., Harel, Y., Trumble, A. C., Jones, D. H., Overpeck, M. D., & Bijur, P. E. (1995). The epidemiology of nonfatal injuries among U.S. children and youth. *American Journal of Public Health, 85,* 932–938.

Seibold, E., & Kennel, S. (1997). Mental retardation. In J. A. Fox (Ed.), *Primary health care of children* (pp. 939–942). St. Louis: Mosby-Year Book.

Shiono, P. H., Rauh, V. A., Park, M., Lederman, S. A., & Zuskar, D. (1997). Ethnic differences in birthweight: The role of lifestyle and other factors. *American Journal of Public Health, 87,* 787–793.

Stepans, M. B. F., & Wilkerson, N. (1993). Physiologic effects of maternal smoking on breast-feeding infants. *Journal of the American Academy of Nurse Practitioners, 5*(3), 105–112.

Stoddard, J. J., & Gray, B. (1997). Maternal smoking and medical expenditures for childhood respiratory illness. *American Journal of Public Health, 87,* 205–209.

Stratton, K., Howe, C., & Battaglia, F. (Eds.). (1996). *Summary—Fetal alcohol syndrome.* Washington, DC: National Academy Press.

Stutman, H. R. (1996, Winter). Varicella vaccine. *Perinatal Care Matters, 1,* 4.

U.S. Department of Commerce. (1996). *Statistical abstract of the United States, 1996* (116th ed.). Washington, DC: Government Printing Office.

U.S. Department of Health and Human Services. (1991). *Healthy people 2000: National health promotion and prevention objectives.* Washington, DC: Government Printing Office.

U.S. Department of Health and Human Services. (1993). *Health United States, 1992, and healthy people 2000 review.* Washington, DC: Government Printing Office.

U.S. Department of Health and Human Services. (1995). *Healthy people 2000: Midcourse review and 1995 revisions.* Washington, DC: Government Printing Office.

U.S. Department of Health and Human Services. (1996a). *Health United States, 1995.* Washington, DC: Government Printing Office.

U.S. Department of Health and Human Services. (1996b). *Fact sheet—Attention-deficit/hyperactivity disorder in children and adolescents.* Washington, DC: Government Printing Office.

U.S. Department of Health and Human Services. (1996c). *Healthy people 2000: Progress review—Immunization and infectious diseases.* Washington, DC: Government Printing Office.

U.S. Department of Health and Human Services. (1996d). *Healthy people 2000: Progress review—Maternal & infant health.* Washington, DC: Government Printing Office.

U.S. Department of Health and Human Services. (1997). Immunization . . . Not just kids' stuff. *Prevention Report, 12*(2), 1–4.

U.S. Preventive Health Services Task Force. (1995). *Guide to clinical preventive services* (2nd ed.). Washington, DC: U.S. Government Printing Office.

Waitzman, N. J., Romano, P. S., Scheffler, R. M., & Harris, J. A. (1995). Economic costs of birth defects and cerebral palsy—United States, 1992. *MMWR, 44,* 695–699.

Weitzman, M., Gortmacher, S. L., & Sobol, A. (1992). Maternal smoking and behavioral problems of children. *Pediatrics, 90,* 342–349.

RESOURCES FOR FAMILIES OF CHILDREN WITH SPECIAL NEEDS

Arthritis

American Juvenile Arthritis Organization
1314 Spring Street, NW
Atlanta, GA 30309
(404) 879-7100

Asthma

Jewish Center for Immunology and Respiratory
    Medicine
1400 Jackson Street
Denver, CO 80206
(303) 388–4461

Birth Defects

Association of Birth Defects in Children
827 Irma Avenue
Orlando, FL 32803
(407) 245–7035

March of Dimes Birth Defects Foundation
1275 Mamaroneck Avenue
White Plains, NY 10605
(914) 428–7100

Blindness

Carroll Center for the Blind
770 Centre Street
Newton, MA 02158
(617) 969–6200

Leader Dogs for the Blind
1039 Rochester Road
Rochester, MI 48307
(810) 651–9011

National Association for Visually Handicapped
22 West 21st Street
 New York, NY 10010
(212) 889–3141

National Braille Association
3 Townline Circle
Rochester, NY 14623–2513
(716) 427–8260

Cancer

Candlelighters Childhood Cancer Foundations
7910 Woodmont Avenue, Ste. 460
Bethesda, MD 20814
(301) 657–8401

United Ostomy Association
36 Executive Park, Ste. 120
Irvine, CA 92714
(714) 660–8624

Cystic Fibrosis

Cystic Fibrosis Foundation
6931 Arlington Road, No. 200
Bethesda, MD 20814
(301) 951–4422

Diabetes

Juvenile Diabetes Foundation International
120 Wall Street
New York, NY 10015–3904
(212) 889–7575

Down Syndrome

National Association for Down's Syndrome
PO Box 4542
Oak Brook, IL 60522–4542
(708) 325–9112

Epilepsy

Epilepsy Foundation of America
4351 Garden City Drive
Landover, MD 20785
(301) 459–3700

Growth Disorders

Human Growth Foundation
7777 Leesburg Pike
Falls Church, VA 22043
(703) 883–1773

Handicapped

Association of Maternal and Child Health Programs
1350 Connecticut Avenue, NW, Ste. 803
Washington, DC 20036
(202) 775–0436

National Easter Seal Society
230 W. Monroe
Chicago, IL 60606
(312) 726–6200

Shriner's Hospital for Crippled Children
2900 Rocky Point Drive
Tampa, FL 33607
(813) 281–0300

Hemophilia

National Hemophilia Foundation
110 Greene Street, Ste. 303
New York, NY 10012
(212) 219–8180

Mental Retardation

The ARC
500 East Border Street, Ste. 300
Arlington, TX 76010
(817) 261–6003

Mental Retardation Association of America
211 East 300 South Street, Ste. 212

Salt Lake City, UT 84111
(801) 328–1575

Pilot Parents
3610 Dodge Street, Ste. 101
Omaha, NE 68131
(402) 346–5220

Multiple Sclerosis

National Multiple Sclerosis Society
733 3rd Avenue
New York, NY 10017
(212) 986–3240

Muscular Dystrophy

Muscular Dystrophy Association
3300 East Sunrise Drive
Tucson, AZ 85718
(520) 529–2000

Phenylketonuria

PKU Parents
c/o Dale Hillard
Eight Myrtle Lane
San Anselmo, CA 94960
(415) 457–4632

Sickle Cell Disease

National Association for Sickle Cell Disease
200 Corporate Pointe, Ste. 495
Culver City, CA 90230–7633
(310) 216–6363

RESOURCES FOR CHILDHOOD NUTRITION

La Leche League
1400 Meacham
Schaumburg, IL 60173
(708) 519–7730

U.S. Department of Agriculture
Food and Consumer Services
Food and Nutrition Services
3101 Park Center Drive, No. 803
Alexandria, VA 22302
(703) 305–2062

U.S. Department of Agriculture
Food and Consumer Services
Human Nutrition Information Service
6506 Belcrest Road, No. 306
Hyattsville, MD 29782

U.S. Department of Agriculture
Food and Nutrition Service

Child-care Food Program
Park Office Building, Rm. 512
3101 Park Center Drive
Alexandria, VA 22302
(703) 305–2276

RESOURCES FOR PROMOTING CHILD SAFETY

American Association of Poison Control Centers
c/o Dr. Ted Long
Arizona Poison and Drug Information Center
Health Science Center, Rm. 3204K
1501 North Campbell
Tucson, AZ 85725
(520) 626–1587

American National Red Cross
431 18th Street, NW
Washington, DC 20006
(202) 737–8300

Boy Scouts of America
1325 Walnut Hill Lane
Irving, TX 75015
(214) 580–2000

National Safety Council
1121 Spring Lake Drive
Itasca, IL 60143–3201
(708) 285–1121

United Cerebral Palsy Association
3 4518 Warren Road, Ste. 264
Westland, MI 48185
(313) 425–8961

U.S. Consumer Product Safety Commission
East West Towers
East West Highway
Bethesda, MD 20814
(301) 504–0580

RESOURCES FOR NURSES AND FAMILIES DEALING WITH CHILD ABUSE

Child Abuse Listening Mediation, Inc.
PO Box 9074
Santa Barbara, CA 93190–0754
(805) 965–2376

Childhelp, USA
1345 N. El Centro Avenue, Ste. 630
Los Angeles, CA 90028–8216
(800) 423–4453

Local child protective services or law enforcement agencies

National Committee for Prevention of Child Abuse
332 South Michigan Avenue, Ste. 1600
Chicago, IL 60604–4357
(312) 663–3520

Parents Anonymous
675 Foothill Blvd., Ste. 220
Claremont, CA 91711–3416
(909) 621–6184

Village of Childhelp
PO Box 247
14700 Manzanita Park Road
Beaumont, CA 92223
(909) 845–3155

COUNSELING AND HEALTH EDUCATION RESOURCES FOR FAMILIES

Counseling

American Academy of Child and
  Adolescent Psychiatry
3615 Wisconsin Avenue, NW
Washington, DC 20016
(202) 966–7300

American Association for Marriage
  and Family Therapy
1133 15th Street, NW, Ste. 300
Washington, DC 20005
(202) 452–0109

American Association of Psychiatric Services
  for Children
1200-C Scottsville Road, Ste. 225
Rochester, NY 14624
(716) 235–6910

Autism Society of America
7910 Woodmont Avenue, Ste. 650
Bethesda, MD 20814
(301) 657–0881

Learning Disabilities Association of America
4156 Library Road
Pittsburgh, PA 15234
(412) 341–1515

National Consortium for Child Mental
  Health Services
601 13th Street, NW, Ste. 400 North
Washington, DC 20005
(202) 347–8600

SIDS Alliance
1314 Bedford Avenue, Ste. 210
Baltimore, MD 21208
(410) 653–8226

Health Education

Council for Sex Information and Education
2272 Colorado Blvd., No. 1228
Los Angeles, CA 90041

National Parents Resource Institute
  for Drug Education
3610 De Kalb Technology Parkway, Ste. 105
Atlanta, GA 30340
(770) 458–9900

Sex Information and Education Council
  of the United States
130 West 42nd Street, Ste. 350
New York, NY 10036–7802
(212) 819–9770

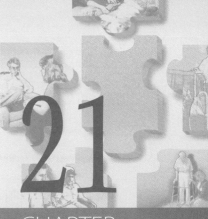

21
CHAPTER

CARE OF WOMEN

Patricia Caudle
Susan Chen

► KEY TERMS

coming out
female genital mutilation
  (FGM)
homophobia
infertility
menarche
menopause
osteoporosis
patriarchy

Women have unique health care needs, not only because of their anatomy and reproductive functions, but also because of their vulnerability within society. Traditionally, women have been wives and mothers, submissive to males and, yet, an essential member of the family. Community health nurses working with women have opportunities to improve not only the health status of women but also women's abilities to care for themselves and their families.

The importance of improving the health of women in the United States is reflected in the national health objectives for the year 2000 (see Appendix A). Several objectives address issues specifically targeting the health needs of nonpregnant women (U.S. Department of Health and Human Services, 1991).

In this chapter the Dimensions Model is applied to the care of adolescent, young adult, and middle adult women. The health needs of older women are the focus of Chapter 23.

► Chapter Objectives

After reading this chapter, you should be able to:

- Identify at least two factors in each of the dimensions of health as they relate to the health of women.
- Identify at least four health problems common to women.
- Describe at least three unique considerations in assessing the health needs of the lesbian client.
- Identify at least five concerns in primary prevention for women.
- Describe three areas of secondary prevention activity with women.
- Describe two dimensions of secondary prevention of physical abuse of women.
- Describe at least two actions that the community health nurse can take to provide more sensitive and effective care to the lesbian client.

► FACTORS AFFECTING HEALTH CARE FOR WOMEN

Women in the United States remain comparatively disadvantaged in society at large and in the health care delivery system. Women have higher rates of diagnosed illness than men, although they have lower mortality rates (Mann, 1996). Women also experience more days of disability per person than men (U.S. Department of Commerce, 1996). Women are also more likely to require medical intervention as a result of rape, physical assault, or battering by spouses. Not only are they more often recipients of health care for themselves, but women make most decisions regarding the need for health care for family members. Finally, because women, as an aggregate, live longer than men (life expectancy of 79 years compared with 72.3 years for men) (U.S. Department of Commerce, 1996), they are more likely to live the latter portion of their lives in a nursing home.

Women not only use health care services more often than men but they are often more hard-pressed to pay for these services. More women live in poverty than men. Women are also less likely to be covered by medical insurance as a job benefit because they are more likely to hold part-time jobs. More women than men are heads of single-parent households and are the sole support of their children. For all of these reasons, women are more likely to be dependent on such programs as Medicaid and Medicare.

These conditions are the result of social traditions and age-old prejudices that have been legitimized through religion, law, and culture. Not sur-

prisingly, the health care system reflects and perpetuates many sexist attitudes and beliefs within the culture at large. At the turn of the century, men and some women believed that a woman's primary functions were procreation and taking care of the home and family. As a result of a prevailing culture of sexism, physicians tended to perceive women as creatures totally controlled by their womb, ovaries, and hormones. Everything from headache to arthritis in women was attributed to sexual disorders. This tradition lingers today to the extent that discussions of women's health issues are often limited to reproductive and gynecologic concerns.

During the formative years of the U.S. health care system, physicians converted female reproductive functions into medical conditions and encouraged women to depend on a male-dominated profession for care. In keeping with the medicalization of normal female responses, the current Diagnostic and Statistical Manual includes as diseases two conditions that some authors consider expected responses to typical female socialization: premenstrual syndrome and masochistic syndrome (Crook, 1995). Because of prevailing paternalistic attitudes, it also became normal for physicians to withhold information about medical conditions and to treat women as if they were intellectually, emotionally, and physically inferior to men. Regrettably, many women are still subjected to such treatment, especially women who are poor, uneducated, or members of minority groups.

► THE DIMENSIONS MODEL AND CARE OF WOMEN

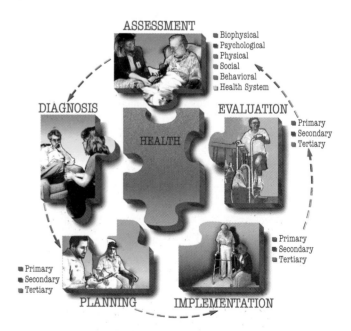

Critical Dimensions of Nursing in the Care of Women

In one study, women identified several characteristics they would like to see in health care providers. These include being heard, receiving complete and accurate information and appropriate and competent help, efforts to advise rather than control, respect for them and for the other demands on their time, a safe environment, the time of the provider, and independence from drug companies (Crook, 1995). Most of these requirements can be met by nurses operating effectively in the interpersonal dimension of nursing. Through interpersonal interactions, nurses can convey an attitude of respect for women and the demands on their lives and time by listening and attending to their concerns and by refraining from attempts to control their behavior. Because the majority of nurses are women, they have an advantage over many other providers in their understanding of women's needs. Sensitive and understanding care can prevent the misdiagnosis of many women's health problems as psychological in origin, a common response of many health care providers.

In the ethical dimension, advocacy by community health nurses can help to assure safe environments for women both in their interactions with providers and in the larger social sphere. For example, women have been found to receive a better response from medical providers when accompanied by an advocate (Crook, 1995); the community health nurse can be that advocate. Advocacy can also promote the use of interventions other than medication to more effectively meet women's needs. For instance, while many women are effectively using alternative treatment strategies rather than hormone replacement therapy to address problems associated with menopause, information about these alternative therapies is not always readily available.

In the reflective dimension, there is a profound need for research related to the health needs of women and the interventions best suited to meet those needs. Much of the medical care currently provided to women is based on research findings related to men. Community health nurses can be actively involved in designing and conducting research on women's health issues.

Assessing the Dimensions of Health in Women

Use of the Dimensions Model with the female client begins with an assessment of health status. Factors influencing health status are examined according to the six dimensions of health: the biophysical, psychological, physical, social, behavioral, and health system dimensions. Aggregates of women, like other groups within communities, can be assessed as described in Chapter 19.

The Biophysical Dimension

Biophysical factors are of concern to the community health nurse assessing the female client. The nurse would obtain information related to genetic inheritance, maturation and aging, and physiologic function.

Genetic Inheritance. Women are prone to a number of genetically related or genetically linked conditions. For example, cancers of the breast have been shown to occur more frequently among women whose mothers, sisters, aunts, or grandmothers have had similar cancers. Similarly, diseases of the thyroid gland seem to occur more frequently among women than men, as do diabetes, asthma, various forms of dermatitis, and hay fever-type allergies, all of which may involve genetic predisposition to disease.

Maturation and Aging. Maturational events affect women throughout their life. Two that are of particular interest are menarche in the adolescent and menopause in the middle-aged to older adult woman.

MENARCHE. *Menarche,* the first appearance of menstrual flow in the adolescent girl, usually occurs between 12 and 13 years of age, but is considered within normal limits unless it occurs before or during the eighth year or after age 18. Menarche that occurs too early (age 8 or younger) is associated with precocious puberty, an anomaly of the endocrine system. Delayed menarche (after age 18) is also a signal that the endocrine system is not functioning properly. Either early or late onset of menses is cause for referral for medical evaluation (Rosenthal & Wilson, 1994).

Before and after menarche, girls experience predictable body changes. These body changes have been described by Tanner and associates as occurring in five stages. For example, girls who are in Tanner stage III usually display an increased amount of dark, curling pubic hair and breasts that are enlarged and have no contour separation between the breast and the areola. It is during Tanner stage III that menarche occurs. With menarche, further changes occur in the appearance of the young female. Her weight, disposition of body fat, breasts, and hair growth patterns change to those of an adult over a period of 4 to 5 years. The stages of sexual maturation in girls are summarized in Table 21–1.

These body changes have the potential to create physical or psychological problems for the adolescent.

TABLE 21–1. STAGES OF SEXUAL MATURATION IN GIRLS

Stage	Pubic Hair Characteristics	Breast Characteristics
1	None present	Preadolescent
2	Sparse, straight, lightly pigmented, present on medial border of labia	Increase in areola diameter, breast and papilla elevated as a small mound
3	Darker pigmentation, increased amount, beginning to curl	Enlargement of breast and areola, no contour separation between breast and areola
4	Dark and curly, abundant, but less than in adult	Areola and papilla form a secondary mound separated from contour of breast
5	Adult female inverted triangle, hair distribution spread to medial aspects of thighs	Nipple projects, areola forms part of general breast contour

Adapted from Litt, I. R., & Vaughan, V. C. (1987). Growth and development during adolescence. In R. E. Behrman & V. C. Vaughan (Eds.), Nelson textbook of pediatrics (13th ed.) (pp. 20–22). Philadelphia: W. B. Saunders.

Community health nurses encounter many young women before, during, and after menarche. Assessment of each 8- to 12-year-old girl should include the client's stage of sexual maturity, knowledge of menstruation, and preparation for the event. If menarche has occurred, other considerations related to menstruation may include menstrual regularity, extent and duration of flow, and the experience of dysmenorrhea, or painful menstruation. The nurse would also inquire about signs and symptoms of premenstrual distress (premenstrual syndrome) such as depression, irritability, nervousness, tension, inability to concentrate, breast tenderness, bloating, edema, fatigue, headache, and food cravings (Hatcher, et al., 1994). Symptoms of premenstrual distress may be severe and require medical referral or may be less severe and respond to dietary changes and exercise.

MENOPAUSE.   Thirty percent of women in the United States, or 40 million women, are considered postmenopausal and at risk for conditions such as heart disease and osteoporosis due to reduction in estrogen levels (Sarrel, 1991). In assessing older women, the nurse should determine whether menopause has occurred. *Menopause* is the cessation of menstruation that occurs with advancing age. Most women experience menopause and its physical and emotional effects between 41 and 59 years of age. The onset of menopausal symptoms and menopause is somewhat determined by heredity. The client's mother's history of menopause will often reveal the pattern the client can be expected to experience.

Physical effects of menopause can include hot flashes or flushes accompanied by perspiration and chills; menstrual irregularity consisting of greater flow and longer times between periods; and vaginal dryness and atrophy. Other effects may be redisposition of body fat, headache, dizziness, insomnia, depression, anxiety, and nervousness and irritability. Symptoms of menopause last an average of 5 to 10 years, but in 10% of women symptoms may persist as long as 17 years (Sarrel, 1991). Each individual responds to these changes differently. Some women are very uncomfortable; others are not. The nurse must assess each individual woman according to symptoms she describes.

Another concern during the perimenopausal years is osteoporosis. *Osteoporosis* is a common metabolic bone disease characterized by a loss of bone minerals that weakens bones so that fractures occur more easily. Although bone mineral loss begins to occur in the fourth decade of life, the loss is gradual until menopause. At menopause, bone loss is accelerated because of declining estrogen levels.

Age may also play a part in the severity of other health conditions. For example, women under 40 years of age or over 80 have worse 5-year survival rates for breast cancer than women in intermediate age groups. With respect to remaining disease-free after treatment, women over age 80 have the worst rates followed by women under 40. These findings appear to be unrelated to the stage of disease at diagnosis suggesting more aggressive tumors in the younger and older age groups (Chung, Chang, Bland, & Wanebo, 1996).

Physiologic Function.   The client's physiologic function is also assessed. Special considerations in assessing the female client include pregnancy, infertility, and presence or absence of specific illnesses such as reproductive cancers and sexually transmitted diseases.

PREGNANCY.   Pregnancy is one of the most prevalent problems related to human physiology in the adolescent girl. In 1991, 74 out of every 1000 girls aged 15 to 17 years became pregnant (U.S. Department of Health and Human Services, 1996a). Ten percent of all pregnancies between 1990 and 1995 were unwanted at the time of conception (National Center for Health Statistics, 1997), and posed ethical and economic dilemmas for many women.

Pregnancy is more often associated with complications, prematurity, and fetal and maternal mortality among adolescents than among older women, but all women are at some risk of complications during pregnancy. In fact, in 1994, 15% of deliveries were associated with serious complications of pregnancy, occasionally resulting in death. The maternal mortality rate for 1993 in the United States was 7.5 deaths per

100,000 live births (U.S. Department of Health and Human Services, 1996b).

Information regarding potential current and past pregnancies is solicited and any related problems should be identified. If the client is pregnant, the nurse assesses fetal growth as well as maternal health. Fetal growth patterns are assessed by measuring fundal height during each visit. The fundal height should increase steadily until just before delivery. Consult Table 21–2 for the expected fundal height at selected weeks of gestation.

Evidence of complications such as pregnancy-induced hypertension and gestational diabetes should also be sought. For example, signs of pregnancy-induced hypertension include increased blood pressure (140/90 or greater or a rise of 30 mm Hg in systolic or 15 mm Hg in diastolic levels over the baseline blood pressure), proteinuria (1+ or greater protein in a clean-catch specimen), and edema (sudden, excessive weight gain or swelling of the hands and face). Gestational diabetes can be suspected if there is a family history of diabetes, history of miscarriage, or history of babies weighing 9 pounds or more, if the pregnant woman is overweight, or if there is positive glycosuria, polyuria, polydipsia, polyphagia, or recurrent monilial infection. Table 21–3 lists some of the most common complications of pregnancy and their signs and symptoms.

INFERTILITY. The incidence of infertility among U.S. women is increasing. *Infertility* is the inability to conceive and have a child. In 1995, 2% of U.S. women (1.2 million) had visited a health care provider regarding infertility in the past year, and 13% had been seen for infertility concerns at some time in their lives (National Center for Health Statistics, 1997). Causes of infertility among women include the occurrence of sexually transmitted diseases that damage fallopian tubes, environmental toxins affecting ova, and a tendency to postpone pregnancy until the late thirties or

TABLE 21–3. SIGNS AND SYMPTOMS OF COMPLICATIONS OF PREGNANCY

Complication	Signs and Symptoms
Gestational diabetes	Polyuria, polydipsia, polyphagia, obesity, large baby, glycosuria (may be asymptomatic)
Iron-deficiency anemia	Fatigue, pallor, hemoglobin below 11 mg/dL, history of poor dietary iron intake
Pregnancy-induced hypertension	BP 140/90, 30 mm Hg rise in systolic pressure of 15 mm Hg rise in diastolic pressure; edema (especially of face and hands); proteinuria (convulsions in severe form)
Hyperemesis gravidarum	Severe vomiting, retching, dehydration, starvation, infant small for gestational age
Rh sensitization	Rh-negative mother, Rh-positive father
Abruptio placentae	Vaginal bleeding
Premature labor	Strong uterine contractions prior to the 35th week of gestation

Adapted from Olds., S., London, M., & Ladewig, P. (1988). Maternal–newborn nursing: A family-centered approach (3rd ed.). Menlo Park, CA: Addison-Wesley.

early forties. Women aged 38 and older tend to ovulate less frequently than younger women, thereby becoming less fertile than they would have been in their twenties (Edge & Miller, 1994).

Infertility can have serious consequences for the individual and the couple who are unable to conceive, among them the following:

- Feelings of guilt, especially among women, who are usually the focus of the search for a cause
- Expense of diagnostic and other procedures
- Obsession with the inability to conceive
- Disapproval and pressure from family to adopt or try other methods to conceive
- In some cultures, perceptions of the female as less than a woman

The community health nurse can assess the client's desire to have children and any attempts made to conceive. Data collected should include the ages of the woman and her partner; her menstrual history (especially information about irregular periods); a medical history that includes information on mumps in the partner, pelvic inflammatory disease in the woman, reproductive or abdominal surgery or serious illness in either partner, and dysmenorrhea or dyspareunia; forms of contraception used in the past (especially use of an intrauterine device, or IUD); diethylstilbestrol (DES) exposure of either partner in utero; and whether or not either partner has ever achieved a pregnancy (Hatcher, et al., 1994). These data form the basis for nursing intervention to be discussed later in this chapter.

ILLNESS.   Assessment of physiologic function also includes the collection of data related to the presence or

TABLE 21–2. FUNDAL HEIGHT AT SELECTED WEEKS OF GESTATION

Weeks of Gestation	Fundal Height
12	At the level of the symphysis pubis
16	Halfway between symphysis pubis and umbilicus
20	At the level of the umbilicus
20–26	Height of fundus in centimeters correlates with weeks of gestation
36–40	1 cm below the xiphoid process until lightening occurs, then decreases; varies with the weight of the baby and maternal parity

Adapted from Olds, S., London, M., & Ladewig, P. (1988). Maternal–newborn nursing: A family-centered approach (3rd ed.). Menlo Park, CA: Addison-Wesley.

absence of physical illness. The community health nurse would obtain a complete health history and physical examination, looking for signs and symptoms of illness. Of particular concern with the female client is evidence of reproductive cancers and possible sexually transmitted diseases.

Cancer is second only to heart disease as a leading cause of death among women. In 1993, women aged 55 to 84 years had far higher death rates from lung cancer than breast cancer (eg, 226 per 100,000 and 146 per 100,000, respectively, among women 75 to 84 years of age) (U.S. Department of Commerce, 1996). The American Cancer Society's 1993 statistics indicated that 18% of cancer deaths among women are due to breast cancer, 5% to cancer of the ovary, and 4% to cancer of the uterus and cervix (Boring Squires, & Tong, 1993). When detected early, these types of cancers can be cured, and their detection is an important component in assessing the health of a female client.

Assessment of each women should include present and past medical history; history of tobacco use; family history of breast, uterine, or ovarian cancer; and use of early detection procedures such as breast self-examination, biannual or annual mammograms (depending on the age of the client), annual Pap smears (for early detection of cervical cancer), and annual pelvic examinations (for early detection of uterine or ovarian abnormalities). Cancer and cancer detection are discussed more fully in Chapter 31.

Problems of sexually transmitted diseases will be addressed in detail in Chapter 30. Here, however, we consider some of the implications of AIDS or HIV disease as it relates specifically to women.

AIDS is a viral disease that destroys the body's immune system, causing the person with AIDS to succumb to opportunistic infections. AIDS is caused by the human immunodeficiency virus type I and type II (HIV-1 and HIV-2). For a person to become infected, the virus must enter the bloodstream. The pathways of transmission that have been identified include sexual contact with an infected person, use of infected needles, use of infected blood or blood products, and transmission of the virus to the fetus during pregnancy. The person infected by HIV may not manifest symptoms of AIDS for 2 to 10 years or more, but can pass the disease to others.

Although once thought to be a disease primarily affecting male homosexuals, HIV disease has proven to be nondiscriminatory with respect to gender. The number of women infected through heterosexual contact has shown a consistent increase since 1985, whereas the percentage of cases among men has decreased. In addition, sexual activity with men in high-risk groups and use of injection drugs also contribute

to increased incidence of HIV infection. This increase in HIV/AIDS mortality among women is a large part of the 31% increase in deaths due to sexually transmitted diseases from 1985 to 1992 (Ebrahim, Peterman, Zaidi, & Kamb, 1997). In 1995, more than 15% of AIDS deaths occurred among women (U.S. Department of Commerce, 1996).

These statistics do not convey the anguish this disease has caused women. AIDS is a physical threat with a tremendous social impact. Single women must enter relationships cautiously and be assertive enough to explore the sexual history of a potential partner. Women are reluctant to do this for fear it may interfere with the relationship. If a woman can convince a male partner to use them, condoms are generally protective, but not foolproof. The only absolute way to avoid HIV infection is to have a mutually monogamous relationship with an uninfected person or to practice sexual abstinence.

Women with HIV disease typically lack the support systems that male homosexuals have been able to build. Often women with HIV disease are ostracized and isolated. Minority women may even avoid treatment for AIDS-related conditions for fear that if it is known that they have AIDS, their children will be taken from them.

Women who are HIV-positive carry a burden that men do not share. An infected pregnant woman can transmit HIV to her unborn child. In 1994, 92% of pediatric AIDS was acquired from infected mothers (Cribsheet, 1995). Infants born with AIDs are usually very ill and have a very short life. For a woman who has dreamed of motherhood and who values children highly, this can be a nightmare. Many of these pregnancies occur during the dormant period of HIV infection, before symptoms of AIDS appear in the mother. Imagine the devastation felt by a mother on learning that her baby is infected with a fatal disease and that she is the cause. Women in these circumstances need assistance to cope.

Because women usually assume caregiver roles within families, they suffer when family members contract and die of AIDS. When a family member is terminally ill, the commitment to care for that individual can be emotionally draining, not only because of the pain and eventual death of the individual, but also because of the ever-present fear of contracting the disease. Women who assume a caregiver role need a strong support system to assist them in working through the fears associated with this role. To provide such assistance, the community health nurse needs to be tactful when eliciting information related to the potential for AIDS in the female client or in family members. Table 21–4 presents some assessment inquiries that can be made by the community health nurse.

TABLE 21–4. ASSESSING AIDS RISK

Question	Response Indicating Risk
• Did you receive a blood transfusion prior to 1984?	Yes
• Are you monogamous?	No
• Is your partner monogamous?	No
• Do you and your partner use a latex condom and nonoxynol-9?	No
• Do you engage in anal intercourse?	Yes
• Do you engage in oral–genital or oral–anal intercourse?	Yes
• Have you or your partner ever used IV drugs?	Yes
• Do you use crack cocaine?	Yes
• Have you or your partner ever tested positive for HIV?	Yes
• Do you share syringes with others for injecting vitamins or other medications?	Yes

In addition to the physiologic conditions discussed earlier, women experience a variety of other diseases. In fact, women experience all chronic and most acute conditions (except injuries) more often than men. Risk factors for some conditions also have differential effects on men and women. For example, an elevated blood cholesterol level is a less significant risk factor for heart disease in women than men, but the presence of diabetes increases women's risk of heart disease more than men's. Similarly, smoking poses a greater risk of lung cancer in women than men. Differential effects in men and women are also noted for some drugs and toxins. For example, women are more susceptible than men to lead poisoning and to hypothyroidism due to lithium use (Mann, 1996). A thorough assessment of women's health will elicit evidence of these and other physiologic conditions.

The Psychological Dimension

Factors in the psychological dimension can have a profound effect on women's health. Areas of particular concern to the community health nurse assessing women's health are stress and coping abilities, life goals, and the psychological implications of sexual identity.

Stress and Coping.   The first area for consideration related to the psychological dimension and its effect on women's health is the extent of the client's exposure to stress and her ability to cope with that stress. It is well known that stress contributes to a variety of illnesses in both men and women. For example, stress plays a part in the development of tuberculosis and hypertension. Severe life events and the stress that accompanies them has also been shown to be related to breast cancer in women. In one study, women exposed to at least one severe life event in the previous 5 years were more than three times as likely as women without stressful life events to have breast malignancies (Chen, David, & Nunnerley, 1995). Women, in general, have been found to be less happy and to experience more stress than men. This is particularly true for married women who experience less life satisfaction and more mental health problems than single women (Mann, 1996). What are the stresses experienced by the woman client? How severe are these stresses and how effectively is the woman able to cope with them?

Learned coping skills are an important facet of the psychological dimension of health that the nurse assesses. How does the client normally handle adversity? What factors in the environment strengthen her ability to cope? What coping strategies does she use and how effective are they? Is the client at risk for suicide or other health problems due to poor coping abilities? Women at all ages are less likely than men to commit suicide, but a significant number of women each year succumb to despair and end their lives. In 1993, the suicide mortality rate for white women was 5 per 100,000 women. Suicide rates for black women were somewhat lower at 2.1 per 100,000 (U.S. Department of Commerce, 1996). Women are also more likely to experience depression than men (Janosik & Green, 1992).

Life Goals.   A second aspect of the psychological dimension that affects women's health status is their ability to establish and accomplish life goals. In assessing the female client, the community health nurse should question the client about her life goals, her plans for achieving them, and factors that may interfere with their attainment. Life goals may include, but are not limited to, finishing one's education, getting married and having three children who grow up to be professionals, being the best high school math teacher, and enjoying a comfortable retirement.

Movement toward retirement as a life goal for middle-aged adult women may present a host of psychological factors that can affect health. Loss of productive work life may result in diminution of self-esteem and onset of depression. As women move toward retirement age, they may find themselves shunted to less challenging jobs (Crook, 1995), which may also contribute to lower feelings of self-worth. Community health nurses can help at this time by assisting women to plan for retirement and for activities to replace work as a foundation for self-esteem. To provide such assistance, the nurse needs to assess the woman's attitudes toward work and retirement and the contribution that productive work provides to her self-esteem.

Sexuality.   Elements of both the psychological and social dimensions affect issues of sexuality in women, but because of the implications of sexuality for women's mental health, they will be addressed under the psychological dimension. Many women are embarrassed to discuss issues of sexuality, and teenagers in particular, may have a number of fears and misconceptions. In assessing the adolescent girl, the community health nurse obtains information related to attitudes and anxieties about menstruation as well as knowledge of menstrual physiology and hygiene. Social factors such as family and cultural attitudes and knowledge and parental education level may affect family readiness to assist the young girl with the physical, emotional, and practical issues posed by menarche.

The nurse cannot assume that older women do not have some of the same concerns regarding menstruation and sexuality as teenagers. Women may have questions about their sexuality, guilt about sexual activity or possible infertility, and difficulty in developing healthy sexual identities. As we will see later in this chapter, these concerns are frequently magnified for the lesbian client. Community health nurses should assess women's comfort with sexuality and their sexual identity and assist them to voice concerns in these areas.

Sexual activity by women, especially teenagers, may have a variety of psychological precursors. For example, the adolescent may think that if she is still a virgin at age 15, there is something wrong with her. Or, if she perceives her mother as asexual or "Madonna-like," she may rebel and seek sexual outlets totally unlike those of her mother. The nurse assesses the client's knowledge and attitudes about her sexual identity and about sexual activity. Sexuality for women is more than a biological drive. Sexual activity may be an attempt to define personal and sexual identity as well as a means of communicating with others. For women, sexuality is a total experience of emotions, relationships, and life experiences.

There is some evidence that both psychological and social factors contribute to the problem of adolescent pregnancy. Teen pregnancy theories include ideas that (1) teens enter into a sexual relationship in search of love and become pregnant accidentally; (2) teens become pregnant to have a baby to love and love them; and (3) teens seek pregnancy to punish their parents (Fogel & Woods, 1994). Research indicates that nearly 95% of teenage pregnancies are unintended (Spitz, et al., 1993).

A number of social factors may also contribute to intended or unintended pregnancy. This is particularly true in the case of adolescent pregnancy. Sexual experimentation by adolescents is expected, but may

come as a shock to parents who have not recognized their son or daughter as a sexual being. Unfortunately, American teenagers are becoming sexually active earlier than was previously the case. In 1988, 27% of girls under age 15 participating in the Youth Risk Behavior Study (YRBS) reported having premarital sexual activity compared with more than 38% in 1995 (U.S. Department of Health and Human Services, 1996a). Such early sexual activity exposes the teen to increased risks for unwanted pregnancy and sexually transmitted diseases.

There are several social theories related to adolescent sexual activity and resultant pregnancy. Learned sexual behavior through interaction and identification with peers, family, and cultural groups is one such theory (Fogel & Woods, 1994). Peer pressure or a need for status and popularity may be the motivation for sexual activity that results in pregnancy.

Some authorities believe that teen pregnancy is a reaction to the dominant American culture in which teens are dependent and have no meaningful role in society (Fogel & Woods, 1994). Furthermore, given the cultural stereotype of the woman's role and function as procreation, the teen who seeks pregnancy may be attempting to fulfill her cultural destiny.

Teens must also negotiate the differences between what society says and does with respect to sexuality. At one level, teens see parents resisting school-based sex education because it is perceived as promoting promiscuity. At another level, teens are exposed to images and messages in the entertainment media in which sexual innuendo and sexual acts are frequently portrayed without even hinting that such activity could lead to pregnancy or sexually transmitted diseases. To condemn the female who becomes pregnant out of wedlock, yet tacitly condone such media exposure, presents teens with conflicting messages about proper sexual conduct.

Finally, a lack of information and knowledge about sexuality, reproduction, and the use of contraception is regarded as a causative factor in unwanted pregnancy, particularly among teenagers. Ultimately, the causes of unintended pregnancy are as complex and as varied as the many women who become pregnant. Research that can capture the essence of the meaning of the pregnancy for the pregnant woman as she experiences it may reveal more reasons that have not been identified as yet. Community health nurses need to assess the psychological and social factors that promote unprotected intercourse by individual clients and by groups in society with an eye toward controlling the problem of unwanted pregnancy.

Menopause, at the other end of the reproductive spectrum, also has psychological implications. In our society, menopausal women have not been held in high esteem. Women have been barred from productive work on the basis of their menopausal symptoms. Society's lack of regard for the older woman adds to her emotional symptoms, thereby limiting her abilities to cope with physical and psychological changes occurring at this time (Office of Technology Assessment, 1992).

One last area of sexuality that may have profound effects on the psychological health status of some women is female genital mutilation. *Female genital mutilation* (FGM), also called female circumcision, is the alteration of female genitalia ostensibly to promote virginity, but in reality to maintain male dominance. An estimated 85 to 140 million women in the world may be affected. A variety of religious groups practice FGM, including some Christian and Jewish sects as well as some Muslim groups. It has been reported in 25 African countries, Malaysia, Yemen, Indonesia, Brazil, Mexico, and Peru, and may also be found in Europe, Canada, and the United States, primarily among immigrant groups (Doyal, 1995).

The community health nurse working with women who have experienced FGM may discover three levels of mutilation. The least severe is *clitoridectomy* in which the tip of the clitoris and surrounding skin are removed. *Excision* involves removal of the entire clitoris and the labia minora. *Infibulation,* the most extensive form of FGM, involves removal of the clitoris, labia minora, and parts of the labia majora and stitching the sides of the area together to leave only a small opening for passage of urine and menstrual blood. The effects of FGM may include wound infection, urinary tract and vaginal infections, and serious complications of childbirth including severe perineal tears and increased incidence of stillbirth (Doyal, 1995). Community health nurses should ask women clients about their exposure to FGM. Gynecologic and urologic referrals may be needed for these clients, as well as referrals to mental health professionals to help these women deal with the psychological effects of this abusive practice.

The Physical Dimension

Physical dimension factors also influence the health of women. They are exposed to physical environmental hazards both at home and in the work setting. In the home, environmental hazards include household chemicals used to clean, inhalants such as powders and sprays, and the potential for falls related to stools, stairs, and throw rugs. The effects of the workplace on women's health are covered later in this chapter during the discussion of the occupational component of

the social dimension. Physical dimension factors are particularly evident in rates for accidental injuries. Although women have far lower injury rates than men, significant morbidity and mortality are related to unintentional injuries in women. In 1993, for example, the overall injury mortality rate was 31.5 per 100,000 population for white women and 38.2 per 100,000 for black women. Motor vehicle accidents accounted for a large portion of mortality in both groups (U.S. Department of Commerce, 1996).

The Social Dimension

Many social dimension factors affect the health status of women. Among these are societal pressures regarding roles and relationships, violence and abuse, and occupational and economic issues.

Roles and Relationships. As noted earlier, women often define themselves in terms of relationships with others. Women tend to invest more in their relationships and exhibit a greater commitment to those relationships than do men (O'Hanlon, 1995). Women's roles in these relationships are culturally defined by the society in which the woman lives. Society even specifies how women should look, and women experience significant "pressure to be ornamental" (Crook, 1995). This often means that women engage in health risk behavior to attain the "perfect" image. This is exemplified in excessive dieting, cosmetic surgery, breast augmentation, and other attempts to alter one's appearance. Social expectations for thinness have also been correlated with increased smoking in women (Chesney & Nealey, 1996).

Marriage and childbearing are prevalent societal expectations of women. Although marriage confers some health benefits for both sexes, this effect is more evident for men. Married men tend to express more life satisfaction and fewer mental and physical health problems than either married women or single men. Married women, on the other hand, have more stress and mental health problems and less satisfaction than single women (Mann, 1996). Many of women's relationships entail what have been called "caregiving careers" (Barusch, 1994) in which they have primary responsibility for the care of children, spouses, aging parents, and ill family members (Doyal, 1995) that compound the stress of daily life. Community health nurses should assess the effect of women clients' relationships on their health and the extent to which those relationships create additional stress.

Relationships often provide social support as well as additional sources of stress. For women, however, social support is less of a protective factor than it is for men. For example, presence of adequate social support networks decreases the incidence of coronary heart disease more in men than in women (Hegelson, 1995). The social support available to women clients should be assessed as well as the extent to which social support assists them in coping with the stresses encountered in their lives.

Violence and Abuse.   Abuse of women is the product of many psychological and social dimension factors, and it fosters a psychological environment detrimental to women's health. Because it is primarily social conditions that allow abuse to continue, the issue is addressed here within the discussion of the social dimension. Psychological dimension factors contributing to abuse of women are also addressed. Psychological dependence on males and poor self-esteem on the part of both the victim and the abuser are some of the psychological causes resulting in abuse. Feelings of shame and worthlessness may hamper the woman's ability to seek help while in an abusive situation.

The community health nurse assesses clients for risk factors for and evidence of violence. Violence against women is a pervasive, underrecognized, and culturally condoned phenomenon in our society. Women, especially single women between the ages of 16 and 24, are more likely to be victims of violence than are women of other ages. Minority and poor women are more often victims of violence than white middle- and upper-class women. The most common acts of violence against women are rape, assault, robbery, incest, and sexual and physical abuse (Furniss, 1993). Statistics indicate that 20% of women in the United States have been physically abused by a man in an intimate relationship. From 22 to 35% of women's visits to emergency departments are related to battering (Doyal, 1995).

Domestic violence such as spouse abuse is rarely a one-time event. By the time injuries are identifiable as inflicted by a batterer, a woman may have been abused for several years. If the woman does not ask for help or injuries are not discovered, battering usually increases in severity and frequency. Violence against women in its most deadly form is reflected in homicide statistics. In 1993, the homicide mortality rate for white women was 3 per 100,000 compared to 13.6 per 100,000 for black women (U.S. Department of Commerce, 1996).

Many causative factors have been postulated for domestic violence and abuse of women. Some are deeply rooted in cultural beliefs that have existed for centuries. Several underlying factors are reviewed here to demonstrate that spouse abuse is not a new or simple problem.

Some of the oldest teachings on how women should be treated are found among the writings of the world's religions, specifically Judaism, Christianity, and Islam. Many of these tenets support *patriarchy,* a hierarchical arrangement of society and family in which the leader is always male. These religious beliefs support the inferiority of women, depicting them as the "private property of men" (Eisler, 1994).

Until 1899, in the United States, men had the legal right to beat their wives to maintain their authority. Even with legislation to prevent spouse abuse, domestic squabbles today are often viewed by police and courts as private matters, and intervention does not always occur.

The socialization of female children also contributes to patterns of violence. Many females are raised to be dependent on males for approval, to be inferior and inadequate. They have been taught that they have little control over what happens in their lives. Males often are taught to be aggressive, domineering, and independent. Where these conditions exist, the dichotomy between male and female socialization extends to form a sexist family structure where men dominate and women submit. Such an arrangement may encourage male-to-female domestic violence.

Other factors contributing to violence against women include a sociocultural tolerance of family violence and violence against women that is sustained by the media; childhood experiences of abusive situations that serve as role models for future generations; and economic insecurity resulting in female dependence on men. Social factors such as lack of equal access to employment, housing, and resources can trap women in abusive situations that they might otherwise flee.

The plight of abused women in the United States has improved somewhat in the last few years. The women's movement stimulated a national "battered women's movement" in the 1970s. Wife abuse and violence against women were identified as social and political issues, not merely private domestic concerns. Among the accomplishments of the battered women's movement was the passage of the Family Violence Prevention and Services Act of 1984 that earmarked federal funds for programs to protect women. Today there are formal shelters, hotlines, and safe-home networks for victims of abuse throughout the country.

The movement continues to work for changes in the criminal justice system so abusers are punished and battered women gain the right to be protected. Where there are still law enforcement agencies that see domestic violence as a private matter and practice a policy of nonintervention, such attitudes are being increasingly challenged by studies that demonstrate that arrest is the best deterrent to repeated violence. In many areas of the country, public safety personnel receive special training in dealing with domestic abuse situations and information provided by these officers has resulted in some women being able to remove themselves from an abusive situation (Coffin-Romig, 1997).

Lawsuits, injunctions, and the use of lawyers to help protect victims against abuse cost money. Unfortunately, the legal system still does not offer much in the way of protection for low-income and minority women. In addition, many lawyers, judges, and health care professionals believe myths that have surrounded violence against women. Table 21–5 presents some of the myths and truths associated with abuse of women.

Community health nurses assessing female clients should be alert to evidence of physical or sexual abuse. Bruises, burns, fractures, or other injuries that are poorly explained or recurrent may suggest abuse. Because battered women are frequently afraid or ashamed to admit to being beaten, the nurse may need to suggest tactfully the possibility of battering as a cause for such injuries. Exploration of such areas requires an atmosphere of trust that is free of value judgments on the part of the nurse.

In assessing a potentially abused woman, the nurse needs to ask the client about depression, the possibility of suicide, and her risk of being killed by her partner. Another important consideration is the woman's willingness to leave the situation. Many women in such situations continue to hope that their partner will change or are fearful that the partner will hunt them down and further injure them if they try to leave. Another common fear is that the partner will attempt to win custody of the children if the woman leaves.

Occupational and Economic Issues. Occupation is a social dimension factor that has profound effects on the health of many women. In fact, it is believed that the decreasing mortality differences between men and women are attributable to increased participation by women in the work force (Waldron, 1991). Most women in the paid labor force continue to work in traditional "women's jobs" such as nursing, teaching, the garment industry, and secretarial/clerical and service jobs. Although considered "women's work," these jobs are not without health risks. Physical risks arise from chemicals, radiation, infectious disease, noise, vibration, and repetitive movements. For example, nurses and other hospital personnel experience occupational illness and injury rates 55% higher those in other service industries (Doyal, 1995).

As more women enter the world of "men's work" such as heavy industry, construction, mining, and factory work, they face a different set of physical hazards. Health risks arise from heavy lifting, use of dangerous machinery, and tools that were designed for larger men rather than smaller women. Minority women are at higher risk than white women for job-related injury because they often take jobs that others will not. Their economic need prevents them from saying no or quitting.

High-tech employment, once touted as safe, also entails health risks. The scrupulously clean area needed to produce a computer chip or to work with computers contains threats to human reproduction posed by radiofrequency or microwave radiation, video display terminal radiation, and arsine and chlorine gases (Rose, 1990). Some of the physical hazards encountered by women in the work setting are pre-

TABLE 21–5. MYTHS AND TRUTHS ABOUT ABUSED WOMEN

Myth	Truth
Battering occurs in a small percentage of the population.	An estimated 3 to 4 million women are beaten annually. Battering often goes unreported.
Violence among family members is a private matter and it is a man's right to keep his woman in line.	Violence is not allowable in society. No one has the right to beat or rape a woman.
The abuse is not bad or the woman would leave. It is easy to leave an abusive situation.	Home is not unbearable all the time. Home offers comfort, memories, and shelter for the children. Many women are economically dependent on the abuser and have nowhere to go. The woman's culture or religion may prohibit separation or divorce. The legal system may also make it hard to leave an abusive situation. Women may fear the loss of their children or further abuse if they leave. Women endure abuse to keep the family together for the sake of the children.
Women tend to become helpless in abusive situations.	Abused women come to believe that they are worthless and that they have no one to turn to but the abuser. Health care workers perceive women as powerless and themselves as "rescuers."
Abused women are masochistic and enjoy being abused.	Abused women may feel that they deserve abuse, but they do not enjoy being abused.
Alcohol causes wife abuse.	Sober men do more damage than those who are drunk. Alcoholism is used as an excuse for abuse.
Battering is limited to minorities and the poor.	Abuse of women occurs in all socioeconomic and racial groups.
Women provoke men to beat or rape them.	Abusers and rapists lose control because of their own inadequacies, not because of the woman's behavior.
Batterers and abused women cannot change.	Batterers and abused women can be resocialized and can learn more effective ways to interact and relate to others.

TABLE 21–6. PHYSICAL HAZARDS BY TYPE OF OCCUPATION

Type of Occupation	Hazards
Clothing, laundry, and textile work	Chemicals, dyes, solvents, synthetic and cotton dust and fiber, bleaches, heat, contamination from dirty clothing
Hospital workers, nurses, laboratory assistants, x-ray technicians	Infection, lifting and falls, radiation, chemical hazards
Service work, waitress, flight attendant	Noise, lifting, falls
Teachers and child care workers	Respiratory infections, viruses, influenza, noise
Clerical and secretarial work	Chemicals from copy and correction fluid, noise, poor lighting and chair design, sedentary work, repetitive-use syndrome

sented in Table 21–6. Working women today face essentially the same physical hazards as working men. They have the same risks for reproductive failure, respiratory ailments, skin disorders, and cancer. The health risks of the work setting are discussed in more detail in Chapter 26.

The psychological environment of the workplace can be as detrimental to women's health as its physical hazards. For example, studies have shown that it is not the female administrator who suffers the most from stress and depression, but women in the more traditional positions of secretary and clerk. It is postulated that stress is intensified by the lack of freedom to control one's work that secretaries and clerks experience. The "dead-end" quality of these jobs with little possibility of advancement may decrease incentive. In addition, the low salaries available for secretaries and clerks add stresses related to financial insecurity.

Social factors in the work environment also affect women's health. The world of work for women differs from that for men in several ways. First, more jobs are open to men than to women. In addition, those jobs that are open to women often provide unequal pay and levels of benefits compared with men in similar jobs. Finally, until a 1991 Supreme Court ruling, women were more often barred from work based on reproductive capacities than were men. Childbearing has also been blamed for women's late entry into the work force and women's lack of training and education.

Once having gained entry into the workplace, women frequently continue to have primary responsibility for maintaining the household and caring for children. Half of married women with children under one year of age work outside the home, and women today engage in simultaneous enactment of family and work roles rather than sequential enactment which was more common in the past. This role proliferation adds tremendous stress to a woman's life and

often leads to feelings of frustration, inadequacy, anxiety, and depression. In one study of professional women, 75% of the women experienced daily role conflict; whereas their husbands reported role conflict between home and family on average of once a week (Wortman, Biernat, & Lang, 1991). In addition, family responsibilities may lower a woman's market value as an employee.

There are no uniform policies for paid maternity leave for U.S. women despite federal mandates for a minimum of 4 months (unpaid) leave for childbirth. Consequently, when a woman must have time off from work because of pregnancy, she must often take it without pay.

Child care is another social environmental factor that creates problems for the working woman. Employer or community assistance with child care is practically nonexistent. Invariably, women must find quality child care on their own. If children are sick, it is usually the mother who stays home, often without pay, to care for them.

Disproportionate pay between traditional women's jobs and such "men's work" as road construction is a strong incentive for women to seek such jobs. Women who enter male-dominated jobs often feel pressure to prove they are equal to men in ability. They may not speak out against safety hazards because they do not want to appear weak or "unable to take it." Sexual harassment is another problem that may be encountered by women in the work setting. Although there are laws prohibiting such abuse, women may not complain because they need work so badly.

It is important to note that minority women must contend with a higher degree of discrimination and lack of job opportunity than white women. They are particularly subject to dead-end and hazardous jobs with low pay and few benefits. Minority women are also less likely to finish high school, more likely to become the head of a single-parent household, and more likely to have job-related illnesses than their white counterparts.

Social factors related to approaching retirement may affect the health status of the middle-aged woman. The woman who is nearing retirement needs to be aware of and plan for the financial shortfalls that are likely to occur with retirement. Leaving the work force means living in poverty for many older people, and women constitute 72% of all older poor (Barusch, 1994). Retirement assets are usually tied to lifetime income. Women who worked for low pay and poor benefits will have neither pensions nor full Social Security benefits. A divorced woman may draw Social Security from her ex-husband's account if they were married at least 10 years, but widows face declining incomes following the death of a spouse. The community health nurse assesses the woman's occupational and economic status and the effects of these factors on health.

The Behavioral Dimension

Behavioral dimension factors also affect the health of women clients. Areas of particular concern include consumption patterns, sexual lifestyle, and attendant concerns with fertility control.

Consumption Patterns. The nurse assesses consumption patterns of the female client in the same terms as assessing any client. Specific areas for consideration include diet, smoking, and substance abuse. Dietary concerns may be particularly problematic among women, many of whom are obese or overweight or who engage in fad diets to attain or maintain a fashionably slim figure. Fad dieting is especially prevalent among adolescent females who also have high incidence rates for eating disorders such as bulimia and anorexia nervosa.

Smoking is another consumption pattern that is problematic for women. Although the number of male smokers has declined rather dramatically in the last few years, the number of women who smoke has increased, leading to corresponding increases in lung cancer and heart disease among women. In addition to the increase in the number of female smokers, women are starting to smoke at younger ages and are less likely to stop smoking than men (Chesney & Nealey, 1996). The nurse assessing the female client obtains data about smoking, including the number of years the client has smoked and the number of cigarettes or other forms of tobacco smoked per day. Motivation to quit smoking should also be explored as part of the assessment.

Substance abuse among women is the third area of concern related to consumption patterns. Although women still tend to abuse alcohol and drugs less often than men, the incidence of such problems among females is increasing. Problems of drug and alcohol abuse are addressed in Chapter 33.

Sexual Lifestyle and Fertility Control. Assessment of the female client's sexual lifestyle may provide information related to potential health problems. For example, clients who are not sexually active and those who engage in homosexual activity have no need for contraceptive assistance, whereas the heterosexually active client who is not ready to have children may need such services. Information about the client's sexual activity may also suggest what form of contraception is most appropriate for those clients who do not wish to become pregnant. For example, the client with multi-

ple sexual partners may prefer to use a barrier method of contraception rather than birth control pills to provide protection against sexually transmitted diseases as well as pregnancy.

Every woman from menarche to menopause has a right and responsibility to choose a method of fertility control that is effective, safe, and compatible with her lifestyle. The right to information on contraception and access to birth control agents is mandated by Title X of the Public Health Services Act and Titles V, XIV, and XX of the Social Security Act. The decision to use contraceptives reflects personal feelings about sexuality, self-concept, sense of autonomy and control, value system, relationship with the significant other, and the personal, social, and political power of women.

The ideal contraceptive method would be absolutely safe, 100% effective, easy to use, immediately reversible, free, and readily accessible to all. It would be acceptable to all religious and social groups and its use would be independent of coitus. No single method available today meets all these criteria. In addition, there is no single method today that will meet the needs of an individual woman throughout her fertile years. The nurse should assess the need for contraception and biological and other factors that influence the need for contraceptive services. Information about various forms of contraception available to clients is presented in Table 21–7.

Fertility control is particularly important for adolescents, for whom pregnancy poses greater disruption of life and potential for adverse physiological effects. Community health nurses can be especially effective in promoting contraception in this age group. Among participants in the 1995 Youth Risk Behavior Survey, more than 17% of sexually active girls 15 to 17 years of age were not using any form of contraception (U.S. Department of Health and Human Services, 1996a). In another study, more than one third of girls age 17 and younger requesting a preg-

TABLE 21–7. TYPES OF CONTRACEPTION AND RELATED CONTRACEPTIVE METHODS

Type of Contraception	Related Contraceptive Methods
Abstinence	Abstinence from sexual intercourse
Barriers	Condom, diaphragm, cervical sponge, cervical cap
Fertility awareness	Basal body temperature, cervical mucous changes, position of cervix
Hormonal	Oral contraceptives, Norplant Progestasert (IUD) injections, post-coital contraception
Intrauterine device	Cooper T, Progestasert, Paragard
Sterilization	Tubal ligation (female), vasectomy (male)

nancy test had had a least one prior negative test indicating a missed opportunity for contraceptive counseling (Zabin, Emerson, Ringers, & Sedivy, 1996).

Vaginal douching is another behavior related to female sexuality that may have adverse health effects. Douching has been associated with pelvic inflammatory disease, ectopic pregnancy, and cervical cancer (Zhang, Thomas, & Leybovich, 1997). The community health nurse should assess this and other behaviors among sexually active women in order to educate them regarding healthy sexuality.

Health System Dimension

Lack of attention to women's health needs, lack of illness prevention and health promotion resources, health insurance discrimination, and lack of support for the informal caregiver in the home are health care system issues that adversely affect women.

As noted earlier, the medical system tends to focus on female reproductive problems, frequently to the exclusion of other health problems faced by women. Failure to recognize and deal with physical abuse is just one example of failure of the health care system to meet the needs of women. By and large, the health care system has only recently come to recognize the special health needs of the female client.

Services provided by the health care system tend to focus on secondary and tertiary prevention of injury and disease. Few efforts are made to provide preventive health care, particularly for women. On a more personal level, those preventive health services that are available are not always offered at a time when busy working women can take advantage of them. Compounding this problem is the lack of provision for child care while women seek preventive health care services (Johnson, Primas, & Coe, 1994).

Another handicap for women is the cost of health care. Women are less likely than men to have employment based health insurance, and they are more likely to work in part-time jobs or jobs that do not offer this benefit. Some insurance companies will not insure single women because of the likelihood of pregnancy and the more frequent occurrence of diagnosed disease among women than among men. Single women are also less likely to be able to pay the monthly insurance premiums. This situation is particularly hard on divorced and separated women with children who are already faced with financial difficulties. For information on economic assistance from Medicaid refer to Chapter 14.

Another problem for working women attributable to the health care system is the lack of support for the informal caregiver. Women may be forced to quit their jobs to care for a sick child or elderly family member but cannot expect the financial support that might be available for institution-based care of the loved one.

The health care system has provided some services to deal with health problems posed by menopause. These have consisted primarily of hormone supplementation. Estrogen therapy, for example, reduces the occurrence of "hot flashes," reduces the rate of bone loss, and decreases cardiovascular risks (Stampfer, et al., 1991). Controversy about estrogen replacement safety persists, however, and more research is needed. Considerations in assessing health system influences on the health of women are summarized in Table 21–8. A guide for assessing factors unique to the health status of women can be adapted from Appendix N, Health Assessment Guide—Adult Client.

Special Focus: Assessing the Lesbian Client

Lesbians are a segment of the female population with whom the community health nurse will knowingly or unknowingly come in contact. According to various studies, an estimated 5% of U.S. women are homosexual (McNaught, 1996). Lesbians have specific health care needs that nurses can be sensitive to and assist

TABLE 21–8. ASSESSING HEALTH SYSTEM INFLUENCES ON WOMEN'S HEALTH

Health Concern	Related Assessment Questions
Need for secondary prevention— screening	• Have you ever had a Pap smear? When? What were the results? • Have you ever had a mammogram? When? What were the results? • When was your last eye examination? What were the results? • Have you had an ECG? When? What were the results? • Have you had a TB skin test? When? What were the results? • Have you had a breast examination? When? What were the results? • Have you had recent blood tests? What were they for? What were the results?
Need for respite	• Is there anyone who can relieve you so you can have a break from caring for your children (elderly parents)?
Access to health care	• Do you have health insurance? • If yes, do you know what services are covered? • Where do you usually go for health care? • How do you usually pay for health care? • Are health care services provided at a time that is convenient for you? • Do you have transportation to receive health care services? • Are child care services available while you seek health care? • Are there any barriers that prevent you from getting the health care you need? If so, what are they?

with. For this section, the terms *lesbians, gay women,* and *homosexual women* are used to indicate women whose preferred sexual partner is another woman. The term *straight* is used to refer to women who prefer heterosexual intimacy. *Bisexual* indicates women who seek sexual intimacy with both males and females.

The American Psychiatric Association recognizes that homosexuality is neither a choice nor a psychiatric disorder; it is a normal variant and an inherent part of a person's identity. Sexual orientation is not chosen; it is discovered. Being a lesbian means that a woman's primary affectional and sexual preferences are for other women. Lesbians exist in all cultures, races, religions, and classes. They cannot be identified by appearance, assumed role, or mannerisms. Lesbians are at high risk for misunderstanding and discrimination because they share the homosexual label with men, yet they have much in common with heterosexual women.

In examining lesbianism from a dimension of health perspective, the goal is for the nurse to become better able to meet the lesbian client's needs by gaining greater understanding and insight into the similarities and differences between lesbians and the heterosexual population. Using this knowledge, the nurse is then able to formulate a more sensitive and effective plan of care for the client.

The Biophysical Dimension

There is some evidence that homosexuality may arise from biophysical causes. For example, homosexual men have structural changes in the hypothalamus more consistent with female anatomy than male (Barinaga, 1993). Alternatively, a portion of the X chromosome may transmit the tendency to homosexuality through the mother (Hamer & Copeland, 1994). Twin studies in both gays and lesbians suggest a genetic component to homosexuality (Griffin, Wirth, & Wirth, 1993; Hamer & Copeland, 1994; O'Hanlon, 1995).

There are no differences in the maturational or aging processes between homosexual and heterosexual women (Hamer & Copeland, 1994). Although it is sometimes assumed that the needs of lesbians are similar to those of gay men, their needs are actually quite different. There have been no medical problems identified that are specifically attributable to being a lesbian, but there are some differences in morbidity between gay and heterosexual women that need to be addressed.

From a gynecologic viewpoint, the woman who engages in sexual activity exclusively with other women is at lower risk for sexually transmitted diseases, including gonorrhea, syphilis, herpes, and

AIDS, than her heterosexual counterpart. Pelvic inflammatory disease is unlikely. A lesbian rarely needs treatment for genital trauma, and she may have a lower incidence of sexual dysfunction and greater sexual satisfaction than her heterosexual counterpart (O'Hanlon, 1995). Although the mode of transmission for monilial or nonspecific vaginitis infections is not necessarily sexual, the lesbian is less likely to develop such infections. Because slightly more than half of all lesbians remain childless, they are at above-average risk for developing endometriosis and severe dysmenorrhea and endometrial, ovarian, and breast cancers (O'Hanlon, 1995; 1996). In addition, 78 to 80% of lesbians have had sexual experiences with men at some time in their lives placing them at risk for a variety of sexually transmitted diseases. Although at present there are no documented cases of female-to-female HIV transmission, there are several cases in which transmission between lesbians is suspected (O'Hanlon, 1995). Gay women who are sexually active exclusively with other women are less likely to contract gonorrhea or chlamydia, however, a herpesvirus-shedding lesion on the lips or genitals of a lesbian can cause the herpes infection to occur in her lesbian lover. Hepatitis B and HIV may have been transmitted woman to woman, although reports of such transmission are infrequent and primarily anecdotal. The incidence of sexually transmitted diseases rises sharply if the lesbian has had recent heterosexual contact. Many bisexual women do not use condoms or other barriers to sexual disease transmission because of their perception of being at "low risk" (AIDS Office, 1993).

Should the lesbian client develop symptoms of disease, it is important for the nurse to obtain a medical history pertinent to those symptoms. If the symptoms indicate a possible sexually transmitted disease, then information about any recent heterosexual contacts should be elicited. Treatment is diagnosis dependent and identical to that for heterosexual women; when an infection occurs, the woman should be counseled to stop activities that are uncomfortable until the infection is treated.

Routine Pap smears are as important for the lesbian client as for heterosexual women. Studies have shown that lesbians have cervical dysplasia and carcinoma in situ. The incidence of these cervical disorders rises sharply if the lesbian has had several heterosexual lovers, just as for her heterosexual counterpart. The screening interval for Pap smears should be determined on an individual basis depending on risk factors. Most lesbians need a Pap smear at least every 3 years or more often if abnormalities have been noted on prior screenings (O'Hanlon, 1995).

Psychological Dimension

Psychological factors affecting lesbians are closely entwined with social factors. A woman who realizes that she has a same-sex orientation has three basic choices. She can live openly as a lesbian, thereby setting herself up for potential rejection by her family, loss of her job or professional reputation, and societal labeling and abuse. Second, she can deny her identity and put her energy into fulfilling the accepted female role. Third, she can live a lesbian life but maintain a heterosexual appearance.

The lesbian who does not live openly as a lesbian must deal, on a daily basis, with the fear that someone will discover who she really is. This involves the complex task of vigilance about how she looks and acts, where she is, who she is with, and what she says. This means that the lesbian must constantly monitor her responses and change pronouns to misrepresent the identity of her partners. She must hide from coworkers, family, or friends important life events such as a new relationship or the break-up of an old one. Recently, both lesbians and gay men have also had to deal with increased fears of being "outed" by other, more militant homosexuals. *Outing* involves publicizing another's homosexuality without their consent (Card, 1995).

An important emotional event the lesbian experiences is "coming out." A lifelong process, *coming out* can be roughly defined as a woman's realization and admission to herself and to others of her same-sex orientation. Although the process of coming out usually occurs in the tumultuous years of the late teens and early twenties, it can happen at any phase in the lesbian's life. Coming out usually (but not always) includes stages of denial, decreased self-esteem, learning, growth, and, eventually for some, self-acceptance (McNaught, 1996). Once the initial coming out is accomplished, the question of how open to be with others becomes a constant underlying source of pressure or tension.

How does a woman discover her sexual orientation? She can begin having vague feelings that she is somehow different from others as early as age 4 or 5. The feelings turn into suspicions during the teen years. At this point, many women with lesbian feelings begin to date, have heterosexual experiences, and try to pass as "straight." After a woman "comes out," homosexual behavior becomes predominant, and the lesbian typically begins to search for a supportive community (McNaught, 1996).

The coming out process deals also with the contradictory feelings of excitement and relief at having found an inner answer to guilt, sadness, and anger about what the lesbian is losing or giving up. She must come to terms with any guilt she experiences for being different and for not fulfilling her role in the heterosexual lifestyle to which she has been socialized. She may also mourn the loss of her relationship with a husband or male lover, the fact that she will not fulfill parental expectations of a wedding and grandchildren, and that she will never be totally socially acceptable. Additionally, it has been found that many women go through the coming out process without the influence or support of the lesbian subculture, thereby adding isolation to the difficulty of the task. The community health nurse should assess for feelings of guilt or depression among lesbians who have recently declared their preference.

From a mental health perspective, although mental health is of concern among lesbians, they are no more likely to be diagnosed with psychiatric disorders than heterosexual women. Their level of social and psychological functioning is indistinguishable from that of their heterosexual counterparts. The community health nurse must be aware, however, of the medical and psychological implications of the emotional stresses that arise from the moral and social stigma of being lesbian. As a result of these stresses, lesbians are more likely to abuse substances such as alcohol and nonprescription drugs than heterosexual women (Mann, 1996). Homosexuals may also experience a greater inclination to suicide, especially during the period of coming to grips with one's sexual orientation. In fact, it is estimated that homosexuals may constitute nearly one third of youth suicides (Mirken, 1993; Vaid, 1995).

The Social Dimension

Elements of the social dimension create problems that the lesbian deals with on a daily basis. The discrepancy between socially prescribed behaviors and homosexual needs automatically sets up a conflict between the lesbian and her environment. Society tends to react to lesbianism as a personal identity rather than merely a sexual behavior. Thus, lesbians are identified in unidimensional terms. The routine conflict with the environment, homophobia, and religious, legal, familial, and economic constraints all combine to make life more difficult for the homosexual woman.

Homophobia, an irrational fear, hatred, or intolerance of homosexuals, encompasses a belief system that justifies discrimination against gays and lesbians. Generally speaking, homophobia arises from three sources: experiential attitudes, defensive attitudes, and symbolic attitudes. Homophobia arising from experiential attitudes is based on generalizations from a past bad experience with a homosexual person. Homophobia related to defensive attitudes usually occurs among people who are insecure in their own sexual identities, and homophobia due to symbolic attitudes arises because homosexuality is perceived to threaten cherished values (eg, the traditional family structure) or to maintain conformity with a desired peer group (McNaught, 1996).

Homophobia is used to justify discrimination and abuse of homosexuals. In studies, roughly one third of gays and lesbians reported being physically assaulted (O'Hanlon, 1996), and more than 7000 hate crimes against homosexuals have been reported to the National Gay and Lesbian Task Force. Many more such crimes probably go unreported due to poor responses by law enforcement agencies (Peters, 1993).

Lesbians may also experience violence, called *horizontal violence,* from their partners. Both battering and stalking are occurring with increasing frequency in the lesbian community. Because battered lesbians tend to fight back more often than their heterosexual sisters, they may lose their credibility as victims, and police may view the battering as a mutual occurrence (Card, 1995). In one study, 11% of lesbians reported experiencing violence at the hands of their partners (O'Hanlon, 1995).

From a religious perspective, many Christian denominations advocate sexual activity only in the context of procreation. Most, especially fundamentalist denominations, consider homosexuality biologically unnatural, sinful, and condemned by the Bible. In a study in the mid-1980s, for example, two thirds of Americans viewed homosexuality as a "sin" (Herek, 1991). Homosexual feelings, no matter how weak, are undesirable. Many religious organizations are becoming increasingly active socially and politically against homosexuals and gay rights groups (Vaid, 1995), leading to greater social polarization on this issue. Consequently, the community health nurse should be sensitive to any feelings of guilt, abandonment, or anger or suicidal tendencies the lesbian client may be experiencing as a result of attitudes and values of the religious denomination to which she may belong.

Homosexuals are denied legal sanction for their pairings and are often discriminated against in housing, employment, or social services (Coles, 1993). They are denied the right to serve openly in the military or to be named as beneficiaries of some insurance policies. Often homosexuals are denied the right to make or to have input into medical decisions for their incapacitated partner because they are not "blood relatives" (O'Hanlon, 1995). In the event of the death of a partner who has left no will, lesbians have no rights to inheritance. The community health nurse can assess for any legal problems the couple may be having and determine whether some legal counseling may be needed. A durable power of attorney and a current will can be suggested to address some of these issues.

Many women realize and act on their same-sex preferences after they are married and have children. In fact, as many as one third of lesbians have been married, and many have children. Their fitness as mothers is often questioned in the courts if their sexual preference becomes known. Because of the threat of custody battles and the inherent difficulties of adoption, many lesbian couples are opting to have their own children, either by artificial insemination or through the participation of a gay or straight male partner. This decision must involve careful planning and negotiation on the part of the lesbian (and possibly her partner) to ensure acceptance by the biological family, the health care provider, and both gay and nongay society. Guidelines the community health nurse can use in assessing the lesbian's adaptation to parenting are found in Table 21–9.

Another potential social issue facing the lesbian client is the lack of social outlets or places other than bars to meet other gay women, particularly outside of large metropolitan areas. This can be a contributing factor in substance abuse and poor self-esteem. Economically, lesbians usually earn lower wages than men or their heterosexual female counterparts despite higher education levels (O'Hanlon, 1995). Those with children from a prior marriage have particularly little disposable income or time to engage in social activities. Also, because homosexuality is such a taboo subject, women in general are socialized to have a negative view of homosexuality. Although there are now several prominent public lesbian role models, many lesbians still begin with a very negative self-image.

For the majority of lesbians, disclosure of sexual preference in the work setting could lead to being passed over for promotion, subtle or overt harassment, or termination, particularly if they work with children or young women. As was mentioned under psychological factors, the ever-present fear of discovery adds immeasurable anxiety and tension to the inherent stress of work.

Nevertheless, the economic and occupational achievements of lesbians are similar to those of their heterosexual counterparts. Although they exhibit more job instability, and earn less income, lesbians work productively, and many tend to be high achievers. They often display a greater degree of assertiveness and aggressiveness in their jobs. One study found that a higher concentration of lesbians had a bachelor's or graduate-level degree than women in general (O'Hanlon, 1995).

TABLE 21–9. ASSESSING THE ADAPTATION OF THE SINGLE LESBIAN OR LESBIAN COUPLE TO PARENTHOOD

Adaptive Task	Assessment Question
Acceptance of pregnancy	• What is the support system? Is there a partner involved? • What is the response of the partner to the pregnancy? • What is the response of the mother's/couple's families, social network, and support system to the pregnancy? • What is the legal relationship of the biological father to the baby? • If a partner is involved, does the partner plan a long-term legal or social relationship as a coparent (eg, through adoption)?
Binding-in	• How was the pregnancy achieved? • Did the partner have a role in the pregnancy? • Are the characteristics of the biological father known? • Has a sex preference for the baby been expressed? If yes, does the couple agree? • What are the couple's views of the baby? Are they congruent?
Safe passage	• If donor's sperm was used to achieve pregnancy, what health screening criteria were used to select donor sperm (eg, was the donor screened for HIV infection)? • Are natural childbirth methods to be used during delivery? Who will serve as the pregnant woman's coach? • Will the couple feel comfortable acknowledging their relationship to prospective birth attendants?
Self-giving	• What do the couple perceive as the costs and benefits (emotional, legal, economic, and social) of having this baby? • How do the couple replenish each other's emotional reserves?
Role development	• How will the tasks of the maternal role be allocated? • Who are the couple's role models for the maternal role? Are these role models adequate? • Will the couple have assistance in developing the facets of the maternal role? From whom? • How is the pregnancy affecting the couple's relationship? • What will the child call the coparent?

Adapted from Wismont, J., & Reame, N. (1989). The lesbian child-bearing experience: Assessing developmental tasks. Image, 21, 137–141.

The Behavioral Dimension

Although lesbianism does not cause alcohol or substance abuse, there is a perception among researchers, clinicians, and lesbians themselves that such problems may be more prevalent and severe among lesbians than in the general population. It has been estimated that homosexuals (male and female) have two to five times more problems with substance abuse than their heterosexual counterparts (Hamer & Copeland, 1994). Lesbians may also be involved in injection drug use increasing their risk of HIV and hepatitis infection. In one study in Northern California, for example, as many as 10% of lesbians reported injection drug use (Lemp, et al., 1995).

Several theories have been advanced to explain this phenomenon. Although the behavior may be a reflection of uncontrolled drinking or the result of growing up in a dysfunctional or alcoholic family, some researchers speculate that because lesbians live under conditions of increased stress and limited social alternatives, they are more vulnerable to the use of alcohol as a coping mechanism (Hall, 1993). The use of alcohol (or other drugs) could be construed as an attempt to alleviate emotional pain and bolster self-esteem, or to ease social and sexual relations with other women.

The nurse can assist the lesbian client by being alert to cues that would indicate patterns of substance abuse, by not assuming that the alcoholism is related to sexual preference, by respecting the woman's reluctance to enter a traditional treatment program, by being familiar with gay resources in the community, and by involving the significant other in the treatment plan (Hall, 1994).

The Health System Dimension

Although women's health care concerns have, in general, tended to be ignored in the health care system, this propensity tends to be heightened when the woman is of color, a rape victim, addicted to drugs or alcohol, a lesbian, or otherwise stigmatized. In fact, in one study, 72% of lesbians reported experiencing a negative reaction from a health care provider (O'Hanlon, 1996).

The basic difference in the way the lesbian interacts with the health care system centers around the issues of acceptance and confidentiality. When the lesbian client senses discomfort or disapproval on the part of the health care provider, she is more likely to hide her sexual orientation for fear of receiving judgmental, nonsupportive, or suboptimal care. Such repercussions might include treatment that is nonresponsive, callous, or unnecessarily painful, or that involves an inappropriate referral for mental health services. The woman may find that her partner either is not allowed to visit (because she is not blood kin), is harassed, or is not allowed input into treatment decisions.

Potential repercussions of loss of confidentiality also arise when sexual orientation is revealed to health care providers. As noted earlier, a breach of confidentiality could negatively affect the client's status at her place of employment, with her family, or with the remainder of the health care team if she was not previously "out" to those persons. A phenomenon that is seen among lesbians as a result of their lack of trust in and alienation from the conventional medical system is that substantial numbers are more holistic in

ASSESSMENT TIPS: Assessing Women's Health

Biophysical Dimension

Age

What is the woman's age? Has she experienced menarche? Menopause?

If she has not yet experienced menarche or menopause, is she knowledgeable about these developmental stages?

Is the woman experiencing any difficulties with menarche or menopause? If so, what are they?

Genetic Inheritance

Does the woman have a family history of genetic predisposition to disease? If so, to what diseases?

Physiologic Function

Is the woman pregnant?

Is the woman experiencing fertility problems?

Does the woman have any existing physical health problems? If so, what are they?

Does the woman have any physical limitations?

Psychological Dimension

Stress and Coping

What is the level of stress to which the woman is exposed?

How effective are the woman's coping strategies?

Does the woman have a history of mental illness? Are there indications of current mental illness?

Is the woman depressed? Is she suicidal?

Life Events

What are the woman's life goals? What are her plans for achieving them?

Is the woman approaching any major life events? How prepared is she for these events? What is her attitude to the approaching event?

Sexuality

What is the woman's attitude toward sexuality? Toward childbearing? Toward menopause?

Does the woman have access to social support in sexual issues?

If the woman is pregnant, what are her feelings about the pregnancy?

What is woman's level of satisfaction with her sexuality and sexual orientation?

Has the woman been subjected to female genital mutilation?

Physical Dimension

Where does the woman live? Is she homeless? If housed, is housing safe and adequate to meet the woman's needs?

Is the woman exposed to environmental health hazards? If so, what are they?

Are there safety hazards in the woman's environment? If so, what are they?

Social Dimension

Roles and Relationships

What roles does the woman play? Is she satisfied with the roles she plays?

Is the woman married, partnered, single, divorced?

Is the woman involved in an intimate relationship? Is the relationship satisfactory from the woman's perspective?

What is the extent of the woman's social support network? Is it adequate to the woman's need for support?

Does the woman have opportunities for social interaction with other adults?

Is the woman responsible for the care of children? What effect does this responsibility have on her health?

Violence and Abuse

Is the woman at risk for abuse? If so, what risk factors for abuse are present?

Is there evidence of current abuse? What action has the woman attempted to avoid abuse, if any? What barriers to such action are present in the situation?

What is the woman's attitude to abuse?

Occupation and Economic Status

Is the woman employed? If so, what is her occupation?

Are there occupational health hazards present in the woman's work setting?

How does the woman manage work and home responsibilities?

Is there a need for child care? If so, has the woman made adequate child care arrangements? Does she have contingency child care plans if the child is sick?

Has the woman experienced sexual harassment in the work setting?

What is the woman's education level?

What is the woman's income level? Is her income adequate to meet her needs and those of dependent family members?

(continued)

ASSESSMENT TIPS: Assessing Women's Health (cont.)

Behavioral Dimension

Consumption Patterns

What are the woman's usual food preferences and consumption patterns?

Does the woman smoke? Does she use alcohol or other drugs?

Is there evidence of substance abuse?

Sexual Practices

What is the woman's sexual orientation? Is she comfortable with this orientation?

To what extent has the lesbian client disclosed her sexual orientation? Is confidentiality a particularly important issue?

Is the lesbian client exposed to homophobia and discrimination?

Does the woman engage in unsafe sexual practices?

If the woman is sexually active, is there a need for contraceptives?

Does the woman engage in monthly breast self-examination?

Does the woman engage in vaginal douching?

Health System Dimension

What is the woman's usual source of health care? Is she satisfied with the care received?

How does the woman finance health care? Does she have health insurance? Is it adequate to meet her health needs?

Does the woman receive routine screening measures (eg, Pap smear, mammogram)?

Does the woman receive health care support in the caretaker role, if needed?

What is the reaction of health care providers to the lesbian client?

---

their approach to health, choosing alternative forms of health care.

Most lesbians believe that their care providers are not well versed on lesbian health care issues, and many are put off by questions about marital status, birth control, and sexual activity. Such issues put the woman in the constant position of having to decide whether to withhold information about her sexuality or to be honest. Because there is no routine or comfortable way for the client to reveal her lesbianism, the decision about disclosure of her lesbian identity can be a source of significant stress. Consequently, the lesbian may be subjected to unwarranted lectures on birth control, prescriptions for contraceptives, and treatment for sexually transmitted diseases, or may be denied the support of her partner when she needs her the most.

There are several suggestions that could be of value to community health nurses assessing lesbian clients. First, nurses need to examine their own attitudes toward sexuality and homosexuality. Studies of both nursing faculty and students have found unfavorable attitudes toward lesbians (O'Hanlon, 1996). Although it is not necessary to sanction homosexual behavior, it is not ethical to discriminate against or deny the gay client supportive professional care that

will assist in strengthening her self-esteem and realizing optimal wellness. As one observer has noted, "passing moral judgments is not a nursing function: such judgments can only impede the ability to give quality care" (Lawrence, 1975). If the nurse is unable to provide such care, the client should be referred to another provider.

Further suggestions are to refrain from recording a client's sexual preference on the record without her approval, to provide an atmosphere of openness and tolerance, and, most importantly, to involve the partner or designated other in the plan of care.

Another peculiar problem arises when the practitioner automatically assumes the client is heterosexual. Assessment questions can be less alienating if differently phrased. Nongender-typed nouns such as "lover" and "partner" can be used. "Are you sexually active?" and "Do you use contraceptives?" are more appropriate than "When was the last time you had intercourse?" or "What kind of birth control are you using?" A question such as "Who would you like contacted in an emergency?" can also go a long way toward helping the lesbian client feel more comfortable.

A lesbian client is more likely to be satisfied with her care if she is able to safely disclose her sexual orientation to health care providers. Additionally, studies show that although most lesbians are more comfortable with female health care providers (O'Hanlon, 1996), it is more important to have a caring, knowledgeable, nonjudgmental provider, regardless of sex or sexual preference.

Diagnostic Reasoning and Care of Women

Based on information obtained during client assessment, the nurse develops nursing diagnoses that direct further interventions. These diagnoses reflect both positive health states and potential or existing health problems and the factors contributing to them. Nursing diagnoses might relate to health problems experienced by an individual woman such as "role overload due to employment, single parenthood, and lack of a social support network." Or diagnoses may be made at the aggregate level regarding the health needs of groups of women. An example of a nursing diagnosis at this level might be a "need for adequate and inexpensive child care due to the number of single-parent working women and a lack of affordable child care." Below are some examples of nursing diagnostic statements for women, both individual and aggregate:

Individual Client
- Strong social support system due to close relationship with parents and siblings
- Lack of knowledge of menarche in adolescent attributable to mother's discomfort with discussing sexuality
- Hot flashes and menstrual irregularity due to menopause
- Guilt over inability to conceive
- Risk for HIV infection stemming from IV drug use
- Risk for repetitive-use syndrome due to assembly line job

Aggregate
- Risk for assault due to lack of safe transportation from factory to home for female workers
- Inadequate access to health care due to lack of health services after working hours
- Risk for occupational injury in construction industry attributable to lack of safety equipment scaled to women's smaller stature
- Risk for unwanted pregnancy stemming from lack of contraceptive counseling for women of childbearing age

Planning and Implementing the Dimensions of Health Care for Women

In planning to meet the identified health needs of female clients, the community health nurse incorporates the general principles of planning discussed in Chapter 7. It is important to keep in mind the unique needs of the female client. Participation by the client in planning for health care is particularly important in view of the passive and dependent role expected of the female client by health care providers of the past. Women need to be encouraged to be active participants in health care decision making. Both community health nurses and their female clients may need additional resources in dealing with the woman's identified health care needs. Some potential resources are listed at the end of this chapter.

Planning and implementing care for groups of women also need to be based on women's unique circumstances. Services should be offered at times when women, especially working women, can take advantage of them. Provision for transportation and child care services during appointments might also need to be considered. Financing of such programs can be problematic, given the lower earning capacity of many women, and political activity to ensure program funding may need to be part of the planning process. Planning to meet the health needs of female clients may involve developing primary, secondary, or tertiary preventive interventions.

Primary Prevention

Primary preventive measures for the female client generally include health education, health appraisal, modifying risk factors, providing a healthy environment, and developing adequate coping skills. Specific needs of female clients include preparation for menarche, sexuality education, fertility control, and prenatal care. Other primary preventive measures for women include preparation for menopause, facilitating access to care, primary prevention in the work setting, preventing sexually transmitted diseases, and developing coping skills and assertiveness.

Preparation for Menarche. Traditionally, the health care system has not been concerned with menarche unless pathology is involved. Many potential problems can be avoided, however, with preventive care. For example, negative feelings toward menstruation, premenstrual tension, emotional lability, the tendency to overeat just before menses, and water weight gain are all controllable with diet, rest, and exercise.

Preventing problems surrounding menarche and menstruation is an important consideration for community health nurses working with preteens and teenagers. The community health nurse can provide direct care, counseling, and teaching in a school-based clinic, in the home, or through community health agencies that offer guidance and information at this time.

Nurses can teach parents to explain menstruation to their daughters or may provide the explanation themselves if parents are unwilling or uncomfortable in doing so. Nurses can also assist girls in the practical aspects of menstruation, for example, how to use tampons or sanitary napkins, the potential dangers inherent in tampon use, and effective hygiene. They can also provide opportunities for girls to discuss fears and anxieties related to this physiologic change. Instruction on dealing with premenstrual tension or menstrual cramps may also be needed.

Sexuality Education.   The community health nurse can provide anticipatory guidance, teaching, and counseling concerning sexuality for adolescent and preadolescent girls. Such issues as giving up one's virginity, romantic love and sex, pregnancy, and contraception can be discussed in a nonthreatening atmosphere that may serve to increase self-confidence and dispel myths related to sexuality. In addition, the nurse may prepare the teen for her first pelvic examination, explaining the procedure in terms that decrease fear and embarrassment. These actions require that nurses be comfortable with their own sexuality and that they be adequately informed about sexual issues.

Community health nurses may also need to educate older women about sexuality and assist them in the formation of healthy sexual identities. This frequently involves correcting past misinformation. Women may also need assistance with sexuality issues during pregnancy. Changes in libido can be discussed and practical suggestions for more comfortable sex as the pregnancy progresses may be helpful. Nurses can also function as advocates for older clients who are attempting to meet their sexual needs, while reassuring them that sexual activity by older persons is a normal phenomenon.

Advocacy and reassurance may also be required by the lesbian client. Community health nurses may need to take an active role in societal changes that protect the rights of lesbians and ensure their freedom of choice in their sexual lifestyle. Advocacy for these clients is particularly needed in the realm of health care services. Lesbian clients may need support and

reassurance in the process of coming out. This is particularly true of the adolescent homosexual who is doubly confused and anxious in the process of developing a sexual identity.

Fertility Control.   Primary prevention related to fertility control usually involves contraceptive education and referral for contraceptive services. In the case of a nurse practitioner, the community health nurse may also provide the physical examination and dispense various contraceptive methods.

The nurse and client together select the type of contraceptive best suited to meet the client's needs based on her sexual lifestyle. It is important to remember that some clients neither want nor need contraceptives. The client may wish to become pregnant. Even if this does not seem to be a wise decision to the nurse in light of client circumstances, it *is* the client's decision. Lesbian clients also have no need of contraceptives; however, they are frequently badgered by health care professionals regarding contraception to the point that they are forced to reveal their sexual preference at the risk of disapproval and discrimination on the part of the health care provider.

Prenatal Care.   Community health nurses are frequently actively involved in the provision of prenatal care to pregnant women. Initial activity frequently involves case finding and referral to a source of care. Nurses may also be involved in monitoring the status of the client during and after the pregnancy and, in the case of the nurse midwife, may actually deliver the baby.

Counseling at the point of recognition of the pregnancy should include the options available to the woman including termination of the pregnancy, adoption, and keeping the child. Women may choose different options depending on their age, marital status, and life goals. The community health nurse should be prepared to support the client's decision regardless of the option chosen and the nurse's personal value system.

Direct care in the form of prenatal teaching and physical care during the pregnancy are other avenues of primary prevention. The goal of care is a healthy infant and mother. Therefore, instruction in the areas of lifestyle such as nutrition, rest and exercise, and avoidance of teratogens is important. Careful assessment for signs of impending complications is also essential.

Home visits to the pregnant woman can be used to assess environmental conditions and their suitability for mother and infant. What provisions have been made for the child? Will the birth of the child present an economic strain on the mother and family? How involved is the father of the child? Answers to these questions assist the nurse to identify potential health problems posed by the pregnancy.

The nurse can assist the pregnant client to deal with common discomforts of pregnancy such as nausea, vomiting, heartburn, constipation, hemorrhoids, urinary frequency, backache, and vaginal discharge. The nurse can also teach and counsel the client regarding clothing, sexual activity, childbirth preparation, baby supplies, signs of labor, danger signs, and fertility control after delivery. In addition, the nurse can encourage the client to voice feelings and concerns about the pregnancy and to explore role changes that will occur with the birth of the child.

Primary prevention of child abuse and problems with the new infant can be started during the last trimester of pregnancy through anticipatory guidance and education in parenting skills. This form of primary prevention can prevent potentially serious problems for the infant. Parenting skills were discussed more fully in Chapter 20.

Preparation for Menopause.   Primary prevention is also warranted for the middle-aged woman in anticipation of menopause. The community health nurse can be of assistance in helping women to accept and cope with menopause and the physical changes that occur with age. Anticipatory guidance, counseling, and referral may be needed depending on the individual's response to the event. These interventions should be geared to allowing the client to make informed decisions regarding medical regimens, nutrition, and exercise.

Preparation for menopause and the changes it causes should begin early in the woman's life. Dietary and exercise habits affect bone structure and the immune system. Community health nurses can help mothers and daughters to adopt a diet high in calcium, protein, complex carbohydrates, and vitamins and low in fat. The nurse can also encourage exercise patterns that include aerobic exercises that place moderate stress on bones so minerals are retained and osteoporosis is delayed indefinitely. These measures greatly enhance health and slow the aging process.

Diet and exercise programs for the prevention of osteoporosis are especially important for the teenage girl. Teens have the poorest nutritional habits of any group studied. In addition, they tend to use alcohol and tobacco, both of which contribute adversely to bone structures leading to osteoporosis. They are also among the most difficult to convince that preventive measures will help them in later years.

Critical Thinking in Research

Johnson, Primas, and Coe (1994) conducted a study to identify factors that prevented low-income pregnant women from seeking prenatal care. Both internal and external barriers to care were identified. Internal barriers included poor motivation for seeking care, lack of awareness of the importance of prenatal care or knowledge of service availability, fear (eg, of deportation), and fatigue. External barriers to obtaining care included financial difficulties, lack of transportation, previous negative experiences or difficulties with enrollment procedures, lack of family support, lack of child care, need to take time off from work, or no time to obtain care.

1. Given the type of findings reported above, what type of research design to do you think the authors used? How else might you obtain data in this area?
2. What are the community health nursing implications of these findings? Which set of barriers would be more amenable to nursing intervention? Why?
3. What additional questions might you want to ask in the area of motivation to obtain prenatal care? How might you go about answering those questions?
4. Do you think your findings would be similar if you repeated this study with middle-class pregnant women? Why or why not?

Primary prevention among women who are nearing menopause includes anticipatory guidance on what to expect as changes occur and information about their options in estrogen replacement therapy. Counseling and teaching should be temporized to be of benefit to all women whether or not they have symptoms that require estrogen replacement. Diet and exercise, avoidance of caffeine and alcohol, and encouragement to quit smoking are also helpful.

Facilitating Access to Care.   A primary preventive intervention requiring political activity is facilitating adequate

CONSIDERATIONS IN PRIMARY PREVENTIVE CARE FOR WOMEN

- Preparation for menarche
- Sexuality education
- Fertility control
- Prenatal care
- Preparation for menopause
- Facilitation of access to health care
- Primary prevention in the work setting
- Development of coping skills and assertiveness

access to health care services for women. Action is needed to ensure the availability of such services and the financial resources that allow women to take advantage of them. Again, advocacy may be required on the part of the nurse to ensure that ancillary services such as transportation and child care are also available to women who need them.

Primary Prevention in the Work Setting. The psychosocial environment of the work setting can be changed by means of several strategies. These strategies include educating and socializing women to expect wage equity and to believe that their work is as important as a man's; promoting legislation to prevent job discrimination; educating women about their rights; and encouraging women to challenge sexual harassment. Additional strategies include supporting women running for political office, influencing the legislative process, and promoting collective bargaining, mentoring, and networking among women. A final strategy is active participation in organizations working for changes to benefit women.

The community health nurse working in the occupational setting can provide primary preventive care for women by identifying and understanding stressors affecting women in the work setting, counseling regarding work options, encouraging women to report safety hazards (or the nurse can report them personally), encouraging organization of women in the work setting, fostering personal preventive measures such as the use of protective devices, and keeping a log of jobs and exposure to hazardous materials and health changes. Another major contribution can be made by community health nurses who have clients experiencing role proliferation. These nurses can assist clients to plan efficient use of time, to use outside help when possible, and to let go of minor household duties that can wait. Single parents particularly need help in this area.

Preventing Sexually Transmitted Diseases. A growing number of women are exposed to sexually transmitted diseases (STDs), including HIV/AIDS, through sexual intercourse with a heterosexual or bisexual carrier of infection. Safer sex practices, monogamous relationships with an uninfected partner, and abstinence are the primary means of preventing infection.

Condom use during sexual intercourse has been shown to reduce the risk for STDs, including HIV infection. Knowing that condoms reduce risk does not, however, mean that a woman will insist on condom use by her partner. The community health nurse can suggest that the woman use a diaphragm and nonoxynol-9 spermicidal jelly, which offer some protection from gonorrhea and chlamydia if used correctly; however, this approach does not prevent HIV infection (Hatcher, et al., 1994).

The community health nurse should teach and counsel regarding STDs in a realistic and nonjudgmental way. Specific information about unsafe sexual practices such as anal sex and the increased risk of HIV infection must at times be explicit. Nurses should let clients know that they are comfortable with the information and that they are properly informed.

Adolescent females may be particularly difficult to reach with education on STDs. Strategies for educating adolescents include recognizing the teen as a sexual being; teaching skills such as condom or diaphragm use needed to reduce risk; instructing in a manner that gives the teen a sense of personal control; using concrete, simple terminology; employing visual aids as much as possible; and involving the teen in the learning process through games and other strategies. Other strategies include making use of role-play and decision-making exercises that help teens rehearse safe-sex scenarios. Peer counseling is also effective because teens are more likely to rely on peers for information and role models than they are to seek adult advice.

Developing Coping Skills and Assertiveness. Primary prevention for female clients also involves assistance in the development of coping skills and assertiveness. Community health nurses can help families to raise their children so little girls are no longer taught to be dependent and passive, but assertive and in control. Boys must be taught that abusiveness, violence, and overcontrolling behavior are not acceptable ways of acting. Societal norms, at present, make these changes in socialization of children very difficult. Even if the family does succeed in raising children this way, schools (from elementary through college) still reward girls who are passive and boys who are aggressive. Community health nurses can begin some more permanent changes in these attitudes by increasing the awareness of parents and teachers about this issue and encouraging them to change the way they view girls and boys.

Older women can also be assisted by the nurse to develop skills in assertiveness. Interventions can be designed to improve women's self-esteem and to teach them how to cope with life stress in effective ways. These strategies along with political activity are effective primary preventive measures for abuse and violence against women. Prevention of family violence and abuse is addressed in more detail in Chapter 34.

► ROUTINE SCREENING PROCEDURES
RECOMMENDED FOR WOMEN
....

- Pap smear
- Tuberculin skin test
- Chest x-ray
- Mammogram
- Vision test
- Hearing test
- Serum cholesterol test
- Serum glucose test
- Blood pressure screening
- Urine test for bacteria, glucose, and protein
- Testing for chlamydia, gonorrhea, syphilis, and genital herpes

(Source: U.S. Preventive Health Services Task Force, 1995.)

Secondary Prevention

Secondary prevention focuses on screening and diagnosis and treatment for existing health problems.

Screening. Screening procedures specifically recommended for women include those used to detect breast and cervical cancer and STDs. Women should, of course, also be screened for other health problems such as hypertension, diabetes, and skin cancers.

Community health nurses can be particularly effective in educating women on the need and procedure for regular breast self-examination (BSE). The nurse can demonstrate the techniques involved in BSE and recommend that women examine their breasts monthly about 1 week after their menstrual period or, in the case of menopausal women, on the same day of each month. Nurses can also recommend periodic mammography and Pap smears for detection of breast and cervical cancers, respectively. Community health nurses may also refer clients to agencies that provide such services as well as educate them on the need for screening. Recommended screening procedures are also presented in Appendix K.

Women at risk for STDs should be screened periodically for gonorrhea, syphilis, and HIV infection. Women in high-risk groups include those with multiple sexual partners, intravenous drug users, and those who have sexual contact with IV drug users or bisexual men. Pregnant women in these high-risk groups should be particularly encouraged to undergo screening for STDs. This subject is discussed in more detail in Chapter 30.

Diagnosing and Treating Existing Problems. Community health nurses refer female clients for medical or social assis-

tance with any identified health problems. Problems unique to female clients for which secondary prevention may be required include infertility, fertility control, menopause, and physical abuse.

INFERTILITY. Treatment for infertility generally requires referral to a fertility specialist. The role of the community health nurse with respect to infertility centers around case finding, referral, and support during a fertility work-up. The nurse can also assist the client and her significant other in considering alternative options such as adoption, artificial insemination, and in vitro fertilization. The nurse may also refer couples to self-help groups for assistance in dealing with problems of infertility.

FERTILITY CONTROL. Helping women who are having difficulty using a contraceptive method is another aspect of nursing care at the level of secondary prevention. Some women discover that they cannot use the method they have chosen and just stop using it. This can lead to unwanted pregnancy. The nurse can counsel, teach, and refer as needed to help each woman or couple find the best way to control fertility or to plan for children. Occasionally, secondary prevention in this area may entail presenting the client with options for dealing with the problem of an unintended pregnancy.

MENOPAUSE. Once menopause has occurred, referral to a physician or nurse practitioner for estrogen replacement therapy can take place if the client expresses discomfort related to hot flashes or has risk factors predisposing her to osteoporosis. These risk factors include white race, small skeleton and lean body, sedentary lifestyle, poor diet, decreased calcium intake, fair complexion, thin skin, and sparse hair (Office of Technology Assessment, 1992).

If the client decides to be evaluated for estrogen replacement therapy, the nurse should describe what to expect during the initial visit. Generally, this visit entails a complete history and physical and several laboratory tests including a fasting blood glucose, complete blood count, blood lipids, liver function tests, and Pap smear. Some physicians also do an endometrial biopsy to determine the potential for endometrial cancer. This procedure is painful for the client and should be discussed by the nurse to alleviate fear and to assist the client to cope with the procedure.

Menopause may cause vaginal dryness and discomfort during sexual intercourse. The nurse can counsel women concerning longer foreplay and the use of vaginal lubricants to relieve the problem.

Some women also experience a decreased sexual desire. The community health nurse can help the client explore some of the contributing factors in this experience such as depression, a feeling of being at the end of the reproductive years, and acceptance of a new phase of life. Self-help groups for women who are having similar problems are extremely beneficial during this stage of life. If there is no such group in the local community, the nurse can start one by inviting clients to meet and begin discussions.

PHYSICAL ABUSE. Secondary prevention related to physical abuse of women has two dimensions. The first of these is dealing with the physical and psychological effects of physical abuse, and the second is dealing with the source of the problem itself. Recognizing the problem is a prerequisite to either dimension of treatment. Female clients should be asked in a caring and sensitive manner about any violence in their lives. Careful recording of the history and of information regarding old and new injuries is important in the diagnosis of abuse. Such a record may reveal a pattern the woman is unwilling or unable to admit to the nurse. If there is evidence of abuse, it is unethical for the nurse not to confirm this diagnosis with the client. Allowing the woman to describe what is happening to her through open-ended questions is therapeutic and can serve as the first step in stemming the cycle of abuse.

It is important that the nurse convey to the client that she does not deserve to be abused and that the nurse is sorry that this has happened to her. These critical statements are needed to reveal to the client that someone cares and that she is not worthless, helpless, or deserving of abuse.

It is not easy for a community health nurse to intervene in an abusive relationship. Inherent in such situations are reasons to fear that intervention will not be successful, that the woman may become depressed and suicidal or resent the nurse for interfering in a private family matter, or that the male abuser may punish the woman or the nurse. Such fears have kept health care professionals from pursuing evidence and attempting to help women in abusive situations.

When the nurse is able to work through and conquer personal fear and is able to identify a client in an abusive relationship, the nurse should encourage the client to discuss the circumstances of her abuse. It is important that the client realize the danger inherent in her situation.

Once the diagnosis of abuse is made, the primary goal is to assist the woman to reestablish a feeling of control and to empower her to change the situation. Supportive counseling and reassurance are essential. The nurse should let the woman work out her problems at her own pace. Each woman has the capacity to change when she is ready. The nurse must realize that the victim will feel ambivalence in the relationship she has with her partner. The nurse should support realistic ideas for change and assist the client in altering unrealistic ideas. The nurse should help the client to clarify her beliefs about the situation. The nurse should also help to identify myths about abuse that the client may have internalized. For example, if the victim believes that she deserves the beatings, the nurse can assure the client that her partner is totally responsible for his own actions.

The nurse can help the client explore alternative plans for solutions to her problem. What are her personal supports? Is there anyone to whom she can go for help? The client may want to go home. If the client can do this without risk of suicide or homicide, the nurse should help her plan strategies for managing at home and provide her with resources for assistance or escape should the need arise. If necessary, however, the community health nurse can also help the woman to plan a quick getaway. The client needs to accumulate extra money, collect necessary documents like birth certificates and immunization records for children, pack a change of clothing, and carry a few emergency supplies. If the client has children, she should take them with her if she leaves or risk losing them to the abuser if he should claim that the client abandoned them.

It is important to remember that the nurse should avoid becoming another controller in the life of the client. The physically abused woman needs every opportunity to develop independence. Nurses tend to want to rescue victims to stop the violence. They cannot make decisions for the woman. Although nurses can provide information on shelters and other resources, they must allow the woman to make the call.

Nurses should be familiar with the resources they recommend. Are they reliable? Will they assist the woman to become independent while providing a safe haven for her and her children?

Community health nurses can also provide assistance in referrals for medical care for injuries and for counseling to deal with contributing factors and psychological effects of abuse. Such services may be needed for children as well as the woman. The woman should also be cautioned that her children may resist being removed from their home and/or father. If this should be the case, the community health nurse can help the client cope with grief and hostility on the part of the children. The client may also need help in dealing with her own grief over the loss of a significant relationship.

Tertiary Prevention

As with all clients, tertiary prevention in the care of women focuses on rehabilitation and preventing the recurrence of health problems. Areas in which tertiary prevention are particularly warranted for the female client include pregnancy, abuse, and STDs. Tertiary prevention may also be needed to deal with some of the effects of menopause.

Tertiary prevention with respect to pregnancy involves the use of an effective contraceptive to prevent subsequent pregnancies. Again, the nurse may be involved in education, counseling, and referral for contraceptive services.

In the case of abuse, tertiary prevention necessitates the rebuilding of the woman's life and that of her family. This may involve developing new financial resources as well as ways of coping with problems. The woman needs to become self-sufficient. Again, referrals to a variety of agencies to help with employment skills and to provide counseling may be of assistance.

Women can also be helped to prevent recurrence of STDs or to cope with the life changes necessitated by a diagnosis of AIDS. Tertiary prevention related to STDs is discussed more fully in Chapter 30.

Evaluating Health Care for Women

Health care provided to women should be evaluated using the evaluative process described in Chapter 7. Once more, it is important to evaluate both the quality of the care given and its outcomes. Because of the dependent role of many women, it is particularly important that they play an active role in evaluating the health care they are given. At the national level, the year 2000 objectives for the health of women can provide criteria for evaluating women's health care services. Table 21–10 presents evaluative information on selected national objectives related to women's health.

TESTING YOUR UNDERSTANDING

1. Describe at least two biophysical factors, two phsychological, two social, two behavioral, and two health system dimension factors that influence the health status of women. (pp. 492–504)
2. Identify at least four health problems common to women. (pp. 493–497)
3. Describe at least three specific considerations that are unique in assessing the health needs of the lesbian client. (pp. 504–511)
4. Identify at least five general concerns in primary prevention for women. (pp. 511–514)
5. Describe three areas for consideration in secondary preventive activities in the care of women. (pp. 515–516)
6. What are the two dimensions of secondary prevention of physical abuse of women? (p. 516)
7. Describe at least two actions that the community health nurse can take to provide more sensitive and effective care to the lesbian client. (pp. 510–517)

TABLE 21–10. STATUS OF SELECTED NATIONAL OBJECTIVES FOR WOMEN'S HEALTH

	Objective	Base	Most Recent	Target
2.10	Reduce iron-deficiency anemia among women of childbearing age	5% (1976–1980)	NDA[a]	3%
3.4	Reduce the prevalence of smoking	27% (1987)	21.1% (1993)	15%
5.1	Reduce adolescent pregnancy (per 1000 girls aged 15–17 years)	71.1 (1985)	74.6 (1991)	50
5.2	Reduce unintended pregnancy	56% (1988)	10% (1990–1995)	30%
7.5	Reduce partner abuse (per 1000 couples)	30 (1985)	NDA	27
7.7	Reduce incidence of rape (per 100,000 women)	120 (1986)	100 (1991)	108
7.15	Reduce proportion of battered women turned away from shelters	40% (1987)	NDA	10%
14.3	Reduce maternal mortality (per 100,000 live births)	6.6 (1987)	7.5 (1993)	3.3
14.11	Increase receipt of prenatal care in the first trimester	76% (1987)	78.9% (1993)	90%
15.10	Reduce overweight prevalence	27% (1976–1980)	24.4% (1993)	20%
16.11	Increase receipt of breast examination and mammography	25% (1987)	50% (1995)	60%
16.12	Increase receipt of Pap smear in last 3 years	75% (1987)	75% (1995)	85%

[a]NDA, no data available.

(Sources: Centers for Disease Control, 1996; U.S. Department of Health and Human Services, 1993; 1995; 1996a; 1996b.)

Critical Thinking in Practice: A Case in Point

Susan is 25 years old, married, and the mother of two girls. She is pregnant for the third time. You have scheduled a home visit with her following a referral from the community clinic where she is receiving prenatal care. According to the referring agency, Susan does not always keep her appointments, and the baby is small for gestational age. The prenatal clinic requests that you teach nutrition and encourage her to keep her appointments.

When you arrive at the home, Susan is reluctant to allow you inside. She turns her face away and does not look at you as she answers your questions.

Because you know that every women has the potential for being a victim of physical abuse, you ask Susan if someone has hurt her. In a nonthreatening, caring, and sensitive manner you say, "I see many women in my practice who are in a relationship with a person who hits or abuses them. Did someone hurt you?" Susan begins to cry and says, "My husband hit me last night." She allows you to come in, and you observe that she has a black eye and a swollen jaw. Her two small children are thin and poorly clothed. The house, though neat, is sparsely furnished.

In speaking with Susan, you find out that her husband works in a local factory and has been denied a promotion and a raise in the last week. He seems to blame Susan for becoming pregnant again and causing more financial worries. Susan tells you that she has been missing appointments at the prenatal clinic because of her black eye and the lack of transportation when her husband is at work.

1. What are the biophysical, psychological, social, behavioral, and health system factors operating in this situation?
2. What are your nursing diagnoses in this situation?
3. How would you address the two dimensions of secondary prevention of physical abuse of women in this case?
4. What other secondary preventive measures seem to be warranted in this situation?
5. What primary and tertiary preventive interventions might be appropriate in working with Susan?
6. How will you evaluate whether intervention has been successful?

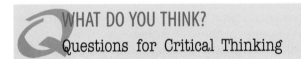

WHAT DO YOU THINK?
Questions for Critical Thinking

1. Why are women more likely than men to live in poverty? How does this state of affairs affect their health status?
2. How can women influence the type of health care they receive?
3. Do you think health care services provided for women are inferior to those provided to men? Why or why not?
4. Should homosexual unions be legally recognized? Why or why not? What would the implications of this recognition be for the couple? For society?

REFERENCES

AIDS Office, Prevention Services Branch. (1993). *Health behaviors among lesbian and bi-sexual women: A community-based women's health survey.* San Francisco: San Francisco Department of Public Health.

Barinaga, M. (1993). Differences in brain structure may cause homosexuality. In W. Dudley (Ed.), *Homosexuality: Opposing viewpoints* (pp. 17–22). San Diego: Greenhaven Press.

Barusch, A. S. (1994). *Older women in poverty: Private lives and public policies.* New York: Springer.

Boring, C., Squires, T., & Tong, T. (1993). *Cancer statistics, 1993.* Atlanta: American Cancer Society.

Card, C. (1995). *Lesbian choices.* New York: Columbia University Press.

Centers for Disease Control. (1996). State and sex-specific prevalence of selected characteristics—Behavioral Risk Factor Surveillance system, 1992 and 1993. *MMWR, 45*(SS-6), 1–36.

Chen, C. C., David, A. S., Nunnerley, H. (1995). Adverse life events and breast cancer: Case-control study. *British Medical Journal, 311,* 1527–1530.

Chesney, M. A., & Nealey, J. B. (1996). Smoking and cardiovascular disease risk in women: Issues for prevention and women's health. In P. M. Kato & T. Mann (Eds.), *Handbook of diversity issues in health psychology* (pp. 199–218). New York: Plenum Press.

Chung, M., Chang, H. R., Bland, K. I., & Wanebo, H. J. (1996). Younger women with breast carcinoma have a poorer prognosis than older women. *Cancer, 77*(1), 97–103.

Coffin-Romig, N. A. (1997). *The process of ending domestic violence among Latinas: Aguantando no mas.* Unpublished doctoral dissertation, University of San Diego.

Coles, M. A. (1993). Homosexuals need civil rights protection. In W. Dudley (Ed.), *Homosexuality: Opposing viewpoints* (pp. 78–86). San Diego: Greenhaven Press.

Crib Sheet. (1995). The littlest legacy, 7, 3–4.

Crook, M. (1995). *My body: Women speak out about their health care.* New York: Plenum Press.

Doyal, L. (1995). *What makes women sick: Gender and the political economy of health.* New Brunswick, NJ: Rutgers University Press.

Ebrahim, S. H., Peterman, T. A., Zaidi, A. A., & Kamb, M. L. (1997). Mortality related to sexually transmitted diseases in US women 1973 to 1992. *American Journal of Public Health, 87,* 938–944.

Edge, V., & Miller, M. (1994). *Women's health care.* St. Louis: Mosby Year Book.

Eisler, R. (1994). *The chalice and the blade: Our history, our future* (2nd ed.). Magnolia, MA: Peter Smith.

Fogel, C., & Woods, N. (1994). *Women's health care.* Newbury Park, CA: *Sage.*

Furniss, K. (1993). When home isn't so sweet: Recognizing and treating domestic abuse. *Advances for Nurse Practitioners, 2,* 10–12.

Griffin, C. W., Wirth, M. J., & Wirth, A. G. (1993). Parent–child relationships do not cause homosexuality. In W. Dudley (Ed.), *Homosexuality: Opposing viewpoints* (pp. 36–44). San Diego: Greenhaven Press.

Hall, J. M. (1994). How lesbians recognize and respond to alcohol problems: A theoretical model of problematization. *Advanced Nursing Science, 16*(3), 46–63.

Hall, J. M. (1993). Lesbians and alcohol: Patterns and paradoxes in medical notions and lesbians' beliefs. *Journal of Psychoactive Drugs, 25*(2), 109–119.

Hamer, D., & Copeland, P. (1994). *The science of desire: The search for the gay gene and the biology of behavior.* New York: Simon & Schuster.

Hatcher, R., Stewart, F., Trussel, J., et al. (1994). *Contraceptive technology, 1992–1994* (16th ed.). New York: Irvington.

Hegelson, V. S. (1995). Masculinity, men's roles, and coronary heart disease. In D. Sabo & D. F. Gordon (Eds.), *Men's health and illness: Gender, power, and the body* (pp. 68–104). Thousand Oaks, CA: Sage.

Herek, G. M. (1991). Stigma, prejudice, and violence against lesbians and gay men. In J. C. Gonsoriek & J. D. Weinrich (Eds.), *Homosexuality: Research implications for public policy* (pp. 60–80). Newbury Park, CA: Sage.

Janosik, E., & Green, E. (1992). *Family life: Process and practice.* Boston: Jones and Bartlett.

Johnson, J. L., Primas, P. J., & Coe, M. K. (1994). Factors that prevent women of low socioeconomic status from seeking prenatal care. *Journal of the Academy of Nurse Practitioners, 6,* 105–111.

Lawrence, J. (1975). Homosexuals, hospitalization, and the nurse. *Nursing Forum, 14,* 305–317.

Lemp, G. F., Jones, M., Kellogg, T. A., et al. (1995). HIV seroprevalence and risk behaviors among lesbians and bisexual women in San Francisco and Berkeley, California. *American Journal of Public Health, 85,* 1549–1552.

Mann, T. (1996). Why do we need a health psychology of gender or sexual orientation? In P. M. Kato & T. Mann (Eds.), *Handbook of diversity issues in health psychology* (pp. 187–198). New York: Plenum Press.

McNaught, B. (1996). *Gay issues in the workplace.* New York: St. Martin's Press.

Mirken, B. (1993). School programs should stress acceptance of homosexuality. In W. Dudley (Ed.), *Homosexuality: Opposing viewpoints* (pp. 106–112). San Diego: Greenhaven Press.

National Center for Health Statistics. (1997). *Fertility, family planning, and women's health: New data from the 1995 National Survey of Family Growth.* Washington, DC: Government Printing Office.

Office of Technology Assessment. (1992). *The menopause, hormone therapy, and women's health.* Washington, DC: Government Printing Office.

O'Hanlon, K. A. (1995, July/August). Lesbian health and homophobia: Perspectives for the treating obstetrician/gynecologist. *Current Problems in Obstetrics, Gynecology, and Fertility,* 100–129.

O'Hanlon, K. A. (1996). Homophobia and the health psychology of lesbians. In P. M. Kato & T. Mann (Eds.), *Handbook of diversity issues in health psychology* (pp. 261–284). New York: Plenum Press.

Peters, J. (1993). Society should accept homosexuality. In W. Dudley (Ed.), *Homosexuality: Opposing viewpoints* (pp. 63–68). San Diego: Greenhaven Press.

Rose, M. (1990). Reproductive hazards for high-tech workers. In S. Rix (Ed.), *The American Woman, 1990–1991* (pp. 277–285). New York: W. W. Norton.

Rosenthal, S. M., & Wilson, D. M. (1994). Pediatric endocrinology. In A. M. Rudolph & R. K. Kamei (Eds.), *Rudolph's fundamentals of pediatrics* (pp. 583–615). Norwalk, CT: Appleton & Lange.

Sarrel, P. M. (1991). Women, work, and menopause. In M. Frankenhaeuser, U. Lundberg, & M. Chesney (Eds.), *Women, work, and health: Stress and opportunities* (pp. 225–237). New York: Plenum Press.

Spitz, A. M., Ventura, S. J., Koonin, L. M., et al. (1993). Surveillance for pregnancy and birth rates among teenagers by state—United States, 1980 and 1990. *MMWR, 42*(SS-6), 1–27.

Stampfer, M. J., Colditz, G. A., Willett, W. C., et al. (1991). Postmenopausal estrogen therapy and cardiovascular disease: Ten-year follow-up from the nurses' health study. *New England Journal of Medicine, 325,* 756–762.

U. S. Department of Commerce. (1996). *Statistical abstract of the United States—1996* (116th ed.). Washington, DC: Government Printing Office.

U. S. Department of Health and Human Services. (1991). *Healthy people 2000: National objectives for health promotion and disease prevention.* Washington, DC: Government Printing Office.

U. S. Department of Health and Human Services. (1993). *Health United States and healthy people 2000 review.* Washington, DC: Government Printing Office.

U. S. Department of Health and Human Services. (1995). *Healthy people 2000: Midcourse review and 1995 revisions.* Washington, DC: Government Printing Office.

U.S. Department of Health and Human Services. (1996a). *Healthy people 2000: Progress review—Family planning.* Washington, DC: Government Printing Office.

U. S. Department of Health and Human Services. (1996b). *Healthy people 2000: Progress review—Maternal and infant health.* Washington, DC: Government Printing Office.

U. S. Preventive Health Services Task Force. (1995). *Guide to clinical preventive services* (2nd ed.). Washington, DC: Government Printing Office.

Vaid, U. (1995). *Virtual equality.* New York: Anchor Books.

Waldron, I. (1991). Effects of labor force participation on sex differences in mortality and morbidity. In M. Frankenhaeuser, U. Lundberg, & M. Chesney (Eds.), *Women, work, and health: Stress and opportunities* (pp. 17–38). New York: Plenum Press.

Wortman, C., Biernat, M., & Lang, E. (1991). Coping with role overload. In M. Frankenhaeuser, U. Lundberg, & M. Chesney (Eds.), *Women, work, and health: Stress and opportunities* (pp. 85–110). New York: Plenum Press.

Zabin, L. S., Emerson, M. R., Ringers, P. A., & Sedivy, V. (1996). Adolescents with negative pregnancy test results: An accessible risk group. *JAMA, 275,* 113–117.

Zhang, J., Thomas, A. G., & Leybovich, E. (1997). Vaginal douching and adverse health effects: A meta-analysis. *American Journal of Public Health, 87,* 1207–1211.

RESOURCES FOR NURSES CARING FOR FEMALE CLIENTS

Advocacy

Learning How
PO Box 35481
Charlotte, NC 28235
(704) 376–4735

Mothers Without Custody
PO Box 36
Woodstock, IL 60098
(800) 457–MWOC

National Organization for Women (NOW)
1000 16th Street, NW, Ste. 700
Washington, DC 20036
(202) 331–0066

Women's Rights Commission
c/o American Federation of Teachers, Human Rights Department
555 New Jersey Avenue, NW
Washington, DC 20001
(202) 879–4400

Women's Rights Project
c/o American Civil Liberties Union
132 West 43rd Street
New York, NY 10036
(212) 944–9800

AIDS

Lesbian AIDS Project
c/o Gay Men's Health Crisis
129 W. 20th Street
New York, NY 10011
(212) 337–3532

Childbirth

American Society for Psychoprophylaxis in Obstetrics
1200 19th Street, NW, No. 300
Washington, DC 20036–2422
(202) 857–1128

Association of Women's Health, Obstetric, and Neonatal Nurses
c/o communications Department
700 14th Street, NW, Ste. 600
Washington, DC 20005–2019
(202) 622–1600

Childbirth Education Foundation
PO Box 5
Richboro, PA 18954
(215) 357–2792

Childbirth Without Pain Education Association
20134 Snowden
Detroit, MI 48235–3816
(313) 341–3816

Healthy Mothers, Healthy Babies
409 12th Street, SW, Room 309
Washington, DC 20024
(202) 863–2458

Drug and Alcohol Abuse

Gay Alcoholics Anonymous World Service Office
457 Riverside Drive
New York, NY 10115
(212) 777–1800

Mothers Against Drunk Driving (MADD)
511 East John Carpenter Fwy., No. 700
Irving, TX 75062
(214) 744–6233

Women's Drug Research Project
c/o Beth G. Reed
University of Michigan
School of Social Work
1065 Frieze Bldg.
Ann Arbor, MI 48109–1285
(313) 763–5958

Fertility and Fertility Control

American Academy of Natural Family Planning
615 South New Ballas Road
St. Louis, MO 63141
(712) 279–2048

Association for Voluntary Surgical Contraception
79 Madison Avenue, 7th Floor
New York, NY 10016–7802
(212) 561–8000

Fertility Research Foundation
1430 2nd Avenue, Ste. 103
New York, NY 10021
(212) 744–5500

International Planned Parenthood Foundation
Western Hemisphere Region
902 Broadway, 10th Floor
New York, NY 10010
(212) 995–8800

Sexuality

Council for Sex Information and Education
2272 Colorado Blvd., No. 1228
Los Angeles, CA 90041

Homosexual Information Center
115 Monroe
Bossier City, LA 71111–4539
(318) 742–4709

Integrity
PO Box 5255
New York, NY 10185–5255
(908) 220–1914

International Gay and Lesbian Human Rights
    Commission
1360 Mission Street, Ste. 200

San Francisco, CA 94103
(415) 255–8680

Lesbian Feminist Liberation
Gay Community Center
208 W. 13th Street
New York, NY 10011
(212) 924–2654

Lesbian Resource Center
1808 Bellevue Avenue, Ste. 204
Seattle, WA 98122
(206) 322–3953

National Gay and Lesbian Task Force
2320 17th Street, NW
Washington, DC 20009–4039
(202) 332–6483

New Ways Ministry
4012 29th Street
Mt. Ranier, MD 20712
(301) 277–5674

Sex Information and Education Council of United
    States
130 West 42nd Street, Ste. 350
New York, NY 10036–7802
(212) 819–9770

Universal Fellowship of Metropolitan Community
    Churches
5300 Santa Monica Blvd., Ste. 304
Los Angeles, CA 90029
(213) 464–5100

Violence and Abuse

Batterers Anonymous
1850 N. Riverside Avenue, No. 220
Rialto, CA 92376
(909) 355–1100

Emerge: Counseling and Education to Stop Male
    Violence
2380 Massachusetts Avenue, Ste. 101
Cambridge, MA 02140
(617) 547–9879

National Coalition Against Domestic Violence
PO Box 18749
Denver, CO 80218
(303) 839–1852

People Against Rape
PO Box 5876
Naperville, IL 60567–5876
(708) 717–0310

Women Against Rape
PO Box 02084
Columbus, OH 43202
(614) 291–9751

22

CARE OF MEN

► KEY TERMS

antisocial personality
  disorder
biological sex
denial
disclosure
gender identity
homosexuality
hydrocele
impotence
joblessness
juvenile conduct disorder
posttraumatic stress
  disorder (PTSD)
reframing
sexual orientation
social sex roles
unemployment

A great deal of health-related literature has been written about specific problems that influence men's health status (eg, cardiovascular disease). Very little, however, is written about the overall health needs of men. The health care of men has been fragmented, approached from an episodic perspective. Little effort has been made to provide comprehensive, holistic health services. Indeed, men are one of the few major population subgroups that have not been explicitly targeted in the national health objectives for the year 2000. (Women, children, and the elderly are among the populations that are targeted.) (U.S. Department of Health and Human Services, 1991.) The current objectives do not address the prevention of or screening for testicular or prostatic cancers, despite the fact that prostatic cancers alone result in more deaths each year than all female cancers combined. Although specific interventions to improve men's health status are not enumerated in the national objectives, many objectives will benefit men. (See Appendix A for a summary of the national objectives.) The lack of attention to the total health of men, however, is a justifiable concern of community health nurses. The focus of this chapter is to help prepare community health nurses to provide holistic care to male clients.

Chapter Objectives

After reading this chapter, you should be able to:

- Describe at least five considerations in assessing the biophysical dimension of health in men.
- Describe four areas for consideration in assessing the behavioral dimension of health in men.
- Identify at least two effects of the health care system on men's health.
- Describe at least three factors that contribute to adverse health effects for male homosexual clients.
- Identify at least four areas for primary prevention with male clients.
- Describe at least four secondary prevention considerations for male clients.
- Identify at least three areas of emphasis in tertiary prevention for male clients.

► COMMUNITY HEALTH NURSING AND MEN'S HEALTH

In 1995, there were nearly 99 million men over 15 years of age in the United States (U.S. Department of Commerce, 1996). Clear differences exist between these men and their female counterparts in the epidemiology of certain health problems and health-related behaviors. These epidemiologic and behavioral differences are reflected in life expectancy, which in 1994 was 79 years for women and only 72.3 years for men (U.S. Department of Commerce, 1996). The gap in life expectancy between men and women is an ironic reflection of the fact that our health care system—created by and still largely controlled by men—apparently does not serve men's health care needs well. Further evidence of this fact is noted in figures indicating that men have higher mortality than women from all ten leading causes of death. In 1993, for example, men were six times more likely to die of AIDS, four times more likely to commit suicide, and almost twice as likely to die of heart disease as women (Mortality Statistics Bureau, 1996).

Just as women's health is not defined solely in terms of reproductive problems, men have unique health needs over and above those related to the male reproductive system. They are both biological and social and include the need to discuss health care concerns; the need to consider health risks posed by lifestyle and gender roles as well as by occupational, leisure, and interpersonal activities; the need for health education and information regarding their bodies and self-care; the need for comprehensive

health assessment; the need for assistance with interpersonal relationships and parenting; and the need for health care services that take into account employment constraints in scheduling and location. Selected national health objectives reflect some of the health needs of men.

► THE DIMENSIONS MODEL AND CARE OF MEN

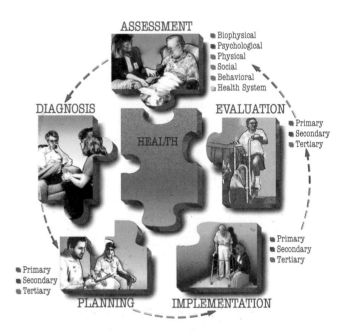

Men differ from women in their patterns of physical health disorders and health-related needs. These differences are attributable to (1) the physiologic differences between men and women (eg, testicular cancer in men); (2) the differences in health-related habits and health-seeking behavior between men and women (eg, men have fewer contacts with health care providers than women); (3) differences in social roles, stress, and coping; and (4) lifestyle differences between the sexes (eg, men consume more alcohol and are more likely to resolve conflicts by resorting to violence) (Mann, 1996). The Dimensions Model provides a useful framework for the community health nurse to account for these differences when assessing and working with men as individuals or as aggregates.

Critical Dimensions of Nursing in the Care of Men

Community health nurses are well placed to meet the health needs of men. Men tend to encounter the health care system on an episodic basis, whereas women are more apt to be regular recipients of health care services. For this reason, community health nurses, who may encounter men in the work setting or in the course of caring for other family members, are in a position to identify unmet health care needs and to provide avenues for men's access to appropriate health care services.

In order to meet the needs identified, community health nurses require cognitive knowledge of health problems encountered by men and of interventions appropriate to their resolution. Motivational skills will be particularly important in the interpersonal dimension since men are generally less cognizant of signs of ill health and less likely to take action even when these signs are recognized (Copenhaver & Eisler, 1996). Motivational abilities and interpersonal skills may also be required to assist men to change socially inculcated attitudes and values that promote high-risk behaviors common among men (Mann, 1996).

In the ethical dimension, advocacy for changes in social factors such as unemployment, occupational hazards, and male socialization can help to create a healthier environment where men may be less inclined to self-destructive behaviors designed to demonstrate their masculinity. Personal and social advocacy is particularly relevant to the care of homosexual clients. Manipulative skills from the skills dimension may be required in the provision of direct care to male clients. Analytic and diagnostic skills will also be needed, particularly in view of men's frequent failure to recognize evidence of health problems. Process dimension skills employed in the care of men may include health education, change, leadership, and political processes as well as the nursing process. Each of these processes may be required in the care of individual men and in designing care delivery systems for groups of men. Finally, although much health care research has focused on men, there is a continuing need for research within the reflective dimension to provide a knowledge base for effective care of male clients.

Assessing the Dimensions of Health in Men

The Biophysical Dimension

Genetic Inheritance.   Genetic factors play a significant role in the physical health of male clients and are an important area for nursing assessment relative to cardiovascular disease, hypertension, and cerebrovascular disease. Genetic factors also may play a role in testicular and prostatic cancer (and cancer generally), as well as in tendencies toward alcoholism and violence. Genetic factors may also influence a man's psychological health. They are, for example, suspected as a con-

tributing factor in various mood disorders (which, in turn, often precipitate suicide among males).

The community health nurse assesses potential genetic contributions to a client's health status by obtaining a family history of the occurrence of physical and psychological disorders. It may be necessary to interview both the client and older family members and relatives to secure an accurate picture of genetically mediated health problems.

Physiologic Function

CARDIOVASCULAR DISORDERS.   Morbidity and mortality rates for cardiovascular disorders, particularly for ischemic heart disease, are significantly higher among men than among women. In 1993, the death rate for heart disease among men was 292.1 per 100,000 population, whereas that for women was 284.9 per 100,000. These differentials exist across racial groups as well, although African American males and females both have higher rates of heart disease mortality than white males and females (U.S. Department of Commerce, 1996). These differences are understandable in the light of the reported presence of cardiovascular risk factors among men and women. For example, in 1992, more than 87% of males 35 to 49 years of age included in the Behavioral Risk Factor Surveillance System (BRFSS) survey reported at least one major risk factor for coronary heart disease compared with only 82% of women in the same age group. In fact, fewer women than men in all age groups studied reported cardiovascular risk factors (Cardiovascular Health Studies Bureau, 1994). As we will see later, men smoke far more often than women, the primary behavioral risk for heart disease.

Given these figures, it is essential that the community health nurse assess the cardiovascular status of male clients. Assessment would include checking blood pressure, pulse, and respirations, as well as auscultating for abnormal heart sounds (such as murmurs) and sounds suggesting pulmonary congestion.

White males have a higher incidence of hypertension than do white females (25.6% vs. 20.5%). Similar differences in the male to female ratio of hypertension incidence are found among black, white, and Latino populations (U.S. Department of Health and Human Services, 1996). The community health nurse needs to monitor the blood pressure of male clients on a regular basis to detect consistently elevated pressures (above 140 systolic or 95 diastolic for males over 40, and above 130 systolic or 90 diastolic for males under 40).

CANCERS.   The incidence and mortality rates for all cancers combined are significantly greater among men than among women. In fact, men are one and a half times more likely than women to die of cancer (Mortality Statistics Bureau, 1996). The leading causes of cancer death among men include lung cancer, colorectal cancer, pancreatic cancer, leukemia, cancers of the brain and central nervous system (CNS), stomach cancer, prostate cancer, testicular cancer, and malignant melanoma.

Testicular cancer is the most common malignancy among males aged 20 to 24 years and the second most common cancer in the 35- to 39-year-old group (Gordon, 1995). Although easily detected by regular testicular self-examination (TSE), research has shown that few young men are familiar with TSE techniques, and even fewer actually perform TSE. In addition, few health care providers teach TSE to men in this high-risk age group.

Cancer of the prostate killed 38,000 men in the United States in 1994 (Albertsen, Fryback, Storer, Kolon, & Fine, 1995). Prostate cancer is most common in men over 50 and is often asymptomatic until late in the course of the disease. For this reason, it is important that community health nurses working with men over age 50 assess clients for signs of bladder obstruction, hematuria, and pyuria, and encourage males to obtain annual prostatic examinations.

Mortality for a variety of smoking-related cancers is higher for men than for women precisely because of the differences in the percentage of each group who smoke. For example, men are twice as likely as women to die of lung cancer. Men are also more likely to die because of esophageal cancers and cancers of the larynx (Division of Cancer Prevention and Control, 1993).

Most of the theories offered to explain gender differences in cancer rates focus on lifestyle factors. Explanations include the higher rates of tobacco and alcohol consumption among men, greater exposure to dietary carcinogens (eg, from eating larger amounts of well-cooked meat), greater exposure to occupational carcinogens, physiological and psychosomatic differences in men's immune responses, and different patterns of health promotion and maintenance among men.

In addition to assessing for cancer risk factors related to lifestyle, the community health nurse should carefully note any symptoms that might suggest impairment or change in a particular organ. Changes of particular importance in the male client would include respiratory difficulty (persistent coughs, blood-tinged sputum, shortness of breath, coughing on exertion); changes in bowel or bladder habits (persistent diarrhea, bloody or dark tarry stools, ribbon-shaped stools); diminished activity tolerance; and unexplained changes in either weight or appetite.

OTHER REPRODUCTIVE SYSTEM DISORDERS.   A variety of disorders involving the male reproductive system may also be encountered by the community health nurse. The prostate gland, for example, is subject to infection (prostatitis), carcinoma, and nonmalignant hyperplasia (benign prostatic hyperplasia). The testes and surrounding structures also are prone to carcinomas and inflammatory diseases.

The symptoms of prostatitis, an inflammation of the prostate, typically include urinary flow restriction in association with fever, burning on urination, and perineal pain. The condition may also be accompanied by pyuria or hematuria. Prostatitis often accompanies cystitis. The condition may result as a consequence of sexually transmitted diseases and may develop into a chronic, recurring form. Because of this risk, it is especially important for the community health nurse to assess for the symptoms of this condition.

Benign prostatic hyperplasia (BPH) commonly occurs in men over age 50, and approximately 40% of men over 70 years of age have some degree of BPH (Barry, Fowler, Bin, Pitts, Harris, & Mulley, 1997). Presenting signs and symptoms include urinary flow restriction (urinary frequency, hesitancy, terminal dribbling, bladder fullness or distension, or urinary incontinence). Nurses should assess male clients over the age of 50 for these symptoms and facilitate follow-up evaluation.

Epididymitis, or inflammation of the epididymis, is the most common form of intrascrotal inflammation. It usually presents as painful swelling within the scrotum and is frequently accompanied by urethritis. Complications include infertility, abscesses, and testicular atrophy. The condition may be idiopathic or result from sexually transmitted pathogens (most frequently, *Chlamydia trachomatis* and *Neisseria gonorrhoeae*) (Kaler, 1990). Assessment by the community health nurse should include a review of the client's sexual habits for factors that would increase the risk of acquiring this infection (frequent sexual partners, failure to use condoms) in addition to assessing for the presence of signs or symptoms.

A *hydrocele* is an abnormal collection of fluid within the tunica vaginalis of a testicle or along the spermatic cord. Males with this disorder typically note a swelling and may report that they have found a scrotal mass. The pain and discomfort associated with this condition can be considerable. Community health nurses assess for this disorder by asking whether the male client has noted any changes in his scrotum or has experienced scrotal pain.

Impotence is another area of reproductive dysfunction experienced by a significant number of men. *Impotence* is a broad term for male sexual dysfunction and encompasses diminished sexual desire, inability to obtain or maintain an erection, premature ejaculation, absence of emission, or inability to achieve an orgasm. Erectile dysfunction alone affects approximately 7 million men in the United States (National Institutes of Health, 1992). Impotence may arise from a variety of causes including male hormonal deficiencies, brain tumors, diseases of the spinal cord, diabetes, medication use (eg, phenothiazines, imipramine, reserpine, fluoxetine [Prozac]), drug and alcohol use, surgical procedures (such as prostatectomy, rectosigmoid surgery, or aortic bypass), or stress. Whatever its cause, impotence, whether transient or long term, can be a devastating experience for the male client. Because men may be reluctant to volunteer information regarding sexual dysfunction to a nurse (especially a female nurse), the community health nurse needs to tactfully probe for evidence of problems in this area, assessing not only for the problem of impotence, but also for its effects on the client and his interaction with others.

INGUINAL HERNIA.   Occurring primarily among men, this disorder is relatively common. Usual symptoms include lower abdominal or groin pain on straining (when lifting and sometimes during bowel movements). Although typically manageable on a symptomatic level, inguinal hernias may require surgical repair. In some cases herniation of the intestine through the inguinal canal(s) may lead to bowel obstruction and necrosis, a life-threatening situation. For this reason, the community health nurse working with a male client who is diagnosed with an inguinal hernia should carefully assess for the presence of persistent pain in the inguinal area, particularly if accompanied by persistent intestinal symptoms such as abdominal rigidity, pain, and cramping.

RESPIRATORY CONDITIONS.   Mortality due to chronic obstructive pulmonary disease (COPD) is twice as high for black men as for black women and more than one and a half times as high for white men compared to white women (U.S. Department of Health and Human Services, 1996), despite the fact that more middle-aged women than men experience chronic respiratory conditions such as chronic bronchitis. Similarly, the incidence rate for influenza is higher among women (U.S. Department of Commerce, 1996), but combined mortality for influenza and pneumonia is higher among men (Mortality Statistics Bureau, 1996).

DIABETES.   Morbidity and mortality patterns for diabetes are similar to those for chronic respiratory conditions. Middle-aged women have higher incidence

rates for diabetes than men, but men have somewhat higher diabetic mortality (Mortality Statistics Bureau, 1996). This is explained largely by gender differences in the occurrence of diabetic complications. Men, for instance, are more likely to experience extremity amputation due to diabetes than women, and African American men, in particular, experience higher mortality from diabetic ketoacidosis. Until recently, African American men also had higher incidence rates for end-stage renal disease related to diabetes than their female counterparts (Geiss, et al., 1993). These findings suggest that men with diabetes receive less care for their disease or are less compliant with recommended treatment regimens, both situations amenable to community health nursing intervention. Community health nurses assessing male clients should be alert to family history and overweight as risk factors for diabetes as well as signs and symptoms of active disease. The nurse should also assess the degree of control of their disease achieved by known diabetics.

LIVER DISEASE.   Men are more than twice as likely as women to die of chronic liver disease and cirrhosis of the liver (Copenhaver & Eisler, 1996). This is true of all age groups through age 65. Women are also one third as likely to be hospitalized for chronic liver disease as men (Chronic Disease Surveillance Bureau, 1993). Community health nurses should assess male clients for problem drinking behaviors as well as symptoms of active liver disease.

OVERWEIGHT.   Although men are slightly less likely than women to be overweight for height, obesity is a significant problem among men as well as women. Nearly one fourth of American men over 20 years of age are overweight. Only 19% of these overweight men were actively engaged in diet and exercise programs to control their weight in 1991, far short of the national target of 50%. In addition to the higher percentage of overweight males, 19% of American men over age 20 tested from 1988 to 1990 had high serum cholesterol levels (U.S. Department of Health and Human Services, 1993).

HIV INFECTION AND AIDS.   Despite increased incidence among women, HIV infection and AIDS continue to be found primarily in men. Eighty-four percent of AIDS mortality in 1995 occurred among males, and the incidence rate was more than six times higher for males over age 13 than females (Mortality Statistics Bureau, 1996). Community health nurses should be alert to the presence of risk behaviors related to HIV infection (and other sexually transmitted diseases) among male clients. Nurses should also assess clients for signs and symptoms of marker diseases for AIDS.

UNINTENTIONAL INJURY AND SENSORY IMPAIRMENT. The final area to be addressed in assessing men's physiologic function is the presence of adverse effects related to accidental injury. Males at all ages have higher rates of unintentional injuries than females. This is particularly true for motor vehicle accidents. In 1993, for example, the motor vehicle accident fatality rate for men was more than twice that for women, and similar gender differences were noted for other types of accidents (U.S. Department of Commerce, 1996). As we will see later, many of these differences arise from risk behaviors engaged in by men. Other factors that may contribute to accidental injuries and should be assessed by the community health nurse are sensory impairments. Both young and middle-aged men have higher incidence rates for visual and hearing impairments than women (U.S. Department of Commerce, 1993). These impairments, if undetected and uncorrected, may contribute to a variety of physical and psychological health problems.

As noted throughout this section, the community health nurse should assess male clients for risk factors for physiologic dysfunction as well as signs and symptoms of existing disorders. In addition, when existing conditions are noted, the nurse should assess the degree of limitation posed by the problem. As men are often reluctant to seek care for health problems, conditions tend to be more severe when help is sought. This leads to greater limitation of function and contributes to a slightly higher percentage of men than women who are unable to work because of disabling conditions.

Maturation and Aging. Because maturation and aging play a significant role in many health risks and problems experienced by male clients, the community health nurse needs to assess these factors when providing care. Certain physical disorders are associated with advanced age in men: cardiovascular disease, cerebrovascular disease, prostate cancer and hypertrophy, and hypertension. Other physical health concerns are more frequently associated with younger male clients: trauma, violence, and testicular cancer.

Physical sexual maturation in the male typically begins between ages 9.5 and 14 years and is completed between ages 14 and 18 years. At age 10 years the preadolescent male is devoid of pubic and underarm hair and has genitals in proportion to their childhood size. As development progresses, testicular enlargement is followed by sparse growth of light-colored, straight pubic hair at the base of the penis. Subsequently, enlargement of the penis begins and fur-

ther growth occurs in the scrotum and testes, accompanied by the growth of darker, curly coarse pubic hair that begins to spread out from the base of the penis. Next the penis and testes enlarge in girth, with further spread of the pubic hair (though still less than in adults) (Chantry, 1994).

In the final period of development the genitals reach adult proportion, and pubic hair continues to spread. More generalized changes are also taking place: Underarm hair develops, followed in many males by hair on the upper legs and later on the lower legs. Most males begin to develop chest hair growth in late adolescence, but this is highly variable. Facial hair can become evident at any time during adolescence but is most typical after age 15. As the adolescent male approaches adulthood he experiences an increase in muscle mass, resulting in a broadening of the shoulders relative to the waist; this, too, is highly individualized. It should be noted that the adolescent male is typically very concerned with his sexual and physical development, often comparing himself to other males and many times experiencing anxiety about the possibility that his development is delayed or inadequate. In some cases this anxiety can be sufficient to cause social impairment or serious emotional distress, and the community health nurse should make a special effort to be supportive and accepting. The community health nurse can also benefit the adolescent male client by offering information and reassurance about the normal patterns and variations in growth and development. In the majority of adolescent males a degree of transient gynecomastia (enlargement of the breasts) occurs. This is variable in degree, but can be a source of significant concern to the adolescent; again, reassurance, explanation, and acceptance are of benefit.

During this period the adolescent becomes increasingly concerned with the values of his peers and is increasingly focused on achieving acceptance from his peer group. He is prone to value peers over parents at this stage, and his attitudes are more reflective of peers than family. He often experiences uncertainty about his identity, and may engage in a variety of behaviors that, although perhaps disconcerting to his family or other adults, are necessary experiments in determining what type of person and life he will incorporate into his self-concept. Hormonal changes result in increased growth and libido, confronting him with the possibility of new (and perhaps anxiety-provoking) roles; these changes are also mirrored in the behavior of his peers, on which he tends to model his own behaviors and choices.

The adolescent male may feel embarrassed about the physical and emotional changes he experiences. For example, he may have spontaneous and ill-timed erections, or nocturnal emissions. His physical development and social circumstances, coupled with peer pressure and a desire to conform, may lead to varying degrees of sexual activity, presenting the risks of unwanted pregnancy and sexually transmitted diseases. It is not unusual for some of the adolescent male's sexual exploration to involve sexual contact with other males; approximately 50% of all males have had such contact at some point, and there is no correlation between such sexual activity and later sexual orientation (though the adolescent may again experience significant anxiety, guilt, or shame about this experimental behavior).

Over time, the adolescent male's preoccupation with sexual performance and activity as the major parameters of a relationship are increasingly replaced by romantic attributes and genuine caring; initially these romantic views are often stereotypical and exaggerated, but this also changes as he progresses through early adulthood. Again, the nurse's role involves assessing the young male's development relative to existing norms and providing education about growth, development, sexuality, and related risks and safety precautions and providing reassurance and guidance relative to the changes he is experiencing.

Psychological maturity or the lack thereof is a significant contributing factor to trauma, substance abuse, and suicide. Additionally, certain health-related life experiences can also be viewed from a maturational perspective, particularly divorce (married males tend to live longer than divorced or never-married males) and retirement (which can result in a higher risk of isolation or depression), both of which are associated with poorer health and higher risk of suicide. Divorce is discussed more fully as a sociological factor later in this chapter.

The nurse assesses the male client's maturational level by observing his behavior or interviewing him to elicit information about his concerns, interests, habits, and judgment. The nurse may also gather assessment data about a client's maturity level from indirect sources, such as reports from significant others and other health care professionals.

The Psychological Dimension

Two related elements of the psychological dimension are of concern to community health nurses caring for men. These elements include socialization, stress, and coping abilities, as well as suicide as an outcome of ineffective coping.

Socialization, Stress, and Coping. Men, like women, have several basic psychological needs. These include the needs to know and be known to others, to be mutually interdependent, to love and be loved, and to live meaningful lives. Society, however, has socialized both men and women to accept a stereotypical male role that makes it difficult to meet these needs. General dimensions of this stereotyped role include a need to actively differentiate oneself from women and refrain from behaviors ascribed to women (such as demonstrating affection or seeking help) and a need to see oneself as superior to others. Other dimensions include the need to be strong and self-reliant and to be more powerful than others, even if this means resorting to violence to demonstrate one's power.

Because of this stereotyped view of the masculine role, men experience social pressures to conform that sometimes conflict with health. Socialized to view the male role as strong or invulnerable, a man may have difficulty admitting health-related frailties to a community health nurse. Similarly, men who believe that taking physical risks is fundamental to their masculinity may experience more frequent health impairment from trauma. As seen from these examples, as societal messages about male roles become internalized by men, they become psychological factors influencing male health behaviors.

Men may also have a stronger psychological need than women to see themselves as healthy and even invulnerable. Because men tend to value strength and endurance more than women, they are more likely to conceal or suppress pain and other perceived indicators of frailty. An example of this state of mind can be seen in the male postmyocardial infarction client who resumes shoveling snow against the recommendations of health care professionals and his family, and who continues it despite the return of the now-familiar angina. As a result of this need for strength in his self-image, the male client minimizes the importance of the problem. Consequently, when shoveling snow causes further angina, he may seek health care less readily and use it less effectively than would a female client in a similar situation.

Conversely, it should be noted that male values of strength and endurance do not always adversely affect a male client's health. Some men who value strength actually may be more motivated to exercise and maintain a higher level of general fitness and to seek preventive health care to preserve their sense of themselves as strong and invulnerable.

Another psychological barrier to men's health is the male client's inconsistent response to feelings attending a health problem. For example, a man who values strength may exercise regularly, but he may avoid having a swelling in his groin examined because he cannot cope effectively with the fear that the swelling may represent a threat to his sexuality. Despite widespread beliefs to the contrary, men may respond with surprising depth of emotion to perceived threats to health and self-sufficiency.

Men are exposed to different kinds of stress than women and their ways of coping with stress differ. Much of the stress experienced by men may arise from their need to live up to societal expectations of masculine behavior. Men with nonextreme measures of trait masculinity have been shown to have better health, engage in more health-promoting behaviors, and have more extensive social support than those who exhibit extreme trait masculinity. Those with more extreme conceptions of masculinity are more likely to engage in risk behaviors and fewer health-promoting behaviors. They also tend to delay seeking treatment longer and exhibit more type A behavior than those with nonextreme trait masculinity. Extreme trait masculinity is also associated with depression and anxiety and with increased severity of myocardial infarction and poorer adjustment after infarction (Hegelson, 1995). Men may also experience more stress than women in similar situations due to cultural expectations and their own perceptions of their ability to cope with certain situations. For example, men may experience more stress when faced with a crying baby or serious illness in the family because they have been socialized to perceive themselves as unable to deal with these kinds of events (Copenhaver & Eisler, 1996).

Masculine expectations and socialization also lead to differences in approaches to coping between men and women. Men tend to be more oriented to action coping which may be reflected in independent and aggressive behavior or suicide (Hegelson, 1995).

Suicide.   Although some sources report that females attempt suicide more frequently than males, males are much more likely to be successful in their suicide attempts. Both men and women view completed suicide as strength and attempted suicide as weakness, so successful suicide may be another aspect of masculinity (Stillion, 1995). The death rate for suicide for males of all ages is three to four times that of females (U.S. Department of Commerce, 1996).

It is important for community nurses to appreciate the often-concealed prevalence of suicide in a community. Suicide claims more lives annually than many of the diseases that health care professionals combat so effectively. Because suicide is such a high source of mortality for males, it is important that the community health nurse directly address the issue with those male clients most at risk:

- Clients 15 to 24 years of age or older than 65 years
- Clients with chronic physical or mental disorders (particularly those that are progressively debilitating or that lead to deterioration in function)
- Clients who are depressed or who feel hopeless or helpless
- Clients with a recent history of significant loss (death of a family member, end of a marriage)
- Clients who are intoxicated
- Clients with a history of recent or remote suicides among peers or family members
- Clients with impaired muscle control

Clients who appear to be at risk for suicide should be directly but empathetically questioned about this possibility. For example, a nurse could state, "It would not be unusual for a person who's been through what you have to be thinking about suicide. Is that something you have considered?" Suicide assessment would further include distinguishing thoughts about suicide from actual intent and plans to initiate it, determining the client's access to lethal means of suicide (guns, heights, drugs), and the presence or absence of support persons who can ensure the client's safety. It is important that the community health nurse not allow his or her own denial of the reality of suicide to limit assessment of this important threat to a male client's well-being.

The Physical Dimension

With the exception of the occupational environment, which is addressed in the discussion of the social dimension, the effects of the physical environment on men's health are much the same as they are on women's health. Pollution, overcrowding, and safety hazards adversely affect both. Men, however, may have increased exposure to environmental hazards due to occupational and leisure activity choices.

The Social Dimension

Many influences of men's health arise from the social dimension. Some social dimension considerations in caring for men are violence and trauma, military service, criminal justice issues, family interactions, sexual abuse, and occupation and employment issues.

Violence and Trauma.   Violence and trauma are often the effects of psychological and sociological factors. A male's socially reinforced aggressiveness and cultural role models that promote risk taking are frequently cited explanations for the significantly greater trauma-related morbidity and mortality rates among males. *Juvenile conduct disorder,* involving a pattern of chronic antisocial behavior during childhood, is approximately four times more common in males than in females. *Antisocial personality disorder,* characterized by a chronic pattern of irresponsible and antisocial behavior that frequently involves criminal acts, is known to be three times more common among men than among women. Both of these disorders predispose males to higher risks of trauma through physically violent behavior, involvement in dangerous activities such as drug dealing, retribution from intended victims or coconspirators, and exposure to prison-based violence when incarcerated.

The death rate from homicide is nearly three times greater for white males than females, with a fivefold difference between African American men and women. Motor vehicle accident mortality for white men is double that for women, and the difference is even greater (approximately 3:1, males vs. females) between black men and women (U.S. Department of Commerce, 1996).

Military Service.   Military service, whether during war or during times of peace, can powerfully influence a man's identity and view of the world around him. Although military service is becoming more common among women, the community health nurse is most likely to encounter men with a prior history of military service. Many military veterans continue to base their network of friends and their social activities in veterans organizations and among peers who are also veterans. As a result of this ongoing military identity, veterans sometimes demonstrate military-based behaviors in civilian settings, such as using military slang that is unfamiliar to civilians.

Another behavior sometimes seen among veterans is claiming entitlement to services. This behavior may provoke a negative reaction in community health nurses, who may view attitudes of entitlement as inappropriate, self-centered, or needlessly demanding. It is important to realize that the armed forces do reward military duty by providing various benefits (entitlements) after discharge. Consequently, a veteran's attitude of entitlement may simply reflect his military values and expectations.

Community health nurses working with veterans exhibiting this attitude may find it helpful simply to remind the veteran of the differences between the military and civilian worlds so that expectations become more realistic and misunderstandings are avoided. Nurses working with veterans, whether on an individual level or on an aggregate basis, also may benefit from familiarizing themselves with the Veterans Administration health care system to assist in their referrals and other efforts to meet the clients' health care needs.

Veterans who have experienced combat may suffer from an insidious and debilitating disorder that requires exceptional understanding and patience on the part of the nurse. ***Posttraumatic stress disorder***

(PTSD) is caused by exposure to traumatic events with which an individual is profoundly unable to cope. This disorder is characterized by disturbances in sleep (insomnia, nightmares), poor interpersonal relationships, modulation of emotions, vivid recollections of the traumatic episode, and periods of profound depression. Other reactions may include rage, homicidal impulses, and suicidal tendencies. Although this disorder can occur equally readily in men or women in the same circumstances (eg, as a result of childhood sexual abuse), the much greater involvement in military combat by men and the resulting disproportionate exposure to the severe trauma of war (particularly the Vietnam War) have led to a significant number of American men with PTSD. As a measure of the magnitude of this problem, some have estimated that more Vietnam veterans have died from suicide since the war (over 100,000) than died from combat injuries during the conflict, and that more than a half million Vietnam veterans may suffer from this disorder (Mullis, 1984).

Community nurses often encounter undiagnosed cases of PTSD, and they can be of tremendous value by case finding and by helping PTSD sufferers to seek or accept treatment. Community health nurses should assess clients who have experienced major psychological or physical trauma for the signs and symptoms of PTSD. These can occur at any time after the trauma, ranging from days to years later. Nurses should also assess for health issues frequently accompanying PTSD, including substance abuse, violence, and risk of suicide.

Another aspect of active-duty military service that may require the community health nurse's intervention is the reallocation of roles during periods of deployment away from home. In two-parent families, roles shift when the military spouse leaves and returns to the family, which may create confusion and strain for the whole family. Role allocation can be even more problematic for military men who are single parents. In both family situations, the community health nurse can assess the extent and use of family support systems and assist families in reallocation decisions. The nurse may also make referrals to both civilian and military sources for counseling and/or material support as needed.

Criminal Justice Issues.   Although men are not alone in their involvement with criminal justice issues, they comprise 80% of arrestees (U.S. Department of Commerce, 1996). In 1992, there were 1.4 million men in prison, three times the number of inmates in 1975. The prison system in general has been referred to as a "pocket of risk" (Polych & Sabo, 1995). Many inmates have been imprisoned for behaviors that put them at higher risk for health problems (eg, substance abuse). The prison environment further enhances the risk of conditions like tuberculosis, hepatitis, and HIV infection. Not only are inmates themselves at increased risk of infection; the 2.2 million annual admissions and discharges from prison systems create a steady flow of infection into the system and back out into the general population. This risk to the general public is a concern for all community health nurses and nurses working with male clients should seek information regarding recent incarceration and be alert for signs of infection. Community health nurses may also be involved in follow-up activities with recently discharged inmates who have tuberculosis or HIV infection. In these cases, the community health nurse promotes continuity of care and continued therapy. Community health nurses may also be involved in care of men within the correctional system itself. This aspect of care is addressed in Chapter 28.

Family Interactions. By far the largest proportion of men live within a family situation, which may create both positive and negative health effects. Marriage has been shown to have a protective health effect for men and less so for women; however, because of socialization to a stereotyped male role, men may have difficulty interacting within the family in ways that effectively meet the psychological needs discussed earlier. Differing role expectations between husband and wife may lead to marital conflicts and, in some cases, spouse or child abuse. Family violence and its effects on health are discussed in more detail in Chapter 34. It is, however, important for the community health nurse dealing with male clients to assess marital interactions and to engage in appropriate interventions.

Parenting is another aspect of family interaction that may prove problematic for men. Again, because of typical male socialization, many men have little or no child care experience. The increase in the number of working women has led to greater assumption of child care duties by men. The community health nurse should assess the male client's involvement in child care as well as the extent of his knowledge of effective parenting skills.

Divorce is another possible aspect of family interactions that can profoundly affect the health of the male client. Divorce is one of the most significant stressors a person can experience, and it frequently has a profound effect on physical and psychological health. Divorced men, in particular, have been shown to experience increased morbidity and mortality as compared with married men. Men may respond to divorce or its aftermath with intense anger, a profound sense of loss, or significant depression. Suicidal be-

havior occasionally occurs as the man reacts to the divorce as an assault against his self-image and self-worth, or homicidal behavior if he directs his anger toward his ex-spouse.

Divorce may also mean stressful battles for custody of any children born to the couple or part-time fatherhood if joint custody is the outcome. More and more divorced fathers have at least partial custody of their children. In 1995, more than 1.3 million U.S. households consisted of an adult male with children. Single parenthood may contribute to stress as well as economic deprivation. The community health nurse should assess the men in these families for needed assistance with parenting as well as for health effects of stress and reduced economic status.

Assessment appropriate to the issue of divorce includes evaluating the client's style of coping with stress, for example, drinking alcohol as contrasted to talking with support persons. The nurse also assesses the client's access to support personnel of adequate quality as well as the client's psychological responses such as depression, suicidal behavior, and anger. Given the impact of divorce on physical health, it is also important to assess for stress-related physiological health problems such as exacerbation of hypertension, infectious illnesses, and cardiovascular disturbances.

Sexual Abuse of Males. Although society tends to think of males as abusers rather than victims, the incidence of sexual abuse of male children is surprisingly high, with studies reporting ranges of 3 to 31% (Draucker, 1992). Male children and adolescents typically experience significant shame and have great difficulty reporting sexual abuse and dealing with its psychological and social effects. Sexually abused males typically experience the same negative societal and professional responses that female sexual abuse victims might encounter (such as "blaming the victim" and disbelief). Additionally, many male victims of abuse either experience—or at least fear—accusations that they are homosexual. As a result, maintaining confidentiality is essential to the nursing care of the male victim of sexual abuse.

Assessment should focus on symptoms of abuse: persistent acting-out behavior, aggression, and withdrawal from family members or peers. Many males, like females, do not disclose or deal with their abuse until years later as adults (Draucker, 1992). Community health nurses can facilitate the disclosure of abuse by the male victim through education, supportive behavior, empathy, and actively conveying acceptance (abuse victims typically fear rejection and/or punishment).

Occupation and Employment. Although the increase in the number of women in the American work force has been significant, most hazardous occupations (such as mining and agriculture) are still performed by men. In 1994, 4 of every 100,000 workers, most of them male, died of injuries incurred on the job, and 3.5 million disabling injuries occurred (U.S. Department of Commerce, 1996). Men have five times the risk of occupational fatality of women (Waldron, 1991). Males are also exposed to workplace toxins such as lead, resulting in impaired fertility and sexual functioning, anorexia and gastrointestinal distress, and (rarely in adults) encephalopathy. Other occupational hazards that men typically face more frequently than women include exposure to chemical agents, physical agents (temperature extremes, sunlight), mechanical agents (vibration, repetitive-use syndromes), and psychosocial agents (stress and burnout, role models of poor health habits such as smoking).

Assessment of occupational health pertaining to the male client would include determining the physical, chemical, and psychosocial hazards existing in the client's work environment. Whenever possible, the community health nurse would collaborate with the occupational health nurse in determining which risks would be most likely in a given work setting and in using those data to determine which health disorders or needs would be appropriate for further evaluation. For example, a nurse working with a male client who had been a coal miner for two decades would consult with occupational health nurses or other professionals to determine that "black lung" (pneumoconiosis) is a significant occupational hazard for miners. The community health nurse would then use this information to assess the client's respiratory function and activity tolerance. Additional assessment recommendations are presented in Chapter 26.

A final social environmental factor that may have a profound influence on the health of male clients is unemployment. Some authors make a distinction between the societal experience of unemployment and the individual experience of "joblessness." From this perspective, *unemployment* is the proportion of the work force that is not employed at a specific point in time and is a statistical measure reflecting the general state of the economy. *Joblessness,* on the other hand, is the personalized experience of being out of work (Abraham & Krowchuk, 1986).

In 1995, 3.9 million men or 5.6% of the American male population over age 16 were without a job. Unemployment rates were highest among adolescent males (18.4%), but ranged from 3.5 to 9.2% for men aged 20 to 64 years (U.S. Department of Commerce, 1996).

The effects of joblessness on health can be many and varied. At the societal level, increased cardiovascular and cerebrovascular mortality has been associated with increased unemployment levels as has cirrhosis mortality. Suicide and psychiatric hospitalization rates also increase in periods of marked unemployment. For the jobless individual, common health effects may include hypertension, cardiovascular disease, myocardial infarction, stroke, depression, aggression, psychosis, drug or alcohol abuse, and child abuse.

The community health nurse should assess male clients' employment status. He or she should also assess jobless males for signs of these and other health problems. In addition, the nurse can assess the strength of coping skills and support systems for helping the male client deal with his joblessness. A further area for consideration is the potential for reentry into the work force via job retraining and similar programs.

The Behavioral Dimension

Consumption Patterns. Five times as many males as females are described as heavy users of alcohol (those consuming more than an ounce of pure alcohol each day). Alcohol abuse is widely known for its negative affect on physical and emotional health. For example, 44% of all traffic fatalities in 1993 were alcohol-related (Division of Unintentional Injury Prevention, 1994). With respect to drug abuse, 15% of men over age 18 used marijuana in 1994 compared to 10% of women, and men were three times more likely than women to report use of cocaine (U.S. Department of Health and Human Services, 1996). Drug abuse is strongly correlated with criminal behavior, physical trauma, and homicide, all of which are significant social and health risks disproportionately evident among males.

Assessment by the community health nurse for alcohol abuse includes observation for signs of intoxication (slurred speech, ataxia, unexplained behavioral changes), presence of an alcohol odor on the client's breath, or evidence of empty alcohol containers. It is also important to assess the client's family history and social circumstances for evidence that alcohol use is prevalent or supported by others. The nurse should also assess the client for the possible presence of depression, as this disorder may either predispose to, or result from, alcoholism.

When assessing for physiologic changes suggesting substance abuse, the nurse should look for unexplained sedation or hyperactivity, dilated or constricted pupils, or elevated vital signs. The community health nurse also should be observant for signs that a client who abuses substances may be experiencing withdrawal: elevated vital signs, hallucinations (particularly tactile and visual forms), irritability, unexplained pain, diaphoresis, psychomotor restlessness or hyperactivity, delirium, and seizures. It is also helpful to assess the client's knowledge of the risks attendant on substance abuse, as well as his motivation to alter his behavior. Detailed assessment information concerning drug and alcohol use appears in Chapter 33.

Cigarette smoking is considered the single most preventable cause of death in the United States. In 1993, nearly 28% of males over age 18 smoked compared with 22.5% of females (U.S. Department of Commerce, 1996). Males clearly dominate in the use of chewed forms of tobacco and experience an increased risk of oral cancers as a result. Tobacco use has also been associated with erectile dysfunction (National Institutes of Health, 1992). Assessment focuses on determining the form and frequency of the client's tobacco use, his knowledge of the health-related risks of smoking, and his motivation to quit smoking or other tobacco use.

Diet is the final consumption pattern to be considered in assessing male clients. As noted earlier, a significant proportion of men are overweight and/or have elevated serum cholesterol levels, in part associated with dietary fat intake. Many men skip breakfast or snack heavily suggesting the potential for a variety of dietary inadequacies. The community health nurse should assess the male client's dietary patterns for adequate balance and nutrient intake. Caloric intake should be assessed in light of the client's size and activity level, and specific dietary deficiencies should be identified.

Leisure. Men and women increasingly share similar leisure patterns in American culture. Nevertheless, men still tend to be more active in competitive contact sports and, more often than women, to choose leisure activities involving some degree of physical risk (skydiving, white-water rafting, rock climbing). Participation in athletic sports is closely linked with images of masculinity and reinforces tendencies to aggressiveness and violence increasing the potential for injury. Expectations of masculinity may also lead men to downplay the severity of injuries, delay treatment, and take insufficient time for healing (White, Young, & McTeer, 1995). Men also tend to choose leisure activities associated with alcohol consumption. For these reasons, men experience relatively greater incidence of recreation-related trauma. Community health nurses should assess male clients' leisure pursuits relative to their risk of producing injury. The nurse should also assess the client's understanding of the risks involved in his leisure behaviors and his knowledge and use of safety techniques or equipment to reduce health risks (eg, eye shields and helmets during contact sports and bicycling).

Sexuality. Once separated by a double standard that encouraged sexual activity by men while discouraging it for women, male and female sexual behavior has grown to have more similarities than differences in many respects. Consequently, the psychosocial aspects of the sexually related health needs of men and women are very similar. For male clients, the differences often involve their physiology. For example, although cystitis is less common in men, males do develop prostatitis and urethritis. Community health nurses should assess male clients' sexual behaviors as they relate to health in a manner similar to that used for female clients, determining the client's knowledge and use of safer sexual practices, the presence or absence of symptoms of sexually transmitted diseases, and the presence of behaviors that may increase the risk of sexually related disorders. The nurse should also address issues of sexual satisfaction and impotence and explore clients' use of safe sexual practices.

The Health System Dimension

Men tend to define health very differently from the way women define it, often viewing health as the ability to complete certain functions rather than as the presence or absence of specific symptoms. For example, a man who is obese, hypertensive, and diabetic may nonetheless feel in good health because he is able to perform what he considers to be necessary role functions at work and home. Moreover, men tend to have fewer contacts with the health care system than women, perhaps because of psychological and sociological factors such as a reluctance to see themselves as needing assistance. This is all the more surprising in that the majority of physicians are male, so male clients typically would have little difficulty obtaining services from someone of the same gender.

The U.S. health care system tends to focus on health from an illness perspective, with relatively little attention afforded to prevention. This state of affairs parallels the health-seeking behaviors of many male clients, who tend to focus on their health only when symptoms are significant enough to interfere with role function. Consequently, the relative lack of concern for prevention seen among many men is reinforced by the prevailing attitudes and operation of the health care system.

As is true of the population at large, men who are unemployed or employed in low-paying or part-time jobs typically lack health insurance and, there-

ASSESSMENT TIPS: Assessing Men's Health

Biophysical Dimension

Age

What is the man's age?

Has he accomplished the developmental tasks relevant to his present and previous developmental stages?

Has the man achieved sexual maturity?

Genetic Inheritance

Does the man have a family history of genetic predisposition to disease? If so, to what diseases?

Physiologic Function

Does the man have any existing physical health problems? If so, what are they?

Is the man experiencing impotence or other sexual problems?

Psychological Dimension

What is the extent of stress in the client's life? What conditions cause stress for him?

How has the man been socialized to deal with stress? What level of trait masculinity does he exhibit?

How effective are the man's coping strategies?

Does the man have a history of abuse as a child?

What is the man's attitude toward health? How does he respond to the possibility of illness?

Is the man depressed? Is he suicidal?

Does the man have a history of mental illness? Does he exhibit current signs of mental illness?

Physical Dimension

Where does the man live? Is he homeless? If housed, is housing safe and adequate to meet the man's needs?

Is the man exposed to environmental health hazards? If so, what are they?

Are there safety hazards in the man's environment? If so, what are they?

Social Dimension

Interpersonal Relationships

How does the man deal with conflict? Is he at risk for homicide?

Is the man married? How satisfied is he with his marriage?

Is the man divorced? If so, what is his response to the divorce? What is the nature of his relationship with his former wife?

Is the man a victim or perpetrator of family violence?

Does the man have children? If so, what is the extent and nature of his interaction with his children? How knowledgeable and comfortable is he regarding child care activities?

What is the extent of the man's social support network? How well does he utilize available support?

Employment and Economic Status

What is the man's education level?

What is the man's income? Is it adequate to meet his needs?

Is the man employed? If so, what is his occupation? Does the work setting pose health hazards for the man?

If the man is unemployed, what is his reaction to being unemployed?

Is the man retired? If so, what is his reaction to retirement?

Does the man have a history of military service? If so, does he exhibit any signs of PTSD?

Behavioral Dimension

Consumption Patterns

What are the man's usual food preferences and consumption patterns?

Does the man smoke? Does he use alcohol or other drugs?

Is there evidence of substance abuse?

Exercise and Leisure Activity

What is the extent of the man's physical activity?

What kind of leisure activities does he pursue?

Do leisure activities pose any health hazards?

Sexual Practices

Is the man sexually active?

What is the man's sexual orientation? Is he comfortable with this orientation?

To what extent has the gay client disclosed his sexual orientation? Is confidentiality a particularly important issue?

Is the gay client exposed to homophobia and discrimination?

(continued)

Does the man engage in unsafe sexual practices?

Does the man engage in regular testicular self-examination?

Health System Dimension

How does the man define health? What is his attitude to health and health care?

What is the man's usual source of health care? Is he satisfied with the care received?

To what extent does the man utilize health care services?

Does the man engage in preventive health care practices?

How does the man finance health care? Does he have health insurance? Is it adequate to meet his health needs?

What is the reaction of health care providers to the gay client? How does this reaction influence attitudes to and use of health care services?

---

fore, experience a barrier to health care services. Men who are employed, however, may also find it difficult to access health care services because their work hours conflict with those of health care providers. Overall, a slightly higher percentage of men than women (16.6% vs. 13.7%) were not covered by any form of health insurance in 1994 (U.S. Department of Commerce, 1996).

Community nurses should assess male clients for self-images (eg, invulnerability) that reduce the motivation to use health care services. Nurses should also assess male clients for other factors that serve as barriers or motivators related to obtaining health care services, such as work hours, value placed on health, ability to function in important roles despite health problems, and financial resources such as insurance.

Special Focus: Assessing the Gay Male Client

Approximately 9% of males are believed to be homosexual in their sexual orientation (McNaught, 1996). Male homosexuals (gay men) are at increased risk of experiencing certain health problems compared with heterosexuals, may have different health care needs, and may benefit from different approaches to nursing care. Appendix N, Health Assessment Guide—Adult Client, can be modified to direct assessment of the homosexual client as well as the heterosexual male client.

Earlier perspectives on homosexuality held that it was the result of the Devil's influence, hostility toward the opposite sex, incomplete psychological development, inadequate parenting, or some noxious environmental influences (eg, being sexually assaulted). Current thinking on the causes of homosexuality fall into biological, social, learning, and psychodynamic categories of theory (Miller & Waigandt,

1993). In biological theories, brain structure or hormone levels are believed to be strong contributors to homosexuality. Social theories posit that the pleasure derived from normal same-sex play in children reinforces attraction to members of the same sex. In learning theory, homosexuality is believed to be rooted in negative heterosexual experiences, and, finally, psychodynamic theory suggests that homosexuality arises from certain types of parent–child interactions. Although the origins of homosexuality are not yet known, it is certain that there exists a range of sexual orientations among individuals, with many being neither exclusively heterosexual nor exclusively homosexual. Research also suggests that most homosexually oriented persons do not differ in any psychological, social respect from their heterosexual peers. These views often conflict with those held by some people, and these conflicts may significantly affect the health behavior and status of gay men.

Internal conflict may also pose problems for homosexual males. In part, these conflicts arise out of incongruences between four identified components of sexual identity. These often confused components of sexual identity are biological sex, gender identity, social sex role, and sexual orientation. *Biological sex* is the sexual component of one's genetic makeup, the arrangement of X and Y chromosomes. *Gender identity* is one's own personal perception of being male or female. *Social sex roles* are societal expectations of behavior appropriate to males and females. For the individual, this component of sexual identity is reflected in the degree of adherence to traditional gender roles. *Sexual orientation* is the feeling of attraction to members of one gender group over another (Gonsoriek & Weinrich, 1991). *Homosexuality* is essentially a matter of sexual orientation in which attraction is to members of one's own sex rather than those of the opposite sex.

Estimates of the extent of homosexuality in the population, however, depend on one's definition of sexual orientation. Sexual orientation defined by involvement in same-sex sexual activity will result in different figures than when it is defined by self-identification as gay or lesbian or by active membership in a gay or lesbian community (Mann, 1996). Homosexuality is also defined differently in different cultures. For example, in Turkish culture, some activities that would be considered homosexual behavior in other cultures, such as mutual masturbation between members of the same sex, are not considered to be homosexual. Turkish homosexuality is also defined by the role of one partner vis-à-vis the other. For example, a man who plays the active inserter role is not considered homosexual while the partner who plays the passive receptor role is. For the active partner, sexual activity with another male is considered an acceptable secondary sexual outlet. Similarly, men who have sex with other men but who consider themselves heterosexual are not considered homosexual (Tapinc, 1992). When sexual orientation is seen as incongruent with one's perceptions of gender identity or social sex roles, internal conflict results. This conflict must be effectively resolved if health is to be maintained.

Myths of Homosexuality

The response of many people to homosexuality is based on a variety of myths and misconceptions:

- Homosexuals are easily identified by their appearance.
- Homosexuals do not marry.
- Homosexuals are antifamily.
- Homosexuals dislike children or are incapable of reproducing.
- Children of homosexuals are also likely to be homosexual.
- Homosexuals dislike members of the opposite sex.
- Homosexuality occurs because of parental dominance or abuse (dominant mother, aloof father).
- Homosexuality is contagious.
- Homosexuals will attempt to seduce "straight" males.
- Homosexuals sexually molest children.
- Bisexual individuals have relationships with males and females at the same time.

These myths lead to some of the discriminatory behaviors experienced by homosexuals. For example, beliefs by some people that homosexuals are poor role models for young boys has led to prohibiting their functioning as adult leaders in the Boy Scouts of America. Other fears voiced are that homosexual leaders may sexually molest boys. Neither of these assertions has any basis in fact. The reality of homosexual existence and its implications for health are presented in the following discussion.

The Biophysical Dimension

Although research findings are inconclusive, some studies suggest genetic or physiologic origins for homosexual orientations, including an imbalance in male and female hormones during the prenatal period or differences in the structure of X chromosomes (Hamer & Copeland, 1994). Hypothalamic differences have also been noted between homosexual and heterosexual men (Barinaga, 1993). Homosexual activities are associated with significantly higher risks of selected physical health disorders. A major concern relative to the health of gay men is that of sexually transmitted diseases (STDs), particularly HIV and AIDS. From 1989 to 1994, rates of AIDS-defining opportunistic infections in men who have sex with other men increased from 12.1 per 100,000 males to 15.9 per 100,000, and more than 150,000 new cases of AIDS were reported in this population (Division of HIV/AIDS Prevention, 1995). The relative proportion of AIDS due to homosexual behavior, however, has declined from 70% of new cases in 1987 to 46.6% of cases in 1993 (Polych & Sabo, 1995). Gay clients experience a significantly greater risk of STDs because of the nature of their sexual practices and physiology. For example, anal-receptive intercourse readily traumatizes the highly vascularized intestinal mucosa, leading to increased susceptibility to entrance of infectious organisms. For this reason the community health nurse needs to assess carefully the safety of the sexual practices of gay clients, the client's experience of symptoms suggesting STDs, and the client's history of exposure to high-risk sexual partners.

Homosexual males are also vulnerable to other physiologic conditions found among their heterosexual counterparts. Due to discriminatory attitudes of some health care professionals and prior unpleasant experiences with the health care system, however, many homosexuals may not volunteer information about problems or seek assistance. For this reason, community health nurses should carefully assess the homosexual client for evidence of physical illness.

The Psychological Dimension

Psychologically, gay men may find themselves unable to access the usual support systems heterosexual men use to cope with health and social concerns. This may result in increased stress in some circumstances, though the research suggests that most gay men adjust well to their circumstances and are no less uncomfortable in their circumstances than are their heterosexual male counterparts. One psychological factor is known to be a great concern for gay men: fear and anxiety related to encounters with homophobia and other potentially dangerous responses to their sexual orientation. As noted in Chapter 21, homophobia is an irrational fear of homosexuality that may manifest as discriminatory behavior, demeaning or derogatory comments and humor, or actual physical assaults. Some homophobics feel they have a right to assault homosexuals owing to their belief that homosexuals are criminals or deviants. Approximately one-third of homosexuals have been robbed or assaulted at least once because of their sexual orientation, and 25% have been threatened with blackmail (Janosik & Green, 1992).

Some gay men may feel compelled to conceal their sexual orientation from the heterosexual world to such an extent that they experience significant isolation; they cannot reveal their romantic joys or losses, share their longing for children, or display affection for another man. This latter problem is more acute for gay men than for lesbians because people are more likely to perceive hugs, hand holding, or dancing between men as homosexual behavior (and, therefore, unacceptable) than if it were to occur between females.

As a result of these psychological factors, community health nurses should assess the gay male client's coping skills and access to support systems, his self-esteem (it is difficult to maintain self-esteem in the face of widespread societal rejection), and his preferences relative to privacy and confidentiality.

Another sensitive area for assessment with respect to the psychological environment is "coming out." As noted in Chapter 21, coming out is a process of acknowledging one's homosexuality to self and others. Some authors reserve the term *coming out* for one's personal acceptance of homosexuality, and use the term **disclosure** to describe the explicit revealing of one's sexual orientation to others (Cass, cited in McDonald & Steinhorn, 1990).

Six stages have been identified in the coming out process, four are related to personal recognition and acceptance and two are related to disclosure:

Stage 1   Confusion
Stage 2   Denial and comparison
Stage 3   Tolerance
Stage 4   Acceptance
Stage 5   Pride
Stage 6   Synthesis

Stage 1 is characterized by confusion regarding one's attraction to persons of the same sex. Because coming out tends to occur earlier for gay males than lesbians (about 18 or 19 years of age), this confusion may be superimposed on unresolved identity confusion in later adolescence and may compound the client's feelings of distress. In stage 2, the homosexual reacts with denial and comparisons of himself to others. Denial may take the form of active pursuit of members of the opposite sex. Stage 3 is characterized by an acceptance and tolerance of homosexuality in general and of other homosexuals. Stage 4 involves self-acceptance. At stage 5, the gay male exhibits pride in himself and engages in selective disclosure. Finally, stage 6 is characterized by a synthesis of one's homosexual identity with other aspects of life (Cass, cited in McNaught, 1996). Although this description of the stages of coming out implies a linear process with a defined beginning and end, coming out is an ongoing, lifelong process. Disclosure, in particular, tends to occur incrementally, beginning with persons to whom the homosexual is emotionally closest and who are perceived as least likely to be rejecting. Even at stage 6 of the coming out process, the gay male may not engage in indiscriminate disclosure to all and sundry.

The community health nurse explores with the gay male client where he is in the coming out process and how he feels about himself and his sexual identity. Because disclosure is frequently selective, confidentiality is a particularly important consideration, and the gay male client should be assured of the confidential nature of all information revealed. To maintain confidentiality, the nurse determines who else in the client's milieu is aware of his homosexuality.

The Social Dimension

A variety of social dimension factors have the potential to adversely affect the health of gay male clients. Beliefs that gay men are psychiatrically ill, deviants, sinners, or criminals have been, and continue to be, anything but rare in the United States. The American Psychiatric Association defined homosexuality as a psychiatric disorder up until 1973, and many states still maintain laws prohibiting homosexual behavior. In 1992, twenty-one states and a few large cities had laws prohibiting discrimination against homosexuals (Dudley, 1993).

Gay men live in a social environment that often considers their behavior unacceptable and overtly and covertly discriminates against them. Gay males experience significant amounts of social stigmatization. They may fear loss of career potential or jobs, shunning by heterosexual peers, or loss of their civil rights. Rarely do homosexual relationships have the legal status accorded to traditional male–female marriages;

this results in discrimination in awarding health care benefits or custody of children, distributing communally acquired property, and abrogating rights of inheritance. Consequently gay men may prefer to conceal their sexual orientation to avoid experiencing discrimination in work or social settings. Community health nurses must make a special effort to establish a high degree of trust so as to enhance their effectiveness in assessing the health-related behaviors and concerns of this population. Nurses should again emphasize the confidential nature of the nurse–client relationship and convey empathy regarding the stigma faced by gay men.

Family interaction is another element of the social dimension that affects the health of gay males. Disclosure of homosexuality to family members and their response, homosexual relationships, and homosexual parenting are the three primary aspects of family interaction to be assessed by the community health nurse.

Disclosure.   Two different themes occur in families' responses to disclosure of a family member's homosexuality, loving acceptance or conventionality, which results in rejection of the homosexual family member. Two processes appear to be involved in the latter negative response. First, family members begin to apply their negative attitudes toward homosexuals in general to the disclosing family member. Second, they negate prior family roles fulfilled by the homosexual member (Strommen, 1989). For example, parents may deny the existence of a homosexual son or may refuse to let him interact with younger siblings.

For those families that are able to accept homosexuality in one of their members, acceptance appears to come about in stages similar to those experienced by the homosexual in coming out. Early stages include an unconscious awareness, an impact stage during which discovery or disclosure occurs, and an adjustment stage during which the family encourages the homosexual member to change to a heterosexual orientation or to keep his activities secret. Later stages include a resolution stage in which the family mourns the loss of traditional hopes for children and begins to dispel negative myths about homosexuality and, finally, a stage of integration in which the homosexual member is given new family roles consistent with his sexual orientation (Strommen, 1989).

Parental response to the disclosure of homosexuality is strongly influenced by a variety of factors: the strength of traditional gender role conceptions, perceptions of the probable attitudes of significant others in the family's social network, and parental age and education level (younger and better educated parents are more accepting). Affiliation with conservative religious ideologies and intolerance of other stigmatized groups are other factors that suggest a negative response to disclosure.

Gay males may face decisions about disclosure to wives as well as parents and siblings. Contrary to popular belief, many homosexual men are or have been married, and about half of these men have children. Some gay men do not become aware of their homosexuality until after marriage. Others marry in an attempt to deny or hide their sexual orientation. Responses of wives to the disclosure of homosexuality vary considerably and may include feelings of living with a "stranger," guilt, development of an asexual friendship or a semi-open relationship in which both husband and wife are free to take outside lovers, or a desire for divorce. The community health nurse should assess the extent of the client's disclosure of his homosexuality and the effects of the responses received to provide needed support. The nurse should also assess the needs of family members for assistance in dealing with the disclosure.

Homosexual Relationships.   Homosexuals, like other individuals, desire human relationships that involve closeness and intimacy. Generally speaking, these relationships fall into five categories: closed-couple and open-couple relationships, functional and dysfunctional singles, and asexual relationships (Janosik & Green, 1992). Closed-couple relationships are monogamous and marital in nature and may or may not have legal standing, depending on the legal status of homosexual unions as marriages recognized under the law. Approximately 28% of lesbians and 20% of gay men are involved in such unions. Open-couple relationships are quasi-marital, but each partner may have sexual involvement with others outside the union. Functional singles have short-term relationships with several partners, and differ from dysfunctional singles in that they have a better level of adjustment to their own sexual orientation. Dysfunctional singles have multiple partners, sometimes as "one night stands" and display poor adjustment to their homosexuality. In asexual relationships, members are attracted to persons of the same sex and may have close relationships with them that do not involve sexual activity.

Homosexual relationships are subjected to the same kinds of stress as heterosexual relationships, but this stress may be exacerbated by the absence of marital role models for same-sex unions and by isolation from the family of origin (O'Hanlon, 1996). In addition, homosexuals may be reluctant to form friendships with other homosexuals because of the potential for jealousy in one's partner, which further reduces the support available to the homosexual couple.

Parenthood. Parenthood poses several additional problems for the male homosexual. Contrary to popular belief, homosexuals do not dislike children, and homosexual fathers frequently feel more positive about themselves as fathers than their heterosexual counterparts. Homosexual fathers also tend to be more flexible in assuming parental roles than heterosexual men. Homosexual parents may have the additional stress of conflict between their parental role and their roles as lovers if their partners are not interested in or accepted by their children (Janosik & Green, 1992). Disclosure of homosexuality to children usually occurs during adolescence, if at all. Fathers who have disclosed their sexual orientation to their children have frequently reported greater satisfaction with their lives than those who have not (Strommen, 1989). Gay fathers may also have problems related to obtaining custody of their children, and the nurse should assess the need to refer clients to other sources of services, as well as identify other health problems related to family relationships and parenthood.

Occupation. The occupational risks and concerns experienced by gay men relate primarily to avoiding discrimination and rejection in the workplace. No clearly established occupational health risks pertain to homosexual lifestyles. It should, however, be noted that in occupational settings where masculine roles are stereotypical and exaggerated (eg, steel mills), there may be an increased incidence of acting out of homophobic thinking, resulting in an increased risk to a gay man's safety due to either assault or failure to provide assistance. Nursing assessment should focus on such potential safety risks and should consider the possibility that gay men who are unable to accept their sexual orientation may themselves enact exaggerated masculine roles and experience the related safety risks these behaviors may entail.

The Behavioral Dimension

Among the many myths about the lifestyles of gay men are that they are very different from heterosexual men in nonsexual matters as well as sexual ones; that they have very different longings and romantic needs; and that they are highly promiscuous. In reality, the majority of gay men maintain lifestyles not significantly different from those of their heterosexual male counterparts. Even "cruising," the active seeking of new and varied sexual partners, is shunned by at least 40% of gay men (Davies & Janosik, 1991). Furthermore, cruising is almost always limited to gay social settings, with no effort to "seduce" heterosexuals into homosexual lifestyles (another myth). For those gay men who do frequently change sexual partners, there is clearly a greater risk of STDs.

In terms of social habits, some research suggests that gay men may have more close friendships and interpersonal support than heterosexual men (Davies & Janosik, 1991). In addition, although a small number of gay men may behave in an overtly or even exaggeratedly feminine manner, the great majority do not appear physically or behaviorally different from heterosexual men. Finally, no clearly established difference has been shown in the consumption patterns of gay men, especially with respect to substance abuse. Prior findings related to the levels of alcohol abuse among homosexuals may be a function of sampling bias when subjects are recruited from gay bars (O'Hanlon, 1996).

In terms of nursing assessment and client behavior, the major area for assessment involves sexual behaviors. It is beneficial to stress the rationale for seeking this information, emphasizing that the community nurse's concern is based solely in the client's health risks and needs. Factors to evaluate include patterns of sexual activity, sexual exposure, and knowledge of sex-related risks and safety procedures. Bisexual men with female spouses may be even more concerned with privacy and confidentiality issues in order to maintain their concurrent heterosexual relationships; this may require significant amounts of reassurance and empathy from the nurse.

The Health System Dimension

Gay men may encounter homophobia among health care workers, and the perception of homophobia represents a significant barrier to health care. Even when the health care provider, whether an individual or an institution, is devoid of homophobia, various circumstances may threaten the gay client and act as health barriers. For example, assessment questions about birth control practices, if answered truthfully, might have the effect of requiring that a client disclose his homosexuality. For the client who fears loss of health care benefits (due to assumed higher risk of AIDS for all gay men), this is very much a situation to be avoided. To best serve gay clients it is necessary to ensure that U.S. health care institutions and personnel do not in any way discriminate or limit services to this population. Unless U.S. society is able to overcome its biases and its homophobic responses (now heightened by the AIDS epidemic), the health care system may remain as much a threat to gay men as it is a benefit. Community health nurses can improve these circumstances by challenging their own prejudices and subconscious fears, by seeking to enlighten themselves about homosexuality and sexuality in general, by actively conveying acceptance of all persons, and by working to make all assessments and interventions sexually neutral (neither presuming nor eliciting a particular sexual orientation) wherever feasible.

Diagnostic Reasoning in the Care of Men

Community health nurses use data from their client assessments to identify health needs and determine appropriate nursing diagnoses. Nursing diagnoses for individual male clients may relate to educational deficits (eg, "increased health risk due to lack of knowledge of TSE technique"), to barriers to health care utilization (eg., "failure to cope with stress related to belief that men should not need help in coping"), to consequences of specific health problems (eg, "pain due to overuse of strained ligaments," or "diminished self-esteem due to lost erectile functioning related to prostatectomy"). Nursing diagnoses may also relate to males as aggregates. For example, many young adult males living in poverty might merit the community health nurse's diagnosis of "increased health risk related to socioeconomic pressures to participate in drug use and sales."

Planning and Implementing the Dimensions of Health Care for Men

Primary Prevention

Although it is difficult to generalize about male clients' attitudes toward health promotion activities, there are some commonly encountered patterns of health behavior among men. One such behavior is a tendency to view exercise as sufficient to compensate for unhealthy behaviors such as a high intake of fats in the diet. Men also tend to attribute greater significance to health changes they can sense than to those they cannot (eg, they can sense pain, but not elevated blood pressure). Because men tend to rate their health as very good or excellent more often than women, they may feel they do not need to be actively involved in health promotion activities. They may also err in their health appraisal efforts, stemming from a tendency to believe that their past athletic or current work activities may provide for their present health needs ("When I was a teenager I would run all day." "I work hard all day in the fresh air. What could be healthier than that?")

One technique that can be used to promote positive behavioral change is *reframing*, which focuses on helping the client to see the same situation in a different light. A second technique for promoting change involves emphasizing alternate ways of coping with anxiety or fearfulness. Education, of course, is a crucial aspect of any primary prevention strategy. Education is perhaps most effective when teaching is initiated with school-age male youngsters, as this is the stage when lifelong health values and habits are forming. Health promotion by the client's family members is known to be a significant motivator and predictor of client compliance and outcomes, and involvement of family members in educational efforts and treatment planning is usually of significant benefit.

Primary prevention for health concerns specific to male clients focuses on increasing the client's use of health-promoting behaviors in the areas of cardiovascular and cerebrovascular disorders, hypertension, cancer, occupational disorders, substance abuse, violence and trauma, suicide, and posttraumatic stress disorder (PTSD).

Cardiovascular disorders involve education as a major primary prevention measure. The community health nurse provides education in home, school, or occupational settings, and emphasizes knowledge of risk factors and preventive strategies. The nurse also emphasizes methods to produce behavioral changes, recognizing that knowledge alone does not determine behavior. For example, most male clients *know* the importance of limiting fat-derived calories, but they fall short in being able to change their behavior because they lack understanding of their own behavioral dynamics (such as eating more when anxious).

Cerebrovascular disorders also involve education as a major preventive strategy. The community nurse educates clients about the relationship between other health problems, such as hypertension and diabetes, and cerebrovascular disease. The nurse educates and motivates the client to maintain a weight and blood pressure appropriate to his age to control hypertension and minimize the risk of developing some forms of diabetes.

Hypertension can be minimized for many male clients by promoting a weight appropriate for the client's body build and by promoting regular exercise. A diet that excludes excessive sodium may have preventive value as well. For some clients, knowledge and use of stress management techniques such as stress compensators (relaxing walks, vacations) and relaxation techniques (progressive muscle relaxation, guided imagery) may assist in minimizing hypertensive changes. It is helpful to focus on the fact that the hypertensive client is typically asymptomatic, as this feature encourages *denial* (a way of responding to fear) and avoidance (which are already prominent among many male clients). Again, it is helpful to link efforts to control hypertension with the client's own values about health, such as invulnerability or physical activity. For example, the nurse could take advantage of the client's interest in sports by noting famous athletes with hypertension.

Primary prevention interventions for cancer include education regarding recognizing and limiting exposure to carcinogens in the workplace (such as chemicals and sunlight), around the home, or in the diet. The possibility of a link between stress and immune system function supports the promotion of effective stress management techniques. Lifestyle choices such as smoking and consuming large amounts of meat are believed to have a significant effect on an individual's risk of cancer. Ascribing healthy behaviors to masculine role images can increase cancer-preventive behaviors in male clients by tying such behaviors to male values such as strength and power. For example, a nurse could state, "Men do what makes them strong, not what makes them weak, and smoking weakens the body." It may also be helpful to reframe male clients' poor health habits as being the result of manipulation by advertisers (eg, "I wonder whether eating all that meat might be because all your life the commercials have made eating meat seem like the right thing to do").

Primary prevention interventions for substance abuse focus on education at all age levels regarding the risks of substance abuse and on alternate means of coping with stress. Also important are efforts to assist males to redefine their social roles in healthier ways so that, for example, teenage males do not feel as compelled to drink or to behave as their peers might wish. In addition, community health nurses' activities that help reshape societal norms held by males, such as the antidrinking publicity campaign undertaken by Mothers Against Drunk Driving, are also appropriate primary prevention measures.

Trauma and violence are complicated issues with many potential levels of nursing interventions. Primary interventions include educating male children on methods of coping with their feelings and countering social demands to take unnecessary risks or to participate in unhealthy behaviors. Teaching males nondestructive ways to express their feelings and initiating political activity on behalf of safety-related legislation (motorcycle helmet laws, enforcement of driving under-the-influence statutes) are also appropriate as primary prevention interventions.

Important nursing interventions related to sexually abused male clients include educating key persons about the realities of male sexual abuse (school teachers, case managers, school nurses) and detecting families at risk. It is also important to facilitate referrals to treatment agencies specializing in sexual abuse of children or adults. Finally, although pairing male nurses with male clients for the purposes of providing care for issues involving male sexuality can be a very helpful strategy, this may not be the case with the child or adolescent male abuse victim, who may instead feel more secure working with a female nurse.

Primary prevention measures for suicide include helping a male client to avoid or cope with feelings of despair, hopelessness, or anger. Interventions that help a male avoid or cope with such feelings include role modeling, teaching disclosure of one's feelings, and prompting expression of a client's concerns through the use of empathy and acceptance. Also helpful are interventions designed to promote self-esteem and a positive self-image. Such interventions should begin with young males, prior even to school age. The community health nurse can promote the use of mental health resources that provide services to individuals or groups. Nurses can also educate families, children, workers, and other groups about the risk of suicide, factors that contribute to its occurrence, and appropriate ways to detect and respond to persons who are at increased risk of becoming suicidal. Males, especially those younger than 24 and over age 65, should be educated about their high degree of risk.

Posttraumatic stress disorder involves primary prevention of a more immediate sort—aiding the male victim to express his feelings about the traumatic experience in a supportive and accepting environment. By aiding the client to work through his feelings about the trauma rather than being overwhelmed by them, the community health nurse can prevent or minimize the severity of this disorder. In that PTSD is a complex psychological disorder, the community health nurse usually works in an adjunctive capacity with more expert or specialized providers within the mental health care system. Vietnam veterans with PTSD may benefit greatly from referral to peer-run "Vet Centers" and other support groups. A list of these is available from the Veterans Administration or local veterans organizations. Nurses should also understand that Vietnam vets with PTSD, and veterans in general, are distrustful of government-related providers. For this reason, a veteran may respond more favorably when the nurse relates to him as an individual rather than as an agent of a health care organization. A willingness to accept the veteran and a high level of trustworthiness are characteristics highly valued by Vietnam vets.

Primary prevention interventions for adolescents include aiding the adolescent to reevaluate images he holds regarding the male role; assisting the client to express his feelings through role modeling; teaching communication and social skills; conveying empathy and acceptance; and raising issues experienced by most male adolescents. Nurses can also intervene at the primary prevention level by promoting effective parent–child relationships via education about growth and development and communication skills, provided to both the client and his family.

Primary prevention measures for newly divorced men include referrals to peer support groups, encouragement of socialization and activities, and referral to mental health professionals when indicated (some mental health agencies sponsor special programs for newly divorced persons). It is also helpful for the community health nurse to provide support, assist the client to express his feelings, and guide him in coping with periods of crisis that may ensue.

For the gay or bisexual male client, providing education to increase the safety of sexual practices is an extremely important primary prevention measure. Community health nurses can perform a very valuable function by promoting safer sexual practices such as condom use and encouraging clients to reduce the number of sexual partners. These efforts are enhanced by conveying openness, showing acceptance of the client, and displaying an intent to address issues in a confidential and professional manner.

Community health nurses may sometimes find themselves in a position wherein a health-promoting intervention (such as reporting an adolescent substance abuser) may also have repercussions within the client's family or result in the client becoming enmeshed in the criminal justice system. The nurse should remember that it is not his or her actions that produce these consequences; rather, it is the actions of the individual that have led to such an outcome. Instead of experiencing guilt, the nurse should reframe nursing actions so that they can clearly be perceived as health promoting.

Secondary Prevention

Secondary prevention involves the earliest possible detection of health needs, using the assessment techniques described earlier in this chapter. It also encompasses the actual treatment of the health needs or disorders themselves. Secondary prevention roles for community health nurses working with male clients are appropriate for all disorders discussed in this chapter via special efforts to assess male clients in high-risk categories such as agricultural workers (trauma, skin cancer), teenagers (trauma, suicide, substance abuse), gay or bisexual males (AIDS), and those over age 50 (prostate cancer, cardiovascular disorders).

Community health nurses may also participate in health screening activities by providing or encouraging the client's use of such health measures as blood pressure screening and cardiovascular risk-assessment programs in public, educational, or occupational settings. Nurses can also facilitate the offering and use of screening examinations by other health care professionals within the community, such as rectal examinations and blood testing for prostate cancer and chest x-rays for lung cancer. Early detection of both prostate and testicular cancer is a very important area for secondary prevention by community health nurses.

One intervention that facilitates detection of testicular cancer is teaching the testicular self-examination (TSE) technique. Because testicular cancer occurs primarily in young men, the community health nurse can often educate and motivate clients efficiently (and minimize individual embarrassment in the process) by working with groups of males in school or work settings.

The TSE technique involves a gentle but thorough palpation of each testis, repeated monthly and akin to the procedure for breast self-examination. The male client should rotate each testis gently, moving his fingers so that all portions of the organ are palpated. He should feel uniform smoothness, without indentations, lumps, or dissymmetry within an individual testis. Abnormal findings, along with any other changes noted since the last TSE, should be promptly reported to his physician. It is helpful for the nurse to inform the client that it is normal for one testis to be larger than the other, and that the client may encounter other intrascrotal structures apart from the testes themselves, so that the client, for example, will not presume the epididymis is an abnormal finding. The ideal source of instruction for this technique would be direct guidance by a physician or nurse

---

Critical Thinking in Research

Hahn, Brooks, & Hartsough (1993) studied the relationship of tendency to self-disclosure and coping style to blood pressure reactivity among men with borderline hypertension and normotensive men who did and did not have family histories of hypertension. Limited self-disclosure was associated with increased blood pressure reactivity in both borderline hypertensive men and normotensive men. These men were also less likely to use emotion-focused coping strategies. Normotensive men with a family history of hypertension were less disclosive than those without a family history. Men with hypertension were more disclosive than normotensive men with a family history of hypertension.

1. Do the findings of this study support either a "nature" (heredity) or "nurture" (learned behavior) perspective on causal factors in hypertension? If so, which perspective is supported?
2. How might you explain why men with greater blood pressure reactivity were less self-disclosing than those with less reactivity? How might you go about testing the accuracy of your explanation?
3. Do you think the findings of this study would be similar if it was replicated with a female sample? Why or why not?

practitioner during a physical examination. Referrals to these providers are an appropriate form of secondary intervention.

Younger male clients may experience even more embarrassment about sexually related issues than their older counterparts, and significant attention to averting this embarrassment and anxiety is indicated. Humor may be a very helpful tool in that it is a common coping mechanism used by males in this age group for dealing with anxiety. Three-dimensional models, slides, and other teaching devices can be quite beneficial by giving the anxious male client something to focus on other than the (usually) opposite-sex nurse. Assignment of male nurses to this population may also reduce clients' hesitancy or embarrassment, as can creating an environment where male clients can feel free to face and voice their fears about their own mortality.

The community health nurse is not usually directly involved in the detection and screening of prostate cancer. Detection is usually achieved by digital rectal examination or by ultrasound examination. In addition, blood screening for a prostate-specific antigen promises to be more effective than rectal screening alone at early identification of prostate cancer. Early detection of prostate cancer can also be aided by psychosocial nursing interventions. For example, education about the risk of this disorder among older males helps counter the denial experienced by many men (due to a need to perceive oneself as invulnerable, perhaps), and informing the client of the importance of annual digital rectal examinations increases health-promoting behavior. Many times such teaching can be effectively enacted with male clients in work or social settings (eg, a senior citizens' organization). It is important to stress the very positive prognosis that accompanies early detection to help motivate the client by compensating for the uncomfortable, but necessary, rectal examination.

Community health nurses do participate in the treatment of other illnesses experienced by male clients. In the case of ischemic and certain other cardiac disorders, for example, stress has been shown to impact negatively on treatment outcomes, in some cases leading to a threefold increase in mortality (eg, postmyocardial-infarction clients). Treatment programs that identify high-stress clients during hospitalization, that track and reduce their stress levels after discharge, and that provide prompt assistance from nurses in the community when episodes of increased stress occur can result in significant reduction of the stress-related mortality experienced by postmyocardial-infarction clients.

Prostatitis is another disorder with implications for secondary prevention by the community health nurse. Prostatitis is usually responsive to a regimen of antibiotics, and education about the nature of the disorder (particularly when sexually transmitted) and its treatment is the major area of nursing intervention. In that it is a personally intimate and uniquely male phenomenon, however, male clients are likely to exhibit embarrassment and avoidance. The nurse can manage this response pattern by being straightforward and matter-of-fact when discussing the issue and by noting that, although perhaps embarrassing, the disorder is not unlike having cystitis or other common infections. In effect, the nurse is using reframing. Interventions for prostatitis also apply to the rare epididymitis.

Benign prostatic hyperplasia (BPH) also involves the nurse at the secondary level of prevention. Here the nurse can educate the male client about his risk of developing this disorder, and by being straightforward and professional in demeanor, the nurse can reduce the client's embarrassment about assessment questions and examinations used to screen older male clients for this disorder. An important part of the detection process involves noting that rectal examination is essential for early detection of BPH as well as prostatic cancer. The nurse should instruct the client that, although this examination may not be pleasant, it serves a double purpose and is, therefore, doubly valuable. In terms of treatment, community health nurses may find themselves assisting the client with postoperative catheter care at home, and interventions to reduce embarrassment apply here as well.

Nurses can assist male clients with mild inguinal hernias to succeed in conservative treatment strategies and avert the need for surgery. One intervention involves education and encouragement to motivate the client's compliance with wearing supportive trusses, limiting exertion, and using proper body mechanics (to reduce straining and increased intraabdominal pressure). Inguinal hernias involve both an intimate area of the body and an image of weakness rather than power. As a result, many men may delay treatment because of embarrassment or fear of surgery. Nurses can assist the client by helping him to overcome his embarrassment and reframing his interpretation of this disorder as a weakness. By being open and upfront about this condition the nurse can demonstrate that it does not require embarrassment, and in fact for many males is part of being a man. These interventions also promote compliance with conservative treatment approaches.

Tertiary Prevention

Tertiary prevention for male clients is directed at those disorders that influence the client in some ongoing manner or that have a likelihood of recurrence.

The goals of tertiary prevention are to assist the client in coping with the continuing manifestations of his illness and to reduce the likelihood of future episodes of an illness. To this end, it is useful to group tertiary prevention measures into care directed toward those disorders that affect a male's sexual functioning or sexual identity or as they present a threat to notions about male strength. Tertiary prevention measures also would be directed at supporting a client's compliance with a long-term course of treatment.

One area for tertiary prevention measures by the community health nurse involves those disorders that affect the male client's sexual functioning or sexual identity, such as testicular and prostate cancers and any male reproductive system disorder. Male clients with testicular or prostate cancer may face significant emotional distress owing to the effect surgical treatment may have on their sexuality. Prostate cancer is treated by surgical removal of the gland in most instances. Although the prognosis is often excellent when discovered early, the surgery itself may result in impotency (though recent nerve-sparing surgical techniques have reduced this problem). Similarly, the treatment for testicular cancer is surgical removal of the affected testes followed by hormonal therapy. These treatments, along with their side effects (loss of fertility, emasculation), can have a profound impact on the client's self-image and psychosocial functioning.

An important area of tertiary prevention in this regard involves encouraging the male client to join support groups. Interaction with other men who have experienced the same problems can be very effective in facilitating the client's adjustment to a treatment that has so tangibly affected his sense of masculinity. On a one-to-one basis, the nurse can be accepting, supportive, and facilitative of the male client's expression of his feeling of loss.

Some disorders may affect the male client's sense of strength; this is particularly true of cardiovascular disorders. The heart is a symbol of masculine strength for some men. Consequently, cardiovascular disorders not only can leave residual symptoms and physiological impairment, but can also threaten a man's self-image. Men with cardiovascular disease often benefit from interventions that support their self-image as masculine and by discussing their feelings about their illness. As noted elsewhere, stress management training also can have a significant positive effect on the outcome of a male client who has cardiovascular disease. These interventions are essential to promote the client's adjustment and compliance with treatment.

Of course, community health nurses should also support and reinforce the male client's positive responses to cardiac rehabilitation efforts initiated in other treatment settings. Foremost among these would be weight control, limiting intake of saturated fats, maintaining regular exercise, compliance with follow-up examinations and medications, and control of other disorders that exacerbate cardiovascular disorders (hypertension, diabetes).

In the case of some chronic disorders, especially those producing no overt symptoms, male clients tend to be lax about complying with long-term treatment recommendations. This is especially true for male clients with hypertension. Interventions that help the male client understand the importance of controlling this disorder and that build on his perceptions of masculinity are very helpful. Maintaining a regimen of antihypertensive medications may be especially difficult for male clients owing to side effects that interfere with what the client judges to be necessary masculine roles. Examples of such side effects could include impotence, dizziness, and decreased tolerance for physical activity. Nurses can assist the male client by teaching ways to compensate for these side effects, thereby helping him to maintain a sense of control over his own circumstances. In cases where the side effects are not manageable and are affecting the client's masculinity (impotence), collaborating with the client's physician or assisting the client to discuss the problem with the physician can lead to acceptance of the treatment for hypertension.

Preventing recidivism, or rehospitalization, in instances of substance abuse is a major tertiary intervention in working with male clients. Interventions that decrease the likelihood of recidivism include encouragement of the client's use of therapeutic support groups (Alcoholics Anonymous) and education regarding factors that predispose the client to continued substance abuse (poor coping skills, codependent relationships, maintaining social contacts with abusers). It is also important for the community health nurse to consider the client's family and significant others when caring for the substance-abusing male. Families and significant others can be either enablers of substance abuse or corrective forces leading to its elimination. Education of family and support persons as to those behaviors that produce improvement and those that permit further substance abuse is essential, and referrals to family treatment and support services are also of value.

Evaluating Health Care for Men

As when working with other individual clients or aggregates, community health nursing plans and interventions are evaluated by determining the degree to

TABLE 22–1. STATUS OF SELECTED NATIONAL OBJECTIVES FOR MEN'S HEALTH

	Objective	Base	Most Recent	Target
1.2	Reduce overweight prevalence	24% (1976–1980)	26.9 (1993)	20%
3.4	Reduce prevalence of smoking	31% (1987)	23.9 (1993)	15%
3.9	Reduce smokeless tobacco use among			
	Males 12–17 years	6.6% (1988)	3.9% (1993)	4%
	Males 18–24 years	8.9% (1987)	7.8% (1993)	4%
5.5	Increase sexual abstinence in males under 17	33% (1988)	44% (1991)	40%
5.6	Increase contraceptive use by sexually active adolescent males	78% (1988)	83% (1991)	90%
6.1	Reduce suicide incidence in men aged 20–34 (per 100,000 men)	25.2 (1987)	25.1 (1991)	21.4
7.1	Reduce homicide among black men aged 15–34 years (per 100,000 population)	91.1 (1987)	130.5 (1991)	72.4
9.1	Reduce unintentional injury deaths (per 100,000 population)			
	Among black males	64.9 (1987)	62.4 (1991)	51.9
	Among white males	53.6 (1987)	46.4 (1991)	42.9
9.5	Reduce drowning deaths in men aged 15–34 years (per 100,000 population)	4.5 (1987)	4.0 (1991)	2.5
15.4	Increase blood pressure control	6% (1976–1980)	16% (1991)	40%

(Sources: Centers for Disease Control, 1996; U.S. Department of Health and Human Services, 1993, 1995.)

which client goals have been met. It is also important to determine whether the interventions were efficient. Could the same results have been accomplished with less expense of time or other resources?

The community health nurse also needs to consider the client's reaction to nursing interventions. Is the client satisfied with the nurse's efforts and with the manner in which interventions were planned and implemented as well as with their results? The goal of

evaluation is to ensure that client needs are met and to improve the nurse's abilities; inviting the critique of one's clients and colleagues is an excellent source of feedback.

The effects of intervention at the aggregate level can be assessed in terms of the level of accomplishment of national health objectives. The current status of selected objectives related to men's health is presented in Table 22–1.

Critical Thinking in Practice: A Case in Point

You are a community health nurse working with a hypertensive, diabetic, middle-aged single mother for the past year. Her 17-year-old son has had hand surgery and has been added to your caseload for wound and cast care. On your next meeting with the mother you discover that she is very upset about her son's behavior. He broke his hand when he punched a wall in a fit of anger, and the necessary care has hurt the family's very limited finances. The mother reports that she believes her son is drinking, and she is especially angry and upset about this because her ex-husband had deserted the family largely because of his own alcohol abuse. While the mother answers a phone call you attempt to speak to the son. He seems wary but does concede he punches walls when angry. His view at present is that "It's no big deal—the cast will handle it." When asked about alcohol, he replies, "It's what we do . . . a little doesn't hurt anyone." When you begin to address the risks involved in this behavior, he cuts you off by angrily retorting, "It's none of your damn business! Get lost and leave me alone!"

1. What psychological and social dimension factors are influencing the son's behavior?
2. What actual and potential health issues are raised by the lifestyle of the son and his past and present family situation?
3. What primary interventions are indicated for the health risks present in the son?
4. What secondary interventions are indicated for the health issues present in the son?
5. How should the nurse respond to the client's denial and anger?
6. How should the nurse's interventions be evaluated?

TESTING YOUR UNDERSTANDING

1. Describe at least five considerations in assessing the effects of biophysical factors on the health of men. (pp. 525–529)
2. Identify at least three social and psychological dimension influences on men's health. (pp. 529–533)
3. Describe four areas for consideration in assessing behavioral dimension factors influencing men's health. (pp. 533–534)
4. Identify at least two effects of the health care system on the health of male clients. (pp. 534–536)
5. Describe at least three factors that contribute to adverse health effects for male homosexual clients. (pp. 536–541)
6. Discuss the stages of coming out for homosexual clients. (p. 538)
7. Identify at least four areas for primary prevention with male clients. How might the community health nurse be involved in each? (pp. 541–543)
8. Describe at least four secondary prevention considerations for male clients. Give an example of at least one community health nursing intervention related to each consideration. (pp. 543–544)
9. Identify at least three areas of emphasis in tertiary prevention for male clients. How might the community health nurse be involved in each? (pp. 544–545)

Q WHAT DO YOU THINK?
Questions for Critical Thinking

1. Why do you think men evolved as hunters and warriors rather than women?
2. In what ways were you socialized into gender roles? How closely do your internalized gender roles conform to those expected of society? What problems, if any, has gender created in your life?
3. What can nurses do to facilitate health-promoting behaviors among men?
4. How might health care services be modified to better meet the needs of gay men?

REFERENCES

Abraham, I. L., & Krowchuk, H. V. (1986). Unemployment and health: Health promotion for the jobless male. *Nursing Clinics of North America, 21*, 27–37.

Albertsen, P. C., Fryback, D. G., Storer, B. E., Kolon, T. F., & Fine, J. (1995). Long-term survival among men with conservatively treated localized prostate cancer. *JAMA, 274*, 626–631.

Barinaga, M. (1993). Differences in brain structure may cause homosexuality. In W. Dudley (Ed.), *Homosexuality: Opposing viewpoints* (pp. 17–22). San Diego: Greenhaven Press.

Barry, M. J., Fowler, F. J., Bin, L., Pitts, J. C., Harris, C. J., & Mulley, A. G. (1997). The natural history of patients with benign prostatic hyperplasia as diagnosed by North American urologists. *Journal of Urology, 157,* 10–15.

Cardiovascular Health Studies Bureau. (1994). Prevalence of adults with no known major risk factors for coronary heart disease—Behavioral Risk Factor Surveillance System, 1992. *MMWR, 43,* 61–63, 69.

Cass, cited in McDonald, H. B., & Steinhorn, A. I. (1990). *Homosexuality: A practical guide to counseling lesbians, gay men, and their families.* New York: Continuum.

Cass, cited in McNaught, B. (1996). *Gay issues in the workplace.* New York: St. Martin's Press.

Centers for Disease Control. (1996). State- and sex-specific prevalence of selected characteristics—Behavioral Risk Factor Surveillance System, 1992 and 1993. *MMWR, 45*(SS-6), 1–36.

Chantry, C. J. (1994). Adolescence. In A. M. Rudolph & R. K. Kamei (Eds.), *Rudolph's fundamentals of pediatrics.* Norwalk, CT: Appleton & Lange.

Chronic Disease Surveillance Bureau. (1993). Deaths and hospitalizations from chronic liver disease and cirrhosis—United States, 1980–1989. *MMWR, 41,* 969–973.

Copenhaver, M. M., & Eisler, R. M. (1996). Masculine gender role stress: A perspective on men's health. In P. M. Kato & T. Mann (Eds.), *Handbook of diversity issues in health psychology* (pp. 219–235). New York: Plenum Press.

Davies, J., & Janosik, E. (1991). *Mental health and psychiatric nursing: A caring approach.* Boston: Jones and Bartlett.

Division of Cancer Prevention and Control. (1993). Mortality trends for selected smoking-related cancers and breast cancer—United States, 1950–1990. *MMWR, 42,* 857, 863–866.

Division of HIV/AIDS Prevention. (1995). Update: Trends in AIDS among men who have sex with men—United States, 1989–1994. *MMWR, 44,* 401–404.

Division of Unintentional Injury Prevention. (1994). Update: Alcohol-related traffic fatalities—United States, 1982–1993. *MMWR, 43,* 861–863.

Draucker, C. B. (1992). *Counseling survivors of childhood sexual abuse.* Newbury Park, CA: Sage.

Dudley, W. (1993). Introduction. In W. Dudley (Ed.), *Homosexuality: Opposing viewpoints* (pp. 12–14). San Diego: Greenhaven Press.

Geiss, L. S., Herman, W. H., Goldschmid, M. G., et al. (1993). Surveillance for diabetes mellitus—United States, 1980–1989. *MMWR, 41*(SS-2), 1–20.

Gonsoriek, J. C., & Weinrich, J. D. (1991). The definition and scope of sexual orientation. In J. C. Gonsoriek & J. D. Weinrich (Eds.), *Homosexuality: Research implications for public policy* (pp. 1–12). Newbury Park, CA: Sage.

Gordon, D. F. (1995). Testicular cancer and masculinity. In D. Sabo & D. F. Gordon (Eds.), *Men's health and illness: Gender, power, and the body* (pp. 246–265). Thousand Oaks, CA: Sage.

Hahn, W. K., Brooks, J. A., & Hartsough, D. M. (1993). Self-disclosure and coping in men with cardiovascular reactivity. *Research in Nursing & Health, 16,* 275–282.

Hamer, D., & Copeland, P. (1994). *The science of desire: The search for the gay gene and the biology of behavior.* New York: Simon & Schuster.

Hegelson, V. S. (1995). Masculinity, men's roles, and coronary heart disease. In D. Sabo & D. F. Gordon (Eds.), *Men's health and illness: Gender, power, and the body* (pp. 68–104). Thousand Oaks, CA: Sage.

Janosik, E., & Green, E. (1992). *Family life: Process and practice.* Boston: Jones and Bartlett.

Kaler, S. (1990). Epididymitis in the young adult male. *Nurse Practitioner, 15*(5), 10–16.

Mann, T. (1996). Why do we need a health psychology of gender or sexual orientation. In P. M. Katon & T. Mann (Eds.), *Handbook of diversity issues in health psychology* (pp. 187–198). New York: Plenum Press.

McNaught, B. (1996). *Gay issues in the workplace.* New York: St. Martin's Press.

Miller, D. A., & Waigandt, A. (1993). The causes of homosexuality are uncertain. In W. Dudley (Ed.), *Homosexuality: Opposing viewpoints* (pp. 45–51). San Diego: Greenhaven Press.

Mortality Statistics Bureau. (1996). Mortality patterns—United States, 1993. *MMWR, 45,* 161–164.

Mullis, M. (1984). Vietnam: The human fallout. *Journal of Psychosocial Nursing, 22*(2), 27–31.

National Institutes of Health. (1992). Impotence. *NIH Consensus Statement, 10*(4), 1–33.

O'Hanlon, K. A. (1996). Homophobia and the health psychology of lesbians. In P. M. Kato & T. Mann (Eds.), *Handbook of diversity issues in health psychology* (pp. 261–284). New York: Plenum Press.

Polych, C., & Sabo, D. (1995). Gender politics, pain, and illness: The AIDS epidemic in North American prisons. In D. Sabo & D. F. Gordon (Eds.), *Men's health and illness: Gender, power, and the body* (pp. 139–157). Thousand Oaks, CA: Sage.

Stillion, J. (1995). Premature death among males: Extending the bottom line of men's health. In D. Sabo & D. F. Gordon (Eds.), *Men's health and illness: Gender, power, and the body* (pp. 46–67). Thousand Oaks, CA: Sage.

Strommen, E. F. (1989). You're a what? Family member reactions to the disclosure of homosexuality. In F. W. Bozett (Ed.), *Homosexuality and the family* (pp. 37–58). New York: Haworth.

Tapinc, H. (1992). Masculinity, femininity, and Turkish male homosexuality. In K. Plummer (Ed.), *Modern homosexualities: Fragments of lesbian and gay experience* (pp. 39–49). New York: Routledge.

U.S. Department of Commerce. (1993). *Statistical abstract of the United States, 1993* (113th ed.). Washington, DC: Government Printing Office.

U.S. Department of Commerce. (1996). *Statistical abstract of the United States, 1996* (116th ed.). Washington, DC: Government Printing Office.

U.S. Department of Health and Human Services. (1991). *Healthy people 2000: National health promotion and disease prevention objectives.* Washington, DC: Government Printing Office.

U.S. Department of Health and Human Services. (1993). *Health United States, 1992, and healthy people 2000 review.* Washington, DC: Government Printing Office.

U.S. Department of Health and Human Services. (1995). *Healthy people 2000: Midcourse review and 1995 revisions.* Washington, DC: Government Printing Office.

U.S. Department of Health and Human Services. (1996). *Health United States, 1995.* Washington, DC: Government Printing Office.

Waldron, I. (1991). Effects of labor force participation on sex differences in mortality and morbidity. In M. Frankenhaeuser, U. Lundberg, & M. Chesney (Eds.), *Women, work, and health: Stress and opportunities.* New York: Plenum Press.

White, P. G., Young, K., & McTeer, W. G. (1995). Sport, masculinity, and the injured body. In D. Sabo & D. F. Gordon (Eds.), *Men's health and illness: Gender, power, and the body* (pp. 158–182). Thousand Oaks, CA: Sage.

RESOURCES FOR NURSES WORKING WITH MALE CLIENTS

Advocacy

Dads Against Discrimination
PO Box 8525
Portland, OR 97207
(503) 222–1111

Fathers for Equal Rights
PO Box 010847
Flagler Station
Miami, FL 33101
(305) 895–6351

Male Liberation Foundation
701 Northeast 67th Street
Miami, FL 33138
(305) 756–6249

Men's Resource Center
2325 East Burnside
Portland, OR 97214
(503) 235–3433

National Congress for Men
4511 Marathor Heights
Adrian, MI 49221–9240
(202) 328–4377

Handicapped Men

Learning How
PO Box 35481
Charlotte, NC 28235
(704) 376–4735

Impotence

I-Anon
119 South Ruth Street
Maryville, TN 37803
(423) 983–6092

Impotence Institute of America
119 South Ruth Street
Maryville, TN 37803
(423) 983–6092

Potency Restored
8630 Fenton Street, Ste. 218
Silver Spring, MD 20910
(301) 588–5777

Recovery of Male Potency
27211 Lasher Road, No. 208
Southfield, MI 48034
(810) 357–1314

Men in Nursing

American Assembly for Men in Nursing
437 Twin Bay Drive
Pensacola, FL 32534–1350

RESOURCES FOR ASSISTING HOMOSEXUAL CLIENTS

Council for Sex Information and Education
2272 Colorado Blvd., No. 1228
Los Angeles, CA 90041

Dignity/USA
1500 Massachusetts Avenue, NW, Ste. 11
Washington, DC 20005
(202) 861–0017

Gay Men's Health Crisis
129 W. 20th Street
New York, NY 10011
(212) 807–6664

Homosexual Information Center
115 Monroe
Bossier City, LA 71111–4539
(318) 742–4709

Integrity
PO Box 5255
New York, NY 10185–5255
(908) 220–1914

International Gay and Lesbian Human Rights
    Commission
1360 Mission Street, Ste. 200
San Francisco, CA 94103
(415) 255–8680

National Gay and Lesbian Task Force
2320 17th Street, NW
Washington, DC 20009–4039
(202) 332–6483

New Ways Ministry
4012 29th Street
Mt. Ranier, MD 20712
(301) 277–5674

Parents, Families, and Friends of Lesbians and Gays
    (PFLAG)
PO Box 96519
Washington, DC 20038
(202) 638–4200

Sex Information and Education Council of United
    States
130 West 42nd Street, Ste. 350
New York, NY 10036
(212) 819–9770

Universal Fellowship of Metropolitan Community
    Churches
5300 Santa Monica Blvd., Ste. 304
Los Angeles, CA 90029
(213) 464–5100

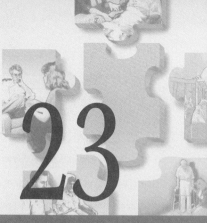

23

CARE OF OLDER CLIENTS

In 1994, there were more than 360 million people over 65 years of age in the world and that figure was increasing by about 800,000 persons per month. It is estimated that by 2025, the world's elderly will number more than 850 million (Kinsella, 1994). This same level of growth in the older population is occurring in the United States with an increase of approximately 60,000 individuals each year (Ginsberg, Gage, Martin, Gerstein, & Acuff, 1994). In 1970, people over 65 years of age constituted just under 10% of the U.S. population. In 1995, the proportion of people over 65 was slightly less than 13%, or 33.5 million people. Most of the elderly fall into the 65- to 74-year-old group, but 1.4% of Americans were over 85 years of age in 1995, and 53,000 of them were more than 100 years old. The proportion of those over age 65 in the United States is expected to rise to 18.5% by the year 2025, and more than 2%, or 7 million people, will be 85 years old or older (U.S. Department of Commerce, 1996).

In part, the growth in the elderly as a percentage of the population is due to a lower birth rate and fewer young persons than in previous years. Another major contributing factor is increased longevity. Improvements in medical treatment and the use of advanced medical technologies to sustain life have resulted in a life expectancy of 72.3 years for men and 79 years for women. Projected life expectancy by the year 2010 is 74.1 years for men and 80.6 years for women (U.S. Department of Commerce, 1996). Although life expectancy has increased, the quality of life for the elderly is often questionable. In working with older adults, individually or as an aggregate, community health nurses must be concerned with quality-of-life concerns as well as longevity.

This emphasis on quality of life can be seen in the focus of the national health objectives for the year 2000 addressing the health needs of the elderly (see Appendix A). A major thread throughout these objectives is to reduce activity limitations that impair the quality of life for older persons (U.S. Department of Health and Human Services, 1991).

▶ Chapter Objectives

After reading this chapter, you should be able to:

- Identify four myths related to aging.
- Describe at least five theories of aging.
- Describe at least two changes in each body system that occur with normal aging.
- Identify three major themes in assessing the physical dimension of health for older clients.
- Describe at least four considerations in assessing the influence of behavioral dimension factors on the health of older clients.
- Identify at least six areas for primary prevention in the care of older adults.
- Describe secondary preventive measures for at least four health problems common among older clients.
- Identify at least three factors related to older clients that may influence the community health nurse's approach to health education.
- Describe four considerations unique to older clients that influence the evaluation of nursing care.

▶ MYTHS OF AGING

Aging is a normal human phenomenon. Although much research has been conducted recently on the aging process, aging itself remains a mystery surrounded by myths. Among the myths surrounding aging are beliefs that aging is a time of tranquility and that aging is synonymous with senility. For many older adults, however, aging is a time of increased problems and decreased resources for dealing with those problems. Moreover, senility is not an inevitable consequence of aging. Many older persons retain their mental faculties well beyond the ninth decade of life.

Another myth is that old age is a time of reduced productivity. This is misleading. Many older adults remain productive throughout life. Societal factors, however, may limit opportunities for older adults to demonstrate their productivity. For example, many older adults are forced to retire at a specific age despite continued abilities to perform their jobs capably. Continued productivity among older persons is seen among those who do continue to work as well as among those who channel their energies into other areas after retirement. Retirees may continue to contribute to society through volunteer activities, artistic endeavors, or other pursuits.

Older persons are also thought by many to be resistant to change—again, a myth. Resistance to change tends to be a lifelong characteristic, not one developed with advancing age. Persons who have been relatively resistant to change throughout life will probably continue to resist change in their older years, whereas those who have welcomed change will probably continue to do so.

Finally, that aging is purely a matter of chronology, a uniform process that progresses at the same rate and with the same results for all, is a myth. The truth is that aging affects each individual differently, and the outcomes of aging may be very different from one individual to another.

▶ THEORIES OF AGING

Aging and circumventing aging are topics that fascinated humanking long before Ponce de Léon's search for the fountain of youth. Science cannot fully explain why aging occurs, but several theories have been advanced to explain the process. These theories tend to fall into four categories: stochastic, genetic, psychological, and sociological theories.

Stochastic Theories

Stochastic theories of aging are based on the assumption that the cumulative effects of environmental assaults eventually become incompatible with life. One of these theories, the *somatic mutation theory,* holds that prolonged exposure to background radiation of several types results in cell mutations that eventually lead to death (Ebersole & Hess, 1994).

The *error theory,* a second stochastic theory, is based on the belief that environmental changes interfere with cell function and protein synthesis, thus causing errors in reproduced cells. These errors multiply in a geometric progression until cells are no longer viable (Ebersole & Hess, 1994).

Genetic Theories

Genetic theories of aging are based on the assumption that aging is a part of the developmental process, with differences in that process genetically programmed from conception. *Neuroendocrine theory* holds that aging is the result of functional decrements in neurons and their hormones (Ebersole & Hess, 1994). In one version of this theory, for example, changes in the hypothalamic–pituitary system, over time, lead to changes in other body systems, possibly due to diminished responsiveness of neuroendocrine tissue to various signals.

Intrinsic mutagenesis theory holds that each person has a genetic constitution that regulates the replication of genetic materials. Over time, regulatory activity diminishes, creating mutations in cells that result in the effects of aging.

Immunologic theory holds that aging is an autoimmune process. As cells change with age, the body's immunologic mechanisms perceive them as foreign bodies and destroy them. Finally, the *free radical theory* is aging is based on the belief that most physiologic changes of aging are due to damage caused by the action of free radicals, which are highly chemically reactive by-products of metabolism. Generally speaking, these free radicals are rapidly destroyed by protective enzyme systems. Over time, however, it is believed that those radicals not destroyed accumulate to cause cell damage (Ebersole & Hess, 1994). Despite the stochastic and genetic theories of aging and related research, the physiologic processes involved in aging and the variability of aging among individuals remain unexplained.

Psychological Theories

A number of theories have also been advanced to explain the psychological aspects of aging. Jungian *psychoanalytic theory* regards aging as a time of developing self-awareness through reflective activity. Harry Stack Sullivan's *interpersonal theory* is developmental in nature. Maturity, in this theory, involves the development of satisfactory interpersonal relationships. The loss of these relationships over time is believed to result in a loss of interpersonal security and the consequent psychological aspects of aging.

In Abraham Maslow's *human needs theory,* physical aging and environmental changes contribute to difficulty in meeting basic human needs. These difficulties contribute, in turn, to the psychological effects sometimes seen with age. The greater the difficulty in meeting basic needs, the greater the impact of aging (Maslow, 1968). Maslow arranged these human needs in a hierarchy:

Survival needs	Oxygen, food, water, sleep, sexual activity
Safety and security needs	Protection from physical hazards, emotional security
Love and belonging needs	Affection from others, ability to feel and express affection for others, group identification, companionship
Esteem and recognition needs	Sense of self-worth, recognition of accomplishments by others
Self-actualization needs	Achievement of personal potential
Aesthetic needs	Order, harmony, and achievement of spiritual goals

Finally, in Erik Erickson's *theory of psychosocial development,* the degree of success experienced in accomplishing the developmental tasks in stages 1 through 7 influences the accomplishment of the tasks of the older adult in stage 8 (Erickson, 1963):

Stage 1: Trust versus mistrust	Focuses on developing a sense of trust in oneself and others
Stage 2: Autonomy versus shame and doubt	Focuses on ability to express oneself and cooperate with others
Stage 3: Initiative versus guilt	Focuses on purposeful behavior and the ability to evaluate one's own behavior
Stage 4: Industry versus inferiority	Focuses on developing belief in one's own abilities
Stage 5: Identity versus role confusion	Focuses on developing a clear sense of self and plans to actualize one's abilities
Stage 6: Intimacy versus isolation	Focuses on developing one's capacity for reciprocal love relationships
Stage 7: Generativity versus stagnation	Focuses on creativity and productivity and developing the capacity to care for others
Stage 8: Ego identity versus despair	Focuses on acceptance of one's life as worthwhile and unique

Sociological Theories

Sociological theories have also been advanced to explain the effects of aging. From the perspective of the *disengagement theory,* the older person recognizes death as inevitable and so begins a process of withdrawal from society that permits the individual to enjoy old age and to prepare for death without causing social disruption when death occurs. The process may actually work in reverse, however, with society disengaging from and isolating older individuals (Gibson, 1992).

Activity theory, on the other hand, posits continued engagement with society and the assumption of new roles and responsibilities by the older person. According to *continuity theory,* one's behavior becomes more predictable with age (Ebersole & Hess,

1994). For instance, the conservative person becomes more conservative and the adventurous person becomes more adventurous. Also, a change occurs in roles and relationships as the older adult becomes more concerned with introspection and self-reflection.

None of the theoretical perspectives presented here completely explains the aging process and its effects, and although nurses need a theory base for gerontologic nursing practice, it may be advisable to adopt more than one theory in working with older persons. Nurses must assess the individual needs of each client and select a theoretical perspective that best fits those needs. Theories of aging are summarized in Table 23–1.

► THE DIMENSIONS MODEL AND CARE OF OLDER CLIENTS

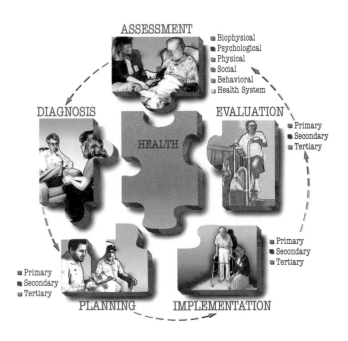

The Dimensions Model can be used to design nursing interventions to meet the health care needs of older clients. Using the model, the community health nurse conducts an in-depth assessment of the older client's health status; derives nursing diagnoses from the data obtained; plans and implements primary, secondary, and tertiary preventive care; and evaluates the effects of nursing intervention.

Critical Dimensions of Nursing in the Care of Older Clients

Elements of each of the dimensions of nursing are brought to bear in community health nursing care of older clients. Knowledge of both normal and abnormal aspects of aging is a critical aspect of the cognitive dimension. Other knowledge required by the nurse working with older clients includes interventions designed to meet the health needs of the elderly and how interventions used for other age groups may need to be modified for use with older populations. Interpersonal skills are particularly important in work with older clients who often have diminished self-esteem and are at increased risk of depression and suicide. Advocacy at both the level of the individual client and at the aggregate level is essential to assure adequate resources and health care for older segments of the population. Abuse of older persons is a particularly important area for nursing advocacy. Other considerations in the ethical dimension may include decisions related to self-determination and compliance issues and to prolonging life in the face of chronic or terminal illness.

A number of manipulative skills may be needed in the provision of direct care to older clients. The nurse may also be involved in teaching manipulative skills, such as assisting with ambulation or catheter care, to family caregivers or to clients themselves. Excellent diagnostic and analytic skills will also be needed when working with older clients because of the atypical presentation of many health problems in this population. In the process dimension, the health education process and case management processes may be particularly relevant to meeting the needs of older adults. The health education process may need to be modified, however, to address sensory changes and learning capabilities in the older person. At the aggregate level, the political process will be critical in the formulation of health care policy that adequately addresses the needs of older Americans. Community health nurses may also be actively involved in helping groups of older clients organize to influence policy formation.

 Assessing the Dimensions of Health in Older Clients

Effective nursing care for older clients requires an accurate assessment of the client's health status. Biophysical, psychological, physical, social, behavioral, and health system factors may influence that health status. Consequently, the community health nurse explores factors in each of these six dimensions of health.

In addition to the routine aspects of any client assessment, there are some special considerations in assessing older clients. The most important considera-

TABLE 23–1. SELECTED THEORIES OF AGING

Perspective	Theory	Description of Theory
Stochastic	Somatic mutation theory	Cumulative exposures to background radiation cause cell mutations incompatible with life.
	Error theory	Aging is the cumulative effects of errors in cell reproduction.
Genetic	Neuroendocrine theory	Aging is due to the effects of diminished response of neuroendocrine tissue to stimuli.
	Intrinsic mutagenesis theory	Genetic regulatory activity diminishes over time, resulting in cell mutations that eventually lead to cell death.
	Immunologic theory	Aging is an autoimmune process.
	Free radical theory	Aging is due to the accumulation of free radicals, by-products of cell metabolism that interfere with cell function.
Psychological	Psychoanalytic theory	Aging leads to a focus on introspection and self-reflection.
	Interpersonal theory	The psychological effects of aging are due to the loss of satisfactory interpersonal relationships and consequent loss of interpersonal security.
	Human needs theory	Difficulty in meeting basic human needs results in the psychological effects of aging.
	Theory of psychosocial development	The degree of success achieved in developmental tasks in earlier stages affects one's response to aging.
Sociological	Disengagement theory	Recognizing death as inevitable, the older person begins to separate from society to provide for the continuity of the social order.
	Activity theory	Interaction with society continues with assumption of new roles and responsibilities.
	Continuity theory	Previous personality traits become more pronounced with age and behavior becomes more predictable.

tion is the need to differentiate normal effects of the aging process from evidence of pathology. Research has indicated that inaccurately attributing health problems to aging (done by both older clients and health care providers) is associated with increased mortality because of resultant delays in obtaining needed care (Rakowski & Hickey, 1992). Some of the common physical effects of the aging process that must be differentiated from organic disease are listed in Table 23–2 along with their implications for the health of older clients. Additional physiologic effects of aging are reflected in changes in normal values for a variety of laboratory tests. For example, older clients may exhibit lower hematocrit and hemoglobin levels and higher blood glucose levels than younger people (Berman, 1994). Typical values for selected laboratory procedures are presented in Table 23–3.

In assessing older clients, the community health nurse must also keep in mind that illnesses may present with atypical symptoms and that dysfunction in one organ system may exacerbate existing problems in another. Particular signs that should lead the community health nurse to suspect illness in an elderly person include cognitive changes or agitation, loss of bladder control, changes in dietary patterns, changes in activity or energy levels, and recurrent falls (Bender, 1992).

Because longevity may contribute to a variety of life experiences that increase resilience and coping abilities, the community health nurse should expect to find strengths as well as problems when assessing older clients. Longevity also means that most older clients have experienced a variety of losses (health, social roles, loved ones). Consequently, the nurse must consider the persistent theme of loss and the extent of the older client's ability to adjust to the losses experienced.

Considerations related to older clients' communication may also influence assessment of their health status. For example, older people tend to underreport symptoms of illness or may describe vague or nonspecific symptoms. Therefore, the community health nurse needs to be particularly thorough in the review of systems with an older client and will elicit specific

GENERAL CONSIDERATIONS IN ASSESSING OLDER ADULTS

- The normal effects of aging must be differentiated from pathology.
- Normal effects of aging are constantly being redefined.
- Normal laboratory values and other findings may differ between younger and older adults.
- Older clients may exhibit atypical signs and symptoms of illness.
- Older clients may exhibit a decreased tolerance for stress.
- Strengths that result from an older client's life experiences may provide a basis for health interventions.
- Loss is a persistent theme in the lives of older adults.
- Older clients usually exhibit multiple health problems that have complex interactions.
- Older clients may underreport symptoms of illness.
- Older clients may have multiple, nonspecific complaints that require explication.
- Older clients may have difficulty communicating their health needs.

TABLE 23–2. COMMON PHYSICAL CHANGES OF AGING AND THEIR IMPLICATIONS FOR HEALTH

System Affected	Changes Noted	Implications for Health
Integumentary system		
Skin	Decreased turgor, sclerosis, and loss of subcutaneous fat, leading to wrinkles	Lowered self-esteem
	Increased pigmentation, cherry angiomas	
	Cool to touch, dry	Itching, risk of injury, insomnia
	Decreased perspiration	Hyperthermia, heat stroke
Hair	Thins, decreased pigmentation	Lowered self-esteem
Nails	Thickened, ridges, decreased rate of growth	Difficulty trimming nails, potential for injury
Cardiovascular system	Less efficient pump action and lower cardiac reserves	Decreased physical ability and fatigue with exertion
	Thickening of vessel walls, replacement of muscle fiber with collagen	Elevated blood pressure, varicosities, venous stasis, pressure sores
	Pulse pressure up to 100	
	Arrhythmias and murmurs	
	Dilated abdominal aorta	
Respiratory system	Decreased elasticity of alveolar sacs, skeletal changes of chest	Decreased gas exchange, decreased physical ability
	Slower mucus transport, decreased cough strength, dysphagia	Increased potential for infection or aspiration
	Postnasal drip	
Gastrointestinal system	Wearing down of teeth	Difficulty chewing
	Decreased saliva production	Dry mouth, difficulty digesting starches
	Loss of taste buds	Decreased appetite, malnutrition
	Muscle atrophy of cheeks, tongue, etc	Difficulty chewing, slower to eat
	Thinned esophageal wall	Feeling of fullness/heartburn after meals
	Decreased peristalsis	Constipation
	Decreased hydrochloric acid and stomach enzyme production	Pernicious anemia, frequent eructation
	Decreased lip size, sagging abdomen	Change in self-concept
	Atrophied gums	Poorly fitting dentures, difficulty chewing, potential for mouth ulcers, loss of remaining teeth
	Decreased bowel sounds	Potential for misdiagnosis
	Fissures in tongue	
	Increased or decreased liver size (2–3 cm below costal border)	Potential for misdiagnosis
Urinary system	Decreased number of nephrons and decreased ability to concentrate urine	Nocturia, increased potential for falls
Reproductive system		
Female	Atrophied ovaries, uterus	Ovarian cysts
	Atrophy of external genitalia, pendulous breasts, small flat nipple, decreased pubic hair	Lowered self-esteem
	Scant vaginal secretions	Dyspareunia
	Vaginal mucosa thinned and friable	
Male	Decreased size of penis and testes, decreased pubic hair, pendulous scrotum	Lowered self-esteem
	Enlarged prostate	Difficulty urinating, incontinence
Musculoskeletal system	Decreased muscle size and tone	Decreased physical ability
	Decreased range of motion in joints, affecting gait, posture, balance, and flexibility	Increased risk of falls, decreased mobility
	Kyphosis	Lowered self-esteem
	Joint instability	Increased risk of falls, injury
	Straight thoracic spine	
	Breakdown of chondrocytes in joint cartilage	Osteoarthritis, joint pain, reduced ability for activities of daily living
	Osteoporosis	Increased risk of fracture
Neurological system	Diminished hearing, vision, touch, and increased reaction time	Increased risk for injury, social isolation
	Diminished pupil size, peripheral vision, adaptation, accommodation	
	Diminished sense of smell, taste	Decreased appetite, malnutrition
	Decreased balance	Increased risk of injury
	Decreased pain sensation	Increased risk of injury
	Decreased ability to problem solve	Difficulty adjusting to new situations
	Diminished deep tendon reflexes	
	Decreased sphincter tone	Incontinence (fecal or urinary)
	Decreased short-term memory	Forgetfulness
Endocrine		
Thyroid	Irregular, fibrous changes	
Female	Decreased estrogen and progesterone production	Osteoporosis, menopause
Male	Decreased testosterone production	Fatigue, weight loss, decreased libido, impotence, lowered self-esteem, depression

TABLE 23–3. CHANGES IN NORMAL LABORATORY VALUES IN OLDER CLIENTS

Test	Young Adult Normal	Older Adult Normal
Urine		
Protein	0–5 mg/100 mL	Up to 30 mg/100 mL
Glucose	0–15 mg/100 mL	Declines slightly
Specific gravity	1.032	1.024
Blood		
Hemoglobin	*Men:* 13–18 g/100 mL	*Men:* 10–17 g/100 mL
	Women: 12–16 g/100 mL	*Women:* No change
Leukocytes	4300–10,800/mm^3	3100–9000/mm^3
Lymphocytes	T: 500–2500/mm^3	Declines
	B: 50–200/mm^3	Declines
Platelets		Increased platelet release factors, decreased granular consistency, no change in absolute number
Beta globulin	2.3–3.5 g/100 mL	Increases slightly
Sodium	135–145 mEq/L	134–147 mEq/L
Potassium	3.5–5.5 mEq/L	Increases slightly
Blood urea nitrogen (BUN)	*Men:* 10–25 mg/100 mL	69 mg/100 mL
	Women: 8–20 mg/100 mL	69 mg/100 mL
Creatinine	0.6–1.5 mg/100 mL	*Men:* 1.9 mg/100 mL
		Women: No change
Glucose tolerance (GTT)	1 h: 160–170 mg/100 mL	Rises faster in first 2 h, then declines more slowly
	2 h: 115–125 mg/100 mL	
	3 h: 70–110 mg/100 mL	
Triglycerides	40–150 mg/100 mL	20–200 mg/100 mL
Cholesterol	120–220 mg/100 mL	*Men:* Decreases after age 50
		Women: Increases from age 50–70, then decreases
Thyroxine (T$_4$)	4.5–13.5 µg/100 mL	Declines by 25%
Triiodothyronine (T$_3$)	90–220 mg/100 mL	Declines by 25%
Thyroid-stimulating hormone (TSH)	13–39 IU/L	Increases 8–10 IU/L
Creatinine kinase (CK)	17–48 U/L	Increases slightly
Lactate dehydrogenase (LDH)	45–90 U/L	Increases slightly

(Source: Gardner, 1989.)

information about symptomatology. In addition, the multiple concerns commonly voiced by older clients may make it difficult for the nurse to sort out relevant information and to complete a comprehensive assessment. Finally, older clients may have difficulty with the actual process of communication due to sensory or other neurologic deficits. In that case, the nurse may need to find alternate means of obtaining assessment data (eg, a 20-questions, yes–no approach or obtaining information from family members).

The Biophysical Dimension

Maturation and Aging.   Aging affects the function of all body systems. Many of the changes brought about by the aging process are contributing factors in health problems frequently experienced by older persons.

INTEGUMENTARY CHANGES.   Normal changes in the integumentary system include decreased skin turgor and perspiration and increased pigmentation. The hair thins, and nails grow more slowly. The thinning of scalp hair predisposes older individuals to sunburn. Sclerosis and loss of subcutaneous fat result in loss of skin elasticity and wrinkling. Concerns over body image due to increased skin pigmentation, loss of hair, and wrinkling may make some older adults susceptible to the claims of quackery in these areas. Nurses may want to explore what types of creams, lotions, or other treatments clients are using on hair and skin, as some of these products can cause damage and most are ineffective and expensive. Loss of skin elasticity also contributes to drooping lower eyelids and increased potential for conjunctivitis. Consequently, the nurse should be sure to assess the client's conjunctivae for signs of irritation.

Dry skin and increased skin fragility are other changes that may cause itching and contribute to skin injuries. Dry, itching skin may also contribute to loss of sleep at night. Decreased perspiration in older persons may predispose them to the effects of hyperthermia (Hogstel & Keen-Payne, 1993) and heat stroke.

CARDIOVASCULAR CHANGES.   Reduced cardiac reserves due to less efficient pump action of the heart result in a decreased ability to meet oxygen needs, leading to diminished physical abilities. Increased fatigue and diminished contractility of vessels resulting in orthostatic hypertension may predispose clients to falls. Systolic blood pressure rises, and the pulse pressure widens in the older adult, creating an increased risk for myocardial infarction. Peripheral vascular changes also include varicose veins and venous stasis.

RESPIRATORY CHANGES.   Structural changes in the respiratory system reduce the efficiency of the respiratory process. As alveolar sacs enlarge and lose their elasticity, they may rupture and fuse with adjacent sacs, resulting in greater residual volume. Arteriole changes lead to reduced gas exchange, and skeletal changes produced by osteoporosis and kyphosis can restrict chest movement, thus lowering vital capacity. All of these changes result in less efficient gas exchange and greater difficulty in meeting oxygen needs. Furthermore, slower mucus transport, reduced cough strength, and dysphagia increase the client's susceptibility to respiratory infection and choking due to aspiration of food.

GASTROINTESTINAL CHANGES.   Gastrointestinal system changes also affect the older adult's ability to maintain usual body function. As teeth wear down, the client may be less able to chew food properly. Decreased volume and acidity of saliva result in less moisture added to food and intolerance to some foods. Decreased salivation also results in dry mouth. Loss of taste buds may contribute to poor appetite and malnutrition.

As muscles in the mouth, cheeks, and tongue atrophy, older persons begin to require more time to eat and to speak. Thinning of the esophageal wall and a reduction in protective mucin, along with reduced peristalsis, may contribute to a sense of fullness or heartburn after eating. Reductions in hydrochloric acid content and enzyme production within the stomach may lead to decreased vitamin B_{12} levels and pernicious anemia. Calcium deposits within the lumen of arterial vessels may reduce the blood supply to the intestines and contribute to intestinal problems. Decreased muscle strength in the intestines can lead to formation of polyps and diverticuli. Many of these changes along with restricted activity, less sleep, and less dietary fiber contribute to constipation.

URINARY CHANGES.   In the urinary system, a reduction in the number of nephrons in the kidney results in a decreased ability to concentrate urine and a need to urinate more frequently. Renal arteriole constriction due to arteriosclerosis leads to decreased filtration. In younger persons, the kidneys automatically lower filtration rates at night. In older persons, however, decreased filtration rates have already reduced kidney efficiency so that this physiologic change no longer occurs. For this reason, many older persons normally experience one or more episodes of nocturia per night. Frequent episodes of nocturia are cause for concern because urinary tract infection is a common occurrence among older clients, especially older women, due to decreased acidity. Nocturia also increases the risk of falls and insomnia (Kennie, 1993).

REPRODUCTIVE CHANGES.   The reproductive system in both male and female clients is also subject to the effects of aging. In the woman, ovarian atrophy leads to an increased potential for development of cysts. Aging also brings about further reductions in progesterone and estrogen levels begun in the fourth and fifth decades of life, respectively. Other reproductive changes in the woman include reduction in uterine size and thickness of uterine walls, loss of subcutaneous fat in external genitalia, loss of pubic and axillary hair, and drooping of breast tissue.

In the man, there is a decrease in the number of sperm produced and changes in the size and shape of sperm, resulting in decreased potential for fertilization. Decreased testosterone levels also occur. Erectile impotence is not a normal consequence of aging; however, erections may take longer to achieve and the refractory period between erections is prolonged in older males.

For both men and women, a reduction in the frequency of intercourse seems to result in lowered response levels. Clients who maintain sexual activity on a regular basis do not appear to experience any loss of libido. The extent of activity, however, is highly dependent on one's psychology and on conditions in the social environment. The sexual changes that occur with aging may have a detrimental effect on a client's self-image. As discussed in Chapter 22, male impotence is a relatively common problem that may distress both older and younger men.

MUSCULOSKELETAL CHANGES.   In the musculoskeletal system, reductions in muscle tone and size usually lead to avoidance of heavy activity. Decreased range of motion in joints affects posture, gait, balance, and skeletal flexibility, thus increasing the potential for falls and injury. The kyphosis that occurs with aging leads to diminished stature and poor use of respiratory muscles, which predisposes clients to respiratory infection. Breakdown of chondrocytes in joint cartilage leads to osteoarthritis with consequent pain, reduced mobility, and diminished ability to accomplish activities of daily living.

▶ COMMON PHYSICAL HEALTH PROBLEMS AMONG OLDER CLIENTS

Cardiovascular System
- Angina
- Atherosclerosis
- Congestive heart failure
- Hypertension
- Myocardial infarction

Gastrointestinal System
- Constipation
- Diverticulosis
- Fecal impaction
- Gallbladder disease
- Hemorrhoids
- Hiatal hernia

Hematopoietic System
- Anemia

Integumentary System
- Basal cell carcinoma
- Decubitus ulcers
- Herpes zoster infection
- Squamous cell carcinoma

Musculoskeletal System
- Arthritis
- Hip and other fractures
- Osteoporosis

Neurological System
- Alzheimer's disease
- Cerebrovascular accident
- Organic brain syndrome
- Parkinson's disease

Reproductive System—Female
- Breast cancer
- Cervical cancer
- Vaginitis

Reproductive System—Male
- Benign prostatic hypertrophy
- Impotence
- Prostatic cancer

Respiratory System
- Emphysema
- Influenza
- Pneumonia
- Tuberculosis

Urinary System
- Bladder cancer
- Incontinence
- Urinary tract infection

NEUROLOGICAL CHANGES.   Neurological changes also occur with age. The slower pace of electrical impulses in the brain reduces sensory ability and slows reaction time, thus increasing the potential for injury. Increased reaction time affects mental as well as physical responses. Intelligence is not diminished, but increased reaction time leads to decreased performance in some mental skills, although some research has indicated similar and even better performance on age-relevant mental tasks for older than younger persons.

Changes in sensory function are particularly noticeable in older clients. Problems with vision may result from changes in focal accommodation, cataracts, and decreased color sensitivity. Older persons also take longer to adapt to change in light, which makes nighttime activities such as driving and moving about the home in darkness particularly dangerous. Reduction in lacrimation results in dry eyes and, combined with lid inversion or the drooping of eyelids mentioned earlier, contributes to irritation and conjunctivitis.

Hearing becomes less acute, particularly for higher-pitched sounds. Cerumen becomes more tenacious and tends to block the ear canal, further reducing the ability to hear. Hearing loss can result in social isolation and withdrawal from interpersonal interaction. Reductions in the senses of taste and smell may add to loss of appetite and lead to inadequate nutrition. Because eating is also a social function, loss of appetite may further impair social interaction. Finally, reduced sense of touch can increase an older person's potential for injury.

DEVELOPMENTAL ISSUES.   The developmental issues faced by many older adults are another aspect of maturation. Some of these issues include adjustment to diminished health and strength, devaluation of social roles, a meaningless daily routine, and reduced autonomy and independence. Other potential developmental issues for the elderly include loneliness, self-absorption, and fear of chronic illness. In assessing an older client, the community health nurse should try to determine the extent to which such issues are a problem and their effects on the client's health and quality of life.

Retirement and preparation for death are two other developmental issues that merit special attention. Retirement is an event avidly anticipated by many, but for some older clients retirement is a source of stress. This stress may be of two different types, retirement transition stress and retirement state stress (Bosse, Levenson, Spiro, Aldwin, & Mroczek, 1992). *Retirement transition stress* occurs during the first year of retirement and is created by the retirement event itself. Retirees who are more extroverted or whose retirement was unplanned or involuntary tend to experience this form of retirement stress and frequently respond with depression. People who experience significant stress on the job are less likely to experience transition stress than those with less stressful occupations.

Retirement state stress is a long-term effect of retirement created by the daily hassles of retired life (eg, boredom, reduced income). State stress occurs more often among extroverts, persons with high general energy levels, and those in white collar occupations. Experience of a variety of life crisis events prior to retirement is associated with both retirement transition stress and retirement state stress. The community health nurse should assess older clients' responses to retirement and the presence of either transition stress or state stress.

Preparing for death is a developmental task of the "old old" age group (people over age 85), but may be a significant issue for others with serious or terminal health conditions. In this area, the community health nurse considers the client's attitude toward death and acceptance of the inevitability of death, as well as the extent to which clients have put their affairs in order. Knowledge of the client's belief or nonbelief in an afterlife also enables the nurse to effectively assist clients with this task. Other issues that the nurse might explore with clients are provision of a durable power of attorney delegating to a significant other the power to make health-related decisions in the event of the client's incapacitation and the making of funeral arrangements. The nurse determines whether or not the client has made such arrangements or desires to do so.

Physiologic Function.   In addition to assessing clients for commonly occurring age-related changes and their effects and developmental issues, community health nurses should assess older clients for the presence of acute and chronic illnesses. Although most older persons are in basically good health, 80% of those over 65 have one or more chronic conditions (Schlenker, 1993).

Assessment for the presence of acute and chronic conditions is best done using a systems approach. Nurses should keep in mind that, when assessing clients for signs of these conditions, symptomatology may differ markedly in younger and older persons. For example, older persons with pneumonia may not exhibit pain or fever, but only confusion and restlessness. Similarly, emphysema may present with weakness, weight loss, and loss of appetite.

Cardiovascular problems are also frequently encountered in the elderly. Myocardial infarction in the older person can occur without symptoms or with only jaw pain or a vague indigestion. Congestive heart failure is also seen relatively frequently, manifesting with confusion, insomnia, wandering at night, peripheral and presacral edema, cough, distended neck veins, and rapid increase in weight. Other cardiovascular problems to be considered include hypertension, angina, and anemias. Hypertension may be evidenced by a dull headache, difficulties with memory, and epistaxis. Angina may only be signaled by vague discomfort after meals.

Anemia may be related to iron-deficient diet, chronic blood loss, or inability to absorb vitamin B_{12} (pernicious anemia). The nurse should assess the client for weakness and fatigue and, in the case of pernicious anemia, for sore tongue and numbness and tingling of the extremities. A thorough diet history should also be obtained and evidence of any bleeding (eg, bleeding gums or blood in the stool) should be sought.

Urinary incontinence is common among older adults, with as many as 15 to 30% of noninstitutionalized people over age 60 affected (Division of Chronic Disease Control and Community Intervention, 1995b). Incontinence may be either acute or chronic. Acute urinary incontinence is a short-term problem with a relatively sudden onset, whereas chronic incontinence is an ongoing problem. Causes of acute incontinence include urinary tract infections, fecal impaction or severe constipation, prostatic hypertrophy, and use of medications (eg, diuretics, tranquilizers, sedatives). Chronic urinary incontinence may be categorized as stress incontinence, urge incontinence, overflow incontinence, or functional incontinence. *Stress incontinence* is involuntary loss of urine in response to pressure exerted on the bladder with coughing, laughing, and sneezing. Urge incontinence involves urine leakage accompanied by a sudden and severe urge to urinate. Overflow incontinence is involuntary loss of urine resulting from overdistention of the bladder and may be characterized by frequent or constant dribbling or manifestations of urge or stress incontinence

(McCormick, Newman, Colling, & Pearson, 1992). Finally, functional incontinence is incontinence due to organic problems existing outside the genitourinary system. Causes of functional incontinence may involve physiologic dysfunction such as neurological trauma or cognitive dysfunction as in organic brain syndrome. In addition to being distressful in itself, urinary incontinence is a risk factor for skin breakdown. Both incontinence and nocturia have been associated with fall-related injuries.

Reproductive system problems in older women include vaginitis with discharge or vaginal soreness and itching. Vaginal prolapse may also occur as evidenced by protrusion, low back pain, and pelvic pulling. Another problem that may occur as a result of scanty vaginal lubrication is dyspareunia, or painful intercourse (Gibson, 1992).

Osteoporosis is a common musculoskeletal problem among older women. This condition causes increased porosity and fragility of bones, contributing to 850,000 fractures a year and costing $13.8 billion in 1995 (National Center for Chronic Disease Prevention and Health Promotion, 1996). More than 300,000 hip fractures occur in the elderly each year, and one fourth of these fracture victims die within a year (Wolinsky, Fitzgerald, & Stump, 1997). Wrist fractures and compression fractures of the spine are also common occurrences (Galsworthy, 1996). The potential for osteoporosis increases with chronically low calcium intake, lack of exercise, smoking, alcohol abuse, and underweight.

Problems commonly encountered in the neurological system include cerebrovascular accidents, Parkinson's disease, and acute or chronic organic brain disease. Cognitive impairment in the elderly has been associated with depression (Devanand, et al., 1996), mid-life hypertension (Launer, Masaki, Petrovitch, Foley, & Havlik, 1995), and genetic predisposition to Down syndrome (Schupf, Kapell, Lee, Ottman, & Mayeux, 1994). Ten percent of persons over 65 years of age and 47% of those over 85 have Alzheimer's disease (Kindig & Carnes, 1993). It has been predicted that by the year 2000 Alzheimer's disease will be the most common health problem in the United States. This condition frequently presents with memory loss and disorientation, leading to confusion and sometimes to wandering. Some clients with Alzheimer's become severely depressed or begin to hallucinate. As the disease progresses, clients become more and more in need of complete care.

There are four major categories of Alzheimer's effects including cognitive or intellectual losses, personality changes, loss of the ability to plan, and progressive lowering of the stress threshold. Of these, personality changes and lower stress threshold leading to violence, anxiety, and agitation may be the most difficult aspects of the disease for family members.

The disease itself progresses in a series of stages, although progression from one stage to another is neither uniform nor predictable. In the first stage, the client is forgetful, realizes this, and attempts to compensate. The second stage is characterized by increasing confusion, diminished capability for performing instrumental activities of daily living such as shopping and housekeeping, and need for moderate supervision. In the third stage, the client is said to have "ambulatory dementia"; he or she is still mobile but has lost most capabilities for performing basic activities of daily living. In the fourth, or terminal, stage, the client is incapable of ambulation or volitional activity. He or she has forgotten such basic skills as swallowing and chewing and eventually dies of malnutrition or the results of other hazards of immobility (Kindig & Carnes, 1993).

The Psychological Dimension

Examination of factors in the psychological dimension includes assessing the client's psychological health status and related problems. A psychological assessment involves considering the client's cognitive and affective status. In assessing the client's cognitive status, the nurse evaluates long- and short-term memory and orientation, powers of concentration and judgment, and ability to engage in mathematical calculations. Considerations in the assessment of affective status include the presence of depression, dementia, and saddened mood states. Commonly noted psychological problems among older adults are confusion, depression, and grief. Information to be obtained in assessing clients for depression includes anniversary dates, recent changes in relationships, changes in physical health status or sleep patterns, fatigue, guilt, social isolation, alterations in mood or behavior, depressive symptoms such as depressed affect and apathy, history of depression, and recent losses or crises (Valente, 1994). Depression in the elderly may manifest in one of several forms: apathy, worry and agitation, somatization, or paranoia and resentment of others for failing to help. Older clients with depressive personalities have displayed a negative attitude throughout life that continues in later adulthood. Those with an existential form of depression frequently display no symptoms, but decide that life is no longer worth living and commit suicide (Satin, 1994).

It is particularly important for the nurse working with older clients to distinguish depression from signs of delirium. In one study, nearly half of older persons referred for psychiatric treatment for depression were found to be delirious (Farrell & Ganzini, 1995). Delirium usually has a rapid onset and is characterized by limited attention span and ability to concentrate, disorganized thinking, diminished consciousness, disorientation, increased or decreased psychomotor activity, or perceptual difficulties (eg, hallucinations). Potential causes of delirium include adverse or toxic effects of medications, infection (eg, urinary tract infection), electrolyte imbalance, small strokes, poor oxygenation, myocardial infarction, increased or decreased blood sugar levels, or hypotension. Delirium is usually reversible once the cause is eliminated, but may pose a medical emergency and requires prompt referral for treatment (Kindig & Carnes, 1993).

It is also important to keep in mind that sensory deficits may interfere with the assessment of psychological status and that such deficits must be compensated for to obtain an accurate assessment. To compensate for sensory deficits, the nurse should face the client, eliminate background noise, provide good lighting, speak clearly and slowly, and keep questions short.

The nurse should also try to reduce the client's anxiety, as this may interfere with obtaining an accurate picture of the client's abilities. The nurse can help to reduce anxiety by establishing rapport, explaining the purpose of the psychological evaluation, providing privacy, and limiting distractions. Other factors that may affect a psychological assessment include the client's use of medications, communication impairments, ethnic and cultural differences, and language barriers. Nurses may want to validate their findings regarding an older client's psychological status with family members to be sure that findings are consistent with typical behavior and not the product of the present situation.

The client's psychological status may be affected by abuse by family members. This is an area in which the nurse's careful observation, assessment, and documentation are essential. Nurses should assess clients for signs of both physical and psychological abuse or neglect. Signs of physical abuse include injuries with questionable explanations, poor hygiene, and poor nutritional status. Psychological abuse is more difficult to determine, but the nurse should observe family interactions with the client. Some signs of abuse or neglect might include social isolation, lack of needed assistance with activities of daily living, evidence of tampering with the client's finances, and failure to assist the older person to maintain his or her independence. Failure of family members to visit institutionalized clients may also indicate neglect, a milder form of elder abuse. Many states have laws requiring mandatory reporting of the abuse of older persons, and community health nurses may be called on to make reports and present testimony in abuse cases. For this reason, the nurse should carefully document all findings when assessing the client, including reports by the client and significant others explaining bruises, burns, or other possible indicators of abuse.

Suicide is a relatively common result of psychological stress, particularly among elderly, white men. In 1992, nearly 20% of suicides in the United States occurred among people 65 years of age and older (Division of Violence Prevention, 1996). Potential suicide victims have been characterized by marriage, having several siblings, retirement, low income, recent loss of a close friend or relative, social isolation, chronic sleep problems, somatic illness associated with pain, depression, and feelings of uselessness. In many instances, suicide victims have been seen by health care providers within a month of committing suicide, suggesting a failure of health care professionals to identify risk factors for suicide (Mellick, Buckwalter, & Stolley, 1992). Suicide in the elderly has also been associated with a diagnosis of cancer, moderate to heavy alcohol use, and mental illness (Grabbe, Demi, Camann, & Potter, 1997). Older clients are more likely than younger people to be successful in suicide attempts, in part because of the use of more lethal methods (Satin, 1994).

The Physical Dimension

Physical dimension concerns with older clients include the adequacy of housing, the existence of safety hazards in the home or community, and the availability of necessary goods and services. The community health nurse assesses the adequacy of living conditions to meet clients' needs. For example, do living arrangements provide adequate space? Is there provision for privacy for the older person? Are living quarters adequately heated and ventilated? The nurse would also note whether there are adequate facilities for food storage and preparation.

A major concern in the assessment of the older client's physical environment is the presence of safety hazards. The community health nurse notes the presence of stairs, rugs, or other objects that might lead to falls and injuries. The nurse also assesses the adequacy of lighting and the presence or absence of tub rails and other safety features. Because of poor circulation, many older clients frequently feel cold and may use space heaters or kerosene stoves that present safety hazards. (See Appendix D, Home Safety Assessment—Older Adult.)

The neighborhood is another area of concern. Are fire and police services adequate to meet the needs of older clients? Is the neighborhood safe? Is transportation available if needed? Finally, does the older person have access to shopping facilities and health care providers within a reasonable distance?

The Social Dimension

In the social dimension, the nurse assesses the client's social network and the extent of available social support. The client's *social network* is the web of social relationships within which the client interacts with other people and from which he or she receives social support. Social support includes emotional, instrumental, or financial assistance that the client receives from the social network.

In assessing the client's social network, the community health nurse identifies those persons with whom the client has frequent contact and whom the client feels able to call on for assistance. The nurse also explores with the client the types and adequacy of support available from members of the social network.

Institutionalization is another important consideration in the social assessment of the client. For many clients there is a need to determine whether institutional care is appropriate. Families caring for older members may need assistance in making such a determination. There is also a need to decide what type of institution is appropriate based on the extent of self-care in which the client can engage. Is placement in a nursing home appropriate? Or would the client do as well or better in a retirement community? Whatever the choice, the institutionalized client needs assistance in adjusting to altered living circumstances. Nurses should assess the extent of the client's adjustment to the institution and attempt to assist in that adjustment. Research has indicated that institutionalization may not necessarily reduce the burden of care for family caregivers and may actually increase emotional stress for family members (Dellasega, 1991). For this reason, the nurse should carefully assess the needs of both client and caregivers relative to the decision to institutionalize.

Another potential source of stress in the social environment is care of grandchildren. With increases in substance abuse, poverty, homelessness, and AIDS, more and more older Americans are faced with the task of raising their grandchildren. In 1993, 360,000 children were in foster care, most frequently with family members, particularly grandparents. The acquisition of a second family at a time when many people look forward to slowing down and need to give more attention to their own health may create considerable stress. In one study, care of grandchildren led to social isolation and loss of important social roles that contributed to increased stress in elderly caregivers (Kelly, 1993).

Poverty is another social dimension factor that can profoundly affect the health of older adults. In 1994, almost 12% of people over the age of 65 had incomes below the poverty level, and nearly 14% of those 75 years of age and older were poor (U.S. Department of Commerce, 1996). Reduced income leads to decreased access to health care as well as reduced ability to provide for necessities such as nutrition and housing.

The elderly are more financially vulnerable than other segments of the population for several reasons. Many older clients are without health insurance, in spite of the Medicare program, and may not be able to afford the cost of health care for catastrophic or chronic conditions. In 1994, for example, approximately 1% of the population over 65 years of age had no health insurance coverage (U.S. Department of Commerce, 1996). Older clients also tend to have fixed incomes that do not allow for increases in the cost of living, particularly increased housing costs. In addition, many older persons lack the financial assets to support long-term care if needed. Finally, the Social Security benefits received by many older clients are inadequate for meeting their needs but make them ineligible for many other forms of financial assistance (Barusch, 1994). One of the major effects of poverty among the elderly is a growing rate of homelessness in older age groups. In Boston, for example, the proportion of elderly among the homeless increased by 50% in a 2-year period (Bissonnette & Hijjazi, 1994).

The community health nurse should assess the adequacy of the client's income for meeting basic needs as well as special needs arising from specific health conditions (eg, the ability to pay for prescription medications). The nurse can also assess clients' abilities to budget their money and prioritize expenditures.

Family interactions are another consideration in the social dimension of elderly clients. As noted earlier, impaired family interactions may lead to abuse of older members or grandparents assuming responsibility for the care of grandchildren. Another area that may affect the health of older clients is the loss of loved ones, particularly a spouse. Older men typically are married until they die, but approximately half of older women are widows (Schlenker, 1993). Among those men who do become widowers, most remarry and experience greater longevity than those who do not remarry and men whose wives are still living. Because older women outnumber men, they have less opportunity for remarriage after the death of a spouse and may seek other types of opportunities for companionship and sexual gratification including affairs with married men, with much older or much younger men, or even with other women. These alternative relationships, as well as remarriage, are frequently resisted by grown children and may lead to family strife and conflict (Gibson, 1992).

One final aspect of the social dimension to be addressed is occupation. Although many older clients will be retired, many more are continuing employment at later ages than was previously the case, particularly among the "young" elderly. For example, it is estimated that between 1990 and 2005, the number of working men aged 55 to 64 years will increase 43% and the number of working women will increase 65%. This aging of the work force has implications for occupational injury incidence which tends to increase with age (Zwerling, Sprince, Wallace, Davis, Whitten, & Heeringa, 1996).

The Behavioral Dimension

Considerations to be addressed in the behavioral dimension include diet, exercise, personal habits including medication use, sexuality, and the client's level of independence and ability to perform activities of daily living. With respect to diet, the nurse should assess eating patterns and the adequacy of nutritional intake. Overall nutritional status, as well as intake of specific nutrients, is an important consideration. Both underweight and overweight increase mortality risks. In fact, older persons who are 25 to 35% underweight are at greater risk of death than those who are proportionally over their desired weight (Schlenker, 1993).

Older persons may have diets deficient in a variety of nutrients. In one study of Medicare recipients, 38% of older persons received less than three fourths of the recommended daily allowance (RDA) for three or more nutrients (Posner, Jette, Smith, & Miller, 1993). In the Health and Nutrition Examination Survey (HANES), a periodic national survey of health and nutrition status, none of the participants aged 65 to 75 years met the RDA for any vitamin, and as many as 50% did not even get two thirds of the RDA for thiamine, riboflavin, niacin, and vitamin C (Russell, 1992). In another study, protein intake was deficient in 50% of older clients (Payette, Gray-Donald, Cyr, & Boutier, 1995).

Even those clients who do obtain the RDA for most nutrients may have nutritional deficiencies. Research has indicated that changes in vitamin metabolism occurring with age increase daily needs for vitamins D, B_6, and B_{12} above the RDA for other age groups. Vitamin A requirements, on the other hand, decline with advancing age (Russell, 1992). The diets of older adults are most likely to be deficient in calcium, zinc, potassium, folates, fiber, and complex carbohydrates, as well as vitamins, and too high in fats, refined sugars, and sodium (Van Stavesen, Burema, De Groot, & Vorrips, 1992).

Some elderly clients may go for periods without eating at all. In one study of meal program recipients, as many as 17% of older clients reported not eating for one or more days prior to starting the program. Factors associated with not eating included living alone, multiple health problems, and limited mobility. Additional contributing factors included nausea and poor appetite, diarrhea, and difficulty swallowing (Frongillo, Rauschenbach, Roe, & Williamson, 1992). The nurse should also evaluate compliance with specific dietary recommendations. Many clients need to restrict sodium intake or increase calcium. The older client with diabetes may or may not comply with a diabetic diet. Particular attention should be given to the amount of fluid and fiber in the diet.

Nurses should also explore with clients how foods are prepared and by whom. Many older clients have inadequate diets because they are not physically able to prepare some foods. Other problems impeding nutrition include lack of adequate cooking facilities, difficulties in chewing or swallowing, and poor dietary habits throughout life. In addition to assessing dietary intake, therefore, the nurse needs to identify factors contributing to poor nutritional status.

Exercise is another lifestyle factor addressed in a comprehensive assessment. In the 1992 Behavioral Risk Factor Surveillance System (BRFSS) survey, the percentage of people over age 65 who engaged in no leisure time physical activity ranged from 27 to 62% in various states, with a median of 38.5% (Division of Chronic Disease Control and Community Intervention, 1995a). Many older clients mistakenly believe that their need for exercise diminishes with age. Lack of exercise, however, has been associated with many of the physiologic changes experienced by the elderly as well as the development of specific health problems (Kennie, 1993). Research has shown that moderate to high levels of recreational activity in the elderly are associated with decreased mortality and maintenance of functional status (Young, Masaki, & Curb, 1995). Furthermore, low- to moderate-intensity exercise has actually resulted in improved functional ability and sleep patterns in older adults (Hunger, et al., 1995; King, Oman, Brassington, Bliwise, & Haskell, 1997). Again, the nurse should assess not only the extent of exercise but also factors that impede adequate exercise such as pain, fatigue, and weakness.

One of the consequences of most chronic illnesses is the need for prolonged use of medication. Consequently, community health nurses assessing older clients with chronic illnesses need to assess medication use carefully. The large majority of the noninstitutionalized elderly use an average of two to

EVALUATING MEDICATION USE IN OLDER CLIENTS

- Is the client taking prescribed medications?
- Is the client taking over-the-counter (OTC) medications?
- Are any of the client's medications contraindicated by existing health conditions?
- Do OTC medications potentiate or counteract prescription medications?
- Do prescription medications potentiate or counteract each other?
- Does the client take prescription and OTC medications as directed (eg, correct dose, route, time)?
- Does the client comply with other directions regarding medications (eg, not taking with dairy products)?
- Is the client aware of potential food–drug interactions or drug–drug interactions?
- Are medications achieving the desired effects?
- Is the client experiencing any medication side effects?
- What is the client doing about medication side effects, if any?
- Is the client exhibiting symptoms of any adverse medication effects?

three prescription drugs daily in addition to a variety of over-the-counter medications. The number and the variety of drugs increase the potential for drug toxicity and drug interactions.

Nurses need to assess older clients to determine what medications they take, when and how these medications are taken, and the client's knowledge of side effects and signs of toxicity. Nurses should also explore with clients their use of nonprescription drugs and acquaint them with those that are contraindicated by their health status or because of other medications they are taking. Clients should also be assessed for signs of side effects or toxicity. Several drugs that pose health hazards for older clients are presented in Table 23–4.

Nurses should determine the extent to which clients engage in other personal habits such as smoking, drinking, and caffeine consumption as well as the extent of motivation to change such habits. Nonsmoking and moderate alcohol intake are two factors found to be highly predictive of healthy aging. Despite the evidence that nonsmoking promotes health, 13.5% of men and 10.5% of women over age 65 smoke (U.S. Department of Commerce, 1996). Caffeine consumption is another personal habit to be addressed. Occult caffeine in medications has also been implicated in sleep problems among the elderly (Brown, et al., 1995).

TABLE 23–4. INAPPROPRIATE DRUGS FOR OLDER CLIENTS

ANALGESICS/NSAIDS
Indomethacin (Indocin)
Pentazocine (Talwin)
Phenylbutazone (Butazolidin)
Propoxyphene (Darvon, Darvocet)

ANTI-ANXIETY AGENTS
Chlordiazepoxide (Librium)
Diazepam (Valium)
Flurazepam (Dalmane)
Meprobamate (Equanil, Miltown)
Pentobarbital (Nembutal)
Secobarbital (Seconal)

ANTIDEPRESSANTS
Amitriptyline (Elavil, Triavil, Etrafon)
Doxepin (Sinequan)
Imipramine (Tofranil)
Nortriptyline (Pamelor, Aventyl)

ANTIEMETICS
Trimethobenzamide (Tigan)

ANTIHYPERTENSIVES
Propranolol (Inderal)
Methyldopa (Aldomet, Amodopa, Dopamet)
Reserpine (Novoreserpine)

ANTISPASMODICS
Cyclobenzaprine (Flexeril)
Methocarbamol (Robaxin)
Carisprodol (Soma)
Orphenadrine (Banflex, Norflex, Neocyten)

HYPOGLYCEMICS
Chlorpropamide (Diabinese)

VASODILATORS
Dipyridamole (Persantine)

(Sources: Delong, 1995; Lee, 1996; Willcox, Himmelstein, & Woolhandler, 1994.)

Alcohol abuse is one more concern that may be identified in the elderly population. Both alcohol abuse and abuse of other drugs occur in two forms in the elderly population, prior abusers who are aging and older adults who seek escape from loneliness, depression, and social isolation (Satin, 1994). Because of metabolic changes, detoxification of alcohol, as well as other substances, is slowed, making the older person increasingly susceptible to the toxic effects of alcohol. Older individuals may also take a number of medications that interact with alcohol, thus increasing the dangers of abuse. Alcohol contributes to deleterious effects on a number of body systems that may already be impaired by age and chronic disease. For example, a definite

► EVALUATING ACTIVITIES OF DAILY LIVING

BASIC ACTIVITIES OF DAILY LIVING

Feeding
- Can the client feed him- or herself?
- Does the client have difficulty chewing?
- Does the client have difficulty swallowing?

Bathing
- Can the client get into or out of the bathtub or shower?
- Can the client manipulate soap and wash cloth?
- Can the client wash his or her hair without assistance?
- Can the client effectively dry all body parts?

Dressing
- Can the client remember what articles of clothing should be put on first?
- Can the client dress him- or herself?
- Can the client bend and reach to put on shoes and stockings?
- Can the client manipulate buttons and zippers?
- Are modifications in clothing required to facilitate dressing (eg, front opening dresses)?
- Is arm and shoulder movement adequate to put on and remove sleeves?
- Can the client comb his or her hair?
- Can the client apply make-up if desired?

Toileting
- Is the client mobile enough to reach the bathroom?
- Is there urgency that may lead to incontinence?
- Can the client remove clothing in order to urinate or defecate?
- Can the client position him- or herself on or in front of the toilet?
- Can the client lift from a sitting position on the toilet?
- Is the client able to effectively clean him- or herself after urinating or defecating?
- Can the client replace clothing after urinating or defecating?

Transfer
- Is the client able to get from a lying to a sitting position unassisted?
- Is the client able to stand from a sitting position without support or assistance?
- Is the client able to sit or lie down without help?

INSTRUMENTAL ACTIVITIES OF DAILY LIVING

Shopping
- Is the client able to transport him- or herself to shopping facilities?
- Can the client navigate within a shopping facility?
- Can the client lift products from shelves?
- Can the client effectively handle money?
- Can the client carry purchases from store to car and from car to home?
- Is the client able to store purchases appropriately?

Laundry
- Can the client collect dirty clothes for washing?
- Is the client able to sort clothes to be washed from those to be dry cleaned?
- Can the client sort clothes by color?
- Can the client access laundry facilities?
- Can the client manipulate containers of soap, bleach, etc.?
- Can the client lift wet clothing from washer to dryer?
- Is the client able to hang or fold clean clothes as needed?
- Can the client put clean clothing in closets or drawers?

Cooking
- Is the client capable of planning well-balanced meals?
- Can the client safely operate kitchen utensils and appliances (eg, stove, can opener, knives)?
- Can the client reach dishes, pots, and pans needed for cooking and serving food?
- Can the client clean vegetables and fruits, chop foods, etc.?
- Is the client able to carry prepared foods to the table?

Housekeeping
- Can the client identify the need for housecleaning chores (eg, when the bathtub needs to be cleaned)?
- Is the client able to do light housekeeping (eg, dusting, vacuuming, cleaning toilet)?
- Is the client able to do heavy chores (eg, scrub floors, wash windows)?
- Is the client able to do yard maintenance if needed?

Taking Medication
- Can the client remember to take medications as directed?
- Is the client able to open medication bottles?
- Can the client swallow oral medication, administer injections, etc., as needed?

Managing Money
- Can the client effectively budget his or her income?
- Is the client able to write checks?
- Can the client balance a checking account?
- Can the client remember to pay bills when due and record payment?

▶ EVALUATING ACTIVITIES OF DAILY LIVING (cont.)

ADVANCED ACTIVITIES OF DAILY LIVING

Social Activity

- Does the client have a group of people with whom he or she can socialize?
- Is the client able to transport him- or herself to social events?
- Can the client see and hear well enough to interact socially with others?
- Does the client tire too easily to engage in social activities?
- Is social interaction impeded by fears of incontinence or embarrassment over financial difficulties?

Occupation

- Can the client carry out occupational responsibilities as needed?

Recreation

- Does the client have the physical strength and mobility to engage in desired recreational pursuits?
- Does the client have the financial resources to engage in desired recreational pursuits?
- Does the client have a group of people with whom to engage in recreation?
- Does the client have access to recreational activities (eg, transportation)?

---

dose–response relationship exists between the amount of alcohol ingested and blood pressure. For the client who is already hypertensive, alcohol abuse compounds the problem and impedes hypertension control.

The meeting of sexual needs is another important, but often overlooked, component of the assessment of social function. As noted earlier, older clients continue to have sexual needs. These may be fulfilled by a spouse if the couple is afforded the privacy necessary for sexual activity. For example, if older parents live with their children, their opportunities for sexual intimacy may be somewhat limited. The same may be true of older people in institutional settings. For clients who have no living spouse or whose spouse is unable to meet these needs, alternative methods of meeting sexual needs include masturbation and fantasizing.

Because most older people grew up in an era when sexuality was not a topic for discussion, they may find it difficult to talk about such needs with the nurse. Before addressing such intimate issues, the nurse should first develop a rapport with the client. The nurse should also assure clients that sexual problems are not uncommon. For the older male client, the nurse should be aware that many of the medications taken for chronic illnesses, especially antihypertensives, may cause impotence.

Nurses should assess clients for problems with sexuality and identify any underlying factors. Nurses should also explore clients' satisfaction with their sex life. Another consideration in assessing this area is the potential for exposure to sexually transmitted diseases. Sexually transmitted diseases, including HIV infection, are a growing problem among older clients.

In 1994, for example, nearly 2000 new cases of AIDS were diagnosed in people over 60 years of age (U.S. Department of Commerce, 1996), and approximately 3% of all cases diagnosed by 1992 occurred in this age group (Gordon & Thompson, 1995). The incidence of syphilis is also increasing in this population (Berenstein & De Hertogh, 1992).

Nurses should also assess the environment of the older person to see whether it is conducive to sexual intimacy if this is desired. Finally, nurses should be aware of the potential for sexual abuse of older clients, particularly in institutional settings.

Older clients' functional status is the last area for consideration in lifestyle assessment. *Functional status* is the ability to perform tasks and fulfill expected social roles. Assessment of functional status includes exploration of abilities at three levels of task complexity: basic, intermediate or instrumental, and advanced activities of daily living. *Basic activities of daily living (BADLs)* are personal care activities and include abilities to feed, bathe, and dress oneself, and toileting and transfer skills (getting in or out of a chair or bed). Intermediate or *instrumental activities of daily living (IADLs)* are tasks of moderate complexity including household tasks such as shopping, laundry, cooking, and housekeeping, as well as abilities to take medications correctly, manage money, and use the telephone or public transportation. *Advanced activities of daily living (AADLs)* involve complex abilities to engage in voluntary social, occupational, or recreational activities (Reuben & Siu, 1992).

An estimated 10% of older persons living in the community experience physical limitations in ADLs (Gill, Williams, & Tinetti, 1995). Cognitive impairments are experienced by approximately 15% of older clients (Callahan, Hendrie, & Tierney, 1995). In 1994, people over 65 years of age reported an average of 35 days per person of restricted activity and 6 days per person of bed-disability (U.S. Department of Commerce, 1996). Conditions associated with disabilities in the elderly include obesity, arthritis, hip fracture, low back pain, diabetes, hypertension, heart disease, congestive heart failure, chronic obstructive pulmonary disease, leg cramps, depression, stroke, visual impairment, cancer, and cognitive deficits (Guiccione, et al., 1994). The community health nurse should be particularly alert to the potential for functional impairment in older clients with these conditions.

► ## EVALUATING COGNITIVE FUNCTION

ATTENTION SPAN
- Does the client focus on a single activity to completion?
- Does the client move from activity to activity without completing any?

CONCENTRATION
- Is the client able to answer questions without wandering from the topic?
- Does the client ignore irrelevant stimuli while focusing on a task?
- Is the client easily distracted from a subject or task by external stimuli?

INTELLIGENCE
- Does the client understand directions and explanations given in everyday language?
- Is the client able to perform basic mathematical calculations?

JUDGMENT
- Does the client engage in action appropriate to the situation?
- Are client behaviors based on an awareness of environmental conditions and possible consequences of action?
- Are the client's plans and goals realistic?
- Can the client effectively budget income?
- Is the client safe driving a car?

LEARNING ABILITY
- Is the client able to retain instructions for a new activity?
- Can the client recall information provided?
- Is the client able to correctly demonstrate new skills?

MEMORY
- Is the client able to remember and describe recent events in some detail?
- Is the client able to describe events from the past in some detail?

ORIENTATION
- Can the client identify him- or herself by name?
- Is the client aware of where he or she is?
- Does the client recognize the identity and function of those around them?
- Does the client know what day and time it is?
- Is the client able to separate past, present, and future?

PERCEPTION
- Are the client's responses appropriate to the situation?
- Does the client exhibit evidence of hallucinations or illusions?
- Are explanations of events consistent with the events themselves?
- Can the client reproduce simple figures?

PROBLEM SOLVING
- Is the client able to recognize problems that need resolution?
- Can the client envision alternative solutions to a given problem?
- Can the client weigh alternative solutions and select one appropriate to the situation?
- Can the client describe activities needed to implement the solution?

PSYCHOMOTOR ABILITY
- Does the client exhibit repetitive movements that interfere with function?

REACTION TIME
- Does the client take an unusually long time to respond to questions or perform motor activities?
- Does the client respond to questions before the question is completed?

SOCIAL INTACTNESS
- Are the client's interactions with others appropriate to the situation?
- Is the client able to describe behaviors appropriate and inappropriate to a given situation?

Mobility limitation is another factor contributing to functional impairment for older clients. The potential for mobility limitation increases with age. Factors affecting mobility include client's cognitive, sensory, cardiovascular, neurological, and musculoskeletal status. Consequences of immobility that affect functional status include diminished muscle strength and range of motion, sleep disturbances, changes in self-image and mood, and depression. Again, the community health nurse should be alert to the presence of mobility limitation and its consequences and its potential effects on older client's functional abilities.

Another consideration in assessing functional status is the older client's ability to function cognitively. Areas of cognitive function to be addressed include attention, concentration, intelligence, judgment, learning ability, memory, orientation, and perception. Other considerations related to cognitive function are problem solving and psychomotor abilities, reaction time, and social intactness (Ebersole & Hess, 1994). Specific questions that the nurse might ask in assessing cognitive function are presented on page 568.

The Health System Dimension

Health system dimension factors also influence the health of older clients. The advent of the Medicare program has improved elderly clients' access to health care services. In 1994, 75% of those aged 65 to 84 years had health insurance coverage under both Medicare and private insurance, and 67% of those over 85 years of age had dual coverage of this type. Other older clients may have combined coverage under Medicare and Medicaid (5%) or coverage under Medicare only (15%) (U.S. Department of Health and Human Services, 1996a); however, slightly less than 1% of American elderly had no health insurance coverage at all (U.S. Department of Commerce, 1996).

Even for those older people with health insurance coverage, preventive services are often neglected. Many health care providers do not see any point in prevention at the far end of the age continuum. For instance, older women often do not receive Pap smears or referrals for mammography (National Cancer Institute, 1996). Immunization is another often neglected preventive strategy in the elderly (Advisory Committee on Immunization Practices, 1995). In 1993, for example, only 50% of people over age 65 received influenza immunizations. Figures for pneumococcal immunization are even worse with fewer than 30% of this population immunized in 1993 (Adult Vaccine Preventable Disease Bureau, 1996).

In assessing the influence of health system factors on older clients' health, the community health nurse ascertains whether the client has a regular source of health care. Are health services sought to promote health as well as cure illness? Does the older client have adequate financial resources to afford health care? To what extent are health services used effectively? In addition to determining the source and adequacy of the client's health care funds, the community health nurse explores the distance to health facilities used and the means of transportation. Health care system factors and other factors affecting the health of older clients can be assessed using the Health Assessment Guide for the Older Client in Appendix O.

Diagnostic Reasoning and the Health Care Needs of Older Clients

Based on the data derived from the in-depth assessment of the older client's health status, the community health nurse derives nursing diagnoses or statements of health care needs that require nursing action. Nursing diagnoses may be derived relative to each of the areas of assessment described above. For example, the client may have problems related to the normal aging process such as constipation and dry skin. There may also be nursing diagnoses related to existing chronic and communicable diseases.

In addition, the client may encounter factors in the physical, psychological, or social dimensions that give rise to nursing diagnoses. For example, a nursing diagnosis related to the physical environment is "safety hazard due to loose handrail on stairs." "Feelings of worthlessness since retirement" and "social isolation due to death of family and friends" are sample nursing diagnoses related to the psychological and social dimensions.

Behavioral factors may also give rise to nursing diagnoses. The diagnosis "shortness of breath due to emphysema and smoking" indicates the contribution of smoking, a lifestyle behavior, to a physiologic problem. The nurse may also derive nursing diagnoses reflecting health care system factors, for example, "lack of health promotion services due to inadequate finances."

Planning the Dimensions of Health Care for Older Clients

Community health nurses must be particularly mindful to involve clients and their families in the planning of care. Because older clients are particularly vulnera-

ASSESSMENT TIPS: Assessing Older Clients' Health

Biophysical Dimension

Age

What is the client's age?

What physiologic effects of aging has the client experienced?

How has the client responded to the effects of aging and decreased function?

How has the client responded to events like retirement or approaching death?

Genetic Inheritance

Does the client have a family history of genetic predisposition to disease? If so, to what diseases?

Physiologic Function

Does the client have any chronic physical health problems? If so, what are they? How well are they controlled? What effects do these problems have on the client's quality of life?

Does the client exhibit any symptoms of acute health problems?

Does the client have sensory deficits that affect health?

Is the client experiencing urinary or fecal incontinence?

Does the client have any mobility limitations that increase the risk of falls?

Does the client have any evidence of Alzheimer's disease?

What is the client's immunization status?

Psychological Dimension

What is the extent of stress in the client's life? What conditions cause stress for the client?

What is the client's cognitive status? Is the client confused or disoriented?

What is the client's usual mood? Is he or she depressed? Suicidal?

Does the client have a history of mental illness? Is there any evidence of current mental illness?

Is the client anxious? What causes anxiety for the client?

Has the client recently lost spouse, friends, or relatives?

Physical Dimension

Where does the client live? Is he or she homeless? If housed, is housing safe and adequate to meet the client's needs?

Does the client's environment provide for privacy?

Are the client's living quarters adequately heated and cooled? Is there adequate ventilation?

Does the client use space heaters of kerosene stoves that present a fire hazard?

Is the lighting adequate for the client to see?

Are there adequate facilities for food storage and preparation?

Are there safety hazards in the client's environment? If so, what are they?

Does the client have to climb stairs? If so, do the stairs have railings in good repair?

Is the bathroom easily accessible to the client? Is it equipped with tub and shower rails?

Does the home have a smoke alarm?

Is the neighborhood safe? Are there shopping facilities accessible to the client?

Social Dimension

Interpersonal Relationships

Does the client live alone? If not, with whom does the client live?

What is the client's level of social interaction? With whom does the client interact?

What is the extent of the client's social support network? Is it adequate to meet the client's need for support? What kinds of support are available?

Is the client at risk for or experiencing abuse? If so, what form does the abuse take?

Is the client responsible for the care of grandchildren? If so, what is the effect of this responsibility on the client's health?

Who is responsible for the care of the client? Is the care provided adequate?

What is the quality of the client's interactions with family members?

Is the client married? divorced? widowed?

Socioeconomic Status

What is the client's education level?

What is the client's income? Is it adequate to meet his or her needs?

Is the client employed? If so, what is his or her occupation? Does the work setting pose health hazards for the client?

Is the client retired? What effect has retirement had on the client's life?

Does the client have access to transportation?

ASSESSMENT TIPS: Assessing Older Clients' Health (cont.)

Behavioral Dimension

Consumption Patterns

What are the client's usual food preferences and consumption patterns?

Who prepares food for the client? How are foods usually prepared?

Does the client have any difficulties in preparing or eating food?

What is the quality of the client's diet? Is his or her diet deficient in any particular nutrients?

Does the client smoke? Does he or she use alcohol or other drugs?

Is there evidence of substance abuse?

Exercise and Leisure Activity

What is the extent of the client's physical activity?

What are the client's rest and activity patterns?

Does the client get sufficient rest? Does he or she have difficulty sleeping?

What kind of leisure activities does the client pursue?

Do leisure activities pose any health hazards?

Medication Use

Does the client use any medications on a regular basis? If so what medications are used?

Is the client taking medications correctly?

Sexual Practices

Is the client sexually active? Are the client's sexual needs effectively met?

Does the client employ safe sexual practices?

Functional Status

What is the client's level of function? Is the client able to perform activities of daily living at all levels?

Health System Dimension

What is the client's usual source of health care?

To what extent does the client utilize health care services when needed?

Does the client receive routine screening and health promotion services?

How does the client finance health care? Does he or she have health insurance? Is it adequate to meet health needs?

Are health care services easily accessible to the client?

---

ble to loss of independence, their involvement in planning their own health care is an important way to foster their sense of independence. Client involvement in planning is also likely to enhance compliance with the plan. Planning to meet the health care needs of older clients may take place at the primary, secondary, and tertiary levels of prevention.

Whatever the level of prevention involved, health care for the elderly has three common goals: (1) improved functional ability, (2) increased longevity, and (3) increased comfort and decreased suffering (O'Malley & Blakeney, 1994). Interventions to achieve these goals should be systematic and may need to be innovative. Case management services are one approach to providing systematic and comprehensive care for older adults and has been shown to improve the health outcomes of recipients (Burns, Nichols, Graney, & Cloar, 1995). Because of older clients' increased health needs, diminished resources, and, occasionally, mobility limitations, innovative approaches to care may be required. For example, telephone care is one such innovation that can provide

many of the services needed by the elderly (Guy, 1995). Telephone care has the advantages of minimal access barriers, immediate access, and client acceptability. Telephone care is also cost-effective and can address many of the health problems of the population that makes the greatest use of health care services.

Primary Prevention

As with other groups of clients, the most cost-effective means of providing health care to older clients involves primary prevention—preventing health problems before they occur. Areas of concern in planning health promotion for older clients include nutrition, hygiene, safety, immunization, rest and exercise, maintaining independence, and preparing for death.

Nutrition. Adequate nutrition is important for the older person to maintain health and prevent disease and further effects of existing chronic conditions. Nurses can assist older clients in choosing a diet that helps them attain and maintain health.

Adequate nutrition for health promotion frequently entails a reduction in caloric intake. Caloric needs decrease roughly 7.5% for each decade after 25 years of age. Recommended daily caloric intake for women aged 50 to 75 years is approximately 1800 calories, whereas for women over 75, the recommendation is 1600 calories. For men, approximately 2400 calories per day are recommended from ages 50 to 75, dropping to 2050 calories daily after age 75. Of course, specific caloric needs vary from person to person, and the nurse should assess the needs of each individual client.

Despite reduced caloric needs, older adults continue to require a balance of all other nutrients. As noted earlier, nutritional deficits are most frequently noted for calcium, iron, vitamins A, D, and C, and the B vitamins riboflavin and thiamine, as well as for dietary fiber. Community health nurses can promote the health of older clients by encouraging diets high in these nutrients as well as other essential nutrients.

Older persons are frequent targets for food faddists promoting supplements. Unfortunately, dietary supplements are most often taken by those clients with relatively healthy diets who do not need them. Nurses can assist clients to obtain adequate nutrition by educating them regarding a well-balanced diet and can discourage expenditure of limited finances on dietary fads. Nurses can also educate clients as to the harmful nature of some food fads.

Other, more general interventions may also be needed to improve older client's nutritional status by eliminating impediments to good nutrition. For example, social isolation may need to be addressed because people tend to eat better in company with others. Older clients can be referred to senior meal programs or family members can be encouraged to drop by at meal times to eat with older clients who live alone. Interventions may also be required to deal with nausea, poorly fitting dentures, or other factors that may impede good nutrition (Phaneuf, 1996).

Hygiene. Promoting adequate hygiene is another aspect of health maintenance in the older adult. Skin care can be maintained by periodic bathing with mild soaps and the use of lotions to prevent drying and cracking of the skin. Clients should be discouraged from using water that is too hot and from using alcohol or powders that may further dry or irritate skin. Nails can be protected by a weekly manicure including a massage with oil and shaping with an emery board. Dry and split nails can also be prevented by advising the clients not the keep their hands in water

or to wear protective gloves while performing household cleaning chores.

Adequate hygiene and hydration can protect the older client's remaining teeth and prevent dry mouth. Special toothpastes (such as Sensodyne) may be needed by clients who have sensitive gums. Toothbrushes should be firm enough to clean teeth, but not so hard as to injure gums. Clients should be encouraged to use a softer toothbrush on their own remaining teeth than they use on dentures.

Community health nurses can also educate older clients on the care of their hair and protection from sunburn. Hair should be brushed and combed daily with a weekly shampoo and monthly conditioning. Care should be taken in the use of dyes or permanent solutions that may irritate fragile skin. Wearing a hat while outdoors will prevent sunburn due to thinning hair.

Wearing apparel may be another area for client education to promote health. Properly fitted clothing and shoes can prevent skin irritation and breakdown. Close-toed shoes and low heels are recommended for everyday wear. Shoes should always be worn with stockings and socks should be changed daily.

Safety. Three aspects of safety should be addressed when planning primary preventive measures for older clients: elimination of environmental hazards, home and neighborhood security, and prevention of elder abuse and neglect. Plans can be made to ensure the interior and exterior repair of the client's home. Modifications can be planned to accommodate special needs. For example, graduated ramps can replace steps to facilitate access by wheelchair or walker.

The community health nurse can also plan to educate older clients on home safety, and plans can be made to eliminate safety hazards in the home. All areas of the home, especially stairs, should be well lighted and furniture should be placed so as to prevent falls. Because many elders experience nocturia, they may need to be encouraged to keep a nightlight burning to avoid disorientation or falls in the dark. Or, the client can keep a flashlight close to the bed for nighttime use as needed.

Clients should be encouraged to keep electrical cords as short as possible and to tack them along baseboards to prevent tripping over them. If throw rugs must be used, they should be of the nonskid variety. Bathrooms can be equipped with tub rails or seats and hand-held shower fixtures to make bathing safer and less arduous for the older person.

The use of space heaters and other portable heating devices should be discouraged because of the danger of burns and residential fires. Nurses should also encourage clients or their landlords to install smoke detection devices, as the elderly are particularly likely to be trapped by a fire and need sufficient warning to get out. To prevent burns, community health nurses can encourage clients to use electric blankets rather than hot water bottles in cold weather.

Older clients should also be warned about the potential for hypothermia. Persons over 60 years of age account for about half of deaths due to hypothermia each year. Clients with hypothyroidism and those using sedative–hypnotic drugs are particularly at risk for hypothermia and should be cautioned accordingly. Nurses should make sure that these and other elderly clients have an adequate caloric intake and that the homes of older persons are adequately heated.

Older clients should be educated regarding other health-promoting behaviors that minimize the risks of falls or their consequences. For example, weight bearing forms of exercise (eg, walking), maintaining body weight, and limiting caffeine intake decrease the risk of fractures when falls do occur (Cummings, et al., 1995). Regular exercise programs, including Tai Chi training, can prevent falls from occurring by improving strength and balance (Province, et al., 1995; Wolf, et al., 1996).

Promoting home and neighborhood security is also of concern. Older clients should be cautioned to be careful about admitting strangers into the home and to refrain from walking along in high-crime areas. Doors and windows should have secure locks, and cars should be locked even when kept in the garage.

In many neighborhoods, police and fire personnel can be notified of homes where older persons live. If this is the case, the nurse can encourage clients to provide such notification. Clients can also arrange for "disaster signals" to neighbors. For example, if neighbors do not see the kitchen window shade raised by a certain time in the morning, they may decide to investigate.

Motor vehicles are a cause for concern in the safety of older adults. Although many older persons would like to retain their independence and continue to drive, they may not be able to do so safely because of a variety of sensory impairments. In this type of situation, the nurse can encourage older clients to find other ways of remaining mobile and maintaining their independence. Perhaps they can be encouraged to drive in the daytime, but not at night. Or the nurse might acquaint the older client with local bus routes and schedules. Many local organizations provide transportation at little or no cost to older people. Or the older adult can be encouraged to ride along with a younger friend.

Motor vehicles are also problematic when older people are pedestrians. In many areas the bulk of pedestrian fatalities occur among elderly individuals. In areas where there are large numbers of elderly, nurses can campaign for traffic signals at heavily used crossings, strict enforcement of speed limits, and public awareness of the presence of older adults.

The last area of concern in promoting the safety of older clients is preventing abuse and neglect. Elder abuse and neglect frequently occur when those caring for elderly clients are unable to cope with the resulting stress. Providing support for these caretakers, teaching positive coping skills, and providing periodic respite care may help to prevent abuse. Assisting older clients to maintain their independence may also help prevent the development of a potentially abusive situation.

Immunization. Immunization of older adults is a special safety issue. Many adults in the United States, particularly older adults, have never been immunized for tetanus and are also unprotected against diphtheria. Current Immunization Practices Advisory Committee (ACIP) recommendations for adult immunization indicate a need for completion of the primary series of diphtheria and tetanus toxoids and boosters every 10 years. Annual immunization for influenza is recommended for all healthy adults over 65 years of age. Immunization against pneumococcal pneumonia is also recommended for older persons. Adults may also require immunization for hepatitis B, measles, mumps, rubella, and varicella if they do not have previously acquired immunity (Centers for Disease Control, 1996). Older clients may need to be referred to sources of inexpensive immunization. For example, many local health departments offer influenza and pneumococcal immunizations free or for a small charge.

Rest and Exercise. Many people believe that the need for exercise decreases with age; however, older people need exercise as much as their younger counterparts. Community heath nurses should encourage older clients to engage in moderate exercise on a regular basis. Encouraging clients to elevate the legs and refrain from crossing the legs will help to prevent venous stasis and skin breakdown.

Older clients also need adequate rest. Older people tend to sleep fewer hours at night than when they were younger. They continue to need rest, however, so daily activity patterns may need to be planned to accommodate an afternoon nap. Clients should also be encouraged to arrange activities to allow for rest periods throughout the day.

Maintaining Independence. Because of physical and economic limitations, it is sometimes difficult for older persons to maintain their independence. Decreased

Critical Thinking in Research

Wolfson and colleagues (1996) conducted a study of the effects of balance or weight training followed by Tai Chi training on balance and strength using healthy older subjects randomly assigned to one of four groups: a balance training group, a strength training group, a group that received both interventions, and a control group. Balance training was associated with improved balance on several measures and strength training with improved lower extremity strength. These improvements were maintained after 6 months of Tai Chi with only minimal losses. The combination of both balance and strength training did not produce any greater improvement in either strength or balance than either intervention separately.

1. How might you use the findings of this study in community health nursing practice?
2. What additional research questions might be generated as a result of this study? For example, one might ask if balance and strength training would result in improved performance in older clients with activity limitations, or what factors might motivate older people to participate in such programs. What additional questions might be explored in these areas?
3. What type of research design was used in the two studies described? What kind of design might you use to study the additional questions raised above?
4. Where might you recruit subjects for studies addressing the additional questions raised? Be specific about how you might identify potential subjects in your community?

income and physical inability to care for oneself sometimes force older clients to give up their own residence and live with family members. Whatever the living arrangements of the older client, community health nurses should assist them to maintain the highest degree of independence possible. Some older clients may be able to continue to live alone if referred to supportive services such as homemaker aides, transportation services, and Meals-on-Wheels. When older persons are living with family members, the nurse can encourage family members to foster independence in the client. This may mean encouraging them to assign specific roles within the household to the older family member.

Life Resolution and Preparation for Death.   As noted earlier, one of the developmental tasks to be accomplished by the older adult is preparation for death. This entails developing a personal set of goals and the ability to view one's life as having been meaningful and productive. Reminiscence is one way of accomplishing life resolution and achieving positive feelings about

one's own life. The community health nurse must recognize and foster the older client's need to reminisce and should encourage other family members to do so as well. This is sometimes difficult given the nurse's busy schedule and the number of clients who need to be seen; however, nurses should be able to find some time during interactions with older clients to listen to these reminiscences and to help clients reflect on their lives.

Preparation for death usually also entails a number of practical activities involved in getting one's affairs in order. Older clients may need to make decisions about funeral arrangements or the disposition of their belongings. Both nurses and family members should be encouraged to listen to clients in their reflections on such matters, rather than put them off with assurances that they "won't die for a long time yet." Nurses may also need to refer clients for legal assistance with wills, burial plans, and other financial arrangements. Many communities have low-cost legal aid services available to elderly clients. Primary preventive interventions for older clients are summarized in Table 23–5.

Secondary Prevention

Secondary preventive measures are undertaken when health problems have occurred and primary prevention is no longer possible. As noted earlier, older clients experience a variety of health problems related to the effects of aging. They are also subject to problems stemming from chronic and communicable diseases. Secondary prevention for communicable diseases and chronic conditions is addressed in detail in Chapters 30 and 31.

Skin Breakdown.   Because of the fragility of older skin, skin breakdown is a common difficulty. The initial plan of care should be to prevent skin breakdown using the primary preventive strategies discussed earlier. Extremities should be inspected regularly for evidence of skin breakdown, and any breakdown noted should be cleansed properly and examined for signs of infection. Adequate dietary intake contributes to maintaining skin integrity and to healing when breakdown does occur. Care should also be taken to relieve pressure on bony prominences by frequent changes of position. When skin breakdown has already occurred, the nurse should make sure that the area is kept clean and dry. If healing does not occur, the client should be referred to a physician for evaluation.

Constipation.   Constipation is another common problem in older clients. Again, the primary consideration is prevention through adequate fluid and fiber in the

TABLE 23–5. PRIMARY PREVENTION STRATEGIES FOR OLDER CLIENTS

Area of Concern	Primary Prevention Strategies
Nutrition	• Educate clients regarding nutritional needs. • Promote caloric intake adequate to meet energy needs. • Encourage well-balanced diet high in nutrient content (especially calcium, iron, vitamins A and C, riboflavin, and thiamine, and fiber). • Discourage participation in food fads. • Maintain hydration.
Hygiene	• Bathe periodically with mild soaps. • Use lotion to prevent drying of skin. • Keep hands out of water or wear gloves. • Maintain oral hygiene with good toothbrush. • Maintain hydration to prevent dry mouth. • Brush and comb hair daily. • Shampoo weekly with mild soap and condition monthly.
Safety	• Wear hat to protect scalp from sunburn. • Wear properly fitted clothes and shoes. • Use electric blanket rather than hot water bottles. • Provide adequate lighting, especially on stairs. • Use a nightlight at night and keep a flashlight handy. • Place furniture to prevent falls. • Keep electrical cords short and tack along baseboards. • Eliminate throw rugs if possible or use nonskid type. • Install tub rails and other safety fixtures. • Discourage use of space heaters, kerosene stoves, and similar devices. • Install smoke alarms. • Notify policy and fire personnel of older person in home. • Promote adequate and safe heating and ventilation of home. • Provide door and window locks and keep car locked. • Do not admit strangers to home. • Ride with others or use public transportation rather than drive if senses are impaired. • Use care in crossing streets. • Promote family coping abilities and relieve stress to prevent abuse of older persons.
Immunization	• Encourage adequate immunization for diphtheria and tetanus. • Provide annual influenza immunization. • Provide pneumonia vaccine.
Rest and exercise	• Encourage moderate exercise on a regular basis. • Arrange activities to accommodate rest periods as needed.
Maintaining independence	• Provide support services that allow clients to live independently if possible. • Encourage family members to foster independence. • Encourage client participation in health care planning. • Advocate for client independence as needed.
Life resolution and preparation for death	• Encourage reminiscence. • Assist client to discuss death with family members. • Assist client to put affairs in order.

diet as well as adequate exercise. But when constipation does occur, the nurse can suggest the use of mild natural laxatives such as prune juice. Clients should be cautioned against the overuse of laxatives. Bulk products such as Metamucil or stool softeners should also be used with caution.

If necessary, the nurse or a family member can administer an enema. Nurses working with older clients who are constipated should determine agency policy regarding whether an enema requires a physician's order. If an order is required, the nurse can call the physician to request the authorization. Care should be taken that the enema solution is not too hot and that the client is close to the toilet, as poor sphincter control occurring with age may result in the inability to hold the enema. Again, overuse of enemas is contraindicated. Fecal impaction that is unrelieved by enema should be referred to the physician.

Urinary Incontinence.   Urinary incontinence is a particularly distressing problem for some older adults. Incontinence may result in social withdrawal because of fear of embarrassing accidents in public. For clients with incontinence, not only are there the problems of hygiene and odor, but self-image is threatened by the inability to control one's bodily functions. Clients with stress incontinence should be referred for a urological consultation. Nursing interventions that may help urinary incontinence include encouraging clients to void frequently and teaching them Kegel pelvic floor exercises. Bladder training may also help to resolve the problem. Biofeedback techniques have been found to relieve both urinary and fecal incontinence in older adults. Environmental modifications that increase access to the toilet may also help, as can loose-fitting and easily removed clothing.

In some instances, incontinence becomes a chronic problem. For clients in this situation, the nurse needs to ensure that skin, clothing, and linens remain clean and dry. Urinary incontinence increases the risk of pressure sores sixfold (Kennie, 1993). Sanitary pads, disposable underpants, or panty liners may prevent clothing and linens from becoming wet and may increase the client's confidence in going out in public. Frequent changes in such sanitary aids should be encouraged to prevent skin breakdown.

For bedfast clients, ready availability of a bedpan or urinal, or assistance to a bedside commode at frequent intervals, may reduce the frequency of linen changes. A bedside commode may also be of use to clients who are able to get up but have mobility limitations. The community health nurse may help arrange for the purchase or rental of these devices from durable medical equipment companies.

Sensory Loss.   Planning to provide adequate lighting is particularly important in compensating for loss of visual acuity. If clients wear glasses, nurses should make sure that the degree of correction is appropriate and that glasses are kept clean. Nurses and clients should also take care that when glasses are removed they are placed in a safe, but accessible, location.

The use of large-print books, a magnifying glass, or books on tape can assist older clients to continue reading as a leisure activity. Taking medications may also be hampered by loss of visual acuity. When clients have difficulties reading medication labels, the nurse can color-code the labels. Colors used should be easily distinguishable, as there may be a loss of color discrimination with age, particularly with the colors blue, green, and violet.

The community health nurse can also suggest several measures that help to compensate for diminished hearing. Speaking clearly (not loudly) and at a lower pitch improves the older client's ability to hear. Properly functioning hearing aids also help some clients. Clients who are concerned about the unsightliness of old-fashioned hearing aids can be assured that there are many less noticeable devices available today. Speech should be slower, as many older persons have problems hearing rapid speech and have difficulty discriminating several specific sounds, among them *s, z, t, f, g,* and *th.* These auditory problems can be overcome by the use of multisensory input (eg, using visual as well as auditory techniques in teaching older clients).

Eliminating background noise may also enhance the older person's ability to hear. Nurses working with older clients should always obtain feedback to be sure that clients have accurately heard and interpreted verbal messages. For clients living alone or others who must be able to use a telephone, the nurse can suggest voice enhancement devices that enable older people to hear better.

Because of older clients' diminished sense of touch, nurses should discourage clients from using hot water for bathing and from wearing open-toed shoes. Clients should be encouraged to check extremities periodically for injuries and to use extreme caution in working with sharp or other potentially harmful objects.

Decreased senses of smell and taste pose problems for older adults in that they may lead to diminished appetite. Older individuals can be encouraged to add additional spices and herbs to flavor foods; however, care should be taken that such condiments are not contraindicated (eg, additional salt for the client with hypertension). Loss of the sense of smell is also problematic in that older clients may not be as easily able to tell when foodstuffs are spoiled or may not be able to smell smoke or a gas leak. Nurses may want to encourage clients using gas for cooking or heating periodically to check that pilot lights remain lit. They should also encourage the purchase of small amounts of perishable foods and rapid use before they spoil. Smoke detectors are also necessary devices in the homes of older clients.

Mobility Limitation. Related problems for older clients involve limitation of mobility and consequent impairment in the ability to carry out activities of daily living. Nurses can explore options for assisting older clients to perform activities of daily living. Referral to a home care agency that has homemaker services may help with tasks such as housekeeping and grocery shopping. Home care agencies may also provide assistance with personal care services such as bathing and hair washing. There are also a number of mechanical devices that make it easier for older clients to care for themselves (eg, special devices for clients with arthritis that make it easier to open jars or reach objects on shelves).

For clients who need outside assistance but do not have insurance coverage or cannot afford special services, volunteer services may be available through local churches or other social groups. Student workers are sometimes a good source of assistance with instrumental activities. Both high school and college students may be willing to provide services for small fees or for a room. The community health nurse can also explore service projects undertaken by sororities or fraternities at local colleges or universities that may provide assistance for older clients.

The nurse may refer clients who cannot cook for themselves to a Meals-on-Wheels program. For clients who are mobile, a referral for a lunch program at the local senior citizen center may be more appropriate. Such centers may also provide assistance with transportation to and from the center, for shopping, and for physician appointments.

Pain. The management of chronic pain is another common problem among older adults. For clients with arthritis, pain may be controlled with the use of anti-inflammatory and analgesic agents such as aspirin. When a mild analgesic is not effective, stronger medication may be prescribed by the physician. Nurses should evaluate the appropriateness of any pain medication being taken by clients and should educate clients on the correct use of medications. They may also need to caution clients regarding overuse of some medications and discourage the use of medications that are contraindicated by the client's condition. For example, clients taking anticoagulants should not take aspirin for pain, because aspirin further increases clotting time and may lead to serious bleeding.

Clients with arthritis pain may do better if they do not attempt strenuous activity immediately after awakening when joints tend to be stiff and sore. Clients can be helped to plan activities for when their pain is at a minimum. Warm baths or soaks may also help to relieve pain. For other forms of pain, medication may again be used and the nurse should monitor its effectiveness. Nurses should also educate clients as to the adverse effects of specific pain medications and make sure that clients are familiar with the symptoms of adverse effects.

Confusion. Confusion is a problem encountered in some older clients. Confusion may be either a transient or a persistent condition. Transient confusion frequently occurs in new situations or in the dark. It may also occur when clients are moved away from familiar surroundings, as might occur following a move to a residential community or nursing home. In this case, confusion may be referred to as *relocation trauma.* Relocation trauma may even occur when the client is moved from one hallway or one bed to another.

Continuing confusion is sometimes called *dementia,* a global impairment of intellectual functioning that may include such symptoms as failing attention, failing memory, and declining mathematical ability. Confusion is a frequent side effect of many medications, and nurses should monitor a client's state of orientation with respect to medication use. Other nursing interventions include improving sensory input, preventing malnutrition and dehydration, and preventing falls.

In working with confused older clients, the nurse should plan for consistent intervention to reorient clients to their environment. Reality orientation interventions are based on several general principles:

- Provide a calm environment without excessive stimulation.
- Establish and maintain a regular routine.
- Phrase questions and answers clearly and concisely.
- Speak directly to the client.
- Provide clear instructions or directions.
- Provide frequent reminders of date, time, and place.
- Refocus the client on reality and prevent rambling speech.
- Be firm, but gentle.
- Be sincere.
- Be consistent.

Reality orientation may not be appropriate for clients with Alzheimer's disease who have lowered stress thresholds, as it may result in argument or agitation (Nagley, 1990).

Confusion is a symptom frequently encountered in clients with Alzheimer's disease. Although Alzheimer's is no longer considered a natural part of aging, its cause is, as yet, not well understood. It is, however, a debilitating disease that places a heavy burden on the client and his or her family. Nurses working with families of clients with Alzheimer's need to provide a great deal of support. Families may need to consider nursing home placement and may need help in making arrangements. They may also need assistance in dealing with the guilt engendered by their inability to care for a family member, especially a spouse, at home.

For families who choose to care for the client with Alzheimer's at home, the nurse can help arrange home care or respite care. Nurses can also encourage families of clients who wander to use an identification kit similar to that used for identifying lost children. Families can also create environments that permit wandering within safe parameters. Other interventions that may help families cope with clients with Alzheimer's disease include creation of a calm, consistent environment with minimal changes, provision of frequent rest periods with nocturnal restlessness, and encouraging reminiscence (Nagley, 1990).

Depression. Depression is another area in which the nurse working with older clients may need to take action. Mild transient depression is a relatively normal phenomenon for most people. Depression may occur with the loss of familiar people and places or on anniversaries of those losses. It is normal, for example, for the older person to become somewhat depressed on the anniversary of a spouse's death or on the deceased person's birthday. In these instances, nurses can help clients to recognize their depression as a normal feeling. Encouraging them to discuss the loved one and to relive happy memories while acknowledging their feelings of sadness may help to alleviate the depression.

Severe depression, on the other hand, requires referral for counseling or other forms of therapy. Severe depression may be marked by continued inattention to personal hygiene, failure to take part in normal activities such as dressing or combing one's hair, and poor appetite. Depression may also be signaled by withdrawal from interaction with others. Again, the nurse should encourage the client to ventilate feelings regarding the cause of the depression, but should also refer the client for additional help as needed. The nurse should also clearly distinguish between clients who are depressed and those experiencing delirium. Evidence of delirium should prompt a referral for medical care.

Social Isolation. Social isolation is a relatively common problem among older adults, especially the "old elderly." Isolation may stem from a variety of circumstances mentioned earlier, including sensory deficits, communication difficulties, and loss of mobility.

Loss of family and friends is a significant contributor to social isolation in the elderly. As spouses and other family members or friends die, the social support system for the older person is reduced. In this instance, nurses can help older clients establish new social support systems by helping them get involved with other groups. Referral to an active senior center may be appropriate. Many religious groups also have a variety of social activities for older persons. Special interest groups that incorporate people of all ages may provide an avenue for social interaction. For example, a local bridge club or garden club may be of interest to a particular client. The nurse can also encourage remaining family and friends to include the older person in their activities.

Loss of family and friends also leads to the problem of grief. Grief may also be engendered by anticipation of client's own death, particularly when the client has a terminal illness. The nurse can assist clients to deal with grief by exploring with them their feelings about death. Acceptance of possible anger may be necessary as well. Clients can be assisted to deal with their own feelings of anger and depression regarding death.

If the client is willing, referral to a pastor or other source of spiritual counsel may be appropriate. Family and friends should be encouraged to talk with the client about the client's impending death and the client should be allowed to make arrangements for disposition of personal property or plans for burial. As much as possible, dying clients should be allowed to continue in accustomed roles and should have control over decisions affecting their own life or death. If the client has a living will or durable power of attorney (see Chap. 15), the nurse should see that a copy of the document is placed in the client's record and that the document is adhered to by both family members and health care professionals.

Abuse and Neglect.   Abuse or neglect of older persons is another problem for which nursing intervention may be required. Nurses should be alert to situations that have potential for abuse. Dependent elders who place a serious burden on caretakers or who were abusive parents themselves are at risk for abuse and neglect. Other situations in which potential for abuse is increased include reduced social status, other sources of stress for caregivers (eg, unemployment or illness in other family members), and family dysfunction.

Resolving an abusive situation may require assisting caretakers to develop adequate mechanisms for coping with the frustrations of caring for an older adult. Persons in abusive situations can also be referred for counseling. Respite care can help to reduce the burden of care of an older family member, and the nurse may need to help families arrange for such care. Removal of the older person and nursing home placement may reduce the potential for abuse. Finally, in situations where abuse cannot be controlled, the nurse may arrange for placement of the older person in a temporary shelter while arrangements are made for other care. Abuse of older adults is discussed in more detail in Chapter 34.

Alcohol Abuse.   Abuse of alcohol may warrant referral for a variety of services. Initially, the nurse may need to refer the client to a detoxification facility. Because of their diminished capacity to detoxify alcohol and other substances, older clients are at high risk for complications during detoxification and should be in a facility where adequate supervision is possible. Once detoxification has been accomplished, the client should be referred for ongoing counseling for his or her drinking problem. Referral to such groups as Alcoholics Anonymous may also be appropriate. Families with older alcoholic members may also need assistance in dealing with the problem, and referral to Al-Anon may help.

Older clients and their families should also be educated regarding the effects of alcohol and its potential for interaction with medication. Overuse of preparations containing alcohol should be discouraged as well.

Inadequate Financial Resources.   Another common problem of older adults is inadequate financial resources. Many older people have reduced incomes that may not be sufficient to meet their needs. Nurses can refer clients to sources of financial assistance as appropriate. Clients who are receiving minimal Social Security benefits may be eligible for Supplemental Security Income (SSI). Referrals may also be made for food and other general assistance programs. Some utility companies provide reduced rates for older adults, something that the client can inquire about. The nurse should become familiar with other local sources of financial assistance for older persons and make referrals to these agencies as appropriate.

The community health nurse may also be of assistance to older persons living on reduced incomes by helping them to prioritize expenditures and budget their income accordingly. The nurse may also provide information about lower-cost foods that provide adequate nutrition. Clients should be encouraged to buy staple goods in quantities that reduce prices. Perishable foods, however, should be purchased only in quantities that can be used before spoiling. The nurse may also encourage several older clients to buy items in bulk and split the costs to reduce expenditures for each individual.

Chronic Illness. As noted earlier, older persons experience a variety of chronic illnesses. Among these are arthritis, heart disease, hypertension, diabetes, and chronic lung conditions. Secondary prevention for these conditions would include screening for specific diseases, diagnosis, and treatment. Community health nursing involvement in secondary prevention for these illnesses includes referral for medical services as needed, as well as supportive therapy during treatment. Community health nurses frequently educate clients regarding their conditions and the treatment recommended. Older persons may need instruction regarding their medications and possible side effects. In addition, the nurse monitors clients for treatment effects and for side effects and toxic effects of medications. They may also educate clients in other forms of symptom relief, for example, warm soaks for arthritic joints. Clients may also need emotional support in dealing with their disease and its effects. Additional secondary preventive measures for specific chronic diseases are addressed in Chapter 31.

Communicable Diseases. Older clients are at higher risk than younger people for communicable diseases such as influenza and pneumonia. Primary prevention of these diseases through immunization is desirable, but when this fails, the community health nurse may be involved in referring clients for medical care for these conditions as needed. Nurses also instruct clients in self-care during illness and monitor the effects of communicable conditions on health status. The nurse working with older clients with these diseases should be particularly alert to signs of complications, as these are more common in older individuals than in their younger counterparts. Controlling fever and maintaining hydration are two particularly important aspects of secondary prevention for communicable diseases in the elderly. Other aspects of secondary prevention in communicable diseases are addressed in Chapter 30.

Advocacy for Older Clients. Many times nursing interventions for older clients involve advocacy. Advocacy may take place at the individual or aggregate level. At the individual level, the nurse may encourage family members to respect the client's need for privacy or allow the client to make his or her own health care decisions. Advocacy may also be needed in interactions with other health care providers. Advocacy may involve encouraging families to allow the client as much independence as possible. Intervention on behalf of the abused client is also a form of advocacy.

At the aggregate level, nurses can see that the needs of the older population are made known to public policy makers. They can become politically active to see that the needs of this group are being met by government agencies. They may also need to work with nongovernment agencies to ensure that the needs of older clients are met. For example, community health nurses might work with a coalition of religious groups to provide shelter for abused elders, or they might help a group of older adults establish some type of cooperative buying effort to decrease expenditures. There may also be a need to point out the needs of older persons to transportation authorities. Table 23–6 summarizes secondary preventive activities that may benefit older clients.

Tertiary Prevention

Tertiary preventive activities for older clients focus on preventing complications of existing conditions and preventing their recurrence. Tertiary prevention for the individual client depends on the problems experienced by the client. For example, tertiary prevention for an abused older client may include long-term counseling for family members, whereas prevention related to financial inadequacies may involve assistance with budgeting.

In many instances, tertiary preventive measures are similar to those used for primary prevention. For example, primary and tertiary prevention for constipation both involve increasing fluid and fiber intake and exercise. Similarly, primary preventive measures to prevent skin breakdown can also be used to prevent a recurrence of the problem. Tertiary prevention measures used with older adults are presented in Table 23–7.

In planning health care to meet the needs of older clients, the nurse frequently makes referrals or obtains assistance for clients from outside agencies. In making referrals for older clients, the nurse should consider carefully the client's ability to follow through on the referral. The nurse should also explain carefully to the client what services may be provided by the referral agency and how to go about obtaining those services. In some instances, it may be necessary for the nurse to make arrangements for the client if the client is not able to do so. For example, some social service agencies make arrangements to visit a client's home if the client is unable to get to them.

 Implementing Nursing Care for Older Clients

Nurse and client together implement the plan of care. Some activities of implementation may also be carried out by members of the client's family or by significant others. The extent of responsibility of each depends

TABLE 23–6. SECONDARY PREVENTION FOR COMMON PROBLEMS IN OLDER CLIENTS

Client Problem	Secondary Preventive Strategies	Client Problem	Secondary Preventive Strategies
Skin breakdown	• Inspect extremities regularly for lesions. • Keep lesions clean and dry. • Eliminate pressure by frequent changes of position. • Refer for treatment as needed.		• Install ramps, tub rails, etc., as needed. • Promote access to public facilities for older persons. • Assist clients to find sources of transportation. • Make referrals for assistance with personal care or instrumental activities.
Constipation	• Encourage fluid and fiber intake. • Discourage ignoring urge to defecate. • Encourage regular exercise. • Encourage regular bowel habits. • Use mild laxatives as needed, but discourage overuse. • Administer enemas as needed; discourage overuse. • Administer bulk products or stool softeners as indicated.	Pain	• Plan activities for times when pain is controlled. • Encourage warm soaks. • Encourage adequate rest and exercise to prevent mobility limitations.
		Confusion	• Apply principles of reality orientation.
		Depression	• Accept feelings and reflect on their normality; encourage client to ventilate feelings. • Refer for counseling as needed.
Urinary incontinence	• Refer for urological consult. • Encourage frequent voiding. • Teach Kegel exercises. • Assist with bladder training. • Encourage use of sanitary pads, panty liners, etc., with frequent changes of such aids. • Keep skin clean and dry; change clothing and bed linen as needed. • Offer bedpan or urinal frequently or assist to bedside commode at frequent intervals.	Social isolation	• Compensate for sensory loss; enhance communication abilities. • Improve mobility; provide access to transportation. • Assist client to obtain adequate financial resources. • Refer client to new support systems. • Assist client to deal with grief over loss of loved ones.
Sensory loss	• Provide adequate lighting. • Keep eyeglasses clean and hearing aids functional. • Eliminate safety hazards. • Use large-print books or materials. • Use multisensory approaches to communication and teaching. • Avoid using colors that make discrimination difficult. • Speak clearly and slowly, at a lower pitch. • Eliminate background noise. • Assist clients to obtain voice enhancers for phone. • Use additional herbs and spices, but use with discretion. • Purchase small amounts of perishable foods. • Check pilot lights on gas appliances frequently. • Encourage the use of smoke detectors.	Abuse or neglect	• Assist caretakers to develop positive coping strategies. • Assist families to obtain respite care or day care for older members. • Refer families for counseling as needed. • Arrange placement in temporary shelter. • Assist families in making other arrangements for safe care of older clients.
		Alcohol abuse	• Identify problem drinking by older clients. • Refer for therapy, Alcoholics Anonymous or Al-Anon as appropriate. • Observe for toxic effects of alcohol ingestion. • Maintain hydration and nutrition.
		Inadequate financial resources	• Refer for financial assistance. • Assist with budgeting and priority allocation. • Educate for less expensive means of meeting needs. • Function as an advocate as needed.
Mobility limitation	• Provide assistance with ambulation, transfer, etc. • Assist clients to obtain equipment such as walkers and wheelchairs.		

on the client's level of function and the ability of the client or others to carry out the actions required.

Frequently, implementing the plan of care involves educating the client (or significant others). Health education for older clients is based on the general principles of teaching and learning discussed in Chapter 9. There are also some unique considerations in implementing an education plan for the older adult.

Sensory losses need to be taken into consideration when teaching the older client. Strategies to circumvent hearing loss include using a lower-pitched

voice; facing the client while speaking; employing nonverbal teaching techniques; using clear, concise terminology; and having the client use a hearing aid when possible. The effects of hearing loss can also be minimized by limiting background noise, reemphasizing important points, and supplementing verbal with written materials (Bastable, 1997).

The use of glasses, a magnifying glass, and large print may help to minimize visual deficits. Learning can also be enhanced by visual materials using black lettering on white or yellow paper and providing ade-

TABLE 23–7. TERTIARY PREVENTION STRATEGIES FOR OLDER CLIENTS

Client Problem	Tertiary Preventive Strategies
Inadequate nutrition	• Educate clients regarding nutritional needs. • Promote caloric intake adequate to meet energy needs. • Encourage well-balanced diet high in nutrient content (especially those with prior deficits). • Discourage participation in food fads. • Maintain hydration.
Skin breakdown	• Bathe periodically with mild soaps. • Use lotion to prevent drying of skin. • Keep hands out of water or wear gloves. • Elevate legs and refrain from crossing legs. • Wear loose-fitting clothing and properly fitted shoes. • Inspect extremities regularly for lesions. • Relieve pressure on bony prominences by frequent change of position.
Constipation	• Encourage fluid and fiber intake. • Discourage ignoring urge to defecate. • Encourage regular exercise. • Encourage regular bowel habits. • Use mild laxatives as needed, but discourage overuse. • Administer enemas as needed; discourage overuse. • Administer bulk products or stool softeners as indicated.
Sensory loss	• Provide adequate lighting. • Keep eyeglasses clean and hearing aids functional. • Eliminate safety hazards. • Use large-print books or materials. • Use multisensory approaches to communication and teaching. • Avoid using colors that make discrimination difficult. • Speak clearly and slowly, at a lower pitch. • Eliminate background noise. • Assist clients to obtain voice enhancers for phone. • Use additional herbs and spices, but use with discretion. • Purchase small amounts of perishable foods. • Check pilot lights on gas appliances frequently. • Encourage the use of smoke detectors.
Confusion	• Apply principles of reality orientation.
Abuse or neglect	• Provide support for victim and caretakers. • Assist families to obtain respite care or day care for older members. • Refer families for counseling as needed. • Monitor family situation closely. • Assist families in making other arrangements for safe care of older clients as needed. • Promote self-image of victim and abuser. • Foster independence of victim and abuser.
Alcohol abuse	• Provide support for abstinence. • Refer to support group. • Provide support to family in dealing with problem. • Provide assistance in dealing with stress. • Promote positive self-image.
Accidental injury	• Eliminate safety hazards from environment. • Encourage use of safety aids. • Provide supervision for confused older person.
Social isolation	• Assist client to build social support network. • Refer to church or other groups for social activities. • Provide means of transportation.

quate lighting and eliminating glare in the learning environment.

In implementing health education plans for the older client, the nurse may need to repeat material more frequently. Because of decreases in short-term memory, it may take longer for an older client to learn new material. Once material is learned, however, older clients retain it as well as younger ones. With age, memory for information that is heard is better than that for information seen, so multisensorial presentation of information is desirable (Arden, Cox, & Schonberger, 1994). Multiple repetitions, reinforcement of verbal content with written materials, and use of memory aids (eg, a calendar for taking medications) may also assist learning in the older client.

Because response times are longer for older people than for their younger counterparts, lessons should proceed at a slower pace and the nurse should allow increased time for responses on the part of the client (Bastable, 1997). Self-paced instruction is helpful. Motivation to learn can be heightened by increasing client participation in the lesson and by setting easily attainable, progressive goals that enhance success and satisfaction. Irrelevant material can confuse clients and should be eliminated from the presentation.

Endurance may be somewhat limited in the older client, so teaching sessions should be kept short (10 to 15 minutes per session). Lessons should be scheduled at times of the day when the client is rested and comfortable. Health education for the older client should not be time limited, as the client may need more or less time to learn specific material. Again, learning should be broken down into small, progressive steps so that periodic success will motivate the client to further effort. The teaching–learning process should also allow for rest periods as needed.

 Evaluating Nursing Care for Older Clients

The last aspect of the use of the epidemiologic prevention process model with older clients is evaluation. Evaluation should include an assessment of the current status of all identified health problems and the effectiveness of nursing interventions in resolving them. Evaluation should also consider the overall health status of the client and the quality of his or her life.

Some specific constraints need to be considered in evaluating the effectiveness of nursing intervention with the elderly. One of these is that the etiology of some problems may lie in other problems caused by

TABLE 23–8. STATUS OF SELECTED NATIONAL HEALTH OBJECTIVES FOR OLDER ADULTS

Objective		Base	Most Recent	Target
1.5a	Reduce the lack of physical activity	43% (1985)	29% (1991)	22%
2.18	Increase home-delivered meals	7% (1991)	NDA[a]	80%
6.1c	Reduce suicide in white men over 65 (per 100,000)	46.7 (1987)	38.4 (1992)	39.2
9.3c	Reduce motor vehicle fatalities (per 100,000)	22.6 (1987)	23.9 (1991)	20
9.4	Reduce fall-related deaths			
	People aged 65–84 (per 100,000)	18.1 (1987)	17.8 (1991)	14.4
	People over age 85	133.0 (1987)	149.5 (1993)	105.0
9.6b	Reduce residential fire deaths (per 100,000)	4.9 (1987)	3.7 (1993)	3.3
16.12b	Increase proportion of women who have had a Pap smear	76% (1987)	82% (1992)	95%
17.1	Increase years of healthy life	11.9 (1990)	NDA	14
17.3	Reduce proportion of people with difficiulty in two or more ADLs (per 1000)	371 (1984–1985)	NDA	90
17.6a	Reduce hearing impairment (per 1000)	203 (1986–1988)	210 (1992–1994)	180
17.7a	Reduce visual impairment (per 1000)	87.7 (1986–1988)	90 (1992–1994)	70.0
17.18	Increase estrogen therapy counseling	NDA	NDA	90%
20.2	Reduce pneumonia and influenza deaths (per 100,000)	19.9 (1979–1987)	31.8 (1994)	15.9
20.11	Increase pneumonia and influenza immunization	14–30% (1989)	22–52% (1993)	60%

[a]NDA, no data available.

(Sources: National Cancer Institute, 1996; Natoinal Center for Infectious Diseases, 1995; Division of Violence Prevention, 1996; U.S. Department of Health and Human Services, 1993; 1995; 1996b.)

aging itself and that these problems may not be capable of complete resolution. In this case, the nurse should evaluate the extent to which the effects of the problem on the client's life have been ameliorated. For example, it is not possible to eliminate arthritis pain. The nurse and client can, however, evaluate the extent to which nursing interventions have limited the effects of pain on the client's ability to perform activities of daily living.

The second consideration is that the prognosis for one problem may be affected by the presence of other problems. For example, the existence of a terminal condition may make pain control increasingly difficult. In some cases, orientation and alertness might need to be sacrificed so as to control pain with the use of more powerful analgesics.

Evaluation must also take into account the possibility that one problem may diminish while another gets worse. Again, the example of pain control in terminal illness may lead to increasing confusion and disorientation that will entail other nursing interventions. Finally, the nurse and client must consider that deterioration in one area might lead to the development of additional problems that will need to be addressed. For example, decreased mobility leads to greater potential for constipation and skin breakdown. Therefore, while the status of individual problems needs to be assessed, there is a need to allow for a give-and-take or a realistic assessment of the ups and downs that may be involved in the care of the older person.

At the aggregate level, evaluation of the effects of care on the health of the elderly can be measured, in part, by the level of accomplishment of relevant national health objectives. The status of selected national objectives for the year 2000 related to the health of older clients is reflected in Table 23–8.

TESTING YOUR UNDERSTANDING

1. What are four common myths related to aging? What is the reality related to each myth? (p. 552)
2. Describe at least five theories of aging. Be sure to identify the category in which each theory belongs. (pp. 552–554)
3. Describe at least two changes in each body system that occur as a normal result of the aging process. What are the implications of these changes for the health of older clients? (pp. 554–561)
4. What are the three major factors in assessing the physical environment of an older client? (pp. 562–563)
5. Describe at least four considerations in assessing the influence of behavioral factors on the health of older clients. Give an example of the influence on health of factors in each area. (pp. 564–569)
6. Describe at least six areas for primary prevention in the care of older clients. (pp. 571–574)
7. Describe at least one secondary preventive measure for each of four common health problems encountered among older clients. (pp. 574–579)
8. Identify at least three factors related to older clients that may influence the community health

Critical Thinking in Practice: A Case in Point

Henrietta Walker is a 68-year-old African American woman who has been referred for community health nursing services following her discharge from the hospital. She was hospitalized after being found unconscious in her room by her 50-year-old daughter. A diagnosis of diabetes mellitus was made, and Mrs. Walker was placed on 15 units of NPH insulin daily. She and her daughter were instructed on injection technique and a diabetic diet at the hospital.

Mrs. Walker lives with her daughter and son-in-law and their three teenage boys (ages 18, 15, and 13). They live in a lower-class neighborhood and the son-in-law works at the local textile plant. His income is barely enough for the family to live on. Mrs. Walker does not know how she will pay her hospital bill. She has Medicare, Part A, and a small Social Security income, but she does not have any supplemental health insurance.

Mrs. Walker's vision is failing, probably as a result of undiagnosed diabetes of longstanding. She hears well, but is 80 pounds overweight, so is unsteady on her feet. The family lives in a second-floor apartment and there is no handrail on the stairs outside the apartment. Mrs. Walker tries to help out around the house because her daughter works. She says she does not want to be a burden to her daughter and her son-in-law. Mrs. Walker's husband died of a heart attack 8 months ago, and that was when she came to live with her daughter. Mrs. Walker's daughter says that her mother's presence has caused some friction among the boys because the two younger ones now have to share a room.

1. What are the biophysical, psychological, physical, social, behavioral, and health system factors influencing Mrs. Walker's health?
2. What nursing diagnoses can be derived from the information presented in the case study? Be sure to include the etiology of Mrs. Walker's problems where appropriate. How would you prioritize these diagnoses? Why?
3. How would you go about incorporating client participation in planning interventions for Mrs. Walker's health problems?
4. List at least three client care objectives that you would like to accomplish with Mrs. Walker.
5. Describe some of the primary, secondary, and tertiary prevention strategies that would be appropriate in resolving Mrs. Walker's health problems. Why would they be appropriate?
6. How would you evaluate your nursing intervention? What criteria would you use to evaluate care?

---

nurse's approach to health education. What nursing interventions might modify the influence of these factors? (pp. 579–581)

9. Describe four considerations in evaluating the effects of nursing care that are unique to older clients. (pp. 581–582)

WHAT DO YOU THINK?
Questions for Critical Thinking

1. Which theory of aging do you think best explains the aging process? Why?
2. In what ways, if any, does the saying "You can't teach an old dog new tricks" apply to the care of older clients?
3. In fostering independence, what kinds of health risks do you think would be acceptable for an older client? Is there a point at which you would curtail some aspects of independence? If so, when?

4. How would you help an older client work through the development task of preparing for death?

REFERENCES

Adult Vaccine Preventable Diseases Bureau. (1996). Pneumococcal and influenza vaccination levels among adults aged ≥ 65 years—U.S., 1993. *MMWR, 45,* 853–859.

Advisory Committee on Immunization Practices. (1995). Assessing adult vaccination status at age 50 years. *MMWR, 44,* 561–563.

Arden, N. H., Cox, N. J., & Schonberger, L. B. (1994). Prevention and control of influenza: Part I, vaccines. *MMWR, 43*(RR-9), 1–13.

Barusch, A. S. (1994). *Older women in poverty: Private lives and public policies.* New York: Springer.

Bastable, S. B. (1997). Teaching strategies specific to developmental stages of life. In S. B. Bastable (Ed.), *Nurse as educator: Principles of teaching and learning* (pp. 91–123). Boston: Jones and Bartlett.

Bender, P. (1992). Deceptive distress in the elderly. *American Journal of Nursing, 92,* 29–32.

Berenstein, D., & De Hertogh, D. (1992). Recently acquired syphilis in the elderly population. *Archives of Internal Medicine, 152,* 330–332.

Berman, L. D. (1994). Uses and misuses of laboratory tests. In F. Homberger (Ed.), *The rational use of advanced medical technology with the elderly.* New York: Springer.

Bissonnette, A., & Hijjazi, K. H. (1994). Elder homelessness: A community perspective. *Nursing Clinics of North America, 29,* 409–416.

Bosse, R., Levenson, M. R., Spiro, A., III, Aldwin, C. M., & Mroczek, D. K. (1992). For whom is retirement stressful? Findings from the normative aging study. In B. Vellas & J. L. Albarede (Eds.), *Facts and research in gerontology 1992* (pp. 223–237). New York: Springer.

Brown, S. L., Salive, M. E., Pahor, M., et al. (1995). Occult caffeine as a source of sleep problems in an older population. *Journal of the American Geriatrics Society, 43,* 860–864.

Burns, R., Nichols, L. O., Graney, M. J., & Cloar, F. T. (1995). Impact of continued geriatric outpatient management on health outcomes of older veterans. *Archives of Internal Medicine, 155,* 1313–1318.

Callahan, C. M., Hendrie, H. C., & Tierney, W. M. (1995). Documentation and evaluation of cognitive impairment in elderly primary care patients. *Annals of Internal Medicine, 122,* 422–429.

Centers for Disease Control. (1996). National Adult Immunization Awareness Week. *MMWR, 45,* 853.

Cummings, S. R., Nevitt, M. S., Browner, W. S., et al. (1995). Risk factors for hip fracture in white women. *New England Journal of Medicine, 332,* 767–773.

Dellasega, C. (1991). Caregiving stress and community caregivers for the elderly: Does institutionalization make a difference? *Journal of Community Health Nursing, 8,* 197–205.

Delong, M. F. (April 2, 1995). Caring for the elderly, Part 4: Medication use and abuse. *NURSEweek,* pp. 8–9.

Devanand, D. P., Sano, M., Tang, M., et al. (1996). Depressed mood and the incidence of Alzheimer's disease in the elderly living in the community. *Archives of General Psychiatry, 53,* 175–182.

Division of Chronic Disease Control and Community Intervention. (1995a). State-specific changes in physical inactivity among persons aged ≥ 65 years—United States, 1987–1992. *MMWR, 44,* 663–673.

Division of Chronic Disease Control and Community Intervention. (1995b). Urinary incontinence in persons aged ≥ 65 years—Mass. and Okla., 1993. *MMWR, 44,* 747, 753–754.

Division of Violence Prevention. (1996). Suicide among older persons—United States, 1980–1992. *MMWR, 45,* 3–6.

Ebersole, P., & Hess, P. (1994). *Toward healthy aging: Human needs and nursing response* (4th ed.). St. Louis, Mosby.

Erickson, E. (1963). *Childhood and society* (2nd ed.). New York: W. W. Norton.

Farrell, K. R., & Ganzini, L. (1995). Misdiagnosing delirium as depression in medically ill elderly patients. *Archives of Internal Medicine, 155,* 2459–2464.

Frongillo, E. A., Rauschenbach, B. S., Roe, D. A., & Williamson, D. F. (1992). Characteristics related to elderly persons' not eating for 1 or more days: Implications for meal programs. *American Journal of Public Health, 82,* 600–602.

Galsworthy, T. D. (1996). Osteoporosis: It steals more than bone. *American Journal of Nursing, 96*(6), 27–33.

Gardner, B. C. (1989). Guide to changing lab values in elders. *Geriatric Nursing, 10*(3), 144–145.

Gibson, H. B. (1992). *The emotional and sexual lives of older people: A manual for professionals.* London: Chapman & Hall.

Gill, T. M., Williams, C. S., & Tinetti, M. E. (1995). Assessing risk for the onset of functional dependence among older adults: The role of physical performance. *Journal of the American Geriatrics Society, 43,* 603–609.

Ginsberg C., Gage, L., Martin, V., Gerstein, S., & Acuff, K. (1994). *America's urban safety net hospitals: Meeting the needs of our most vulnerable populations.* Washington, DC: National Association of Public Hospitals.

Gordon, S. M., & Thompson, S. (1995). The changing epidemiology of human immunodeficiency virus infection in older persons. *Journal of the American Geriatrics Society, 43,* 7–9.

Grabbe, L., Demi, A., Camann, M. A., & Potter, L. (1997). The health status of elderly persons in the last year of life: A comparison of deaths by suicide, injury, and natural causes. *American Journal of Public Health, 87,* 434–437.

Guiccione, A. C., Felson, D. T., Anderson, J. J., et al. (1994). The effects of specific medical conditions on the functional limitations of elders in the Framingham study. *American Journal of Public Health, 84,* 351–358.

Guy, D. H. (1995). Telephone care for elders: Physical, psychological, and legal aspects. *Journal of Gerontological Nursing, 21*(12), 27–34.

Hogstel, M. O., & Keen-Payne, R. (1993). *Practical guide to assessment through the life span.* Philadelphia: F. A. Davis.

Hunter, G. R., Treuth, M. S., Weinsier, R. L., et al. (1995). The effects of strength conditioning on older women's ability to perform daily tasks. *Journal of the American Geriatrics Society, 43,* 756–760.

Kelly, S. J. (1993). Caregiver stress in grandparents raising grandchildren. *Image, 25,* 331–337.

Kennie, D. C. (1993). *Preventive care for elderly people.* New York: Cambridge University Press.

Kindig, M. N., & Carnes, M. (1993). *Coping with Alzheimer's disease and other dementing illnesses.* San Diego: Singular.

King, A. C., Oman, R. F., Brassington, G. S., Bliwise, D. L., & Haskell, W. L. (1997). Moderate-intensity exercise and self-rated quality of sleep in older adults. *JAMA, 277,* 32–37.

Kinsella, K. G. (1994). An aging world population. *World Health, 47*(4), 6.

Launer, L. J., Masaki, K., Petrovitch, H., Foley, D., & Havlik, R. J. (1995). The association between midlife blood pressure levels and late-life cognitive function. *JAMA, 274,* 1846–1851.

Lee, M. (1996). Drugs and the elderly: Do you know the risks? *American Journal of Nursing, 96*(7), 5–31.

Maslow, A. (1968). *Toward a psychology of being* (2nd ed.). New York: Van Nostrand Reinhold.

McCormick, K. A., Newman, D. K., Colling, J., & Pearson, B. D. (1992). Urinary incontinence in adults. *American Journal of Nursing, 82,* 75–92.

Mellick, E., Buckwalter, K. C., & Stolley, J. M. (1992). Suicide among elderly white men: Development of a profile. *Journal of Psychosocial Nursing, 30*(2), 29–34.

Nagley, S. J. (1990). Cognitive functioning. In D. M. Corr & C. A. Corr (Eds.), *Nursing care in an aging society* (pp. 178–201). New York: Springer.

National Cancer Institute. (1996). Trends in cancer screening—United States, 1987 and 1992. *MMWR, 45,* 57–61.

National Center for Chronic Disease Prevention and Health Promotion. (1996). Incidence and costs to Medicare of fractures among Medicare beneficiaries aged ≥ 65 years. *MMWR, 45,* 877–883.

National Center for Infectious Diseases. (1995). Pneumonia and influenza death rates—United States, 1979–1994. *MMWR, 44,* 535–537.

O'Malley, T. A., & Blakeney, B. A. (1994). Physical health problems and treatment of the aged. In D. G. Satin (Ed.), *The clinical care of the aged person: An interdisciplinary perspective* (pp. 27–61). New York: Oxford University Press.

Payette, H., Gray-Donald, K., Cyr, R., & Boutier, V. (1995). Predictors of dietary intake in a functionally dependent elderly population in the community. *American Journal of Public Health, 85,* 677–683.

Phaneuf, C. (1996). Screening elders for nutritional deficits. *American Journal of Nursing, 96*(3), 58–60.

Posner, B. M., Jette, A. M., Smith, K. W., & Miller, D. R. (1993). Nutrition and health risks in the elderly: The Nutrition Screening Initiative. *American Journal of Public Health, 83,* 972–978.

Province, M. A., Hadley, E. C., Hornbrook, M. C., et al. (1995). The effects of exercise on falls in elderly patients: A preplanned meta-analysis of the FICSIT trials. *JAMA, 273,* 1341–1347.

Rakowski, W., & Hickey, T. (1992). Mortality and the attribution of health problems to aging among older adults. *American Journal of Public Health, 82,* 1139–1141.

Reuben, D. B., & Siu, A. L. (1992). New approaches to functional assessment. In B. Vellas & J. L. Albarede (Eds.), *Facts and research in gerontology 1992* (pp. 191–202). New York: Springer.

Russell, R. M. (1992). Vitamin requirements in old age. In B. Vellas & J. L. Albarede (Eds.), *Facts and research in gerontology 1992* (pp. 61–66). New York: Springer.

Satin, D. (1994). Emotional and cognitive issues in the care of the aged. In D. G. Satin (Ed.), *The clinical care of the aged person: An interdisciplinary perspective* (pp. 62–107). New York: Oxford University Press.

Schlenker, E. D. (1993). *Nutrition in aging* (2nd ed.). St. Louis: Mosby.

Schupf, N., Kapell, D., Lee, J. H., Ottman, R., & Mayeux, R. (1994). Increased risk of Alzheimer's disease in mothers of adults with Down's syndrome. *Lancet, 344,* 353–356.

U.S. Department of Commerce. (1996). *Statistical abstract of the United States, 1996* (116th ed.). Washington, DC: Government Printing Office.

U.S. Department of Health and Human Services. (1991). *Healthy people 2000: National health promotion and disease prevention objectives.* Washington, DC: Government Printing Office.

U.S. Department of Health and Human Services. (1993). *Health United States, 1992, and healthy people 2000 review.* Washington, DC: Government Printing Office.

U.S. Department of Health and Human Services. (1995). *Healthy people 2000: Midcourse review and 1995 revisions.* Washington, DC: Government Printing Office.

U.S. Department of Health and Human Services. (1996a). *Health United States, 1995.* Washington, DC: Government Printing Office.

U.S. Department of Health and Human Services. (1996b). *Healthy people 2000: Progress review, Older adults.* Washington, DC: Government Printing Office.

Valente, S. M. (1994). Recognizing depression in elderly patients. *American Journal of Nursing, 94*(12), 19–24.

Van Stavesen, W. R., Burema, J. A., De Groot, L. C., & Vorrips, L. E. (1992). Nutrition in the elderly. In B. Vellas & J. L. Albarede (Eds.), *Facts and research in gerontology 1992* (pp. 61–66). New York: Springer.

Willcox, S. M., Himmelstein, D. U., & Woolhandler, S. (1994). Inappropriate drug prescribing for the community-dwelling elderly. *JAMA, 272,* 292–296.

Wolf, S. L., Barnhart, H. X., Kutner, N. G., et al. (1996). Reducing frailty and falls in older persons: An investigation of Tai Chi and computerized balance training. *Journal of the American Geriatrics Society*, *44*, 489–497.

Wolfson, L., Whipple, R., Derby, C., et al. (1996). Balance and strength training in older adults: Intervention gains and Tai Chi maintenance. *Journal of the American Geriatrics Society, 44*, 498–506.

Wolinsk, F. D., Fitzgerald, J. F., & Stump, T. E. (1997). The effect of hip fracture on mortality, hospitalization, and functional status: A prospective study. *American Journal of Public Health, 87*, 398–403.

Young, D. R., Masaki, K. H., & Curb, J. D. (1995). Associations of physical activity with performance-based and self-reported physical functioning in older men: The Honolulu Heart Program. *Journal of the American Geriatrics Society, 43*, 845–854.

Zwerling, C., Sprince, N. L., Wallace, R. B., Davis, C. S., Whitten, P. S., & Heeringa, S. G. (1996). Risk factors for occupational injuries among older workers: An analysis of the Health and Retirement Study. *American Journal of Public Health, 86*, 1306–1309.

RESOURCES FOR NURSES WORKING WITH OLDER CLIENTS

Aging

American Society on Aging
833 Market Street, Ste. 512
San Francisco, CA 94103–1824
(415) 974–9600

Gerontological Society of America
1275 K. Street, NW, Ste. 350
Washington, DC 20005
(202) 842–1275

National Institute on Age, Work, and Retirement
c/o National Council on Aging
409 3rd Street, SW, Ste. 200
Washington, DC 20024
(202) 479–1200

National Institute on Aging
9000 Rockville Pike
Bethesda, MD 20892
(301) 496–1752

Airway Disease

American Lung Association
1740 Broadway
New York, NY 10019–4374
(212) 315–8700

Emphysema Anonymous
PO Box 2644
Clearwater, FL 34617

Alcohol Abuse

Al-Anon Family Group Headquarters
PO Box 862
Midtown Station
New York, NY 10018–0862
(212) 302–7240

Alcoholics Anonymous World Services
475 Riverside Drive
New York, NY 10163
(212) 870–3400

Alzheimer's Disease

ADEAR Center—Alzheimer's Disease Education and Referral
PO Box 8250
Silver Spring, MD 20907–8250
(800) 438–4380

Alzheimer's Association
919 North Michigan Avenue, Ste. 100
Chicago, IL 60611
(800) 272–3900

National Caregiving Foundation
401 Wythe Street, Ste. A3
Alexandria, VA 22314
(800) 930–1357

National Family Caregivers Association
9621 E. Bexhill Drive
Kensington, MD 20895–3104
(800) 804–6604

Athritis

Arthritis Foundation
1314 Spring Street NW
Atlanta, GA 30309
(404) 872–7100

National Arthritis and Musculoskeletal and Skin Disease Information Clearinghouse
9000 Rockville Pike
PO Box AMS
Bethesda, MD 20892–2903
(301) 495–4484

Cancer

American Cancer Society
1599 Clifton Road, NE
Atlanta, GA 30329
(404) 320–3333

Cancer Care, Inc.
1180 Avenue of the Americas
New York, NY 10036
(212) 221–3300

United Ostomy Association
36 Executive Park, Ste. 120
Irvine, CA 92714
(714) 660–8624

Death and Dying

Hospice Education Institute
190 Westbrook Road
Essex, CT 06426
(203) 767–1620

Living/Dying Project
75 Digital Drive
Novato, CA 94949
(415) 884–2343

Make Today Count
1235 E. Cherokee Street
Springfield, MO 65804–2203
(417) 885–3324

Dental Problems

American Society for Geriatric Dentistry
211 East Chicago Avenue, Ste. 948
Chicago, IL 60611
(312) 440–2661

Diabetes

American Diabetes Association National Center
PO Box 25757
1660 Duke Street
Alexandria, VA 22314
(703) 549–1500

Diet/Nutrition

Local Meals-on-Wheels
Local senior citizens' centers
Area Office on Aging

Health Promotion

Health Promotion Institute
409 3rd Street SW, 2nd Floor
Washington, DC 20024
(202) 479–1200

Hearing Loss

Alexander Graham Bell Association for the Deaf
3417 Volta Place, NW
Washington, DC 20007–2778
(202) 337–5220

American Speech–Language–Hearing Association
10801 Rockville Pike
Rockville, MD 20852
(301) 897–5700

Deafness Research Foundation
9 East 38th Street, 7th Floor
New York, NY 10016
(212) 684–6556

Hearing Industries Association
515 King Street, Ste. 420
Alexandria, VA 22314
(703) 684–5744

National Association of the Deaf
814 Thayer Avenue
Silver Spring, MD 20910
(301) 587–1788

Heart Disease

American Heart Association
7272 Greenville Avenue
Dallas, TX 75231–4596
(214) 373–6300

Mended Hearts, Inc.
7272 Greenville Avenue
Dallas, TX 75231–4596
(214) 706–1442

Home Care/Nursing Homes

American Association of Homes for the Aging
901 East Street NW, Ste. 500
Washington, DC 20004–2037
(202) 783–2242

CHAP Program of the National League for Nursing
100 Columbus Circle
New York, NY 10014

Foundation Aiding the Elderly
PO Box 254849
Sacramento, CA 96865–4849
(916) 481–8558

International Council of Homehelp Services
c/o LVT Postbus 100
NL 3980 CC
Bunnik, Netherlands

Nursing Home Advisory and Research Council
PO Box 18820
Cleveland Heights, OH 44118
(216) 321–4499

Menopause

International Menopause Society
c/o Monique Boulet
8 Avenue Don Bosco
B1150 Brussels, Belgium

Safety

American Red Cross National Headquarters
One-in-a-Million Program
431 18th Street, NW
Washington, DC 20006
(202) 737–8300

Social Welfare

American Association of Retired Persons
601 East Street NW
Washington, DC 20049
(202) 434–2277

Gray Panthers
PO Box 21477
Washington, DC 20009–9477
(202) 466–3132

Medicare Hospital Insurance
Medicare Supplemental Hospital Insurance
Meadows East Building
6300 Security Building
Baltimore, MD 21207
(410) 966–3000

National Indian Council on Aging
6400 Uptown Blvd., NW
Center City, Ste. 510–W
Albuquerque, NM 87110
(505) 888–3302

Social Security Administration
6401 Security Building
Baltimore, MD 21235
(410) 965–7700

U.S. Department of Health and Human Services
Administration on Aging
330 Independence Avenue SW
Washington, DC 20201
(202) 619–0554

U.S. House of Representatives Select Committee
   on Aging
Subcommittee on Health and Long-term Care
H2-377 House Office Building
Annex II
Washington, DC 20515
(202) 226–3381

U.S. Senate Committee on Labor
   and Human Resources
Subcommittee on Aging
SH-404 Hart Senate Office Building
Washington, DC 20510
(202) 224–3239

Visual Impairment

Christian Record Services
4444 South 52nd Street
Lincoln, NE 68526
(402) 488–0981

Eye Bank for Sight Restoration
210 East 64th Street
New York, NY 10021
(212) 980–6700

John Milton Society for the Blind
475 Riverside Drive, Room 455
New York, NY 10115
(212) 870–3336

Local Lions Club

National Association for Visually Handicapped
22 West 21st Street
New York, NY 10010
(212) 889–3141

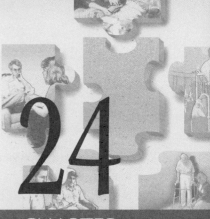

24

CARE OF HOMELESS CLIENTS

benign homelessness
deindustrialization
deinstitutionalization
gentrification
homeless individual
malignant homelessness
marginal homeless
means-tested income
  transfers
noninstitutionalization
safe havens
structural unemployment

Who are the people that make up the growing homeless population? Contrary to popular belief, the typical homeless person is not the "skid row bum," a perpetually drunk male vagrant inhabiting a rundown district of a large city. Today, homeless people include families, single women with children, and the elderly, as well as single men. Most are poor, but some are not. Many have little education, but some are well educated. Many are mentally ill, but, again, many are not. African Americans, Latinos, and Native Americans are all overrepresented among the homeless population in the United States particularly in rural areas (Flynt, 1996).

A community health nurse may encounter homeless clients in a variety of ways. When going to visit another client at home, the nurse may be approached by homeless individuals asking for work, shelter, or food. Or the nurse may provide health care services for the homeless in shelters or in clinics. Or, when following up contacts of persons with a communicable disease, the nurse may meet homeless persons. In addition, community health nurses may participate in task forces mounted by local governments or religious groups to address the problems of homelessness. Wherever they encounter homeless clients, community health nurses must be prepared to assist them to deal with a variety of health and social needs.

▶ ## Chapter Objectives

After reading this chapter, you should be able to:

- Identify at least three biophysical problems common among homeless individuals.
- Describe at least three social dimension factors that contribute to homelessness.
- Identify two behavioral dimension factors that influence the health of homeless clients.
- Describe two ways in which health systems factors contribute to homelessness.
- Describe at least three approaches to primary prevention of homelessness.
- Identify at least three areas in which secondary preventive interventions may be required in the care of homeless individuals.
- Identify at least two strategies for tertiary prevention of homelessness at the aggregate level.
- Describe two considerations in implementing care for homeless individuals.
- Identify the primary focus of evaluation for care of homeless clients.

▶ ## DEFINING HOMELESSNESS

Homelessness can be defined in various ways. For the most part, the definition used is that included in the McKinney Homeless Assistance Act of 1987 in which a *homeless individual* is one who (1) lacks a fixed, regular, and adequate nighttime residence and who (2) has a nighttime residence that is a shelter, an institution, or a place not intended as sleeping accommodations (Jahiel, 1992a). Although technically accurate, this definition ignores people who are forced to live with friends or family because of a lack of other housing alternatives (Jencks, 1994).

For the individual client, the designation of "homeless" has three primary aspects: a physical aspect, a social aspect, and a psychological aspect. The physical aspect is being without regular shelter. The social aspect involves the loss of family support great enough to meet the client's needs for shelter and other forms of support. Finally, the psychological aspect reflects the stigma attached to the social role of homelessness (Snow & Anderson, 1993).

Homeless people can be categorized in different ways and the importance of these three aspects of homeless varies with the type of homelessness encountered. Homelessness has sometimes been classified as

benign or malignant (Jahiel, 1992a). *Benign homelessness* is homelessness of short duration, with minimal effects, the resolution of which is long-lasting. Spending the night in your car because all the local hotels are filled and sleeping a day or two in a tent in the backyard while the house is fumigated are examples of benign homelessness. *Malignant homelessness* is of longer standing and may be divided into subcategories also based on length of time involved. The first category is one of temporary, but recurrent homelessness that occurs in a regular pattern. For example, seasonal workers may be able to afford housing when they are steadily employed and not during seasons of unemployment. A second category of malignant homelessness is experienced by those who are between housing situations, but who have potential for regaining long-term housing. For example, a family whose home has burned or who have been evicted due to building condemnation. The last category, which is the most difficult to address, is that of long-term homelessness (Marsh, 1996). People in this category are, for a variety of reasons, homeless for extended periods of time and are the ones most likely to be unable to meet needs other than shelter that having a home supports. Some of these needs and the hardships created by not meeting them are listed in Table 24–1.

▶ ## THE PROCESS OF HOMELESSNESS AND ITS RESOLUTION

Malignant homelessness is a process of disconnection. Conversely, its resolution involves a progressive reconnection. Disconnection begins with some precipitating event or "violation," such as an eviction, destruction of one's residence, or rent increase beyond one's ability to pay (Francis, 1992). For many homeless individuals, violation is preceded by a long period of economic marginality in which they are less and less able to afford life's basic necessities including housing (Rosenthal, 1994). This vulnerable group has sometimes been called the *marginal homeless* (Davis, 1996) because of their high risk for homelessness. Violation frequently leads to a period of what has been termed temporary private connections, in which the homeless individual or family moves in with friends or family members. This is usually followed by a period of "temporary" public connections in which help is sought from public institutions and agencies such as shelters and welfare, housing, or employment agencies. This period may entail a lengthy wait for assistance. Finally, resolution of homelessness, if it occurs, involves the rebuilding of societal connections in obtaining permanent housing and other needed services.

TABLE 24–1. NEEDS MET BY HAVING A HOME AND CONSEQUENCES OF UNMET NEEDS

Needs Met by a Home	Consequences of Unmet Needs
• Protection from the elements	• Hypothermia/hyperthermia
• Protection from crime	• Criminal victimization
• A place to rest, wash	• Fatigue, skin disorders, lowered self-esteem due to decreased hygiene
• Storage for possessions	• Potential for theft/loss
• Privacy	• Increased stress
• A place to interact with friends	• Social isolation
• A place to raise and interact with family	• Family stress
• A place to be reached	• Missed opportunities for employment, decreased eligibility for aid
• Symbol of community integration	• Alienation, decreased social participation/influence
• Social status	• Loss of identity, self-esteem
• Economic investment	• Lack of economic reserve
• A reflection of self	• Loss of self-identity

(Source: Jahiel, 1992a.)

During the actual period of homelessness, people also experience several stages which Kuhlman (1994) likened to the three stages of Selye's Stress Adaptation Syndrome. In the first stage, immediately following dislocation from one's previous housing situation, the homeless person experiences homelessness as a traumatic threat, but continues to identify with the mainstream of society. Agency assistance is readily sought, and the focus of energy is on "getting off the streets." People in this stage actively distance themselves from the rest of the homeless population, and reconnection is relatively easy. In the second stage, the homeless individual begins to see homelessness less as an isolated episode and more as a way of life and establishes a beginning identification with the population of homeless individuals. This stage may be characterized by feelings of shame, hostility, and bitterness. Plans for getting off the street are less concrete and assistance programs may be actively avoided. If reconnection does not occur, clients may pass into the third stage in which homelessness has been accepted as a basic identity and the focus of effort is on survival (Snow & Anderson, 1993; Kuhlman, 1994).

Although the needs of the homeless population are not specifically addressed by the national health objectives for the year 2000, the majority of objectives targeted to low-income individuals also address the needs of homeless individuals. These objectives are summarized in Appendix A.

▶ **THE MAGNITUDE OF HOMELESSNESS**

There are no exact figures on the number of homeless persons in the United States, and estimates vary from 250,000 to 3 million (Jezewski, 1995). A 1994 study by

Link and associates (1994) indicated that approximately 14% of the U.S. population, 26 million people, had been homeless at some time in their lives and more than 7% had been literally homeless with the remainder moving in with friends and family. Just over 3% (5.7 million people) had been literally homeless in the previous 5 years. Homeless individuals can be found in almost any major city, in affluent suburbs, and in rural areas, and the number of homeless nationwide is growing each year. In fact, the annual increase in the homeless population in the United States may be as much as 10 to 38% (Kuhlman, 1994).

Who are the homeless? The homeless are by no means a homogeneous group. Recent literature speaks to the difference in composition between the homeless population of today and that of several years ago. In the past, most homeless individuals were men over the age of 45. Today, however, the average age of homeless individuals is 34 years, and approximately a third of the homeless population consists of women and children (Davis, 1996). Roughly 5% of the homeless population was over age 60 in 1991 (Hales & Magnus, 1991), and this population is growing. For example, over a 2-year period the homeless elderly population in Boston increased by 50% to represent nearly one quarter of Boston's homeless (Bissonnette & Hijjazi, 1994).

Many more families are becoming a part of the homeless population, which in the past was composed primarily of single individuals. It is estimated that families with children constitute as much as 40% of the homeless population nationwide (Shinn & Weitzman, 1996). In 1994 alone, requests for shelter from families increased by 21% (Hatton, 1997). Many of these homeless families are headed by single women and include preschool children (Davis, 1996; Hatton, 1997).

▶ THE DIMENSIONS MODEL AND CARE OF THE HOMELESS

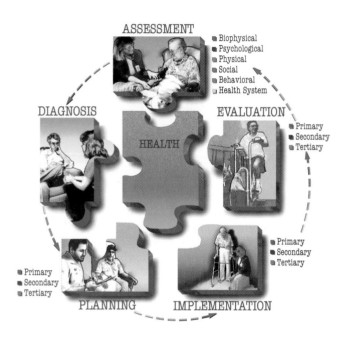

Efforts of community health nurses to resolve problems of homeless people can be guided by use of the Dimensions Model. Nurses can use the model to identify factors contributing to homelessness and the effects of homelessness on health, and to plan, implement, and evaluate interventions to resolve some of these problems.

Critical Dimensions of Nursing and Care of the Homeless

Each of the six dimensions of nursing are important in caring for homeless and poor clients. In the cognitive dimension, the nurse must have a clear grasp of the risks for and causes of homelessness as well as its probable effects on clients' health. The nurse must also have specific knowledge of resources available to homeless clients and how these resources can be obtained. In the interpersonal dimension, the nurse will need to be able to motivate clients who are often bitter and hostile toward service agencies after frustrating attempts to get help (Jezewski, 1995). Interpersonal skills will also be critical to the nurse's ability to network with other providers to achieve the array of services needed by many homeless clients. Within the ethical dimension, advocacy will be required at both the individual and societal levels, and community

health nurses must be actively involved in the development of social policies that prevent and ameliorate poverty and homelessness (Porter-O'Grady, 1993).

Both manipulative and intellectual skills will be needed in the skills dimension to address the many needs of the homeless clientele. The nurse may need to be particularly creative in developing ways to maintain asepsis in wounds when clients have no access to facilities for normal hygiene. Analytic skills will also be needed to identify client problems and the most appropriate sources of care for the homeless. Necessary elements of the process dimension that are needed in the care of the homeless include the change, leadership, and political processes. The nurse may need to employ the change process to motivate clients to make behavioral changes conducive to better health. This may be particularly difficult until the nurse has assisted clients to meet basic survival needs. This assistance most often entails the use of the referral and case management processes so comprehensive, rather than fragmented, care is provided. Change, leadership, and political skills will be required to engage in the societal advocacy activities mentioned above. Finally, research is needed to further identify risks for homelessness and to evaluate the effectiveness of interventions designed to minimize risk of homelessness and to ameliorate homelessness when it occurs.

 Assessing the Dimensions of Health Among the Homeless

The first step in the use of the Dimensions Model is assessing the health status of homeless clients and the factors that influence their health. The community health nurse examines factors in the client's situation that contribute to homelessness as well as the health effects of their homeless state.

The Biophysical Dimension

Biophysical factors, in conjunction with factors in other dimensions, may lead to homelessness. Conversely, homelessness has serious consequences for biophysical health that vary with age and prior health status.

Age and Homelessness.   The health effects of homelessness are exacerbated for both the young and the elderly. Homeless children are twice as likely as other children to experience anemia, parasitic infestations, dental problems, seizures, and circulatory or dermatologic conditions. They also have a high incidence of asthma and other respiratory conditions and gastroenteritis (Riemer, Van Cleve, & Galbraith, 1995; Shinn & Weitz-

▶ TWO HOMELESS WOMEN

Angela

Angela is a good-looking woman in her late 30s. She and her 6-year-old daughter are staying temporarily at a shelter for homeless women with children. She has a college education and had her own business in New York. She has been divorced for a year, but her ex-husband still beat her regularly, so she decided to take her daughter and move to California. She sold her business and left without letting her ex-husband know what she was doing. When Angela arrived in California, she used the money from her business to buy inventory and rent a place to begin again. She used the little money left over to pay the rent on a small apartment. After living in the apartment for a week, she discovered that the building housed an illegal drug lab run by the building's owner and that most of the other tenants were substance abusers. She decided that this was not an appropriate environment for her child, so she left. She was afraid to ask the landlord for her money back for fear that he would think she was going to the police. She had no other funds, so she and her daughter were homeless.

Angela was very close to her parents, but her father had recently had heart surgery and her parents could barely afford their mortgage payments. Angela did not think she could ask them for help. Fortunately, Angela knew that there were usually shelters available for homeless women with children, so she contacted the health department and was referred to the shelter.

Nancy

Nancy is also staying in the shelter. Nancy is in her early 30s and is tall, gaunt, and emaciated. She describes living for a year in a Volkswagen with her boyfriend and her 7-year-old son.

Nancy and her boyfriend were drug abusers and occasionally gave drugs to her son when he began to "snivel about being hungry." Nancy and her boyfriend worked odd jobs, but used the bulk of their income to support their drug habit.

Nancy's son was enrolled in public school but was frequently absent, and his school performance was poor. When school personnel began to investigate his absences, his circumstances were discovered, and he was placed in a foster home. Nancy voluntarily entered a drug detoxification center, but had no place to go when she was discharged. The social worker at the center made arrangements for Nancy to stay at the women's shelter. Nancy is currently trying to regain custody of her son.

man, 1996). Homeless children may also experience significant developmental delays (Wagner, Menke, & Ciccone, 1995).

The elderly are at particular risk of health problems stemming from homelessness. All of the usual problems of the elderly that are discussed in Chapter 23 are intensified by homelessness. The homeless elderly are particularly susceptible to the effects of communicable diseases, exposure, burns, and trauma due to alcoholic, physical, or mental impairment or assault. The elderly homeless population is also more likely than younger groups to experience chronic disability due to physical, mental, or emotional impairment. In fact, in one study 79% of older homeless individuals had at least one impairment (Bissonnette & Hijjazi, 1994).

Physiologic Function.   As noted earlier, elements of physiologic function may actually cause homelessness. For example, catastrophic illness, particularly in conjunction with a lack of health insurance, may catapult those who are already financially vulnerable into homelessness. Conversely, homelessness contributes to increased mortality and morbidity. The average life expectancy of homeless persons has been reported as 51 years compared to more than 70 years for the general population (Davis, 1996). In addition, nonfatal health problems encountered among the homeless

population are many and varied and are compounded by their lack of income and residence. Accidental and violence-related trauma is a common occurrence, as are skin diseases and ulcerations. Upper respiratory infections and influenza are easily spread among poorly nourished persons congregating in crowded shelters and food lines. Infestations of lice are prolonged by the inability to shower or wash clothes. Extensive walking and standing in line for prolonged periods, coupled with an inability to recline, leads to venous statis and edema that contribute to foot and leg ulcerations and cellulitis. Such problems are further complicated by poorly fitted or rundown shoes (Gelberg, 1997).

Other problems seen among homeless individuals include hypothermia; burns from sleeping on hot grates in an effort to keep warm; hypertension; neurological diseases; injuries and poisoning (including food poisoning); circulatory diseases; gastrointestinal disease; and chronic respiratory problems (Davis, 1996; Heffron, Skipper, & Lambert, 1997; May & Evans, 1994). It is estimated that one third to one half of the homeless population experience one or more health conditions (Gelberg, 1997), with hypertension present in many homeless adults. Prevalence rates for tuberculosis are up to 300 times higher than those of the general population, with 968 cases of active tuberculous disease per 100,000 homeless persons (Advisory Council for the Elimination of Tuberculosis, 1992). Nearly 6% of all new cases of tuberculosis diagnosed in 40 reporting areas in 1994 occurred among the homeless (Division of Tuberculosis Elimination, 1995). In addition, to the increased prevalence of disease in this population, homeless individuals are more likely than the general population to exhibit drug-resistant tuberculosis. In part, the increased incidence of tuberculosis among the homeless is due to a concurrent increase in the prevalence of HIV infection. This is particularly true among those homeless individuals who turn to prostitution as a means of survival.

Chronic health problems are compounded by the homeless person's difficulty in following a prescribed treatment regimen. For example, exposure to cold exacerbates the effects of chronic respiratory diseases, and an unstable diet places the diabetic at higher risk. In addition, because insulin syringes are highly valued by IV drug users, the homeless person with diabetes faces the risk of being attacked for the syringes in his or her possession. The homeless person with diabetes also might be tempted to sell the syringes.

Physiologic problems experienced by homeless children include respiratory and ear infections, dental problems, poor vision, musculoskeletal problems, abdominal pain and ulcers, seizures, sickle cell disease, trauma, and renal disease. Other problems seen in homeless children include lead poisoning, sleep disorders, and malnutrition (Attala & Warmington, 1996). In addition, these children are less likely to be adequately immunized. For example, 24% of children in one study were not up-to-date on their immunizations (Halbach & Shortridge, 1993). In another study as many as 38% of homeless children were not adequately immunized. On average, homeless children in this study had 1.8 diagnosed health problems each, and 8.5% had four or more diagnoses (Evans, 1993).

Problems frequently encountered among the homeless elderly include hypothermia, malnutrition, parasitic infestations, peripheral vascular disease, and tuberculosis. Other common conditions are cardiac disease, diabetes, hypertension, and pulmonary disease.

The community health nurse working with a homeless individual would be particularly alert for these commonly encountered health problems. In addition, the nurse would assess the client for the presence of any other chronic or communicable diseases.

Pregnancy is a physiologic condition that has particular implications for homeless women. In general, homeless women have a pregnancy rate twice as high as nonhomeless women (Killion, 1995). In part, this is the result of sexual activity while homeless. Sexual activity may result from attempts to earn money or to solicit protection, a need for intimacy, or rape or coercion. Pregnancy may also be the result of inability to afford contraceptives. Both poor and homeless women are at risk for having low birth weight babies (Infant and Child Health Studies Bureau, 1995). In fact, low birth weight is more than twice as common among babies of homeless women as poor women with regular housing (Gelberg, 1997).

In addition to the risk of poor pregnancy outcomes, homeless women have more difficulty managing the normal discomforts of pregnancy which are often made worse by homelessness. Few homeless women receive ongoing prenatal care. Urinary tract infections are experienced more frequently because of lack of access to clean and safe toilet facilities. The increase in vaginal discharge that accompanies pregnancy, in conjunction with lack of facilities for adequate hygiene, leads to skin irritation. In addition, it is often impossible for the pregnant homeless woman to eat small frequent meals as a remedy for morning sickness. In fact, maintaining adequate nutrition at all is a challenge for these women. The usual mood swings of pregnancy may be exacerbated by depression and consequent substance abuse among homeless women. Homeless pregnant women may be tempted to (and often do) use cocaine to bring on labor when the discomforts of the third trimester become insupportable (Killion, 1995). Pregnant homeless women are a subpopulation that is clearly in need of early and ongoing community health nursing intervention.

The Psychological Dimension

Psychological factors can lead to homelessness when people are unable to cope with the demands of daily life and have limited support systems. Estimates of the extent of psychiatric illness in the homeless population vary. The Federal Task Force on Homelessness and Severe Mental Illness (1992) estimated that one third of homeless adults (or about 200,000 persons) experience serious mental illness. Approximately 12% have dual diagnoses of mental illness and substance abuse (Gelberg, 1997). Homeless clients with psychiatric illnesses are often noncompliant with therapeutic medications. Reasons given include medication side effects and inability to purchase medications (Mason, Jensen, & Boland, 1992).

History of mental illness is less prevalent among homeless families than single adults, but more common than among the housed poor. Prior hospitalization for mental illness occurs among 4 to 16% of homeless families compared to an average of 24% of homeless single adults across studies and 1 to 6% of the housed poor (Shinn & Weitzman, 1996). Homeless children, however, are at risk for mental health problems, sometimes reflecting poor mental health on the part of parents. In one study, for example, homeless women with children were quite articulate regarding their own mental health concerns, but were often unaware of their own or their children's other health problems (Hatton, 1997). In another study, 15% of homeless children over 4 years of age were in need of psychiatric evaluation (Wagner, Menke, & Ciccone, 1995). Homeless children are more likely than other children to display behavior problems. Homeless children also tend to do less well in school than their agemates. In one study, for example, 52% of homeless children exhibited behavior problems, 37% had poor school performance, and 21% had attempted suicide (Halbach & Shortridge, 1993). In some studies, nearly half of homeless children in shelters met criteria for special education evaluations, but only 22% had been referred for these services (Zima, Bussing, Forness, & Benjamin, 1997). Many preschool children were also believed to be at risk for mental health problems, but were never referred for services because child care workers felt referral was unrealistic in view of other family problems (Stokley, 1993).

Mentally ill persons tend to swell the homeless populations of large urban areas. This may be due in part to a migration of individuals with psychiatric illness from rural to urban areas. Large metropolitan centers have been shown to be more tolerant of bizarre behavior than rural areas. In rural areas, mentally ill persons tend to be cared for by family members and are less likely to become homeless. Homeless mentally ill persons in rural areas, on the other hand, are frequently incarcerated for unusual behavior or encouraged to move on (Belcher & McLeese, 1988).

Other psychological environmental factors besides mental illness may contribute to homelessness. For example, homeless individuals have reported almost three times as many stressful life events as their domiciled counterparts (Jahiel, 1992b). A significant number of recurrently homeless people have a history of multiple foster placements in childhood and consequently have never experienced a stable home environment (Koegel, Burnam, & Baumohl, 1996). Divorce, child abuse, and other forms of violence and family conflict also contribute to homelessness.

Psychological and physical abuse are contributing factors in the homelessness of many women with children. These women may experience symptoms of posttraumatic stress disorder (PTSD) including depression, somatic complaints, and suicidal ideation. Abandonment of one's home and significant others to escape abuse, although justified, may engender feelings of guilt, shame, grief, fear, and loneliness. Other emotions that may be experienced include anger, helplessness, and diminished self-esteem (Attala & Warmington, 1996). For many abused women, however, the decision to become homeless rather than suffer abuse can be seen as a strength that can be a positive focus for intervention by the community health nurse (Montgomery, 1994).

As noted, psychological factors can contribute to homelessness. Conversely, homelessness can result in a variety of psychological problems. Homelessness is a source of great anxiety and stress and may lead to depression, sadness, and loneliness. Loss of meaningful social roles may contribute to low self-esteem and low motivation. Desperation and hopelessness may also be seen among homeless clients (Davis, 1996).

The Physical Dimension

Physical dimension factors also contribute to the effects of homelessness on health. Exposure to cold, even in the mildest climates, can lead to hypothermia. This is particularly true when people are lying on concrete or are clothed in wet garments. Overcrowding and poor sanitary conditions in shelters contribute to the spread of communicable diseases among a population that is already debilitated by exposure and poor nutritional status. In fact, in one study, length of shelter stay was directly correlated with the rate of tuberculosis infection (Paul, Leibowitz, Moore, Hoven, Bennet, & Chen, 1993).

Unsafe physical environments also present health hazards for young children. In addition to the potential for physical injury, the restrictions placed by parents on children's activities in unsafe surroundings may result in developmental delays.

The Social Dimension

Social dimension factors play a major role in the development of homelessness and in its effects on the health of homeless individuals and families. Changes in family structure and support, widespread unemployment, poverty, and urban redevelopment are some of the societal conditions that contribute to homelessness. As noted by one observer, "Poverty may beget homelessness, but it seems to do so more often when social and economic conditions limit housing resources or when they promote population mobility" (Chafetz, 1988).

In some cases, homelessness may occur as a result of a breakdown in family ties. Mobility within the population has led to the break-up of extended family systems. This, in turn, results in a restricted social support network for families facing psychological and/or economic crises. High unemployment rates in some areas have led large numbers of individuals and families to move to other parts of the country in search of work. Others have fled countries plagued by poverty and violence. Many of these people arrive in a new locale to find the job market closed and a lack of available low-cost housing. Without an established social support network, they have no recourse but to live in cars, on the street, or in "welfare hotels."

Increases in poverty and consequent homelessness in the United States are, in part, the result of declining family income. From 1970 to 1988, the number of Americans living below the poverty level increased 26% (Koegel, Burnam, & Baumohl, 1996). By 1994, 14.5% of the U.S. population had incomes below the poverty level (U.S. Department of Health and Human Services, 1996). The increases are the result of several social environmental factors, including changes in government assistance programs and increased taxes.

Changes in government programs to assist the poor have contributed to increased poverty and homelessness in two ways. First, the level of assistance provided has not kept pace with the rate of inflation. Consequently, individuals and families receiving aid fall deeper into poverty. For example, the purchasing power of families receiving Aid to Families with Dependent Children (AFDC) declined by one third at the same time that rents increased by the same amount (Koegel, Burnam, & Baumohl, 1996).

Second, budgetary cutbacks have actually reduced benefits in some instances and stiffened eligibility requirements so that fewer of the working poor are eligible for aid. At the same time, taxes paid by the poor have increased. A further problem with the current system of public assistance is a need for persons to rid themselves of most of their resources to be eligible for help. In some instances, this also means breaking up family units and suffering the degradation often involved in the application and verification processes. When family members do obtain work in an attempt to add additional income, assistance benefits are frequently reduced by a similar amount, placing these families in a no-gain situation from which escape is impossible (Woodson, 1996). Some social assistance programs also create incentives to become homeless, because homeless individuals frequently receive priority for services (Marsh, 1996).

Unemployment is another major social factor contributing to homelessness. Although many people remain employed, there has been a shift in the job market from relatively well-paid manufacturing jobs to lower-paid employment in service industries (eg, janitorial work). This phenomenon is referred to as *structural unemployment* or *deindustrialization* because it arises from changes in the nation's economic and occupational structure, such as the shifts from heavy to light industry and from manufacturing to service occupations (Snow & Anderson, 1993). The emergence of high-technology occupations requires new sets of skills that many displaced workers do not have. Such changes in the structure of the job market have resulted in a situation in which 7.4 million people were unemployed in 1994 (U.S. Department of Commerce, 1996). An additional 8 million people were underemployed (Hardin, 1996).

The percentage of homeless people who are jobless varies from group to group. In some studies, as many as 99% of the homeless population is unemployed; in others, many of the homeless were working or had worked recently. Whether employed or not, almost all homeless individuals and families in these studies had low incomes and anywhere from 13 to 65% had no income at all (Jahiel, 1992b).

Finding employment is difficult for most homeless individuals. Those with mental illness find it hard to maintain a job, if they can get one, because of their instability. Homeless single women with children, who account for almost half of homeless families, have problems of child care while they work.

Even those homeless persons with employable skills in areas where jobs are available may have difficulty negotiating the employment process. Lack of transportation may make it difficult to go to an interview or to get to work when a job is found (Woodson, 1996). Another factor is a lack of available jobs. In one study, there were 14 applicants for every job opening (Newman, 1996). In addition, job application and interviews take time, which may prevent the individual from securing food or shelter for the night when these are obtained only after long waits in line in competition with many other homeless persons. Moreover, the homeless person may also find that he or she is penalized for working by reduction or even loss of assistance benefits and publically financed health care coverage (Hatton, 1997). Homeless individuals who cannot find regular work may engage in day labor or "shadow work." Shadow work may involve selling junk, personal possessions, or plasma; begging or panhandling; scavenging food, salable goods, or money; and theft (Snow, Anderson, Quist, & Cress, 1996).

Homelessness is not necessarily correlated with the social factor of low education levels. In various populations of homeless persons, those with at least a high school education constituted 41 to 65% of the group (Jahiel, 1992b).

Loss of affordable housing for low-income individuals and families is a major contributing factor in homelessness. Eviction is a common precipitating cause and may result from inability to pay rent or mortgage. Furthermore, the redevelopment of urban areas with a consequent loss of many low-cost housing units also fosters homelessness (Kuhlman, 1994). This process, called *gentrification,* occurs when more affluent members of society move into and rehabilitate areas inhabited by the poor. Since 1970 more than 1 million single-room occupancy units, one half of the available supply, have been lost, eliminating many low-cost housing alternatives (Dolbeare, 1996).

The cost of housing in relation to income is another factor contributing to homelessness among the poor. The amount of family income spent on housing has steadily increased over the last few years. In 1989, there were 7.8 million renters in the lowest income quartile vying for the 2.8 million housing units affordable on their income (Dolbeare, 1996). It is estimated that by 2003 the number of housing units renting for less than $325 a month will be 9.4 million, while the need for low-income housing units will increase to 17.2 million (Marsh, 1996).

Other social factors that contribute to homelessness in certain populations are divorce or separation and flight from abuse. Many women and their children are forced from their homes by abusive partners/fathers; another sizable group of homeless individuals are teenage runaways fleeing abusive home situations.

The effects of homelessness on health status are compounded by social factors such as lack of transportation and residential requirements for public assistance programs. Lack of transportation limits the ability of the homeless to secure housing, employment, and health care, among other things. Other contributing factors include lack of knowledge about entitlements, inability to produce required documentation, complexity of application forms, and frequent changes in eligibility requirements from place to place and over time.

Crime is another effect of homelessness. Homeless men are twice as likely to report arrest as a comparable group of nonhomeless. They are also more likely to report multiple arrests. Often the arrests of the homeless are for theft of items sold to purchase food or shelter. Other reasons for arrest include violation of vagrancy laws, the stigma of just being homeless, and the substitution of incarceration for needed treatment for mental illness (Federal Task Force on Homelessness and Severe Mental Illness, 1992). The extent of criminalization of homelessness is reflected in the 21,000 arrests for vagrancy in 1994 (U.S. Department of Commerce, 1996). The homeless are also at risk for robbery and assault. This is particularly true of homeless women and the elderly, who are less able to protect themselves and their belongings than homeless adult men.

Provision of shelter for the homeless may create problems in and of itself. The number of shelter beds available is often unequal to the needs of the population, especially in areas with large numbers of homeless. Competition for beds often results in intimidation of women and older persons in an attempt to force them to give way to stronger and more dominant males. Unless shelters are segregated by age or sex, or special shelters provided for homeless women, families, and the elderly, these groups may be prevented from making use of available shelter resources.

The Behavioral Dimension

Substance abuse is a behavioral factor that may contribute to homelessness when the abuser is unable, because of his or her addiction, to meet, or even care about, needs for shelter. Substance abuse may also lead to expenditure of money for alcohol or drugs that could be used for shelter. Alcohol abusers constitute about 33% of the overall homeless population (Kuhlman, 1994), and 6 to 31% of the homeless in some studies report abuse of other drugs (Robertson, Zlotnick, & Westerfelt, 1997; Susser, Betne, Valencia, Goldfinger, & Lehman, 1997). Cocaine use, in particular, has contributed to the increase in homelessness in many U.S. cities.

Prostitution is a lifestyle that may arise as a result of homelessness in an effort to earn enough money for food and shelter. Prostitution is particularly prevalent among adolescent runaways who find no other way to earn enough money to support themselves.

Prostitution and intravenous drug abuse among some members of the homeless population place this group at risk for communicable diseases such as AIDS and hepatitis B. AIDS in and of itself may be a contributing factor in homelessness when persons with AIDS lose their jobs and their ability to provide shelter for themselves or their families. In many instances, avenues of assistance such as shelters and nursing homes that might otherwise assist terminally ill people may be closed to people with AIDS because of fear of the disease.

Homelessness also influences behavioral factors related to nutrition and rest, further compounding the health problems of this population. Inadequate nutrition among the homeless is a lifestyle factor leading to ill health. Even those homeless persons housed in shelters rarely have access to kitchen facilities. Some shelters do provide meals, but they are rarely adequate to meet the nutritional needs of those served. This is particularly true in the case of homeless children, who frequently exhibit anemia or serious growth failure. Homeless persons may also obtain foods from soup kitchens, fast food restaurants, or trash cans and tend to have diets high in sodium and fat and low in vitamins and minerals (Carter, Green, Green, & Dufour, 1994). The homeless often have difficulty meeting special dietary needs posed by chronic illness and pregnancy.

The inability to rest frequently places homeless individuals at greater risk for a variety of health problems and worsens existing health conditions. For example, the inability to lie down to rest may lead to venous stasis and contribute to leg and foot ulcers. These adverse effects on circulation are made worse if the homeless individual smokes. Smoking also intensifies the effects of respiratory infections contracted from others in crowded shelters. Smoking has been reported in 63 to 80% of homeless adults (Skelly, Getty, Kemsley, Hunter, & Shipman, 1993; Halbach & Shortridge, 1993).

The Health System Dimension

Deinstitutionalization of the mentally ill has been described as a major health care system factor in the growing number of homeless people. *Deinstitutionalization* is the process of discharging large numbers of mentally ill persons from mental institutions in an attempt to enable them to live in the least restrictive environment possible (Jencks, 1994). This move was prompted by recognition of the appalling conditions prevalent in many institutions for the mentally ill. Although the intent of deinstitutionalization was laudable, the results were not. Unfortunately, there was no concurrent move to provide the community services needed for the mentally ill to live in noninstitutional settings, and many mental health providers prefer to work with the "worried well" rather than severely disturbed clients who often become homeless (Kuhlman, 1994). Many deinstitutionalized persons were virtually left to fend for themselves. Without the social or personal resources to provide adequate care for themselves, many of the deinstitutionalized became part of the homeless population.

A related social phenomenon is *noninstitutionalization* of the mentally ill. This refers to a lack of hospitalization of persons with mental problems who are in need of care (Jencks, 1994). Often, particularly in urban areas, people with mental illness are not hospitalized until they have deteriorated to the point where they are a danger to themselves or others. Such tolerance of deviant behavior prevents mentally ill individuals from obtaining help when they need it and when they could most easily benefit from it (Belcher & McLeese, 1988).

Health care system factors also contribute to homelessness when overwhelming medical bills cause an individual or family to be unable to continue to afford paying rent or making mortgage payments. The effect of medical expenses on one's ability to provide shelter is particularly noticeable in the case of clients with catastrophic illness. These clients are already at risk for a variety of health problems and homelessness further complicates their needs.

More often than causing homelessness, however, health care system factors make it more difficult for homeless individuals to obtain health care and to prevent or resolve health problems. Three types of barriers to health care for homeless individuals have been identified: system barriers, provider barriers, and personal barriers (Stark, 1992). Financial costs are one system barrier to health care for the homeless. Up to 89% of the homeless in one study had no health insurance coverage and many cannot afford the out-of-pocket costs of health care (Stark, 1992).

Cost is not the only system barrier to health care access. Other problems include lack of transportation, long waits for service (which may mean missing a meal at the soup kitchen or being unable to obtain shelter for the night), fragmentation of services due to lack of case management, and billing practices that result in attaching the wages of those who make next to nothing. In one study, homeless clients with frequent difficulties meeting subsistence needs were significantly less likely to have a regular source of health care and more likely to have gone without needed care than those without subsistence difficulties (Gelberg, Gallagher, Andersen, & Koegel, 1997). Provider barriers include insensitivity to the needs and circumstances of the homeless and unwillingness to provide care to those with no means of payment. Personal barriers posed by homeless persons themselves include priority placed on survival over health needs, denial of illness, fears of loss of personal control, lack of money, and embarrassment over personal appearance and hygiene. Homeless individuals and families may also lack the expertise or the energy to complete the processes involved in registration or application for services.

Lack of preventive care is a common problem among this population. Few pregnant homeless women receive prenatal care. These women and their offspring are at higher risk for complications of pregnancy than is the general population (Melnikow & Alemagno, 1993). Homeless women are also less likely to receive Pap smears and other preventive services (Gelberg, 1997).

Preventive care is also lacking for young children. Homeless youngsters use emergency room services as a regular source of health care two to three times more frequently than the general pediatric population, suggesting a focus on crisis care rather than prevention. These children are also likely to receive immunizations, particularly measles immunization.

Compliance with treatment recommendations may also be difficult. Homeless clients may be unable to afford prescribed medications or may not have a watch to time doses correctly. They may not have access to water to take oral medications, and syringes for insulin may be lost or stolen. Other difficulties include retaining potency in medications exposed to frequent temperature changes and obtaining prescription refills (Carter, et al., 1994).

Mental health services for the homeless population are also lacking. Some observers have noted a

---

ASSESSMENT TIPS: Assessing Homeless Clients' Health

Biophysical Dimension

Age

What is the age composition of the homeless population?

What is the proportion of children among the homeless? What is the proportion of elderly?

What proportion of the homeless population is comprised of adolescent runaways?

What effects has homelessness had on growth and development among homeless children?

What effects has homelessness had on elderly homeless individuals?

Physiologic Function

What is the extent of chronic illness among the homeless population?

What is the prevalence of tuberculosis and other communicable diseases among the homeless population?

What other physiologic health problems are found among the homeless population?

What is the immunization status of the homeless population (particularly children)?

What contribution does physical illness make to homelessness in the population?

Do homeless individuals exhibit signs and symptoms of disease? If so, what are these signs and symptoms?

What is the prevalence of pregnancy among homeless women?

Psychological Dimension

What is the extent of mental illness in the homeless population?

What stressful life events in the population contribute to homelessness?

What is the level of coping exhibited by the homeless individual?

What is the individual client's response to being homeless? What is the attitude toward obtaining help from social service agencies?

Is the homeless client depressed? Suicidal?

What is the psychological effect of homelessness on children? Do they display behavior problems? Anxiety?

Physical Dimension

What is the climate like? What health hazards does the climate pose for homeless individuals in the community?

Where do homeless individuals in the community seek shelter?

How adequate are shelter facilities in the community? Are they overcrowded? Poorly ventilated?

What hygiene facilities are available to homeless persons in the community?

Do environmental conditions pose other health hazards for homeless individuals (eg, flooding under bridges used for shelter)?

Social Dimension

Social Interaction and Support

What is the community attitude to the problem of homelessness? To homeless individuals?

What is the extent of family support available to the homeless individual?

What is the extent of community support available for the homeless population?

To what extent does family violence contribute to homelessness in the community?

Economic Factors

What is the education level of the homeless population in the community?

To what extent do economic factors contribute to homelessness in the community?

What is the level of unemployment in the community?

What proportion of the homeless population is employed? What is their income level?

What types of employment are available to the homeless population?

What source(s) of income, if any, does the homeless individual have?

What proportion of the eligible homeless population are receiving financial assistance?

Other Social Factors

What is the homeless individual's education level? Does he or she have employable skills?

What child care resources are available to homeless women with children?

What education programs are available for homeless children?

How does the individual homeless child perform in school?

Is transportation available to the homeless individual?

What is the availability of low-cost housing in the community?

(continued)

ASSESSMENT TIPS: Assessing Homeless Clients' Health (cont.)

What is the availability of shelter for homeless persons? For individuals with special needs?

What proportion of the homeless population consists of families?

What proportion of homeless families are headed by women?

What is the extent of crime victimization among homeless individuals?

Behavioral Dimension

Consumption Patterns

What food resources are available in the community for homeless individuals?

What nutritional deficits do homeless individuals experience?

How adequate is the nutritional value of food served in shelters?

What is the extent of drug and alcohol abuse in the homeless population?

What is the prevalence of smoking in the homeless population?

Rest and Exercise

Are there facilities available in the community for homeless individuals to rest during the day?

What health effects does lack of rest have on the homeless individual?

Medication Use

Does the homeless individual take prescription medications? Can he or she afford medication?

Is the homeless individual able to take medications as directed?

Sexual Practices

What is the extent of sexual activity in the homeless population? What is the extent of prostitution?

What is the prevalence of unsafe sexual activity in the homeless population?

Health System Dimension

To what extent have health care system factors contributed to homelessness in the community?

What health care services are available to homeless persons in the community?

Where do homeless persons usually go for health care?

What is the attitude of health care providers to homeless individuals?

What proportion of the homeless population has Medicaid or other health care coverage?

To what extent are preventive health services available to and utilized by the homeless population?

Are health care services easily accessible to homeless persons? How fragmented are available services?

What is the availability of mental health services for homeless individuals? Drug and alcohol treatment services?

---

mismatch between traditional community mental health services and the needs of the homeless population. Comprehensive services are seldom offered at one location, and mental health services seldom address the social factors contributing to homelessness.

 Diagnostic Reasoning and the Health Needs of Homeless Clients

Based on the assessment of the health status of homeless clients and factors contributing to that status, nursing diagnoses may be derived at any of several levels. At the individual client level, the community health nurse may make diagnoses related to the existence of homelessness. As discussed before, the diagnostic statement includes underlying factors if identifiable, for example, "homelessness due to inability to pay for shelter" or "homelessness due to mental illness and inability to care for self."

Other kinds of diagnoses made at the individual or family level might relate to specific health problems resulting from or intensified by homelessness. As an example, the nurse might make a diagnosis of "stasis ulcers due to excessive walking and standing and inability to lie down at night" or "malnutrition due to inability to afford food and lack of access to cooking facilities."

Nursing diagnoses may also be made at the group or community level. For example, the community health nurse may diagnose a significant problem of homelessness in the community. Such diagnoses might be stated as an "increase in the homeless population due to recent closure of major community employer" or an "increase in the number of homeless families due to unemployment and reductions in public assistance programs." Diagnoses may also be made at the aggregate level relative to specific problems engendered by homelessness, for example, "increased prevalence of tuberculosis due to malnutrition and crowding in shelters for the homeless" or "increased incidence of anemia among homeless children due to poor nutrition."

 ## Planning the Dimensions of Health Care for Homeless Clients

Planning done to meet the needs of homeless clients should focus on long-term as well as short-term solutions to problems. Planning should also reflect the factors contributing to the needs of the homeless in a particular locale. For example, if most of the homelessness in one community is due to unemployment, long-term interventions would most likely be directed toward improving employment opportunities in the area or increasing the employability of those involved. If, on the other hand, a significant portion of homelessness in the area is due to mental illness and inability to care for self, attention would be given to providing supportive services for the mentally ill.

Planning should address the underlying factors contributing to homelessness as well as its health consequences. For example, providing shelter on a nightly basis may decrease the risk of exposure to cold for homeless persons but does nothing to relieve homelessness. In planning to meet the health needs of homeless clients, community health nurses may work independently or in conjunction with other health care and social service providers. When planning to address factors contributing to homelessness, however, the community health nurse frequently is part of a group of government officials and concerned citizens who have assumed responsibility for dealing with the overall problem of homelessness.

Efforts to alleviate homelessness and its consequences may take place at the primary, secondary, or tertiary level of prevention. Community health nurses may be involved in activities at any or all three levels. Whatever the level of prevention undertaken, nurses working with the homeless may be in need of assistance in resolving the problems engendered by homelessness. Resources to assist community health nurses working with homeless clients are provided at the end of this chapter.

As is true in caring for any client, planning care for a homeless client begins with giving priority to the client's health needs. In many instances, for example, the first priority would be obtaining shelter, a secondary preventive measure. Other health needs could then be addressed in terms of their priority. For each of the health care needs identified for the homeless client, the community health nurse would develop specific outcome objectives and design interventions at the primary, secondary, or tertiary level of prevention. Planning efforts should be a joint function of the community health nurse and the homeless client, who best knows his or her situation and the kinds of interventions that are likely to be successful in that situation.

Primary Prevention

Primary prevention may be directed at either preventing homelessness or preventing its health consequences. Primary prevention can occur at the individual or family level or at community levels. Community health nurses can help prevent individuals and families from becoming homeless by assisting them to eliminate factors that may contribute to homelessness. For example, if a family is threatened with eviction because of a parent's unemployment, the nurse can assist family members to obtain emergency rent funds from local social service agencies. The nurse can also encourage the family to apply for ongoing financial aid programs or assist the parent to find work.

As noted earlier, some people become homeless because of underlying psychiatric illness and an inability to deal with the requirements for maintaining shelter. Severely disturbed people may just wander away from home and take up residence on the streets. Homelessness in this group can be prevented by referrals for psychiatric therapy and counseling. A case management approach to the transition from hospital to home has been found to be helpful in preventing recurrent homelessness among the mentally ill (Susser, Valencia, Conover, Felix, Tsai, & Wyatt, 1997). Nurses may also provide support services to families caring for mentally ill members to prevent these persons from becoming part of the homeless population. Placement in a sheltered home might also be an approach to preventing homelessness in the mentally disturbed person when family members either cannot or do not wish to care for the client. In addition, the community health nurse can monitor the effectiveness of therapy and watch for signs of increasing agitation or disorientation that may precede wandering. The nurse can also assist the disturbed person by giving concrete direction in such tasks as paying one's rent.

Runaway children and teenagers are another segment of the homeless population for whom homelessness could have been prevented through primary preventive interventions. Efforts of community health nurses to promote effective communication in families and to enhance parenting skills may prevent young people from feeling a need to run away. Similarly, efforts to prevent or deal with child abuse may prevent runaways.

Primary prevention at the community level to reduce the incidence of poverty and homelessness requires major changes in societal structure and thinking. Some suggested avenues for intervention include federal support for low-cost housing, increases in the minimum wage, and access to supportive services for the mentally and physically disabled to allow them to function effectively in society. Another suggestion aimed at reducing the incidence of poverty in families with children to prevent their homelessness is to provide child care assistance and paid parental occupational leaves as needed. It has been suggested that unemployed parents could be effectively employed providing subsidized child care to allow other welfare recipients to obtain work (Woodson, 1996).

Creating employment opportunities and programs to train people with employable skills is another possible primary preventive measure for both poverty and homelessness. Current public job training programs, however, have been criticized for their failure to facilitate job placement for those who complete the programs. Job training programs directed specifically toward the local job market have been suggested as more appropriate approaches to unemployment. Child care and transportation to and from work are other essential considerations if welfare-to-work programs are going to be effective (Woodson, 1996). Another societal intervention could be to provide a guaranteed annual income to all citizens. Such an approach is exemplified in part by social insurance programs such as Social Security and unemployment insurance that are not restricted to the poor but available to all eligible participants. Other social programs that may help to prevent homelessness include legal assistance to prevent evictions as well as increased housing subsidies including direct payments to landlords. Changes in housing codes and tax laws to prevent loss of welfare benefits or allowing tax credits in shared housing situations may also be helpful. There is also a need for "discharge planning" for housing assistance for people displaced by building condemnation or renovation or release from prisons and other institutions (Lindblom, 1996).

Community health nursing involvement in such activities occurs primarily through advocacy and political action. As advocates, community health nurses can make policy makers aware of the needs of the homeless and can contribute in efforts to plan programs that prevent homelessness. Nurses can also engage in political activities such as those described in Chapter 13 to influence policies that help to eliminate these conditions.

Primary prevention may also be undertaken with respect to specific health problems experienced by homeless persons. Here community health nurses may work with individuals, families, or groups of people. For example, community health nurses working with homeless substance abusers might advocate a program providing clean syringes to intravenous drug users. Failing that, the nurse might provide a simple bleach solution for injection equipment to minimize the risk of bloodborne diseases such as hepatitis and AIDS. Similarly, nurses may provide assistance to families with budgeting and meal planning to provide nutritious meals on limited incomes.

Community-based avenues for preventing homelessness among the mentally ill include providing access to services within the community that enable these persons to maintain themselves adequately without institutionalization. Efforts may also be needed to ensure hospitalization for those persons who cannot be adequately maintained in the community. Treatment for substance abuse and secure places for convalescence after hospital discharge might also serve to prevent homelessness in this subgroup.

Also at the group level, nurses may engage in primary prevention for specific problems by encouraging community groups to provide shelters for homeless individuals. Nurses may also provide basic health care for the homeless, focusing particularly on primary preventive measures such as influenza vaccine and routine immunizations for children. They may suggest the use of a bleach solution in the showers of shelters to prevent the spread of fungal infections. Adequate ventilation, reduced crowding, and use of ultraviolet lights in shelters may also help to prevent the spread of communicable disease.

Another area for primary prevention of the health consequences of homelessness is adequate nutrition. Community health nurses can advocate food programs for the needy, including the homeless. They can also serve as consultants to existing food programs to ensure that meals are nutritionally adequate to meet the needs of the population served. Community health nursing activities in this area may also include attempts to arrange diets for homeless clients with special needs (eg, assisting a diabetic client to select foods from those prepared in a shelter that approximate a diabetic diet as closely as possible).

Community health nurses can also work with other concerned citizens to initiate programs to provide adequate clothing and shoes for homeless clients. Efforts may also be needed to arrange mechanisms for the homeless to bathe and wash their clothing. In some cities, day shelters that do not provide sleeping accommodations often provide homeless individuals an opportunity to shower and wash their clothing. These shelters may also provide a clean change of clothing on a periodic basis.

Another aggregate approach to preventing specific health problems among the homeless is providing universal access to health care through national health insurance or similar programs at the state level. Nurses can promote such programs through political activity and advocacy and may also be involved in implementing them by providing direct services to the homeless.

One approach to dealing with the many health problems experienced by the homeless would be to separate Medicaid eligibility from eligibility for other forms of public assistance. Although such action would not prevent homelessness per se, it would certainly mitigate its effects on health and on access to health care.

Secondary Prevention

Secondary prevention is designed to alleviate existing homelessness and its health effects. At the individual level, secondary interventions may include referral for financial assistance via "means-tested income transfers." *Means-tested income transfers* involve the distribution of cash or noncash assistance to individuals and families on the basis of income. As noted earlier, such programs frequently serve only the poorest of the poor and may necessitate loss of all resources before eligibility can be confirmed. Community health nurses may need to function as advocates to assist clients through the bureaucratic process frequently involved. This is particularly true for elderly clients and those with mental health problems. At the community level, nurses can advocate a review of eligibility criteria for means-tested income transfer programs so that a greater proportion of the homeless population are served.

Shelter is an immediate need for homeless individuals. The community health nurses can assist the homeless client to locate temporary shelter. This may be accomplished by means of referrals to existing shelters. If the nurse is not aware of homeless shelters provided in the community, he or she can contact a local YMCA or YWCA, a Salvation Army service center, or local churches for information on shelter avail-

ability. When organized shelter facilities are not available, the nurse may try contacting local houses of worship to see if members of religious congregations can provide shelter for a homeless person on a short-term basis. In making a referral for emergency shelter, the community health nurse would consider the needs of the particular client. Ideally, for example, the elderly and women and children would be referred to shelters where they are protected from victimization. Similarly, homeless persons with chronic health problems should be referred to shelters where health services are available and their conditions can be monitored on an ongoing basis.

At the group level, community health nurses can work with governmental officials and other concerned citizens to develop shelter programs for homeless individuals or families. Avenues that might be pursued include school gymnasiums, churches, and public buildings. Many cities have used these and other buildings as temporary nighttime shelters for the homeless during cold weather. Plans might also be developed for more adequate shelters that provide other services as well as a place to sleep. In designing a shelter program, the community health nurse and other concerned individuals would employ the principles of program planning presented in Chapter 19.

For homeless persons with significant mental health problems, it may be necessary to create specialized shelters called "safe havens." *Safe havens* are secure, stable places of residence that place few demands on those receiving help. Many mentally ill homeless individuals are not able to deal with the behavioral restrictions and other policies imposed by many typical homeless shelters. They need a place with limited restrictions that offers the same bed each night, a place to stay during the day, and a place to store their belongings. Because of the special needs of this segment of the homeless population, safe havens do not limit the length of stay for those served. Safe havens then become a stage in clients' progressive movement toward permanent housing in which they can learn to trust and relearn skills needed to maintain a permanent residence while unlearning the distrust required for survival on the streets (Federal Task Force on Homelessness and Severe Mental Illness, 1992).

Shelters are an emergency resource, not a solution to the problem of homelessness. Community health nurses should help homeless clients find ways to meet long-term shelter needs. For individual clients, this may mean referrals for employment assistance or other services to eliminate factors that resulted in homelessness. At the community level, nurses can participate in planning long-term solutions to the problems of homelessness. Unfortunately, such planning has not often been the focus of community attempts to deal with the problem. As noted by one observer, "We are, as a society, in danger of creating a shelter system that contains—even warehouses—a deviant and troubling group of people" (Chafetz, 1988). Community health nurses can advocate and participate in planning efforts to provide low-cost housing, employment assistance, job training, and other services needed to resolve community problems of homelessness. Initiating these planning activities may require political activity on the part of the community health nurse.

Planning for long-term resolution of the problem of homelessness for runaways involves a different set of strategies. The community health nurse can explore with the youngster his or her reasons for running away from home. Nursing interventions are then directed toward modifying factors that led the child to run away. For example, if the child was abused, the nurse can institute measures to prevent further abuse if the youngster returns to the home, or foster home placement can be arranged. If problems stem from poor family communication, the nurse can make a referral for family counseling or other therapeutic services. The nurse can also serve as a liaison between the child and his or her family, negotiating for changes that make the child's return possible.

Particular care should be taken to involve the child in planning interventions to resolve his or her situation. A child returned to his or her family unwillingly will probably run away again. In addition, such actions on the part of the community health nurse may also destroy any faith the child may have had in health care providers as a source of assistance.

At the aggregate level, community health nurses should alert community policy makers to the need for coordinated services for the homeless offered in a single location to meet the health and social needs of homeless clients. They should also make sure that planning groups in which they participate plan services to address the needs of the homeless for housing, food, clothing, employment, child care services for working parents, and adequate preventive and therapeutic health care services. Planning should also include avenues for outreach and follow-up services, particularly for the homeless who may be lost to service. Such comprehensive programs require changes in health care and social systems that may necessitate legislation and public policy formation that can be guided by nursing input.

Community health nurses can also provide curative services for a variety of health problems experienced by the homeless. For example, they may make referrals for food supplement programs or provide treatment for skin conditions or parasitic infestations. They will also be actively involved in educating clients for self-care. Homeless clients may have difficulty with simple aspects of treatment regimens. For example, if the homeless client does not have access to a clock or watch, it may be difficult to take medications as directed. Nurses can suggest the use of medications that can be taken in conjunction with set activities, such as on arising or at bedtime.

The special needs of homeless children and older persons require particular attention. One sug-

Critical Thinking in Research

Marsh (1996) conducted a study to determine the composition and needs of a homeless population and the services available to them in a county undergoing a rural to urban transformation. The study consisted of survey questionnaires completed in interviews with 50 homeless clients, key informants in local churches, and service providers. Homeless individuals were interviewed at a free lunch program, the department of social services office, evictions court, the county housing agency, and a shelter for women and children. Based on the findings, the typical homeless person in this population was a single unemployed female under 30 years of age. Many of the women had children with them and virtually all of the homeless were seeking work. Nearly half of the homeless persons interviewed had monthly incomes less than $400, and more than three fourths were seeking permanent housing. The most common causes of homelessness were unemployment and job loss, income insufficient to afford housing, or divorce. Needs identified by participants included jobs, housing, rental assistance, food, clothing, and education.

Members of local churches were interviewed to determine the kinds of services they provided to homeless individuals. Most provided financial help with rent or motel rooms, but only 10% actually provided shelter through church members. Other forms of assistance included food, clothing, gas, transportation, money for electric bills or medication, and referral to other agencies.

Service providers included the housing agency, Red Cross, a juvenile services department, county mental health agency, police, community services, a local abuse resource, and the department of social services. Perceptions of needs among the homeless included food, shelter, transportation, counseling, mental health services, jobs, education or training, financial assistance for the disabled, and referrals for medical, dental, child care, and other needs.

1. How did perceptions of need by homeless clients differ from the perceptions of service providers? What implications do these differences have for meeting the needs of homeless individuals?
2. How might you design a study to get more information about differences in perceived needs between homeless clients and providers?
3. If you wanted to replicate this study, where would you go to find a representative sample of homeless individuals in your community?
4. What service agencies would you survey? What would you want to ask them about services for the homeless?

gestion is age-segregated shelters or services specifically designed for older persons and families with children to prevent their victimization by other subgroups within the homeless population. Special attention also needs to be given to meeting the nutritional needs of these vulnerable groups as well as those of pregnant women.

Tertiary Prevention

Tertiary prevention may be aimed at preventing a recurrence of poverty and homelessness for individuals, families, or groups of people affected. Or the emphasis may be placed on preventing the recurrence of health problems that result from conditions of poverty and homelessness.

Community health nursing involvement in tertiary prevention may entail political activity to ensure the provision of services to relieve poverty and homelessness on a long-term basis. This means involvement by nurses in efforts to raise minimum wages or to design programs to educate the homeless for employment in today's society. Advocacy and political activity may also be needed to ensure the adequacy of community services for the mentally ill to allow them to care for themselves or to support their families as caregivers.

At the individual or family level, community health nurses may be involved in referral for employment assistance or for education programs that allow homeless clients to eliminate the underlying factors involved in their homelessness. Moreover, nurses might assist clients to budget their incomes more effectively or engage in cooperative buying efforts to limit family expenses. Community health nurses may also be actively involved in monitoring the status of mentally ill clients in the home and in assisting families of these clients to obtain respite care and other supportive services needed to prevent the mentally ill client from returning to a state of homelessness. In such cases, nurses also monitor medication use and encourage clients to receive counseling and other rehabilitative services.

Implementing Care for Homeless Clients

Acceptance of clients and their circumstances is an essential function of community health nurses working with the homeless. Dirty bodies and unwashed clothing are most likely the result of inadequate opportunities for hygiene rather than an indication that the client does not value cleanliness.

Another area in which understanding and acceptance may be required is failure to keep appointments. In the absence of timepieces and calendars, which may not be available to the homeless client, keeping appointments for health care and other services may be difficult. One suggestion is to provide clients with a photocopy of a date book on which they can keep track of days until their next appointment. Providing services on a walk-in basis is another way in which clients can be seen when the need arises, rather than at the convenience of the health care facility.

Evaluating Care for Homeless Clients

Evaluating the effects of nursing interventions with homeless clients can take place at two levels: the individual level and the group or community level. At the individual level, evaluation of the effectiveness of interventions reflects the client care objectives developed by the nurse and client in planning care. For example, if an objective for a homeless family was to provide them with an income sufficient to meet survival needs, the nurse and family would determine whether this objective has been achieved. Does the family now have sufficient income to provide adequate housing, appropriate nutrition, and other needs? If the objective was to find employment for the mother or father, has this been accomplished?

Evaluation of group interventions must also be undertaken. For example, nurses and other concerned individuals will want to determine whether shelter programs are sufficient to meet the needs of the homeless population, or are there still people sleeping under bridges and in doorways? Evaluation of tertiary prevention programs focuses on the extent to which interventions prevent people from returning to poverty and again becoming homeless. Are job training programs effective in increasing the income of participants above the poverty level? Criticism of current welfare programs seems to indicate that such programs do not effectively relieve the problems of the poor and homeless. If current programs are not effectively alleviating the problem, other solutions must be sought; community health nurses must be actively involved in developing those solutions.

The Working Group on Homeless Health Outcomes (1996) of the Bureau of Primary Health Care suggested that evaluation of programs for the homeless address both systems-level and client-level outcomes. Systems-level outcomes to be considered

► EVALUATING PROGRAMS FOR HOMELESS CLIENTS

Systems-level Outcomes

Access to care:

    Are services provided in a location that is accessible to homeless individuals?

    Are services provided at times that do not interfere with the ability of homeless individuals to meet other needs?

Comprehensiveness of services:

    Do services address the wide spectrum of needs experienced by the homeless population?

    Can the agency provide or arrange for the full array of services needed?

Continuity of care:

    Do services provide for long-term involvement with clients rather than episodic assistance?

    Do services include an effective referral network?

    Is there provision made to follow up on the effectiveness of services provided to clients?

    Are case management services available to promote continuity of service?

Systems integration:

    Do homeless clients experience the service system as seamless?

    Are there gaps and overlaps between services provided?

    Are there multiple ways for clients to gain entry to the full range of services provided?

Cost-effectiveness:

    Do services make efficient use of available resources?

    Do services result in cost savings to society in the form of reduced emergency room visits or hospitalizations, etc.?

Prevention focus:

    Are preventive services available?

    Are preventive services appropriate to clients in terms of age, gender, etc.?

    Are preventive services effectively utilized by the homeless population?

Client involvement:

    Are clients active participants in their own treatment planning?

    Are clients involved in the planning and implementation of services provided?

    Do clients function as role models, peer advocates, and outreach workers?

Client-level Outcomes

Involvement in treatment:

    Are clients committed to the treatment plan?

    Are clients compliant with treatment plans?

    Do clients continue to request services as long as they are needed?

Improved health status:

    Have specific client health problems been resolved or ameliorated?

    Do clients perceive their own health status as improved?

Improved level of function:

    Are clients better able to function emotionally and socially?

    Has the client's level of physical function improved?

Disease self-management:

    Are clients able to effectively engage in self-care?

    Can clients minimize the effect of disease on everyday life?

Improved quality of life:

    Do clients describe improvement in their quality of life?

Client choice:

    Do clients have choices among relevant treatment options or social service plans?

    Are these choices perceived by clients?

Client satisfaction:

    Have services provided met clients' expectations and addressed perceived needs?

    Do clients express satisfaction with services provided?

(Source: Working Group on Homeless Health Outcomes, 1996.)

include ease of access to programs; the comprehensiveness of services offered; continuity of care including appropriate referrals, follow-up, and case management; the degree to which an integrated set of services is provided; cost-effectiveness; focus on prevention; and client involvement in the design and implementation of services. Client-level outcomes include client involvement in and commitment to treatment, improved health status, improved func-

tional status, effective disease self-management, improved quality of life, client choice of providers, and client satisfaction. These areas and related evaluative questions are summarized above.

An additional focus for evaluation is the achievement of those national health objectives that relate to low-income individuals and families. The current status of some of these objectives is presented in Table 24–2.

TABLE 24–2. **STATUS OF SELECTED NATIONAL OBJECTIVES FOR LOW-INCOME INDIVIDUALS**

	Objective	Base	Most Recent	Target
2.4	Reduce growth retardation	11% (1988)	met (1995)	10%
2.10b	Reduce iron deficiency in children	4% (1976–1980)	NDA[a]	3%
8.3	Achieve access to preschool programs	47% (1990)	55% (1991)	100%
16.11b	Increase receipt of clinical breast examination and mammography	15% (1987)	41% (1991)	60%
16.12d	Increase receipt of Pap smear	85% (1987)	NDA	95%
17.2a	Reduce activity limitation	18.9% (1988)	19.6% (1991)	15%
21.3c	Increase access to primary care	71% (1991)	72% (1993)	95%

[a]NDA, no data available.

(Sources: U.S. Department of Health and Human Services, 1991; 1993; 1995.)

Critical Thinking in Practice: A Case in Point

Crystal is a 16-year-old girl with a 3-month-old baby boy. She has been referred for community health nursing services by her teacher at a special program for adolescents with children. In this program, the girls attend school while child care services are provided for the children. During the day, the girls participate in the care of their infants and learn about child care as well as the usual high school subject material. Crystal has been referred because she has not been coming to school and her teacher is concerned. The school does not have a home address or phone number for Crystal, but the teacher gives you the phone number of Crystal's grandmother. After several attempts, you finally contact the grandmother, who agrees to give Crystal a message to get in touch with you. The grandmother says that Crystal does not live with her and that she only sees her occasionally.

The following week you receive a call from Crystal. She is reluctant to give you an address, but agrees to come to the health department with the baby. When she arrives, she tells you that she has not been going to school because the baby was ill and cannot return to the child care center without a doctor's note that the baby is well. Crystal says she cannot afford to see a doctor. She has no health insurance and no money for health care. She began the application process for Medicaid but never followed through because it was "too much hassle." She lives with her mother and stepfather in a camper shell at a construction site where her stepfather is temporarily employed. She refuses to give you the location of this construction site, saying that they will probably move to a new site soon. Crystal says her parents provide her with food and formula for the baby, who appears clean and well nourished. The baby has not begun his immunizations, again because of lack of funds for health services.

Crystal says she is in good health, but has not had a postpartum check-up. Although not currently sexually active, she has a steady boyfriend and is contemplating sexual intimacy with him. She asks about various types of contraceptives.

The father of her baby is no longer in the area and is not aware that Crystal had a baby. Crystal's own father is also removed from the picture and she does not know where he is. When asked about her grandmother, Crystal says that they do not get along well and that her grandmother hardly speaks to her since she got pregnant.

Crystal is anxious to complete high school and go into a program to become a beautician. She tried recently to get a part-time job in a fast-food restaurant, but was told they wanted someone with experience. She socializes somewhat with the girls at school and goes with several of them to take their babies to the park and similar outings.

1. What health problems are evident in this situation? What are the biophysical, psychological, physical, social, behavioral, and health system factors influencing these problems?
2. What considerations are important in planning care for Crystal?
3. What primary prevention measures would you undertake with Crystal and her son?
4. What secondary prevention measures would be warranted to deal with existing health problems? Describe specific actions that you would take to resolve these problems.
5. What could be done in terms of tertiary prevention to prevent further consequences or recurrence of health problems in this situation?
6. How would you evaluate the effectiveness of your interventions with Crystal? Describe the specific evaluative criteria you would use and how you would obtain the evaluative data needed.

TESTING YOUR UNDERSTANDING

1. Identify at least three physiologic problems common among homeless individuals (pp. 592–594)
2. Describe at least three social dimension factors that contribute to homelessness. (pp. 595–597)
3. What are two behavioral factors that influence the health of homeless clients? (pp. 597–598)
4. Describe two ways in which health system dimension factors have contributed to homelessness and its health effects. (pp. 598–600)
5. Describe at least three approaches to primary prevention of homelessness. How might community health nurses be involved in each approach? (pp. 601–604)
6. What are three areas in which secondary preventive activities may be appropriate in the care of homeless clients? What kinds of secondary preventive measures might a community health nurse employ in these areas? (pp. 604–605)
7. Identify at least two strategies for tertiary prevention of homelessness at the aggregate level. How might community health nurses be involved in implementing these strategies? (pp. 605–606)
8. What are two primary considerations in implementing care for homeless clients? (p. 606)
9. What is the primary focus in evaluating care for homeless clients? Is this focus the same for evaluating care for individuals and families and care for groups of homeless people? (p. 606)

WHAT DO YOU THINK?
Questions for Critical Thinking

1. What factors in your local community contribute to homelessness? What contributions might community health nurses make to modify these factors?
2. Are there elements of the local health care delivery system that would make it difficult for homeless people to get health care?
3. Why are some health care providers reluctant to care for homeless clients? What strategies can you suggest to minimize their reluctance to deal with this vulnerable population?

REFERENCES

Advisory Council for the Elimination of Tuberculosis. (1992). Prevention and control of tuberculosis among homeless persons. *MMWR, 41*(RR-5), 13–23.

Attala, J. M., & Warmington, M. (1996). Clients' evaluation of health care services in a battered women's shelter. *Public Health Nursing, 13,* 269–275.

Belcher, J. R., & McLeese, G. (1988). The process of homelessness among the mentally ill: Rural and urban perspectives. *Human Services in the Rural Environment, 12*(2), 20–25.

Bissonnette, A., & Hijjazi, K. H. (1994). Elder homelessness: A community perspective. *Nursing Clinics of North America, 29,* 409–416.

Carter, K. F., Green, R. D., Green, L., & Dufour, L. T. (1994). Health needs of homeless clients assessing nursing care at a free clinic. *Journal of Community Health Nursing, 11,* 139–147.

Chafetz, L. (1988). Perspectives for psychiatric nurses on homelessness. *Issues in Mental Health Nursing, 9,* 325–335.

Davis, R. E. (1996). Tapping into the culture of homelessness. *Journal of Professional Nursing, 12,* 176–183.

Division of Tuberculosis Elimination. (1995). Tuberculosis morbidity—United States, 1994. *MMWR, 44,* 387–389, 395.

Dolbeare, C. N. (1996). Housing policy: A general consideration. In J. Baumohl (Ed.), *Homelessness in America* (pp. 34–45). Phoenix, AZ: Oryx Press.

Evans, K. (1993). Health needs of infants and children in homeless families in Houston, Texas. In J. K. Hunter (Ed.), *Nursing and health care for the homeless* (pp. 95–105). Albany, NY: State University of New York Press.

Federal Task Force on Homelessness and Severe Mental Illness, National Institutes of Mental Health. (1992). *Outcasts on Main Street.* Washington, DC: Interagency Council on the Homeless.

Flynt, W. (1996). Rural poverty in America. *National Forum, The Phi Kappa Phi Journal, 76*(3), 32–34.

Francis, M. B. (1992). Eight homeless mothers' tales. *Image, 24,* 111–114.

Gelberg, L. (1997). Homelessness and health. *Journal of the American Board of Family Practice, 10*(1), 67–70.

Gelberg, L., Gallagher, T. C., Anderson, R. M., & Koegel, P. (1997). Competing priorities as a barrier to medical care among homeless adults in Los Angeles. *American Journal of Public Health, 87,* 217–220.

Halbach, J. L., & Shortridge, L. M. (1993). Characteristics of homeless families: A research report. In J. K. Hunter (Ed.), *Nursing and health care for the homeless* (pp. 71–77). Albany, NY: State University of New York Press.

Hales, A., & Magnus, M. H. (1991). Feeding the homeless. *Journal of Nursing Administration, 21*(12), 36–41.

Hardin, B. (1996). Why the road off the streets is not paved with jobs. In J. Baumohl (Ed.), *Homelessness in America* (pp. 46–62). Phoenix, AZ: Oryx Press.

Hatton, D. (1997). Managing health problems among homeless women with children in transitional shelter. *Image: Journal of Nursing Scholarship, 29*(1), 33–37.

Heffron, W. A., Skipper, B. J., & Lambert, L. (1997). Health and lifestyle issues as risk factors for homelessness. *Journal of the American Board of Family Practice, 10*(1), 6–12.

Infant and Child Health Studies Bureau. (1995). Poverty and infant mortality—United States, 1988. *MMWR, 44,* 922–927.

Jahiel, R. I. (1992a). The definition and significance of homelessness in the United States. In R. I. Jahiel (Ed.), *Homelessness: A prevention-oriented approach* (pp. 1–10). Baltimore: Johns Hopkins University Press.

Jahiel, R. I. (1992b). Empirical studies of homeless populations in the 1970s and 1980s. In R. I. Jahiel (Ed.), *Homelessness: A prevention-oriented approach* (pp. 40–56). Baltimore: Johns Hopkins University Press.

Jencks, C. (1994). *The homeless.* Cambridge, MA: Harvard University Press.

Jezewski, M. A. (1995). Staying connected: The core of facilitating health care for homeless persons. *Public Health Nursing, 12,* 203–210.

Killion, C. M. (1995). Special health care needs of homeless pregnant women. *Advances in Nursing Science, 18*(2), 44–56.

Koegel, P., Burnam, M. A., & Baumohl, J. (1996). The causes of homelessness. In J. Baumohl (Ed.), *Homelessness in America* (pp. 24–33). Phoenix, AZ: Oryx Press.

Kuhlman, T. L. (1994). *Psychology on the streets: Mental health practices with homeless persons.* New York: John Wiley & Sons.

Lindblom, E. N. (1996). Preventing homelessness. In J. Baumohl (Ed.), *Homelessness in America* (pp. 187–200). Phoenix, AZ: Oryx Press.

Link, B. G., Susser, E., Stueve, A., Phelan, J., Moore, R. E., & Struening, E. (1994). Lifetime and five-year prevalence of homelessness in the United States. *American Journal of Public Health, 84,* 1907–1912.

Marsh, C. E. (1996). *Harford County, Maryland Homeless and Shelter Survey: Housing and shelter in a community in transition.* Lanham, MD: University Press of America.

Mason, D. J., Jensen, M., & Boland, D. L. (1992). Health behaviors and health risks among homeless males in Utah. *Western Journal of Nursing Research, 14,* 775–790.

May, K. M., & Evans, G. G. (1994). Health education for homeless populations. *Journal of Community Health Nursing, 11,* 229–237.

Melnikow, J., & Alemagno, S. (1993). Adequacy of prenatal care among inner-city women. *Journal of Family Practice, 37,* 575–582.

Montgomery, C. (1994). Swimming upstream: The strengths of women who survive homelessness. *Advances in Nursing Science, 16*(3), 34–45.

Newman, K. S. (1996). Job availability: The Achilles heel of welfare reform. *National Forum, The Phi Kappa Phi Journal, 76*(3), 20–23.

Paul, E. A., Lebowitz, S. M., Moore, R. E., Hoven, C. W., Bennet, B. A., & Chen, A. (1993). Nemesis revisited: Tuberculosis infection in a New York City men's shelter. *American Journal of Public Health, 83,* 1743–1745.

Porter-O'Grady, T. (1993). Nursing care for the underserved: Crisis and opportunity. In J. K. Hunter (Ed.), *Nursing and health care for the homeless* (pp. 7–16). Albany, NY: State University of New York Press.

Riemer, J. G., Van Cleve, L., & Galbraith, M. (1995). Barriers to well child care for homeless children under age 13. *Public Health Nursing, 12,* 61–66.

Robertson, M. J., Zlotnick, C., & Westerfelt, A. (1997). Drug use disorders and treatment contact among homeless adults in Alameda County, California. *American Journal of Public Health, 87,* 221–228.

Rosenthal, R. (1994). *Homeless in paradise: A map of the terrain.* Philadelphia: Temple University Press.

Shinn, M., & Weitzman, B. C. (1996). Homeless families are different. In J. Baumohl (Ed.), *Homelessness in America* (pp. 109–122). Phoenix, AZ: Oryx Press.

Skelly, A. H., Getty, C., Kemsley, M. J., Hunter, J. K., & Shipman, J. (1993). Health perceptions of the homeless: A survey of Buffalo's City Mission. In J. K. Hunter (Ed.), *Nursing and health care for the homeless* (pp. 51–63). Albany, NY: State University of New York Press.

Snow, D. A., & Anderson, L. (1993). *Down on their luck: A study of homeless street people.* Berkeley, CA: University of California Press.

Snow, D. A., Anderson, L., Quist, T., & Cress, D. (1996). Material survival strategies on the street: Homeless people as bricoleurs. In J. Baumohl (Ed.), *Homelessness in America* (pp. 86–96). Phoenix, AZ: Oryx Press.

Stark, L. R. (1992). Barriers to health care for homeless people. In R. I. Jahiel (Ed.), *Homelessness: A prevention-oriented approach* (pp. 151–164). Baltimore: Johns Hopkins University Press.

Stokley, N. L. (1993). Providing quality child-care for homeless children: A descriptive study of the Seattle experience. In J. K. Hunter (Ed.), *Nursing and health care for the homeless* (pp. 107–115). Albany, NY: State University of New York Press.

Susser, E., Betne, P., Valencia, E., Goldfinger, S. M., & Lehman, A. F. (1997). Injection drug use among homeless adults with severe mental illness. *American Journal of Public Health, 87,* 854–856.

Susser, E., Valencia, E., Conover, S., Felix, A., Tsia, W., & Wyatt, R. J. (1997). Preventing recurrent homelessness among mentally ill men: A "critical time" intervention after discharge from a shelter. *American Journal of Public Health, 87,* 256–262.

U.S. Department of Commerce. (1996). *Statistical abstract of the United States, 1996* (116th ed.). Washington, DC: Government Printing Office.

U.S. Department of Health and Human Services. (1991). *Healthy people 2000: National health promotion and disease prevention objectives.* Washington, DC: Government Printing Office.

U.S. Department of Health and Human Services. (1993). *Health United States, 1992, and healthy people 2000 review.* Washington, DC: Government Printing Office.

U.S. Department of Health and Human Services. (1995). *Healthy people 2000: Midcourse review and 1995 revisions:* Washington, DC: Government Printing Office.

U.S. Department of Health and Human Services. (1996). *Health United States, 1995.* Washington, DC: Government Printing Office.

Wagner, J. D., Menke, E. M., & Ciccone, J. K. (1995). What is known about the health of rural homeless families. *Public Health Nursing, 12,* 400–408.

Woodson, R. L. (1996). Welfare reform: A message from the "receiving end." *National Forum, The Phi Kappa Phi Journal, 76*(3), 15–19.

Working Group on Homeless Health Outcomes, Bureau of Primary Health Care. (1996). *Meeting Proceedings.* Rockville, MD: Health Resources and Services Administration.

Zima, B. T., Bussing, R., Forness, S. R., & Benjamin, B. (1997). Sheltered homeless children: Their eligibility and unmet needs for special education evaluation. *American Journal of Public Health, 87,* 236–240.

RESOURCES FOR HOMELESS CLIENTS

Community for Creative Non-violence
425 2nd Street, NW
Washington, DC 20001
(202) 393–1909

Families for the Homeless
c/o John Ambrose
National Mental Health Association
1021 Prince Street
Arlington, VA 22314–2971
(703) 684–7722

Health Care for the Homeless
Information Resource Center

John Snow, Inc.
44 Farnsworth Street
Boston, MA 02210–1211
(617) 482–9485

Homeless Information Exchange
1830 Connecticut Avenue, NW, 4th Floor
Washington, DC 20009
(202) 462–7551

Interagency Council on the Homeless
U.S. Department of Housing and Urban Development
451 7th Street, NW
Washington, DC 20410
(202) 708–1422

Legal Services Homelessness Task Force
c/o National Housing Law Project
1815 H Street, NW, #501
Washington, DC 20006
(202) 783–5140

National Alliance to End Homelessness
1518 K Street, NW, Ste. 206
Washington, DC 20005
(202) 638–1256

National Coalition for the Homeless
1621 K Street, NW, Ste. 1004
Washington, DC 20006
(202) 777–1322

National Coalition for Homeless Veterans
918 Pennsylvania Avenue, SE
Washington, DC 20003–2140
(800) 838–4357

National Low Income Housing Coalition
1012 14th Street, NW, #1200
Washington, DC 20005
(202) 662–1530

National Resource Center on Homelessness and Mental Illness
Policy Research Associates
262 Delaware Avenue
Delmar, NY 12054
(518) 439–7415

National Runaway Switchboard
3080 North Lincoln Avenue
Chicago, IL 60657
(800) 621–4000

Operation PUSH (People United to Save Humanity)
930 East 50th Street
Chicago, IL 60615
(312) 373–3366

Runaway Hotline
Governor's Office
PO Box 12428
Austin, TX 78711
(512) 463–1980

Salvation Army
615 Slater's Lane
PO Box 269
Alexandria, VA 22313
(703) 684–5500

Save the Children Federation
54 Wilton Road
Westport, CT 06880
(203) 221–4000

United Way of America
701 North Fairfax Street
Alexandria, VA 22314–2045
(703) 836–7100

GOD AND THE TELEPHONE

Why don't you come
when I phone?

I come once a week—
sometimes more.
Some days you're
calling me every
few minutes. How
can I come every time?

When I call you
it's always important.
Last night I slid
out of my chair
and had to sit there
on the floor for hours.

It couldn't have been
as bad as you say
because when you phoned
for me to come
what you asked for
was chicken and ice cream.

Well, I have to think
about Lady Jane Jackson!
You're young and
you have your strength.
You have to come.

But phone calls every day
and all night long?

Well, if you can't
be called, you ain't
gonna hold a job for long.
You don't have
that many patients.

Do you know when you call
you always yell
and say I have to
come right away?

I don't want to hear—
Who yells?
Look here Sweetheart.
There are only two things
Lady Jane needs—
God and this pink telephone.
But God is a spirit
and sometimes I need
a flesh and blood person.
That's you.

Reprinted with permission from V. Masson (1993). just who. *Washington, DC: Crossroads Health Ministry.*

THE DIMENSIONS MODEL IN SPECIALIZED SETTINGS

People typically think of community health nursing as nursing care that is provided in public agencies such as state and county health departments. Community health nursing, however, is carried out in any setting where the focus of care is health promotion and illness prevention for groups of people. Indeed, the work of community health nurses may include case management and discharge planning in hospitals or other acute care settings.

Some specialized settings offer opportunities for community health nursing. When community health nurses work in such settings, for example the school or workplace, they incorporate principles of community health practice to improve the health status of individual clients and groups of people in that setting, as well as the total population.

School nursing addresses the health care needs of individual children in the school. But when school nurses are also community health nurses, interventions are targeted to the school population as a whole and to the larger community (Chapter 25). In work settings, community health nurses may also influence behaviors and conditions that contribute to ill health in a large segment of the population (Chapter 26).

Rural settings present unique problems. Health care services may be less accessible or facilities less adequate than in urban settings. Moreover, rural populations are exposed to unique environmental factors that make their health care needs different from urban populations. Community health nurses may be among only a few health care providers available in rural communities. Their role in that setting is discussed in Chapter 27.

Crime is a growing problem in the United States and throughout the world, and correctional facilities are filled to overflowing. Provision of health care for this segment of society is a challenging task that may involve the skills of community health nurses. Special issues in the care of clients in correctional settings are addressed in Chapter 28.

Not infrequently, natural or manmade disasters cause tremendous loss of life and property and disrupt the day-to-day routines of many. Working with individuals, families, and communities, the community health nurse has a primary role in helping to prevent manmade disasters and in working with victims following catastrophic events. A discussion of community health nurses' involvement in planning, implementing, and evaluating health care services in the event of a natural or manmade disaster is presented in Chapter 29.

In each specialized setting described in Unit V, the Dimensions Model is used to adapt nursing care to the needs of the individual and setting.

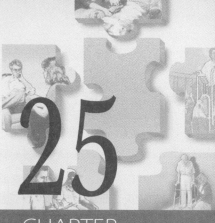

CARE OF CLIENTS IN THE SCHOOL SETTING

Education and health have a reciprocal relationship. Health factors influence one's ability to learn. Education affects one's ability to engage in healthful behaviors. This reciprocal relationship makes the school setting an ideal place to provide health care. Most school nurses are community health nurses practicing in a specialized setting. Given their community health preparation, school nurses retain their concern for the health of the community and apply the principles of community health nursing to the needs of the overall community as well as to the needs of the school population.

Community health nurses working in school settings have a threefold concern for the health of schoolchildren. First, the health of schoolchildren influences the health status of the community at large. Second, health promotion and illness prevention efforts directed at youngsters will improve their health status as adults. Finally, healthy children learn better and can take greater advantage of the educational opportunities provided to them.

The importance of the school health program as an avenue for improving the health of the population is evident in the number of national health objectives for the year 2000 that reflect health measures in schools (U.S. Department of Health and Human Services, 1991). These objectives are included in Appendix A.

► Chapter Objectives

After reading this chapter, you should be able to:

- Identify three goals of a school health program.
- Describe the components of a modern school health program.
- Describe at least two considerations in assessing physical dimension factors influencing the health of the school population.
- Identify at least four areas to be assessed in the psychological dimension of school health.
- Describe at least two areas to be addressed in assessing social dimension influences on the health of the school population.
- Identify at least five areas of emphasis in primary prevention in the school setting.
- Describe at least three approaches to secondary prevention in the school setting.
- Describe at least two areas of emphasis in tertiary prevention in the school setting.

► HISTORICAL PERSPECTIVES

School nursing is one of several traditional roles for community health nurses. It originated with a concern for the number of children being excluded from school owing to communicable diseases. In New York City in 1902, 15 to 20 children per school were being sent home daily. In response to this problem, Lillian Wald assigned nurses from the Henry Street Settlement to four New York City schools in a pilot project in school nursing. In the first month of the program's operation, the number of school exclusions declined 90%. Because of the success of the project, the New York City Board of Health hired additional nurses to continue this type of work (Pollitt, 1994).

Early school nursing focused on preventing the spread of communicable disease and treating ailments related to compulsory school attendance. By the 1930s, however, the focus had shifted to preventive and promotive activities including case finding, integration of health concepts into school curricula, and maintenance of a healthful school environment. Treatment of any health problems by the nurse was strongly discouraged to prevent infringement on the private medical sector. School nurse activities at this time consisted of screening for vision, hearing, and orthopedic defects, as well as detecting developmental difficulties and providing minor first aid (Igoe, 1994b).

School health nurses, dissatisfied with such a minimal role, continued to provide clandestine diagnostic services and treatment of minor ailments in addition to engaging in classroom teaching related to health. More recently, school nurses have begun to return to activities related to the diagnosis and treatment of health problems. Several factors account for current changes in the school nurse role. Among these are the number of families of school-age children in which both parents work. In these families neither parent may have time to deal with routine health problems of their children. Other factors include the interest of school nurses in expanding their role, the failure of government programs (eg, the Early and Periodic Screening, Diagnosis, and Treatment Program, EPSDT) to resolve the health problems of school-age children, enrollment of handicapped youngsters in regular school programs, and consumer demands for alternative sites for providing health care to children. One other major factor is that approximately one third of school-age children in the United States have no regular source of health care except for care rendered in emergency rooms (Passarelli, 1994). For these children, in particular, the school nurse may be the only source of health care.

► THE SCHOOL HEALTH PROGRAM

Health care is provided in schools for a number of reasons: the school environment itself may create hazards from which students must be protected; children need to be healthy to learn effectively; maintaining the health of children today produces healthier adults in years to come; and finally, there is a need to protect and enhance the health of the overall community. The national health objectives reflect these points.

The overall goal of a school health program is to enhance the health of members of the school community (Redican, Olsen, & Baffi, 1993). More specific goals of a school health program include promoting health and preventing illness, identifying and resolving existing health problems, and educating students and families for a healthier lifestyle.

These goals traditionally have been achieved through the three basic components of a school health program: health services, health instruction, and a healthy environment (Yates, 1994). More recently, other aspects of school life have also been considered integral features of a comprehensive school health program. According to the Joint Commission on Health Education Terminology, a *comprehensive school health program* is defined as the policies, procedures, and activities designed to protect and promote the health and well-being of students and school personnel (Henderson, 1993). Components of this comprehensive program include the traditional elements of health services, health education, and a healthy environment, as well as physical education activities, guidance and counseling services, food services, social work services, psychological counseling, employee health promotion and parent and community involvement (Resnicow & Allensworth, 1996). Components of a comprehensive school health program are depicted in Figure 25–1.

The health services component of a school health program should provide a wide variety of health care services. Broadly categorized, these services include assessment and screening, case finding, counseling, health promotion and illness prevention, case management, remedial or rehabilitation services, specific nursing procedures, and emergency care. Examples of activities in each of these categories are presented in Table 25–1.

The focus of the health education component of the school health program is educating students for health awareness and healthful behavior. Health education in the school setting focuses on both cognitive and affective learning. *Cognitive learning* involves acquisition of facts and information related to health and healthy behavior. *Affective learning,* on the other

hand, refers to developing attitudes toward health and health behaviors that foster a healthy lifestyle. Recommended content areas for health education curricula include:

Nutrition	Growth and development
Personal health	Weight control
Exercise and fitness	Communicable disease
Safety and injury	prevention and control
prevention	Chronic disease prevention
Sexuality	and control
Family life	Mental and emotional health
Interpersonal	Stress management
relationships	Substance use and abuse
Violence	Consumer health
Community health	Aging and death
Environmental health	

The environmental component of the school health program includes activities directed toward improving the physical, psychological, and social environment of the school and the surrounding community. In the area of physical education, the emphasis is on promoting physical activity among school-age chil-

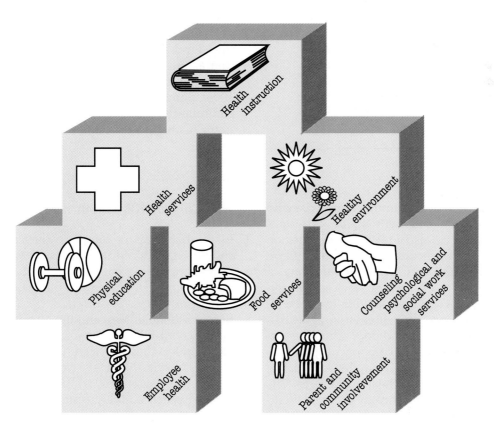

Figure 25–1. Components of the school health program.

TABLE 25–1. SAMPLE ACTIVITIES RELATED TO SCHOOL HEALTH SERVICE CATEGORIES

School Health Service Category	Related Activities
Assessment and screening	• Preschool entry assessments • Transfer student health assessments • Special appraisals for high-risk students or students referred by other school personnel • Routine screening • Home visiting for comprehensive assessment • Monitoring chronic conditions and treatment effects
Case finding	• Identification of communicable disease • Identification of chronic disease • Referral for diagnostic and treatment services
Counseling	• Counseling to decrease health risks • Counseling regarding existing health problems • Anticipatory counseling for students, parents, staff
Health promotion/illness prevention	• Exclusion of students with communicable diseases • Immunization of unimmunized students, staff • Health teaching in and outside of classrooms • Health promotion activities for students/staff (eg, smoking cessation, weight control)
Case management	• Liaison with community services • Referral to outside services as needed • Follow up on referrals • Fostering parental involvement • Arranging transportation
Remedial/rehabilitative services	• Speech therapy • Physical therapy • Behavior modification
Nursing procedures	• Development of student care plans • Administration of medications • Specialized nursing procedures • Teaching procedures to other staff
Emergency care	• Development of emergency protocols • First aid services • Postemergency assessment

dren, as well as developing attitudes to exercise and fitness that will continue throughout life. Attitudes and good food habits are also a focus of the nutrition component of the school health program in addition to provision of healthful diets while children are at school. Counseling and social work services are provided to assist students and their families to deal with changes and problem areas in their environments that may contribute to poor health and poor school performance. The employee health component provides similar types of services for school employees in addition to assistance with physical health problems. The final component of the school health program is directed toward fostering partnerships between school, family, and community that enhance the health of the overall community. Each component of the school health program will be addressed in more detail in the area of the Dimensions Model to which it relates.

► EDUCATIONAL PREPARATION FOR SCHOOL HEALTH NURSING

Depending on the requirements of the particular jurisdiction, nurses working in school settings may have varying levels of education. In some parts of the country, for example, the Southeast, a person designated as a "school nurse" may not even be a registered nurse. Because of the autonomy of nursing practice in the school setting and the complexity of health problems addressed, ideally the school nurse should be prepared at least at the baccalaureate level. This level of educational preparation guarantees that the nurse has the community health nursing background to deal effectively with the health needs of the school population.

In some states, employment as a school nurse requires advanced preparation beyond a baccalaureate degree in nursing. In California, for example, school nurses must complete a state-approved *school nurse credential program.* This is a nondegree program offered in an institution of higher learning that meets state requirements for educating school nurses.

Other school nurses may be prepared at the master's level in nursing. These nurses frequently function as nurse practitioners, promoting health and diagnosing and treating minor illnesses (Rajsky-Steed, 1996). Some, however, have advanced preparation in community health nursing and are involved in program planning rather than primary care of minor illnesses.

► STANDARDS FOR SCHOOL HEALTH NURSING

Like other areas of nursing practice, school nursing should be practiced in accordance with a set of minimum care standards. The first national *Standards for School Nursing Practice* were published in 1983 by the American Nurses Association, the National Association of School Nurses, and the National Association of state School Nurse Consultants (Passarelli, 1994). In 1993, these standards were updated in the document *School Nursing Practice—Roles and Standards* (Proctor, Lordis, & Zaiger, 1993). The standards for school nursing practice, like the standards for nursing practice in other specialty areas, reflect the use of the nursing process.

▶ STANDARDS FOR SCHOOL
NURSING PRACTICE

1. The school nurse uses a clinical knowledge base in practice.
2. The school nurse uses a systematic approach to problem solving.
3. The school nurse contributes to the education of students with special needs through use of the nursing process.
4. The school nurse uses effective communication skills.
5. The school nurse establishes and maintains a comprehensive school health program.
6. The school nurse collaborates with other school personnel and caregivers to meet students' needs.
7. The school nurse collaborates with community members in designing health care delivery systems and functions as a liaison between school and community.
8. The school nurse assists clients (students, families, and communities) to achieve optimal wellness via health education.
9. The school nurse contributes to nursing and school health through research and innovative practice.
10. The school nurse defines the nursing role, promotes quality care and professional growth, and demonstrates professional conduct.

(Adapted from Proctor, et al., 1993 currently under revision.)

▶ THE SCHOOL HEALTH TEAM

Health problems identified in individual children or in the community served by the school are frequently beyond the capabilities of the community health nurse acting independently. To meet the needs of the school population and the community, the school health nurse often needs to participate as a member of a team.

Because identified health problems may be the consequence of factors beyond the control of health care professionals, the school health team often consists of a variety of individuals, not all of whom have a health or medical background. The team acts to design a school health program that meets the health needs of students and of the larger community.

The school health team should use the strategies discussed in Chapter 12 to create an effective team that can address the health needs of the population. One of the critical features of group development for the school health team is negotiating member roles. Group members should clarify for themselves the roles that each will play, so that infringement on anyone's professional territory is avoided.

Specific members of the team will vary with the identified needs of the population, but some of those who may be involved, in addition to the nurse, are parents, teachers, administrators, counselors, psychologists, social workers, physicians and dentists, a health coordinator, food service personnel, janitorial and secretarial staffs, public health officials and other public officials, and students. Additional team members in some school settings include nurse practitioners; physical, occupational, and respiratory therapists (Healthcare Trends and Transition, 1994); and speech pathologists (Igoe, 1994a).

Parents, of course, have the primary responsibility for the health of their children. With respect to the school health program, parents have a responsibility to reinforce health teaching at home and to follow up on referrals for assistance with health problems identified in their children. They should also provide input into the planning and evaluation of the school health program. Parents may also provide volunteer services for first aid or "sick room duty" when there is not a nurse employed full-time.

Teachers also have a variety of responsibilities for the health of their students. Among these are the need to motivate students in the development of good health habits, to encourage student responsibility for health, and to observe them for signs of health problems. Teachers have a responsibility to model healthy behavior and to provide health instruction. Other responsibilities include assisting with screening efforts and measures to control the spread of disease and helping to identify factors in the physical, psychological, and social environments that are detrimental to the health status of students and coworkers. In addition, teachers may counsel students with health problems and may make referrals for assistance as appropriate.

School administrators include principals, district superintendents, and school board members. Administrators are responsible for the implementation of the school health program and should provide both material and nonmaterial support. They also function as a liaison between the school and the larger community. In collaboration with other team members, administrators participate in planning and evaluating the school health program. Other administrative responsibilities include hiring and evaluating health service employees and fostering collegial relationships among school health team members. Finally, administrators have the ultimate responsibility for the creation of a healthy and safe environment.

Some schools employ counselors, psychologists, or social workers or contract for their services as consultants. Counselors may provide emotional counseling or assistance to students in career decisions. Psychologists may also be involved in counseling for emotional problems. In addition, they may conduct psychological testing on selected youngsters to identify emotional problems or learning disabilities. Or, they may be called on to administer tests of school readiness to all incoming children. Social workers may likewise counsel students regarding problems and may provide referrals for students and families to assist with socioeconomic problems. When the services of these specialists are not available in a particular school setting, many of these functions may be assumed by the school nurse, if he or she is educationally prepared to carry them out. Or, the nurse might make a referral to an outside source of assistance.

Physicians and dentists usually are not employed by a school system, but they may provide services on a contract or referral basis. Under a contractual arrangement, physicians and dentists may spend a certain amount of time in the school assessing health and dental needs or making treatment recommendations. In other instances, students may be referred to their own physicians or dentists for follow-up treatment of identified health problems. Physical, occupational, or respiratory therapists may be employed in some school systems that provide comprehensive health services or may serve as outside consultants in the care of individual children. School systems may also have similar kinds of interactions with speech pathologists.

The school nurse may function as the school's health coordinator, or the school health team may include a health coordinator who is not a nurse. The health coordinator may be a parent, teacher, or other person with some health-related preparation. Responsibilities of the health coordinator include serving as a liaison with families and with the community, arranging in-service education for staff, facilitating team relationships, and coordinating the health instruction program. Other areas of responsibility include planning for speakers on health topics, arranging health-related learning experiences such as field trips or health fairs, and reviewing materials for use in health education.

In schools where meals are provided, food service personnel are responsible for preparing and serving nutritious meals. They may also be responsible for planning menus, depending on their background and knowledge of the nutritional needs of school-age children.

The janitorial staff is usually responsible for maintenance of the physical environment. Remediation of physical health hazards usually comes under their jurisdiction as well. They also ensure the cleanliness of kitchen and sanitary facilities to prevent the transmission of disease.

Clerical personnel are responsible for maintaining student records and for processing family notification of screening test results and recommendations. They may also be responsible for notifying families in the case of student injury or illness.

Public health officials are not employed by the school, but still form part of the school health team in that they are responsible for inspection of school sanitation, cooking facilities, and immunization status. They also act to establish local health policy related to schools and other institutions and to safeguard the health of the overall community. Other public officials may also be involved in planning a school health program to meet the needs of the school's population. Fire or police personnel might be involved, for example, in designing safety education programs for children and their parents.

In older age groups, students within the school may also be part of the school health team. Student responsibilities include helping to maintain a healthful and safe environment and providing input regarding student health needs and planning to meet those needs. Older students should also be involved in evaluating the effectiveness of the school health program.

▶ THE DIMENSIONS MODEL AND CARE OF CLIENTS IN THE SCHOOL SETTING

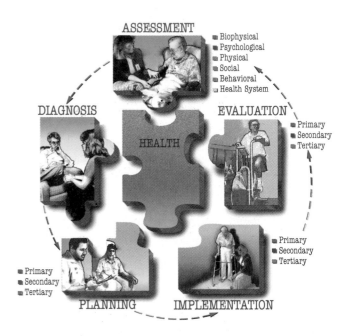

The community health nurse in the school setting will find the Dimensions Model a useful framework for directing nursing care. Components of the model remain the same as in any other setting and include assessing the school population and setting in terms of an epidemiologic perspective; diagnosing health problems; planning and implementing care at primary, secondary, and tertiary levels of prevention; and evaluating the care given.

Critical Dimensions of Nursing in the School Setting

School nurses carry out roles and responsibilities to three types of care recipients: students and their families, school personnel, and the community. Elements of each of the six dimensions of nursing will be employed in carrying out responsibilities to each of these client groups. In the cognitive dimension, the nurse will require knowledge of normal growth and development for the age groups in the school. In addition, the nurse will need a wide range of knowledge related to typical health problems seen in these age groups, both in terms of presenting signs and symptoms and appropriate interventions. Because of the growing numbers of children with chronic or handicapping health conditions in schools, school nurses also need specific knowledge about the conditions experienced by these children. The nurse will also need a thorough grounding in family dynamics to identify influences on child health and to assist families to promote their children's health. Knowledge of community resources for both children and their families is also important.

Many of the roles and responsibilities of the school nurse involve elements of the interpersonal dimension. For example, the nurse often serves as a consultant to teachers, administrators, and parents or as a coordinator of care. All of these roles require interpersonal skills in communication and collaboration. Similarly, the school nurse's educator role requires effective communication skills. In the ethical dimension, advocacy may be required at many levels. For example, the nurse may need to advocate for the special learning needs of a handicapped child in the school setting, or advocate with teachers and administrators for more frequent water breaks for all children to prevent dehydration in hot weather. Similarly, advocacy may be needed for the teacher with health problems who needs to take a leave of absence. At a systems level, the nurse may be called upon to advocate for inclusion of health-related content in school curricula.

Providing first aid for illness and injury is one of the manipulative skills required in the skills dimension. Basic physical assessment skills are also required. Other manipulative skills that the school nurse should possess include screening skills related to hearing and vision problems and scoliosis. In school systems with a high incidence of lead poisoning or tuberculosis, the school nurse may also need to screen for these diseases. Intellectual skills needed include interpretive and analytic skills to identify health problems in individual students and staff, as well as

problems affecting groups of people and the community at large. Critical thinking and program planning skills will also be required to develop an effective school health program.

Elements of the process dimension brought into play in school nursing certainly include the nursing process as executed with individual clients (students or staff) as well as with subgroups within the school and in the community served by the school. Another process element critical to school nursing is the education process. Community health nurses working in schools will also be called upon to employ case management, change, leadership, and group processes. Use of the epidemiologic and political processes may also be needed to identify health problems in the school population and surrounding community and to muster support for programs to meet those needs.

Research related to school health, factors that promote health in school populations, and interventions designed to achieve health in this segment of society is needed to create a basis for effective school nursing. Research in these areas can also lead to the development and testing of theoretical models that can guide and direct care in this setting. Finally, evaluation of school health programs in terms of both process and outcomes is needed to enhance the quality and effectiveness of such programs, as well as to demonstrate their cost-effectiveness in promoting the health of the general public.

 Assessing the Dimensions of Health in the School Setting

Use of the Dimensions Model in the school setting begins with assessing the health needs of the school population and identifying the factors influencing those needs. Areas for consideration include the biophysical, psychological, physical, social, behavioral, and health system dimensions of health.

The Biophysical Dimension

Areas for consideration related to the biophysical dimension include maturation and aging, genetic inheritance, and physiologic function.

Maturation and Aging. School nurses work with students in preschool, elementary school, junior high and high school, and college and university settings. Consequently, the age of the client population influences the types of health problems that may be present. For example, prevention of communicable disease would receive greater emphasis in the preschool population, and sexuality issues and substance abuse would be of greater concern with adolescent populations. For college students, substance abuse and sexuality issues are also pertinent as are stress-related problems stemming from academic pressures and being away from home.

Client maturation also influences the content and process of the health instruction component of the school health program. Basic hygiene conveyed via cartoon films is appropriate to the preschool or early elementary age child; a frank discussion of sexuality and sexually transmitted diseases is appropriate with older groups.

Genetic Inheritance.   Aspects of genetic inheritance of particular interest to the school nurse are the gender and racial composition of the population. A predominance of females in an elementary school increases the frequency with which the nurse will encounter students with symptoms of urinary tract infection as these are common in girls of that age. In adolescent girls, on the other hand, there is increased risk of unwanted pregnancy. Boys of all ages tend to have more sports-related injuries with which the nurse must deal.

Racial composition of the school population also influences the types of health problems encountered. For example, in schools with large African American populations, sickle cell screening might be included as a routine part of the school health program. The nurse must also be alert to the prevalence of other diseases that exhibit genetic predispositions, such as thalassemia and diabetes.

Physiologic Function.   An important aspect of the human biological component of the assessment is the physiologic function of the school population. In assessing physiologic function, the community health nurse looks for general indicators of health in elementary and secondary schoolchildren:

1. A display of energy and development normal for the child's age group, and the ability to participate regularly in physical education activities
2. Ability to carry out normal school and home responsibilities without undue fatigue or emotional upset
3. Normal, progressive gains in weight and height
4. Clear, smooth skin
5. Normal experience of illness or accidents expected for the child's age group
6. Enthusiasm and zest for life
7. Good social health and peer group interactions
8. Emotional control (Cornacchia, Olsen, & Nickerson, 1995)

Many school children may not exhibit these characteristics and suffer from a variety of health problems. These can be categorized as short-lived and self-limiting diseases, environmental and psychological stress, chronic diseases with long-term health and education implications, chronic diseases and handicaps that interfere with function, and fatal irreversible disease.

Examples of self-limiting conditions include communicable diseases such as the common cold, influenza, and chickenpox and injuries such as a fractured arm or leg. Diabetes, seizure disorders, and minor visual or hearing problems are examples of chronic conditions that may have health and education implications. Many of these conditions can be controlled if properly diagnosed and treated and do not necessarily interfere with the child's ability to function in school. Other chronic and handicapping conditions do interfere with school function. Examples are blindness, deafness, mental retardation, attention deficit hyperactivity disorder (ADHD), and long-term effects of fetal drug exposure. Conditions related to environmental or psychological stress may or may not affect physiologic function, although they may affect the child's ability to function effectively in the school situation.

The kinds of physical health problems seen by school nurses among students and staff are many and varied. Acute and chronic conditions commonly encountered in the school setting are listed in Table 25–2.

The majority of health conditions seen in most school populations are acute respiratory illnesses. Ten to fifteen percent of school-age children, however, have some type of chronic condition (Passarelli, 1994), and 10% of children receive specialized services due to one or more handicapping condition (Berkson, 1993). Common chronic conditions in school populations include asthma, migraine, seizure disorder, ADHD, diabetes, cerebral palsy, hearing and vision loss, heart disease, cancer, arthritis, renal disease, muscular dystrophy, cystic fibrosis, sickle cell disease, and AIDS and HIV infection (Williams & McCarthy, 1995). The school nurse should be conversant with the signs and symptoms of common illnesses and other conditions among children. The nurse should be aware of the prevalence of these and other health conditions among the school population so as to plan health care to meet the needs of children with these conditions.

Immunity is another important consideration related to physiologic function in the school population. The community health nurse working in the school setting monitors the immunization status of students and school employees. For example, maintenance personnel are at risk for tetanus because of the potential for dirty injuries, and their immunization status

TABLE 25–2. ACUTE AND CHRONIC PHYSICAL HEALTH PROBLEMS ENCOUNTERED IN THE SCHOOL SETTING

Organ System Affected	Conditions Encountered
Cardiovascular system	Heart murmurs, hypertension
Central nervous system	Mental retardation, blindness, deafness, attention deficit hyperactivity disorder, learning disability, seizure disorder, meningitis, cerebral palsy
Endocrine system	Diabetes mellitus, thyroid disorders
Gastrointestinal system	Encopresis, hepatitis, diarrhea, dental caries, constipation, peptic and duodenal ulcers
Genitourinary/reproductive system	Sexually transmitted diseases, urinary tract infection, enuresis, dysmenorrhea, pregnancy
Hematopoietic system	Anemia, hemophilia, leukemia, sickle cell disease, lead poisoning
Immunologic system	AIDS and related opportunistic infections
Integumentary system	Acne, eczema, impetigo, lice, scabies, dermatitis, tinea corporis
Musculoskeletal system	Arthritis, sprains, fractures, scoliosis, Legg–Calvé–Perthes disease
Respiratory system	Upper and lower respiratory infections, strep throat, influenza, asthma, hayfever, pertussis, diphtheria, pneumonia
Other diseases	Measles, mumps, rubella, scarlet fever, chickenpox, infectious mononucleosis, otitis media, otitis externa, conjunctivitis, Lyme disease, cancer, hepatitis

should also be monitored. For female teachers and other school personnel of childbearing age, the risk of rubella during pregnancy is increased by working with children, and they should also be adequately immunized.

A final health problem frequently encountered in the school population that may have a physiologic basis is learning disability. Approximately 5% of school children experience some form of learning disability. A *learning disability* is operationally defined as being 2 or more years behind classmates in one academic area (Berkson, 1993).

Children with learning disabilities may exhibit any of several characteristics, including poor visual and/or auditory discrimination or the tendency to confuse shapes, letters, or sounds; poor visual memory in which the child has difficulty remembering what is seen or read; and poor kinesthesia or the inability to discriminate objects by touch. Other characteristics that may be evident are poor eye–hand coordination, poor spatial orientation (eg, inability to tell right from left), poor figure–ground discrimination (inability to pick a specific object from a group), perseverance (obsessive repetition of a newly learned skill), and poor self-image. Moreover, it is thought that the hyperactivity characteristic of some of these children is due to their bewilderment that they have not understood what they have seen or heard in their classroom instruction.

The Psychological Dimension

The psychological environment of the school can either foster good health or undermine it. Aspects of the psychological dimension to be assessed include the organization of the school day, the aesthetic quality of the physical environment, the nature of relationships among students and school staff members, discipline and grading practices, and parent–school relationships.

Organization of the School Day. The nurse would determine whether the organization of the school day is conducive to health. Assessment areas to be addressed include the extent to which periods of strenuous physical activity are alternated with periods of quiet study and the extent of opportunities for developing a variety of psychomotor as well as academic skills. The nurse also assesses whether mealtimes are arranged so that students have the energy reserves to handle the tasks of the school day. For younger children, this usually means providing a snack time. Another area for assessment is the scheduling of time for toileting activities. The nurse should determine whether children are given time to go to the lavatory or permitted to go when necessary to prevent chronic constipation or urinary tract infection. There should also be opportunities for children to obtain drinks of water. Such opportunities should increase in frequency with hot weather.

Aesthetic Quality. The appearance of the physical environment is interrelated with the psychological dimension, and the nurse assesses the aesthetic quality of the environment. Are the rooms clean, bright, and cheerful and conducive to good psychological health? Or, are they dark, dingy, and depressing?

Peer Relations. The relationships of a student with his or her peers can create a psychological environment that is either conducive or detrimental to mental and physical health. The community health nurse can assess the extent to which students who have difficulties with peer relationships are encouraged to participate in group activities. Is there adequate adult supervision of student activities to moderate unhealthy peer relationships? If school personnel see that particular children are unable to participate or are even victimized, do they act to stop such behaviors? Are opportunities provided within the school setting and the curriculum for values clarification and learning about healthy interpersonal interactions?

Teacher–Student Relationships. Teacher–student relationships also affect the psychological climate of the school. The nurse assesses the quality of student–teacher relationships within the school in general and also between specific teachers and their students. Ideally, teachers are people who listen, reward appropriate behavior, maximize student assets, allow personal expression, and foster responsibility. Teachers who foster good student relationships tend to be enthusiastic and have a way of making learning fun. They exhibit a sincere concern for students and respect, accept, and trust them. They get to know their students well, encourage participation and curiosity, foster healthy competition, and encourage students to perform to their best potential. They also refrain from harsh or sarcastic comments, and they discipline students appropriately (Redican, Olsen, & Baffi, 1993).

Unfortunately, not all teachers fit this picture. In assessing teacher–student relationships, the nurse identifies any tendencies on the part of teachers to use undue punishment or to make demands that students are incapable of meeting. Inconsistent demands or conflicting expectations on the part of a teacher can also create stress in students and lead to physical and mental health problems. Nurses might note that certain children are singled out for punishment by a particular teacher and may need to function as advocates. School nurses should also be alert to the potential for emotional, physical, or sexual abuse of students by teachers (and, on occasion, of teachers by students).

Teacher–Teacher Relationships. The relationships among teachers in a school and between teachers and other school personnel also influence the psychological environment of students. The nurse should assess the extent to which healthy teacher relationships—those that are supportive, encourage creativity and freedom, and foster cooperation—exist within the school. Effective relationships among teachers foster sharing and self-confidence, recognize achievements, and provide guidance for teacher development. In schools where teacher–teacher relationships are strained, students may get caught in the middle between teachers, or student morale may be undermined by the stress created by strife among teachers. For example, if the basketball coach and a particular high school English teacher do not get along well, the coach may demand that basketball players cut English class for an extra practice before a championship game and the English teacher may threaten to fail any player that cuts class. In this instance, the students cannot win. If they cut class, they may fail English. Conversely, if they miss the practice, they may be dropped from the team.

Discipline. In discussing the characteristics of supportive teachers, the issue of discipline was alluded to. In addition to looking at disciplinary measures employed by individual teachers, school nurses should assess the school's philosophy regarding discipline. In one study of schools in Washington State, 11% of the participating schools permitted corporal punishment and slightly more than 3% reported actual instances of corporal punishment in the prior year (Grossman, Rauh, & Rivara, 1995). Discipline should be used for inappropriate behavior and should not be unduly harsh. The nurse determines whether rules of behavior are clearly communicated to students and whether expectations are realistic. The nurse should also assess whether discipline, when warranted, is administered fairly and in a manner that does not diminish the student's self-respect (Redican, Olsen, & Baffi, 1993).

A particular need in today's society is to prevent violence in and around the school setting. Violence within the school environment can be addressed by explicit codes of conduct that are clearly communicated to students and consistently and uniformly enforced. Weapons should be strictly banned from school campuses and the ban stringently enforced. A 1994 nationwide study indicated that 80% of school districts and 90% of junior and senior high schools have policies prohibiting violence and weapons possession. Despite these policies, however, approximately half of the schools surveyed reported at least one instance of weapons possession in the prior year (Ross, Einhaus, Hohenemser, Greene, Kann, & Gold, 1995). Peer counseling and off-campus counseling sites to address interpersonal problems have been effective means of reducing violence. The community health nurse in the school setting can assess the level of violence on campus as well as the effectiveness of steps taken to prevent violence. The nurse can also examine the inclusion of conflict resolution strategies and content on interpersonal relations in the school's health education curriculum.

Grading. School and teacher grading policies should be clearly understood and should be fairly implemented. Particular grading practices are usually the province of the individual teacher, but the community health nurse can assess whether grading standards are consistent and grades are communicated to students privately to avoid humiliation. If graded work is displayed, the nurse can examine the extent to which student work is exhibited in a way that all students are made to feel good about some of their abilities. This is particularly important in elementary grades when children incorporate perceptions of their school performance into either positive or negative self-images.

Parent–School Relationships.   Another area for assessment is the quality of relationships between school personnel and parents, which can have a strong influence on the psychological climate of the school setting. When this relationship is cooperative, students do not receive conflicting messages about what is expected of them. On the other hand, when relationships between parents and school personnel are adversarial, students may again be caught in the middle of a power struggle. Or, students may attempt to exploit the situation by manipulating both parents and teachers to their own advantage. Other areas that the nurse might explore in assessing the psychological environment are the quality of students' school performance and absenteeism and dropout rates.

The Physical Dimension

The nurse assesses both the internal and external physical environment of the school. The external environment includes the area surrounding the school. Assessment considerations here include traffic patterns, water hazards, use of pesticides, and rodent control in the area. Other environmental concerns include the proximity of hazardous waste dumps or nuclear power plants, industrial hazards, and the presence of various forms of pollution. (See Chap. 17 for a discussion of environmental health issues.)

Several aspects of the school's internal environment, such as fire hazards and sanitation, are the responsibility of official agencies like the fire department and health department; however, there are other aspects of the physical environment that are rarely adequately assessed. The school health nurse needs to be alert to other hazards to physical safety that may be present in the school setting. Examples of these hazards are toxic art supplies, scientific equipment in laboratories, kitchen appliances in home economics classrooms, and chemical substances used either in chemistry labs or by maintenance and janitorial staffs. Animals in classrooms may also present safety hazards in terms of the potential for scratches and bites or disease transmission. Other conditions that may jeopardize safety include asbestos used in building materials, inadequate maintenance of fire hoses and extinguishers, and inoperable communications systems in the event of an emergency.

Other areas of concern are the safety of industrial arts classrooms, the gymnasium, and play areas. As noted in Chapter 20, the safety of outdoor play equipment should be inspected on a regular basis and repairs made as needed. A similar need exists for periodic assessment of sports equipment and practices. Other hazards associated with play areas include broken glass and other refuse on the playground. Hard surfaces below play equipment increase the potential for injuries stemming from falls.

Other assessment considerations with respect to the school's internal physical environment include noise levels within and outside of classrooms and adequacy of lighting, ventilation, heating, and cooling. Food sanitation should also be assessed. If hot meals are provided at school, cooking facilities should be inspected regularly. Such inspections are usually the official responsibility of the local health department, but the community health nurse should also assess these facilities periodically. If students bring their lunches, the potential for food poisoning from spoiled foods should be appraised.

Assessing sanitary facilities in the school is another area for consideration. Here the nurse would examine the adequacy of toilet facilities for the size of the school population. The nurse would also periodically inspect sanitary facilities to make sure they are in good working order and do not pose hazards for the transmission of communicable diseases. Again, this area is usually the responsibility of health department personnel, but official inspections may only occur at lengthy intervals and the nurse should be aware of hazards that might arise in the interim.

Another area of concern with respect to sanitation is the use and cleaning of shower facilities. The nurse should assess that showers are adequately cleaned to prevent transmission of communicable conditions such as tinea pedis (athlete's foot).

Physical facilities for preventing the spread of disease by infected children should also be assessed. Are there places within the school where youngsters with infectious conditions can be isolated? All too often these children are merely kept in the nurse's office until a parent can come for them. This presents opportunities for exposure of all those who visit the nurse while the child is there.

Special consideration should be given to the physical environment as it relates to handicapped children. Many physical barriers may exist, particularly in older schools, that limit the ability of handicapped youngsters to benefit from the education setting. Areas of concern include the presence of ramps, easily opened doors and windows, nonslip flooring, elevators, and curb modifications to eliminate the need to step up. Another consideration is access to toileting facilities by handicapped children. Are toilets accessible to wheelchairs? Are sinks placed so that a wheelchair can be maneuvered beneath them? Placement and height of mirrors, drinking fountains, and telephones is also of concern. Other considerations with respect to the environment of handicapped children are the adequacy of storage for wheelchairs and other special equipment, wheelchair space in classrooms and auditoriums, modification of laboratory and library carrels for wheelchair use, and adequacy of evacuation plans for the handicapped in case of emergency. The intent is to create a school that is barrier-free so that all students, staff, and community members who may use the premises after school hours have access to facilities and equipment.

The Social Dimension

The social dimension also plays a part in influencing the health status of members of the school community. The nurse needs to assess the community's attitudes toward education because these attitudes determine, in large part, the degree of support given to the schools and to health care within the schools. Community attitudes also affect the allocation of funds for both school and health programs.

The extent of crime in the school neighborhood is another aspect of the social environment to be assessed. Is violence a problem for children going to and from school? Is drug dealing going on in the area and will youngsters be pressured to experiment with drugs?

A social factor that influences health in the school setting is the prevalence of families in which both parents work. Unfortunately, children are often sent to school when they are ill because there is no one at home to care for them. The nurse should assess the number of students who come to school ill and explore with parents their reasons for sending sick children to school. It may be a lack of awareness on the part of parents of the signs and symptoms of illness or an absence of other options available to parents.

The social environment within the school is also influential. What is the socioeconomic status of students? Of school personnel? What is the racial or ethnic composition of the school population? Are racial tensions present? Do religious beliefs influence the health of the school population? For example, if there are large numbers of children whose parents object to immunization on religious grounds, the nurse needs to be particularly alert to signs of outbreaks of childhood diseases such as measles, rubella, and diphtheria. Another area for consideration is the cultural backgrounds of students and school personnel. Are they similar? Do cultural practices influence students' health? Do differences in cultural practices create tension among students or between students and staff? Cultural factors may also lead to inappropriate diagnosis of some children as having ADHD, when their behavior is considered perfectly normal within their own culture (Canuso, 1997).

Homelessness is another social dimension factor that can have a profound effect on the health of school-aged children. Homeless children are more likely than their housed peers to be behind in their classes, need remediation, or repeat a grade (Wiley & Ballard, 1993). As a result of the McKinney Homeless Assistance Act, homeless children are guaranteed access to free and public education. Under this act, homeless children may be eligible for other services that must be provided by schools receiving assistance funds. These services may include clothing, a place to bathe and change clothes, free or reduced cost meals, school supplies, tutorial assistance, and access to medical care (Gregory, 1993).

Homelessness is often the result of divorce or violence within families. Children may be homeless because their mothers are fleeing an abusive situation. In such circumstances and in disputes over child custody, the school system needs to be alert to the potential for abduction of school children by the other parent. Similarly, abduction and mistreatment by strangers is an area of concern, and the school nurse should assess school policies designed to prevent such occurrences for their adequacy and the extent to which they are enforced.

The Behavioral Dimension

Enrollment in school is itself a lifestyle factor that influences health. School attendance increases one's risk of exposure to a variety of communicable diseases. Children generally experience an increase in the number of acute illnesses during the first few years of school whether this occurs at the daycare/preschool level or with admission to elementary school.

The rigidity of the school day may also affect the health status of students. Attempts to postpone defecation or urination until prescribed times may lead to chronic constipation or to urinary tract infections. Likewise, inability to get a drink of water except at specific times may lead to dehydration, particularly in hot weather. The nurse should assess the effects of these aspects of regimentation on the health of students.

Nutrition is another behavioral dimension factor that should be assessed in the school population. The adequacy of lunches brought from home should be examined, as should evidence of poor nutrition of meals eaten at home. For example, the nurse would assess children for evidence of anemia or poor growth and development. In those schools without a dietary consultant, the nurse should appraise the nutritional quality of school lunch and/or breakfast programs. Too often, food for such programs is purchased with an eye toward economy rather than nutritional value.

Recreational activities should also be explored. The need to examine recreational and sports equipment for safety hazards has already been touched on, but the nurse should also be aware of the types of recreational and competitive activities engaged in by students. Is there ample opportunity for physical activity? Is it adequately supervised? Are sports and recreational programs appropriate to children's ages and developmental levels? For example, contact sports are not appropriate for children in lower elementary grades because of increased risk of injury. Another question is whether recreational activities are suited to children's interests. Are various opportunities available, or must all children engage in the same activity, whether they choose to or not? Is a gender bias evident in recreational opportunities provided? For example, is soccer restricted to boys while girls are expected to play hopscotch or jump rope? Attention should also be given to the recreational needs of teachers. Are teachers given a break from classroom and playground duties?

The physical education curriculum of the school will also influence students' exercise behaviors. Many schools do not include the exposure to physical education activities required to meet the national health objectives (Kolbe, Kann, Collins, Small, Pateman, & Warren, 1995). The International Consensus Conference on Physical Activity Guidelines for Adolescents recommends daily physical activity of some kind for all adolescents and three or more sessions per week of vigorous physical exercise sustained for a minimum of 20 minutes (Centers for Disease Control and Prevention, 1997). The school nurse should assess the extent to which the school physical education curriculum achieves standards set in the national objectives or by the Consensus Conference.

Rest is another component of the behavioral dimension that is assessed. Nurses and teachers should note whether children appear to be getting sufficient sleep at night. The nurse should also examine the adequacy of rest periods provided for younger children. Are these periods appropriately incorporated into the school day? Are there adequate facilities for rest periods (ie, cots or mats)? Facilities for rest periods are also an important consideration for handicapped children or those with chronic illnesses who may tire easily.

Other lifestyle behaviors should also be assessed, particularly among older students. The extent of tobacco use or use of alcohol or other drugs should be explored as should the extent of sexual activity among preadolescent and adolescent students. Approximately half of all adolescents aged 15 to 19 years are sexually active (Igoe, 1994a), and the nurse should assess the extent of sexual activity in the school population. The nurse must also be alert to signs of pregnancy and sexually transmitted diseases as well as being aware of the potential for sexual assault in the

school population. Similar assessments are needed with respect to substance use and abuse. In spite of the fact that three fourths of health education classes address problems of alcohol and drug use (Kolbe, et al., 1995), and that 97% of schools nationwide have policies prohibiting the use of tobacco, alcohol, and other drugs (Ross, et al., 1995), use of these substances among preadolescents and adolescents remains high. The nurse should assess the extent of substance use and abuse in the school population, ease of access to these substances in the community, and the adequacy and enforcement of school policies regarding their use. The nurse should also be alert to signs of substance use and abuse in individual students and school personnel.

The Health System Dimension

The health of the school population is influenced at both the individual and community levels. At the individual level, the community health nurse assesses the usual source of health care for individual children and their families. Do children have a regular source of health care? Do they make use of health-promotive and illness-preventive services as well as curative services? Or is health care for children crisis-oriented, focusing only on the treatment of acute conditions? Do children have unmet health needs because their families cannot afford care?

At the community level, the nurse assesses the availability of health care services to meet the needs of the school-age population. Are health-promotive and illness-preventive services easily accessible in the community? Are services available for youngsters with special health needs (eg, handicapped children)? Are specific pediatric or adolescent services available? Is there access to contraceptive services or treatment of sexually transmitted diseases for the adolescent population? Is community attention to possible child abuse adequate?

The nurse also assesses the relationship between the school and the health care community. Are private physicians conversant with regulations for excluding children with communicable conditions from school? Do physicians and other health care providers work cooperatively with school personnel to meet the health care needs of individual youngsters? Do health care providers in the community offer services within the school on either a paid or a voluntary basis?

Another consideration is the organizational structure for delivering health services in the school setting. New models of health care delivery in the schools include school-based and school-linked health centers or clinics and their natural extension, family health centers located in or near schools. The goal of these new

Biophysical Dimension

Age

What is the age composition of the school population (staff and students)?

Do any of the students exhibit developmental delays?

Are there specific developmental issues related to the student population (eg, sexual development)?

Genetic Inheritance

What is the relative proportion of males and females in the school population?

What is the racial/ethnic composition of the school population?

What is the prevalence of genetic predisposition to disease in the school population? What diseases are involved?

Physiologic Function

What existing health problems are prevalent in the school population?

What is the incidence of communicable diseases in the school population?

Are there any handicapped students present in the school population?

What are the immunization levels in the school population?

Psychological Dimension

Does the organization of the school day promote health?

What is the aesthetic quality of the school environment?

What is the quality of relationships among the students? Between students and staff? Among staff?

What type of discipline is used in the school setting? Is it appropriate? Is discipline employed fairly and consistently?

Is there undue pressure on students to perform scholastically or athletically?

Are school grading practices fair and consistent?

What is the quality of relationships between parents and school?

Physical Dimension

Where is the school located? Are there health hazards in the school neighborhood (eg, pollution)?

Are there fire or safety hazards in the school environment?

Are any hazardous chemicals appropriately stored and correctly used?

Is hazardous equipment used? If so, is it used correctly?

Are play areas safe? Is play equipment in good repair? Are there resilient surfaces beneath playground equipment?

Are there animals in the school environment? Do they pose a health hazard?

Are there plant allergens or poisonous plants in the school environment?

Does the school environment have adequate heat, light, and ventilation?

What is the noise level in the school environment? Does it pose a health hazard?

Are food sanitation practices adequate to prevent communicable diseases, vermin infestation, etc.?

Are toilet facilities adequate and in good repair?

Are shower facilities (if present) adequately cleaned?

Are there adequate facilities for handicapped students or staff?

Social Dimension

What are the community attitudes toward education? Toward the school?

To what extent does the community support the school program?

What is the extent of crime in the school neighborhood? What is the effect of crime on students and staff?

What is the source of school funding? How adequate is funding?

Is before- and after-school care available for children of working parents?

What is the socioeconomic status of the students? The staff?

What is the cultural background of students and staff? What languages are spoken?

What is the typical home environment of students like? Is there evidence of family violence?

Are any of the students homeless?

What is the education background of students' families and the extent of their health knowledge?

Are there intergroup conflicts in the school population?

Behavioral Dimension

Consumption Patterns

What are the nutritional needs of students and staff? Are there members of the school population with special nutritional needs? If so, what are they?

What is the nutritional quality of school meal programs?

What is the extent of nutrition knowledge among students, staff, and families?

What is the extent of alcohol, tobacco, and other drug use among students and staff?

Exercise and Leisure Activity

What are the rest and activity patterns of the school population? Are they appropriate to the age and health status of the population?

What recreational opportunities are available to the school population? Do recreational activities pose health hazards?

Are appropriate safety equipment and devices used (eg, in sports)?

Medication Use

Do any members of the school population use prescription medications on a regular basis?

Are medications used, stored, and dispensed as directed?

Sexual Practices

What is the prevalence of sexual activity among the school population?

Do students engage in unsafe sexual practices?

Do sexually active students use contraception?

Health System Dimension

What health services are offered in the school setting?

How accessible are needed health services in the community?

To what extent does the school population use available health services?

How are health care services funded? Is funding adequate to meet health needs?

To what extent do health care professionals in the community support the school health program?

What are the attitudes of the school population and the community toward health and health care?

---

models is to provide extended medical and mental health services at present, with the ultimate goal of comprehensive ambulatory health care services (Yates, 1994b). A *school-based health center (SBHC)* is a program of integrated health and social services provided in a school setting and designed to ensure access to necessary services. A *school-linked health center (SLHC)* is a cooperative effort of health and social services personnel to provide coordinated education, health, and social services to a target population of students and their families. Services are usually provided at sites near involved schools (Yates, 1994a).

Both SBHCs and SLHCs are efforts to provide accessible services to the more than 45 million children who attend school (Kolbe, 1994). Family health centers, which are still in the planning stages, extend these services to family members as well (Igoe, 1994b). Because of their centrality to community life, school-based clinics have been found to be a viable means of health care delivery. From 1985 to 1993, the number of SBHCs and SLHCs increased tenfold (Yates, 1994b). In 1994, nearly 12% of all school districts in the United States had at least one SBHC or SLHC (Small, Majer, Allensworth, Farquhar, Kann, & Pateman, 1995). In addition to providing direct care services to students and school staff, clinic personnel may be actively involved in health fairs; crisis intervention teams; classroom, parent, and teacher education; student health

clubs; and other health promotion activities (Lear, 1992). School-based clinics have been associated with more visits to health providers and greater health knowledge (Kisker & Brown, 1996), as well as fewer emergency department visits and significantly lower costs (Jones & Clark, 1997). The intent of the proposed family health centers is to provide these same types of services to families along with a variety of other community services. Programs such as SBHCs and SLHCs may already exist in a particular system, or the community health nurse can assess the potential for their successful development.

Appendix P, Special Assessment Considerations in the School Setting, provides guidelines for assessing health care delivery and other health needs in schools.

Diagnostic Reasoning and Care of Clients in the School Setting

The second aspect of the use of the Dimensions Model in the school setting is deriving nursing diagnoses from assessment data. Diagnoses can be derived at two levels, in relation to individual students and in relation to the school population. Examples of diagnoses related to a population group are "safety hazard due to placement of play equipment on asphalt surface" and "need for drug abuse education due to high prevalence of drug abuse in the surrounding community." Diagnoses related to an individual student are "inability to participate in vigorous physical exercise due to exercise-induced asthma" and "need for referral to child protective services due to suspected physical abuse by father."

Again, each of the sample diagnoses provided above contains a statement of the probable underlying cause of the problem. Such a statement provides direction for efforts to resolve the problem. For example, one approach to the playground safety hazard might be to relocate play equipment in a sandy area. With the individual examples, measures might be taken to provide less strenuous forms of exercise for the asthmatic child or to make a referral for child protective services in the abuse situation.

Planning to Meet Health Needs in the School Setting

Planning to meet health needs identified in the school setting takes place at two levels: the macrolevel, at which the general approach to providing health services in the school is planned, and the microlevel, at which plans are made to meet specific health needs of members of the school population. The community health nurse working in the school setting participates in planning efforts at both levels.

Macrolevel Planning

Health services are provided in keeping with an overall health services plan. The plan should specify the population to be served and the services to be provided. Typical categories of services include assessment of health status, problem management services, acute care services, and other preventive services such as immunizations and safety education. An additional component of the health services plan is specification of the personnel involved and of the resources needed to implement the program.

The health services plan should also address the nature of records to be kept. Categories to be addressed include clinical records related to the health of particular children or staff members, administrative records, and evaluative records. Planning program evaluation should also be included in the plan. Finally, the plan should specify budgetary considerations related to salaries, facilities, and other expenses. Specific elements of the plan in each of these areas are listed in Table 25–3. Initial development of a health services plan in the school setting would entail use of the program planning process described in Chapter 19.

TABLE 25–3. ELEMENTS OF THE SCHOOL HEALTH PLAN AND RELATED CONSIDERATIONS

Health Plan Element	Related Considerations
Population served	Ages and grades of students involved Extent of service to be given to staff
Services provided	Assessment/screening services First aid Acute care services Problem management services Immunizations Safety education Health education Counseling services
Personnel	Categories of health personnel Qualifications of health personnel Functions and responsibilities Staff development needs
Resources	Facilities Equipment Supplies/postage Health records Telephone
Record system	Clinical records for individuals seen Administrative records Immunization records Absenteeism records Program evaluation records
Program evaluation	Focus of evaluation Data collection procedures Data analysis procedures
Budgetary considerations	Salaries Facility construction and maintenance Equipment and supply costs Record-keeping costs Staff development costs

Microlevel Planning

The school health program includes planning for activity at all three levels of prevention: primary, secondary, tertiary.

Primary Prevention. Primary prevention in the school setting involves many of the same planning considerations as those used with children in general. Areas of emphasis in planning primary preventive measures in the school setting are immunization, safety, exclusion from school, health education, diet and nutrition, and exercise. Other concerns in primary prevention include developing a strong self-image, positive coping skills, and good interpersonal skills in students.

IMMUNIZATION. Young children are at particular risk for a variety of communicable diseases for which immunization is possible. Immunizations against measles, mumps, rubella, diphtheria, pertussis, tetanus, and polio are required for school entry. Immunizations are also available for diseases caused by *Hemophilus influenzae* B, hepatitis B, varicella, and influenza. These diseases are discussed in more detail in Chapter 30.

The school nurse may be involved in referring individuals who are not immunized for appropriate services or may provide immunizations in the school setting. In addition to providing for routine immunizations, school nurses may also suggest other immunizations in the event of exposure to certain diseases, such as hepatitis.

SAFETY.   Part of the school nurse's responsibility is to identify safety hazards and report them to those responsible for eliminating them. Safety education may also be the responsibility of the school nurse. In addition, the nurse might collaborate with others within and outside the school setting to reduce safety hazards in the surrounding area. Moreover, the nurse and other school personnel might become involved in cooperative efforts with local police to reduce drug traffic in the neighborhood.

EXCLUSION FROM SCHOOL.   One of the earliest responsibilities of the school nurse was to determine when children should be excluded from school because they had communicable illnesses. Children were also excluded from school as part of an effort to stop the spread of scabies, lice, and other parasites among a highly susceptible population. This responsibility still requires the school nurse to be knowledgeable of the signs and symptoms of communicable disease and infestation and to be aware of state and local regulations regarding school exclusion. Several conditions that usually warrant exclusion and guidelines for readmission are listed in Table 25–4.

The responsibility of the nurse does not stop with excluding the affected child from school. The nurse should also educate parents and children regarding the need to stay home from school when they are ill and about care during illness. The nurse may also make referrals for medical care as needed. In addition, the nurse follows up on children excluded from school to make sure that they are receiving appropriate care and that they are able to return to school when there is no longer any danger of exposure to others.

HEALTH EDUCATION.   Health education in the school setting provides a foundation for healthy behaviors in adulthood. Most states and school districts require some form of health education at the elementary and junior and senior high school level. At the elementary level, health education is most likely to be incorporated into the total curriculum. Separate health courses are more likely at the junior and senior high levels (Kolbe, et al., 1995).

TABLE 25–4. CONDITIONS TYPICALLY WARRANTING EXCLUSION FROM SCHOOL AND GUIDELINES FOR READMISSION

Condition	Readmission Guidelines
Bacterial conjunctivitis	After acute symptoms subside
Chickenpox	5 days after eruption of the first vesicles or after lesions are dried
Diphtheria	Until negative cultures of nose and throat are obtained at least 24 hours after discontinuing antibiotics
Hepatitis A	One week after onset of jaundice
Impetigo (staphylococcal)	24 hours after treatment is initiated
Influenza	After acute symptoms subside
Measles	4 days after onset of the rash
Meningococcal meningitis	24 hours after chemotherapy is initiated or when the child is sufficiently recovered
Mononucleosis, infectious	After acute symptoms subside Delay resumption of strenuous physical activity until spleen is nonpalpable
Mumps	9 days after onset of swelling
Pediculosis	24 hours after application of an effective pediculocide
Pneumonia, pneumococcal and *Mycoplasma*	48 hours after initiation of antibiotics or when child is sufficiently recovered
Pertussis	After 5 days of antibiotic therapy or when child is sufficiently recovered
Respiratory disease (viral) and upper respiratory infection	After acute symptoms subside
Rubella	7 days after onset of the rash
Scabies	24 hours after treatment
Streptococcus (strep throat, scarlet fever, impetigo)	24 hours after treatment is initiated or when child is sufficiently recovered
Tinea corporis	Excluded only from gym, swimming pool, or other activities where exposure of other individuals may occur; activities resume after treatment is completed

The principles of health education discussed in Chapter 9 are particularly relevant to community health nursing in the school setting. The nurse may either serve as a resource for teachers on health content or provide health education classes, or do both. The school nurse is also involved in the development of the health education curriculum. Activities involved in curriculum development in which the nurse may engage include the assessment of needs and resources, review of health curricula from other school systems, development of goals and objectives, and design of specific learning activities. In addition, the nurse may also be involved in preparing teachers to participate in the health education program. Finally, the nurse participates in the implementation and evaluation of the program.

FOOD AND NUTRITION.   Nutrition is another important aspect of health promotion with the school population. As noted earlier, when this function is not performed by a dietician or nutritionist, school nurses assess the nutritional status of children and monitor the nutritional value of school lunches. When nutritional offerings are inadequate, the nurse works with school administrators and food service personnel to improve the nutritional quality of meals served. The nurse may also educate children and their parents regarding nutrition and good dietary habits.

EXERCISE AND PHYSICAL ACTIVITY.   Exercise and physical activity are another important area for primary prevention in the school setting. The school health program must be designed to assure physical activity while students are in school and to promote continued activity throughout life. The Centers for Disease Control and Prevention (1997) has developed the following recommendations for promoting physical activity among young people:

1. Policies should be established that promote enjoyable physical activity throughout life.
2. Schools should provide physical and social environments that encourage physical activity.
3. Schools should implement physical education curricula that promote enjoyable participation in physical activity and enable students to develop the skills and self-confidence to continue to be physically active.
4. Schools should implement health education curricula that assist students to adopt physically active lifestyles.
5. Schools should provide extracurricular programs that emphasize physical activities congruent with students' needs and interests.
6. Parents and guardians should become actively involved in instruction and extracurricular activities related to physical activity.
7. School personnel should be effectively trained to promote physical activity among students.
8. Health services personnel should assess student activity patterns and counsel students regarding the need for physical activity.
9. Communities should provide a range of sports and recreational opportunities for physical activity that are developmentally appropriate.
10. Schools and communities should regularly evaluate physical activity instruction, facilities, and programs. Community health nurses working in school settings can be actively involved in planning to implement these recommendations in their schools.

SELF-IMAGE.   Sound mental health is promoted by a strong self-image developed throughout childhood. Health promotion in the school setting should focus on the development of a healthy self-image as well as a healthy physical self. School nurses can foster self-image development by serving as role models in their dealings with children. They can also suggest to teachers learning activities that enhance development of a positive self-image.

On occasion, school nurses may need to function as advocates for children who do not have a strong self-image or for those who may be emotionally (or physically) abused by family members, peers, or even teachers. As noted earlier, the nurse should be aware of disciplinary measures used in the school and be alert to forms of discipline or unfair exercise of authority that are harmful to a child's self-image. When such circumstances are identified, the nurse might discuss his or her observations with teachers or other personnel involved and suggest other avenues for achieving the goals of disciplinary action. When corrective actions do not result from these interactions, the nurse may need to bring the problem to the attention of the appropriate authorities such as the school principal or members of the school board.

Occasionally this requires filing a report of child abuse. In addition to reporting the situation, however, the nurse has a responsibility to provide counseling or referral for assistance to those involved and to serve as a support person for both victim and abuser. In such cases, referrals may also be needed to address socioeconomic problems that may be contributing to the situation.

COPING SKILLS.   Another aspect of primary prevention that should be fostered in schools is the development of coping skills. Students and personnel can be assisted to develop active problem-solving strategies that promote their abilities to cope with adverse circumstances. School health nurses can serve as role models in this respect and can also provide counseling that assists students and their families or staff to engage in positive problem solving. Nurses can also reinforce evidence of positive coping by making others aware of their abilities to cope. In addition, the nurse can present information on stress, and can offer strategies for dealing with stress that enhance the development of sound coping skills.

INTERPERSONAL SKILLS.   The ability to interact effectively with others is essential to civilized society. Such abilities are not innate and must be learned. Education for effective interpersonal skills is another aspect of primary prevention with the school population. This is because interpersonal skills enhance mental and social health. Again, the nurse can serve as a role model for effective interpersonal skills and can educate students, parents, and staff regarding interpersonal interactions and the development of communication skills. The nurse can also provide information on group dynamics and communication skills that can enhance interpersonal skills within groups. For example, the nurse might promote role-play in a class to which a handicapped child will soon be admitted or help youngsters learn how to express anger at a teacher in an appropriate manner. Aspects of primary prevention in the school setting and related community health nursing responsibilities are summarized in Table 25–5.

Secondary Prevention. Secondary prevention deals with existing problems that require intervention. Generally speaking, secondary prevention involves screening for existing health conditions, referral, counseling, and treatment.

SCREENING. Screening is a major facet of most school health programs and an important responsibility of the school nurse. The goals of screening programs within the school setting include the obvious goal of detecting disease. Other goals include identifying children with special needs that require adjustment of the education program, promoting the importance of primary preventive measures, and evaluating the effectiveness of current measures.

Screening can be used to detect health conditions that are amenable to treatment and that can be resolved with appropriate therapy. For example, vision screening is used to identify children with visual problems, the majority of whom can benefit from corrective lenses. Screening may also help to identify children with particular needs that necessitate adjustments in the education program. For example, developmental screening may help to identify youngsters with learning disabilities who will benefit from special education programs.

A screening program also provides an opportunity to stress the importance of primary prevention. Dental screening, for example, provides an excellent opportunity to educate students on the need for good dental hygiene. Finally, screening efforts provide one measure of the effectiveness of current preventive efforts. For example, hematocrit screening can provide evidence of one aspect of the efficacy of a school lunch program or nutrition education program in promoting good nutrition.

Screening is a cost-effective approach to the identification of health problems. Typical costs of a screening program include those of the screening procedure itself and of retesting those with positive results; time spent by the nurse in referral; costs of diagnostic and treatment services; special education costs; and costs of corrective maintenance (eg, for hearing aids or replacing eyeglasses). These costs tend to be far less than the costs incurred when diagnoses are made later, after problems become more pronounced.

Screening programs typically undertaken in the school setting include screening of vision and hearing,

TABLE 25–5. AREAS OF EMPHASIS IN PRIMARY PREVENTION IN THE SCHOOL SETTING AND RELATED COMMUNITY HEALTH NURSING RESPONSIBILITIES

Area of Emphasis	Community Health Nursing Responsibilities
Immunization	• Refer for immunization services as needed. • Provide routine immunizations. • Suggest additional immunizations as warranted by circumstances (eg, an epidemic of hepatitis A).
Safety	• Report safety hazards to appropriate authorities. • Provide safety education. • Collaborate with others to eliminate safety hazards in the community.
School exclusion	• Determine need for exclusion from school. • Explain need for exclusion to parents. • Refer child for treatment of condition if needed. • Educate children and parents on preventing the spread of communicable diseases. • Follow up on children excluded from school to ensure appropriate care.
Health education	• Participate in designing health education curricula. • Provide consultation to teachers on health education topics. • Provide in-service for teachers related to health education. • Teach health education in the classroom. • Arrange for other health education experiences (eg, field trips or guest speakers). • Arrange or provide health education for families.
Food and nutrition	• Provide consultation on menu planning. • Educate children and families regarding nutrition.
Self-image	• Provide a role model for teachers and others in positive interactions with children. • Provide consultation to teachers on activities to enhance children's self-esteem. • Function as an advocate for children who have poor self-esteem.
Coping skills	• Provide a role model for students and staff for effective problem-solving skills. • Provide counseling regarding problem-solving skills. • Reinforce use of appropriate coping skills. • Educate students and staff on stress and coping.
Interpersonal skills	• Provide a role model for students and staff for effective interpersonal skills. • Educate students, staff, and parents on group dynamics and communication skills.

dental screening, height and weight measurements, and screening for scoliosis (Small, et al., 1995). Other screening tests may also be employed depending on the needs of the population served by the school. For example, tuberculosis, lead, sickle cell, and diabetes screening may be conducted in communities with high prevalence of these conditions.

The community health nurse in the school setting may perform a variety of roles with respect to screening programs. The nurse might arrange for the screening to be done or might conduct the screening tests. Or, the nurse might train volunteers to perform certain screening procedures. Moreover, the nurse is also responsible for informing students and parents of the results of screening tests and for interpreting those results. The nurse may also need to make referrals for follow-up diagnostic or treatment services. In addition, the nurse follows up on these referrals to make sure that students are receiving appropriate health care services.

REFERRAL.   School health nurses make a number of referrals. In addition to referrals for following up on positive screening test results, the nurse may make referrals for a variety of other services. For example, the nurse might refer children who are not immunized to the local health department for immunizations. Or, a referral for counseling might be needed for a child with behavior problems. School personnel may also be referred for health problems that require medical attention. In making these and other referrals, the school nurse uses the principles of referral discussed in Chapter 11.

COUNSELING.   Another important role for the school nurse in secondary prevention is that of counseling. As noted in Chapter 4, counseling involves assisting clients to make informed health decisions. Nurses may counsel individual students regarding personal problems, or they may assist students, families, and staff to engage in problem solving.

TREATMENT.   School nurses may also be involved in the actual treatment of existing health conditions. Treatment can involve emergency care in the event of illness or injury. School nurse practitioners might even engage in medical management of minor illnesses such as antibiotic treatment of otitis media.

Nurses may also be involved in providing specific treatments designed to minimize the effects of acute and chronic conditions. For example, the nurse may need to dispense prescribed medications, assist with physical therapy exercises for some children, or perform tracheostomy suction or catheter irrigations. They may also be involved in programs for bowel or bladder training. Community health nurses working with handicapped children in the school setting may also find it necessary to educate other school personnel in procedures required by the child's condition. In addition, the community health nurse monitors the therapeutic effects and side effects of medications and other treatments. Emphases in secondary prevention in the school setting and related community health nursing responsibilities are summarized in Table 25–6.

Tertiary Prevention.   Tertiary prevention is undertaken to prevent the recurrence of a problem or to minimize the effects of an existing one. To a large extent, tertiary preventive measures depend on the problems experienced by the student or staff member. Generally speaking, however, there are four aspects of tertiary

prevention with which the school nurse is concerned: preventing the recurrence of acute problems, preventing complications, fostering adjustment to chronic illness and handicapping conditions, and dealing with learning disabilities.

ACUTE CONDITIONS.   Preventing the recurrence of acute health problems depends on adequate treatment for existing problems and eliminating conditions that might lead to recurrence. For example, the school nurse might need to educate parents and children regarding the need to complete the course of therapy for otitis media. Or, education might be needed related to toileting hygiene (eg, wiping from front to back) to prevent a recurrent urinary tract infection. The nurse might also engage in efforts to help an abusive parent or unduly harsh teacher find other ways to vent frustrations, or might make a referral to help alleviate financial difficulties that are taxing coping abilities.

PREVENTING COMPLICATIONS.   Tertiary prevention is also directed toward preventing complications of either acute or chronic health problems. For example, the school nurse might encourage parents of a child with strep throat to complete a course of antibiotics to prevent cardiac and urinary complications. Similarly, the nurse might suggest a cushion and frequent changes of position to prevent pressure sores in a student confined to a wheelchair.

TABLE 25–6. AREAS OF EMPHASIS IN SECONDARY PREVENTION IN THE SCHOOL SETTING AND RELATED COMMUNITY HEALTH NURSING RESPONSIBILITIES

Area of Emphasis	Related Community Health Nursing Responsibilities
Screening	• Conduct screening tests or arrange for screening by others. • Train volunteers in screening procedures. • Interpret screening test results. • Notify parents of screening test results. • Make referrals for further tests or treatment as needed. • Follow up on referrals to determine outcomes and to ensure appropriate care for identified conditions.
Referral	• Refer children and families for health care and other services as needed. • Refer other school personnel for needed services.
Counseling	• Assist students, staff, or families to make informed health decisions. • Counsel students, staff, or families regarding personal problems. • Assist students, staff, or families to engage in problem solving.
Treatment	• Provide first aid for illness or injury. • Dispense medications prescribed for acute or chronic illnesses. • Perform special treatments or procedures warranted by identified conditions. • Teach others to perform special treatments or procedures. • Monitor therapeutic effects and side effects of medications and other treatments.

CHRONIC ILLNESS AND HANDICAPPING CONDITIONS.   Tertiary prevention for children with chronic or handicapping conditions involves assisting them to adjust to their condition and preventing complications. Specific measures depend on the condition involved. For example, special arrangements for physical education might be needed to prevent recurrent attacks of exercise-induced asthma, and special attention to diet might be required for the diabetic child or staff member.

Major considerations in dealing with children with chronic illness in the school setting involve money, transportation and facilities, and equipment. Additional considerations include nutrition and psychological well-being. The school nurse may need to refer students and parents to sources of financial assistance as a way to deal with the long-term care requirements of chronic and handicapping conditions.

Transportation and facility considerations in the school setting include issues of physical access to facilities discussed earlier in this chapter. Another area for consideration is that of transportation to and from school and for field trips. The nurse identifies barriers to access in the school setting and serves as an advocate for the removal of those barriers. Likewise, the nurse attempts to arrange transportation and other circumstances so that students with chronic or handicapping conditions can participate in as many regular school activities, including field trips, as possible. Advocacy in this area might also be needed with parents who may have a tendency to overprotect these children.

There may also be a need for special equipment to be used either at home or at school. The school nurse makes referrals to obtain such equipment or sees that necessary equipment is provided by the school itself.

Nutrition may be particularly problematic for schoolchildren with chronic diseases or handicap conditions. Youngsters with diabetes, for example, may need assistance in adapting a school lunch program to a diabetic diet. Severely handicapped children may need assistance with eating or may need to be fed. The school nurse assesses the special nutritional needs of children with these and similar conditions and then assists the child, family, and other school personnel to meet those needs.

The final consideration with children who have chronic illnesses or handicapping conditions is that of psychological well-being. These children should be helped to adjust to their conditions and to participate as normally as possible in the school routine. Parents, teachers, and other children may need to be discouraged from undermining the child's independence by "doing for" them. Values clarification exercises can help other children to understand the problems of the handicapped or chronically ill child rather than to poke fun at them or pity them.

Psychological health may be particularly fragile among those children with AIDS. There is a need to provide emotional support for these children as they deal with a stigmatized illness that may cause others to withdraw from them in fear. Again, the community health nurse in the school setting may need to function as an advocate to prevent social isolation of these and other children with chronic or handicapping conditions. Another concern about the child with AIDS is the need to protect the child from infection and the use of universal precautions when dealing with blood and body fluids; both of these concerns may heighten the child's sense of isolation and alienation. There is also a need to deal with the child's knowledge of his or her own mortality. Thus, the nurse may want to refer the child and family members for counseling. The nurse might also need to help other children, parents, and school personnel deal with their feelings of fear and grief related to AIDS and death.

LEARNING DISABILITY.   Because there does not seem to be any form of primary or secondary prevention available for learning disability, the focus in working with learning-disabled children is on minimizing the effects of their disability.

Some of the interventions that may be planned to assist learning-disabled children are learning by activity; involving multiple senses in learning activities; repetition; providing direction in small steps; and giving directions without irrelevant detail. Teaching at the appropriate level, a level that creates a challenge but does not lead to frustration, may also be helpful. Other useful strategies include avoiding drastic changes in activities, limiting distractions, and creating a climate in which success is ensured and reinforced as often as possible.

The nurse is involved in development of individualized lesson plans that allow children with learning disabilities, as well as those with other chronic or handicapping conditions, to learn as easily as possible. Again, attention must be given to the psychological effects of being tagged "learning disabled." The nurse may need to function as an advocate with parents, teachers, and other children to avoid the application of labels that undermine the child's self-esteem. The nurse can also function as a role model in providing positive reinforcement for the child's strengths and for his or her accomplishments, however small. Considerations related to tertiary prevention in the school setting and related community health nursing responsibilities are summarized in Table 25–7.

In planning primary, secondary, or tertiary preventive measures in the school setting, the community health nurse may need information or assistance from outside sources. Sources of assistance for specific

TABLE 25–7. AREAS OF EMPHASIS IN TERTIARY PREVENTION IN THE SCHOOL SETTING AND RELATED COMMUNITY HEALTH NURSING RESPONSIBILITIES

Area of Emphasis	Related Community Health Nursing Responsibilities
Preventing recurrence of acute conditions	• Eliminate risk factors for the condition. • Teach students, staff, or parents how to prevent recurrence of problems. • Make referrals that can assist in eliminating risk factors.
Preventing complications of and promoting adjustment to chronic and handicapping conditions	• Assist parents with finding sources of financial aid to deal with chronic and handicapping conditions. • Facilitate meeting special nutritional needs. • Assist with meeting special needs for transportation and facilities. • Provide for special equipment needs. • Promote psychological well-being. • Assist students, families, and staff to deal with the eventuality of death in terminal illnesses. • Refer for counseling as needed. • Function as an advocate as needed.
Preventing adverse effects of learning disabilities	• Provide consultation for teachers in dealing with children's learning disabilities. • Participate in the design of individualized learning programs for children with learning disabilities. • Function as an advocate for the learning-disabled child as needed. • Serve as a role model in positively reinforcing the child's accomplishments.

health problems among children were provided in Chapter 20. Additional resources are listed at the end of this chapter.

Implementing Health Care in the School Setting

Implementing health care for individuals or groups in the school setting frequently involves collaboration between the nurse and other members of the school health team. At the individual level, for example, the community health nurse may need to contact the private physician of a child with a chronic illness with information about adverse effects of medications or to request a change in the medical treatment plan based on changes in the child's condition. The nurse also needs to solicit the cooperation of parents in following through on a referral for medical services, testing, counseling, or other services needed by their child.

Implementing care for groups within the school setting also requires collaboration between the nurse and others. For example, the nurse may invite local police personnel to participate in a drug education

program to be presented in the school. Or, the nurse might work with teachers, media specialists, food service personnel, and others to implement an education program on basic nutrition for elementary school children. Parental permission may be required in certain school-based health programs. For example, parents need to grant permission for screening procedures such as hematocrit testing. The nurse may also need to recruit parent or community volunteers to assist with screening programs or with other health-related programs such as a health fair.

Evaluating Health Care in the School Setting

Evaluating the effectiveness of care in the school setting focuses on the outcomes of that care. Evaluation can occur at two levels, the individual child or the total school health program. Evaluative criteria for the

Critical Thinking in Research

Jones and Clark (1997) conducted a study of the effects of care by a pediatric nurse practitioner in an elementary school-based clinic on students' access to health care services. Access to care was defined in terms of Medicaid certification, Early and Periodic Screening, Diagnosis, and Treatment (EPSDT) program participation, and illness encounters. Students in the school-based clinic group had more Medicaid encounters than those in a control group although the differences were not significant. The control groups had significantly higher proportions of emergency department visits and fewer EPSDT health maintenance visits than the school-based clinic group. They also had more hospitalizations, although the number of hospitalizations in either group was too small to test for significant differences. Overall emergency service costs were 50% higher for the control group than for the school-based clinic group. Minor illness encounters with physicians were similar for both groups. The authors suggested that the availability of services in the school-based clinic might have promoted early preventive care and fewer emergent conditions.

1. What other possible explanations might account for the findings of this study (as reported here)? What information would lead you to discard these alternative explanations and support the interpretation of the authors?
2. What other variables might you want to examine regarding the outcomes of care in a school-based clinic? How might you go about collecting data related to these outcomes?
3. Suppose you wanted to compare the cost-effectiveness of care provided in a school-based clinic with that provided in a pediatrician's office. What variables might you consider in your study?

care of the individual child reflect the effects of nursing care on the youngster's health status. For example, if a child is no longer abused by a parent, or no longer has recurrent ear infections, or is now able to interact effectively with peers, the interventions of the nurse have probably been effective.

Evaluation of the overall school health program focuses on indicators of the health status of the total population. For instance, absentee rates might indicate how effective the program has been in preventing disease. Student screening test results may also provide information on the effectiveness of primary preventive efforts.

Changes in the prevalence of certain health problems within the school population may also indicate the efficacy of secondary preventive measures. For example, if alcohol abuse has been a problem among the student population, a declining prevalence of alcohol abuse would indicate that secondary measures are having an effect. Similarly, a decline in the teenage pregnancy rate would indicate that a sex education program is effective. Guidelines for evaluating the effectiveness of school health programs have been developed by a coalition of organizations concerned with school health (see the Recommended Readings at the end of this book) and can be used by the community health nurse to evaluate the health program in a particular school.

TABLE 25–8. STATUS OF SELECTED NATIONAL OBJECTIVES RELATED TO SCHOOL HEALTH

	Objective	Base (%)	Target (%)
1.8	Daily physical education	36	50
3.10	Tobacco use prevention education	75–81	100
4.13	Substance abuse education	63	100
5.8	Discussion of sexuality	66	85
18.10	HIV prevention education	66	95
19.12	Sexually transmitted disease prevention education	95	100

(Source: U.S. Department of Health and Human Services. [1993]. Health United States 1992, and healthy people 2000 review. Washington, DC: Government Printing Office.)

The processes used in evaluating the school health program are those discussed in Chapter 19. The school nurse collaborates with other members of the school health team in designing and implementing an evaluation of the program. Moreover, the nurse may also be involved in data collection related to the evaluation and in interpreting those data. Finally, the nurse should be actively involved in decisions made on the basis of evaluative data.

At the national level, national objectives for the year 2000 related to school health can provide additional evaluative criteria. Information on the current status of some of these objectives is presented in Table 25–8.

Critical Thinking in Practice: A Case in Point

Brandon is a third grader in the school where you work as a school nurse. He comes to see you because he "has a stomachache." This is his third visit to your office in as many days. Each day you have seen him for a similar complaint but have found no physical evidence of illness. According to his teacher, his appetite has been good at lunch, although his lunches are large and not particularly nutritious. Brandon says he is not constipated and has not had any diarrhea or vomiting. His abdominal pain usually disappears after lying down in your office for about 20 minutes.

When you talk to the teacher, she tells you that lately the other children have been making fun of Brandon because he always comes in last in running games and can't run very fast during PE. Brandon is about 35 pounds overweight for his height and becomes short of breath with strenuous physical exercise. Brandon has two younger brothers who are both slender and have no difficulties with physical activity.

The teacher also mentions that Brandon has been talking during class and disturbing the other children. She has tried to take him aside and explain why he should not talk in class, but he continues. His grades are not the best in the world (they're not the worst either), but he has been discouraged lately because he is having trouble mastering long division.

1. What biophysical, psychological, social, behavioral, and health system factors are operating in this situation?
2. What nursing diagnoses would you derive from the information provided above? How would you prioritize Brandon's problems? Why?
3. Write at least two client care objectives for Brandon.
4. What primary, secondary, and tertiary prevention measures would be appropriate in this case?
5. How would you evaluate the effectiveness of your interventions with Brandon? Be specific.

TESTING YOUR UNDERSTANDING

1. What are the three goals of a school health program? (p. 616)
2. What are the basic components of a school health program? (pp. 616–618)
3. Identify at least four areas to be assessed in relation to the psychological dimension in the school setting. Describe the influence of factors in each area on the health of the school population. (pp. 623–625)
4. Describe at least two considerations in assessing physical dimension factors influencing the health of the school population. Give an example of the health effects of factors in each area. (pp. 625–626)
5. Describe at least two areas to be addressed in assessing social dimension influences on the health of the school population. Give an example of the health effects of factors in each area. (p. 626)
6. Identify at least five areas of emphasis in primary prevention in the school setting. Describe at least two nursing activities related to each area. (pp. 630–633)
7. Describe at least three approaches to secondary prevention in the school setting. Identify at least two community health nursing responsibilities related to each approach. (pp. 633–634)
8. Describe at least two areas of emphasis in tertiary prevention in the school setting. How might the community health nurse be involved in each of these areas? (pp. 634–636)

WHAT DO YOU THINK?
Questions for Critical Thinking

1. Are students with handicapping conditions better off in regular or specialized classrooms? Why?
2. How can school nurses motivate parent participation in school health activities?
3. Should health education be provided in the school setting by nurses or by teachers? Why?
4. What are the advantages and disadvantages of school-based health centers (SBHCs) compared to school-linked health centers (SLHCs)?

REFERENCES

Berkson, G. (1993). *Children with handicaps: A review of behavioral research.* Hillsdale, NJ: Lawrence Erlbaum.

Canuso, R. (1997). Rethinking behavior disorders: Whose attention has a deficit? *Journal of Psychosocial Nursing, 35*(4), 24–29.

Centers for Disease Control and Prevention. (1997). Guidelines for school and community programs to promote lifelong physical activity among young people. *MMWR, 46*(RR-6), 1–36.

Cornacchia, H. J., Olsen, L. K., & Nickerson, C. J. (1995). *Health in elementary schools* (8th ed.). St. Louis: Mosby Year Book.

Gregory, E. K. (1993). Nursing practice management. *Journal of School Nursing, 9*(3), 40–41.

Grossman, D. C., Rauh, M. J., & Rivara, F. P. (1995). Prevalence of corporal punishment among students in Washington State schools. *Archives of Pediatric and Adolescent Medicine, 149*, 529–532.

Healthcare and Trends and Transition. (1994). *Who are the school health providers and what do they do?* 6(1), 19.

Henderson, A. C. (1993). *Healthy school, healthy futures: The case for improving school environment.* Santa Cruz, CA: ETR Associates.

Igoe, J. B. (1994a). School health: Extending primary care's reach. *Healthcare Trends and Transition, 6*(1), 9–13, 19, 28.

Igoe, J. B. (1994b). School nursing. *Nursing Clinics of North America, 29*, 443–458.

Jones, M. E., & Clark, D. (1997). Increasing access to health care: A study of pediatric nurse practitioner outcomes in a school-based clinic. *Journal of Nursing Quality Care, 11*(4), 53–59.

Kisker, E. E., & Brown, R. S. (1996). Do school-based health centers improve adolescents' access to health care, health status, and risk-taking behavior? *Journal of Adolescent Health, 18*, 335–343.

Kolbe, L. J. (1994). Our children's future. *Healthcare Trends and Transition, 6*(1), 14–17.

Kolbe, L. J., Kann, L., Collins, J. L., Small, M. L., Pateman, B. C., & Warren, C. W. (1995). The school health policies and programs (SHPPS): Context, methods, general findings, and future efforts. *Journal of School Health, 65*, 339–343.

Lear, J. G. (1992). Building a health/education partnership: The role of school-based health centers. *Pediatric Nursing, 18*, 172–173.

Passarelli, C. (1994). School nursing: Trends for the future. *Journal of School Nursing, 10*(2), 10–21.

Pollitt, P. (1994). Lina Rogers Struthers: The first school nurse. *Journal of School Nursing, 10*(1), 34–46.

Proctor, S., Lordis, S., & Zaiger, D. (1993). *School nursing practice—Roles and standards.* Scarborough, ME: National Association of School Nurses.

Rajsky-Steed, N. (1996). The nurse practitioner in the school setting. *Nursing Clinics of North America, 31*, 507–518.

Redican, K., Olsen, L. K., & Baffi, C. R. (1993). *Organization of school health programs* (2nd ed.). New York: Macmillan.

Resnicow, K., & Allensworth, D. (1996). Conducting a comprehensive school health program. *Journal of School Health, 66*, 59–63.

Ross, J. G., Einhaus, K. E., Hohenemser, L. K., Greene,

B. Z., Kann, L., & Gold, R. S. (1995). School health policies prohibiting tobacco use, alcohol and other drug use, and violence. *Journal of School Health, 65,* 333–338.

Small, M. L., Majer, L. S., Allensworth, D. D., Farquhar, B. K., Kann, L., & Pateman, B. C. (1995). School health services. *Journal of School Health, 65,* 319–326.

U.S. Department of Health and Human Services. (1991). *Healthy people 2000: National health promotion and disease prevention objectives.* Washington, DC: Government Printing Office.

Wiley, D. C., & Ballard, D. J. (1993). How can schools help children from homeless families. *Journal of School Health, 63,* 291–293.

Williams, J. K., & McCarthy, A. M. (1995). School nurses' experiences with children with chronic conditions. *Journal of School Health, 65,* 234–236.

Yates, S. (1994a). The practice of school nursing: Integration with new models of health service delivery. *Journal of School Nursing, 10*(1), 10–19.

Yates, S. (1994b). School health delivery programs throughout the United States. *Journal of School Nursing, 10*(2), 31–36.

RESOURCES FOR COMMUNITY HEALTH NURSES WORKING IN SCHOOL SETTINGS

Health Education

American Alliance for Health, Physical Education, Recreation and Dance
1900 Association Drive
Reston, VA 22091
(703) 476–3400

American Automobile Association
Traffic Safety Department
1000 AAA Drive
Heathrow, FL 32746–5063
(407) 444–7000

American Dental Association
Bureau of Health Education and Audiovisual Services
211 East Chicago Avenue
Chicago, IL 60611
(312) 440–2500

American Health Foundation
320 East 43rd Street
New York, NY 10017
(212) 953–1900

American Medical Association
Department of Health Education
515 North State Street
Chicago, IL 60610
(312) 464–5000

Distilled Spirits Council of the United States
1250 Eye Street, NW, Ste. 900
Washington, DC 20005
(202) 628–3544

Environmental Protection Agency
401 M Street, SW
Washington, DC 20460
(202) 260–2090

Epilepsy Foundation of America
4351 Garden City Drive
Landover, MD 20785
(301) 459–3700

Harcourt Brace & Company Juvenile Books
525 B Street, Ste. 1900
San Diego, CA 92101
(619) 231–6616

Institute of Makers of Explosives
1120 19th Street, NW, Ste. 310
Washington, DC 20036
(202) 429–9280

Mental Health Materials Center
PO Box 304
Bronxville, NY 10708
(914) 337–6596

National Center for Health Education
72 Spring Street, Ste. 208
New York, NY 10012–4019
(212) 334–9470

National Fire Protection Association
1 Batterymarch Park
PO Box 9101
Quincy, MA 02269–9101
(671) 770–3000

National PTA–National Congress of Parents and Teachers
330 N. Wabash Avenue, Ste. 2100
Chicago, IL 60611–3690
(312) 670–6782

Office on Smoking and Health
5600 Fishers Lane, Room 1-10
Park Building
Rockville, MD 20857

President's Council on Physical Fitness and Health
701 Pennsylvania Avenue, NW
Washington, DC 20202
(202) 272–3412

Scott, Foresman, and Company
1900 East Lake Avenue
Glenview, IL 60025
(708) 729–3000

Sex Information and Education Council of the United
 States
130 West 42nd Street, Ste. 2500
New York, NY 10036
(212) 819–9770

Raintree Stech-Vaughn, Publishers
11 Prospect Street
Madison, NJ
(201) 514–1525
(800) 531–5015

Nutrition

American Dairy Products Institute
130 North Franklin Street
Chicago, IL 60606
(312) 782–4888

Consumer Nutrition Center Human Nutrition
 Information Service
U.S. Department of Agriculture
6506 Belcrest Road
Hyattsville, MD 20782
(301) 436–7725

National Dairy Council
1025 Higgins Road
Rosemont, IL 60018
(708) 830–2000

National Livestock and Meat Board
Nutritional Department
444 North Michigan Avenue
Chicago, IL 60611
(312) 467–5520

U.S. Department of Agriculture
Food and Nutrition Service
National School Lunch Program
National School Breakfast Program
Park Office Bldg., Room 512
3101 Park Center Drive
Alexandria, VA 22302
(703) 756–3590

School Health

American School Health Association
7263 State Route 43
PO Box 708
Kent, OH 44240
(216) 678–1601

School Nursing

National Association of School Nurses
Lamplighter Lane
PO Box 1300
Scarboro, ME 04070
(207) 883–2117

School Nurse Achievement Program
c/o Ann Smith
University of Colorado
School of Nursing
PO Box C287
4200 East 9th Avenue
Denver, CO 80262
(303) 270–8733

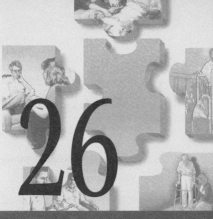

CARE OF CLIENTS IN THE WORK SETTING

► KEY TERMS

company wellness
    policies
employee assistance
    program
ergonomics
job strain
occupational health
    nursing
paraoccupational
    exposure
risk factors

Because half of the U.S. population, or 125 million Americans, is employed, the work setting is an important place for promoting the health of the general population (National Institute for Occupational Safety and Health, 1996a). Although the work environment contributes to a wide variety of health problems, it also provides opportunities to influence a major segment of the population regarding personal health behaviors.

Over the years, employers have come to appreciate that healthy employees are more productive and that it is in the employer's interest to promote and maintain employee health. Moreover, the escalating cost of health insurance makes health promotion increasingly cost-effective. One way that some companies have chosen to decrease health-related costs is to provide on-site health care for employees.

The importance of health care in the occupational setting can be seen in the national health objectives for the year 2000. In fact, one entire section of the objectives deals with health in the occupational setting (U.S. Department of Health and Human Services, 1991). These objectives are summarized in Appendix A.

▶ Chapter Objectives

After reading this chapter, you should be able to:

- Describe at least three advantages in providing health care in the work setting.
- Identify at least six of the ten leading health problems encountered in the work setting.
- Identify at least five types of health and safety hazards encountered in work settings.
- Describe four spheres of social influence on the health of employees.
- Differentiate between internal and external health systems in occupational health.
- Describe four types of internal health care programs in the work setting.
- Describe the three main areas of emphasis in primary prevention in the work setting.
- Describe three major considerations in secondary prevention in the work setting.
- Describe three emphases in tertiary prevention in the work setting.

▶ **ADVANTAGES OF PROVIDING HEALTH CARE IN THE WORK SETTING**

From a community health nursing perspective, there are a number of advantages to providing health care in the work setting. They include the substantial amount of time that people spend in this setting and the fact that this time is spent on a regular basis. In addition, when employees are present, they are essentially a "captive audience," subject to powerful pressures from peers and employers to engage in healthy behaviors. For example, nonsmoking peers may object to smoking in their work or recreation areas, or employers may provide financial or nonfinancial incentives for healthy behavior. Another advantage is that the work force frequently consists of people who may be at risk for a variety of health problems or who may be motivated to maintain their health to ensure their continued ability to work. Because health care personnel are frequently in the setting and mechanisms are in place for communicating health messages, health promotion in the work setting is efficient and cost-effective. More and more companies are acknowledging the advantages of providing health care in the occupational setting. The national health objectives also acknowledge the work setting as an effective location for promoting healthful behavior.

▶ **OCCUPATIONAL HEALTH NURSING**

Not all nurses who practice in occupational settings are community health nurses. The community health nurse, however, is uniquely prepared to meet the health needs of the working population because of his or her knowledge of community health principles. Occupational health nursing is not a new role for the community health nurse. Nurses may have been employed in the work setting as early as 1888 and certainly by 1895 when the Vermont Marble Company employed Ada M. Stewart (Parrish & Alfred, 1995). Since that time, the role of the occupational health nurse has been expanded along with other nursing roles. Several years ago, the U.S. Department of Labor defined *occupational health nursing* as "giving nursing service under general medical direction to ill or injured employees or other persons who become ill or suffer an accident on the premises of a factory or other establishment" (Hughes, 1979).

This definition did not, however, fully describe today's community health nursing role in the work setting. It concentrates on the treatment aspects of care and the nurse's dependent functions and does not acknowledge the promotional and preventive aspects that are paramount in this practice setting. In 1994, the American Association of Occupational Health Nurses (AAOHN) defined occupational health nursing as "the specialty practice that provides for and delivers health care services to workers and worker populations. The practice focuses on promotion, protection, and restoration of workers' health within the context of a safe and healthy work environment."

▶ **EDUCATIONAL PREPARATION FOR OCCUPATIONAL HEALTH NURSING**

Several types of nursing personnel may be found in occupational settings including registered nurses prepared in associate degree and diploma programs in nursing as well as in baccalaureate degree programs; licensed practical nurses; and nurses prepared at the master's level. Because of the need to apply principles of community health nursing, nurses who engage in the full scope of the occupational health nurse's role should be prepared at least at the baccalaureate level in nursing. Advanced preparation in occupational health nursing may result in certification by the AAOHN. Nurses working in occupational settings might also hold master's degrees in nursing. Educational preparation at this level might be in occupational health nursing, in community health nursing, or as a nurse practitioner.

Nurses in other settings may also be involved in providing care for health conditions related to the work setting. In one study, for example, 20% of nurse practitioners working in nonoccupational health settings reported seeing clients with work-related illnesses or injuries at least weekly (Lipscomb, Burgel, McGill, & Blanc, 1994). These findings suggest that all nurse practitioners working in ambulatory care settings where occupational conditions may be seen should have a basic grounding in the principles of occupational health.

► THE OCCUPATIONAL HEALTH TEAM

Community health nurses working in occupational health settings may be part of an occupational health team. In some small companies, the nurse is the only health care professional employed by the company. In such instances, other health care professionals interact with the nurse on a consultant basis. For example, the community health nurse might collaborate with an employee's private physician to plan for the employee's return to work after an illness or injury. In other instances, the company may contract with outside physicians for consultation services related to employee health needs.

Other companies have a well-developed occupational health team present within the facility. In addition to the community health nurse, such teams may include physicians, safety engineers, industrial hygienists, counselors, ancillary nursing personnel (eg, licensed practical nurses), toxicologists, emergency medical technicians, physicians' assistants, epidemiologists, laboratory and x-ray technicians, safety coordinators, and nurse practitioners. The functions and roles of most of these individuals are already familiar to the reader. A few, however, may be unfamiliar. A safety engineer, for example, is responsible for monitoring the safety of the physical environment in the work setting, and an industrial hygienist has similar responsibilities for identifying and controlling physical, biological, and chemical hazards in the work setting (Asfahl, 1995). Toxicologists may be involved in research on the toxic effects of chemical exposures in the work setting, as well as in contributing to plans for the control and treatment of such exposures.

► THE DIMENSIONS MODEL AND CARE OF CLIENTS IN THE WORK SETTING

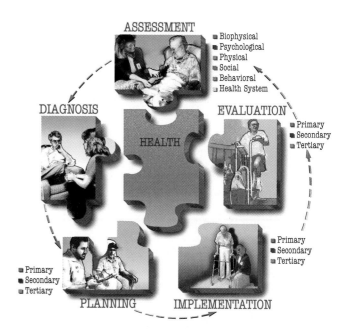

Critical Dimensions of Nursing in the Work Setting

Elements of each of the six dimensions of nursing are necessary to effective occupational health nursing. Particular knowledge required in the cognitive dimension includes information on health problems commonly encountered in the occupational health setting and on appropriate interventions for those problems. The nurse will also need to know about the potential health hazards in the setting in which he or she works. For example, are toxic chemicals used at the worksite? What are their potential health effects? Finally, the nurse will need knowledge of community resources that may be required by employees and their families to address identified health problems.

Communication and collaborative skills will be necessary in the interpersonal dimension. Much of the occupational health nurse's practice involves motivating employees to change health-related behaviors, a role necessitating excellent communication and motivation skills. The nurse must also have well-developed skills in collaboration because of the need to work effectively, not only with other members of the occupational health team, but also with management, in order to modify employment conditions, policies, and procedures that may jeopardize employee health.

Ethical dilemmas may come from a variety of sources in the occupational health setting and the nurse will need to deal with these as they arise. Some of the ethical issues that may be experienced include conflicting loyalties, blaming the victim, paternalism, coercion, reduction of health benefits, confidentiality and privacy issues, and issues of liability (Allegrante & Goldfein, 1995). The nurse may be faced with conflicting loyalties when presented with certain information. For example, if the employee has a substance abuse problem, what is the nurse's responsibility to report this behavior to the employee's supervisor? In a slightly different circumstance, the nurse may need to decide between a course of action that protects employees' health and one that minimizes employer expenses. In this situation, the nurse may need to advocate for employee health over company profits. Similarly, the nurse may need to prevent employers from "blaming the victim" or attempting to foist responsibility for a health condition on the employee and away from the employer.

Other ethical issues revolve around paternalism and coercion. To what extent does the employer have a right to dictate healthful behaviors to employees? And, to what extent should the community health nurse working in an occupational setting advocate for employee self-determination or employer policies that mandate healthy behavior? Similarly, the nurse may become involved in mandatory drug- or HIV-screening programs or genetic risk factor screening that may violate employees' rights to privacy or promote discrimination based on results. The nurse may also need to guard against the tendency of some employers to substitute health promotion programs for other needed health care benefits because of their lower cost. Ideally, employees should have access to both health promotion services and coverage for restorative and curative services. Finally, the nurse might be involved in ethical decisions regarding responsibility for injury or other adverse effects while employees are participating in employer-provided health promotion programs (eg, an injury sustained during an employee exercise program). The importance of the ethical dimension in occupational health nursing is reflected in the code of ethics developed by the American Association of Occupational Health Nurses in 1996. Elements of the code are summarized on this page.

Both manual and intellectual skills will be required in the skills dimension of occupational health nursing. First aid skills are an important example of manual skills that may be required, but the nurse may also be called upon to perform other technical procedures depending upon employees' needs. For example, the nurse may provide immunizations, perform tuberculin skin testing, or execute other diagnostic or treatment procedures. Intellectual skills needed are those required in any community health nursing setting and include critical thinking, analytic, and inter-

> ## OCCUPATIONAL HEALTH NURSING CODE OF ETHICS
>
> The occupational health nurse:
> - Provides care in the work environment with regard for human dignity and client rights, unrestricted by considerations of social or economic status, personal attributes, or health status.
> - Promotes collaboration with other health professionals and agencies to meet the health needs of the work force.
> - Safeguards employees' rights to privacy.
> - Provides quality care and safeguards clients from unethical and illegal actions.
> - Accepts societal obligations as a professional and responsible community member.
> - Maintains personal competence and accepts responsibility for judgments and actions, while complying with laws and regulations influencing health care delivery.
> - Contributes to the development of the profession's body of knowledge while protecting the rights of research subjects.
>
> (Source: American Association of Occupational Health Nurses, 1996.)

pretive skills, as well as program planning and evaluation skills.

Elements of the process dimension that will be particularly relevant to the occupational health setting include the health education process; change, group, and leadership processes; referral and case management processes; and the political process. While most of these processes may be required internally, the political process may be needed both within and outside of the employment setting to create a social milieu that fosters employee health. Research and program evaluation are critical elements of the reflective dimension in occupational health nursing. The National Institute for Occupational Safety and Health (NIOSH) (1996a) has identified three priority areas for occupational health research, including (1) research on disease and injury, (2) research on the work force and workplace factors influencing health, and (3) delineation of research tools and approaches appropriate to the occupational setting. Once research based interventions have been identified and implemented, program evaluation will be required to assess their effects in terms of outcomes, processes, and cost-effectiveness.

 ## Assessing the Dimensions of Health in the Work Setting

Assessment of employee health status and health needs is undertaken from the epidemiologic perspective of the Dimensions Model. Biophysical, psychological, physical, social, behavioral, and health system factors are explored in light of their contribution to health or illness in the working population.

The Biophysical Dimension

Human biological factors to be addressed in assessing employee health status include those related to maturation and aging, genetic inheritance, and physiologic function.

Maturation and Aging.   The age composition of a firm's work force affects its health status. If employees are primarily young adults or adolescents, health conditions that may be noted with some frequency include sexually transmitted diseases, hepatitis, and pregnancy. Younger employees may also be at increased risk of injury due to limited job training and skills. In 1995, there were 2.6 million 16- and 17-year-olds in the work force (National Institute for Occupational Safety and Health, 1996a). If, on the other hand, the workers are middle-aged, problems such as heart attack and cancer are more likely to be seen.

The health needs of older employees should also be considered. Because of prohibitions on forced retirement at specific ages, many employees are continuing in the work force beyond the time when they would have retired. Economic need and a desire for continued productivity are two factors that may influence this trend. In 1995, nearly 12% of the U.S. population over 65 years of age was employed (U.S. Department of Commerce, 1996). This amounted to 3.7 million older people in the work force (National Institute for Occupational Health and Safety, 1996a). Musculoskeletal capacity diminishes and sensory impairments increase with age, placing older employees at higher risk for occupational injury. Economic constraints will force many older workers to continue employment beyond retirement age and to assume jobs requiring strenuous physical activity. Because older workers will be required in the future to perform more strenuous jobs, the potential for serious injury and occupational fatality will increase (Zwerling, Sprince, Wallace, Davis, Whitten, & Heeringa, 1996). Older workers planning to retire in the near future may need assistance with retirement planning and in dealing with both retirement transition stress and retirement state stress (see Chapt. 23 for a discussion of these issues).

Genetic Inheritance.   Genetic inheritance factors likely to be of greatest importance in the work force are those related to race and gender. For example, in a largely African American labor force, hypertension may be prevalent. In an Asian population, particularly if large numbers are refugees, communicable diseases such as tuberculosis and parasitic diseases may be common.

By the year 2000, the proportion of women in the work force will equal that of men (Bellingham & Pelletier, 1995). The sex composition of the employee population affects the types of health conditions seen. For example, if large numbers of employees are women of childbearing age, there may be a need to provide prenatal or contraceptive services. There would also be a need to monitor more closely environmental conditions that may cause genetic changes or damage to an embryo. Occupational reproductive effects to be monitored include infertility, spontaneous abortion, low birth weight, pre- and postmaturity, birth defects, chromosomal abnormalities, preeclampsia, and an increased incidence of childhood cancers (Wegman, 1992).

Physiological Function.   The community health nurse in an occupational setting must be prepared to recognize and deal with the multitude of illnesses and injuries likely to be encountered in the workplace. Although these vary with the occupational setting, the National Institute for Occupational Safety and Health (NIOSH) has established a list of the 10 leading causes of work-related diseases and injuries in the United States:

1. Occupational lung diseases
2. Musculoskeletal injuries
3. Occupational cancers
4. Severe traumatic injuries
5. Cardiovascular disease
6. Disorders of reproduction
7. Neurotoxic disorders
8. Noise-induced hearing loss
9. Dermatologic conditions
10. Psychological disorders (Burgel, 1994)

Community health nurses working in any occupational setting should be aware of the prevalence of these conditions and of the factors that influence the development of these problems. These contributing factors may be related to the work environment itself or to the personal behaviors of employees within and outside the workplace.

Of the common occupation-related conditions reviewed by NIOSH, 52 involve some form of occupational lung disease and include illnesses such as silicosis, byssinosis (due to inhalation of cotton dust), asbestosis, and coal worker's pneumoconiosis. The effects of these conditions range from mild respiratory irritation to lung cancer and asphyxia.

Musculoskeletal injuries are the leading cause of lost workdays among U.S. employees and include injuries due to the cumulative trauma of repetitive activities as well as acute trauma. Cumulative trauma disorders (CTDs) include carpal tunnel syndrome, tendonitis, tenosynovitis, trigger finger, de Quervain's disease (washerwoman's sprain), and vibration syndrome. Diagnosis of CTDs increased 10-fold from 1983 to 1993 and now constitutes approximately 60% of all occupational illness in the United States. CTDs may affect as much as 5 to 10% of the general labor force with as much as 15% of some occupational groups (eg, meat packers) affected. The causes of CDTs include repetitive motions, high force actions, mechanical pressure, awkward posture, and vibration (Dembe, 1996).

Approximately 4% of the 500,000 cancer deaths each year in the United States are attributable to workplace exposures. These include 10% of lung cancer deaths, 21 to 27% of bladder cancers, and nearly 100% of mesotheliomas (National Institute of Occupational Safety and Health, 1996a). Other cancers that may result from occupational exposures include those of the blood, bone, larynx, liver, nasal cavity and sinuses, peritoneum, pharynx, pleura, and skin (including scrotal malignancies).

Serious traumatic injuries are those in which multiple injuries occur as a result of trauma, where musculoskeletal injuries are usually confined to localized areas. In 1994, job-related injuries resulted in 5000 deaths and 3.5 million disabilities. In addition, 410 million days of work were lost because of injuries. Occupations with the highest occupational injury fatality rates are agriculture and mining and quarrying (U.S. Department of Commerce, 1996). Disability rates, on the other hand, are highest for construction workers, followed by transportation, communication, and utilities workers, and then by agricultural and manufacturing employees (U.S. Department of Health and Human Services, 1996). The annual costs of traumatic occupational injuries averages $121 billion (National Institute for Occupational Safety and Health, 1996a).

For the most part, cardiovascular diseases are influenced by personal risk factors of employees; however, evidence suggests that occupational factors may also contribute to the incidence of cardiovascular diseases. Some of these factors include exposure to metals, dust, and chemical inhalants, noise exposure, and psychosocial stress. Exposures to carbon disulfide, ethylene compounds, halogenated hydrocarbons, nitroglycerin, and nitrates have also been associated with cardiovascular disease. The extent of one's control over one's job has also been shown to influence cardiovascular mortality. People with greater control tend to have lower mortality rates (Johnson, Stewart, Hall, Fredlund, & Theorell, 1996). Shift work may also

contribute to cardiovascular disease (Kawachi, et al., 1995).

With greater numbers of women working today, there is growing concern for the reproductive and social effects of working conditions. Thus far, 1000 occupational chemicals have been associated with reproductive effects in animals, but their human effects have not been assessed. Other working conditions also have reproductive effects (National Institute of Occupational Safety and Health, 1996a). Although the primary concern is the impact on the female reproductive system, evidence indicates that exposure to some of these conditions (eg, heat) can also affect the reproductive capabilities of men.

Neurotoxic conditions are another of the 10 leading concerns in occupational health. Some of the conditions encountered include heavy metal poisonings, behavior changes related to chemical exposures, and difficulty concentrating and performing one's job. Specific neurodegenerative diseases, such as presenile dementia, Alzheimer's disease, Parkinson's disease, and motor neuron disease, have also been associated with occupational factors. High prevalence of each of these conditions has been found among teachers, medical personnel, machinists and machine operators, scientists, writers, entertainers, and clerical workers. Selected conditions are also noted with some frequency among workers exposed to pesticides, solvents, and electromagnetic fields (Shulte, Burnett, Boeniger, & Johnson, 1996).

Noise-induced hearing loss is a serious problem both within and outside the occupational setting. According to the National Institute for Occupational Safety and Health (1996a), 30 million workers in the United States are exposed to hazardous noise levels and another 9 million are exposed to other ototoxic conditions such as heat, solvents, metals, and asphyxiants. Noise-induced hearing loss accounts for 28% of all reported occupational conditions (Dembe, 1996).

With respect to dermatologic conditions arising from occupational factors, the nurse is again in a position to assess the health status of employees. As with other types of health problems, the nurse should be aware of outbreaks of dermatologic conditions that indicate the presence of hazards in the environment and a need for control measures. Conditions encountered include a variety of rashes, pruritus, chemical burns, and desquamation. NIOSH recommendations are available for 31 substances and conditions that result in dermatologic problems, and such problems account for more than 13% of reported work-related conditions. From 1983 to 1994, the rate of occupational skin diseases increased more than 25% to 81 per 100,000 workers. The annual cost to business and individual employees for medical care and lost work time resulting from these dermatologic problems is estimated at nearly $1 billion (National Institute for Occupational Safety and Health, 1996a).

The occupational health problems discussed here are only a few of the many physical health problems likely to be encountered by the community health nurse working in an occupational setting. For example, more than one fourth of asthma and significant proportions of communicable diseases and low back pain are work-related (National Institute for Occupational Safety and Health, 1996a). Each occupational setting contains factors unique to that setting that influence the health of employees. The nurse should be cognizant of the factors operating in any given place, their effects, and the appropriate measures of control.

Immunization is the final physiologic consideration in assessing health needs in the workplace. The nurse assesses the immunization status of employees, with special emphasis on groups of employees who may be at increased risk for certain diseases preventable by immunization. For example, employees who may be at risk for dirty injuries should be assessed for immunity to tetanus, whereas women of childbearing age should be assessed for immunity to rubella. Health care workers, on the other hand, should be particularly assessed for immunity to hepatitis B.

The Psychological Dimension

In assessing psychological dimension factors influencing the health of clients in the work setting, the community health nurse identifies psychological health problems prevalent in the population and assesses factors contributing to psychological problems. It is estimated that as many as 20% of employees experience some form of psychological problem that reduces their safety and/or job performance. Psychological health problems may manifest in substance abuse, violence, psychiatric disorders such as psychoses and neuroses, somatic complaints such as ulcers or fatigue, or a general inability to cope. The nurse can assess clients for some of the following indicators of psychological health problems:

- Increased absenteeism (especially on Mondays, Fridays, and the day after being paid)
- Mood changes or changes in relationships with others (especially health care providers)
- Increased incidence of minor accidents on and off the job
- Fatigue, weakness, or a general decrease in energy
- Sudden weight loss or gain
- Increased blood pressure
- Frequent stress-related illnesses (eg, stomach distress, sore throat, chronic gastritis, headache, or other vaguely defined illnesses)
- Bloodshot or bleary eyes
- Facial petechiae (especially over the nose)
- Ulcer (Csiernik, 1990).

Job strain has also been shown to be associated with higher mortality. *Job strain* has been operationally defined as high job demands coupled with low ability to control demands (Curtis, James, Raghunathan, & Alcser, 1997). In one study, men with high levels of job strain and limited support had twice the mortality of those exposed to low levels (Johnson, et al., 1996). Similarly, extremes of decision latitude at work seem to be linked to hypertension, with high decision latitude associated with a 50% decrease in hypertension prevalence (Curtis, et al., 1997). Stress and job strain have also been correlated with atherosclerosis in men with stress-induced blood pressure reactivity (Everson, et al., 1997) and absenteeism (North, Syme, Feeney, Shipley, & Marmot, 1996), and moderately associated with preterm labor in pregnant employees (Brett, Strogatz, & Savitz, 1997).

Occupational health nurses also need to be able to identify sources of stress in and out of the work setting that may contribute to the development of psychological health problems. Psychological stress is the tenth leading occupational disease. Employees particularly prone to work-related psychological stress include health care and other service personnel, blue-collar workers, and those who work nights or who rotate shifts. Nurses who work with these groups should be particularly aware of the potential for stress-related illnesses.

Other sources of stress in the work setting include work overload, the organizational structure of the company, job insecurity, and interpersonal relationships with coworkers or supervisors. Stress may also be created by sexist or racist attitudes of others in the workplace. Perceptions of the source of occupational stress may differ greatly between employees and employers. Sources of stress most frequently identified by workers include lack of control over the content, process, and pace of one's work; unrealistic demands and lack of understanding by supervisors; lack of predictability and security regarding one's job future; and the cumulative effects of occupational and family stressors. Employers, on the other hand, most often perceive employees' lifestyles and health habits as the primary contributors to stress.

The Physical Dimension

Physical environmental factors contribute to a variety of health problems encountered in the work setting.

Categories of health hazards in the physical environment include chemical hazards, physical hazards (radiation, noise, vibration, and exposure to heat and cold), electrical hazards, fire, heavy lifting and uncomfortable working positions, and potential for falls.

Poor lighting or high noise levels may adversely affect vision and hearing, respectively. Heavy objects that must be moved may cause musculoskeletal injuries. In addition, there is the potential for falls or exposure to excessive heat or cold in many workplaces.

The use of toxic substances in work performance is another source of possible health problems related to the physical environment. Toxic substances may be encountered as solids, liquids, gases, vapors, dust, fumes, fibers, or mists (California Occupational Health Program, 1992). As noted earlier, a great number of toxic substances are present in the work environment that may result in respiratory, dermatologic, and other health problems. Of particular concern in this area is exposure to heavy metals (Table 26–1). The adverse effects of occupational exposure to lead, for example, have been known for more than 2000 years. Despite this knowledge and efforts to minimize occupational exposure to lead and other heavy metals, significant numbers of workers in the United States have the potential for work-related lead exposure, and in many industries no mechanism is in place for biological monitoring of lead levels in employees with potential for exposure. Other metals of concern include mercury, arsenic, and cadmium. Exposure to lead and other metals occurs in a variety of occupations including those listed in Table 26–1. Areas to be assessed relative to the potential for toxic exposures in the workplace include substances used in the setting and their level of demonstrated toxicity, portals of entry into the human body, established legal exposure limits, extent of exposure, potential for interactive exposures, and the presence of existing employee health conditions that put the individuals affected at greater risk

for exposure-related illnesses. The nurse and other personnel would also assess the extent and adequacy of controls to prevent or limit exposures and the availability of and compliance with recommended screening and surveillance procedures (California Occupational Health Program, 1992).

Equipment may also constitute an occupational health hazard. The use of heavy equipment or sharp tools can result in injury. There is also the potential for hand–arm vibration syndrome in the use of tools that vibrate or visual disturbance related to the use of computer display terminals. Another relatively recent physical hazard generated by widespread computer use is the potential for tendonitis and other similar conditions stemming from the use of word processors. Extreme or awkward postures have been associated with low back problems and repetitive or high-force movements with carpal tunnel syndrome.

The nurse in the occupational setting identifies the presence of any hazards in the physical environment that contribute to health problems. In addition, the nurse monitors the status of known hazards and their effects on the health of employees.

The Social Dimension

The social environment of the work setting can influence employee health status either positively or negatively. The quality of social interactions among employees, attitudes toward work and health, and presence or absence of racial, sexual, or other tensions can all affect health status as well as employee productivity.

Four spheres of influence in the workplace social environment may affect the health status of individual employees, and the effects of each sphere on health should be assessed by the community health nurse in the occupational health setting. The first sphere of influence involves the health-related behaviors of em-

---

TABLE 26–1. OCCUPATIONAL SOURCES AND HEALTH EFFECTS OF HEAVY METAL EXPOSURES

Metal	Occupational Sources	Health Effects
Antimony	Iron works, red dye manufacture	Irritation, cardiovascular and lung effects
Arsenic	Photographic equipment and supplies	Lung and lymphatic cancer, dermatitis
Cadmium	Soldering, battery manufacture, fuses, paint manufacture and painting, nuclear reactors	Lung cancer, prostatic cancer, renal system effects
Chromium	Steel manufacture, chrome plating, dye and paint manufacture, leather tanning	Lung cancer, skin ulcers, lung irradiation
Lead	Soldering, dispensing leaded gas, cable cutting and splicing; painting, casting, or melting lead; radiator repair, welding, grinding, or sanding lead-painted surfaces; battery manufacture; construction; paper hanging; foundries; plumbing	Kidney, blood, and nervous system effects
Mercury	Metal foil and leaf application, industrial measurement instruments, gold and silver refining	Central nervous system and mental effects
Nickel	Nickel plating, steel manufacture, heating coils, hydrogenation processes	Lung and nasal cancer, skin effects
Tungsten	Steel manufacture, x-ray tubes	Lung and skin effects
Zinc oxide	White paint manufacture	Metal fume fever

EVALUATING OCCUPATIONAL HAZARD POTENTIAL

Substances/Conditions Present

What substances or conditions are associated with production processes (eg, toxic chemicals, heat)?

What substances or conditions are associated with clerical processes (eg, repetitive movements)?

What substances or conditions are associated with other office processes (eg, cleaning products, pesticides)?

What is the typical extent and duration of exposure to hazardous substances or conditions?

What are the designated exposure limits for substances and conditions in the work setting?

Health Effects

What research evidence is there for adverse human health effects (eg, toxicity, teratogenicity, potential for injury) associated with substances used or conditions existing in the work setting?

Do low levels of exposure have a cumulative effect?

What is the usual portal of entry or mechanism of exposure for a specific toxic agent or condition?

What organ systems are typically affected by specific toxic agents or hazardous conditions?

What are the usual signs and symptoms of toxicity/health effects?

Are there synergistic effects among substances or between substances and other conditions (eg, heat)?

Employee Considerations

Do employees have preexisting health conditions that put them at greater risk for toxic effects?

Do employees engage in other behaviors (eg, smoking) that increase their risk of toxic effects?

Do employees use safety equipment and procedures to minimize potential for exposure?

Environmental Considerations

What are the recommended control practices to prevent or minimize potential for exposure?

Are the recommended practices in place in a given occupational setting (eg, ventilation, other engineering controls)?

Are employees provided with education to prevent or minimize exposure potential?

Are employees provided with appropriate personal protective devices (eg, respirators, ear protection)?

What are the recommended surveillance practices for monitoring environmental conditions and hazardous exposures?

Are there surveillance systems in place for monitoring the presence or extent of hazardous conditions in the environment?

Health System Considerations

Are there surveillance systems in place for monitoring employees for evidence of exposure or exposure effects?

Are surveillance procedures implemented in a systematic way to periodically assess all employees at risk for exposure?

Are there processes in place for diagnosing and treating health conditions that arise from employee exposures to hazardous conditions?

---

ployees themselves and is addressed in the discussion of behavioral factors affecting health. The other three spheres are more directly related to the social environment of the work setting.

The second sphere of influence on health in the workplace occurs among groups of coworkers, and the community health nurse should assess the influence of coworker groups on the health of individual employees and on the group as a whole. For example, a group of coworkers may decide that they do not wish to be exposed to smoke in their work area. This decision can lead to formal or informal bans on smoking in certain areas. Formal bans may occur when groups of employees request no-smoking policies from company management. When this is not the case, work groups may enforce the decision infor-

mally by exerting peer pressure on the smokers in the group. In other words, they can make life unpleasant for those who wish to smoke by ostracizing them or using other social sanctions. Another example of this sphere of social influence lies in the influence that more experienced employees have on the use of safety precautions by younger, less experienced workers. Because of their need to become an accepted part of an established work group, new employees often imitate behaviors (either positive or negative) displayed by those who have been on the job for some time (Asfahl, 1995).

The third sphere of influence is the management sphere. The nurse assesses management's attitudes toward health and health-related policies and the effects of these policies (or lack of them) on employee health. For example, management may decide on and enforce a no-smoking policy throughout the company, whether or not employees favor such a policy. Management makes other kinds of policy decisions that affect employee health. For example, the type of health care coverage provided to employees is a management decision. Or, a policy that provides "well leave" or extra vacation for those who have not taken sick leave may prompt employee efforts to promote health and prevent illness.

For employees to value wellness and health promotive efforts, they must perceive them to be valued by employers. This means that wellness programs and other aspects of occupational health must receive the same degree of emphasis as other areas of business. It has been suggested that companies develop *company wellness policies*, statements of administrative commitment to employee health, and expectations of employees related to health promotion and maintenance, to convey the importance given to health issues. These companies must be seen to abide by, as well as create, such policies (Grant & Brisbin, 1992).

The last sphere of influence involves legal, social, and political action that influences the health of employees. A prime example of this is the regulation of conditions in the work setting by agencies such as the Occupational Safety and Health Administration (OSHA). Through legislation, society can mandate that business and industry create specific conditions that enhance the health of employees. Another example of such a mandate is legislation that requires companies over a certain size to offer employees a health maintenance organization (HMO) as one option for health insurance coverage. In assessing health needs in the work setting, the community health nurse examines the extent to which the employer adheres to legislative and regulatory standards and the effect of these standards in promoting employee health.

Legislation may also influence what qualifies as a work-related illness and can be duly compensated (Dembe, 1996). For example, in some states, health care workers who acquire HIV infection through needle sticks at work are not eligible for workers' compensation (Tereskerz & Jagger, 1997). Other social factors that influence what is considered a work-related condition include new production and diagnostic technology, union campaigns, media attention to certain conditions, interest in the effects of similar hazards found in the wider community, marketing efforts of vendors of safety products, and attention drawn to certain conditions by political figures. Medical specialization that benefits from compensation for certain kinds of conditions may influence decisions to consider these conditions work-related. Similarly, conditions experienced in military actions and resulting

health effects may draw attention to similar conditions in civilian industry (Dembe, 1996).

One final social dimension factor in the work setting that is not currently compensable, but is drawing increasing attention, is workplace violence. In 1993, the rate of occupational homicide was 0.64 per 100,000 workers (National Institute for Occupational Safety and Health, 1994). Approximately 20 workers are murdered each week in the United States and 1 million workers are assaulted annually. Homicide is the second leading cause of occupational injury mortality. Contrary to popular belief few of these crimes are perpetrated by fellow employees; most (75%) are robbery-related. The risk of exposure to violence in the workplace is increased in jobs where employees interact with the public, where money is exchanged, or in the delivery of goods or services. Working early in the morning or late at night, working alone, guarding valuables or property, and working with violent people or in volatile situations also increases one's risk of violence. Men and older workers (over 65 years of age) are at higher risk for violence than women and younger people. Taxicab drivers are 60 times more likely to be murdered than any other occupational group (41.4 per 100,000 workers), followed by liquor store employees (7.5), detective or protective personnel (7.0), service station attendants (4.8), and jewelry store clerks (4.7 per 100,000) (National Institute for Occupational Safety and Health, 1996b). Personal safety issues are an important area for occupational health nurses to assess in working with employees.

The Behavioral Dimension

As noted above, behavioral factors exemplified in individual decisions about health-related actions constitute the first sphere of social influence on employee health. Lifestyle factors to be considered here include the type of work performed, consumption patterns, patterns of rest and exercise, and use of safety devices.

Type of Work Performed. The type of work performed by an individual within a company can significantly influence the employee's health. The type of work performed determines the risk of exposure to various physical hazards and level of stress experienced. For example, factory workers in industries using lead may run the risk of lead poisoning, whereas executives in the same companies may be exposed to more stress.

The type of work done also influences the extent of exercise that employees obtain. Construction workers, for example, have ample opportunities for physical activity but also risk serious injury in the use of heavy equipment. Bank tellers, on the other hand, are at risk for cardiovascular and other diseases related to a sedentary lifestyle.

The community health nurse in an occupational setting should be conversant with the variety of jobs performed in that setting. The nurse should also be aware of the health hazards posed by each type of work performed and be alert to signs of health problems deriving from the work itself.

Another aspect of the type of work performed is that of *ergonomics*, the degree of fit between the employee and the job performed. The nurse should assess the degree to which employees are qualified to perform their particular job function and their interest in that job. Employees who work at jobs that do not interest them, that are beyond their capabilities, or that do not provide sufficient challenge may be at greater risk for both emotional and physical health problems than those who are better suited to their jobs. Ergonomics also reflects the design of work stations and their effects on health. For example, the height of a computer keyboard may influence the development of neck and shoulder problems.

Consumption Patterns. Consumption patterns of interest to the occupational health nurse include those related to food and nutrition, smoking, and drug and alcohol use. The influence of nutrition on health is well established, and the occupational health nurse assesses the nutritional patterns of employees with whom he or she works. In addition, the nurse assesses how the work environment affects eating habits. For example, sufficient opportunity may not be provided for employees to eat despite OSHA regulations regarding time and place for breaks and meals.

The nurse also determines whether food service is available to employees. If there is an employee cafeteria, the nurse may need to assess the nutritional quality of the food provided. If no food services are available in the workplace, the nurse would determine whether they are available nearby, or whether adequate storage facilities exist for employees who bring meals from home.

Smoking is another consumption pattern of concern to the occupational health nurse. Smoking is harmful to health in and of itself. In addition, smoking may increase the adverse effects of other environmental hazards in the work setting, particularly those that affect respiration. Many employers have recently begun to prohibit smoking except in carefully controlled areas in the workplace and have been active in promoting programs to help employees quit smoking. The nurse assesses the extent of smoking in the employee population as well as the specific implications of smoking in that particular environment.

As noted earlier, employees may have problems with substance abuse. The prevalence of these problems should be monitored and the nurse should be alert to signs and symptoms of substance abuse in the employee population. Overindulgence in other substances, such as caffeine, may also pose a health hazard to employees.

Rest and Exercise. Work places many physical and psychological demands on people. Sometimes these demands result in inadequate rest and recreation, as with the executive who works constantly, or the blue-collar worker who holds two jobs in an attempt to make ends meet. Conversely, work may also lead to too much sitting and too little exercise.

The nurse in the work setting assesses the amount of activity engaged in by employees and the balance between rest and exercise. He or she also obtains information on the types of recreation used by employees and any potential health hazards posed by recreational choices.

Many companies are recognizing the benefits of exercise in terms of both the physical and psychological health of employees. These companies are promoting physical exercise and may even provide facilities for exercise and recreation in the workplace. If this is the case, the nurse should be alert to potential health hazards and the potential for too much exercise. For example, if there is a company pool, the epileptic employee who swims to relieve tension should be cautioned against swimming alone. Similarly, the overweight executive should engage in physical activity cautiously to lessen the risk of heart attack or injury.

Another consideration with respect to rest and exercise is the influence of rotating shifts on employee health and safety. In one study, for example, employees who rotated shifts were twice as likely as those with stable work shifts to fall asleep while driving to or from work. They were also more likely to report sleep disturbances, falling asleep at work, and increased accidents and errors at work (Gold, et al., 1992). Similarly, women who worked rotating shifts for more than 6 years were more than one and a half times more likely than those who had never rotated shifts to experience coronary heart disease (Kawachi, et al., 1995).

Use of Safety Devices. A last behavioral factor that is particularly relevant to health in the occupational setting is the use or nonuse of safety devices. Hazards present in the workplace frequently can be mitigated by the use of appropriate safety devices; however, this can only occur if employees use these devices consistently and appropriately.

The community health nurse identifies the need for safety devices and also monitors the extent to which they are used. For example, do individuals working in high-noise areas wear earplugs? Are those earplugs correctly fitted? Do people involved in heavy lifting wear weight belts or do they ignore the potential for injury? Are heavy shoes or gloves worn in areas with dangerous equipment? Again, the attitude of management toward health promotion and illness prevention strongly influences employee behaviors. When administrators, for example, fail to use hearing protection in high-noise areas, they convey an attitude of disinterest in health which frequently filters down to employees.

The Health System Dimension

Health system factors influencing employee health relate to both external and internal health care systems. The external system reflects the availability and accessibility of health care services outside the workplace, whereas the internal system consists of those services offered within the workplace.

The External System.

In assessing employee health status, the community health nurse in the occupational setting gathers information about the use of health services in the community at large. The nurse examines the type of services used and the reasons for and appropriateness of their use (Monaghan, 1995). The nurse also assesses the availability of services needed by company employees in the external health care system.

One of the work-related factors influencing use of outside health services is the availability of insurance coverage. Health insurance is an employment benefit for many, but large segments of the working population still do not have health insurance coverage. Many of these uninsured workers do not have sufficient income to afford health insurance themselves or out-of-pocket health care expenses. Even for insured employees, medical benefits have steadily declined due to high insurance costs. Copayments and deductibles have increased at the same time, further limiting access to care for some employees and their families (Allegrante & Goldfein, 1995). The occupational health nurse should become familiar with the insurance status of employees in his or her company and with the kinds of benefits covered under group policies where they exist. As noted earlier, the legal status of a condition as eligible for workers' compensation will also influence care by external and internal providers.

The Internal System.

The internal health care system consists of those health services and programs provided to employees in the work setting. Four general types of occupational health programs can be found in business and industry: programs aimed at controlling exposure to toxic substances; those emphasizing health promotion policies in the workplace; those focusing on limited health promotion efforts; and comprehensive programs that attempt to meet a variety of employee health needs.

PROGRAMS TO CONTROL TOXIC EXPOSURES.   Programs to control or eliminate toxic substances and other hazardous conditions in the workplace usually occur in response to OSHA regulations. Control programs may involve engineering controls, controlled work practices, use of safety equipment or devices, or elimination of toxic substances from the work environment (Burgess, 1995). In industries with this type of program, the community health nurse should assess the efficacy of these control measures and the extent to which they are adhered to in the setting.

HEALTH PROMOTION POLICIES.   The second type of program involves policies that are initiated by employers to keep health care expenditures to a minimum. These policies seek to limit hospitalization and expenses for acute care services by promoting the health of the employee population and by encouraging a less expensive approach to providing services. For example, employers may have policies related to the need for a second opinion before covering employee expenses for elective surgery or encouraging home care rather than hospitalization whenever possible. In this type of an occupational health program, the community health nurse assesses the effect of these and similar policies on the health of the employee population.

LIMITED HEALTH PROMOTION PROGRAMS.   The third type of program provides a limited approach to health promotion. Generally, these programs focus on one aspect of health care and may make use of prepackaged health promotion and education programs that do not meet the specific needs of the employee group. These programs also tend to be illness oriented rather than to focus on the promotion of overall health. For example, there may be emphasis on education for good body mechanics to prevent injuries or first aid for injuries, but little attention to overall health promotion. These programs also focus on the individual employee's responsibility for his or her health and may neglect conditions within the work setting that create health problems. In this type of a system, the community health nurse identifies the types of health promotion programs provided and the extent to which they meet employees' identified health needs.

ASSESSMENT TIPS: Assessing Health in the Work Setting

Biophysical Dimension

Age and Genetic Inheritance

What is the age composition of the employee population?

What is the relative proportion of males and females in the work setting?

What is the racial/ethnic composition in the work setting?

What is the prevalence of genetic predisposition to disease in the employee population? What diseases are involved?

Physiologic Function

What existing health problems are prevalent in the employee population?

What is the incidence of communicable diseases in the employee population?

Are there handicapping conditions present in the employee population?

What are the immunization levels in the employee population?

Psychological Dimension

Do work schedules promote health or create stress?

To what extent does the work environment contribute to stress?

What is the quality of relationships among the employees? Between employees and management?

Do employees encounter role conflicts between work and home?

What is the prevalence of mental illness among employees?

What is the level of employee morale?

What is the extent of absenteeism among employees?

Physical Dimension

Where is the work setting located?

Does the physical environment of the work setting pose any health hazards?

Is there potential for hazardous materials exposures? If so, what kind of exposures?

Is hazardous equipment used? If so, it is used correctly?

Are there animals in the work environment? Do they pose a health hazard?

Are there plant allergens or poisonous plants in the work environment?

Does the work environment have adequate heat, light, and ventilation?

Does the work entail exposure to extreme weather conditions?

What is the noise level in the work environment?

Are food sanitation practices adequate to prevent communicable diseases, vermin infestation, etc.?

Are toilet facilities adequate and in good repair?

Are shower facilities available for dealing with hazardous substance exposures?

Are there adequate facilities for handicapped employees?

Are workstations designed to prevent injury and fatigue?

Is there potential for a disaster in the work setting? Is there a disaster plan in place?

Social Dimension

What is the extent of crime in the area? Does the work pose a high risk for crime victimization?

What assistance, if any, is provided to working parents relative to child care?

What is the education level of employees?

What is the cultural background of employees? What languages are spoken?

Are there intergroup conflicts in the employee population?

What types of work are performed? Does the type of work pose health hazards for employees?

What is the extent of social support among employees?

To what extent do coworkers support healthful behaviors?

What is the potential for violence in the work setting?

Behavioral Dimension

Nutrition and Other Consumption Patterns

What are the nutritional needs of employees? Are there employees with special nutritional needs? If so, what are they? How well are they being met?

Are there food services available in the work setting? What is the nutritional quality of food served?

What is the extent of employees' nutrition knowledge?

What is the extent of alcohol, tobacco, and other drug use among employees?

Are no-smoking policies in place in the work setting? If so, are they enforced?

(continued)

ASSESSMENT TIPS: Assessing Health in the Work Setting (cont.)

Exercise and Leisure Activity

What are the rest and activity patterns of the employee population?

Are there any recreational opportunities available to the employee population? Do recreational activities pose health hazards?

Medication Use

Do any members of the employee population use prescription medications on a regular basis? Are medications used, stored, and dispensed as directed?

Safety Practices

Are safety policies and procedures in place in the work setting? Are they enforced? Do employees use appropriate safety equipment and procedures?

Health System Dimension

What health services are offered in the work setting?

Are primary preventive services available and is their use promoted in the work setting?

How accessible are needed health services in the community?

To what extent does the employee population use available health services?

How are health care services funded? Is funding adequate to meet health needs?

What is the quality of interaction between internal and external health care services?

To what extent are health promotion and illness/injury prevention emphasized in the work setting?

What are employees' attitudes toward health and health care?

What systems are in place to control and monitor toxic exposures in the work setting?

COMPREHENSIVE PROGRAMS.   The fourth type of occupational health program is a comprehensive approach to health care. These programs educate employees so as to promote health and prevent illness, but they also emphasize organizational programs, policies, and environmental changes that are conducive to health. For example, a company with a comprehensive health care approach might provide educational sessions on stress management *and* engage in organizational changes aimed at reducing the amount of stress engendered by the work setting. Again, the nurse assessing the influence of health care system factors on employees' health determines the extent to which the designated program meets employees' health needs.

FAMILY CARE.   In some work settings, comprehensive health care programs go beyond the provision of care to employees to include some form of direct care for family members. Employees who are concerned about their families may be less productive than they would be were their family situation less stressful. As more and more families are supported by two wage earners, employment of both spouses has implications for the life of the family and the well-being of children. Community health nurses who care for clients in the work setting should be aware of the stresses involved in dual-career (or single-parent) families and how work schedules and conditions may affect the health of the family. Work schedules that allow for outside

responsibilities and family life are very helpful, and the nurse may be able to influence management in the creation of flexible scheduling systems. The nurse may also be of assistance in helping employees deal with the stress of role overload.

Some companies are becoming more aware of the interplay of family influences and occupational factors in employee performance and are establishing systems designed to assist families. One recent effort is the establishment of child care centers on company premises. Some centers provide care whether the child is well or ill. In such cases, the community health nurse working in this setting may assume responsibilities relative to the health of the children in the centers. These nurses need to be versed in pediatric as well as adult health care. Elder care services are also provided in a few occupational settings.

Even in occupational settings where there are no child or elder care facilities, nurses are asked for assistance in dealing with health problems of family members. The nurse may counsel the employee regarding resolution of family problems or may provide referrals to outside sources of assistance that can be found in Chapters 20 and 23.

The last aspect of the occupational health nurse's role in the care of employees' families deals with the concept of paraoccupational exposures to hazardous substances. *Paraoccupational exposure* occurs when employees are exposed to hazardous substances and in turn expose their families (usually via contaminated clothing). These exposures may involve metals, chemicals, or biological agents.

Nurses who have knowledge of problems experienced by members of employees' families are in a position to recognize paraoccupational exposure and to take action to correct such exposure. Nurses should be aware of the potential for such exposures and should make it a practice to ask employees questions designed to elicit information about family exposure to hazardous substances.

Diagnostic Reasoning and Care of Clients in the Work Setting

Community health nurses working in occupational settings derive nursing diagnoses from assessment information related to individuals or groups of employees. For example, the nurse might diagnose "inability to sleep due to work pressures" for a company executive or "poor employee morale due to increased tension and stress in the work setting." Other nursing diagnoses related to individual employees are a "need for referral for counseling due to heavy drinking" and "moderate hearing loss due to failure to use hearing protection in high-noise areas." Additional nursing diagnoses at the group level are a "potential for exposure to hepatitis B due to frequent contact with blood" for a group of laboratory technicians in a hospital, and the "potential for falls due to work in elevated areas" for a group of construction workers.

Planning Nursing Care in the Work Setting

Interventions may be developed by the occupational health nurse alone or in conjunction with others in the work setting to address the health needs identified. In the case of individual clients, interventions would be tailored to individual needs and circumstances. When identified health problems affect groups of employees, planned interventions are likely to be more complex. Planning to meet the needs of groups in the workplace will employ the principles of health programming discussed in Chapter 19.

Whether the client is an individual, a group of employees, or the total population in the work setting, interventions may be planned at primary, secondary, and tertiary levels of prevention.

Primary Prevention

Primary prevention in the occupational setting is directed toward minimizing the risk of injury and illness (Martin, 1995) and promoting health and well-being.

Health Promotion.   Community health nurses in occupational settings educate employees to lead healthier lives. A 1992 survey indicated that 81% of worksites offered at least one health promotion activity for employees (U.S. Department of Health and Human Services, 1994). Generally, these activities fall into one of five categories: programs to promote awareness, motivation programs, behavior change programs, maintenance programs, and culture change programs (Bellingham & Pelletier, 1995). Awareness programs are designed to make employees aware of the ill effects of unhealthy behaviors and encourage behavior change. General education efforts by the nurse fall into this category. Motivation programs are also geared toward moving employees to take action on their own to change unhealthy behaviors. For example, employees may be rewarded with additional vacation days for maintaining their health. Behavior change interventions are programs designed to assist employees to make changes in their health-related behavior. Work-based smoking cessation programs and exercise programs are examples of this type of health promotion activity. Maintenance programs provide assistance to employees to continue with healthier behaviors and may include such interventions as coworker support groups as well as increased environmental support for healthy behavior. For example, a nonsmoker support group may be coupled with employer policies prohibiting smoking. Both interventions are designed to help employees who smoke to develop a no-smoking habit. Finally, culture change programs are intended to alter the organizational culture of the work setting to reinforce the importance of health. Actions in these types of programs are directed at both the individual and the organization. For instance, the organization may strive to find effective ways to reduce stress in the work environment, while incorporating a health behavior review as part of regular performance appraisals for employees.

Health promotion programs in the occupational setting have been highly successful. One review of literature in this area found that 47 out of 48 studies indicated positive outcomes of health promotion programs (U.S. Department of Health and Human Services, 1994). Specifically, health promotion programs have been shown to result in behavior change and decrease risks, decrease short-term health care service use, decrease short-term health care costs, and decrease absenteeism. Fitness programs, in particular, have been found to increase productivity and employee performance ratings. They also lead to fewer injuries and more rapid recovery when injury occurs. Employee assistance, stress management, and other similar programs have also been shown to increase productivity and psychological health among employees (Opatz, Chenoweth, & Kaman, 1994). Further research is needed to document the long-term effects and costs of health promotion programs.

Another avenue for health promotion is providing prenatal care to pregnant workers. This could involve referral for prenatal care if this service is not provided by the company health facility. The nurse might also monitor the employee for signs and symptoms of complications of pregnancy. The nurse may find it necessary to function as an advocate for the employee who needs to be relieved of some of her duties as the pregnancy progresses. For example, it may be necessary to move the employee to another position that does not require heavy lifting. The nurse may also be involved in childbirth education for pregnant employees or male employees and their spouses.

Illness Prevention. Preventing illness is the second aspect of primary prevention in the workplace. Illness prevention can involve either employee education or prevention of specific illness through immunization. For example, some industries routinely offer employees influenza immunization to cut down on illness-related absenteeism.

Another aspect of illness prevention involves modifying risk factors. *Risk factors* are personal or group characteristics that predispose one to develop a specific health problem. For example, it is well known that smoking increases one's risk of developing heart disease and lung cancer, so smoking is a risk factor for both of these problems.

Some risk factors can be modified or eliminated, thus decreasing one's chances of developing specific health problems. Again, using smoking as an example, people who quit smoking lower their risk of developing lung cancer. Occupational health nurses can be instrumental in assisting employees to modify risk factors, helping them to prevent health problems. Some risk factors that receive particular attention in the occupational setting are smoking, elevated blood pressure, sedentary lifestyle, stress, and overweight.

Occupational health nurses can work on risk factor modification with individuals or groups of employees. They can also engage in risk factor modification efforts at the company level. One example of this would be efforts to convince company policy makers that a no-smoking policy should be instituted and enforced within the workplace. Nurses can also develop

weight standards for job categories in which being overweight is particularly hazardous.

At the individual level, the nurse can counsel employees regarding the hazards of smoking, particularly in conjunction with occupational exposure to respiratory irritants. They can also provide assistance to individuals who wish to quit smoking.

Restructuring the work environment can help in minimizing occupational stress as a risk factor for health problems. Efforts in this direction include developing flexible scheduling plans to minimize conflicts with employees' outside responsibilities. The nurse can also facilitate employee input into work related decisions and strive to minimize role overload and role ambiguity. The nurse can also promote opportunity for social interaction, job security, and career development.

As is obvious, most of these efforts must be undertaken by management, but the nurse can provide management with evidence of related research and can provide the impetus for change in these areas. At the individual level, the occupational health nurse can be aware of the stressors experienced by employees in various jobs in the work setting. The nurse is also in a position to monitor the effects of stress on the individual employee and to counsel employees in stress management.

Injury Prevention. Injury prevention may again entail employee education in a variety of areas. Employees

> ### PRIMARY PREVENTION IN THE WORK SETTING
>
> *Health Promotion*
> - Awareness
> - Motivation
> - Behavior change
> - Maintenance
> - Culture change
> - Prenatal care for pregnant employees
>
> *Illness Prevention*
> - Immunization
> - Modification or elimination of risk factors
> - Stress reduction and management
>
> *Injury Prevention*
> - Safety education
> - Use of safety devices
> - Safe handling of hazardous substances
> - Elimination of safety hazards
> - Good body mechanics

need to be acquainted with safety procedures to prevent accidents. There may also be a need to educate employees in the correct use of safety equipment. For example, individuals working in some areas should wear protective clothing or use breathing apparatus. The nurse should explain the need for safety equipment and be responsible for monitoring its use. This may entail planning periodic visits to certain areas of the workplace to determine whether employees are indeed using safety equipment as directed.

Employees may also be in need of education in other areas related to injury prevention. Handling of hazardous substances, proper use of machinery, need for fluid replacement in high-heat areas, and good body mechanics are all educational topics that may be appropriate in certain industrial settings. Nurses may also provide education on first aid and cardiopulmonary resuscitation.

One aspect of injury prevention in which the nurse may be involved is monitoring hazardous conditions in the workplace. The nurse should be aware of potential hazards and their appropriate management. In the absence of an industrial hygienist, the nurse may plan and conduct environmental testing to detect hazardous levels of chemicals, heat, or noise.

The nurse may need to acquaint management with the occurrence of injuries due to hazardous conditions and advocate changes designed to protect employees from injuries. Recommendations for dealing with the problem of noise-induced hearing loss include engineering efforts to minimize noise production, use of properly fitted hearing protection devices, education of employees and managers in the use of protective devices and their importance, and periodic audiometric screening. The occupational health nurse may be actively involved in planning and executing the majority of these recommended activities, particularly in screening for hearing loss, fitting protective devices, and educating employees and supervisors. Control of noise-related hearing loss requires commitment on the part of employees and management to the proper use of protective devices. Motivating employees to use these devices and monitoring their use are crucial functions of the occupational health nurse.

Secondary Prevention

Secondary prevention in the work setting is aimed at recognizing and resolving existing health problems. General areas of involvement for occupational health nurses include screening, treatment for existing conditions, and emergency care.

Screening. Screening activities can take any of three directions. Screening efforts begin with preemployment assessment of potential employees. Screening may also be conducted at periodic intervals to monitor employee health status. Finally, the work environment may be screened periodically for the presence or absence of hazardous conditions. The community health nurse would be involved in planning and implementing screening efforts at all three of these levels.

PREEMPLOYMENT SCREENING.   For many employees, their first interaction with an occupational health nurse is the preemployment screening examination. The purpose of this initial screening is to facilitate employee selection and placement. Hiring an employee for a particular job is in part dependent on his or her physical, mental, and emotional capabilities for performing that job. A similar process may be needed when considering an employee for a change of job (Cox & Edwards, 1995). These capabilities can be determined in an initial screening examination. At this time the nurse usually obtains a complete health history from the employee and conducts a battery of routine screening tests. Nurse practitioners in the occupational setting may also conduct the physical examination.

Based on the information derived from the screening, the nurse may make determinations regarding the person's employability in a particular capacity. To make such determinations, the nurse must be familiar with the types of activities involved and stressors encountered in a particular job. The preemployment screening also provides baseline data for determining the effects of working conditions on the health of employees.

PERIODIC SCREENING.   The nurse in the occupational setting also plans periodic screening activities to monitor employees' continuing health status. This is particularly true of employees working under hazardous conditions. For example, monitoring devices are used by personnel working with radiation and are periodically checked for exposure limits. Likewise, blood chemistries may be done at periodic intervals to test for exposure to toxic substances. Periodic blood pressure screenings and pulmonary function tests may also be warranted. In some occupational groups such as the armed forces, employees are routinely screened for overweight and for physical capacity.

The types of screening done depend on the type of job performed, the risks involved, and the capabilities required. Some screenings are routinely performed on all employees in a particular setting. For example, employees may receive a routine physical examination at periodic intervals. Other screening tests are performed only on specific employees. For example, lead screening may be done routinely on in-

▶ EVALUATING FITNESS FOR WORK

Physical Health Considerations

Does the employee have the physical stamina required?

Does the employee have any mobility limitations that would interfere with performance?

Does the employee have sufficient joint mobility to do the job?

Does the employee have any postural limitations that would interfere with performance?

Does the employee have the required strength for the job?

Does the employee have the level of coordination required?

Does the employee have problems with balance that would interfere with performance?

Does the employee have any cardiorespiratory limitations?

Is there a possibility for unconsciousness that would create a safety hazard?

Does the employee have the required level of visual and auditory acuity?

Does the employee have communication and speech capabilities required by the job?

Mental and Emotional Health Considerations

Does the employee have the requisite level of cognitive function (eg, memory, critical thinking)?

Will the employee's mental or emotional state (eg, depression) interfere with performance?

Does the employee have the required motivational level?

Does the employee have a substance abuse problem that would interfere with performance?

Does the employee have effective stress management skills?

Is there any possibility that the employee might endanger self or others?

Health Plan Considerations

Are there treatment effects that will interfere with performance (eg, drowsiness from medications)?

Will subsequent treatment plans interfere with performance (eg, nausea due to future chemotherapy)?

What is the employee's prognosis? Will existing conditions improve or deteriorate further?

Does the employee have any special health needs to be met in the work setting (eg, diabetic diet)?

Are any assistive aids or appliances required? Will work processes or setting need to be adapted to accommodate these aids (eg, space for a wheelchair)?

Task/Setting Considerations

Are there risk factors in the work setting that would adversely affect the employee?

What is the level of stress involved in the job?

Will the employee be working with others or alone? What health effects might this have?

What are the temporal aspects of the job and how will they affect health (eg, shift work, early morning or late evening work, length of shift)?

Is there travel involved in the job? How will this affect employee health?

(Source: Cox & Edwards, 1995.)

dividuals who work in the company plant, but not on clerical personnel.

Occupational health nurses are frequently responsible for conducting these and other screening tests on employees. They may also interpret test results, explain them to employees, and take action when warranted by positive test results.

ENVIRONMENTAL SCREENING. Periodic screening of the environment may also be warranted and, in the absence of industrial hygienists or safety engineers, the nurse may be responsible for planning and conducting environmental screenings. For example, the nurse may measure noise levels in various work areas at specific intervals to determine areas in which hearing protection is required. Similarly, measurements of volatile chemicals or radiation might be done in high-risk areas.

Treatment of Existing Conditions. The second aspect of secondary prevention is the diagnosis and treatment of existing health problems. Community health nurses are actively involved in planning health interventions for individual employees and should also participate in planning health programs to meet the needs of groups of clients.

Many industries go beyond treating only job-related illness and conditions to treating a variety of major and minor conditions. The rationale for the extension of services to nonjob-related conditions is that any health problem, physical or emotional, can serve to impair the employee's performance. Also, treatment of these conditions within the work setting itself limits time lost in pursuing outside treatment, saving the company money in the long run.

Depending on the capabilities of the occupational health unit, employees with existing health problems may be referred to the external health care system for problem resolution, or treatment may be provided within the workplace itself. Those occupational health nurses who are nurse practitioners may treat illness in the work setting. Even those nurses who are not nurse practitioners may treat minor conditions on the basis of protocols established in conjunction with medical consultation.

Occupational health nurses also need to plan to monitor the effectiveness of therapy, whether or not that therapy is provided by the occupational health unit. For example, an employee with hypertension might be followed by his or her private physician, but the occupational health nurse will monitor medication compliance and effects on the employee's blood pressure. In addition, the nurse will educate the employee regarding the condition and its treatment.

In the case of employees with problems related to substance abuse or stress, the community health nurse usually plans a referral to an appropriate source of assistance. The nurse may also need to function as an advocate for impaired employees, encouraging employers to provide coverage for treatment for psychological as well as physical illness. Nurses may also find it necessary to report conditions of abuse to supervisory personnel when either the health or the safety of other employees is threatened.

Community health nurses in occupational settings may be involved in planning and implementing employee assistance programs (EAPs) for employees with psychological problems. An *employee assistance program* is a program within the occupational setting designed to counsel employees with psychological problems and assist them in dealing with those problems (Roman & Blum, 1995). EAP programs are provided by approximately one third of private sector employers with 50 or more employees (Hartwell, Steele, French, Potter, Rodman, & Zarkin, 1996). Employee assistance programs usually focus on motivating individuals to seek help and on referring the person for needed services.

The nurse can plan to motivate the employee to get help through seven feedback steps performed in sequence until the employee (client) is willing to seek assistance (Csiernik, 1990). First, the nurse discusses with the client (employee) his or her observations of the client's behavior or appearance that indicate the existence of a problem. Second, the nurse comments on several instances of the client's behavior that suggest a psychological problem, making connections between discrete behavioral events to show the employee a definite pattern in his or her behavior. Third, the nurse asks the employee to explain the causes for the observed signs and symptoms. Interpreting possible causes for behavior is the fourth feedback step in motivating employees with psychological problems to take action. The fifth step is to provide suggestions for change that would eliminate or modify factors contributing to the problem. Sixth, if the employee has not decided to take action by this point, the nurse may need to provide a warning on the progressive nature of most psychological problems and on the possible consequences if no action is taken. Finally, the nurse may strongly recommend action to correct the problem. The choice of whether or not to take action, however, remains with the employee (client).

Once the individual is motivated to seek help for the problem, the nurse can make a referral to counselors within or outside the organization. In addition to planning the referral, the nurse should plan activities to support and encourage the employee and to monitor the employee's progress in resolving problems. Finally, the community health nurse should plan interventions that help reintegrate the employee into the work setting if an extended absence has been necessary.

Emergency Response. Another aspect of secondary prevention in the work setting is response to emergency situations. Nurses may find themselves dealing with both physical and psychological emergencies and should have a basic plan for dealing with various types of emergencies that may arise. Physical emergencies may result from serious accidents or from physical conditions such as heart attack, stroke, seizure disorder, and insulin reaction. Treatment for these emergencies is usually based on established protocols.

With respect to emergencies due to illness, it is helpful if the nurse has prior information related to the employee's condition. For example, if the nurse has prior knowledge that the client is diabetic, the diagnosis of hypoglycemic reaction will be reached and treatment initiated more rapidly than would otherwise be the case. For this reason, occupational health

SECONDARY PREVENTION IN THE WORK SETTING

Screening
- Preemployment screening
- Periodic screening of employees at risk for health problems
- Environmental screening

Treatment of Existing Conditions

Emergency Response
- Physical emergencies
- Psychological emergencies
- Occupational disasters

nurses should be well acquainted with employees' health histories.

Psychological emergencies may result in homicide, suicide, or both. Of the occupational fatalities occurring each year, 20% are the result of violence (U.S. Department of Commerce, 1996). Although businesses may have generalized protocols for dealing with such emergencies as threatened homicide or suicide, the nurse faced with such situations will probably need to exercise a great deal of creativity in planning to address a psychological emergency. General considerations include remaining calm and removing others from the immediate vicinity. The nurse *should not* plan any heroic measures that may endanger him- or herself, the employee, or others. Additional interventions are dictated by the situation. Again, prior identification of employees under excessive stress may help to prevent psychiatric emergencies.

Another psychological emergency with which occupational health nurses may need to deal is sexual assault. Most victims of sexual assault in the workplace are women, and most assaults occur at night when women are working in isolation from coworkers or the public. The majority of attackers in one study were strangers, and robbery was frequently a concurrent motive for the attack. Occupations with higher rates for sexual assault include convenience store and food service personnel, taxicab drivers, bartenders, janitorial personnel, and nursing home employees (Alexander, Franklin, & Wolf, 1994). The nurse who encounters a female employee who has been sexually assaulted should address immediate physical and psychological needs, assess the client for suicidal tendencies, and refer her for counseling. The nurse may also need to act as an advocate with the legal and criminal justice systems and to provide emotional support.

One further type of emergency that requires an occupational health nursing response is the emergency that affects large numbers of people. Examples of mass emergencies are fires or explosions, radiation exposure, and hazardous substance leaks. In addition to providing treatment for those injured in such emergencies, the nurse may be responsible for assisting in evaluating affected areas and in organizing to provide needed care. Occupational health nurses should be involved in planning the overall company response to

Critical Thinking in Research

The National Institute for Occupational Safety and Health (1996a) developed a set of research priorities for occupational health care. Areas in which a need for further research is needed were grouped into three categories (1) disease and injury, (2) work environment and work force, and (3) research tools and approaches. Priority needs for research in each area included the following:

DISEASE AND INJURY
- Allergic and irritant dermatitis
- Asthma and chronic obstructive pulmonary disease
- Fertility and pregnancy abnormalities
- Hearing loss
- Infectious diseases
- Low back disorders
- Cumulative trauma disorders
- Traumatic injuries

WORK ENVIRONMENT AND WORK FORCE
- Emerging technologies
- Indoor environment
- Mixed exposures
- Organization of work
- Special populations at risk

RESEARCH TOOLS AND APPROACHES
- Cancer research methods
- Control technology and personal protection
- Exposure assessment methods
- Health services research
- Intervention effectiveness research
- Risk assessment methods
- Social and economic consequences of illness and injury
- Surveillance research methods

1. Which of these areas would be appropriate for nursing research? Why?
2. Select two or three of the priority research areas and identify research questions related to each that would be of interest to community health nurses working in occupational health settings.
3. What variables would you study if you designed a study to answer one of the research questions you have identified?
4. In what type of work setting would you conduct a study of the research question selected? Will the type of setting chosen influence potential findings? In what way?

such situations as well as planning health care in such an eventuality. The role of the nurse in disaster preparedness is discussed in greater detail in Chapter 29.

Tertiary Prevention

Tertiary prevention in the work setting is directed toward preventing a recurrence of health problems and limiting their consequences. The types of tertiary intervention measures employed depend on the problems to be prevented. In many instances, primary prevention measures, which would be used to prevent a problem from occurring in the first place, can also be used as tertiary prevention to prevent its recurrence. For example, engineering measures may be used to prevent leakage of a toxic chemical or to prevent subsequent leaks if one has already occurred.

Generally speaking, tertiary prevention is geared toward preventing the spread of communicable diseases, preventing recurrence of other acute conditions, and preventing complications of chronic conditions. Sick-leave policies and employee immunization are examples of tertiary preventive measures that might be taken to stop the spread of influenza in the employee population. By encouraging employees to take advantage of sick-leave benefits when they or family members are ill, the nurse can minimize exposure of others in the occupational setting to communicable diseases and can control the spread of disease. Safety education might prevent a recurrence of accidental injuries due to hazardous equipment, and use of hearing protection might prevent further deterioration of an employee's hearing after noise exposure has already caused some damage. Similarly, treatment of an employee's hypertension can prevent further health problems.

Another aspect of tertiary prevention may be assessing an employee's fitness to return to work after an illness or injury (Cox & Edwards, 1995). Assessment considerations in this case would be similar to those in preemployment assessment.

Implementing Health Care in the Work Setting

Implementing nursing interventions in the work setting frequently involves collaboration with others. Most often, collaboration occurs between the nurse and the employee. In other instances, the nurse may collaborate with health care providers and others within or outside of the occupational setting. For example, the nurse might collaborate with a pregnant employee's private physician to monitor her progress

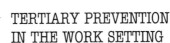

► TERTIARY PREVENTION IN THE WORK SETTING

- Preventing the spread of communicable disease through immunization and sick leave for ill employees
- Preventing the recurrence of other acute conditions
- Preventing complications of chronic conditions
- Assessing fitness to return to work

throughout the pregnancy. Implementing the plan of care for an employee with carpal tunnel syndrome might involve collaboration with the physician and with a supervisor to facilitate movement to a job that does not necessitate repetitive wrist movements.

When health problems affect groups of employees, implementing the plan of care might involve collaboration with other health care providers and with company management and other personnel. For example, the nurse who has documented an increased incidence of respiratory conditions due to aerosol exposures will advocate plans to resolve the problem. These plans need to be approved by management and implemented by engineering personnel, if engineering controls are required, or by company purchasing agents, if special respiratory protective devices are needed. In the latter instance, the nurse may be involved in determining the types of protective devices needed and recommending their purchase to management.

Evaluating Health Care in the Work Setting

As in all other settings for nursing practice, the effectiveness of health care in the work setting must be evaluated. Evaluation can focus on the outcomes of care either for the individual employee or for the total employee population. Evaluation is conducted on the basis of principles discussed in Chapters 7 and 19 and focuses on the achievement of expected outcomes and the processes used to achieve those outcomes. For example, the occupational health nurse may evaluate the effectiveness of body mechanics education in decreasing the incidence of back injuries. At the individual level, evaluation might focus on the impact of no-smoking education on an individual employee's smoking behavior. Achievement of objectives related to occupational health can be used to evaluate efforts at the national level. The status of selected national objectives is presented in Table 26–2.

TABLE 26–2. **STATUS OF SELECTED NATIONAL OBJECTIVES RELATED TO OCCUPATIONAL HEALTH**

	Objective	Base	Most Recent	Target
1.10	Companies with worksite fitness programs			
	50–99 employees	14% (1985)	33% (1992)	20%
	100–249 employees	23% (1985)	47% (1992)	35%
	250–749 employees	32% (1985)	66% (1992)	50%
	750 or more employees	54% (1985)	83% (1992)	80%
2.20	Worksite nutrition/weight management programs			
	Nutrition education	17% (1985)	31% (1992)	50%
	Weight control	15% (1985)	24% (1992)	50%
3.11	Worksite smoking policies	27% (1985)	59% (1992)	75%
6.11	Worksite stress management programs	27% (1985)	37% (1992)	40%
8.6	Worksite health promotion activities	66% (1985)	81% (1992)	85%
10.1	Work-related injury deaths (per 100,000)	6 (1983–1987)	4 (1994)	4
10.2	Nonfatal injuries (per 100)	7.7 (1983–1987)	8.4 (1994)	6
10.3	Cumulative trauma disorder (per 100,000)	100 (1987)	383 (1993)	60
10.4	Occupational skin disorders (per 100,000)	64 (1983)	81 (1994)	55
10.5	Hepatitis B infection (cases)	3090 (1987)	727 (1993)	1250
10.6	Worksite occupant protection systems mandated	82% (1992)	82% (1992)	95%
10.8	Occupational lead exposure	4804 (1988)	30,000 (1994)	0
10.9	Hepatitis B immunization	37% (1989)	71% (1994)	90%
10.10	States with occupational health and safety plans	10 (1989)	32 (1992)	50
10.12	Worksite health and safety programs	64% (1992)	64% (1992)	70%
10.13	Worksite back injury prevention/rehabilitation programs	29% (1985)	32% (1992)	50%
10.14	States with small business safety and health programs	26 (1991)	26 (1991)	50

(Sources: Bellingham & Pelletier, 1995; National Institute for Occupational Safety and Health, 1996a; U.S. Department of Health and Human Services, 1993, 1994, 1995a, 1995b.)

Critical Thinking in Practice: A Case in Point

You are a community health nurse employed by a large manufacturing plant. On Wednesday you see several employees complaining of abdominal cramping and diarrhea. They all state that their symptoms started at home during the night. You get word from one of the plant supervisors that several of her employees called in sick this morning because of similar symptoms. In checking with other departments, you find that there are a number of absences throughout the plant. Two of the older employees and one whom you know has AIDS have been hospitalized with severe dehydration. All of the people with cramps and diarrhea eat regularly in the cafeteria.

1. What are the biophysical, psychological, physical, social, behavioral, and health system factors operating in this situation?
2. What are your nursing diagnoses?
3. What are your client care objectives?
4. What secondary prevention measures will you employ in relation to your diagnoses? Why? What primary preventive measures might have prevented the occurrence of these problems? What tertiary prevention measures are warranted to prevent the recurrence of problems or complications?
5. How will you evaluate the effectiveness of your interventions?

TESTING YOUR UNDERSTANDING

1. Describe at least three advantages in providing health care in the work setting. (p. 642)
2. Identify at least six of the ten leading causes of health problems encountered in the work setting. Give at least one example of how a community health nurse working in an occupational setting might be involved in preventing conditions in each category. (p. 645)
3. Identify at least five types of health and safety hazards encountered in work settings. Describe at least one potential control measure for hazards in each category. (pp. 647–648)
4. Describe four spheres of social influence on the health of employees. (pp. 648–650)
5. Describe four potential types of health care programs in the work setting and the community health nurse's focus in assessing each. (pp. 652–654)
6. What are the three main areas of emphasis in primary prevention in the work setting? Given an example of a community health nursing intervention related to each area. (pp. 655–657)
7. Describe three major considerations in secondary prevention in the work setting. What activities might a community health nurse be involved in with respect to each? (pp. 657–660)
8. Describe three emphases in tertiary prevention in the work setting. Describe at least one community health nursing responsibility related to each area of emphasis. (p. 661)

WHAT DO YOU THINK?
Questions for Critical Thinking

1. Should women of childbearing age be prohibited from working in jobs that pose potential health risks for unborn children? Why or why not?
2. Why might an occupational health nurse be the most qualified person to coordinate an occupational health program?
3. Who should supervise the work of occupational health nurses? Why?
4. Should employee participation in health promotion activities be voluntary or mandatory? Why?
5. Should high-risk health behaviors be used as a reason not to employ someone who is otherwise qualified for a particular job? Why or why not?

REFERENCES

Alexander, B. H., Franklin, G. M., & Wolf, M. E. (1994). Sexual assault of women at work in Washington State. *American Journal of Public Health, 84,* 640–642.

Allegrante, J. P., & Goldfein, K. D. (1995). Ethical problems and related critical issues in worksite health promotion. In D. M. Dejoy & M. G. Wilson (Eds.), *Critical issues in worksite health promotion* (pp. 51–70). Boston: Allyn and Bacon.

American Association of Occupational Health Nurses. (1996). Code of ethics and interpretive statements. *AAOHN Journal, 44,* 432A.

Asfahl, C. R. (1995). *Industrial safety and health management* (3rd ed.). Englewood Cliffs, NJ: Prentice Hall.

Bellingham, R., & Pelletier, K. R. (1995). Health promotion in business and industry: An overview and status report. In D. M. Dejoy & M. G. Wilson (Eds.), *Critical issues in worksite health promotion* (pp. 3–27). Boston: Allyn and Bacon.

Brett, K. M., Strogatz, D. S., & Savitz, D. A. (1997). Employment, job strain, and preterm delivery among women in North Carolina. *American Journal of Public Health, 87,* 199–204.

Burgel, B. J. (1994). Occupational health: Nursing in the workplace. *Nursing Clinics of North America, 29,* 431–442.

Burgess, W. A. (1995). *Recognition of health hazards in industry: A review of materials and processes* (2nd ed.). New York: John Wiley & Sons.

California Occupational Health Program. (1992). *Understanding toxic substances: An introduction to chemical hazards in the workplace.* Berkeley, CA: California Occupational Health Program.

Cox, R. A. F., & Edwards, F. C. (1995). Introduction. In R. A. F. Cox, F. C. Edwards, & R. I. McCallum (Eds.), *Fitness for work: The medical aspects* (2nd ed.) (pp. 1–24). Oxford: Oxford University Press.

Csiernik, R. P. (1990). An EAP intervention protocol for occupational health nurses. *AAOHN Journal, 38,* 381–384.

Curtis, A. B., James, S. A., Raghunathan, T. E., & Alcser, K. H. (1997). Job strain and blood pressure in African Americans: The Pitt County study. *American Journal of Public Health, 87,* 1297–1302.

Dembe, A. E. (1996). *Occupation and disease: How social factors affect the conception of work-related disorders.* New Haven, CT: Yale University Press.

Everson, S. A., Lynch, J. W., Chesney, M. A., et al. (1997). Interaction of workplace demands and cardiovascular reactivity in progression of carotid atherosclerosis: Population based study. *British Medical Journal, 314,* 553–558.

Gold, D. R., Rocagz, S., Bock, et al., (1992). Rotating shift work, sleep, and accidents related to sleepiness in hospital nurses. *American Journal of Public Health, 82,* 1011–1014.

Grant, C. B., & Brisbin, R. E. (1992). *Workplace wellness: The key to higher productivity and lower health costs.* New York: Van Nostrand Reinhold.

Hartwell, T. D. Steele, P., French, M. T., Potter, F. J., Rodman, N. F., & Zarkin, G. A. (1996). Aiding troubled employees: The prevalence, cost, and characteristics of employee assistance programs in the United States. *American Journal of Public Health, 86,* 804–808.

Hughes, H. V. (1979). A view from the top: Today's needs in occupational health service. *Occupational Health Nurse, 27*(2), 13–15.

Johnson, J. V., Stewart, W., Hall, E. M., Fredlund, P., & Theorell, T. (1996). Long-term psychosocial work environment and cardiovascular mortality among Swedish men. *American Journal of Public Health, 86,* 324–331.

Kawachi, I., Colditz, G. A., Stampfer, M. J., et al. (1995). Prospective study of shift work and risk of coronary heart disease in women. *Circulation, 92,* 3178–3182.

Lipscomb, J., Burgel, B., McGill, L. W., & Blanc, P. (1994). Preventing occupational illness and injury: Nurse practitioners as primary care providers. *American Journal of Public Health, 84,* 643–645.

Martin, K. J. (1995). Workers' compensation: Case management strategies. *AAOHN Journal, 43,* 245–250.

Monaghan, M. (1995, November). Company nurses save money and ensure quality care. *NURSEweek,* 11.

National Institute for Occupational Safety and Health. (1994). Occupational injury deaths of postal workers—United States, 1980–1989. *MMWR, 43,* 594–595.

National Institute for Occupational Safety and Health. (1996a). *National occupational research agenda.* Cincinnati: National Institute for Occupational Safety and Health.

National Institute for Occupational Safety and Health. (1996b). *Violence in the workplace: Risk factors and prevention strategies.* Cincinnati: National Institute for Occupational Safety and Health.

North, F. M., Syme, S. L., Feeney, A., Shipley, M., & Marmot, M. (1996). Psychosocial work environment and sickness absence among British civil servants: The Whitehall II study. *American Journal of Public Health, 86,* 332–340.

Opatz, J., Chenoweth, D., & Kaman, R. (1994). Economic impact of worksite health promotion. In J. P. Opatz (Ed.), *Economic impact of worksite health promotion* (pp. 229–241). Champaign, IL: Human Kinetics.

Parrish, R. S., & Alfred, R. H. (1995). Theories and trends in occupational health nursing: Prevention and social change. *AAOHN Journal, 43,* 514–521.

Roman, P. M., & Blum, T. C. (1995). Contrasts and complements of employee assistance and health promotion programs in the worksite. In D. M. Dejoy & M. G. Wilson (Eds.), *Critical issues in worksite health promotion* (pp. 71–94). Boston: Allyn and Bacon.

Shulte, P. A., Burnett, C. A., Boeniger, M. F., & Johnson, J. (1996). Neurodegenerative diseases: Occupational occurrence and potential risk factors, 1982 through 1991. *American Journal of Public Health, 86,* 1281–1288.

Tereskerz, P. M., & Jagger, J. (1997). Occupationally acquired HIV: The vulnerability of health care workers under workers' compensation laws. *American Journal of Public Health, 87,* 1558–1562.

U.S. Department of Commerce. (1996). *Statistical abstract of the United States, 1996* (116th ed.). Washington, DC: Government Printing Office.

U.S. Department of Health and Human Services. (1991). *Healthy people 2000: National health promotion and disease prevention objectives.* Washington, DC: Government Printing Office.

U.S. Department of Health and Human Services. (1993). *Health United States, 1992, and healthy people 2000 review.* Washington, DC: Government Printing Office.

U.S. Department of Health and Human Services. (1994, August/September). Worksite programs target health and cost benefits. *Prevention Report, 1–2,* 4.

U.S. Department of Health and Human Services. (1995a). *Healthy people 2000: Midcourse review and 1995 revisions.* Washington, DC: Government Printing Office.

U.S. Department of Health and Human Services. (1995b). *Healthy people 2000: Progress report for occupational safety and health.* Washington, DC: Government Printing Office.

U.S. Department of Health and Human Services. (1996). *Health United States, 1995.* Washington, DC: Government Printing Office.

Wegman, D. H. (1992). The potential impact of epidemiology on the prevention of occupational disease. *American Journal of Public Health, 82,* 944–945.

Zwerling, G., Sprince, N. L., Wallace, R. B., Davis, C. S., Whitten, P. S., & Heeringa, S. G. (1996). Risk factors for occupational injuries among older workers: An analysis of the Health and Retirement Study. *American Journal of Public Health, 86,* 1306–1309.

RESOURCES FOR NURSES IN OCCUPATIONAL HEALTH SETTINGS

Disease Prevention

National High Blood Pressure Education Program
120/80 National Institutes of Health
Bethesda, MD 20014

Health Promotion

American College of Occupational and Environmental Medicine
55 West Seegers Road
Arlington Heights, IL 60005
(708) 228–6850

American College of Preventive Medicine
1660 L Street, Ste. 206
Washington, DC 20036–5603
(202) 466–2044

Association for Worksite Health Promotion
60 Revere Drive, Ste. 500
Northbrook, IL 60062–1577
(847) 480–9574

Health Education Foundation
2600 Virginia Avenue, NW, Ste. 502
Washington, DC 20037
(202) 338–3501

National Center for Health Education
72 Spring Street, Ste. 208
New York, NY 10012
(212) 334–9470

National Health Information Center
PO Box 1133
Washington, DC 20013–1133
(301) 565–4167

President's Council on Fitness and Sports
701 Pennsylvania Avenue, NW
Washington, DC 20202
(202) 272–3412

U.S. Department of Health and Human Services
Office of Health Information and Health Promotion
Washington, DC 20203

Mental Health

American Institute of Stress
124 Park Avenue
Yonkers, NY 10703
(914) 963–1200

The Other Victims of Alcoholism
PO Box 1528
Radio City Station, NY 10101
(212) 247–8087

Safety

American Industrial Health Council
2001 Pennsylvania Avenue, NW, Ste. 760
Washington, DC 20006
(202) 833–2131

National Institute of Occupational Health
and Safety
Office of Information
4676 Columbia Parkway
Cincinnati, OH 45226–1998
(800) 35–NIOSH

National Safety Council
1121 Spring Lake Drive
Itasca, IL 60143–3201
(708) 285–1121

Public Citizen Health Research Group
2000 P Street, NW, 7th Floor
Washington, DC 20036
(202) 833–3000

Toxic Project Clearinghouse Environmental Action
Foundation
6930 Carroll Avenue, 6th Floor
Takoma Park, MD 20912
(301) 891–1100

Other

American Association of Occupational Health Nurses
50 Lennox Pointe
Atlanta, GA 30324
(404) 262–1162

American Board for Occupational Health Nurses
9944 S. Roberts Road, Ste. 205
Palos Hills, IL 60465–1555
(708) 598–6368

Just One Break
373 Park Avenue, S
New York, NY 10016
(212) 725–2500

National Institute for Occupational Safety and Health
Humphrey Bldg., Room 715-H
Washington, DC 20201
(202) 401–6997

U.S. Department of Labor
Occupational Safety and Health Administration
Room N-3647
200 Constitution Avenue, NW
Washington, DC 20210
(202) 219–8151

U.S. House of Representatives Committee on Education and Labor
Subcommittee on Health and Safety
B 345-A Rayburn House Office Bldg.
Washington, DC 20510

U.S. Senate Committee on Appropriations
Subcommittee on Labor, Health and Human Services,
Education and Related Agencies
SD-186 Dirksen Senate Office Bldg.
Washington, DC 20510
(202) 224–7283

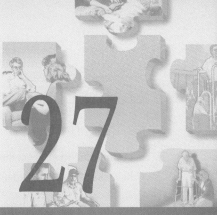

27

CARE OF CLIENTS
IN RURAL SETTINGS

Charlene M. Hanson

► KEY TERMS

advanced practice nurses
(APNs)
Community Nursing
Centers (CNCs)
frontier
nurse generalist
rural
stroke belt
urban

Rural community health nursing requires high levels of skill and competence. Although rural nursing may offer less opportunity for interchange with colleagues, there are many rewards. Nurses who practice in small rural communities form close relationships with clients and their families. They also tend to exhibit higher levels of autonomy and job satisfaction than do their urban counterparts (Bigbee, 1993). The unique relationship with client and family includes "knowing" the family well, understanding some of the strengths and weaknesses of the family structure, and being sensitive to family support systems. Community activities related to helping families prevent illness can be one of the most rewarding aspects of rural community health nursing. Rural community health nursing, with its commitment to health promotion and holistic family-centered primary care, plays a central role in improving the health of rural Americans.

Rural community health nursing offers the nurse unique opportunities to care for clients within a broad practice environment with high potential for autonomy and job satisfaction. The focus of this chapter is to identify the many ways in which community health nurses can provide health care to rural-based people within the context of rural culture and ethnicity. Differences in lifestyle and in the health problems rural populations experience are explored using the Dimensions Model.

▶ Chapter Objectives

After reading this chapter, you should be able to:

- Describe three domains of the concept of rurality.
- Describe at least four barriers to effective health care in rural areas.
- Identify two age groups at particular risk for health problems in rural settings.
- Describe at least five physical dimension concerns unique to rural settings.
- Identify four major occupational and safety risk factors for rural populations.
- Discuss two aspects of the impact of health policy on rural community health care.
- Identify three aspects of primary prevention in rural settings.
- Describe four approaches to secondary prevention in rural settings.

▶ WHAT IS URBAN? WHAT IS RURAL?

There is no generally accepted definition of what is rural or what is urban. Some authors note the existence of three *domains of rurality,* an ecological domain, an occupational domain, and a sociocultural domain (Miller, Farmer, & Clarke, 1994). The focus in the ecological domain is the spatial dispersion of the population which may reflect one of three dominant concepts: (1) the total number of persons living in an area, (2) distance from a large metropolitan area, or (3) density of the population (National Institute for Nursing Research, 1995). In the occupational domain, emphasis is placed on traditional rural occupations such as agriculture and extractive industries (eg, mining, fishing, logging). Finally, in the sociocultural domain, rurality is reflected in a set of shared ideals and values structure (Miller, et al., 1994).

According to the U.S. Census Bureau, rural populations are those inhabited by fewer than 2500 residents (American College of Physicians, 1995) and rural counties are those consisting of open area or counties with no cities larger then 25,000 population (Hospital Research and Education Trust, 1992). The U.S. Office of Management and Budget uses the alternative designations *metropolitan* (counties or groups of counties with populations of at least 50,000 people) and *nonmetropolitan* (American College of Physicians, 1995). Other groups advocate using a continuum to describe rurality. For example, the National Rural Health Association (Miller, et al., 1994) identified adjacent rural areas (those near a metropolitan statistical area, or MSA), urbanized rural areas (those with populations greater than 25,000, but not included in an MSA), frontier areas (those with a population density of less than 6 people per square mile), and countryside rural areas (the rest of the country excepting MSAs). For the sake of consistency, the Census Bureau definition of rural and urban will be used in this chapter. Descriptors of rural and urban areas are summarized in Table 27–1.

▶ THE RURAL POPULATION

Approximately one fourth of the U.S. population lived in rural areas at the time of the 1990 census (U.S. Department of Commerce, 1996). This is a far lower proportion of the population than the 95% found in rural areas in the first census, conducted in 1790 (Miller, et al., 1994). Despite this decrease in the proportion of people living in rural areas, the number of rural residents is actually greater now than at any time in history (Bigbee, 1993).

The popular perception of rural areas includes rolling farms and isolated farm families. The reality of rural life is better exemplified by the axiom, "If you've seen one rural community, you've seen one rural com-

TABLE 27–1. DESCRIPTORS OF RURAL AND URBAN AREAS

Source	Rural Descriptors	Urban Descriptors
U.S. Census Bureau	Rural: areas with populations less than 2500 persons	Urban: areas with populations greater than 2500 persons
U.S. Office of Management and Budget	Nonmetropolitan areas: areas with populations less than 50,000 persons	Metropolitan Statistical Areas (MSAs): areas with populations greater than 50,000 persons
National Rural Health Association	Adjacent rural areas: areas near or in a Metropolitan Statistical Area Urbanized rural areas: areas with populations greater than 25,000 but not part of a Metropolitan Statistical Area Frontier areas: areas with a population density less than six persons per square mile Countryside rural areas: all other areas of the country outside Metropolitan Statistical Areas	Metropolitan Statistical Areas

munity" (cited in Miller, et al., 1994). This axiom highlights the tremendous diversity found in rural populations today. Some rural residents continue to be engaged in agriculture, but other industries are also found in rural areas. Some of these are traditional rural industries such as mining and logging; others reflect the movement of large manufacturing concerns to rural areas. Rural areas also include many small towns with a service economy and, in some parts of the country, have become a haven for retirees who have health needs similar to those of any aging population. The rural population also includes 3 to 5 million seasonal farm workers who have unique health needs characteristic of a migratory lifestyle. A further segment of the rural population lives in rural areas, but works in nearby cities.

▶ RURAL COMMUNITY HEALTH NURSING

Rural nursing has been defined as "the practice of professional nursing within the physical and sociocultural context of sparsely populated communities" (Bigbee, 1993). In one study, less than 9% of 1.6 million RNs in the United States were practicing in rural areas, despite the fact that 25% of the population lives in these areas. Rural community health nursing originated around 1896 with the advent of rural nursing projects such as the one established in Winchester, New York (Bigbee, 1993). In 1912, the American Red Cross founded the Rural Nursing Service which later became the Town and Country Nursing Service. This organization was credited with decreasing infant and overall mortality and improving sanitation, hygiene, and nutrition in rural populations (Anderson & Yuhos, 1993). The Town and Country Nursing Service continued until 1947 when it was disbanded due to the rise of official nursing agencies in state and local health departments. Other rural nursing services were provided by organizations such as the Frontier Nursing Service established by Mary Breckenridge in 1925 (Bigbee, 1993). More recent developments in rural nursing include the Migrant Health Act of 1962 which established the Migrant Health Program (Hibbeln, 1996) and the passage of the Rural Health Clinic Service Act in 1978 (Thornton, 1996). Both of these pieces of legislation provided funding for health care services in rural areas that have addressed some of the health needs of the rural population.

Other needs, however, still remain to be met and provide a fertile ground for community health nursing practice with rural populations. Some of these needs are reflected in specific health objectives for the year 2000 for migrant and seasonal farmworkers (Na-

▶ MIGRANT AND SEASONAL FARMWORKER HEALTH OBJECTIVES

Health Promotion
- Improve nutrition
- Improve mental health and prevent mental illness
- Improve maternal and infant health
- Improve oral health
- Improve reproductive health

Prevention of Illness and Injury
- Reduce environmental health hazards
- Improve occupational safety and health
- Immunize against infectious diseases
- Prevent and control unintentional injuries
- Prevent chronic diseases and other disorders
- Prevent HIV infection

Secondary Prevention
- Reduce alcohol and other drug abuse
- Reduce violent and abusive behavior
- Control HIV infection and AIDS
- Reduce adolescent pregnancy
- Detect and control chronic diseases and other disorders
- Control infectious diseases

Health Care Delivery
- Improve health education
- Improve access to preventive health services
- Improve surveillance and data systems

(Source: National Migrant Resource Program, 1990.)

tional Migrant Resource Program, 1990). These objectives are summarized above in terms of their focus on health promotion, illness and injury prevention, secondary prevention, and health care delivery.

Community health nurses may be the only health care providers in many rural localities (Horner, et al., 1994), so they must be able to function as highly expert generalists to meet the needs of rural populations (Long, Scharff, & Weinert, 1997). In addition to this generalist perspective, rural community health nursing is characterized by close community ties and relationships, role diffusion, autonomy and self-direction, cohesiveness, and increased visibility within the community (Bigbee, 1993). Rural community health nurses may find themselves faced with limited back-up, long hours, and limited opportunities for educational advancement. In addition, many nurses are not educationally prepared for the challenges of rural nursing (American Nurses Association, 1996). For many nurses, however, rural community health nursing can be a rewarding and fulfilling experience.

Health problems encountered in rural community health nursing practice are intensified by several major barriers to effective care. These barriers include few health care providers, distance to existing health care facilities, lack of diversity in services available, poverty and a dwindling rural economy, health policy inequities (American Hospital Association, 1993), and reliance on informal support networks (Wagner, Menke, & Ciccone, 1995). These barriers to care will be addressed in more detail in the application of the Dimensions Model to health care in rural settings described in the remainder of this chapter.

▶ THE DIMENSIONS MODEL AND CARE OF CLIENTS IN RURAL SETTINGS

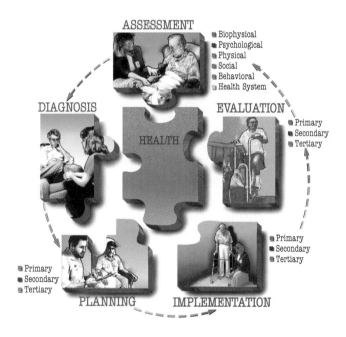

The Dimensions Model lends itself to the assessment of health needs and planning for primary, secondary, and tertiary care in rural settings. Using this model, the community health nurse can identify the health needs of rural residents and explore ways to improve their access to care.

Critical Dimensions of Nursing in Rural Health Care

Special considerations arise in each of the six dimensions of nursing as applied to the care of rural populations. The critical feature of the cognitive dimension is the breadth of knowledge required of the rural community health nurse. As noted earlier, rural nurses are

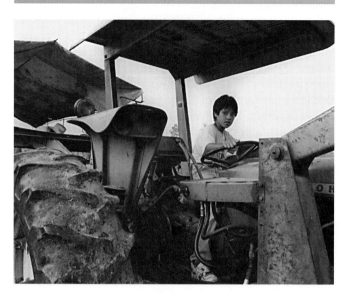

Rural community health nursing offers the nurse unique opportunities to care for clients within a broad practice environment.
Photo courtesy of Charlene Hanson. Photo credit: Denise Wilkerson.

often the only health care providers in many sparsely populated areas and therefore must function as extremely knowledgeable generalists. Some authors note that many tasks performed elsewhere by other health professionals are "by default or design, performed by rural nurses" (Long, et al. 1997) necessitating a broader knowledge base than might be required of nurses in other practice settings.

The close community ties and relationships experienced by rural community health nurses create advantages while also posing potential difficulties. The nurse's increased visibility in the community provides opportunities for assessing health needs and for developing interventions acceptable to community members (Anderson & Yuhos, 1993). This same visibility, however, may lead to burnout when the nurse is expected to help with every health-related and many nonhealth-related community problems (Bigbee, 1993). The nurse's isolation in the community may make it difficult to engage in collaborative relationships with other health care providers, but places the nurse at an advantage in engaging community members in health-related activities. The nurse may also experience difficulty in separating personal and professional relationships.

Increasing visibility and close relationships may also have implications in the ethical dimension of community health nursing. Maintaining confidentiality and rights to privacy may be more difficult in settings where nurses have limited anonymity (Bigbee, 1993). Nurses may also find it more imperative, and simultaneously, more difficult to advocate for the needs of vulnerable and underserved rural subpopulations, such as migrant laborers, the homeless, and persons with HIV infection. Advocacy may be further complicated by the traditionally conservative values held by many members of rural populations (Bigbee, 1993).

In keeping with the role diffusion characteristic of rural nursing, community health nurses may be called on to exhibit a wider variety of skills and employ a broader array of processes than their urban counterparts. Again, because of their visibility and isolation as providers, rural community health nurses often play a significant part in policy development and must be skilled in the political and change processes. Traditional rural reliance on informal helping networks may often require the community health nurse to exercise leadership in coordinating a variety of lay helpers in meeting the needs of rural clients.

Research is critically needed on health care delivery in rural settings. Much of the research on which modern health care is based has been conducted in urban settings and with urban populations. One cannot assume that solutions to health problems that work in urban settings will be equally effective in rural areas. For example, a relatively frequent approach to improving access to care in urban settings is a mobile health facility. This type of solution would not be cost-effective in many rural areas, however, because of the sparsity of the population and the distances between client groups (American Nurses Association, 1996).

 ## Assessing the Dimensions of Health in the Rural Setting

The health care needs of rural populations are assessed using the six dimensions of health (biophysical, psychological, physical, social, behavioral, and health system). These factors are considered within the context of rural culture and rural living patterns.

The Biophysical Dimension

Genetic Inheritance. Genetic factors most prevalent within the rural setting are those associated with rural-based minority aggregates. For example, the genetic predisposition to diabetes mellitus and chronic alcoholism among Native Americans is a well-known and serious health problem. Rural African American families may have unusually strong histories of hypertension, stroke, or sickle cell anemia. Moreover, African American women have a higher risk for breast cancer. As America's rural Asian population continues to increase, genetic disorders related to these ethnic groups will become statistically more evident in the rural population mix of the United States.

The migrant farmworker population is highly diverse, comprised of Latinos, African-Americans, Native Americans, Haitians (Hibbeln, 1996), and some Caucasians. An estimated 16% of this population is female (Maternal and Child Health Bureau, 1997) and rural elders tend to be predominantly women (Miller, et al., 1994).

Maturation and Aging. Compared to urban populations, the very young and the elderly are disproportionately represented in rural areas (National Institute for Nursing Research, 1995). The growth in the rural elderly population is a result of both "aging in place" by many long-time residents and out-migration of younger adults moving to urban areas (Vrabek, 1995). Roughly one third of the elderly population in the United States are rural residents and one of every eight rural citizens is elderly compared to one in ten in urban areas (Bigbee, 1993).

Twenty-eight percent of U.S. children live in rural areas (Bigbee, 1993), and children under 15 years of age constitute 20% of the farm population (Schenker, Lopez, & Wintemute, 1995). Farmworkers' children are not covered by child labor laws and may legally begin work in the fields as early as age 10 (Hibbeln, 1996). Because of their continuing physiologic development, children are particularly susceptible to the effects of many health hazards prevalent in rural areas. Malnutrition, pesticide poisoning, infectious diseases, and injuries are prevalent among migrant farmworkers' children.

Physiologic Function. Although mortality rates are slightly lower in rural than urban settings (Beaulieu, 1994), rural residents have significant health problems related to infectious and chronic diseases, disability, and birth outcomes. Infectious diseases are particularly prevalent among migrant farmworkers who are subjected to crowded living conditions, poor sanitation, and contaminated water. Parasitic infestations are also common in this population. Tuberculosis is six times more prevalent among migrants than in the general population. Sexually transmitted diseases are also prevalent because of limited health knowledge in this area (Hibbeln, 1996). The incidence of HIV infection and AIDS is increasing in rural areas in general and treatment is complicated by the absence, in many areas, of interdisciplinary discharge planning, specialty facilities, treatment options, and home care services (Sowell & Opava, 1995).

Morbidity for most chronic conditions is higher in rural than urban settings. For example, rural populations have higher rates than their urban counterparts for heart disease, hypertension, cerebrovascular disease, chronic bronchitis, asthma, chronic sinusitis, arthritis, gout, and orthopedic impairments. Higher rates are also noted for problems such as visual and hearing impairment, cataracts, glaucoma (Beaulieu, 1994), diabetes, and cancer (American Nurses Association, 1996). Disability figures show similar discrepancies between rural and urban dwellers. For example, almost 11% of rural residents report major activity limitations compared to less than 9% of their urban counterparts, and figures for any limitation of activity are 14.9% and 12.6%, respectively. These discrepancies are even more pronounced among those over 75 years of age, with 45% of rural elders reporting some limitation compared to 41% of urban dwellers of the same age (Beaulieu, 1994).

Birth outcomes are also less favorable for rural residents than for the urban population. The infant mortality rate in rural areas is 15 per 1000 live births compared to a national rate of 11.2 (Bigbee, 1993). The prevalence of low birth weight is also higher, particularly among migrant women for whom low birth weight occurs in 6.7% of pregnancies compared to a national average of 5% (Maternal and Child Health Bureau, 1997).

The Psychological Dimension

Many people think of rural areas as places to get away from the stress of urban life. Persistent economic problems experienced by farmers in the last decade, however, have brought the stress faced by rural farming families to national attention. Crop failures triggered by severe weather conditions, coupled with a declining economy, have caused excessive emotional and physiological stress for farm families nationwide. These factors have contributed to mental and physical disabilities among rural clients as well as to substance abuse and family violence. Increased cases of suicide, situational depression, gastrointestinal diseases, and eating disorders are only a few of the rural health problems arising from economic stress.

Another area needing assessment from a psychological standpoint is that of family violence and neglect. Research indicates that isolation and lack of day care and other support services for the young and the aged are contributing factors in child abuse, spouse and elder battering, and neglect. The close contact that community health nurses have with rural families offers an opportunity for early identification

---

Critical Thinking in Research

Silveira and Winstead-Fry (1997) conducted a study of the physical and psychological needs of rural clients with cancer and their caregivers. Participants were asked to complete needs scales of 104 items (clients) or 90 items (caregivers) indicating whether or not they perceived a particular item as a need, the importance of that need for them, and whether or not the identified needs were met. Most clients identified needs related to personal care issues such as being able to carry out physician orders, relief of anxiety through information about symptoms, receipt of treatments or medicines on time, and good physical care. Clients also identified needs related to their involvement with health care providers such as knowing when to call the provider, getting honest information about their condition, and receiving relevant information about their condition. Interpersonal interactions expected of providers by clients included respect, cheerfulness, consideration for family members, listening, and being well organized. Caregivers identified similar personal care needs including the need to know the client is comfortable and knowing how to observe for treatment effects and symptoms of health status changes. Health care involvement needs reported by caregivers included information about the client's condition and any changes noted, assurance of the availability of services if needed, and available emergency help. Interpersonal interaction needs for caregivers included needs for communication with the client and support from other family members.

1. What nursing interventions might help meet the needs for clients and caregivers? Would the interventions be different for the two groups? Why or why not?
2. How would you test the effectiveness of your interventions in meeting the needs of clients and caregivers? What variables do you think you would examine? How would you go about measuring them?
3. Do you think the needs identified would have been different if an urban population had been studied? Why or why not?

---

of all kinds of family violence. The lack of resources for early referral for mental health problems increases the prevalence of these problems for both individual clients and family members.

In assessing the psychological dimension, the community health nurse examines the effects of the economic climate of the area on residents' psychological health as well as the incidence of indicators of emotional distress such as substance abuse, violence, and depression. In addition, the nurse assesses individual clients and families for evidence of psychological distress.

The Physical Dimension

The rural environment is often thought to be a healthy, stress-free place to live; however the physical dimension presents a variety of health hazards related to weather, housing and sanitary conditions, isolation, and the presence of disease-causing vectors. Weather hazards may include disasters such as tornadoes and drought that may have severe effects on rural families as well as on the rural economy. Other, more routine hazards may also be experienced, particularly by farm families and migrant workers. These hazards include constant exposure to temperature extremes, sun, dust, wind, rain, and pesticides (Hibbeln, 1996). Housing and sanitation hazards may be experienced by migrant farmworkers as well as other rural residents. Migrant families frequently live in substandard housing without ventilation, plumbing, or adequate space. Water sources are often limited to irrigation ditches containing water contaminated with pesticides, fertilizers, and human wastes (National Migrant Resource Program, 1990). Rural elders may also live in inadequate housing. Although they are somewhat more likely than their urban counterparts to own their homes, those homes are more likely to be in disrepair and without indoor plumbing (Beaulieu, 1994). Water is frequently obtained from private wells and natural springs which may also be contaminated with pollutants and infectious agents.

Geographic isolation is another physical dimension factor that influences health. Isolation can contribute to psychological dimension factors such as depression and family violence (American Nurses Association, 1996). Great distances and rugged terrain may also limit rural residents' access to health care services, particularly when coupled with the lack of public transportation typical of rural areas. Approximately 40% of people at a transportation disadvantage live in rural areas (Vrabec, 1995). Distance is a particularly significant factor in the care of clients with conditions that require intensive special care such as cancer treatment (Silveira & Winstead-Fry, 1997). Finally, rural localities increase the potential for exposure to animal and insect vectors of disease.

The Social Dimension

Each rural community is unique and needs to be considered separately from others. Because of the special flavor of the social environment in rural communities, researchers have found that urban models of health care delivery superimposed on rural communities frequently do not work. For this reason the community health nurse needs to know the internal workings of the community to design health care programs that best meet the needs of rural people. Social dimension factors to be considered include traditionalism and self-reliance, education and economic concerns, political inequities, homelessness, and occupational concerns.

▶ **SOCIAL DIMENSION ASSESSMENT CONSIDERATIONS IN RURAL SETTINGS**

- What is the economic status of the community? What are the mean and median salaries of community residents?
- What are the transportation needs of community members? How are they met?
- What education facilities are available to community residents? Are they adequate to meet the education needs of community members?
- What social support services are available within the community? How accessible are these services to the needy? Are services adequate to meet the needs of community members?
- How cohesive is the community? Is there conflict between groups within the community?
- What are the attitudes of community members toward health and healthy behaviors?
- What cultural groups are represented in the community? To what extent does culture influence the health and health practices of community members?
- What religious groups are represented in the community? What is the influence of religion on the health of community members?
- What values are held by members of the community? How do values influence health and health care?
- Who can be relied on to help with finances, transportation, meals, and other needs?
- What child care services are available in the community? Are they adequate to meet community members' needs?

Rural communities are traditionally conservative, both morally and politically. This conservatism tends to increase residents' faith in local institutions, particularly church, family, and friends, and leads to a reliance on self and informal helping networks. Rural families tend to display traditional values and family roles that may lead to early marriage, larger families, and lower divorce rates (Bigbee, 1993). Rural elders, for example, are more likely to be married, live in family households rather than alone, and have more children than their urban counterparts. They also exhibit more frequent interaction with children and neighbors, but it is unclear what level of assistance is provided by these networks. Rural elders are also more likely than urban dwellers to be actively involved in church activities and less likely to participate in other organizations (Stoller & Lee, 1994).

Educationally, rural populations are less highly educated than urban populations. In the most remote rural areas, for example, more than 17% of the population has less than 9 years of education (Miller, et al., 1994). Education level is even lower for migrant and seasonal workers with less than half completing 9 or more years of school (National Migrant Resource Program, 1990) and 30% having fewer than 5 years of education (Hibbeln, 1996).

Rural economic situations also contribute to health problems. The rural economy overall is in a decline due to reductions in agriculture and extractive industries. Unemployment is high, and many rural jobs are low-paying positions (American Hospital Association, 1993). In addition, there is a growing gap in income levels between urban and rural areas (Miller, et al., 1994). Overall, in 1987, 17% of the rural population had incomes below poverty level (Wagner, et al., 1995). Approximately 25% of rural elders have incomes below poverty level compared to 18% of the urban elderly (Vrabec, 1995). Income levels are even lower for migrant and seasonal farmworkers who are hampered by short-term work contracts and lack of eligibility for unemployment compensation. Even during peak work seasons, migrant workers are considered "seriously underemployed" (Hibbeln, 1996).

The economic situation of migrant workers is further complicated by political inequities. Despite the fact that 80% of migrant workers are U.S. citizens, they are not covered by the National Labor Relations Act which governs minimum wages. They are also excluded from workers' compensation and unemployment insurance programs in many states (Hibbeln, 1996). Inequities also occur for other segments of the rural population. For example, rural elders have been shown to receive social security benefits 10% lower than those residing in urban areas and many rural elders are not covered at all, having retired from occupations that are not covered by Social Security. Discriminatory policies also extend to Medicare and Medicaid reimbursement for health care services; limited payments under these programs in rural areas makes it difficult to attract and retain health care providers for rural practice (American Hospital Association, 1993).

Homelessness is a condition usually associated with inner city populations; however, there is a growing problem of homelessness in rural areas. Rural homelessness tends to be more prevalent in agricultural areas and areas with declining extractive industries. Even when rural economies are burgeoning, the possibility of employment attracts more job seekers than the jobs available creating more demand for limited housing. Additional factors in rural homelessness are restrictive land use regulations and prohibitions on living in housing while fixing it for habitation and on the use of used building materials (Aron & Fitchen, 1996).

The final social dimension consideration to be assessed is that of occupation. Primary occupations in rural areas include farming, mining and other extractive industries, and manufacturing (Hospital Research and Education Trust, 1992). Approximately 13% of rural counties are primarily involved in farming activities and 40% in manufacturing efforts (American Nurses Association, 1996). Agricultural work, in particular, is physically demanding and may involve fast-paced repetitive tasks that involve bending and stooping. In addition, 80% of all pesticides are used in agriculture increasing the potential for pesticide exposures and poisoning, particularly for farmworkers' children. Unsafe transportation between worksites and migrant camps also presents a safety hazard (Hibbeln, 1996). Noise-induced hearing loss is another occupational hazard associated with farming, and in one study, 50% of farmworkers had experienced significant hearing loss by age 50 (National Institute for Nursing Research, 1995).

In 1994, mining had the highest rate of occupational fatality in the nation, 27 deaths per 100,000 workers followed by agricultural pursuits at 26 per 100,000. Fatalities occurring in manufacturing, another common rural occupation, amounted to only 4 per 100,000 workers. For nonfatal injuries and illness, manufacturing had the highest rates at 12.2 per 100 workers or 12% of the work force in this occupation. Construction had an injury and illness rate of 11.8 per 100 workers. Injury rates for mining were comparatively low at 6.3 per 100. In 1994, 590,000 disabling injuries occurred in manufacturing throughout the country (urban and rural areas), 140,000 in agriculture, and 20,000 in mining and quarrying (U.S. Department of Commerce, 1996).

Injuries and fatalities are particularly prevalent among farm children. Approximately 300 children die each year and 25,000 are injured in farm accidents (Hibbeln, 1996). In some areas, as much as one fourth of all farm injuries involve children under age 15 (Schenker, et al., 1995).

The Behavioral Dimension

Behavioral assessment considerations in rural settings relate to leisure activity risks, daily consumption patterns, and other health-related behaviors.

Leisure Activity Risks. Some rural families tend to be "tied down" by the need to care for crops and animals. The majority, however, go to work each day in structured nonfarm work settings. Getting together for family outings and church programs is common, and food-oriented activities are prevalent. Obesity, diabetes, and high cholesterol levels are common health problems related to leisure activities in rural areas.

Organized recreational activities are carried out primarily in either schools or churches. There are few job-related or freestanding "health clubs" with professional personnel to oversee exercise programs. Community-sponsored recreation centers and state parks offer other avenues for leisure activities. Exercise may be lacking for rural residents other than those whose occupations entail strenuous physical activity, since members of rural populations are less likely than their urban counterparts to exercise regularly (American College of Physicians, 1995).

Consumption Patterns. Major health-related consumption patterns of rural people include those related to smoking, diet and nutrition, and substance abuse. As noted earlier, many social activities in rural areas center around food consumption and may contribute to problems of obesity and hypercholesterolemia. Adequate nutrition may be particularly problematic for migrant farmworkers who may rely on significant amounts of convenience foods while working and who have limited budgets for providing adequate diets (National Migrant Resource Program, 1990). In addition, English language difficulties may force many families to rely on children to read labels and make food choices with children selecting foods with high sugar content and few vegetables and fruits. The absence of adequate refrigeration and cooking facilities may further hamper efforts to provide adequate family nutrition. Common health problems in migrant workers with nutritional deficits include anemia, diabetes, obesity, and cardiovascular disease (Hibbeln, 1996).

Although rural areas are sometimes considered health and drug-free, being farther from potential sources of illicit drugs, substance abuse is a significant problem in many rural communities. This may be particularly true among young people who have few leisure opportunities and turn to substance use out of boredom. Substance abuse also occurs among migrant and seasonal farmworkers (National Migrant Resource Program, 1990). Tobacco use, in both chewed and smoked forms, is still common in many rural areas (National Institute for Nursing Research, 1995).

Other Health-related Bheaviors. Other risky health behaviors include riding in the back of open pick-up trucks and failure to use seat belts (Bigbee, 1993). The final behavioral consideration to be assessed is that of sexual behavior. Despite more traditional family-oriented value systems that may be prevalent in many rural communities, rural youth have been shown to engage in sexual activity as often or even more often than their urban counterparts. Although rural youth in some studies have greater knowledge in areas such as HIV-prevention, they were more likely to be sexually active and to engage in risky sexual behaviors than urban youth. They were also more apt to combine alcohol use and sexual activity (Polivka, 1996).

The Health System Dimension

Both the external and internal health care systems influence health and illness in rural communities. The goal for successful access to rural health care is to coordinate the efforts of the external federal and state programs with the internal community-based health care system to create a strong collaborative partnership.

The formal health care system in rural settings needs to fit into the informal rural helping system. The use of old and trusted resources rather than "outsider" influence is often the key to success in health care programming in rural areas. It is important to recognize that rural people constitute a large segment of the population who have little or no health insurance coverage. Rural residents without insurance often "fall through the cracks" of the health care system and are in need of health care services. Fixing the health care system from outside the community often does not have lasting effects because of environmental constraints related to distance, poor transportation, and few economic resources.

The External System: National and State Programs. The heightened awareness of health concerns in rural areas has strengthened federal support for rural health care. Federally funded rural health clinics and community health clinics offer primary health care to local residents. In these clinics, nurse practitioners, supported by collaborative physician back-up, assess clients and manage care for a variety of health problems. Mental health clinics, detoxification units, and substance abuse follow-up programs receive funding priorities at both the state and national levels. In addition, new programs for addicted pregnant women are springing up throughout the nation. These federal and state initiatives provide community health nurses with much needed resources to assist high-risk rural clients.

Both Medicare and Medicaid programs provide health care coverage for members of rural population groups. Compared to urban health systems, in fact, rural systems may have proportionally higher numbers of Medicare and Medicaid clients (70% of the clientele in some areas), limiting the ability of rural providers to offset the effects of low reimbursement rates for these programs with fees from privately insured or fee-for-service clients. Rural areas also expe-

ASSESSMENT TIPS: Assessing Health in Rural Settings

Biophysical Dimension

Age and Genetic Inheritance

What is the age composition of the rural population? What is the proportion of children and elderly?

What is the infant mortality rate for the rural community?

What is the relative proportion of males and females in the rural setting?

What is the racial/ethnic composition in the rural setting?

What is the prevalence of genetic predisposition to disease in the rural population? What diseases are involved?

Physiologic Function

What existing health problems are prevalent in the rural population?

What is the incidence of communicable diseases in the rural population?

What is the extent of disability in the rural population?

What are the immunization levels in the rural population?

Psychological Dimension

What sources of stress are experienced by members of the rural population?

What is the extent of family violence in the rural population?

What is the prevalence of mental health problems in the rural population?

Physical Dimension

To what extent are rural residents exposed to extreme weather conditions? What health hazards are presented by weather conditions?

What is the potential for exposure to hazardous substances? What substances are involved?

What is the quality of housing in the rural area? Is housing in good repair or does it present health and safety hazards?

What safety hazards are presented by the rural environment (eg, poor roads, heavy equipment)?

What is the usual source of water? Is the water safe for consumption?

How is waste disposal handled? Does waste disposal pose health hazards?

To what extent is the rural community geographically isolated? What effect does isolation have on the community?

What is the prevalence of disease-causing vectors in the area?

What is the potential for disaster in the rural area?

Social Dimension

Interpersonal Interactions

How cohesive is the rural community?

What values are held by members of the rural community?

What racial, ethnic, and cultural groups are represented in the rural community? Is there evidence of intergroup conflict?

What languages are spoken in the rural community?

What are the primary modes of communication within the community?

What is the extent of social interaction in the rural community? Where does this interaction take place?

What is the extent of social support among rural residents?

Socioeconomic Factors

What is the education level of the rural population? What is the extent of their health knowledge?

What education facilities are available in the rural community? How adequate are they?

What is the state of the local economy?

What is the income level of community members? Is income adequate to meet needs?

What types of work are performed by rural residents? What health hazards are posed by the types of work available?

Is there a migrant or seasonal work force in the area? What social problems do they experience? What is the attitude of other community members to migrant workers?

What is the unemployment level in the rural community?

What is the extent of homelessness in the rural community? What types of assistance are available for homeless persons?

Other Social Factors

What transportation services are available to rural residents?

Does the rural community have a plan for disaster events?

ASSESSMENT TIPS: Assessing Health in Rural Settings (cont.)

Behavioral Dimension

What is the overall nutritional level of the rural population?

What is the extent of alcohol, tobacco, and other drug use in the rural population?

What is the prevalence of substance abuse in the population?

Exercise and Leisure Activity

What is the extent of exercise in the rural population?

What recreational opportunities are available to rural residents? Do recreational activities pose health hazards?

Safety Practices

To what extent are safety measures used by rural residents (eg, seat belts)?

Sexual Activity

To what extent do rural residents engage in unsafe sexual practices?

Health System Dimension

What are rural residents' attitudes toward health and health care? How do they define health and illness?

What health services are available to rural residents? Are the available services adequate to meet needs?

What factors deter health providers from locating in the rural area?

Are primary preventive services available and are they used by community residents?

To what extent are specialty services available in the community? If there are none, where do rural residents obtain care?

How accessible are needed health services in the community? What is the usual distance to health care facilities?

To what extent does the rural population use available health services? What barriers to health service use exist?

Are there folk health practitioners providing services in the area? To what extent are their services used by members of the rural population?

How are health care services funded? Is funding adequate to meet health needs?

What is the extent of the uninsured or underinsured population in the rural community?

---

rience larger populations of underinsured persons, although the proportion of uninsured residents is similar to that found in urban areas. Rural areas also bear the burden of services for many undocumented migrants and seasonal workers (Coburn & Mueller, 1995). Even for those clients who are covered under federal programs such as Medicare and Medicaid, reimbursement rates for comparable services are less than those in urban areas (American Hospital Association, 1993).

The Internal System: Local Community Care and Family-centered Care. Health care services for many rural residents are less accessible, more costly to deliver, narrower in range and scope, and fewer in number than those available to their urban counterparts. This is true for most professional services including those of physicians, dentists, nurses, and social workers and is particularly true of services for the elderly in rural areas.

There is a severe shortage of health care providers in many rural areas. In fact, approximately 20 million rural residents live in designated provider

shortage areas and 92% of all counties with nursing shortages in particular are rural counties. The ratio of nurse to clients drops from 675 per 100,000 population in the United States in general to 349 per 100,000 in the most sparsely populated counties (American Nurses Association, 1996). Many of the nurses who do work in rural areas are older and have less education; more than 77% of nurses in nonmetropolitan areas have a diploma or associate degree in nursing. Historically, rural nurses often assume advanced practice roles due to a dearth of physicians in rural areas. The proportion of nurse practitioners in rural settings, however, has declined from more than 50% of the nation's nurse practitioners in 1980 to 9% in 1988. In addition, nurse practitioners in rural areas are less likely than their urban counterparts to be prepared at the baccalaureate or higher levels in nursing (Bigbee, 1993).

Similar figures are noted for coverage by physicians and other health care providers in rural settings. The National Health Service Corps (NHSC) was established in 1972 to provide health manpower for rural areas. Since its inception, more than 20,000 health professionals have been placed in underserved areas and currently 3.8 million rural residents receive care from NHSC providers. In spite of these efforts, there is still less than one primary care physician per 3500 people in designated shortage areas (Rural Clinician Quarterly, 1995). Among those primary care providers who do function in rural areas, approximately 20 to 30% of physicians are Doctors of Osteopathy compared to 4.5% of the physician population in the country as a whole (Coward, McLaughlin, Duncan, & Bull, 1994).

It is difficult to attract and retain health care providers in rural areas due to diminished financial incentives, lack of back-up coverage and professional isolation, limited opportunities for continued education, and family concerns regarding perceived social and cultural disadvantages of living in isolated areas (Vrabec, 1995). In addition, there may be a dearth of employment opportunities for spouses.

Health care in rural areas is also influenced by the relatively great distances to facilities and the lack of specialized facilities to meet particular needs (eg, facilities for cancer therapy). Furthermore, small rural hospitals are at risk for low patient census and closure further reducing availability of services (Campion, Helms, & Barrand, 1993). During the 1980s, for example, 237 rural hospitals closed (Bigbee, 1993). Limited emergency services and long distances to health care facilities contribute to accidental injury mortality rates in rural settings.

Use of available services may also influence rural health status. Because of the cultural values of self-reliance and neighborliness, rural dwellers may be far more likely to access informal helping networks than formal health care services. Use of traditional healers and alternative therapies is also common among some rural populations. Because of a tendency to define health as the ability to work, rural residents are also less likely than city dwellers to utilize preventive health services. For example, approximately 99% of all immunizable conditions occur in underserved areas including rural areas. Preventive and health-promotive services may also be deemphasized because the few providers available, of necessity, focus on meeting the needs posed by existing illness in the community (National Institute for Nursing Research, 1995).

Diagnostic Reasoning and Care of Clients in Rural Settings

In rural areas, the etiology of nursing diagnoses is frequently related to a lack of resources and limited ac-

cess to health care in the community. A nursing diagnosis of "potential for poor infant outcome due to 3-hour travel time to nearest maternity delivery service" is common in today's rural health system and requires that the rural nurse providing prenatal care be most astute in assessing this client during her pregnancy. A second nursing diagnosis might be "increased suicide risk due to lack of access to mental health services." Again, this diagnosis is attributable to limited access to health care.

The financial pressures of farming in rural America have caused rural mothers to seek outside employment and leave the farm father to care for the children while he is attending to farm chores. This change in child care might suggest a nursing diagnosis of "increased potential for farm accidents due to lack of day care services for rural preschoolers during the absence of working mothers." Rural nurses are often the caregivers who can identify the potential safety problems in this situation and help the family work toward solutions.

Planning the Dimensions of Care in Rural Settings

Planning primary, secondary, and tertiary levels of prevention can be directed toward meeting the needs of individual clients, families, or the community itself. The community health nurse plays a pivotal role in planning preventive strategies for rural communities.

The American College of Physicians (1995) has outlined several strategies for meeting the health care needs of rural populations. These include providing for universal coverage for primary health care services for both urban and rural populations; increasing the number of primary care providers in rural settings through emphasis on educating practitioners specifically for rural practice and increasing rural provider reimbursements; decreasing professional isolation in rural areas via telecommunications; assisting rural hospitals to meet tertiary care needs; and creating innovative networks of providers to deliver care.

Community nursing centers (CNCs) are another strategy suggested for meeting the health care needs of rural populations. **Community nursing centers** have been defined as "organizations which enable clients to contract directly with professional nurses for health care services rendered in community settings" (cited in Lockhart, 1995). CNCs are characterized by nurse management, nurse responsibility and accountability for client care and professional practice, and the use of nurses, frequently advanced practice nurses, as the primary providers of care. While most CNCs involve ambulatory care services in a clinic setting, they may also support nurse-managed home care, and community-based, hospital, or nursing home services. Community nursing centers may be freestanding community outreach clinics, institution-based agencies, wellness centers, or independent practice sites for nurse entrepreneurs (Lockhart, 1995).

One other strategy suggested for improving health care delivery to rural populations is the use of lay health promoters. This is a particularly appropriate strategy given the tendency of some rural populations to rely on informal helping networks. Lay provider programs have been used successfully with migrant and seasonal farmworkers as well as Native Americans. Lay health promoter programs are characterized by the use of workers indigenous to the community, scope of lay training, activity among previous underserved populations, creativity in responding to health needs, and use of "popular education" concepts (Murphy, 1995).

Primary Prevention

In rural settings, primary prevention focuses on preventing high-risk health problems endemic to rural communities. Prevention is achieved through health promotion activities, prevention of common illnesses, and prevention of accidents and injuries related to work and leisure activities.

Health Promotion.   Planning health-promotive activities in selected community agencies is a rewarding task for the community health nurse. One of the items of the national school agenda for the next decade is to introduce health promotion practices to children beginning in kindergarten. Rural school nurses and community health nurses can play major roles in this endeavor. Community health nurses can also plan to teach principles of good nutrition to pregnant women and to cafeteria workers and cooks who plan and serve meals in schools and other institutions.

The lack of access to healthy foods is sometimes apparent in rural communities where elderly persons and migrant workers must shop at "convenience" stores that sell high-cholesterol, high-fat, sodium-laden foods. To alleviate problems of this sort, the community health nurse can help to plan community support for transportation for communal shopping trips to the nearest supermarket to allow rural residents to maintain healthy eating habits.

A strong emphasis on organized athletics in junior and senior high schools provides another opportunity for health promotion. Nurses can also emphasize healthy activities and use of appropriate safety

equipment in organized summer camps sponsored by churches and other organizations.

There is a pressing need for school-based clinics for adolescents for both family planning and prenatal care, and community health nurses can be actively involved in planning and implementing care in such clinics. These clinics offer the rural nurse prime opportunities for teaching women's self-care practices, including breast self-examination, encouraging Pap smears, and explaining safe sexual practices. Community health nurses in rural areas play a critical role in sex education and in helping both girls and boys to develop prudent sexual practices.

In rural communities, there are often few formal programs for cardiovascular fitness, and community health nurses can be instrumental in designing programs of this type. Public health and church-based aerobics classes and diet programs are other ways for nurses to lend their professional expertise to health promotion in the rural community.

Illness Prevention.   Rural community health nurses can plan nursing interventions aimed at modifying risk factors among aggregates of rural clients in several ways. Booths at annual country fairs offer excellent opportunities for children and adults to present projects related to health promotion and illness prevention. The nurse is a resource person in these types of activities. Planning hypertension, cholesterol, breast self-exam, or glaucoma screening opportunities through the auspices of a local church or other community organization is another way to assist the community to focus on the need to lower health risks.

Sitting on school, public health, or mental health boards affords the rural community health nurse an opportunity to help the community set the "health agenda" around illness prevention. Rural community leaders are often not well advised on how to carry out these matters. Speaking at Rotary or Lion's Club meetings, Jaycees, or the local garden club is another way that the rural nurse can encourage clients to assume a role in illness prevention. Many resources are available from national and state groups to support these efforts.

Injury Prevention.   Planning to prevent accidents within the rural community is a major role for the rural community health nurse. Farm and motor vehicle accidents rank as the number-one cause of morbidity and mortality for young people in rural America. Farm accidents, especially those involving children, are receiving national emphasis. Children operating farm equipment, hearing and eye protection, machine safety education, and preventing childhood poisonings are all areas requiring education and preventive strategies. The rural community health nurse serves as both formal and informal educator as well as community planner for accident prevention strategies.

Secondary Prevention

As in other nursing settings, planning for secondary prevention is geared toward resolving health problems identified during assessment. Rural nurses focus on screening for health problems, treating clients with ongoing problems and providing episodic care, performing triage, and referring clients in emergency situations.

Screening. Major screening activities of rural community health nurses may be carried out in one of two settings: the local school system or the public health department. Children, for example, typically are screened for scoliosis, hearing and vision problems, and immunization status. Community health nurses also routinely monitor children's growth patterns and test for anemia. Adults are screened for hypertension and tuberculosis; screening examinations for breast, cervical, and colon cancer may also be performed.

Funding for most of the monitoring and screening activities that nurses provide is derived from state and federal sources. Therefore, it is crucial that rural community health nurses take an active part in the assessment, planning, and decision-making processes to allocate program funds. Coalition building and political activity for a rural health care platform are professional activities of rural community health nurses.

Environmental Screening. Rural community health nurses frequently assist environmentalists to plan for community improvement based on environmental health problems identified during assessment. This includes concerns about indoor plumbing, lack of heat for the elderly, poor or contaminated water supplies, unacceptable care of animals, reporting of animal bites, and outbreaks of infectious illness, for example, gastrointestinal infections caused by *Giardia* or *Salmonella.*

Treatment of Existing Conditions. Community health nurses working in rural settings spend a major portion of their time caring for clients with existing health problems and providing episodic health care. Legislation that allows rural hospitals to expand into primary care centers to provide care management for clients across a continuum of health states will further increase this component of rural nursing care.

In rural areas, where mental health services are severely lacking, it is most often the nurse who assists client and family to deal with the burden of emotional stress and chronic mental illness. Homeless mental health patients are part of the rural extended family, and their health care needs are part of the rural nursing repertoire.

Management of chronic illness is a family affair in rural settings, with the community health nurse acting as a resource person and facilitator. The nurse may plan several strategies to assist family-centered services. For example, encouraging Congress and state legislatures to continue to target health care programs to rural areas, encouraging neighbors and friends to help, and recognizing the diversity that exists among communities and families are some strategies that would assist families in these situations.

Emergency Care, Triage, and Referral. Another important area of rural community health nursing is emergency care. Research has shown that the early hours of care are critical to successful outcomes for emergency situations. Telecommunications networks such as telemetry and facsimile capabilities put the rural nurse in close contact with medical and nursing expertise. Simulations and protocols assist the nurse to implement emergency care until support arrives. Careful planning and coordination of members of the emergency team are essential to successful emergency care services.

Tertiary Prevention

Tertiary preventive efforts of community health nurses who work in rural practice settings are directed toward preventing complications of chronic illness and preventing recurrences of acute health problems. These nursing care measures are carried out primarily by community-based home health nurses who care for elderly and chronically homebound clients who are monitored closely to ensure stability of their disease process. Case management activities to coordinate care and resources can be quite effective in preventing complications.

Community health nurses carefully monitor the nation's health through the administration of immunizations to both children and adults. Pneumonia and influenza vaccines are available for the rural elderly. Rural communities are just seeing the tip of the iceberg with regard to AIDS, and community health nurses are the mainstay of AIDS care both as counselors for HIV-infected individuals and as providers of nursing care for clients with full-blown AIDS.

A great deal of the follow-up care in rural communities is carried out through "being neighborly." The local nurse is viewed as the person to contact before making the return visit to the city physician. In both the school and community settings in rural areas, education about safety and high-risk health behaviors is a key strategy of the community health nurse involved in tertiary prevention.

The last focus for community health nurses involved in tertiary prevention in rural settings is monitoring the health status of clients with chronic health problems. For example, monitoring elderly clients with the triad of diabetes mellitus, hypertension, and renal disease is a common activity in rural care. Patients with chronic illnesses are treated during the acute phase of their illness in tertiary urban settings and then discharged to convalesce at home. The nurse may need to plan to continue chemotherapy and observe for treatment effects for clients with cancer; to monitor cardiac status after coronary bypass surgery; or to monitor clients on respirators or home dialysis.

Implementing Health Care in Rural Settings

Nursing interventions in rural settings usually involve the client and family and any other available resources. The case management approach within the context of continuity of care for the entire family is the desired outcome. The plan of care should be implemented locally whenever possible because distant services are not only expensive but also difficult for clients to manage. A broad understanding of what health services are available and how to obtain these services is critical. Good communication skills and strong interprofessional networks are vital to successful nursing intervention in the rural practice setting.

Evaluating Health Care in Rural Settings

Evaluating health care in the rural setting is done by focusing on outcomes for rural clients and for the rural community. One way that community health nurses can evaluate outcomes is by carrying out clinical research projects within the community. For example, are nursing interventions lowering the teen pregnancy rate in the local high school? Are the infants who receive milk through the rural health department progressing satisfactorily in terms of their growth and development? Is the overweight elderly population in a community-based hypertension clinic losing weight? These and other issues are of concern to community health nurses in rural areas.

Critical Thinking in Practice: A Case in Point

You are a rural community health nurse assigned to the county health department mobile van visiting a large migrant community at a local farm. Mr. Robert Kelbert is a 64-year-old African American migrant worker who comes into the mobile unit to have his blood pressure medication refilled. He will be in the county for the next 3 to 4 weeks to harvest the soybean crop. He usually attends a rural health clinic in the northern part of the state where he has been receiving his care and medications free.

Today his blood pressure is 154/98, pulse 88, height 69 inches, and weight 198 pounds. He states he is "worn out" from the heat. He chews tobacco and drinks alcohol "some." He travels and stays with his son and family. His daughter-in-law does the cooking. During your interview, Mr. Kelbert tells you he is worried because two of the migrant workers have been given medicine for lung congestion and one of them has been coughing up blood.

1. What are some of the biophysical, psychological, physical, social, behavioral, and health system factors operating in this situation?
2. List three nursing diagnoses that you would identify for Mr. Kelbert.
3. What are your objectives for today's visit?
4. How might your care for Mr. Kelbert differ from that provided to a client you see regularly at the rural health department?
5. What primary, secondary, and tertiary prevention measures are appropriate for Mr. Kelbert?
6. How will you follow up on this visit?

TESTING YOUR UNDERSTANDING

1. Discuss differences in the definition of rurality from each of the three perspectives presented. (p. 668)
2. Describe at least four barriers to effective health care in rural areas. What might community health nurses do to eliminate these barriers? (p. 670)
3. What two age groups in rural settings are at particular risk for health problems? Why? (p. 671)
4. Describe at least five physical dimension concerns unique to rural settings. What influence might they have on the health of rural residents? (pp. 672–673)
5. Identify four major occupational and safety risk factors for rural populations. (pp. 673–674)
6. In what two ways do inequities in health policy create barriers to health care in rural settings? (pp. 675–678)
7. Identify three aspects of primary prevention in rural settings. How might community health nurses be involved in each? (pp. 679–680)
8. Describe four approaches to secondary prevention in rural settings. What interventions might community health nurses employ with respect to each? (p. 680)

WHAT DO YOU THINK?
Questions for Critical Thinking

1. Should rural health care be provided by generalists or specialists. Why?
2. How might nursing education institutions help to meet the rural community health nurse's need for an expanded knowledge base? What strategies might work for providing continuing education opportunities for rural nurses? Why?
3. What would be the major advantages and disadvantages of community health nursing in a rural setting?
4. In what ways might health promotion activities for rural populations differ from those designed for urban populations?

REFERENCES

American College of Physicians. (1995). Rural primary care. *Annals of Internal Medicine, 122,* 380–390.

American Hospital Association. (1993). *Working from within: Integrating rural health care.* Chicago: American Hospital Association.

American Nurses Association. (1996). *Rural/frontier nursing.* Washington, DC: American Nurses Publishing.

Anderson, J., & Yuhos, R. (1993). Health promotion in rural settings. *Nursing Clinics of North America, 28,* 145–155.

Aron, L. S., & Fitchen, J. M. (1996). Rural homelessness. In J. Baumohl (Ed.), *Homelessness in America* (pp. 82–85). Phoenix, AZ: Oryx Press.

Beaulieu, J. E. (1994). Services for the rural elderly and disabled. In Beaulieu, J. E., & Berry, D. E. (Eds.), *Rural health services: A management perspective* (pp. 229–257). Ann Arbor, MI: AUPHA Press/Health Administration Press.

Bigbee, J. L. (1993). The uniqueness of rural nursing. *Nursing Clinics of North America, 28,* 131–143.

Campion, D. M., Helms, W. D., & Barrand, N. L. (1993). Health care reform in rural areas. *Health Affairs, 12*(3), 76–80.

Coburn, A. F., & Mueller, K. J. (1995). Legislative and policy strategies for supporting rural health network development: Lessons from the 103rd Congress. *Journal of Rural Health, 11*(1), 22, 31.

Coward, R. T., McLaughlin, D. M., Duncan, R. P., & Bull, C. N. (1994). An overview of health and aging in rural America. In R. T. Coward, C. N. Bull, G. Kukulka, & J. M. Galliher (Eds.), *Health services for rural elders* (pp. 1–32). New York: Springer.

Hibbeln, J. A. U. (1996). Special populations: Hispanic migrant workers. In S. Torres (Ed.), *Hispanic voices: Hispanic health educators speak out.* New York: National League for Nursing.

Horner, S. D., Ambrogne, J., Coleman, M. A., et al. (1994). Traveling for care: Factors influencing health care access for rural dwellers. *Public Health Nursing, 11,* 145–149.

Hospital Research and Education Trust. (1992). *Increasing rural health personnel: Community-based strategies for recruitment and retention.* Chicago: American Hospital Association.

Lockhart, C. A. (1995). Community nursing centers: An analysis of status and needs. In B. Murphy (Ed.), *Nursing centers: The time is now.* New York: National League for Nursing.

Long, K. A., Scharff, J. E., & Weinert, C. (1997). Advanced education for the role of rural nurse generalist. *Journal of Nursing Education, 36,* 91–94.

Maternal and Child Health Bureau. (1997). Pregnancy-related behaviors among migrant farm workers—Four states, 1989–1993. *MMWR, 46,* 281–283.

Miller, M. K., Farmer, F. L., & Clarke, L. L. (1994). Rural populations and their health. In Beaulieu, J. E., & Berry, D. E. (Eds.), *Rural health services: A management perspective* (pp. 3–26). Ann Arbor, MI: AUPHA Press/Health Administration Press.

Murphy, M. (1995). Lay health programs: Public health services that work. *Migrant Health Newsline, 12*(5), 1, 3.

National Institute of Nursing Research. (1995). *Community-based health care: Nursing strategies.* Bethesda, MD: National Institute of Nursing Research.

National Migrant Resource Program. (1990). *Migrant and seasonal farmworker health objectives for the year 2000.* Austin, TX: National Migrant Resource Program.

Polivka, B. J. (1996). Rural sex education: Assessment of programs and interagency collaboration. *Public Health Nursing, 13,* 425–433.

Rural Clinician Quarterly. (1995). *Impact of the National Health Service Corps on rural and underserved health care, 5*(4), 1–2.

Schenker, M. B., Lopez, R., & Wintemute, G. (1995). Farm-related fatalities among children in California, 1980 to 1989. *American Journal of Public Health, 85,* 89–92.

Silveira, J. M., & Winstead-Fry, P. (1997). The needs of patients with cancer and their caregivers in rural areas. *Oncology Nursing Forum, 24*(1), 71–75.

Sowell, R. L., & Opava, W. D. (1995). The Georgia rural-based nurse model: Primary care for persons with HIV/AIDS. *Public Health Nursing, 12,* 228–234.

Stoller, E. P., & Lee, G. R. (1994). Informal care of rural elders. In R. T. Coward, C. N. Bull, G. Kukulka, & J. M. Galliher (Eds.), *Health services for rural elders* (pp. 33–64). New York: Springer.

Thornton, C. L. (1996). Nurse practitioner in a rural setting. *Advanced Practice Nursing, 31,* 495–505.

U.S. Department of Commerce. (1996). *Statistical Abstract of the United States, 1996* (116th ed.). Washington, DC: Government Printing Office.

Vrabec, N. J. (1995). Implications of U.S. health care reform for the rural elderly. *Nursing Outlook, 43,* 260–265.

Wagner, J. D., Menke, E. M., & Ciccone, J. K. (1995). What is known about the health of rural homeless families. *Public Health Nursing, 12,* 400–408.

RESOURCES FOR NURSES IN RURAL HEALTH SETTINGS

Education

AARP Health Advocacy Series
Program Coordination
American Association of Retired Persons
601 E Street, NW
Washington, DC 20049

Health Promotion

Cooperative Extension Service
Local chapter in each state

National Health Information Center
Box 1133
Washington, DC 20013–1133
(301) 565–4167

Migrant Workers

East Coast Migrant Health
1234 Massachusetts Avenue, NW, Ste. C-1017
Washington, DC 20005
(202) 437–7377

Migrant Legal Action Program
2001 South Street, NW, Ste. 310
Washington, DC 20009
(202) 462–7744

National Migrant Resource Program
c/o Roberta Ryder
1515 Capital of Texas Hwy., Ste. 220
Austin, TX 78704
(512) 328–7682

National Migrant Workers Council
502 W. Elm Avenue
Monroe, MI 48161
(313) 243–0711

Rural Elderly

Center on Rural Elderly
University of Missouri
5245 Rockhill
Kansas City, MO 64110
(816) 276–2180

Rural Health

National Rural Health Association
One West Armour Blvd., Ste. 301
Kansas City, MO 64111
(816) 756–3140

Office of Rural Health Policy
U.S. Department of Health and Human Services
5600 Fishers Lane, Room 14-22
Rockville, MD 20857
(303) 443–6152

U.S. Department of Agriculture
Rural Information Center
National Agricultural Library, Room 304
Beltsville, MD 20705
(301) 344–2547

U.S. House of Representatives
Rural Health Care Coalition
2244 Rayburn House Office Bldg.
Washington, DC 20515
(202) 225–2911

U.S. Senate
Rural Health Caucus
511 Hart Senate Office Bldg.
Washington, DC 20510
(202) 224–2551

Rural Health Statistics

California NURSE (Nurses Using Rural Sentinel
   Events) Project
Occupational Inquiry Control Section
Occupational Health Branch
California Public Health Foundation
California Department of Health Services
2151 Berkeley Way, Annex 11, Third Floor
Berkeley, CA 94704
(510) 849–5150

Centers for Disease Control and Prevention
National Center for Health Statistics
6525 Belcrest Road, Room 1070
Hyattsville, MD 20782
(301) 436–7035

Rural Issues

Center for Rural Affairs
PO Box 406
Walthill, NE 68067
(402) 846–5428

State Rural Health Association
State Offices of Rural Health (contact local state
   government)

Rural Mental Health

National Association for Rural Mental Health
P.O. Box 570
Wood River, IL 62095
(618) 251–0589

National Mental Health Association
1021 Prince Street
Alexandria, VA 22314–2971
(703) 684–7722

National Rural Institute on Alcohol and Drug
   Abuse
Arts and Sciences Outreach Office
University of Wisconsin—Eau Claire
Eau Claire, WI 54702–4004
(715) 836–2031

Rural Mental Health and Substance Abuse
   Directory
National Rural Health Association
1 West Armour Blvd., Ste. 301
Kansas City, MO 64111
(816) 756–3140

Rural Nursing

American Nurses Association
600 Maryland Avenue, SW, Ste. 100 West
Washington, DC 20024–2571
(202) 651–7000

Safety

National Institute for Occupational Safety
   and Health
1600 Clifton Road
Atlanta, GA 30333
(404) 639–3771

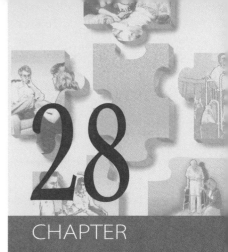

CARE OF CLIENTS IN CORRECTIONAL SETTINGS

▶ KEY TERMS

detainees
jail
juvenile detention
  facilities
prison
TB prophylaxis

The correctional facility is a relatively new practice setting for community health nursing. Correctional nursing, however, is congruent with the primary focus of community health nursing, and offers a challenging position for the community health nurse to expand the frontiers of nursing practice. Corrections nursing involves challenges not encountered in other community health nursing settings. As noted by Squires (1996), "Health in prisons is a product of the demographic characteristics of prisoners and the health behaviors that they bring with them into the prison environment. It is influenced within prison by the built environment, the regime, and the organizational culture of the prison, and is dependent on the connections that prisoners maintain with the environment outside."

Correctional nursing takes place in three general types of facilities; prisons, jails, and juvenile detention facilities (American Nurses Association, 1995). *Prisons* are state and federal facilities that house persons convicted of crimes, usually those sentenced for longer than 1 year. Local facilities, called *jails,* house both convicted inmates and detainees. *Detainees* are people who have not yet been convicted of a crime. They are being detained pending a trial either because they cannot pay the set bail, or because no bail has been set (Kay, 1991). *Juvenile detention facilities* house children and adolescents convicted of crimes and those awaiting trial but who cannot be released to the custody of a responsible adult.

Nurses working in correctional facilities must be committed to the belief that inmates retain their individual rights as human beings despite incarceration. Society does not categorically deprive any other group of individuals access to health care. In fact, there are carefully monitored health care standards in such institutions as nursing homes, and mental health facilities. As recently as 1975, however, a program for accrediting health services in prisons was initiated by the American Medical Association and only since 1985 have published standards for nursing practice in such settings been available (American Nurses Association, 1985).

▶ Chapter Objectives

After reading this chapter, you should be able to:

- Identify at least three reasons for providing health care in correctional settings.
- Describe at least three elements of the ethical dimension of nursing in correctional settings.
- Differentiate between basic and advanced nursing practice in correctional settings.
- Identify at least three biophysical dimension elements influencing the health status of inmates.
- Describe at least four major considerations in assessing the psychological dimension of health in correctional settings.
- Discuss at least three aspects of the behavioral dimension that influence health in correctional settings.
- Identify three aspects of primary prevention in correctional settings.
- Describe two approaches to secondary prevention in correctional settings.
- Discuss two considerations in tertiary prevention in correctional settings.

▶ **THE NEED FOR HEALTH CARE IN CORRECTIONAL SETTINGS**

Health care in correctional facilities is an appropriate endeavor for several reasons. First, the right to adequate health care is a constitutionally recognized right arising from the Eighth Amendment which prohibits "cruel and unusual punishment" of those convicted of crimes. Detainees also have a constitutional right to health care under the Fifth and Fourteenth Amendments which prohibit punishment of any kind without "due process" which means conviction through the normal legal processes of the nation. In the case of both convicted inmates and detainees, "deliberate indifference" to serious illness or injury is interpreted as unusual punishment (*Estelle v. Gamble*, cited in Kay, 1991).

In addition to the constitutional right to health care, correctional care is good common sense for a variety of other reasons. Because of poverty, lower education levels, and unhealthy lifestyles that frequently involve substance abuse, inmates may enter a correctional facility with significant health problems (Shields & de Moya, 1997). Because many of these individuals cannot afford to pay for care on the outside, the cost of care will be borne by society. Societal costs for this care will be less if interventions occur in a

timely fashion, before they become severe. Provision of care within the correctional facility also saves taxpayers the cost of personnel and vehicles to transport inmates to other health care facilities. Primary prevention in correctional settings is also cost-effective.

Another possible societal cost of failure to provide adequate health care to inmates lies in the potential for the spread of communicable disease from correctional facilities to the community. Environmental conditions and behaviors within correctional facilities lend themselves to the transmission of communicable diseases such as tuberculosis (Koo, Baron, & Rutherford, 1997), HIV infection (Polych & Sabo, 1995), hepatitis B (National Commission on Correctional Health Care, 1997b), and other sexually transmitted diseases (Beltrami, Cohen, Hamrick, & Farley, 1997). In fact, correctional facilities have been described as a "pocket of risk" for communicable disease (Polych &

▶ STANDARDS FOR NURSING PRACTICE IN CORRECTIONAL SETTINGS

Standards of Care: The nurse:
- collects client health data
- analyzes assessment data in determining diagnoses
- identifies expected outcomes individualized to the client
- develops a care plan that prescribes interventions to attain expected outcomes
- implements the interventions identified in the care plan
- evaluates the client's progress toward attainment of outcomes

Standards of Professional Performance: The nurse:
- systematically evaluates the quality and effectiveness of nursing practice
- evaluates his/her own nursing practice in relation to professional practice standards and evaluates statutes and regulations
- acquires and maintains current knowledge in nursing practice
- contributes to the professional development of peers, colleagues, and others
- determines decisions and actions on behalf of the client in an ethical manner
- collaborates with the client, significant others, other criminal justice system personnel, and health care providers in providing client care
- uses research findings in practice
- considers factors related to safety, effectiveness, and cost in planning and delivering client care

(Source: American Nurses Association, 1995.)

Sabo, 1995). The more than 22 million admissions and releases from U.S. correctional facilities that occur each year put the general public at significant risk for increased incidence of communicable diseases spread from correctional settings (Polych & Sabo, 1995).

Standards for Nursing Practice in Correctional Settings

As noted earlier, the first standards for nursing practice in correctional settings were promulgated by the American Nurses Association in 1985. These standards were revised in 1995 and address the scope of nursing practice in correctional settings as well as standards of care and standards of professional performance. Nursing standards for correctional settings are summarized on page 686. The designated standards of care reflect the expected level of care to be provided to individual clients in the correctional setting. The standards of professional performance, on the other hand, are more reflective of the aggregate focus of community health nursing as practiced in correctional settings.

► THE DIMENSIONS MODEL AND CARE OF CLIENTS IN CORRECTIONAL SETTINGS

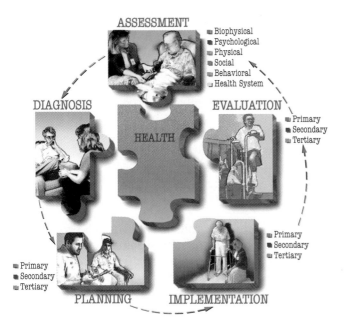

Use of the Dimensions Model in the correctional setting allows the community health nurse to identify the critical dimensions of nursing operating in this setting and provides direction for assessing health needs in each of the six dimensions of health. Finally, the model can be used to plan interventions related to

each of the three levels of health care, primary, secondary, and tertiary, to meet identified health needs.

Critical Dimensions of Nursing in Correctional Settings

There are some critical elements of the dimensions of nursing that are unique to correctional settings. The American Nurses Association (1995) has identified two levels of scope for correctional nursing practice based on the cognitive dimension of nursing and the depth and breadth of the nurse's knowledge and expertise. Basic nursing practice focuses on a full range of nursing services including health promotion, intervention for existing health problems, and evaluation of the care provided to individual clients. Nursing care at this level may be provided independently or in collaboration with other health care professionals. The second level is advanced nursing practice in correctional settings which is characterized by increased breadth and depth of knowledge in an area of specialization and by the ability to incorporate knowledge of corrections into the development of care services. Nurses at this level provide direct client care services at an advanced level and may also be responsible for facility management, direction of other personnel, and evaluation of health care service delivery. Despite the relatively autonomous nature of practice in correctional settings, the education level of many corrections nurses may not reflect adequate preparation for practice in this area. For example, in one study of 146 nurses in 19 facilities in 5 states, 8% of corrections nurses were LPNs/LVNs, 11% were diploma nursing graduates, and 25% were educated at the associate-degree level. An additional 40% had some college education but had not completed a baccalaureate degree. Only 16% of the nurses had baccalaureate degrees (9% in nursing and 7% in other fields), and less than 1% had a master's degree (Shields & de Moya, 1997). Similarly, of the 612 nursing personnel certified as correctional health professionals in 1997, 11% were LVNs/ LPNs, 56% were associate-degree or diploma-prepared RNs, 23% had a baccalaureate degree in nursing or another field, 10% held a master's degree in nursing or another field, and less than 0.5% held a doctorate (National Commission on Correctional Health Care, 1997a).

Skills in the interpersonal dimension of nursing are particularly important in correctional settings. Corrections nurses are often working with clients who are relatively unmotivated regarding their health, whose priorities may differ significantly from those of the nurse. Nurses may need to engage in motivational activities to promote compliance with medical treatment plans or to foster changes in unhealthful behaviors. The attitudes of nurses toward their clientele are a particularly important feature in motivating clients for change. In one study, correctional nurses had less favorable attitudes toward inmates than other groups surveyed including inmates, students, members of the community at large, correctional officers, defense attorneys, and prison rehabilitation teams. The only group that scored lower than the nurses on attitudes toward inmates was one group of law enforcement officers (Shields & de Moya, 1997). Empathetic attitudes on the part of nurses can go far toward motivating behavior change in clients and can also serve to increase satisfaction in a group frequently perceived as litigious.

Excellent communications and collaborative skills will also be required in working with other corrections personnel. Although the focus of nursing in correctional institutions is on the quality of care given and the promotion of inmate health, the major considerations for other corrections personnel are security and control. This divergence of goals may lead to conflicts among health care personnel and others in the correctional setting. Good communications skills on the part of the nurse will help to avoid or resolve these conflicts.

There are several elements of the ethical dimension of nursing that are particularly relevant to nursing in a correctional facility. The right to health care is an ethical, as well as legal, issue that has already been addressed. Other ethical issues include confidentiality and appropriate use of health care personnel, refusal of care, abuse of prisoners, and advocacy. Confidentiality issues may be a source of conflict in correctional settings when health care providers have access to information that may be of use in criminal proceedings against inmates. The standards for correctional health care promulgated by the American Public Health Association (Dubler, 1986) indicate that confidentiality of client health information should be maintained except in instances where there is reason to suggest that the client may pose a danger to him- or herself or to others. Health professionals in correctional institutions, however, may be pressured to divulge client information or to assist with procedures designed to provide evidence for criminal proceedings (eg, body cavity searches, blood alcohol levels). When these procedures need to be performed by trained personnel (eg, venipuncture), they should be the task of personnel hired specifically for these types of responsibilities to prevent conflict of interest for health care providers and to avoid jeopardizing a relationship of trust between provider and client. Similarly, health care professionals should not be called upon to engage in security measures or to witness the application of measures to subdue unruly inmates (American Nurses Association, 1995). Assuring appropriate use

of personnel in the correctional setting may also mean making sure that nonprofessionals (including inmates are not allowed to perform medical tasks or dispense medications (Kay, 1991).

In addition to maintaining confidentiality, nurses may be called upon to support an inmate's refusal of care including forcible administration of psychotherapeutic medications. Inmates have the right to refuse care unless they are determined to be legally incompetent to make that decision. Aggressive or potentially suicidal inmates can, however, be subjected to physical restraint if they are deemed a danger to self or to others. This includes the use of medical isolation when clients suspected of infectious diseases refuse screening procedures or treatment (Dubler, 1986). Medical isolation may also be legitimately employed to protect inmates with symptomatic AIDS from opportunistic infection (National Commission on Correctional Health Care, 1992). In other instances, correctional facilities may mandate involuntary provision of care when they can demonstrate "a compelling state interest" such as protecting others from communicable disease or violent behavior.

Because of the imbalance of power inherent in a correctional setting, there is always the potential for abuse of inmates in the name of punishment. For example, pepper spray is occasionally used as a means of forcing compliance among inmates. Punitive use of such chemicals over and above necessary use for subduing violence has been described as constituting torture and falls within the Eighth Amendment proscription of cruel and unusual punishment (Cohen, 1997). Preventing this and other forms of abuse of inmates (eg, through denial of health care services) is another ethical aspect of nursing in correctional settings. Finally, nurse advocacy may be needed in the correctional setting. Advocacy may be required at the level of the individual client to ensure that rights are upheld and that appropriate health care services are received or at the aggregate level to assure adequate health care delivery systems in correctional institutions.

The corrections nurse will also need to employ the intellectual skills of critical thinking and analysis. Accurate diagnosis of client health problems may be complicated by the interactions of the correctional environment and health behaviors such as substance abuse. In addition, inmates may have incomplete health knowledge or be unable to give an accurate health history. Finally, inmates may attempt to manipulate the health care provider in order to meet other needs (eg, medications for sale to other inmates, respite from work details) (Anno, 1997).

In the process dimension, one critical element of correctional nursing practice is the case management process. Frequently, care provided within the correctional facility may be fragmented and may require the inmate to see multiple providers at different times to resolve a single problem. For example, initial contact may be made with a triage nurse who recommends that the inmate see a physician who is only available at certain times. The physician may order lab work or procedures that may require arrangements for out-of-facility appointments which are complicated by the need to arrange for transportation and security coverage. In addition, correctional facilities are concerned with minimizing both costs to the institution and disruption of facility routine, all of which can make obtaining and coordinating care particularly challenging.

The major consideration in the reflective dimension interfaces with issues in the ethical dimension. There is a definite need for research in correctional settings, both on the effects of incarceration on health and on the effectiveness of health care interventions, and nurses should be actively involved in such research (American Nurses Association, 1995). Inmates, however, are a vulnerable population open to exploitation by the very nature of the correctional setting and the potential for coercion that exists. For this reason, nurses who are working in correctional settings, and particularly those who are conducting research in these settings, must be particularly alert to the need to ensure informed consent when inmates are included as research subjects.

Assessing the Dimensions of Health in Correctional Settings

Factors in each of the six dimensions of health influence the health status of clients and staff in correctional settings. The nurse assesses factors related to the biophysical, psychological, physical, social, behavioral, and health system dimensions to identify health problems and to direct interventions to resolve those problems.

The Biophysical Dimension

Elements of age, genetic inheritance (sex and ethnicity), and physiologic function all influence health status in correctional settings.

Age.   There is considerable concern recently over the increase in inmate populations comprised of very young offenders and the elderly. The case rate for juvenile delinquency per 1000 youth aged 10 to 17 years increased from 38.3 in 1983 to 54.6 in 1993. Over half of juvenile crimes are delinquency offenses related to

vandalism and drug violations, but a growing number of violent crimes are being committed by juveniles. For example, the number of aggravated assaults by juveniles nearly tripled from 1983 to 1993 (U.S. Department of Commerce, 1996). More and more juveniles are being tried as adults and sentenced to extended periods of incarceration. This trend means that correctional health care providers must deal with the developmental needs of this age group as well as addressing their physical and psychological health needs.

There is also a significant increase in the number of elderly inmates in correctional institutions. For example, in 1995 there were 55,000 state and federal inmates over age 50. Even without mandatory sentencing included under "three strikes laws," it is estimated that this number will increase to more than 125,000 by the year 2000 (Holman, 1997). Older inmates experience many of the same chronic conditions as older people in the general population, but they tend to experience them at an earlier age. In fact, appraised ages for inmates have averaged 11.5 years more than their chronological ages (Anno, 1997). The annual cost to society for care for older inmates is approximately $69,000 per person (Holman, 1997) and some people are calling for early release of older inmates who are not a danger to society. The aging of the prison population means that corrections nurses must deal with all of the problems common to the elderly (see Chap. 23) within the constraints of the correctional setting, a daunting task. Both older and younger inmates may also be at greater risk for exploitation and violence than other age groups.

Genetic Inheritance.   Gender and ethnicity are two genetic inheritance factors that also affect health in correctional populations. While men continue to make up 80% of arrestees (U.S. Department of Commerce, 1996), the proportion of women in the correctional population is increasing. From 1983 to 1994, the number of women in correctional facilities tripled (Teplin, Abram, & McClelland, 1997), and in 1994, women constituted 10% of the population in jails and 6% of the federal and state prison population (U.S. Department of Justice, 1996). This amounts to over 64,000 women in correctional systems in the United States (Martin, Kim, Kupper, Meyer, & Hays, 1997).

Generally speaking, correctional facilities are sex-segregated, so nurses working with male prisoners are unlikely to work with females and vice versa. This may not be true, however, in some small local or county facilities. Whichever gender is being cared for, the nurse is apt to encounter problems unique to that group as well as those that are common to both men and women.

Women inmates experience different health problems than men and, because of their relatively small numbers, may have less access to health care resources while incarcerated (Teplin, et al., 1997). Women inmates are twice as likely to have HIV infection as their male counterparts and their health care costs are higher (*CorHealth,* 1996b). Other communicable diseases (eg, rubella) and use of drugs that have teratogenic effects are of greater concern among women. Incarcerated women also experience more severe mental illness and depression than men (Teplin, et al., 1997). The fact that approximately 80% of women inmates have children and 70% are single parents adds to the psychological burden of incarceration for these women whose children may be placed with relatives or in foster homes during their sentence (Jonsen & Stryker, 1993).

Ethnicity is another aspect of genetic inheritance that is reflected in inmate populations. Members of ethnic minority groups are disproportionately represented in correctional facilities (American Nurses Association, 1995). In 1994, black non-Hispanics constituted 39% of the jail population and 51% of the prison population. Hispanics comprise 15% of jail populations. The nurse needs to assess ethnic inmate populations for conditions common in these groups. For example, a high preponderance of Native Americans in many southwestern jurisdictions would suggest a high prevalence of diabetes in the inmate population, whereas sickle cell disease, diabetes, and hypertension would be common among African American inmates. Minority group members are also more likely to be in poor health and are less likely to be immunized presenting risks for communicable diseases in the correctional situation.

Physiologic Function. The nurse in the correctional setting needs to assess individual clients for existing physical health problems. He or she also needs to identify problems that have a high incidence and prevalence in the overall institutional population. Particular areas to be considered include communicable diseases, chronic diseases, injury, and pregnancy.

As noted earlier, environmental conditions and behavioral patterns in correctional settings foster the spread of communicable diseases. Although many communicable diseases are found in this population, four of particular concern in correctional populations are tuberculosis, HIV infection and AIDS, hepatitis B, and other sexually transmitted diseases. Overcrowding and generally poor health status are two of the factors that promote the spread of tuberculosis in inmate populations. Moreover, coinfection with both TB and HIV is occurring in large segments of some correctional populations. A further complicating factor in the problem of tuberculosis in correctional facilities is the prevalence of multidrug-resistant tuberculosis (Wilcock, Hammett, Widom, & Epstein, 1996). Although the overall number of inmates being treated for tuberculosis declined from 1992 to 1995 (Wilcock, et al., 1996), tuberculosis continues to be a significant health problem in correctional facilities. In 1994, for example, 14% of inmates in 31 state prison systems had positive tuberculin skin tests. Approximately 9% of those with positive tests in state and federal prison systems were coinfected with HIV, whereas less than 1% of those in local and county jail systems were coinfected (Wilcock et al., 1996). In one California prison, the incidence of active tuberculosis was 184 per 100,000 inmates with nearly 6% of new cases attributable to transmission within the facility (Koo, et al., 1997). In a New York City facility, the prevalence of active TB in 1993 was 767 per 100,000 population (Layton, et al., 1997). The community health nurse working in correctional settings should assess inmates for signs of tuberculosis as well as provide routine screenings for TB according to agency policy. Tuberculin skin test screening in jails may be inappropriate for many inmates who stay only 1 or 2 days, so the nurse should ask about TB symptomatology and history of exposure during the intake assessment in order to isolate potentially infectious inmates.

HIV infection and confirmed cases of AIDS are another growing problem in correctional facilities. Many inmates are at increased risk of infection because of injection drug use and the potential for exposure during incarceration via continued drug use and homosexual activity is high. Between 1991 and 1993, the number of known cases of HIV infection increased by 22% in state prisons and 52% in federal prisons, and the number of diagnosed cases of AIDS in both types of facilities increased by 125% (*CorHealth,* 1996c). Overall, rates for confirmed cases of AIDS are seven times higher in correctional populations than in the general public. In 1994, 2.3% of all state and federal prisoners were infected with HIV and 0.5% had AIDS diagnoses. Inmate deaths due to AIDS have also risen. In 1994, for example, the death rate for AIDS in state prisons was 104 per 100,000 inmates, or 35% of all inmate deaths (Brien & Beck, 1996). Rates of HIV infection vary from one area of the country to another and nurses should be aware of the overall prevalence of infection in their jurisdictions. In fact, 79% of inmates with AIDS are housed in only seven prison systems (Jonsen & Stryker, 1993). Areas with high prevalences of HIV infection in 1994 included New York, Florida, Texas, California, and the federal prison system (Brien & Beck, 1996). Corrections nurses should assess all inmates for history of HIV infection, high-risk behavior, and history or symptoms of possible opportunistic infections.

Drug use behaviors contribute to the increased incidence of tuberculosis and HIV infection in inmates. Such behaviors also place inmates at risk for other sexually transmitted diseases and hepatitis B. In one study, nearly 2% of arrestees had untreated syphilis, and 13% had tests indicative of gonorrhea and chlamydia (Beltrami, et al, 1997). Women were more likely than men to test positive for syphilis possibly reflecting prostitution for drugs. In 1994, heroin use among arrestees in 23 cities ranged from almost 2% in Omaha, Nebraska, to more than 30% in Manhattan, putting inmates at risk for hepatitis B as well as HIV infection and syphilis (U.S. Department of Commerce, 1996). In one California Department of Corrections study, half of incoming women inmates and one third of men were HBV positive. In addition to drug use, sexual activity and tattooing are other risk factors for HBV common in correctional populations (National Commission on Correctional Health Care, 1997b). In assessing individual inmates for health problems, the nurse should ask about history of sexually transmitted diseases and hepatitis B and should be alert to the presence of physical signs and symptoms of these diseases (see Appendix S for information on signs and symptoms of selected communicable diseases).

Chronic illnesses of particular concern in correctional settings include diabetes, hypertension, heart disease, and chronic lung conditions. Seizure disorders are also common and inmates may also exhibit seizure activity during withdrawal from drugs and alcohol. Diabetes may be particularly difficult to control given the rigid structure of the correctional routine and the need to time hypoglycemic medications, meals, and exercise periods appropriately. The availability of vending machines and the use of commissary privileges as a reward may also complicate dietary control for inmates with diabetes. Many inmates with chronic conditions, particularly those with substance abuse problems, enter the correctional facility after prolonged periods without medications or may not know what medications they have been taking. In many instances, the nurse has to exert considerable ingenuity to obtain an accurate health history from clients, family members, and health care providers in the community. Because of poor overall health status, inmates may also be especially susceptible to exacerbations of chronic conditions. The nurse should assess individual inmates for existing chronic conditions and should also identify problems with high incidence and prevalence in the correctional population with whom he or she works.

Injury is another area of physiologic function that should be assessed by the nurse. Injury may result from activities preceding arrest, from actions taken by arresting officers, or from accidents or assaults occurring during incarceration. The nurse should be aware of the potential for internal as well as visible injuries and should assess inmates for signs of trauma.

The final consideration with respect to physiologic function in assessing the biophysical dimension is that of pregnancy. As noted earlier, the number of female inmates increases annually. Approximately one fourth of women entering prison are pregnant or have recently given birth. A large percentage of these women have been incarcerated for drug-related incidents which puts them at high risk for poor pregnancy outcomes. They also have higher levels of alcohol and tobacco use and poor access to prenatal care. Incarceration of substance-abusing pregnant women tends to occur more frequently than among nonpregnant offenders in an effort to promote a drug-free environment for mother and fetus (Fogel, 1995). In 1994, more than 5000 women gave birth in custody (*Corhealth*, 1996b). Some research actually indicates that incarceration may result in better pregnancy outcomes (Martin, et al., 1997).

In assessing female inmates, the nurse should ask about the last menstrual period and solicit any symptoms of possible pregnancy. Because drug use can interfere with menses, menstrual history is not always reliable for indicating pregnancy or for suggesting length of gestation when pregnancy is confirmed. The nurse should also ask about high-risk behavior that may affect the fetus such as smoking, drug and alcohol use, and so on. The pregnant inmate's nutritional status should also be assessed. In one study, 40% of pregnant inmates experienced anemia and more than one third failed to gain sufficient weight during the pregnancy. Pica is also common in incarcerated pregnant women. Other physical problems common in this population that may affect pregnancy outcomes include urinary tract infections and sexually transmitted diseases (Fogel, 1995), and the nurse should assess for symptoms of these conditions. Depression and anxiety are also common phenomena among these women.

The Psychological Dimension

Assessment in the psychological dimension is particularly important in the correctional setting for a number of reasons. First, many inmates have previously existing mental illness that may have led to their incarceration. In fact, it is not uncommon, since deinstitutionalization, for the mentally ill to be held in jails for lack of any other safe place for them. By law, inmates are entitled to mental health services as well as medical treatment. Mental health services, however, may be lacking in some correctional systems, or the need for these services may go unrecognized. This is particularly true among women inmates. In one study, less than one fourth of women with severe mental illness received mental health services while incarcerated (Teplin, et al., 1997).

Incarceration itself is stressful and can lead to psychological effects including depression and suicide. In one study, nearly a third of inmate requests for services were related to stress. Younger inmates and those incarcerated for shorter periods of time are more likely to manifest stress-related concerns (Anno, 1997). Pregnant inmates are particularly susceptible to depression. In one study, 80% of pregnant inmates exhibited symptoms of clinical depression and 50% displayed signs of anxiety (Fogel, 1995). Correctional nurses should be alert to signs of depression and other mental or emotional distress in inmates, and assessment of suicide potential is a critical part of every intake interview. Suicide currently accounts for 36% of inmate deaths in U.S. jails (Teplin, et al., 1997). Over half of suicide attempts occur in the first 24 hours of incarceration and 27% in the first 3 hours (Dubler, 1986). All correctional facilities must have suicide prevention programs, and suicidal ideation or threats are grounds for immediate referral. Nurses should also maintain close watch on inmates placed in isolation as this may also increase the risk, as well as the opportunity, for suicide.

The correctional environment may also contribute to sexual assault with its attendant psychological consequences. In addition, many women inmates arrested for prostitution and drug use have histories of sexual abuse (Stevens, Zierler, Dean, Goodman, Chalfen, & De Groot, 1995). In one study, 58% of women inmates reported prior sexual abuse. For men, rape while incarcerated is fairly common. While much sexual activity among male inmates is consensual, the nature of correctional systems places some men at risk for forcible assault. In some correctional systems, homosexual or effeminate males are segregated from the rest of the population for their protection, but forced isolation may also have psychological consequences or lead to discrimination and assault by other inmates (Jonsen & Stryker, 1993). In assessing clients, particularly those with symptoms of sexually transmitted diseases, corrections nurses should be alert to signs of assault and should question clients about this issue. If sexual assault has occurred, the nurse will also need to take action to protect the client from further injury.

Finally, state and federal prison systems may house a number of inmates who have been sentenced to death, creating a need for emotional and psychological support. At the end 1994, for example, there were 2890 inmates under sentence of death in state and federal prison systems. Approximately half of these inmates had been awaiting execution of their sentences, pending appeals and so on, for more than 6 years (U.S. Department of Justice, 1996). Corrections nurses working in systems with "death-row" inmates should assess them for evidence of psychological problems and refer them for counseling as appropriate.

The Physical Dimension

The physical dimension of the correctional setting is constrained by the need for security. Inmates may be relegated to specific spaces at specific times of the day. Because of the tremendous growth in the incarcerated population, jails and prisons are extremely overcrowded and few jurisdictions are not in violation of space standards for inmates. Other physical environmental problems common in correctional settings include poor ventilation, lack of temperature control, and unsanitary conditions (Anno, 1997). Lack of funds for maintenance may lead to buildings in poor repair creating safety hazards for both inmates and staff. Other areas that should be assessed by the nurse include the safety of recreational areas, fire protection, lighting, plumbing, solid waste disposal, and safety of the water supply. Additional considerations include vermin control, noise control, and the presence of high levels of radiation. Because correctional facilities are often situated in areas away from the general population, they may be located in sites with disaster potential such as flooding, earthquake, and so on. The nurse should assess the potential for such disasters as well as the adequacy of the facility's disaster response plan. Disaster potential may also arise from prison industries. Inmate occupations may also give rise to other physical hazards for individual clients that need to be assessed.

The Social Dimension

Particular elements of the social dimension that should be assessed in correctional settings include the attitudes of correctional and health personnel toward inmates, the extent of social support available to inmates, the effects of education level and language on the health status of inmates, the potential for violence in the setting, transience, and employment. Security concerns may also hamper provision of health care. The nurse should be alert to the use of excessive force or punitive conditions to which inmates may be subjected. Correctional nurses will also assess the extent of social support available to inmates. Social support may arise from interactions and programs available within the correctional system or from continued interactions with persons or agencies outside the system (eg, family). Development of a continuing social support program may be particularly important for clients about to be released from the facility.

Because members of ethnic minority groups are disproportionately represented among inmate populations, language may prove a significant barrier to providing effective health care for some inmates. Racial and ethnic differences, as well as other factors, may also lead to violence among inmates, and the nurse may need to assess the potential for violence within the population and alert security personnel. Nurses may also need to assess the extent of individual injuries to staff or inmates stemming from inmate violence.

Low socioeconomic level, poverty, and low education levels are all associated with incarceration. All of these factors may adversely affect health status prior to admission to a correctional facility, and education level may influence clients' knowledge of healthful behaviors or understanding of prescribed regimens for existing health problems. Inmate transience is another social dimension factor that may affect inmate health status. Inmates are frequently moved from one facility to another making completion of treatment for some conditions, contact follow-up for communicable diseases, and continuity of other health services difficult to maintain. Release back into the general population is another factor that may impede continuity of care, particularly in the case of communicable diseases like tuberculosis.

Some correctional facilities have assets that promote rehabilitation and permit inmates to earn some money. In some states, there are even provisions for inmates to work to repay victims of their crimes. Such opportunities are less readily available to women inmates than men and are rarely adequate to meet the rehabilitation needs of all inmates. The presence of occupational opportunities, however, may contribute to a variety of occupational risks to health that should be assessed by nurses in correctional facilities. Occupational hazards for correctional facility staff, as well as those for inmates, should also be considered.

Security concerns within the correctional setting are another social dimension factor that may influence health by hampering efforts to provide health care services. In some institutions, nurses do not have immediate access to inmates unless security personnel are present. In other instances, transportation of inmates for outside services may be postponed if there are insufficient security personnel available to accompany them. There is also the potential for violence against health care providers and their use as hostages.

The Behavioral Dimension

Behavioral dimension factors that influence the health of inmates and staff in correctional settings include diet, substance abuse, smoking, opportunities for exercise and recreation, and sexual activity. Inmates are more likely than the general public to engage in tobacco use and alcohol and drug use and abuse. Drug use was reported by 32% to nearly 90% of all arrestees in 23 major cities in 1994 (U.S. Department of Commerce, 1996). Alcohol and tobacco use are also common. With little to occupy their time, inmates may find themselves smoking more after than before incarceration. Smoking, coupled with overcrowding, lack of exercise, and inadequate diet may increase inmates' risk of both communicable and chronic diseases. The correctional nurse should assess substance use and abuse in individual clients as well as in the inmate population as a whole. The nurse should also assess inmates' nutritional status and particular dietary needs for individual inmates (eg, those with diabetes). Other behavioral dimension factors that should be assessed include opportunities for and participation in exercise and recreational activities. Potential safety hazards posed by exercise and recreation activities should also be assessed. Sexual activity in correctional settings has already been touched on, but the nurse should assess the extent to which condoms are available and their use within correctional systems. This is particularly important given the high incidence of sexually transmitted diseases and HIV infection among inmates.

The Health System Dimension

The correctional nurse also assesses the adequacy of the health care system in meeting the needs of the correctional facility population. Depending on several factors, including size and financial capabilities, correctional facilities may take one of two approaches to the provision of health care services for inmates. Services may be provided in-house by staff employed by the facility or the agency may contract with other provider agencies for needed services. In many institutions, a combination of both approaches is used, although recently more facilities are moving to contracting with outside providers (Anno, 1997).

Whatever the approach used, the corrections nurse should assess the adequacy of health services for inmates. Minimum services should include both primary and secondary care services. Primary health care services begin with an initial health screening on admission to the facility. This initial screening is a brief immediate evaluation of whether or not it is safe to admit the inmate to the facility given their current health status. The initial screening also facilitates correct placement of the inmate within the facility, initiates planning to meet identified health needs, and provides aggregate data for use in overall program planning (Dubler, 1986). Minimal areas to be

ASSESSMENT TIPS: Assessing Health in Correctional Settings

Biophysical Dimension

Age and Genetic Inheritance

What is the age composition of the correctional population (inmates and staff)?

What is the relative proportion of males and females in the correctional setting?

What is the racial/ethnic composition of the correctional population?

What is the prevalence of genetic predisposition to disease in the correctional population? What diseases are involved?

Physiologic Function

What existing health problems are prevalent among inmates? Among staff?

What is the incidence of HIV infection in the correctional setting? TB? Hepatitis? Other communicable diseases?

Does HIV infection pose a physical safety hazard for inmates (due to discrimination by other inmates)?

Are there handicapping conditions present among inmates? Among staff? If so, what are they? What activity limitations do they pose?

What is the prevalance of pregnancy among inmates?

What is the extent of physical injury among inmates?

What are the immunization levels in the population?

Psychological Dimension

What procedures are in place for dealing with suicidal ideation or attempts? Are these procedures followed?

What is the psychological effect of incarceration? Does the individual inmate exhibit signs of depression? Does the inmate express thoughts of suicide?

What is the extent of sexual assault among inmates? What are the psychological effects of assault?

Are there inmates in the setting under sentence of death? If so, what psychological effects does this have?

What is the prevalence of mental illness among inmates? How is mental illness manifested?

Physical Dimension

Where is the correctional facility located? Does the location pose any health hazards?

What is the extent of crowding in the facility? What are the effects of crowding?

Are facilities in good repair? Is inmate housing adequate?

Is hazardous equipment used? If so, is it used correctly?

Are recreational facilities and equipment safe and in good repair?

Are there vermin or nuisance factors in the setting? Do they pose health hazards?

Are heating, cooling, lighting, and plumbing adequate?

What is the source of water for the correctional facility? Is the water safe for consumption?

How is waste disposal handled? Does waste disposal pose health hazards for inmates or staff?

Is there potential for disaster in the area? Is there a disaster plan?

Are there other physical health hazards in the setting (eg, related to work conditions)?

Social Dimension

What are the attitudes of health and correctional personnel toward inmates?

What is the attitude of the surrounding community to the correctional facility and to the inmates?

What is the character of interactions between health care personnel and corrections personnel? Between inmates and personnel?

What kinds of sanctions are employed against inmates? Are they excessive?

What is the extent of ethnic group representation in the inmate population? Are there intergroup conflicts? Do these conflicts result in violence?

What is the incidence of violent behavior in the correctional setting? What are the health effects of violence?

What is the education level of the correctional population (inmates and staff)?

What is the income level of inmates?

What is the extent of mobility in the population?

Are inmates employed in the correctional setting? Are they employed outside? What health hazards, if any, are posed by the type of work done?

How do security concerns affect the ability of health care personnel to provide services?

What is the availability of transportation outside the facility?

Behavioral Dimension

Are there inmates with special nutritional needs? If so, what are they? How well are they being met?

ASSESSMENT TIPS: Assessing Health in Correctional Settings (cont.)

What is the nutritional quality of food served in the correctional setting?

What is the extent of alcohol, tobacco, and other drug use among inmates? Among staff?

What is the availability of drugs and alcohol in the correctional setting?

Are no-smoking policies in place in the setting? If so, are they enforced?

Exercise and Leisure Activity

What are the rest and activity patterns of the inmate population?

What recreational opportunities are available to inmates? Do recreational activities pose health hazards?

Medication Use

How are medications dispensed in the correctional setting?

Are there procedures in place to prevent inmates from selling medications or accumulating them for use in a suicide attempt?

Sexual Activity

What is the extent of sexual activity in the correctional setting?

To what extent do inmates engage in unsafe sexual practices?

What is the availability of condoms in the correctional setting?

Health System Dimension

What health services are offered in the correctional setting? Are there sufficient health care personnel to meet needs?

Are primary preventive services available and is their use promoted?

What diagnostic and treatment services are available to inmates?

What screening programs for communicable diseases are in place?

Are there isolation procedures in place for inmates with communicable diseases? Are these procedures followed?

Is substance abuse treatment available to inmates?

How accessible are needed health services in the community?

To what extent does the inmate population use available health services? What was their use of health services prior to incarceration?

How are health care services funded? Is funding adequate to meet health needs?

Are inmates charged a fee for health care services?

What is the quality of interaction between internal and external health care services?

What is the extent of emergency response capability of the correctional facility (eg, to myocardial infarction, stab wound)?

What provisions are made for continuity of care after release from the correctional facility?

---

addressed in this screening include evidence of infectious disease, existing health problems, current medications, evidence of disability or activity limitation, suicide risk, and other special needs (eg, dietary restrictions, pregnancy, need for dialysis).

The correctional health care system should also make adequate provision for diagnostic and treatment services with access assured to health personnel evaluation in a timely fashion. In some situations, this may mean curtailing the discretion of corrections personnel in determining whether or not an inmate should be brought to the attention of health care providers. If needed diagnostic and treatment services are not available within the facility, arrangements should be in place for securing these services elsewhere. The need for diagnostic and treatment services extends to dental health and mental health needs as well as care for physical health problems. The nurse should assess the adequacy of in-house services as well as the effectiveness of procedures designed to accomplish outside referrals.

The extent of emergency response capabilities (including suicide prevention programs) and health promotion activities should also be assessed. Recommended health promotion and education emphases for correctional settings include mental health issues, substance abuse, smoking cessation, sexuality issues, nutrition, disease prevention, women's health, hygiene, safety and first aid, cardiovascular health, dental health, and immunization.

The health care system within a correctional setting should also make adequate provision for efforts to control communicable diseases. This means screening programs, provision for isolation of infectious inmates, and follow up on contacts both within and outside the correctional system.

In order for health care services to be adequate to meet clients' needs, health care personnel must be available in adequate numbers and with adequate preparation for practice in correctional settings. The American Public Health Association has recommended one full-time physician for every 200 to 750 inmates (Dubler, 1986) depending upon the health needs and turnover of the population served. As noted earlier, because of the autonomous nature of practice in correctional settings, nursing personnel should be prepared—at a minimum—at the baccalaureate level.

Another assessment consideration related to the health care dimension is inmates' use of health care services prior to their incarceration. For example, the nurse might ask the female inmate when she had her last Pap smear or mammogram. The nurse would also want to explore prior interactions with health care providers related to existing health problems. For example, was the client being seen for hypertension or other health problems? Or, has the client not been taking antihypertensive medications because he or she did not have the prescription renewed.

One other feature of the correctional health care system that may affect inmates' health status is the growing tendency to require copayments of up to $5 per inmate visit to a health care provider. The intent of this practice is to decrease service utilization rates which are five to six times higher in correctional settings than in the general population. However, the point has been made by some authors that the excess use of services may be a function of the organization of services themselves when inmates may have to make multiple visits to resolve one problem that would be handled in a single visit in the civilian sector (Anno, 1997). Correctional nurses may need to be actively involved in evaluating the effect of copayment systems on the health of inmates and the implications for the health of the general public if legitimate needs for services are not being addressed.

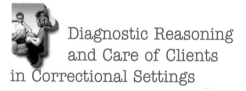

Diagnostic Reasoning and Care of Clients in Correctional Settings

Based on information obtained in assessing the dimensions of health, the nurse in the correctional setting "uses independent judgment and available data to formulate diagnoses" (American Nurses Association, 1995). Diagnoses should be validated with the client, significant others, or other health care providers when possible. Community health nurses

working in correctional settings determine nursing diagnoses relevant to individual clients as well as diagnoses related to the health needs of the total population of inmates and staff. For example, an individual diagnosis might be "uncontrolled diabetes mellitus due to substance abuse." A diagnosis related to the population group might be "increased potential for violence due to racial tensions and unrest." This second diagnosis would affect facility personnel as well as inmates since all might be involved in any violence that occurs.

 ## Planning and Implementing the Dimensions of Health Care in Correctional Settings

Planning to meet identified health problems in correctional settings may be accomplished by the nurse alone, or in conjunction with other personnel within and outside the institution. Interventions may take place at the primary, secondary, or tertiary level of prevention.

Primary Prevention

Primary prevention in correctional settings involves both health promotion and illness prevention. Health promotion emphases include adequate nutrition, rest and exercise, health education, prenatal care, and contraceptive services. Preventive efforts center around prevention of communicable diseases, suicide prevention, and violence prevention.

Health Promotion.   Nutritional intake in correctional settings may be far from adequate. The nurse in this setting may need to monitor the diet of inmates and may need to influence administrative decisions regarding the nutritive value of meals served. There may also be a need to suggest changes in food served to facility personnel if meals are provided for them as well. In addition, the nurse may need to make arrangements to meet the special dietary needs of specific inmates based on their health status. Examples include a diabetic diet or a liquid diet for an inmate recuperating from a broken jaw.

Attention should also be given to provisions for adequate rest and exercise by inmates. Nurses may need to advocate for adequate space and facilities for sleeping in inmate housing units. In addition, the nurse should work to assure that time and facilities are provided for inmates to obtain exercise. In some instances this may mean curtailing certain activities that place inmates at risk because of existing health problems. Nurses can also educate both inmates and staff on the benefits of exercise and suggest forms of exercise congruent with health status and available opportunities.

Both inmates and facility staff may be in need of a variety of health education efforts. Areas of importance include the elimination of risk factors for disease. Education programs that may be planned and implemented by nurses may include smoking cessation campaigns or stress management classes. Education regarding problem solving and positive coping strategies may also benefit both staff and inmates.

Prenatal care is a significant health promotion activity for pregnant female inmates. Areas to be addressed include adequate nutrition, the effects of smoking and other substances on the fetus, parenting skills, discomforts of pregnancy, and planning for child care if the child is delivered while the client is still in custody. Contraceptive education may benefit both pregnant and nonpregnant inmates.

Illness Prevention.   Prevention of the spread of communicable diseases in correctional settings is an important primary prevention activity. Possible approaches include the use of universal precautions in the handling of blood and body fluids (see Chap. 30 for a discussion of universal precautions), isolation of infected persons when appropriate, immunization, TB prophylaxis, and education on condom use during sexual encounters. Isolation is appropriate for diseases spread by airborne transmission such as measles and influenza. Isolation of HIV-infected individuals is not recommended unless there is a need to protect the inmate from exposure to opportunistic infection or to prevent the potential for assault by other inmates (Jonsen & Stryker, 1993). Immunization is particularly recommended for hepatitis B, but other immunizing agents may be needed as well depending on the incidence of specific diseases in the general community. For example, measles immunizations may be warranted for all inmates and staff during a measles outbreak in the community. Corrections staff, particularly health care personnel, should definitely receive HBV immunization (National Commission on Correctional Health Care, 1997b). *TB prophylaxis* is treatment of persons with reactive tuberculin skin tests, but without evidence of active tuberculosis, to prevent their development of disease. Prophylactic treatment is recommended for a minimum of 6 months for persons with positive skin tests who are not HIV-infected and 12 months for those who have HIV infection (Wilcock, et al., 1996). Corrections personnel with positive skin tests should also receive prophylaxis.

Other avenues for illness prevention include suicide prevention and prevention of violence. The primary mode of suicide prevention is identification of inmates at risk for suicide. Suicidal inmates are often placed in close observation settings and stripped of any items that could potentially be used in a suicide attempt. Those at risk for suicide should also receive timely referrals for psychiatric services. Some correctional facilities have instituted the use of inmate "aides" to assist health professionals in maintaining suicide watches on inmates at risk (*CorHealth*, 1996a). This practice is acceptable when inmate aides are used as an adjunct to professional staff rather than in place of them.

Violence prevention activities may need to be directed to both inmates and corrections staff. The purpose of such activities is to teach alternative behavioral responses to violence. Recommended components of violence prevention programs in correctional settings include incorporation of violence assessment (including prior exposure to violence) in intake screening, referral of inmates with a history of personal violence or violence exposures for counseling, education on alternative responses to potentially violent situations for both inmates and corrections staff, and referral of inmates for continued counseling on release (National Commission on Correctional Health Care, 1993a). Primary prevention emphases in correctional health care are summarized in Table 28–1.

Secondary Prevention

Secondary prevention activities in correctional health settings focus on screening and diagnostic and treatment activities.

Screening.   Screening activities center around communicable diseases and suicide risk. As noted earlier, assessment for suicide risk should be an integral part of every intake interview. Screening for certain communicable diseases may also be warranted based on client health status and the incidence and prevalence of specific conditions in the surrounding community. Screening for tuberculosis has been identified by the Centers for Disease Control as a need in correctional health systems (Woods, Harris, & Solomon, 1997). All admissions should be questioned regarding TB exposure, past diagnosis, and current symptoms suggesting active disease. Inmates who will be in custody long enough for the test to be read (48–72 hours) should be given a Mantoux skin test (see Chap. 30 for information on tuberculin skin tests) (National Commission on Correctional Health Care, 1993b). Because of the tendency for HIV-infected individuals to have

TABLE 28–1. PRIMARY PREVENTION ACTIVITIES IN CORRECTIONAL SETTINGS

Health promotion	Provision of adequate nutrition
	Provision of opportunities for adequate rest and exercise
	Health education for self-care, risk factor elimination, stress reduction, etc.
	Prenatal care for pregnant inmates
	Contraceptive education
Illness prevention	Control of communicable diseases
	Immunization
	Isolation of persons with infectious diseases
	Use of universal precautions for blood and body fluids
	TB prophylaxis
	Education for safe sex
	Suicide prevention
	Violence prevention

negative TB skin tests even with active disease, it has been suggested that radiographic testing may be more appropriate in populations with a high prevalence of HIV infection (Layton, et al., 1997). Rapid screening for syphilis, gonorrhea, and chlamydia has also been suggested for all admissions to correctional facilities (Beltrami, et al., 1997), and the National Commission on Correctional Health Care (1997b) recommends screening of all inmates for hepatitis B. Pregnancy screening for female inmates may also be warranted given the erratic nature of menses in the face of abuse of some drugs, particularly narcotics. Nurses in correctional settings will most likely be responsible for conducting these screenings.

Diagnosis and Treatment. Correctional nurses may also be actively involved in the diagnosis and treatment of existing medical conditions. Many minor illnesses are handled exclusively by nurses working under medical protocols. In other instances, nurses are responsible for implementing medical treatment plans initiated by physicians. This may involve giving medications or carrying out treatment procedures. Treatment procedures would be handled in much the same way as in any health care facility. Dispensing medications in a correctional setting, however, requires that the nurse directly observe the client take the medication and only a single dose is dispensed at a time rather than giving the client several doses of medication to be taken at prescribed times. This precaution is necessary because of potential for inmates to sell medications to other inmates or to stockpile certain medications for use in a suicide attempt.

Nurses will also be involved in emergency response to life-threatening situations. Emergency situations likely to be encountered include seizures, car-

diac arrest, diabetic coma or insulin reaction, attempted suicide, and traumatic injury due to inmate violence. The nurse would respond to these situations with actions designed to relieve the threat to life and stabilize the client's condition prior to transportation to a hospital facility either within or outside the correctional system. Correctional nurses may also find themselves involved in emergency care of large numbers of persons injured in manmade or natural disasters involving the correctional facility. Table 28–2 summarizes the major foci in secondary prevention in correctional settings.

Tertiary Prevention

Tertiary prevention in correctional settings focuses on preventing complications of existing conditions, preventing recurrence of problems, rehabilitation, and discharge planning. Tertiary prevention directed toward preventing complications of existing health problems depends upon the conditions experienced by inmates. For example, tertiary prevention for the inmate with diabetes will be directed toward preventing circulatory changes, diabetic ketoacidosis, and hypoglycemia. For the client with arthritis, tertiary prevention will focus on pain management and prevention of mobility limitations. Tertiary preventive activities may also be directed toward preventing the recurrence of problems once they have been resolved. For example, the nurse may educate an inmate who has been treated for gonorrhea on the use of condoms to prevent reinfection. Rehabilitation activities, on the other hand, may be required for clients who have already suffered consequences of acute health problems. Rehabilitation may be physical, as in the case of an inmate whose arm was fractured in a fight with other inmates, or psychological, as exemplified by care for substance abusers.

TABLE 28–2. SECONDARY PREVENTION ACTIVITIES IN CORRECTIONAL SETTINGS

Screening	Screening for communicable diseases
	Tuberculosis
	HIV infection
	Hepatitis B
	Sexually transmitted diseases
	Screening for suicide risk
	Screening for pregnancy
Diagnosis and treatment	Treatment of existing acute and chronic conditions
	Emergency care for accidental and intentional injuries
	Emergency care in the event of a disaster

TABLE 28–3. TERTIARY PREVENTION ACTIVITIES IN CORRECTIONAL SETTINGS

Preventing consequences of acute and chronic health problems

Preventing recurrence of health problems

Rehabilitation

Physical rehabilitation: restoration of normal function after physical illness or injury

Psychological rehabilitation: restoration or creation of abilities to cope with the stress of life

Social rehabilitation: assistance with resumption of life outside of the correctional facility following release

Discharge planning is another tertiary prevention activity for inmates who are about to be released back into the general population. The nurse may need to make arrangements for continuing care or arrange for housing or other survival needs. Nurses may also assist clients to anticipate and deal with some of the difficulties that are likely to arise with reintegration into families or communities after prolonged absences. Discharge planning and continuity of care are particularly important for clients experiencing ongoing chronic conditions or communicable diseases such as tuberculosis and HIV infection. Table 28–3 summarizes tertiary prevention emphases in correctional health care.

Evaluating Health Care in Correctional Settings

The principles that guide the evaluation of health care in correctional settings are the same as those applied in other settings. The nurse evaluates the outcomes of

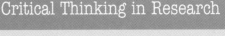
Critical Thinking in Research

Woods and colleagues (1997) conducted a study of tuberculosis knowledge and beliefs among inmates and nonhealth-professional employees (counselors and corrections officers) in correctional facilities for felony substance abusers. Both inmates and counselors were able to correctly answer, on average, three fourths of questions asked, but corrections officers were able to answer only half of the questions correctly. The most common misperceptions among all three groups were related to transmission of tuberculosis, the difference between TB infection and active disease, prevention measures, and treatment. All groups also indicated significant perceptions of stigma related to tuberculosis and expressed fear of contact with someone who has tuberculosis.

1. What are the implications of the findings of this study for tuberculosis control in correctional settings?
2. What nursing interventions could minimize the effects of misperceptions on TB control efforts? Would the interventions differ for the three groups involved? Why or why not?
3. Do you think the findings of this study would be any different if it was conducted with the general public? Why or why not? How might you go about replicating this study with the general public?

care for individual clients in light of identified goals. Correctional nurses may also be involved in evaluating health outcomes for groups of inmates or for the entire facility population, including staff. In addition, the nurse examines processes of care and makes recommendations for improvements in terms of quality, efficiency, and cost-effectiveness.

Critical Thinking in Practice: A Case in Point

You are the only nurse on the night shift in a county jail housing 150 male inmates. A new inmate is admitted to the jail for driving under the influence of alcohol. During your initial history and physical, the inmate tells you that he is on kidney dialysis and missed his last dialysis appointment which was yesterday. It is Sunday night and your facility does not have dialysis capabilities. The dialysis unit at the local hospital does not function on Sundays except in the case of emergencies. The inmate appears to be in no immediate distress and has normal vital signs and no evidence of edema. He is appropriately alert and oriented despite the odor of obvious alcohol consumption. The watch commander tells you he has no one to spare to transport the inmate to the hospital and if he goes, it will have to be by private ambulance. Your back-up physician is out of town for the weekend and the on-call physician is tied up with an emergency.

1. What are the biophysical, psychological, physical, social, behavioral, and health system factors operating in this situation?
2. What are your nursing diagnoses? How would you prioritize those diagnoses?
3. What action would you take in this situation? Why?

TESTING YOUR UNDERSTANDING

1. What are the implications of providing health care in correctional settings for inmates and for the general public? (p. 686)
2. Describe at least three ethical considerations facing nurses in correctional settings? What values are in conflict in each of these areas? (pp. 688–689)
3. Discuss at least two differences between basic and advanced nursing practice in correctional settings. (p. 687)
4. List at least three ways in which the age composition of the inmate population may affect health status. (p. 689)
5. What are the major considerations in assessing the psychological dimension of health in correctional settings? (pp. 691–692)
6. How do behavioral dimension factors influence the health status of inmates? (p. 693)
7. Describe at least three aspects of primary prevention in correctional settings. What activities might nurses perform in relation to each? (pp. 696–697)
8. What are the two main aspects of secondary prevention in correctional settings? How might community health nurses be involved in each? (pp. 697–698)
9. Discuss two considerations in tertiary prevention in correctional settings. (pp. 698–699)

WHAT DO YOU THINK?
Questions for Critical Thinking

1. In one of the studies alluded to in this chapter, correctional nurses had less favorable attitudes toward inmates than corrections officers, defense attorneys, students, and members of the general public. Why do you think the nurses' attitudes were so unfavorable? Why might these nurses continue to work in correctional settings with such unfavorable attitudes?
2. In the same study, the attitudes of jail nurses toward inmates were more favorable than those expressed by prison nurses. What might be some reasons for these differences?
3. If there were no legal mandate to provide health care to inmates in correctional settings, would you choose to spend taxpayers' dollars on care for people convicted of crimes? Would you provide care for some inmates and not for others? If so, who and why?
4. What do you think are some of the possible outcomes of requiring copayment for health care services provided in correctional settings? Do you think copayment is a good idea or not?

REFERENCES

American Nurses Association. (1985). *Standards of nursing practice in correctional facilities.* Kansas City, MO: American Nurses Association.

American Nurses Association. (1995). *Scope and standards of nursing practice in correctional settings.* Washington, DC: American Nurses Publications.

Anno, B. J. (1997). Correctional health care: What's past is prologue. *Correct Care, 11,* 6–11.

Beltrami, J. F., Cohen, D. A., Hamrick, J. T., & Farley, T. A. (1997). Rapid screening and treatment for sexually transmitted diseases in arrestees: A feasible control measure. *American Journal of Public Health, 87,* 1423–1426.

Brien, P. M., & Beck, A. J. (1996, March). HIV in prisons 1994. *Bureau of Justice Statistics Bulletin,* 1–8.

Cohen, M. D. (1997). The human health effects of pepperspray—A review of the literature and commentary. *Journal of Correctional Health Care, 4,* 73–88.

CorHealth. (1996a, January/February). *Do inmate aides prevent suicides?,* 4.

CorHealth. (1996b, January/February). *Females increase; Have more HIV,* 3.

CorHealth. (1996c, January/February). *HIV figures may be too low,* 4.

Dubler, N. N. (1986). *Standards for health services in correctional institutions* (2nd ed.). Washington, DC: American Public Health Association.

Fogel, C. I. (1995). Pregnant prisoners: Impact of incarceration on health and health care. *Journal of Correctional Health Care, 2,* 169–190.

Holman, J. R. (1997, March/April). Prison care. *Modern Maturity,* 31–36.

Jonsen, A. R., & Stryker, J. (Eds.). (1993). *The social impact of AIDS in the United States.* Washington, DC: National Academy Press.

Kay, S. L. (1991). *The constitutional dimensions of an inmate's right to health care.* Chicago: National Commission on Correctional Health Care.

Koo, D. T., Baron, R. C., & Rutherford, G. W. (1997). Transmission of *Mycobacterium tuberculosis* in a California state prison. *American Journal of Public Health, 87,* 279–282.

Layton, M. C., Henning, K. J., Alexander, T. A., et al. (1997). Universal radiographic screening for tuberculosis among inmates upon admission to jail. *American Journal of Public Health, 87,* 1335–1337.

Martin, S. L., Kim, H., Kupper, L. L., Meyer, R. E., & Hays, M. (1997). Is incarceration during pregnancy associated with infant birthweight? *American Journal of Public Health, 87,* 1521–1531.

National Commission on Correctional Health Care. (1992). *Position statement regarding the administrative management of HIV in corrections.* Chicago: National Commission on Correctional Health Care.

National Commission on Correctional Health Care. (1993a). *Correctional health care and the prevention of violence.* Chicago: National Commission on Correctional Health Care.

National Commission on Correctional Health Care. (1993b). *Position statement regarding the management of tuberculosis in correctional facilities.* Chicago: National Commission on Correctional Health Care.

National Commission on Correctional Health Care. (1997a). *Certified correctional health professional directory.* Chicago: National Commission on Correctional Health Care.

National Commission on Correctional Health Care. (1997b). Management of hepatitis B virus in correctional facilities. *Journal of Correctional Health Care, 4,* 87–97.

Polych, C., & Sabo, D. (1995). Gender politics, pain, and illness: The AIDS epidemic in North American prisons. In D. Sabo & D. F. Gordon (Eds.), *Mens' health and illness: Gender, power, and the body* (pp. 139–157). Thousand Oaks, CA: Sage.

Shields, K. E., & de Moya, D. (1997). Correctional health care nurses' attitudes toward inmates. *Journal of Correctional Health Care, 4,* 37–59.

Squires, N. (1996). Promoting health in prisons. *British Medical Journal, 313,* 1161.

Stevens, J., Zierler, S., Dean, D., Goodman, A., Chalfen, B., & De Groot, A. S. (1995). Prevalence of prior sexual abuse and HIV risk-taking behaviors in incarcerated women in Massachusetts. *Journal of Correctional Health Care, 2,* 137–149.

Teplin, L. A., Abram, K. M., & McClelland, G. M. (1997). Mentally disordered women in jail: Who receives services? *American Journal of Public Health, 87,* 604–609.

U.S. Department of Commerce. (1996). *Statistical abstract of the United States, 1996* (116th ed.). Washington, DC: Government Printing Office.

U.S. Department of Justice. (1996). *Correctional populations in the United States, 1994.* Annapolis Junction, MD: Bureau of Justice Statistics.

Wilcock, K., Hammett, T. M., Widom, R., & Epstein, J. (1996, July). Tuberculosis in correctional facilities 1994–95. *National Institute of Justice Research in Brief,* 1–12.

Woods, G. L., Harris, S. L., & Solomon, D. (1997). Tuberculosis knowledge and beliefs among prison inmates and lay employees. *Journal of Correctional Health Care, 4,* 61–71.

RESOURCES FOR NURSES WORKING IN CORRECTIONAL SETTINGS

Bureau of Justice Statistics Clearinghouse
PO Box 179, Dept. BJS
Annapolis Junction, MD 20701–0179

National Commission on Correctional Health Care
2105 N. Southport
Chicago, IL 60614–4044
(312) 528–0818

U.S. Department of Justice
Office of Justice Programs
National Institute of Justice
Washington, DC 20531

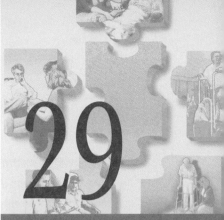

29

CARE OF CLIENTS IN DISASTER SETTINGS

Throughout history, people have been subjected to unexpected events that cause massive destruction, death, and injury. Almost any day of the week, the news media cover some kind of disaster somewhere in the world. Preparation for disasters and effective response when a disaster occurs can help minimize the long-term effects of these events. The United Nations declared the 1990s the Decade for National Disaster Reduction in an effort to combat the sense of fatalism often attached to disasters (Logue, 1996). This chapter explores the role of the community health nurse in proactive efforts before, during, and after disaster events.

▶ Chapter Objectives

After reading this chapter, you should be able to:

- Describe four ways in which disaster events may vary.
- Describe the three elements of a disaster.
- Identify at least three benefits of disaster preparedness.
- Identify at least two factors in each of the dimensions of health to be assessed in relation to disaster.
- Discuss at least six principles of community disaster preparedness.
- Describe four characteristics of a successful disaster plan.
- Identify at least five elements of an effective disaster plan.
- Describe the role of the community health nurse in primary, secondary, and tertiary prevention related to disaster situations.

▶ **DISASTERS**

Disasters are "traumatic events that are so extreme or severe, so powerful, harmful, or threatening that they demand extraordinary coping efforts" (Meichenbaum, 1995). Emergencies, on the other hand, are serious events that fall within the coping abilities of the individual or community. Disasters test the adaptive responses of communities or individuals beyond their capabilities and lead to at least a temporary disruption of function. In the 20 years from 1975 to 1995, disaster events resulted in more than 3 million deaths,

adversely affected 800 million people, and caused over $50 billion in damages worldwide (Meichenbaum, 1995; Noji, 1997b). Each year 2 million households in the United States alone experience the effects of major disasters (Meichenbaum, 1995). Table 29–1 provides an overview of some of the effects of recent disasters.

Types of Disasters

Disasters have traditionally been categorized as natural or manmade (Waugh & Hy, 1990). Natural disasters are those produced by epidemics, famine, and forces of nature such as storms, floods, and earthquakes. Manmade, or human-generated, disasters can be further differentiated as complex emergencies, technological disasters, and other human-caused catastrophes (Noji, 1997b). Complex emergencies are events caused or significantly affected by intense political considerations (Yahmed, 1994) and include war, insurrection, and civil strife. Technological disasters occur as a result of technology gone awry, as in the case of an airplane crash or train derailment. Other such disasters may include a ruptured dam. A third category of disaster combines human and natural causes. For example, toxic substances released in a transportation disaster may be widely dispersed by a windstorm. These combined disasters are sometimes referred to as "NA-TECH" disasters (Noji, 1997b). Whether natural or manmade, disasters vary considerably in terms of their frequency, predictability, preventability, imminence, and destructive potential.

TABLE 29–1. **EFFECTS OF SELECTED DISASTERS DURING THE FIRST HALF OF THE 1990S**

Year	Place	Type of Disaster	Deaths	Injury/Illness	Cost	Other Effects
1990	Iran	Earthquake	50,000	60,000		500,000 homeless
1991	Midwestern United States	Tornadoes	24	200	$250 million	8000 in need of disaster relief
1992	Los Angeles	Rioting	60	2400	$180 million	Health care system and food supplies disrupted 20,000 jobs lost
1992	Florida Louisiana	Hurricane Andrew	55		$30 billion	350,000 homeless 28,000 residences destroyed 107,000 residences damaged
1993	India	Earthquake	10,000			
	Mississippi River Valley	Flooding			$10 billion	
1994	Southern United States	Tornadoes	47	422		
1994	Georgia	Flooding (Tropical Storm Alberto)	30			175 roads closed 100 dams or watersheds damaged or destroyed
1994	Northridge, CA	Earthquake	33	7000		
1995	Kobe, Japan	Earthquake	5500			
	Virgin Islands	Hurricane Marilyn	10	3265	$3 billion	71–92% of residences on St. Thomas, St. Croix, and St. John destroyed
	Southeastern United States	Hurricane Opal	27	2131		

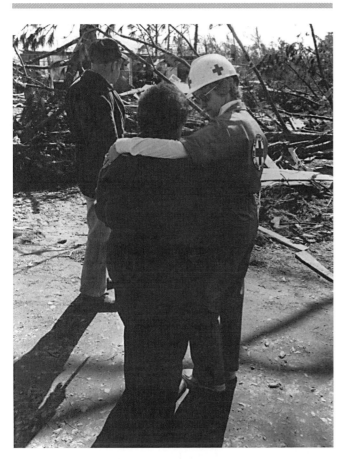

Preparation for disasters and effective response when a disaster occurs can help minimize the long-term effects of these events.
Photo courtesy of the American Red Cross, Falls Church, VA.

Some disasters occur relatively frequently in certain parts of the world. Consequently, people in those areas have some knowledge of what to expect and what can be done to minimize the effects of the event. For example, earthquakes occur periodically in California, and residents in earthquake-prone areas are encouraged to be prepared in the event of a large quake. Similarly, hurricanes and other severe storms are frequently experienced during certain seasons in other parts of the country.

Some disaster events are predictable. The probability of destructive tornadoes increases from April through June in the United States in general, but in North Dakota most tornadoes occur from June to August (Lillibridge, 1997c). Similarly, many rivers are known to flood periodically with heavy spring rains. Other events, such as a plane crash or a fire in a chemical plant, are not predictable.

Some types of disasters are more easily prevented than others. For example, periodic flooding can be prevented by rerouting waterways or by building dams. Others, such as earthquakes, cannot be controlled or prevented.

Disasters also vary with respect to their imminence in terms of their speed of onset, extent of forewarning, and duration. Some disasters provide evidence of their imminent occurrence and allow time for forewarning and preparation prior to impact. For example, hurricanes can be tracked and their probable path determined. People along that path usually have sufficient warning to take preventive actions that minimize the potential for death and destruction. Other disasters such as fires and explosions occur instantaneously, with no prior warning. In some cases, the disaster event itself is of short duration, as in the case of an earthquake or a transportation disaster. At other times, the disaster event lasts some time. Examples of prolonged disasters are epidemics, famine, and war.

Finally, disasters vary in terms of their impact and their destructive potential. Some disasters are fairly limited in scope, affecting a small geographic area or a relatively small number of people. For example, the effects of a mine cave-in are generally restricted to the area where the mine is located. The effects of war or famine, on the other hand, may be more far-reaching. Many experts distinguish between primary and secondary effects of disasters. Primary disaster effects are the immediate effects of the disaster event itself, such as the extent of death, injury, and destruction of property. Rapid-onset natural disasters, such as earthquakes, often have severe primary effects. Secondary disaster effects are those that occur indirectly as a result of the disaster. Examples might be malnutrition due to disruption of food supplies or psychological problems such as posttraumatic stress disorder. In slow-onset natural disasters like famine and manmade disasters such as war, secondary effects often influence health more profoundly than primary effects (Toole, & Malkki, 1992). Disasters also vary in terms of the severity of their effects. Some disasters cause moderate loss of life or property and result in only temporary inability to function, whereas others are devastating. The destructive potential of a nuclear explosion, for example, is far greater than that of a plane crash.

Elements of a Disaster

To plan with other members of the community for an effective response to a disaster, community health nurses need to understand the three elements of a disaster: the temporal, spatial, and role elements.

The Temporal Element: Stages of Disaster Response

Disaster experts characterize disasters as cyclic phenomena unfolding in five stages: the nondisaster or interdisaster stage, the predisaster stage, the impact stage, the emergency stage, and the reconstruction or rehabilitation stage (Noji, 1997b).

The Nondisaster Stage. The nondisaster stage, also referred to as the interdisaster stage, is the period of time before the threat of a disaster materializes. This period should be a time of planning and preparation. During this stage, communities should engage in such activities as identifying potential disaster risks and mapping their locations in the community. Vulnerability analysis is another feature of this stage in which the community assesses the potential consequences of disasters likely to occur within the community and its ability to cope with these consequences. Determination of adaptive capacity involves an inventory of resources that are likely to be needed in the event of specific types of disasters. During this stage, the community should also engage in prevention, preparedness, and mitigation activities. *Mitigation* is action taken to prevent or reduce the harmful effects of a disaster on human health or property (Malilay, 1997a). Retrofitting or reinforcing major highway overpasses is an example of mitigation being used in California to prevent the collapse of highways and bridges in the event of an earthquake. The final area of activity in the nondisaster planning period is education of both professionals and the public regarding disaster prevention and preparation. Unfortunately, many communities deny the need for disaster planning when they are not faced with the direct threat of a disaster.

The Predisaster Stage. The predisaster stage occurs when a disaster event is imminent but has not yet occurred. This stage may also be referred to as the warning (Noji, 1997b) or threat stage (McFarlane, 1995). Major activities during this stage are warning, pre-impact mobilization, and, in some cases, evacuation. The latter two activities are sometimes referred to as pre-impact mobilization. Warning involves apprising members of the community of the imminence of a disaster event and of the actions that should be taken to minimize its consequences. For example, storm warnings are broadcast in many areas when there is potential for a severe storm, but people do not immediately go to a storm cellar or leave the area, because the possibility remains that the storm will bypass the area.

Just as communities may accept or deny the need for disaster planning, members of the community may respond positively or negatively to warnings of possible disasters. Several factors can influence a person's response to warnings of imminent disaster. These factors include the source, content, and channel of the warning message, individual perceptions, warning confirmation, and belief or effect (Burkhart, 1991). Warning messages that are clear, practical, and relevant or that originate from credible sources are more likely to be acted on than vague or impractical warnings. Warnings need to specify the exact nature of the threat and provide specific recommendations for action (World Health Organization, 1989). Warnings should also contain sufficient information to allow people to decide on an appropriate course of action. It is sometimes erroneously believed that detailed information about a disaster will cause panic. In effect, failure to provide information usually leads to failure to act on warnings; providing information does not seem to contribute to panic among individual citizens.

Response to a warning is also affected by each individual's perceptions about the possibility of disaster. These perceptions arise from past experiences with disaster, psychological traits, and sociocultural factors. For example, if people have previously been only on the fringes of a hurricane path, they may not perceive a hurricane as a very frightening event, and they may ignore storm warnings. Or, if the individual has a fatalistic attitude that one's own actions will not make much difference in the outcome of an event, he or she might not act in response to warnings. Such an attitude may be the result of an individual personality trait or a sociocultural norm in the group.

Warning confirmation also influences the way people respond. Warnings tend to be believed if the source of the warning is official, if the probability of the event is increasing, and if one is in close geographic proximity to the area where the disaster is likely to occur. For example, people who live on a recognized geological fault line are more likely to take warnings about potential earthquakes seriously than those who do not live on a fault.

Finally, belief influences action with respect to warnings. Again, belief in the potential for disaster is enhanced if the source of the warning is an official agency and if that agency has credibility. For example, if there have been numerous false alarms in the past, people are less likely to pay attention to warnings. Belief is also enhanced if the medium of the warning is personal rather than impersonal. People are more likely to evacuate their homes if someone comes to their door to warn them than if they hear a warning on the radio. Previous experience also influences the likelihood of belief (Smith & Jervis, 1990). If one has experienced the full force of a hurricane before, one is more likely to believe and act on a hurricane warning than would otherwise be the case.

FACTORS INFLUENCING RESPONSE TO DISASTER WARNINGS

Factors Related to the Warning Message
- Clarity
- Practicality
- Relevance
- Informativeness

Factors Related to Individual Perceptions
- Past experience with disasters
- Psychological traits
- Sociocultural attitudes

Factors Related to Warning Confirmation
- Official source for the warning
- Increasing probability of the disaster event
- Geographic proximity to the expected disaster location

Factors Related to Beliefs
- Credibility of the warning source
- Personal, rather than impersonal, contact
- Previous experience of disaster
- Frequency of warning
- Observable changes in the situation
- Belief and action by others

The frequency with which the warning is received also influences belief, as do observable changes in the situation. For example, if people see evidence of flames on a nearby hill, they are more likely to believe in the danger posed by a brush fire. Perceived behavior of others can influence belief either positively or negatively. When others act in response to the warning, belief is enhanced. If, however, others appear to be ignoring the warning, belief is less likely. People are also more likely to believe warnings if they are with family members than if they are with other groups of people. In fact, the group environment may reinforce disbelief rather than belief. Finally, men and older people tend to place less credence in warnings than do women and younger individuals.

Preimpact mobilization is action aimed at averting the disaster or minimizing its effects. Categories of activity involved in this stage might include efforts to prevent the disaster or its effects, seeking shelter from the effects of the disaster, evacuating people from areas threatened by the disaster, and implementing plans to deal with the effects of a disaster. For example, in the threat of a flood, people may sandbag river banks to divert floodwaters from a town, or board up windows and tie down equipment when a hurricane

is forecast. People may seek shelter from tornadoes or other storms by moving to a basement, a storm cellar, or an interior room of a house. Preimpact mobilization might also involve evacuating people from an area threatened by fire, radiation, or chemical leakage. Finally, the initial phases of a disaster response plan may be implemented. For example, health care personnel may be recalled to health facilities in preparation for treating anticipated casualties.

The Impact Stage. In the impact stage of a disaster, the disaster event has occurred and its immediate effects are experienced by the community. The effects of the disaster impact will vary with the type of disaster, the density of population in the area affected, the predisaster status of the community, and the extent to which mitigating actions have been taken and the community is prepared to deal with the consequences of the specific disaster event that has occurred (Noji, 1997b). One major activity in this stage is the assessment of

STAGES OF COMMUNITY DISASTER RESPONSE

Nondisaster Stage
- Identification of potential disaster risks
- Vulnerability analysis
- Resource inventory
- Prevention and mitigation
- Public and professional education

Predisaster Stage
- Warning
- Pre-impact mobilization
- Evacuation

Impact Stage
- Damage inventory
- Injury assessment

Emergency Stage
- Search and rescue
- First aid
- Emergency medical assistance
- Restoration of communication and transportation
- Public health surveillance
- Evacuation

Reconstruction Stage
- Restoration
- Reconstitution
- Mitigation

the impact of the disaster with an inventory of the immediate needs of the community. *Inventory* is a rapid assessment of the damage to buildings and the type and extent of injuries suffered. This information is used to determine actions needed in carrying out the efforts of the emergency stage.

The Emergency Stage. The emergency stage involves the immediate response to the effects of the disaster and can be divided into two phases, an early *isolation* phase and a later *relief* phase (Noji, 1997b). In the isolation phase, the response to community needs arises from community members themselves because there has not been time for assistance to arrive from outside sources. If the community is geographically isolated or access to the community is impeded by the disaster, this isolation period will be prolonged. In the relief phase, assistance is provided from sources outside of the area affected by the disaster. The activities performed are essentially the same, although performed by different agents in the two phases, and include search and rescue operations, first aid, emergency medical assistance, establishment or restoration of modes of communication and transportation, surveillance for public health effects of the disaster (eg, infectious disease, mental health problems), and, in some cases, evacuation of community members from affected areas.

The Reconstruction Stage. In the reconstruction or recovery stage the focus is on returning the community to equilibrium. This stage can be divided into substages of restoration, reconstitution, and mitigation.

Restoration is the reestablishment of a basic way of life and occurs within the first 6 months of a disaster. Activities of this stage include returning to or rebuilding homes, replacing lost or damaged property, and continuing life without those who were killed in the catastrophe. At the community level, restoration involves reestablishing community services that may have been disrupted by the disaster. After a flood, for example, people may return to their homes, clean up the mud, and replace water-damaged furniture. Schools reopen, and residents return to work. If a prominent community official was killed in the flood, someone is appointed to fill that post until an election can be held.

Reconstitution occurs when the life of the community has returned, as far as possible, to normal. This return to normal may take from several months to several years depending on the degree of damage sustained in the disaster. It may take several years after a flood, for example, to restore the landscape of the community to its former state or to replenish the city treasury after disaster costs have depleted it. It may also take some time for individuals to adjust to

the loss of loved ones or for the community government to be reconstituted.

The final stage of recovery after a disaster is mitigation, which involves future-oriented activities to prevent subsequent disasters or to minimize their effects. For example, a community that has experienced a flood may take engineering action to prevent the likelihood of subsequent floods. Or, a community that was unprepared for disaster may develop a disaster response plan. These activities cycle the community back into the nondisaster stage.

The Spatial Element

The spatial elements of a disaster refer to the extent of its effects on specific geographic regions. These regions include the area of total impact, the area of partial impact, and outside areas (Fig. 29–1).

The area of total impact is the zone where the most severe effects of the disaster are found. In an earthquake, for example, this would include the area where the greatest damage to buildings has occurred and where the greatest number of injuries was sustained.

In the area of partial impact, evidence of the disaster can be seen but the effects are not of the magnitude of those in the total impact area. Using the earthquake example, windows may be broken or objects shaken from shelves in the partial impact area, but buildings are intact and injuries, if any, are infrequent and relatively minor. Or, only telephone and electrical services might be disrupted in the partial impact area.

The outside area is not directly affected but may be a source of assistance in response to the disaster. Areas immediately adjacent to the disaster area are called on first to provide assistance, with further outlying areas being involved later as needed.

Spatial elements of a disaster vary greatly from event to event. For example, the total and partial impact areas affected by a nuclear accident would be far larger than those affected by a fire at an industrial chemicals plant. The area from which assistance might be requested would also be larger given the greater magnitude of the problem, the number of victims involved, and the damage sustained.

Spatial elements of a potential disaster can also be explored prior to a disaster event. The World Health Organization (1989) recommends the use of community risk maps and community resource maps to help delineate spatial dimensions in disaster planning. *Community risk maps* pinpoint the locations of disaster risks within the community. Risk maps also delineate probable areas of effect for different types of disasters. Figure 29–2 is an example of a community risk map. Two primary disaster risks are identified in the

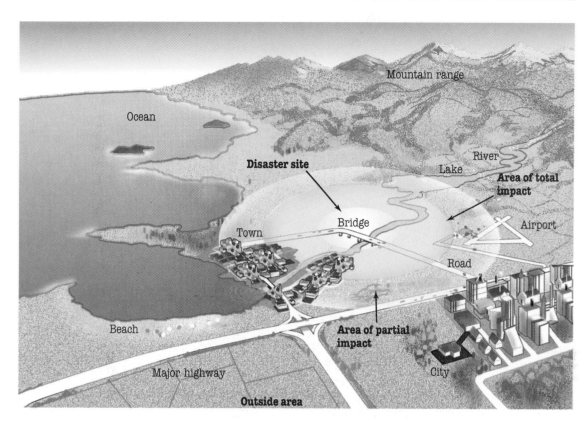

Figure 29–1. Areas of disaster impact.

community risk map in Figure 29–2, a dam and reservoir that could result in flooding and a chemical manufacturing plant on the south side of the river. In addition, this community is in an area that experiences periodic tornadoes. The community risk map delineates the areas of the community likely to be affected by a flood (along the river) and a fire or explosion at the chemical plant. The area affected by a tornado would depend on where the tornado touched down. The map also indicates several pockets of particularly vulnerable populations in areas likely to be affected by disasters. These include residents of a nursing home, prison inmates, and schoolchildren in the vicinity of the chemical plant. These same groups, along with patients at the hospital at F and No. River streets and children in the school just north of the river, would be at risk in the event of a flood on the river.

Community resource maps indicate the locations of resources likely to be needed in the event of each of the types of disasters for which the community is at risk. Notations on a community resource map include, for example, potential shelter locations, designated command headquarters (and alternates if advisable), storage places for supplies, and areas where heavy equipment is available, health care facilities, and proposed emergency morgue areas for the dead. Resource maps also indicate primary and alternate evacuation and transportation routes. Figure 29–3 is a sample resource map related to the community risks identified in Figure 29–2. Looking at Figure 29–3, we see that city hall is adjacent to the river and likely to be affected by a flood. Therefore, the command headquarters has been situated at the television station in the northern part of town. It was believed that placement at the station would facilitate communication because of the equipment available there. A southern command post has also been established in the event that both bridges are impassable and response operations on either side of the river cannot be coordinated. Because of the potential for splitting the community and lack of access across the river, potential shelter sites have been established and supplies have been stored on both sides of the river. Health services are also available on both sides even if the hospital at F and No. River streets has to be evacuated due to flooding. Rescue operations for people stranded along the river would have to be handled from the north side of the river because that is where the boat docks are located. Personnel and supplies can be brought in from other towns in several different directions and could be brought directly to tent shelter sites if necessary. Only the road from Phildon is likely to be im-

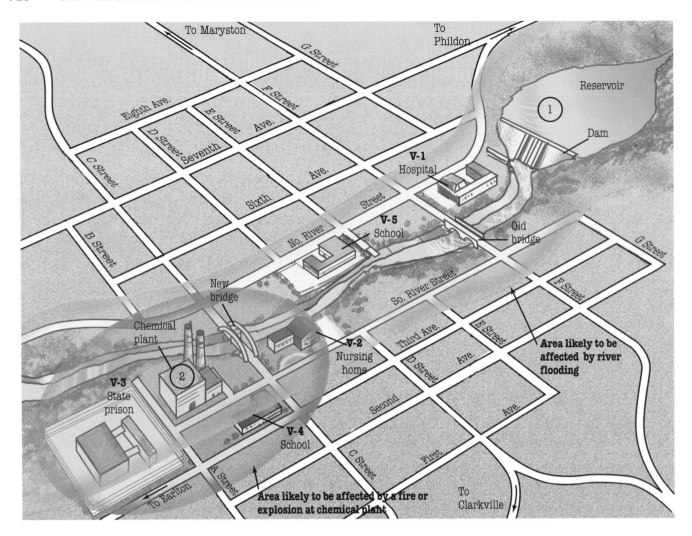

Legend:

Disaster risk
1. dam and reservoir: potential for flooding
2. chemical plant: potential for explosion/fire

V   Vulnerable populations
1. Hospitalized patients
2. Nursing home residents
3. State prison inmates
4. School children
5. School children

Figure 29–2. Sample community risk map.

passable if flooding reaches that far from the reservoir. Both the community risk and resource map allow disaster planners to visualize what is likely to occur in a disaster event and to plan the most effective response to a disaster.

The Role Element

The final element of a disaster is its role element. Two basic roles for people involved in a disaster are *victim* and *helper* roles.

People may be direct or indirect victims of a disaster. ***Direct victims*** are those who experience maximum exposure to and effects of the event. ***Indirect victims*** are friends and family of direct victims. Direct victims may require medical or psychological assistance or help with basic survival necessities. Indirect victims need reassurance and may require help in locating family members affected by the disaster.

Refugees and displaced persons are special categories of direct victims of disasters. ***Displaced persons*** are those who are forced by the disaster to leave their

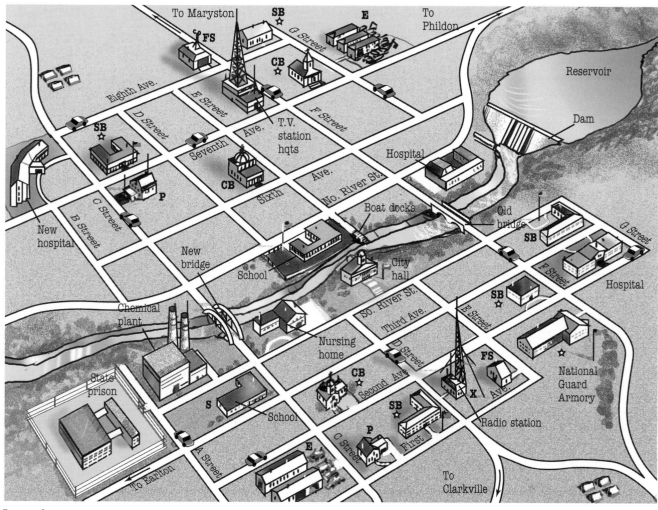

Legend:

☆	Stored supplies	**CB**	Church with basement, shelter site
E	Heavy equipment		Tent shelter site
hqts	Command headquarters	**FS**	Fire station
X	Southern command post	**P**	Police installation
SB	School with basement, shelter site		Evacuation route

Figure 29–3. Sample community resource map.

homes. Displacement may occur for a variety of reasons including destruction of one's home, temporary hazardous conditions, and war, and may persist for varying periods. *Refugees* are a subgroup of displaced persons defined by the United Nations Convention and the Organization of African Unity as those who have fled their own country for fear of war, civil disturbance, or other forms of violence. In 1994, approximately 121,000 refugees sought asylum in the United States alone (U.S. Department of Commerce, 1996) and thousands fled to other countries. Numerous

other people were displaced to other areas within their own nations. These disaster victims constitute populations at high risk for multiple health problems including malnutrition, trauma, communicable diseases, and psychological problems.

Helpers include designated rescue and recovery personnel as well as community members who help provide care or who assist in the provision of necessities such as food, shelter, and clothing. It is important to remember that victim and helper roles may overlap and that rescue and recovery personnel or other community helpers may themselves have suffered injury or loss as a result of the disaster.

Both victims and helpers are under stress as a result of the disaster. Stressors for victims may be quite obvious and include injury and the loss of loved ones or property. Stressors for helpers during the rescue and recovery periods include encounters with multiple deaths that are frequently of a shocking nature, experiencing the suffering of others, and role stress. Frequently the overwhelming nature of role demands or needs for assistance by victims lead to feelings of helplessness and depression. Other sources of role stress include communication difficulties, inadequacies in terms of resources or staff, lack of access to people needing assistance or resources to help them, bureaucratic difficulties, exhaustion, uncertainties regarding role or authority, and intragroup or intergroup conflicts. Stress may also arise from conflicts between demands of the helper's family members and the needs of victims, and between demands of one's regular job and disaster role.

▶ DISASTER PREPAREDNESS

As noted earlier, it is to be hoped that the earlier stages of a community's response to a disaster involve planning for a disaster event. For this to occur, community health nurses and others in the community must have an understanding of the concepts and principles of disaster preparedness.

Benefits of Disaster Preparedness

The need for disaster preparation and plans for disaster response is greater today than at any time in history. Increased population density throughout the world has heightened the potential for widespread effects of disasters. Technologies such as nuclear reactors and dams to provide water and electricity have also contributed to increased potential for disastrous events, as has the increased capacity to wage destructive warfare.

The costs of all types of disasters are staggering in terms of death and human suffering as well as dollars. With adequate preparation and timely response, the monetary costs of disaster could be greatly reduced. The savings in human lives that could result is another strong motivation for concerted community efforts in disaster planning. Paradoxically, while enormous sums are spent each year on disaster relief, little money is available to help communities with disaster preparedness (Waugh & Hy, 1990).

The need for disaster planning is reinforced by observations that there is less confusion regarding responsibilities and communications when specific agencies have been assigned specific functions in keeping with an overall disaster response plan. In addition, the development of interagency linkages that take place in disaster planning increases the smoothness of response in an actual disaster situation. A final reason for concerted disaster planning is that well-developed existing plans can be used in the event of other unforeseen events.

Disaster planning can also increase the adaptive capacity of the community. Planning for a disaster event heightens the community's ability to respond effectively to the aftermath of the disaster. For example, if there is a plan for emergency food and shelter that can be put into operation in the event of a disaster, the number of lives that are disrupted can be minimized. Or, if contingency plans exist for different situations, performance of critical functions will be less disrupted than it would otherwise be. For example, plans may call for casualties to be brought to a certain hospital during a disaster. If that hospital is affected by the disaster and no alternative is planned, the community will be less able to adapt to the situation, care of victims will suffer, and more lives may be lost.

Purposes of Disaster Preparedness

Disaster planning has two major purposes. The first is to reduce the community's vulnerability to the disaster and to prevent it, if possible. For example, when the threat of flood is imminent, work crews may sandbag river banks in an attempt to prevent flooding of homes and businesses. Or, in an area where flooding occurs periodically, a dam might be built to control water flow and prevent flooding. A community's vulnerability to the effects of flooding may also be reduced by locating vital community services on high ground to prevent their disruption by floodwaters.

The second purpose of disaster planning is to ensure that resources are available for effective response in the event of a disaster. This aspect of planning involves determining procedures that will be employed in response to a disaster event and obtaining material and personnel that will be required to implement the disaster plan.

Principles of Disaster Preparedness

Disaster planning should be based on several general principles (Drabek, 1986). First, measures used for everyday emergencies typically are not useful for major disasters. Disasters and everyday emergencies differ in their degree of uncertainty, urgency, and "emergency consensus." They also differ in terms of the role played by private citizens. Disasters typically present a greater degree of uncertainty than do everyday emergencies in that the latter tend to be more predictable. For example, the types of activities needed to respond to the usual residential fire are well known and predictable. The precise needs in a disaster situation are largely dependent on the type and extent of the disaster; although some of this can be predicted, the exact extent of needs is uncertain until the event occurs.

Disasters are also attended by a greater degree of urgency than everyday emergencies. Traffic accidents, for example, occur frequently and pose a need for action. People may be trapped in damaged vehicles, and there is a need to get them out. In a large-scale plane crash or train wreck, however, there is less knowledge of what the status of those trapped may be than when one individual is trapped in a single vehicle. There would be an even greater urgency if the train were carrying hazardous materials that might cause further damage.

In a disaster there is also less of an *emergency consensus,* or agreement, on what must be done and how to do it than is usually true of an everyday emergency. In addition, private citizens may have a very active role in rescue and response activities in a disaster situation, but little or no role in responding to everyday emergencies. In the case of a residential fire, for example, once fire department personnel have arrived, private citizens are expected to stay out of the way rather than assist in fighting the blaze. When a lengthy section of a major highway collapsed during an earthquake in San Francisco, however, residents in the area began immediately to help rescue people trapped in their cars and continued to help with rescue operations after emergency personnel arrived.

A second principle in disaster planning is that plans need to be adjusted to people's needs and not vice versa. If a large portion of the population is non-English-speaking, for example, it is unreasonable to issue disaster warnings only in English in the hope that someone will be available to translate the message. Third, disaster planning does not stop at the development of a written plan. Rather, disaster planning is a continuing process that changes as community circumstances change.

Fourth, the greater the incorporation of disaster "myths" into the plan, the less effective the plan will be. For example, some individuals believe that disasters inevitably trigger widespread looting and theft when this is not usually the case (Noji, 1997b). If disaster planning focuses on such myths, supplies and personnel will be diverted from necessary activities and directed instead toward preventing events that are unlikely to occur.

A fifth principle is that people in the community affected must be informed. All too frequently, some planners believe that providing the public with detailed information about the disaster and its effects will lead to panic. For this reason, vital information may be withheld, actually leading to a lack of response or to an inappropriate response on the part of the public.

Sixth, in the event of a disaster, people are likely to respond without direction, in the absence of a specific disaster plan. The typical response of most community members will be to do what seems best in the circumstances, sometimes even with heroic action. Although such efforts are commendable, they may result in duplication of effort, inefficient use of resources, and confusion.

Seventh, the disaster plan should enlist the support and coordinate the efforts of the entire community. To achieve this end, major components of the community that would be involved in a disaster response should be involved in developing the response plan. Some of those that might be involved include police and fire departments, local governing bodies, major health care facilities, and large corporations. Predisaster incorporation of these various segments of the community limits confusion with respect to authority and direction for disaster-related activities and enhances the smooth operation of a disaster effort.

Eighth, there is a need to link the disaster plan for one area with those of surrounding areas to allow coordination of efforts in the face of widespread catastrophe. Conversely, when help is needed from surrounding areas, that help will better complement local efforts if plans are coordinated. The World Health Organization (1989) refers to this kind of mutual disaster planning between adjacent communities as *twinning.*

Ninth, there is a need for a general plan that addresses all potential types of disasters in the community. When separate plans exist for different types of disasters, there is potential for confusion regarding roles and responsibilities in any particular situation. If, for example, fire personnel are supposed to have primary authority in disasters involving fires and military personnel in disasters related to destruction of property (eg, an earthquake), there may be confusion about authority in any disaster involving both. Conversely, in an unanticipated disaster, neither group may take responsibility for decision making, and the response will be hampered by lack of leadership.

Tenth, disaster plans should be based as much as

possible on everyday working methods and procedures. If one approach to communication is used in dealing with everyday emergencies, the same approach should be used in the event of a major disaster. This eliminates the need for personnel to learn new procedures and prevents confusion about which procedure is applicable in a given situation.

Eleventh, a disaster plan should be flexible enough to fit the specific situation. If the disaster event has eliminated usual means of communication, there should be a contingency plan to adapt to that circumstance. Similarly, if injured victims were to be taken to a specific hospital for treatment after stabilization and that hospital is damaged in an earthquake, there is a need to change the plan to adapt to this situation.

Finally, the plan should not specify responsible persons by name but by position or title. This prevents a need to revise the plan when one person leaves and another takes over the position. For example, the plan may specify that the chief of police be notified of the emergency situation and put the disaster plan into effect. Then, whoever happens to be chief of police will know that it is his or her responsibility to mobilize personnel in the event of a disaster. The principles of disaster planning at the community level are summarized here:

1. Measures used for everyday emergencies are not sufficient for major disasters.
2. Disaster plans should be adjusted to people's needs and not vice versa.
3. Disaster planning does not stop with the development of a written plan, but is a continuous process changing with community circumstances.
4. The greater the incorporation of disaster myths, the less effective the disaster plan will be.
5. Lack of information, rather than too much information, causes inappropriate response by community members.
6. People respond to a disaster situation with or without direction.
7. The disaster plan should coordinate the efforts of the entire community so large segments of the citizenry should be involved in its development.
8. The community's disaster plan should be linked to those of surrounding areas.
9. Plans should be general enough to cover all potential disaster events.
10. As much as possible, plans should be based on everyday work methods and procedures.
11. Plans should be flexible enough to be used in a variety of situations.
12. Plans should specify persons responsible for implementing segments of the plan by position or title rather than by name.

Participants in Disaster Preparedness

Planning community response in the event of a disaster should involve a broad cross-section of the community. Categories of people who should be involved in developing a disaster response plan are those discussed in Chapter 19 and include individuals who have the authority to sanction the plan, those who will implement the plan, beneficiaries of the plan, experts in the area, and those who are likely to resist the plan.

In disaster planning, the people who have authority to sanction a disaster plan are usually local government officials, so local governing bodies should be represented in the planning group. Representatives of those who will implement the plan might include health care professionals (including community health nurses) and personnel from local health care facilities; fire department and police department spokespersons; personnel from major industries in the area; and others who have special capabilities that might be needed in a disaster (eg, representatives of local radio and TV stations). Beneficiaries of the disaster plan are community residents, so members of concerned citizen's groups might be asked to participate in developing a disaster response plan. Consultants in disaster planning may also be invited to participate and to share their expertise. Finally, those who might object to the plan could include people who are concerned with the cost of mounting disaster planning efforts. They should be included in the planning group because they might be able to envision less expensive ways of achieving the ends of disaster planning.

Characteristics of Successful Disaster Plans

Disaster plans can be more or less effective. An effective plan has four basic qualities (Drabek, 1986). First, an effective plan typically is based on realistic expectations of the effects and needs a disaster will generate. Second, a sound disaster plan is brief and concise. A lengthy or complicated plan is unlikely to be properly implemented. Third, an effective plan unfolds by stages. The plan designates activities that must be carried out first and establishes priorities and time lines appropriate to the situation. Finally, a good disaster plan possesses an official stamp of authority. When a plan is officially sanctioned by all of the participating agencies and governing bodies, those agencies are more likely to cooperate in implementing the plan. The characteristics of successful disaster plans are summarized here:

1. The plan is based on realistic expectations of effects and needs

2. The plan is brief and concise
3. The plan unfolds and expands by stages
4. The plan possesses an official stamp of authority

General Considerations in Disaster Preparedness

General considerations in planning the response to a disaster event include designating authority, developing communication mechanisms, providing transportation, and developing a recordkeeping system.

Authority

An effective disaster response plan designates a central authority figure (Meyer & Graeter, 1995) and lays out the responsibilities that are delegated to specific persons and organizations. For example, if it is clear that evacuation decisions are made by the mayor and implemented by members of a local military installation, while police have the responsibility for keeping roads open, there will be less confusion and evacuation efforts will be carried out more smoothly. Central authority may be assigned to several people in a hierarchical order so that in the absence of the first person designated, the second person has authority to implement the plan. In this individual's absence, a third person would assume that authority, and so on.

Communication

Communication is critical to the effective implementation of a disaster response plan. Modes of communication should be established, and disaster personnel and the general public should be familiarized with them. Specific considerations in this area include how warnings of an imminent disaster will be communicated, how communication between various emergency teams and facilities will be handled, and how communication with the outside world will be facilitated. It is important to remember that normal means of communication may be disrupted during an emergency. There should also be some consideration given to facilitating communication among members of the community. For example, there may be a central bulletin board where messages can be left or a specific agency that is responsible for handling personal communications that permit family members separated by a disaster to locate each other.

Transportation

General plans for the provision of necessary transportation must also be considered. There will be a need to transport personnel and equipment to the disaster site as well as to transport victims away from the site. There will also be a need to move personnel to areas where they are most needed. Another consideration with respect to transportation is keeping access roads open so that emergency vehicles can pass. There is a need to provide alternate transportation routes, especially for evacuating people from a high-risk area, in case first-choice routes are blocked.

Records

Records are needed prior to a disaster regarding the availability of supplies and equipment and areas where they are stored. This information should be updated on a regular basis and a systematic process for its updating should be established. Local institutions such as schools and businesses should be encouraged to keep records of all those present at any given time to allow everyone to be accounted for and to permit the identification of those missing as early as possible.

During the disaster itself, there is a need for a variety of other types of records. Victims need to be identified and their condition and treatment documented. Deaths should also be recorded. Records are also needed of the use of supplies and equipment so that additional materials can be obtained if required. Records of the deployment of rescue personnel are needed to ensure the most effective use of personnel. It would be difficult to develop systematic recordkeeping systems during an actual disaster, so it is important that such systems be in place before a disaster occurs.

Critical Health Considerations in Disaster Preparedness

Four critical considerations related to the health aspects of disaster planning are suggested by the World Health Organization. They are closely related to other elements of a community disaster plan and include early warning systems, vulnerability assessment, rescue chains, and disaster-resistant facilities (Pickens, 1992). **Early warning systems** are planned surveillance systems designed to alert health care personnel of potential large-scale health problems resulting from a disaster. For example, an effective early warning system would identify early cases of communicable disease in a refugee camp, permitting immunization or other control measures to prevent an epidemic. **Vulnerability assessment** involves predisaster identification of groups within the population who would be particularly vulnerable to the adverse effects of a disaster. Elderly persons are an example of a highly vulnerable population. The extent and location of vulnerable populations should be determined and plans made for meeting their unique needs in the event of a disaster.

Rescue chains are the logistical component of emergency health care services and reflect plans for moving injured persons to appropriate care facilities. Plans should be made for distribution and transport of persons with specific types of health problems to specific facilities. Rescue chain planning also involves training in mass casualty management for health personnel in designated facilities.

Finally, there is a need for disaster-resistant health care facilities. Disaster-resistant facilities are buildings that can be expected to withstand the effects of most types of disasters without major damage. For this reason, health care and other facilities essential to disaster response should be located above potential flood levels, built to stringent earthquake-resistant building codes, and so on.

Elements of a Typical Disaster Plan

A thorough disaster plan should address notification, warning, control, coordination, evacuation, and rescue. Additional elements of the plan should specify protocols for immediate care, supportive care, recovery, and evaluation.

Notification

A disaster plan specifies in a systematic fashion the means of notifying the person or persons who can set the plan in motion. Persons who might be in a position to have advance warning of a disaster (eg, local weather service personnel) should have a clear understanding of who should be apprised of the potential for disaster. There must also be specific plans for notifying personnel and organizations involved in the disaster response. Notification should always include the fact of occurrence of a disaster, the type of disaster involved, and the extent of damage as far as it is known at the time. Notification should also convey any other relevant information that is known about the situation.

Warning

The disaster plan should also spell out the procedures for disseminating disaster warnings to the general public. Procedures should specify the content of warnings, who will issue the warnings, and the manner in which warnings will be communicated. For example, the plan might specify that warnings include the type of disaster involved, the area affected, and specific directions on actions to be taken by community members. Warnings may be issued by local radio and TV stations and by police vehicles with loudspeakers. Or, sirens may be used to alert people if they have been informed beforehand of the meaning of the siren and where to turn for more information. Sirens have been shown to be effective warning systems for severe weather conditions such as tornadoes (Liu, Quenemoen, Malilay, Noji, Sinko, & Mendlein,

1996). If warnings are to be communicated by media personnel, the plan should specify contact persons at radio and TV stations.

Control

A disaster plan also specifies how the effects of a disaster are to be controlled. Different control efforts are required for different types of disasters, and a community should be prepared to implement a variety of control activities. In the case of an earthquake, for example, control measures are directed at preventing and extinguishing fires before further damage is caused (Bay Area Earthquake Preparedness Project, 1992). Again, the procedures, materials, and personnel needed to carry out control measures must be specified in the plan.

Logistical Coordination

Another element of a community disaster plan deals with logistical coordination. **Logistical coordination** is the coordination of attempts to procure, maintain, and transport needed materials. The disaster plan specifies where and how supplies and equipment will be obtained, where these will be stored, and how they will be transported to the disaster site.

Traffic control is another aspect of logistical coordination. The disaster plan should specify personnel and procedures for controlling access to the disaster site. Traffic control procedures should also specify means by which access to the disaster site is ensured for rescue vehicles and vehicles carrying personnel, supplies, and equipment.

Evacuation

A disaster plan also specifies evacuation procedures. The plan should indicate how those to be evacuated will be notified, what they can take with them, and how the evacuation will be accomplished. The plan may need to specify several contingency evacuation procedures depending on the type of disaster.

The disaster response plan also provides for the logistics of evacuation, including the personnel needed to carry out the evacuation, how they are to be recruited and assigned, and how they will be notified. The plan also specifies the forms of transportation to be used during evacuation, where appropriate vehicles can be obtained, and how they will be refueled.

Rescue

The response plan should specify the process to be used to assess rescue needs and who is responsible for carrying out the assessment. Once the assessment is made, there should be procedures in place for obtaining the appropriate personnel and equipment. For example, in the event of an earthquake, heavy construction equipment and operators are needed, whereas fire department personnel are needed in a fire-related disaster.

The rescue operation should focus on removing victims from hazardous conditions and providing first aid as needed. Rescue personnel should refrain from providing other forms of care as much as possible. This care can be provided by others, thus freeing rescue personnel to carry out the rescue operation.

Immediate Care

Provision of immediate care is another consideration detailed in a disaster response plan. *Immediate care* is care required on the spot to ensure a disaster victim's survival or a disaster worker's continued ability to function. Plans for providing immediate care in four areas in the vicinity of the disaster site (Fig. 29–4) should be detailed in the disaster response plan. Immediate care begins at the actual site of the disaster, with a rapid initial assessment of all victims by the first health care provider on the scene. This phase of immediate care is geared to correcting any life-threatening problems.

The second area of immediate care is the triage area. *Triage* is the process of sorting casualties on the basis of urgency and their potential for survival to determine priorities for treatment, evacuation, and transportation (Duffy, 1990). Triage decisions are intended to maximize the number of survivors of a disaster event. When victims are easily accessible, triage can take place at the site of the disaster. Victims are then removed to treatment areas based on their triage priority. In a disaster occurring in an enclosed environment (eg, in a mine or in a building), victims may not be easily accessible and will probably need to be removed to a more distant triage area as they are found.

The triage process usually involves placing color-coded tags on victims. Typically, black tags are attached to victims who are already dead. Red tags indicate top priority and are attached to victims who have life-threatening injuries but who can be stabilized and who have a high probability of survival. Priority is automatically given to injured rescue workers, their family members, hysterical persons, and children. Yellow tags, indicating second priority, are assigned to victims with injuries with systemic complications that are not yet life-threatening and who are able to withstand a wait of 45 to 60 minutes for medical attention. Yellow tags are also assigned to victims with severe injuries who have a poor chance of survival. Green tags indicate victims with local injuries without immediate systemic complications who can wait several hours for treatment.

The third area of immediate care at the disaster site is the treatment area to which victims are removed after triage. In this area medical stabilization,

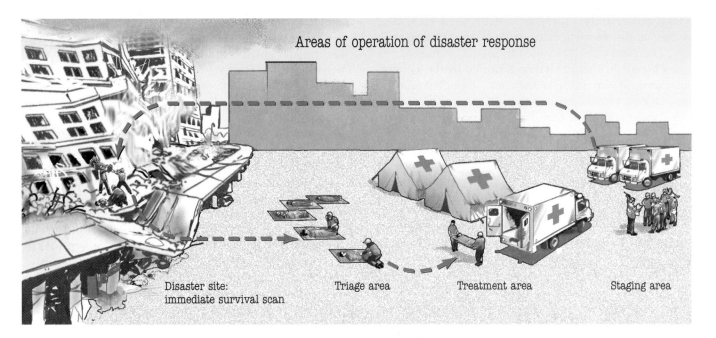

Figure 29–4. Areas of operation in the rescue phase of disaster response.

temporary care, and emergency surgical stabilization are provided as needed. There may also be a need for psychological first aid at this point. The final area at the site of the disaster is the staging area. It is here that immediate care operations are coordinated and vehicles and personnel are directed to areas of greatest need. The disaster plan should specify the procedures for setting up and operating each of the four areas of immediate care. The plan should also address the supplies, equipment, and personnel needed in each area, how they will be obtained, and how they will be transported to the area.

Another area related to immediate care that should be addressed in the disaster plan is care of the dead. Plans should be included for procedures to identify bodies and transport them to a morgue of some sort. Records of deaths should be kept, and procedures for rapid disposal of bodies should be specified should contagion be a problem. Plans should also include where and how body bags and identification tags will be obtained.

Supportive Care

Supportive care must also be addressed in an effective disaster response plan. Supportive care includes providing food, water, and shelter for victims and disaster relief workers. Other considerations in this area are sanitation and waste disposal, providing medications and routine health care, and reuniting families separated by the disaster.

Shelter is required for those who are evacuated from their homes or whose homes are damaged in the disaster. The disaster response plan should specify which community buildings can be used to shelter victims and how victims are to be transported to shelters. There may also be a need to use the homes of private citizens to shelter victims if public shelters are insufficient. When such is the case, the plan should specify how to notify concerned citizens of the need to place victims in their homes and how placement is to be handled. It is helpful to have a list of people willing to provide shelter to others should a disaster occur. In the case of large groups of displaced persons, refugee camps may be set up. Camp sites, for example, should be carefully selected in relation to possible physical hazards or water runoff.

Within the shelter, there is a need for supplies to sustain daily living. Shelters should have adequate sanitation and sleeping facilities. There should be plans for heating shelters and cooking food if area gas and electrical power systems are disrupted. Mechanisms should also be specified for governance and security within the shelter, particularly if the shelter will be in use for some time. Shelter leaders can be ap-

pointed or elected, and persons within the shelter should have a means of providing input into governance in long-term shelter situations.

Food supplies should be planned and obtained prior to a disaster. There should also be a mechanism for obtaining more food and other supplies from outside the community in the event of damage to stores and stockpiled supplies. A source of clean water is needed, and the disaster plan should identify how and where water will be supplied. Equipment for water purification should be stored in case of need (Lillibridge, 1997b). There is also a need to plan for adequate sanitation, waste disposal, and vector control at shelters and throughout the community following a disaster (Malilay, 1997b).

Victims may have other health care needs unrelated to the disaster that need to be met, so plans for providing basic health care in shelters should also be specified. These plans should include stores of medications most likely to be needed by the general public and critical to survival. For example, diabetics will continue to need insulin or oral hypoglycemics, whereas individuals with heart conditions may need a variety of medications. Priority should be given to medications required for serious illnesses rather than for minor conditions. Because communicable diseases spread more rapidly in a debilitated population following a disaster, antibiotics and vaccines should be stored in case of need.

Supportive care also includes psychological counseling for those who are not coping adequately with the situation. Counseling may be required by both victims and disaster workers, and plans should be made to provide crisis intervention services during the response stage of the disaster (Gerrity & Flynn, 1997). Psychological support can be provided by comforting and consoling those in distress and by protecting them from the ongoing disaster threat. The disaster plan should include mechanisms for identifying those in need of counseling and providing them with the services required.

Disaster victims may require goal orientation and guidance, and they can be directed to perform specific tasks that help them achieve a sense of control. Support is needed for those who must identify loved ones among the dead. Expression of feelings should be fostered, and victims should be encouraged to make use of available support networks. Immediate referral to mental health personnel may be required in some instances. Structuring the environment and regularizing schedules, particularly in shelters, can also help to reestablish a sense of security.

Some relief from psychological stress can frequently be obtained if victims can be assured that family members are safe. Disaster plans should therefore include mechanisms for locating people and re-uniting families. Names of persons admitted to shelters or health care facilities should be recorded and communicated to a central location where others can check for word of loved ones. Deaths should also be reported if the dead can be identified, and information should be kept on the assignment of disaster workers to specific areas. It is helpful if institutions, such as schools and businesses, compile the names of those who were present prior to a disaster so that they can be accounted for afterward.

Recovery

Another component of the disaster plan is mechanisms for supporting community rehabilitation. There may be a need to rebuild or repair damaged structures, and plans should be made for obtaining financial and material assistance in these endeavors. Mechanisms should be developed that help victims to process insurance claims as rapidly as possible. There may also be a need for outside assistance in rebuilding, and plans should be made for obtaining that assistance.

Psychological counseling is needed in the aftermath of a disaster, and mechanisms should be developed for identifying and referring those in need of counseling. Postdisaster counseling may be delegated to specific mental health agencies that would plan how postevent counseling will be handled, who will be eligible for care, and procedures for obtaining care. Particular attention should be given to the counseling needs of both disaster workers and victims, because research has indicated the potential for psychological trauma to both as a result of a disaster experience.

Evaluation

Plans should also be made prior to the disaster for evaluating the effectiveness of the disaster plan and its implementation. Again, consideration should be given to procedures, personnel, and materials needed to carry out the evaluation. Records are needed that permit evaluation of the efficiency and effectiveness of the plan, and procedures should be developed for obtaining and storing data. Plans should also be made for follow-up meetings with disaster workers to provide input into the evaluation process. The focus of these meetings would be on what worked and what did not work and what could be done to improve the plan and its implementation in subsequent disasters.

▶ ## ELEMENTS OF A TYPICAL DISASTER PLAN

- Mechanisms exist for notifying individuals responsible for authorizing disaster plan implementation.
- Mechanisms exist for warning individuals likely to be affected by the disaster.
- Mechanisms exist for controlling damage due to disaster.
- Procedures are specified for logistical coordination in traffic control and transportation of equipment, supplies, and personnel to the disaster site.
- Procedures are specified for evacuating individuals in the potential disaster area.
- Plans are in place for rescue operations to remove victims from hazardous situations.
- Plans and procedures have been designed to meet immediate care needs of disaster victims related to triage, first aid, transportation to other facilities, and care of the dead.
- Plans and procedures have been designed to provide supportive care to meet ongoing needs of disaster victims and relief workers related to emergency shelter, food and water, sanitation and waste disposal, health care and medications, and reuniting families.
- Mechanisms are in place to provide assistance to victims during the recovery period.
- Mechanisms exist for evaluating the adequacy of the disaster plan in meeting the community's needs.

▶ ## NURSING RESPONSIBILITIES IN DISASTER PREPAREDNESS

Community health nurses are well suited to assist in the actual development of a disaster plan. Because of their background in program planning and group dynamics, they can help ensure that planning is a systematic rather than a haphazard process. Community health nurses also have knowledge of what the health-related needs of the population would be in a disaster and can provide input regarding needs and vulnerable populations, as well as potential resources for meeting needs.

Another role for community health nurses in disaster preparation is to train rescue workers in triage techniques and basic first aid. Nurses might also help educate personnel who will staff shelters regarding the needs of disaster victims and considerations related to group interactions that will make shelter operations run more smoothly. A final responsibility of community health nurses in the disaster planning stage is educating the public regarding the disaster plan and the need for personal preparation for a disaster.

► THE DIMENSIONS MODEL AND CARE OF CLIENTS IN DISASTER SETTINGS

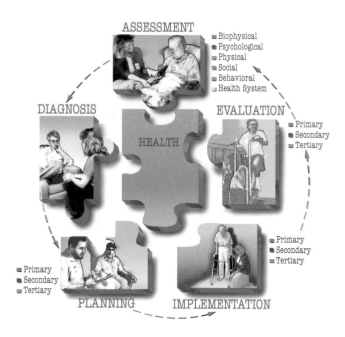

The Dimensions Model can be used by community health nurses and others involved in disaster response planning to guide the development, implementation, and evaluation of the disaster plan.

 Assessing the Health Dimensions of a Disaster

Assessment in providing disaster care has three aspects: assessing the extent of disaster preparedness, assessing the potential for disaster, and assessing possible effects of a disaster. The first task of community health nurses and others involved in disaster planning is to examine the current level of disaster preparedness in the community. How prepared is the community to respond to a disaster, and how effective is that response likely to be? The World Health Organization has developed a preparedness checklist intended for use in assessing national levels of disaster preparation (Pickens, 1992). This checklist has been adapted for use at the community level. Answers to the questions posed in the checklist provide direction for comprehensive community disaster planning.

Identifying the potential for disaster in a particular community involves forecasting the types of disasters possible and the likelihood of their occurrence. The possible types of disasters, of course, vary from community to community. Disaster potential and the probable effects can be systematically assessed by examining factors related to each of the six dimensions of health. The dimensions of health perspective can also be used to assess the effects of an actual disaster.

The Biophysical Dimension

One determinant in forecasting potential disasters is that of human biology. Certain groups of people are more likely than others to be affected by a disaster. For example, if the anticipated disaster is an epidemic of influenza, those most likely to be severely affected are the very young and the elderly; however, there also will be illness among the work force that may impede efforts to halt the spread of disease. On the other hand, if there is potential for an explosion in a local chemical plant, those affected are likely to be company employees and persons in surrounding buildings that might be damaged as well. Again, this might

► COMMUNITY DISASTER PREPAREDNESS CHECKLIST

- Is there a community disaster plan? Is the plan being implemented?
- Is there a person in charge of promoting, developing, and coordinating emergency preparation?
- Are emergency preparedness activities coordinated among relevant community agencies?
- What joint emergency preparedness and response activities are undertaken by community agencies?
- Are there operational plans for health response to a disaster?
- Have mass casualty plans been developed?
- What surveillance measures are in place for early detection and response to health emergencies?
- What steps have been taken by environmental health services to prepare for disaster response?
- Have facilities and safe areas been designated as shelter sites in the event of a disaster? What health care provisions have been made?
- What disaster preparedness training has been undertaken with health care personnel?
- What resources are available for rapid health response to disaster (eg, communications, financing, transport, supplies)?
- Is there a system for updating information on supplies and personnel?
- What opportunities exist to test the effectiveness of the disaster plan?

include children if there is a school nearby. In disasters requiring evacuation, the elderly are at particular risk because of potential mobility limitations.

Human biology is also a factor in predicting the types of effects expected as a result of the disaster. In the case of an influenza epidemic, illness potentially accompanied by dehydration and electrolyte imbalance may be expected. In an explosion, expected injuries may consist of burns and trauma (Lillibridge, 1997a), whereas a flood results primarily in drownings (Malilay, 1997a).

The overall health status of the community also influences disaster planning requirements. For example, if hypertension is prevalent in the community, provisions need to be made in a disaster plan for ongoing treatment of hypertension or other prevalent diseases. Possible biophysical effects of several types of disasters are presented in Table 29–2.

In the event of disaster, the community health nurse assesses the physiologic effects of the event on human biology. The nurse appraises the extent of injuries incurred by victims and relief workers and may also assess other needs for health care. For example, the nurse might need to assess the health status of a disaster relief worker with diabetes or of a child with a fever. The nurse assists in assessing the health status of groups of people. For example, the nurse may note an increased incidence of diarrhea among evacuees in a shelter or identify nutritional needs in war refugees.

The Psychological Dimension

Components of the psychological dimension can also influence the effects of a disaster on health. As noted earlier, a number of psychological factors can affect the way people respond to a warning of disaster. Similarly, psychological factors can influence responses once a disaster has occurred. For example, familiarity with earthquakes may limit panic in some people, whereas those new to the area, who have never before experienced an earthquake, may panic and respond

TABLE 29–2. BIOPHYSICAL EFFECTS OF SELECTED DISASTERS

Type of Disaster	Considerations Related to Human Biology
All disasters	• Greater loss of life and injury among the elderly, young children, and chronically ill and disabled persons
Avalanches	• May result in asphyxiation
	• May result in frostbite and other effects of exposure to cold
	• May result in fractures or other forms of trauma
Chemical spills	• May result in chemical burns of the skin
	• May result in respiratory irritation and illness
	• May result in poisoning with a variety of symptoms depending on the chemical involved
	• May result in eye irritation
Earthquake	• May result in crushing injuries and fractures from falling bricks, masonry, and other objects
	• May result in burns suffered in fires and explosions due to ruptured natural gas mains
	• May result in waterborne diseases because of ruptured water mains and lack of safe drinking water
	• May result in electrocutions from fallen power lines
Epidemics	• May result in communicable diseases with a variety of symptoms depending on the disease involved
Explosions	• May result in burns due to associated fires
	• May result in fractures or crushing injuries due to explosion impact or falling masonry, bricks, and other debris
Famine	• May result in developmental delay in young children
	• May result in failure to thrive in nursing infants because of inadequate lactation by mothers
	• May result in protein–energy malnutrition and other nutritional deficiencies
Fire	• May result in minor to severe burns
	• May result in respiratory problems due to inhalation of smoke and hazardous fumes from burning objects
Floods	• May result in drownings
	• May result in waterborne and insectborne diseases from contaminated water supplies and insect breeding grounds
Radiation leakage	• May result in radiation burns or radiation sickness
	• May result in later cancer
	• May result in later infertility, spontaneous abortion, or fetal defects
Storms	• May result in crushing injuries due to windblown objects and debris
	• May result in minor to severe lacerations due to flying glass from broken windows
Transportation disasters	• May result in crushing injuries and other trauma
	• May result in burns with associated vehicle fires
	• May result in drownings or asphyxiation if disasters occur over water or in tunnels
	• May result in exposure to the elements if disaster occurs in a remote area

inappropriately. Communities and persons with good coping skills usually respond more effectively in a disaster situation than those who have poor coping skills.

The community health nurse should assess the attitudes of community members toward disaster preparedness. To what extent are individuals and families in the area prepared for potential disasters? Have families in an earthquake-prone region, for example, gathered supplies that will be needed in the event of an earthquake and placed them in an accessible location? Have emergency escape routes from homes, schools, and other buildings been identified? Have families discussed an emergency contact person who can relay messages for and about family members separated in a disaster? Or, are these types of preparation largely ignored?

In the event of an actual disaster, the community health nurse assesses the psychological effects of the disaster event. As noted earlier, both victims and relief workers may experience stress related to a disaster, and the nurse should be alert to signs of emotional distress in both groups. Signs of psychological distress might include confusion, inability to make decisions, excessive crying, aggressive behavior, restlessness, inability to sleep, and nightmares.

Various factors influence psychological responses to disaster events. In particular, characteristics of the community response to the disaster event can influence the number and type of mental health problems exhibited in the population (Quarantelli, cited in Weaver, 1995). Factors that influence the development of mental health problems include the proportion of the population directly involved in the disaster and the social centrality of the population involved. For example, psychological responses to a disaster are likely to be more extreme if large segments of the population have been affected or if those most affected are central to the community such as a large number of community leaders or small children as in the Oklahoma bombing disaster. Length, rapidity, and predictability of involvement in the disaster also influence the propensity for adverse psychological reactions. In addition, lack of familiarity with the type of disaster involved may increase the potential for mental health effects. For example, in a population that is somewhat accustomed to earthquakes, the incidence of psychological problems following a severe earthquake is likely to be less than in a community that has never experienced an earthquake before. The depth of involvement of an individual also influences mental health effects. Members of the community who have experienced personal loss are at greater risk of psychological problems than those who have not experienced losses themselves.

▶ FACTORS INFLUENCING PSYCHOLOGICAL RESPONSES TO DISASTER
· Proportion of the population affected
· Social centrality of population affected
· Length of involvement
· Rapidity of involvement
· Predictability of involvement
· Familiarity with type of disaster
· Depth of involvement
· Frequency of recurrence

Finally, the frequency of recurrence of the disaster may influence psychological responses. For instance, if this is the third year in a row that a particular community has experienced severe flooding, community members may be at greater risk for mental health effects. Similarly, repeated aftershocks of an earthquake can intensify fear and anxiety in many community members.

Types of immediate psychological responses to disasters range along a continuum from calm, collected action to confusion and hysteria. Plans should be made for services to address each level of response. Health care providers should also keep in mind that psychological responses change with time and with the progression of the disaster event. The sequence of psychological responses to a disaster parallel the stages of the disaster itself (Gerrity & Flynn, 1997). For example, the typical response in the warning stage of a disaster is fight or flight, either of which may be appropriate or inappropriate in a given situation. In the alarm stage, the most likely response is one of anxiety, whereas a feeling of being stunned is typical of the impact stage. During the rescue stage, many people may exhibit mood and attitude extremes. Ambivalence is common in the recovery stage as the reality of loss is acknowledged. Finally, psychological responses in the reconstruction stage may be quite varied. These responses are basically normal unless they are extreme in nature. Even normal response, however, can place one at risk for harm. For example, the feeling of being stunned during the impact stage may lead one to disregard personal safety and to fail to avoid environmental hazards like unsafe masonry in an earthquake area. Psychological recovery occurs for most people within 6 to 12 months of the disaster, but a small segment of the population may exhibit chronic anxiety, depression, or interpersonal difficulties at home or at work (Cohen, 1992).

The Physical Dimension

Many disasters arise out of features of the physical environment. For example, the presence of a river near the community and the likelihood of heavy rainfall both contribute to the potential for flooding, as does the construction of homes and businesses on floodplains. A geological fault, a nuclear reactor, and a chemical plant are other examples of factors in the physical environment that may increase the potential for a disaster.

Elements of the physical dimension can either help or hinder efforts to control the effects of a disaster. For example, limited traffic access to the part of town where an explosives plant is located could hinder movement of emergency vehicles in the event of a fire or explosion. Similarly, the physical isolation of a mountain community may impede rescue efforts in the event of a forest fire or flood. On the other hand, such isolation might spare the community from the effects of an epidemic in the surrounding area.

In conducting a community assessment, the community health nurse identifies physical environmental factors that might contribute to the occurrence of a disaster. The nurse also determines whether the community is prepared for potential disasters. When the community is not prepared, the nurse would advocate the planning activities described earlier in this chapter.

The nurse also identifies factors that might impede the community's response in the event of a disaster. The nurse can then share these observations with others involved in disaster planning, and interventions to modify or circumvent these factors can be incorporated into the community's disaster response plan.

The Social Dimension

Social dimension factors can also influence the way people respond to a disaster and may even give rise to one. For example, the presence of racial tensions could trigger outbreaks of violence in some communities. War is another disaster arising out of social environmental conditions. In assessing a community, the nurse identifies social factors that might contribute to disasters and to the way people respond to them.

Elements of the social dimension also may increase or limit the effects of a disaster on a community. For example, the economic status of community members and of the community at large may limit the ability of people to prepare for potential disasters or to recover after a disaster event. Language barriers may hamper evacuation or rescue efforts. Strong social networks in the community that can be tied into disaster planning aid in effective disaster response, whereas intragroup friction hampers response effectiveness. Surprisingly, strong family social support networks within the population may actually hamper disaster response efforts. Cultural groups with strong family ties may be willing to interact with other family members to provide mutual aid and support but may be resistant to communitywide activities (Cohen, 1992). The nurse identifies social factors present within the community that may decrease the effectiveness of the community's response to a disaster and participates in planning efforts to modify these factors. The nurse also identifies social factors that enhance the community's ability to respond effectively in the event of a disaster. Planning groups could then capitalize on these factors in designing an effective disaster plan. For example, well-established cooperative relationships between groups and agencies in the community are an asset in designing and implementing a disaster plan, whereas the presence of relatively isolated cultural groups may impede planning and response efforts.

Another aspect of the social environment that should be assessed is community attitudes toward and participation in disaster planning. Are local government agencies supportive of planning efforts? Do community members exhibit concern for disaster planning and do they follow through on recommendations for disaster preparedness?

Occupational factors are another element of the social dimension that can contribute to the potential for disaster in a community and should be assessed by the nurse. For example, the community health nurse should be aware of industries in the area that pose hazards related to fire or explosion. The potential for radiation exposure or leakage of toxic chemicals in the community should also be determined. The nurse may also want to appraise the extent to which local industries adhere to safety regulations related to hazardous conditions. Community health nurses working in industrial settings would be particularly likely to have access to this type of information. Other community health nurses may need to advocate regular inspection of industrial conditions by the appropriate authorities.

The community health nurse also identifies occupational factors that may enhance a community's abilities to respond effectively in the event of a disaster. The nurse and others involved in disaster planning would explore the adequacy of rescue services and personnel for dealing with potential disasters. Is the number of firefighters in the community, for example, adequate to deal with an explosion and fire in a local chemical plant? Do firefighting units possess the equipment needed to deal with such an event? Planners also assess the existence of other occupational groups that may assist with disaster response. For example, are there construction companies in the community that could supply heavy equipment that might be needed for rescue operations?

In the event of an actual disaster, the nurse might also assess social factors influencing the community's disaster response. For example, the nurse might identify growing intergroup tensions in shelters for disaster victims or disorganization in efforts to reunite families separated by the disaster. Other areas for consideration include the degree of cooperation among groups providing disaster relief and, following the disaster, the availability of recovery assistance to individuals and families.

The Behavioral Dimension

Behavioral factors related to consumption patterns and even leisure pursuits can also influence the occurrence of disasters and their effects on the health of community members.

Consumption Patterns. Consumption patterns such as smoking, drinking, and drug use can contribute to disasters. Smoking, for example, is often the cause of residential fires and forest and brush fires that result in loss of life as well as extensive property damage. Drinking and drug abuse have both been known to contribute to transportation disasters, and they may also contribute to industrial disasters when the abuser is working in a setting with disaster potential. For example, if a person responsible for monitoring the safety of a nuclear reactor is drunk, he or she is unlikely to recognize or respond appropriately to signs of danger. The community health nurse assesses the extent of smoking and substance abuse in the community in relation to the potential for disaster. The nurse may also want to assess (or encourage others to assess) the effectiveness of substance abuse policies in transportation services and industries where there is potential for disaster. Another area for assessment is the extent of safety education in regard to smoking (eg, not smoking in bed) that occurs in the community.

Consumption patterns may also intensify the effects of a disaster on the health of a population. A community whose members are poorly nourished, for example, is at greater risk for consequences of disaster such as communicable diseases. Substance abuse may limit one's potential for appropriate behavior in an emergency and lead to injury and even death due to failure to respond appropriately. For example, intoxication may prevent someone from fleeing a burning building.

Consumption patterns and their effects are particularly relevant in disasters involving famine and large displaced or refugee populations. *Famine* is a populationwide condition involving substantial mortality from malnutrition. Common nutritional effects of famine among refugee populations include *protein-energy malnutrition (PEM),* a severe state of undernutrition that may be either acute or chronic, and deficiencies of specific micronutrients such as vitamin A, iron, vitamin C, niacin, and thiamine. Acute PEM is associated with wasting and diminished weight-for-height measures. Chronic undernutrition, on the other hand, results in stunted growth and decreased height-for-age measures (Toole & Malkki, 1992).

Lack of exercise in the population can limit the ability to engage in strenuous labor that might be demanded in a disaster situation. Unaccustomed activity may result in exhaustion or heart attack. The nurse assesses the levels of exercise engaged in by the general population. Community health nurses in occupational settings may also be responsible for determining the physical fitness of personnel who would be involved in rescue operations in the event of a disaster (eg, firefighters).

Leisure Pursuits. The leisure pursuits of community members may, on occasion, contribute to the occurrence of a disaster event. Careless campers, for example, could ignite a forest fire, or skiers might trigger an avalanche. Fires can be started by sparks from recreational vehicles. The community health nurse and others involved in disaster planning assess the extent of such leisure pursuits in the community, the existence of safety regulations related to these pursuits, and the degree of adherence to safety regulations. Do campers, for example, refrain from lighting fires in fire-prone areas, or do skiers avoid restricted areas where avalanches are possible?

Leisure pursuits can also enhance the community's response to a disaster event, and the nurse assesses the presence of leisure pursuits that may have this effect. For example, the existence of a group with an interest in wilderness survival may be an advantage in the event of an avalanche or a plane crash in a remote area. Or, people with citizen-band radios may assist with communications in the event of an emergency.

The Health System Dimension

The adequacy of the health care system's response capability in the event of a disaster influences the extent to which a disaster affects a community and the health of its members. Assessing the ability of the health care system to respond to a disaster includes examining facilities and personnel as well as the organizational

ASSESSMENT TIPS: Assessing Health in Disaster Settings

Biophysical Dimension

Age and Genetic Inheritance

What is the age composition of the population involved in the disaster? Are the effects of the disaster likely to be worse for some age groups than others? If so, which age groups are most likely to be affected?

What is the racial/ethnic composition of the group affected by the disaster?

Physiologic Function

What is the extent of injury resulting from the disaster?

What chronic health problems are prevalent among those involved in the disaster?

What is the potential for communicable diseases as a result of the disaster? What is the extent of existing communicable disease among those affected? What diseases are involved?

Are there pregnant women involved in the disaster?

Psychological Dimension

How does the population respond to disaster warnings?

What is the extent of community/individual ability to cope with the disaster?

What is the effect of the disaster on rescue workers? On victims? Do individuals exhibit signs of distress?

What is the extent of existing mental illness among those involved in the disaster?

What are the long-term psychological effects of the disaster on the community?

What is the extent of damage or loss of life involved in the disaster?

Does the disaster present the potential for continuing damage or loss of life?

Physical Dimension

What physical features of the community create the potential for disaster? Is there potential for flooding? Forest or brush fires? Earthquake?

What structures are likely to be threatened by a disaster? To what extent are vital structures likely to withstand a disaster?

What structures could be used as emergency shelters?

Will weather conditions influence the effects of the disaster? If so, how?

Are there elements of the physical dimension that will hinder response to the disaster (eg, blockage of roads)? If so, what are they?

Have buildings been structurally damaged? Is there potential for additional structural damage? Does structural damage pose further risk to victims? To rescuers?

Is there a need for sources of shelter for persons displaced by the disaster?

Is there a safe water source available to victims of the disaster?

To what extent are animals involved in the disaster? What health effects might this have?

Social Dimension

Interpersonal Relationships

Do relationships in the community have the potential to create a disaster (eg, civil strife, war)?

How cohesive is the community? Are community members able to work together for disaster planning? What is the attitude of community members to disaster planning?

Is there potential for conflict among disaster victims? Rescuers?

What provisions have been made for reuniting families separated by disaster?

What is the extent of social support available to disaster victims?

What is the extent of collaborative interaction among relief agencies involved in the disaster?

Communication

Has the community disaster plan been communicated to residents?

How are disaster warnings communicated to residents?

Are there language barriers that impede communication in the disaster setting?

What is the effect of disaster on normal channels of communication?

Leadership

What community groups are responsible for disaster planning?

Who is available to provide leadership in responding to the disaster?

What is the level of credibility of leaders among those affected by the disaster?

Occupational and Economic Issues

What community industries pose disaster hazards? What type of hazards are present?

(continued)

ASSESSMENT TIPS: Assessing Health in Disaster Settings (cont.)

To what extent do local industries adhere to safety procedures that would prevent a disaster? Is adherence monitored by regulatory bodies?

What occupational groups in the community are available to respond to the disaster?

How adequate is the number of rescue personnel available to meet disaster needs?

What is the extent of property damage and loss resulting from the disaster?

What is the economic status of those affected by disaster? Do they have economic resources available to them?

What is the effect of the disaster on the local economy?

Other Social Factors

What is the effect of the disaster on transportation?

What is the effect of the disaster on community services?

What community services are available to assist with recovery?

Is equipment needed to deal with the disaster available and in good repair?

Behavioral Dimension

Consumption Patterns

To what extent do consumption patterns (eg, drugs or alcohol) create the potential for disaster in the community?

What is the availability of food and water to disaster victims? To rescuers?

Are there special dietary needs among those affected by the disaster? If so, what are they? What provisions have been made to meet these needs?

What is the extent of drug and alcohol abuse among disaster victims?

Leisure Pursuits

Do community members engage in leisure pursuits that pose a disaster hazard?

To what extent do community members engage in recreational safety practices that can prevent disasters?

What leisure pursuits by community members could enhance the community's disaster response?

Health System Dimension

How well prepared are health service agencies to respond to a disaster?

What health care facilities are available to care for disaster victims? What are their capabilities?

What is the extent of basic first aid and other health-related knowledge in the community?

What health care personnel are available to meet health needs in a disaster? How can they best be mobilized?

What is the effect of a disaster on health care facilities? Health care services?

What health care services are needed as a result of disaster? Are available services adequate to meet the need?

---

framework in which they operate. A community that has a variety of health care facilities joined in a cooperative network can respond more effectively to the health care demands of a disaster situation than can a community with limited facilities or where there is no existing system for coordinating joint efforts.

The nurse and other disaster response planners identify the types of health care facilities available in the community and the number and type of health care personnel that could be called on in the event of a disaster. Planners might also determine the existence and adequacy of disaster plans developed by health care facilities. For example, has a local hospital developed a plan for evacuating patients if the hospital is involved in the disaster? Or, is there a plan for handling mass casualties of various types in the event of a disaster? Assessment of potential avenues for obtaining health care

personnel is also important. For example, local professional organizations might serve as a means of contacting and organizing health care providers. Or, area educational programs for health care professionals may provide a source of manpower.

In the event of an actual disaster there is also a need to assess the effects of the disaster on the health care system and its ability to respond effectively. For example, are facilities badly damaged or unusable for other reasons? During the Los Angeles riots in 1992, for instance, ambulances were unable to reach victims due to fears of violence, and many health care facilities burned or were inaccessible because of the rioting. In addition, food supplement programs became ineffective when grocery stores were burned or closed. Finally, the loss of 20,000 jobs created a large newly uninsured population who had no means of paying for health care (*The Nation's Health,* 1992). In other instances, health care facilities have collapsed in earthquakes or become inaccessible due to flood waters or highway damage.

Diagnostic Reasoning and Care of Clients in Disaster Settings

Based on the assessment of biophysical, psychological, physical, social, behavioral, and health system factors, the nurse derives nursing diagnoses related to disaster care. These diagnoses may reflect the potential for disaster occurrence, the adequacy of disaster preparation, or the extent of effects in an actual disaster. A diagnosis related to forecasting is "potential for major earthquake damage and injury due to community location on a geological fault." A diagnosis of "inadequate disaster planning due to fragmentation of planning efforts among community agencies" is a possible nursing diagnosis related to disaster preparedness. A diagnosis derived from information about the effects of an actual disaster is "need for additional shelter sites due to destruction of planned shelters by fire."

In the event of an actual disaster, nursing diagnoses might relate to individual clients as well as to the status of the overall community. For example, individual diagnoses include "grief due to loss of husband" and "pain due to leg fracture suffered in the collapse of a wall." Nurses may derive diagnoses related to both helpers and victims, such as "role overload due to need to rescue disaster victims and care for own family" and "stress related to constant exposure to death."

Planning the Dimensions of Health Care in a Disaster

Activities related to disaster care take place in several areas. Two of these areas, prevention and education, involve primary prevention. The third area of activity, the actual emergency response, reflects secondary prevention, whereas recovery, the fourth area of activity, involves tertiary prevention.

Primary Prevention

Primary prevention is geared toward preventing the occurrence of a disaster or limiting consequences when the event itself cannot be prevented. Activities to prevent or minimize the effects of a disaster take place during the pre-impact mobilization stage of the disaster. Community health nurses may be involved

in eliminating factors that may contribute to disasters to the extent that they identify these factors and report their existence to the appropriate authorities. For example, the community health nurse working in an occupational setting may note that an employee who is responsible for monitoring pressure levels in a boiler may be drinking heavily. This employee's drinking problem may lead to lack of attention to rising pressures and an explosion and fire in the plant. In such a case, the nurse would call the employee's drinking behavior to the attention of a supervisor.

Community health nurses may also become politically active to ensure that risk factors for potential disasters present in the community are eliminated or modified. For example, the nurse might campaign for stricter safety regulations for nuclear power plants (Whitcomb & Sage, 1997) or stricter building safety codes (Noji, 1997a) or serve as a mediator in an attempt to defuse social unrest in the community.

Community health nurses are more often involved in educating the public about how to prevent disasters and minimize their consequences. This may involve planning education for individuals, families, or groups of clients on home safety practices to prevent fires and explosions (Sanderson, 1997), how to prepare for a possible community disaster, and what to do in the event of a disaster situation.

The nurse would plan to acquaint clients with whom he or she works with the types of disasters possible in their community and about actions they can take to minimize the consequences should an emergency arise. The nurse can also guide clients to resources that help them prepare for the possibility of a disaster. A variety of government agencies publish literature containing guidelines for emergency preparation by individual citizens. One such publication, *In Time of Emergency: A Citizen's Handbook,* is published by the Federal Emergency Management Agency. The American Red Cross publishes the *Family Disaster Plan and Personal Survival Guide.* These and similar publications offer general guidelines for emergency preparation as well as more specific recommendations for certain common types of disasters.

Secondary Prevention

Secondary prevention involves the response to a disaster occurrence. Implementing the community's disaster plan is a secondary preventive measure. Secondary prevention is geared toward halting the disaster and resolving problems caused by it. Secondary prevention may take place at the community level or at the level of individual victims. For example, efforts to provide food and shelter are secondary preventive measures taken at the group level, whereas treatment of burns and other injuries is secondary prevention related to specific individuals.

Community health nurses are actively involved in the response to an actual disaster event. Areas for involvement include triage, treatment of injuries and other health conditions, and shelter supervision. Community health nurses may be some of several health care providers who perform triage activities described earlier and who determine priorities for treatment, evacuation, and transportation of disaster victims. In planning for triage responsibilities, community health nurses would familiarize themselves with criteria for assigning priority.

Community health nurses may also be involved in treating injuries or other health conditions. This may occur in "definitive care sites" (hospitals or other health care facilities removed from the disaster site itself) or in shelters. Nurses involved in first aid for victims should plan to update their skills in basic first aid on a periodic basis. Community health nurses, particularly those working in shelters, need to plan to deal not only with existing health conditions, such as hypertension and diabetes, but also with acute conditions. For example, the nurse may encounter a child with a middle ear infection that requires treatment or a woman in labor. In planning for these and similar activities, the nurse should be familiar with procedures included in the disaster plan for care of minor illnesses and dispensing medications for clients with chronic diseases. The nurse needs to know to whom to refer those in need of services and how to arrange for transportation or other needs. The disaster plan may call for nurses to treat minor illnesses on the basis of protocols developed in conjunction with medical personnel. If such is the case, the nurse should become familiar with those treatment protocols. Finally, the nurse needs to plan for activities to monitor clients' health status. For example, the nurse might schedule periodic blood pressure measurements for a disaster relief worker with hypertension.

Community health nurses may also be responsible for supervising and coordinating shelter activities. Responsibilities might include supervising the meeting of health care and other needs by other disaster relief workers; supervising recordkeeping related to people brought to and released from the shelter; assisting people housed in shelters on a long-term basis to develop some form of governance; and using interpersonal skills to keep the shelter running smoothly. Secondary preventive activities by community health nurses in a disaster setting are summarized in Table 29–3.

Tertiary Prevention

Tertiary prevention with respect to a disaster has two major goals. The first is recovery of the community and its members from the effects of the disaster and

TABLE 29–3. SECONDARY PREVENTIVE ACTIVITIES BY COMMUNITY HEALTH NURSES IN DISASTER SETTINGS

Secondary Prevention Focus	Related Nursing Activities
Triage	• Assess disaster victims for extent of injuries. • Determine priority for treatment, evacuation, and transportation. • Place appropriate colored tag on victim depending on priority.
Treatment of injuries	• Render first aid for injuries. • Provide additional treatment as needed in definitive care areas.
Treatment of other conditions	• Determine health needs other than injury. • Refer for medical treatment as required. • Provide treatment for other conditions based on medically approved protocols.
Shelter supervision	• Coordinate activities of shelter workers. • Oversee records of those admitted and discharged from the shelter. • Promote effective interpersonal and group interactions among those housed in the shelter. • Promote independence and involvement of those housed in the shelter.

return to normal. The second aspect of tertiary prevention is preventing a recurrence of the disaster.

Community health nurses have responsibilities in both of these areas after the disaster is over. Community health nurses may be called on to provide sustained care to both victims and disaster workers following the disaster. They may also be involved in identifying health and psychosocial problems that require further assistance. Community health nurses should plan to provide counseling or referral for persons with psychological problems stemming from their experiences during the disaster. There may also be a need to refer disaster victims to continuing sources of medical care. Community health nurses may also need to plan referrals for clients in need of social and financial assistance. For example, disaster victims may require help in finding housing or in getting financial aid to rebuild homes or businesses.

Community health nurses may also provide input into interventions designed to prevent future disasters or to minimize their effects. For example, if the disaster involved rioting by minority groups, the community health nurse might advocate measures to meet the needs of minority group members to prevent further rioting. Or, community health nurses might campaign for stronger building codes to prevent the collapse of buildings in subsequent earthquakes. Community health nurses can also help to educate the public on disaster preparedness to minimize the effects of subsequent disasters. Tertiary prevention foci in disaster settings and related community health nursing activities are summarized in Table 29–4.

TABLE 29–4. **TERTIARY PREVENTIVE ACTIVITIES BY COMMUNITY HEALTH NURSES IN DISASTER SETTINGS**

Tertiary Prevention Focus	Related Nursing Activities
Follow-up care for injuries	• Provide continued care for people injured as a result of the disaster or during rescue operations. • Monitor response to treatment.
Follow-up care for psychological problems resulting from the disaster	• Provide counseling for those with psychological problems resulting from the disaster. • Refer clients for counseling as needed. • Monitor progress in resolving psychological problems.
Recovery assistance	• Refer clients for financial assistance. • Provide assistance in finding housing.
Prevention of future disasters and their consequences	• Advocate measures to prevent future disasters. • Educate the public about disaster preparation to minimize the effects of subsequent disasters.

Implementing Disaster Care

Prior to the occurrence of a disaster, the community health nurse may be involved in activities preliminary to implementing a disaster plan, particularly in disseminating the plan to others. Dissemination needs to occur among persons and agencies who will have designated responsibilities during a disaster. The community health nurse participating in disaster planning is responsible for communicating elements of the plan to members of the nurse's employing agency. They may also ensure that the plan is disseminated to nursing organizations in the area (eg, to members of a district nurses' association). The nurse who assumes this responsibility should be sure that the general plan, as

► **AREAS FOR CLIENT EDUCATION RELATED TO DISASTER PREPAREDNESS**

- Install and maintain smoke detectors in homes.
- Bolt bookcases and cabinets to walls in areas with earthquake potential.
- Seek shelter in a reinforced area (eg, a doorway) during an earthquake and face away from windows. Stay indoors.
- Seek shelter from hurricanes or tornadoes in basements or inner rooms without windows.
- Seek high ground in the event of a flood.
- Drop to the ground and roll about to extinguish flaming clothing, or smother flames with a rug.
- Close doors and windows to prevent the spread of a fire, and place wadded fabric beneath doors to prevent smoke inhalation.
- Determine avenues of escape from the home or other buildings.
- Install fire escape ladders as needed at upper windows.
- Keep stairways and doors free of obstacles to permit easy egress.
- Identify a place for family members to meet after escape from the home.
- Designate a person living outside the area as a family contact if family members are separated during a disaster.
- Learn community disaster warning signals and their meaning.
- Keep a battery-operated radio and extra batteries available (replace batteries periodically).
- Collect and store, in an accessible location, sufficient emergency supplies for 1 week, including:
    Nonperishable foods (including pet foods)
    Drinking water
    Warm clothing
    Bedding (blankets or sleeping bags)
    Tent or other type of shelter
    Source of light (flashlights or lanterns)
    Chlorine bleach for treating suspect water supplies to prevent infection
    First-aid supplies and first-aid manual
    Medications needed by family members
- Replace stored food, water, and medications periodically.
- Know where natural gas and water valves are located and how to turn them off. Attach a wrench close to valves.
- Determine what valuables are to be taken if evacuation is required.
- Assign activities related to evacuation (eg, designate the person responsible for taking the baby or family pets).
- Know the general plan for evacuating the community.
- Know where proposed shelters will be located.
- Know what actions should be taken when warning is given.
- Know where to seek additional information.

well as the specific part to be played by members of the agency or organization, is understood.

The essential features of the community's disaster response plan should also be communicated to the general public so residents will be prepared to follow the plan in the event of a disaster. The community health nurse may be involved in helping to communicate the plan to the public by apprising clients with whom he or she works of relevant aspects of the plan. The public should be alerted to mechanisms that will be used to inform them of a disaster and where to go for additional information. Community members should also know the general procedures to be followed in terms of caring for disaster victims and setting up shelters. They should also be informed of the locations of proposed shelters. Finally, community members should be told of specific disaster preparations that should be undertaken by individuals and families.

Evaluating Disaster Care

The final responsibility of community health nurses with respect to disaster care is evaluating that care. Nurses and others involved in the disaster participate in evaluative activities outlined in the disaster plan. Evaluation focuses on the adequacy of the plan for curtailing the disaster and meeting the needs of those involved in it.

In this effort it may be helpful to examine the disaster response in light of the six dimensions of health. Did the plan adequately provide for the needs of the people affected and the kinds of health problems that resulted? Did physical, psychological, or social dimension factors impede implementation of the

> ### Critical Thinking in Research
>
> Community health nurses have the knowledge of the community and the expertise in program planning to make significant contributions to community disaster preparedness. In many instances, however, the only involvement that community health nurses have is in practicing and executing the emergency health care services components of a local disaster plan.
>
> 1. To what extent do you think community health nurses are involved in disaster planning in your local community? How would you go about discovering if your perceptions of their involvement are correct?
> 2. What do you think might be the barriers that prevent community health nurses from participating in disaster planning? How might you design a study to answer this question?
> 3. How often do community health nurses educate members of the general public regarding disaster preparedness? How might you determine what approaches to community disaster education are most effective?

plan or limit its effectiveness? What influence did behavioral factors have on plan implementation, if any? Were health care services adequate to meet the health needs posed by the disaster itself as well as those encountered in the period after the disaster? Data obtained in the evaluative process are used to assess the adequacy of the community disaster plan and to guide revisions of the plan to better deal with future disasters.

The effectiveness of care provided to individual disaster victims should also be assessed. Evaluation in this area focuses on the degree to which individual needs were met and the extent to which problems resulting from the disaster were resolved.

Critical Thinking in Practice: A Case in Point

Two commuter trains have collided in a tunnel at rush hour. Both trains derailed and one of them struck the side of the tunnel, causing it to collapse on two of the derailed cars. Approximately 300 people were passengers on the two trains, with 50 or more people trapped in the two buried cars. The accident occurred approximately one-quarter mile from the west end of the tunnel and 2 miles from the east end. Most of both trains lie on the west side of the collapsed portion of the tunnel.

One of the passengers is a community health nurse. The nurse was not injured in the accident and was able to get out of the wreckage to the west end of the tunnel, where most of the survivors are gathered.

1. What are the biophysical, psychological, physical, social, behavioral, and health system factors that may be influencing this disaster situation?
2. What role functions might the community health nurse carry out in this situation?
3. What primary, secondary, and tertiary preventive activities might be appropriate in this situation? Why?

TESTING YOUR UNDERSTANDING

1. Describe four ways that disaster events can vary. (pp. 704–705)
2. Describe the three elements of a disaster. (pp. 705–712)
3. Identify at least three benefits of disaster preparedness. (p. 712)
4. Identify at least two factors in each of the six dimensions of health to be assessed in relation to a disaster. Describe how each of the factors identified might influence a disaster or a community's response to a disaster. (pp. 720–727)
5. Discuss at least six principles of community disaster preparedness. (pp. 712–714)
6. Describe four characteristics of a successful disaster plan. (pp. 714–715)
7. Discuss at least five elements of an effective disaster plan. (pp. 716–719)
8. Describe the role of the community health nurse in primary, secondary, and tertiary prevention related to disaster situations. (pp. 727–728)

WHAT DO YOU THINK?
Questions for Critical Thinking

1. What factors in your community contribute to the potential for a disaster event? What interventions could be taken to prevent a disaster? What actions could mitigate the effects of a disaster if one occurs?
2. How prepared are you and your family in the event of a disaster? Why doesn't everyone engage in personal disaster preparation?
3. Who is involved in disaster planning in your community? What role do community health nurses have in disaster planning? Should that role be expanded? If so, how?

REFERENCES

Bay Area Earthquake Preparedness Project. (1992). *Earthquake preparedness guidelines for large retirement complexes and large residential care facilities.* Oakland, CA: Bay Area Earthquake Preparedness Project.

Burkhart, F. N. (1991). *Media, emergency warnings, and citizen response.* Boulder, CO: Westview.

Cohen, R. C. (1992). Training mental health professionals to work with families in diverse cultural contexts. In L. S. Austin (Ed.), *Responding to disaster: A guide for mental health professionals* (pp. 69–80). Washington, DC: American Psychiatric Press.

Drabek, T. E. (1986). *Human systems responses to disaster.* New York: Springer/Verlag.

Duffy, J. C. (Ed.). (1990). *Health and medical aspects of disaster preparedness.* New York: Plenum Press.

Gerrity, E. T., & Flynn, B. W. (1997). Mental health consequences of disasters. In E. K. Noji (Ed.), *The public health consequences of disasters* (pp. 101–121). New York: Oxford University Press.

Lillibridge, S. R. (1997a). Industrial disasters. In E. K. Noji (Ed.), *The public health consequences of disasters* (pp. 354–372). New York: Oxford University Press.

Lillibridge, S. R. (1997b). Managing the environmental health aspects of disasters: Water, human excreta, and shelter. In E. K. Noji (Ed.), *The public health consequences of disasters* (pp. 65–78). New York: Oxford University Press.

Lillibridge, S. R. (1997c). Tornadoes. In E. K. Noji (Ed.), *The public health consequences of disasters* (pp. 228–244). New York: Oxford University Press.

Liu, S., Quenemoen, L. E., Malilay, J., Noji, E., Sinks, T., & Mendlein, J. (1996). Assessment of a severe-weather warning system and disaster preparedness, Calhoun County, Alabama, 1994. *American Journal of Public Health, 86,* 87–89.

Logue, J. N. (1996). Disasters, the environment, and public health: Improving our response. *American Journal of Public Health, 86,* 1207–1210.

Malilay, J. (1997a). Floods. In E. K. Noji (Ed.), *The public health consequences of disasters* (pp. 287–301). New York: Oxford University Press.

Malilay, J. (1997b). Tropical cyclones. In E. K. Noji (Ed.), *The public health consequences of disasters* (pp. 207–227). New York: Oxford University Press.

McFarlane, A. C. (1995). Stress and disaster. In S. E. Hobfol & M. W. de Vries (Eds.), *Extreme stress and communities: Impact and intervention* (pp. 247–265). Boston: Kluwer Academic.

Meichenbaum, D. (1995). Disasters, stress and cognition. In S. E. Hobfol & M. W. de Vries (Eds.), *Extreme stress and communities: Impact and intervention* (pp. 33–45). Boston: Kluwer Academic.

Meyer, M. U., & Graeter, C. J. (1995). Health professional's role in disaster planning. *AAOHN Journal, 43,* 251–262.

The Nation's Health. (1992, July). *L.A. riot aftermath: Damage to public health in myriad ways,* p. 1.

Noji, E. K. (1997a). Earthquakes. In E. K. Noji (Ed.), *The public health consequences of disasters* (pp. 135–178). New York: Oxford University Press.

Noji, E. K. (1997b). The nature of disaster: General characteristics and public health effects. In E. K. Noji (Ed.), *The public health consequences of disasters* (pp. 3–20). New York: Oxford University Press.

Pickens, S. (1992). The decade for natural disaster reduction: The role of health care workers. *Nursing & Health Care, 13,* 192–195.

Sanderson, L. M. (1997). Fires. In E. K. Noji (Ed.), *The public health consequences of disasters* (pp. 373–396). New York: Oxford University Press.

Smith, L. B., & Jervis, D. T. (1990). Tornadoes. In W. L. Waugh & R. J. Hy (Eds.), *Handbook of emergency management: Programs and policies dealing with major hazards and disasters* (pp. 106–128). New York: Greenwood Press.

Toole, M. J., & Malkki, R. M. (1992). Famine-affected, refugee, and displaced populations: Recommendations for public health issues. *MMWR, 41*(RR-13), 1–76.

U.S. Department of Commerce. (1996). *Statistical abstract of the United States, 1996* (116th ed.). Washington, DC: Government Printing Office.

Waugh, W. L., & Hy, R. J. (1990). Introduction to emergency management. In W. L. Waugh & R. J. Hy (Eds.), *Handbook of emergency management: Programs and policies dealing with major hazards and disasters* (pp. 1–10). New York: Greenwood Press.

Weaver, J. D. (1995). *Disasters and mental health interventions.* Sarasota, FL: Professional Resource Press.

Whitcomb, R. C., & Sage, M. (1997). Nuclear reactor incidents. In E. K. Noji (Ed.), *The public health consequences of disasters* (pp. 397–418). New York: Oxford University Press.

World Health Organization. (1989). *Coping with natural disasters: The role of local health personnel and the community.* Geneva: World Health Organization.

Yahmed, S. B. (1994). Population growth and disasters. *World Health, 47*(3), 26–27.

RESOURCES IN DISASTER PLANNING AND RESPONSE

Agency for International Development
Office of External Affairs
Bureau for Program and Policy Coordination
Washington, DC 20523–0001
(202) 647–1850

Agricultural Stabilization and Conservation Service
Department of Agriculture
PO Box 2415
Washington, DC 20013
(202) 720–5237

American Red Cross National Headquarters
431 185th Street, NW
Washington, DC 20006
(202) 737–8300

Doctors for Disaster Preparedness
2059 North Campbell
Box 272
Tucson, AZ 85719
(520) 325–2680

Emergency Shelter Grants Program
Office of Block Grant Assistance
Department of Housing and Urban Development
451 7th Street, SW
Washington, DC 20410
(202) 708–1422

Emergency Response Coordination Group (F-38)
National Center for Environmental Health
Centers for Disease Control and Prevention
4770 Buford Hwy.
Atlanta, GA 30341–3724
(404) 488–7100

Farmers' Home Administration
Department of Agriculture
Washington, DC 20250
(202) 720–4323

Federal Crop Insurance Corporation
Department of Agriculture
Washington, DC 20250
(202) 254–8460

Federal Emergency Management Agency
500 C Street, SW
Washington, DC 20472
(202) 646–4600

National Flood Insurance Program
Federal Insurance Administration
Washington, DC 20472
(202) 646–4600

Office of Disaster Assistance
Small Business Administration
409 3rd Street, SW
Washington, DC 20416
(202) 205–6734

Office of Emergency Transportation
Department of Transportation
400 7th Street, SW
Washington, DC 20590
(202) 366–5270

Office of U.S. Foreign Disaster Assistance
Washington, DC 20011
(202) 647–8924

U.S. Fire Administration
Federal Emergency Management Agency
500 C Street, SW
Washington, DC 20472
(202) 646–4600

ON HEARING THE NEWS OF A PATIENT'S DEATH

Morning light glances off the chrome
   of a stripped down car in the alley
slices through window panes
   along the edges of drawn shades
Opens fire on sheets pulled up
   to shield the eyes of sleepers.

This summer the sun won't light your eyes.
Not even the cries of the baby reach you.
It's too late, for you went early
just as we thought you might
   but not like this
   manacled to a bed
   in the maternity ward
   of D.C. General Hospital.

Hearing the news, I call up your face
a wide-open face with a slow shy smile
as if the shock of life had somehow dazed
   you.
You took each day
   each man
   each child
   each welfare check
   each jail cell
   as it came.

It just wasn't in you to ask why or why not
to look ahead or behind.
Since when does someone like you get to
   choose?
Since when do poor ignorant women take
   charge of their lives?

The judge decided to keep you in jail
those last few months of your pregnancy—
the best he could do for your unborn child.
Why bring another addict into the world?

Oh, it isn't that you never tried to kick.
You'd come to us in pain
   with abscesses from dirty needles.

You'd come when the drug supply dried up.
You'd come when there was no money to
   buy.
You'd come when you felt too tired to sell.
I can do it alone, you said
   I can kick.
Just give me a few Valiums.
A little help is all I need.

I suppose we'll never know just how you
   died.
It was after the baby was born
after they'd taken you back to the ward.
Some people said they heard calls for help.
When they found you, you were hanging
   over the side of the bed
   dangling by the foot
   they'd shackled to the bedframe.
Your family set up a wail that went on for
   days
   alleged foul play
   hinted at revenge.
There was gunfire at the wake, they say
and eight motherless children destined for
   your mother's house
   the street
   the welfare office
   hospital &
   jail.

The last light you saw in the blank night
   of your life
was your newborn girl
Is that why you named her Star?

Excerpted with permission from V. Masson (1993). just who. Washington, DC: Crossroads Health Ministry.

THE DIMENSIONS MODEL AND SELECTED COMMUNITY HEALTH PROBLEMS

Community health nurses frequently confront several categories of health problems that impair an individual's health and that of the family and the society as a whole. To deal effectively with these conditions, community health nurses must be knowledgeable about contributing factors and control strategies.

In recent years the destructive power of communicable diseases has been somewhat limited by advances in medical science and improved sanitation. Acquired immunodeficiency syndrome (AIDS) and other sexually transmitted diseases (STDs), however, persist. Preventable childhood diseases also contribute to morbidity and mortality. Chapter 30 addresses the epidemiology of childhood diseases, AIDS and other STDs, viral hepatitis, tuberculosis, and influenza, and the community health nurse's role in controlling them.

Many people suffer the debilitating consequences of chronic health problems; they are the primary focus of epidemiologic research and control efforts. Control strategies focusing on heart disease and stroke have had success; however, chronic physical illnesses contribute to increased morbidity and mortality throughout the world. Chapter 31 presents epidemiologic factors and control strategies for accidental trauma that results in chronic disability, and for diabetes, cancer, heart disease, arthritis, chronic respiratory disease, and obesity.

Chronic mental health problems, such as schizophrenia and depression, are also encountered relatively frequently by community health nurses. The conditions are described in Chapter 32 in terms of epidemiology and control. Mental distress is reflected in the drug abuse and violence evident in our society today. These abuses are concerns confronting community health nurses. The addictive behaviors of many clients who abuse alcohol and other drugs may profoundly affect families, as well as society as a whole. Long-term ramifications of abuse are seen in the growing number of children with health problems that result from fetal exposure to drugs. The community health nurse's role in dealing with substance abuse is discussed in Chapter 33. The problems of violence against self and others are explored in Chapter 34.

Action is necessary at the individual, family, group, and societal levels to resolve these major deterrents to health in contemporary society.

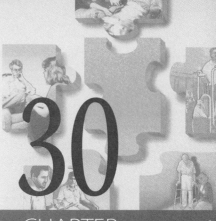

30

COMMUNICABLE DISEASES

For many years progress has been made in controlling communicable diseases. Smallpox is officially eradicated and polio is following, at least in the Western Hemisphere. Control has occurred, in part, because vaccines were developed, and antibiotics have provided miraculous cures.

Yet, we continue to be faced with communicable diseases. Infectious diseases are among the top contributors to death in the United States. New diseases are emerging; others thought to be controlled are resurfacing; and now we are faced with a group of emerging infectious diseases (Centers for Disease Control, 1994). *Emerging infectious diseases* are those for which the incidence has increased significantly in the past two decades, or is expected to.

Several factors contribute to the emergence of disease. For example, societal changes, such as war, population growth, and urban deterioration, have increased people's susceptibility; environmental changes, such as deforestation, expose previously hidden animal reservoirs of disease. Human behaviors, such as global travel, sexual promiscuity, and drug use, also lead to exposure to infectious agents. Moreover, within the health care system the use and abuse of antimicrobial agents is a factor, as is reduced funding for control programs.

Community health nurses work to prevent, identify, and control communicable diseases. General concepts of communicable disease and control measures are addressed in this chapter, as well as the responsibilities of community health nursing. Specifically, childhood diseases, AIDS and other STDs, hepatitis, tuberculosis, and influenza are discussed.

▶ Chapter Objectives

After reading this chapter, you should be able to:

- Describe trends in the incidence of at least five major communicable diseases.
- Identify six major modes by which communicable diseases are transmitted.
- Identify at least four roles for community health nurses in controlling communicable diseases.
- Identify the two major approaches used to control communicable diseases.
- Discuss the influence of at least two factors in each of the six dimensions of health as they relate to childhood diseases.
- Describe at least two nursing interventions for controlling childhood diseases at each level of prevention.
- Compare and contrast the epidemiologic factors contributing to the development of HIV infection and other major sexually transmitted diseases.
- Describe at least two nursing interventions for controlling HIV infection and other sexually transmitted diseases at each level of prevention.
- Discuss the influence of at least two factors in each of the six dimensions of health as they relate to hepatitis.
- Describe at least two nursing interventions for controlling hepatitis at each level of prevention.
- Discuss the influence of at least two factors in each of the six dimensions of health as they relate to tuberculosis.
- Describe at least two nursing interventions for controlling tuberculosis at each level of prevention.
- Discuss the influence of at least two factors in each of the six dimensions of health as they relate to influenza.
- Describe at least two nursing interventions for controlling influenza at each level of prevention.

▶ GENERAL CONCEPTS OF COMMUNICABLE DISEASES

Communicable diseases are those diseases spread by direct contact with an infectious agent. Communicable diseases affecting humans arise from both human and animal sources. In some instances, however, there is an extended period between the excretion of the organism by the *reservoir* and infection of a new *host*. (For a complete discussion of these terms, see Chapter 8.) Thus, it may sometimes be difficult to identify the immediate source of infection in a particular person.

Several communicable disease concepts must be understood prior to examining specific diseases. These include concepts related to the "chain of infection," such as modes of transmission and portals of entry and exit, and the concepts of incubation and prodromal periods.

Chain of Infection

In communicable diseases, epidemiologic factors related to biophysical, psychological, physical, social, behavioral, and health system dimensions create what may be termed a chain of infection. A *chain of infection* is a series of events or conditions that lead to the development of a particular communicable disease. The "links" in the chain are the infected person or source of the infectious agent, the reservoir, the agent itself, the mode of transmission of the disease, the agent's portals of entry and exit, and a susceptible new host. The concepts of reservoir, agent, and host were introduced in Chapter 8. This discussion focuses on the remaining links in the chain: modes of transmission and portals of entry and exit.

Modes of Transmission

The *mode of transmission* of a particular disease is the means by which the infectious agent that causes the disease is transferred from an infected person to an uninfected one. Communicable diseases may be spread by any of several modes of transmission: airborne transmission, fecal–oral (gastrointestinal) transmission, direct contact, sexual contact, direct inoculation, insect or animal bite, or via inanimate objects or soil.

Airborne Transmission. Airborne transmission occurs when the infectious organism is present in the air and is inspired (inhaled) by a susceptible host during respiration. Diseases transmitted by the airborne route include the exanthems (diseases characterized by a rash, such as measles and chickenpox), infections of the mouth and throat (such as streptococcal infections), and infections of the upper and lower respiratory system (such as tuberculosis, pneumonia, influenza, and the common cold). Certain systemic infections are also products of airborne transmission. Examples of these are meningococcal meningitis and pneumococcal pneumonias, hantavirus pulmonary infections, and coccidioidomycosis.

Fecal–Oral Transmission. Fecal–oral transmission of an infectious agent may be either direct or indirect. Direct transmission occurs when the hands or other objects (fomites) are contaminated with organisms from human feces and then put into the mouth. Indirect transmission occurs via contaminated food or water. For example, a person with hepatitis A may defecate, fail to wash his or her hands properly, and then prepare a sandwich for someone else. The second person would ingest the virus with the sandwich and, if susceptible, might develop hepatitis A. Additional examples include Salmonella- or Shigella-caused diarrheas.

Direct Contact.   Direct contact transmission involves skin-to-skin contact or direct contact with mucous membrane discharges between the infected person and another person. Diseases typically spread by this route include infectious mononucleosis, impetigo, scabies, and lice. Scabies, lice, and other parasitic diseases also may be transmitted through contact with clothing and other items containing the eggs of the parasites.

Sexual Transmission.   Transmission of diseases via sexual contact is a special instance of direct contact transmission. Diseases spread by this mode of transmission are usually referred to as sexually transmitted diseases (STDs). Diseases spread during sexual intercourse include (but are not limited to) AIDS, gonorrhea, syphilis, genital herpes, and hepatitis B and D. These diseases may also be spread by other modes of transmission. For example, hepatitis B, C, and D and AIDS may be spread by direct inoculation.

Transmission by Direct Inoculation.   Direct inoculation occurs when the infectious agent (a bloodborne pathogen) is introduced directly into the bloodstream of the new host. Direct inoculation can occur transplacentally from an infected mother to a fetus, via transfusion with infected blood or blood products, through the use of contaminated hypodermic equipment, or through a splash of contaminated body fluid to mucous membrane or nonintact skin. With the advent of several screening tests for blood donors, transmission via transfusion has been significantly decreased (National Institutes of Health, 1995). Health care workers are particularly at risk for several communicable diseases caused by bloodborne pathogens. Diseases commonly spread by direct inoculation include AIDS and hepatitis B, C, and D. Some evidence suggests that hepatitis A can also be spread by injection drug use with contaminated needles.

Transmission by Insect or Animal Bite.   Insect and animal bites can also transmit infectious agents. For example, the bite of the *Anopheles* mosquito is the mode of transmission for malaria. Similarly, rabies frequently is transmitted via a bite from infected, warm-blooded animals such as dogs, skunks, and raccoons. Lime disease is transmitted by the bite of an infected tick.

Transmission by Other Means.   Some communicable diseases are transmitted through contact with spores present in the soil or with inanimate objects. For example, exposure to the bacillus that causes tetanus frequently occurs through a dirty puncture wound. Modes of transmission and typical diseases most often transmitted by each mode are summarized in Table 30–1.

Portals of Entry and Exit

Communicable diseases differ in terms of the portals through which the infectious agent causing the disease enters and leaves an infected host. Portals of entry include the respiratory system, the gastrointestinal tract, and the skin and mucous membranes.

Portals of exit also differ among communicable diseases. Infectious agents may leave an infected host through the respiratory system or through feces passed from the gastrointestinal tract. Blood and other body fluids such as semen, vaginal secretion, and saliva are the portals of exit for infectious agents causing diseases such as AIDS, gonorrhea, and hepatitis B. The skin acts as a portal of exit as well as a portal of entry for conditions such as impetigo and syphilis. Portals of entry and exit and related modes of disease transmission are summarized in Table 30–2.

Incubation and Prodromal Periods

The *incubation period* of a communicable disease is the interval from exposure to an infectious organism to development of the symptoms of the disease. The length of the incubation period for a particular disease may influence the success of efforts to halt the spread of the disease. Some diseases, such as influenza and scarlet fever, have incubation periods of less than a week. Others typically require incubation periods of 1

TABLE 30–1. MODES OF DISEASE TRANSMISSION AND TYPICAL DISEASES

Mode of Transmission	Diseases Transmitted
Airborne	Measles, mumps, rubella, poliomyelitis, *Hemophilus influenzae* type B (HiB) infection, tuberculosis, influenza, scarlet fever, diphtheria, pertussis, hantavirus, coccidioidomycosis
Fecal–oral	Hepatitis A and E, salmonellosis, shigellosis, typhoid, polio (in poor sanitary conditions)
Direct contact	Impetigo, scabies, lice
Sexual contact	Chlamydia, gonorrhea, hepatitis B, C, and D, HIV infection, herpes simplex virus (HSV) infection, syphilis
Direct inoculation	Syphilis, hepatitis A, B, C, and D, HIV infection
Insect or animal bite	Malaria, plague, rabies, Lyme disease
Other means of transmission	Tetanus, hookworm

TABLE 30–2. PORTALS OF ENTRY AND EXIT FOR EACH MODE OF DISEASE TRANSMISSION

Mode of Transmission	Portal of Entry	Portal of Exit
Airborne	Respiratory system	Respiratory system
Fecal–oral	Mouth	Feces
Direct contact	Skin, mucous membrane	Skin, mucous membrane
Sexual contact	Skin, mouth, urethra, vagina, rectum	Skin lesions, vaginal or urethral secretions
Direct inoculation	Across placenta, bloodstream	Blood
Animal or insect bite	Wound in skin	Blood, saliva
Other means of transmission	Wound in skin, intact skin	Animal feces, soil

to 2 weeks (gonorrhea, measles, pertussis, and polio), 2 to 3 weeks (rubella, chickenpox, and mumps), or months (viral hepatitis, syphilis). In some diseases, such as AIDS, the incubation period can be years.

The *prodromal period* of a communicable disease is the period between the first symptoms and the appearance of the symptoms that typify the disease. For example, prior to appearance of the jaundice that is characteristic of viral hepatitis, the client may experience prodromal symptoms of nausea, fatigue, and malaise. Similarly, a cough, runny nose, and watery eyes are prodromal symptoms for measles.

▶ PRINCIPLES OF COMMUNICABLE DISEASE CONTROL

The interventions of community health nurses and other health care providers in the control of specific communicable diseases are determined by the nature of the disease. Two basic approaches are used to control communicable diseases: preventing the spread of the disease and increasing the resistance of the host.

Preventing the Spread of Infection

Preventing the spread of infection may be accomplished through measures aimed at the agent or at the source of the infection. For example, the use of ultraviolet light and adequate ventilation in areas where *Mycobacterium tuberculosis* is found is an attempt to control or kill the infectious agent that causes tuberculosis. Interventions aimed at the source of infection include eradicating the mosquito that spreads malaria and isolating persons with disease to prevent infection of others. Other specific methods of preventing

the spread of infection from one person to another are contact notification and chemoprophylaxis.

Contact Notification

Contact notification is the process of identifying persons who have been exposed to a communicable disease, informing them of exposure, testing them for the particular disease, and, in some cases (eg, syphilis, gonorrhea, tuberculosis, and hepatitis), offering treatment to prevent them from becoming symptomatic and exposing others to the disease. Who is considered a contact to a particular disease depends on the mode of transmission of that disease. For AIDS and hepatitis B, for example, contacts would include past and present sexual partners, persons who shared needles in injection drug use, and young children born to infected women. For tuberculosis and hepatitis A, people living with the infected person are considered contacts.

Contact notification is usually handled in such a way that individuals notified of their potential exposure to a communicable disease are not told the source of that exposure, thereby protecting the anonymity of the infected person. In fact, in many jurisdictions, legislation prohibits subpoenaing client records of communicable disease treatment so as to ensure confidentiality.

Contact notification can be carried out in one of two ways: client referral and provider referral. In client referral, individuals who are known to have a communicable disease notify their contacts themselves and refer them for testing and possible treatment. In provider referral, designated health care personnel solicit names of contacts from infected persons and notify the contacts of potential exposure. When given the option, many people with communicable diseases select provider referral as the preferred mechanism of contact notification. In other instances, they may prefer to notify their contacts themselves.

Community health nurses are frequently involved in the provider referral approach to contact notification. The process used is systematic and begins with an interview of the client with a communicable disease. In this interview, the community health nurse explains the need for notification, testing, and possible treatment of contacts, and then elicits names, addresses, and other information that will allow contacts to be located and informed of their exposure. Depending on how the notification system is organized, this same nurse may follow up on contacts whose names were elicited or communicate this information to another health care provider (frequently another community health nurse) who will get in touch with the individuals named. The identity of the client with the communicable disease from whom the names were elicited is not included in the information communicated.

Nurses involved in contact follow up may make home visits or approach contacts at work or any other place where they can be located. When they approach contacts, nurses should speak to them in a setting that ensures privacy and inform them that they have been exposed to a communicable disease. Nurses frequently need to exercise creativity to prevent others from knowing why the person is being contacted by a nurse.

The nurse who approaches the contact never divulges information about the source of the exposure, but explains that the person has potentially been exposed to a communicable disease. In addition to notifying the contact regarding the exposure, the nurse educates the client about the potential for developing the disease and for spreading it to others and refers the client for testing and treatment for the condition as needed.

Chemoprophylaxis

Chemoprophylaxis is the use of medications to prevent the onset of disease in exposed individuals. When individuals are prevented from developing symptomatic disease, they are usually also prevented from spreading the disease to others. Chemoprophylaxis is used for a variety of communicable diseases including tuberculosis, gonorrhea, syphilis, hepatitis A and B, *Hemophilus influenzae* type B (HiB) infection, diphtheria, and tetanus. Chemoprophylaxis has also been shown to be effective in slowing the development of AIDS in persons with HIV infection and in preventing some of the opportunistic infections that occur in people with AIDS.

Increasing Host Resistance

The second approach to the control of communicable disease is to increase the resistance of the host. Means of achieving this include promoting general health, producing immunity, and preventing complications of communicable diseases, all of which involve nursing action. Chapter 8 addressed measures that can be used to promote health. Measures to prevent complications of communicable diseases are addressed for each of the diseases presented later in this chapter. Here, the focus is on developing host immunity to disease.

Immunity to communicable diseases can occur in three ways: transplacental transfer of maternal antibodies, having the disease, or immunization. Transplacental transfer provides short-term immunity in young infants, but depends on the mother having antibodies to a particular infectious agent. If the mother

has antibodies to certain diseases, the newborn will have some degree of short-term immunity to these same diseases.

Having the disease is an effective, though sometimes dangerous, means of developing immunity to some diseases. Immunity seems to be conferred in measles, diphtheria, pertussis, mumps, varicella, and hepatitis A and B. Having other diseases such as gonorrhea and early stages of syphilis, however, does not appear to protect against reinfection.

Immunization is available for many communicable diseases including polio, measles, mumps, rubella, diphtheria, pertussis, tetanus, hepatitis A and B, diseases caused by HiB varicella, influenza, and pneumococcal pneumonia. In the United states, routine immunization of all persons (preferably in childhood) is recommended for measles, mumps, rubella, diphtheria, pertussis, tetanus, and polio. Immunization of children, especially those in day care centers, against HiB is also recommended, as is hepatitis B vaccine. In developing countries, bacille Calmette–Guérin (BCG) immunization for tuberculosis is also suggested. Immunization for other diseases is recommended for certain groups at higher risk of developing them (discussed later in sections on individual diseases). Recommendations for routine immunization are summarized in Table 30–3.

TABLE 30–3. RECOMMENDATIONS FOR ROUTINE IMMUNIZATION

Immunizing Agent	Recommendations for Administration
Diphtheria, tetanus, pertussis vaccine (DTP)	2, 4, 6, and 18 months, school entry
Tetanus, diphtheria (Td)	Children over 7; adults; booster every 10 years
Trivalent inactivated poliovirus vaccine (IPV)	All children, 2 and 4 months
	Immunocompromised children, 18 months, school entry
Trivalent oral poliovirus vaccine (OPV)	Healthy children, 18 months, school entry
Measles, mumps, rubella (MMR) vaccine	15 months, booster at school entry
Hemophilus influenzae type B (HiB)	2, 4, and 6 months; booster at 15 months
Hepatitis B vaccine (HBV)	Birth, 1 month, 6 months
	Health care workers, prostitutes, others with multiple sexual partners, injection drug users
Varicella vaccine	One dose at 12–18 months for young children or one dose from 19 months to 12 years or two doses, 4–8 weeks apart for persons 13 years of age and older
Influenza vaccine	Annually for persons over age 65 and those with debilitating physical illness
Pneumonia vaccine	Persons over age 65 and those with debilitating physical illness

Other Control Measures

Other measures that aid in the control of communicable diseases include legislation requiring screening for specific diseases in high-risk groups and mandatory reporting of cases of communicable disease. Additional control measures include compulsory immunization prior to school entry, compulsory examination of contacts and treatment of infected persons, and regulation of vehicles of transmission such as secondhand mattresses and pillows. Use of these and related measures is addressed in more detail later in this chapter.

► THE DIMENSIONS MODEL AND CONTROL OF COMMUNICABLE DISEASES

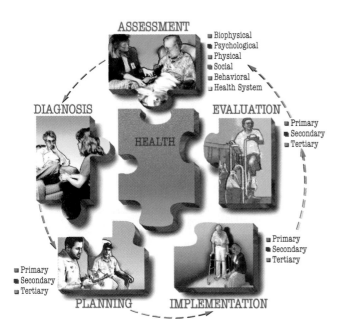

The Dimensions Model can be used to enhance the control of communicable diseases. General questions derived from the model that can be used to assess risk for any communicable disease are presented on page 743. In the remainder of this chapter, the model is applied to childhood illnesses, AIDS, hepatitis, other sexually transmitted diseases, tuberculosis, and influenza.

Critical Dimensions of Nursing in Communicable Disease Control

The dimensions of community health nursing incorporate a variety of roles and responsibilities in efforts to control communicable diseases. These roles generally fall into the categories of contact notification, chemoprophylaxis, education, immunization, case finding, referral, treatment, supportive care, and political activity. The roles of the nurse in notifying contacts and providing chemoprophylaxis are addressed later in the chapter.

The nurse's educational role involves educating the general public about means to prevent communicable diseases, signs and symptoms of existing diseases, and where to seek help for possible communicable diseases. The nurse may also be involved in educating other health care providers on the appropriate diagnostic and screening procedures for certain communicable diseases, particularly sexually transmitted ones. It is the responsibility of community health nurses in some public health agencies, for example, to contact private physicians who report cases of gonorrhea and syphilis to educate them regarding appropriate treatment measures.

Community health nurses also educate the public regarding the need for immunizations. They are frequently involved in planning, implementing, and evaluating immunization campaigns and in giving immunizations to susceptible individuals.

Community health nurses are also actively involved in case finding for communicable diseases. Because they serve large segments of the population who may not receive care from other health care providers, community health nurses are in a unique position to identify possible cases of communicable diseases. Once a person with a potential communicable disease has been identified, the community health nurse may make a referral for further diagnosis and treatment. Or, in some cases, the nurse may be involved in diagnosing and treating communicable diseases on the basis of medically approved protocols. Community health nurses may either refer contacts (those exposed to communicable diseases) for chemoprophylaxis as appropriate or provide chemoprophylaxis themselves.

Another role for community health nurses related to communicable diseases is providing supportive care for clients with these conditions. Supportive care may include educating clients and families about measures to reduce fever or enhance comfort until the disease has run its course, or providing emotional support and assistance during clients' adjustment to the long-term consequences of some communicable diseases. Supportive care might also involve helping clients and their families to deal with the psychological implications of incurable diseases such as genital herpes and AIDS.

Finally, the role of the nurse in controlling communicable diseases may involve political activity and advocacy. For example, the nurse might be actively engaged in efforts to ensure access to health care for

ASSESSMENT TIPS: Assessing Risk for Communicable Diseases

Biophysical Dimension

What age groups are most likely to develop the disease?

Are there differences in disease effects among age groups?

Are there racial or gender differences in disease incidence?

Are there other physiologic conditions that increase the risk of disease? If so, what are they?

What are the signs and symptoms of the disease?

What are the physiologic effects of the disease?

What is the effect of the disease in pregnancy?

What is the mode of disease transmission? What are the physiologic portals of entry and exit?

Psychological Dimension

Does exposure to stress increase risk of the disease?

Do psychological factors play a part in the risk of exposure to disease?

Does the disease have potential psychological consequences (eg, suicide risk with HIV infection)?

Physical Dimension

What effect, if any, do crowded living conditions have on the incidence of the disease?

Can the disease be transmitted to humans by animals or insects?

What physical dimension factors contribute to the presence of disease vectors (eg, mosquito breeding areas)?

Is the disease spread by contaminated food or water?

Social Dimension

Does society condone behaviors that increase the risk of disease (eg, sexual activity)?

Does social interaction increase the risk of the spread of disease?

What are societal attitudes to the disease? Do they hamper control efforts?

Is there social stigma attached to having the disease?

Do occupational factors influence the incidence of the disease?

Does socioeconomic status affect risk of the disease? Consequences of the disease?

What effect, if any, do cultural beliefs and behaviors have on incidence of the disease?

Behavioral Dimension

Does diet play a part in the incidence of the disease (eg, malnutrition as a risk factor for TB)?

Does nutritional status influence the consequences of the disease?

Does alcohol or drug use contribute to the incidence of the disease?

Does sexual activity increase the risk of the disease?

Do specific sexual behaviors increase the risk of the disease? If so, what are these behaviors?

Health System Dimension

What primary preventive measures are available for the disease? Are they widely used?

To what extent do health care providers educate the public on primary prevention of the disease?

Is there a vaccine available for the disease?

Is there a screening test for the disease? If so, are persons at risk for the disease adequately screened?

How is the disease diagnosed?

Is there an effective treatment for the disease?

Are diagnostic and treatment services for the disease available and accessible to infected persons?

What is the attitude of health care providers to persons with the disease?

---

persons with AIDS or in promoting legislation to make immunization for HiB infections mandatory for day care admission.

Childhood Diseases

Childhood diseases are so named because, in the past, the incidence of these diseases was higher among chil-

dren than adults. These diseases were also the major source of mortality among children. They are not, however, experienced exclusively by children. A growing number of young adults are susceptible to measles and pertussis, and older adults are frequently unprotected against tetanus. Although adults develop these diseases relatively infrequently, consequences of infection in adults are often more severe than in children. The childhood diseases to be discussed here include measles, mumps, rubella, diphtheria, pertussis (whooping cough), tetanus, poliomyelitis, diseases caused by the HiB virus, and varicella (chickenpox). Unless otherwise specified, incidence rates reflect the total population, not just cases of disease among children.

The importance of community health efforts to deal with the problems posed by the continued incidence of childhood diseases is reflected in the national objectives for the year 2000 related to control of these conditions (U.S. Department of Health and Human Services, 1991). A summary of these objectives is presented in Appendix A.

Trends in Childhood Diseases

Measles is a highly communicable viral disease that used to be common in childhood in the United States and still is in developing countries. Following the development of a vaccine, there was a significant decline in the incidence of measles in the United States. During the late 1980s and early 1990s, however, measles incidence again increased to a period high of 11 cases per 100,000 population in 1990. Since that time measles incidence has again begun to decline to a rate of 0.12 per 100,000 in 1995 (Centers for Disease Control, 1996). In spite of recent declines in the United States and elsewhere, measles incidence continues to be a global problem. For example, in 1995, 44 million cases and 1.1 million measles deaths occurred worldwide. Measles remains responsible for approximately one tenth of all deaths among children under 5 years of age (Centers for Disease Control, 1997b).

Rubella is a relatively mild disease in itself, but poses serious consequences to children who are exposed in utero. The incidence of both rubella and congenital rubella syndrome has declined consistently since the advent and widespread use of the rubella vaccine in the United States. In 1995, for example, there were 128 cases of rubella (an incidence rate of 0.05 per 100,000 population) and six cases of congenital rubella syndrome (Centers for Disease Control, 1996; U.S. Department of Health and Human Services, 1996).

Mumps, also called infectious parotitis, is an acute viral disease characterized by swelling and tenderness of salivary glands, especially the parotid gland. The incidence of mumps decreased significantly following the development of a vaccine. For instance, from 1968 to 1993 there was a 99% decline in reported cases (van Loon, Holmes, Sirotkin, et al., 1995). This decline has continued to a low of 0.35 cases per 100,000 in 1995 (Centers for Disease Control, 1996).

Deaths due to mumps are rare, but approximately 20 to 30% of adult males infected develop orchitis (inflammation of the testes), with subsequent potential for infertility. Other complications include oophoritis (inflammation of the ovaries) in females, pancreatitis, nephritis, arthritis, mastitis, thyroiditis, and pericarditis. Meningitis may also occur (Benenson, 1995).

Diphtheria, pertussis, and *tetanus* are three more childhood diseases for which the availability of vaccines has resulted in a marked decline in incidence. Since 1980, the incidence rate for diphtheria has been negligible, with only an occasional case occurring throughout the population (Centers for Disease Control, 1996). The decline in the incidence of pertussis is not quite so dramatic, and cases continue to occur. In 1970, the incidence of pertussis had declined 99% from a record high of 260,000 cases in 1934. Subsequently, however, pertussis has shown cyclic peaks even among highly immunized groups, suggesting the need for a vaccine that can be used for people over age 7 who demonstrate waning immunity (Centers for Disease Control, 1997c). In 1996, there were 2.9 cases of pertussis per 100,000 population (Childhood Vaccine Preventable Diseases Bureau, 1997b). Both pertussis and measles display cyclical incidence patterns with peaks every 3 to 4 years, which may explain recent increases. Tetanus incidence has also decreased, with the use of available vaccines, to 0.02 cases per 100,000 population (Centers for Disease Control, 1996). Cases continue to be reported, however, and carry a high rate of fatality (25% of cases from 1991 to 1994) (Izurieta, et al., 1997).

Incidence rates for *poliomyelitis* have been stable at zero per 100,000 population each year since 1979 (Centers for Disease Control, 1996). In 1994, the International Commission for the Certification of Poliomyelitis Eradication in the Americas certified the elimination of the disease in its wild form from the Americas (National Immunization Program, 1994c). Similar, but not yet as successful, efforts are being made to eradicate polio throughout the world by the year 2000 (National Center for Infectious Diseases, 1996). **Eradication** involves eliminating the causative organism of a disease from nature. **Elimination,** on the other hand, is more circumscribed and may involve eliminating a disease from a single country or region or controlling manifestations of the disease so it is no longer a public health problem (International Task Force for Disease Eradication, 1993).

Varicella virus infection, or *chickenpox,* is another communicable disease that occurs primarily in children. Approximately 4 million cases of chickenpox occur each year (Stutman, 1996), and the chickenpox mortality rate among infants is 6.23 deaths per 100,000 infants. Because of the vast number of cases, the annual cost of this disease (including parental work absences) may be as high as $399 million. In addition, approximately 2% of babies born to women who have chickenpox in the first or second trimester of pregnancy develop congenital varicella syndrome (Committee on Infectious Diseases, 1995), further adding to the cost of this disease.

Prior to the advent of vaccine, *Hemophilus influenzae* type B, or *HiB,* caused thousands of cases of invasive disease each year. HiB is the causative agent in most pediatric cases of meningitis and is the most frequent cause of epiglottitis, both highly fatal diseases. Other related conditions include otitis media, sinusitis, septic arthritis, pericarditis, pneumonitis, and buccal, facial, or periorbital cellulitis (Schulman, McKendrick, & Atamos, 1993). From 1987 to 1995, however, the incidence of HiB disease declined 96% from 41 cases per 100,000 children to 1.6 cases (Childhood and Respiratory Diseases Bureau, 1996).

 Assessing the Dimensions of Health in Childhood Diseases

The Biophysical Dimension

Biophysical factors can increase one's risk of developing childhood diseases. Factors to be assessed by the community health nurse include the age and sex composition and physical health status of the population.

The nurse assesses the age of population groups in a community to determine their susceptibility to childhood diseases. Young children tend to be more susceptible to many childhood diseases and their effects than older children. Many of the cases in recent measles outbreaks have occurred in children too young to have received routine immunizations (Mortimer, 1994). There is, however, increasing incidence of measles in older age groups. In 1995, for example, nearly 40% of cases occurred among people over 20 years of age (Measles Virus Section, Respiratory and Enteric Viruses Bureau, 1996). Children aged 5 to 14 years have the highest incidence of mumps (van Loon, et al., 1995), but adults are more likely than children to experience complications. Children under 2 years of age frequently have subclinical cases of mumps (Benenson, 1995). Because of high immunization levels among young children, recent rubella outbreaks have tended to occur in groups of young adults (Childhood Vaccine Preventable Diseases Bureau, 1997b). Women of childbearing age may also be at risk for rubella increasing the potential for congenital rubella syndrome in their offspring. Approximately 90% of infants exposed to rubella virus during the first trimester will develop congenital rubella syndrome, but risk of congenital anomalies drops to 10 to 20% after the 16th week of gestation and effects are rare after the 20th week (Benenson, 1995).

The risk of fatality due to diphtheria is highest among infants and young children and case fatality rates have been stable at 5 to 10% of cases for several decades. There are increasing cases of diphtheria in adults throughout the world as well. From 1980 to 1992, for example, two thirds of diphtheria cases in the United States occurred in people over 20 years of age and as much as 40% of the adult U.S. population may lack protective antibody levels due to waning immunity and failure to obtain boosters at the recommended 10-year intervals in adulthood (Benenson, 1995). Pertussis, once a disease chiefly of young children, is also increasingly common in older age groups. From 1992 to 1994, 28% of cases of pertussis occurred in people over 10 years of age. Risk of complications, however, remains highest among children under 6 months of age (Childhood Vaccine Preventable Diseases, 1995), and increased adult transmission increases the potential for infection in the very young (Nennig, Shinefield, Edwards, Black, & Fireman, 1996). More than half of the cases of tetanus reported in the United States from 1991 to 1994 were in people over 60 years of age and those over 80 years of age have ten times the risk of persons aged 20 to 29 years. Tetanus fatality rates also increase with age with death occurring in 54% of cases of tetanus in persons over 80 years of age, compared to no deaths among those under 30 years of age who have contracted the disease (Izurieta, et al., 1997). These figures are due to failure of older persons to be immunized against tetanus or to obtain regular boosters as recommended. In developing nations, a significant number of cases of neonatal tetanus continue to occur as a result of infection during delivery in unsanitary conditions.

Infants and young children are at the greatest risk for poliomyelitis. In fact, in countries where poliomyelitis is still endemic, 70 to 80% of cases occur in children under 3 years of age. Adults are more likely than children to experience paralysis due to poliomyelitis (Benenson, 1995). School-age children comprise most of cases of varicella with 95% of cases occurring before 15 years of age, two thirds of which are among elementary school children (Mortimer, 1994). Varicella-related fatalities occur primarily among infants and adults with fatality rates above 25 per 100,000 population in those aged 30 to 49 years (Holmes, Reef, Hadler, Williams, & Wharton, 1996). In fact, adults, who experience only 2% of cases, account for 50% of deaths (Stutman, 1996). Adults are also at greater risk of nonfatal complications than children

(Choo, Donahue, Manson, & Platt, 1995). Invasive disease due to HiB occurs almost exclusively in children under age 5, and younger children seem to be at greater risk for complications of these diseases (Benenson, 1995).

Because sex may also be an influencing factor in the development of childhood diseases and their consequences, the nurse determines the sex composition of the population to determine the extent of risk for specific childhood diseases. Complications of mumps, for example, are more common in adult males than females. Morbidity and mortality for pertussis, on the other hand, are higher among females than among males of all ages. Males, however, more frequently develop tetanus, probably as a result of occupational exposure.

Physical health factors can increase both susceptibility to disease and complications of childhood illnesses, and the community health nurse assesses the community for the prevalence of conditions that increase susceptibility to childhood diseases. For example, malnutrition and immunosuppression place young children at higher risk of death and complications from measles. Malnutrition in children with measles may contribute to diarrhea and dehydration, severe skin infections, and vitamin A deficiency, resulting in blindness. Tonsillectomy predisposes one to bulbar involvement and motor center-mediated paralysis caused by polio. In addition, increased susceptibility to polio is noted in pregnancy (Benenson, 1995). Certain physical conditions, including asplenia, sickle cell disease (which occurs primarily in African Americans), and immunodeficiency, also contribute to the incidence of HiB-related diseases. In addition, immunodeficient children may not develop adequate immunity in response to HiB immunization. Disseminated chickenpox, with fatality rates of 5 to 10%, occurs more commonly in immunocompromised children with acute leukemia or HIV infection (Benenson, 1995). Pregnancy also increases the risk of complications of chickenpox (Advisory Committee on Immunization Practices, 1993).

The Physical Dimension

Physical dimension factors influence the development of childhood diseases and should be assessed by the community health nurse. Crowded living conditions, particularly in inner-city areas, enhance the spread of airborne diseases such as measles, mumps, rubella, pertussis, polio, and HiB infection. College campuses and military installations experience frequent outbreaks of measles among young adults in close quarters who are not immunized or whose immunity levels have declined over time.

Sanitation and disposal of both human and animal feces are other factors in the physical dimension that affect the development of childhood diseases, particularly tetanus and polio. The organism causing tetanus is found on a variety of surfaces and is more common in areas where there is animal excrement. In addition, home delivery births and poor hygiene on the part of untrained midwives in developing countries and some parts of the United States contribute to the development of tetanus in neonates and, occasionally, in postpartum women. Poor sanitation also fosters the spread of polio in underdeveloped countries (Global Program on Vaccines and Immunization, 1996). The polio virus is excreted in the feces of an infected person and then contaminates food and water supplies ingested by others, spreading the disease.

The Social Dimension

Social dimension factors that influence the incidence and consequences of childhood diseases include poverty, unemployment, lower education levels, and religion. Poverty and unemployment, with consequent loss of health insurance, may limit the ability of parents to have their children immunized or to provide prompt medical care when illness does occur, resulting in more serious consequences of disease. Pregnant women with low incomes might not receive prenatal care, thus denying them the opportunity to obtain screening and counseling for congenital rubella syndrome.

Racial and ethnic group differences are factors in the incidence of childhood illnesses. The incidence of childhood illnesses is higher, for example, among minority group children than their white counterparts, although these findings probably reflect access to health care rather than increased susceptibility among these minority groups. Native Americans and Alaskan Natives have higher rates of HiB infection than do their white counterparts, and in recent rubella outbreaks, incidence was highest among Latino children (Childhood Vaccine Preventable Diseases Bureau, 1997c).

Language barriers and lower education levels among some ethnic and socioeconomic groups may impede awareness of the need for immunization against childhood diseases. In addition, the beliefs of some religious sects prohibit immunizations, thus increasing the size of the susceptible population among members of these sects and the community at large (National Immunization Program, 1994a; 1994b). Because of reduced herd immunity (see Chap. 8 for a discussion of herd immunity), the presence of these unimmunized individuals increases the potential for the spread of disease throughout the community.

School attendance and occupation are additional social dimension factors that play a part in the development of some childhood diseases. Pertussis and varicella, for example, have high incidence rates among school-age children because of the ease of transmission in such group settings (Childhood Vaccine Preventable Diseases Bureau, 1997b; Holmes, et al., 1996). Occupation may be a factor in tetanus incidence which occurs more frequently among people who work outdoors, particularly those working around animals or in outdoor occupations in which there is a high potential for puncture wounds, such as trash collection and construction work. Pertussis and varicella occur with some frequency among health care workers who have low immunity levels.

Children of working parents who are placed in day care are at higher risk for HiB infection than children cared for at home. Although HiB immunization is required for preschool entry in many states, it is not required in all jurisdictions, nor does the requirement apply to family day care settings in some states. Social and economic conditions that require both parents to work or that limit support networks, particularly for single-parent families, contribute to the incidence of HiB-related disease. This trend is likely to continue as welfare reform requires more single parents of young children to become employed.

Other social factors that can increase the incidence of childhood diseases include homelessness and other forms of social upheaval and media communications. The fatigue, malnutrition, exposure to cold and crowding, and general debilitation associated with homelessness have contributed to increased pertussis and other communicable diseases in homeless populations. Large population movements may result in sanitation problems (Global Program on Vaccines and Immunization, 1996) or tax the capabilities of local health services to provide immunizations or diagnostic and treatment services. This is particularly true of large influxes of refugee populations in times of war or civil strife. Similarly, breakdown of the social order, as occurred with the disintegration of the former Soviet Union, may disrupt provision of health care services or abilities to procure vaccines (Childhood Vaccine Preventable Diseases Bureau, 1996). Finally, media reports of adverse reactions to immunization have led some parents to put off immunizing their children.

The Behavioral Dimension

The community health nurse also assesses for behavioral factors that might increase the susceptibility of a population to childhood diseases. Individuals and families in lower socioeconomic groups tend to engage in a "present-oriented" lifestyle in which energies are focused on dealing with current problems. Consequently, immunization of young children may

not be assigned a high priority in light of other needs. Moreover, inattention to routine health care needs and poor nutrition also contribute to increased susceptibility to childhood diseases. Overexertion and fatigue are also risk factors for childhood diseases, particularly polio.

Injection drug use is another lifestyle factor that contributes, on occasion, to the development of childhood diseases. Use of injection drugs contaminated with tetanus bacilli has been implicated in some cases of tetanus (Benenson, 1995).

The Health System Dimension

The community health nurse assesses the effects of health care system factors on the incidence of childhood diseases in the population. Health care system factors have contributed in several ways to the continued incidence of childhood diseases. Some contributing factors related to the health care system are errors in recommendations for routine immunizations and predictions of their efficacy; limiting access to immunizations; failure to educate the public adequately on the need for immunization; and failure to plan effective immunization strategies for groups at risk for disease.

Because of incomplete knowledge of the efficacy of various vaccines, health care providers have sometimes failed to give routine immunizations at appropriate times and have erroneously assured the general public of protection from disease when such may not have been the case. In the past, for example, measles immunization was given to many children prior to the first birthday. These children frequently did not develop adequate levels of immunity, leaving them susceptible to measles. Even when the first dose of measles vaccine is delayed to 15 months of age (the current recommendation), it appears that immunity is not lifelong and that a booster dose is required at school entry or adolescence (Benenson, 1995).

The health care system also may have contributed to the rise in the incidence of some childhood illnesses by limiting the availability of immunization services. The increasing practice in the public health care system of charging fees for immunization services that were formerly free deters economically disadvantaged clients from seeking immunizations for young children, thus limiting their ability to protect their youngsters from disease. In addition, health care providers in some areas have, in the past, been reluctant to provide rubella immunization to women of childbearing age, despite evidence that no harm has come to children of women inadvertently immunized during pregnancy. Furthermore, failure to monitor immunization rates among schoolchildren in some areas may also contribute to increased incidence of disease. Missed opportunities for immunizations and failure to give immunizations because of mythical contraindications also increase the risk of childhood illness. For example, many providers withhold immunizations for children with minor illnesses. Research indicates, however, that mild illness does not interfere with development of immunity (King, et al., 1996).

Failure of health care providers to educate the public in the appropriate treatment of wounds and failure to stress the need for immunization are factors contributing to the occurrence of tetanus. Also, relatively little attention has been given to educating the general public regarding the need for and availability of a vaccine for diseases caused by HiB virus (particularly compared with education campaigns related to both the Salk and Sabin polio vaccines).

Health care providers may also fail to recognize atypical forms of childhood illnesses and treat them effectively. For example, because of its relative infrequency in modern society, providers may lack clinical experience with pertussis or consider it as a possible diagnosis (Childhood Vaccine Preventable Disease Bureau, 1997b). Similarly, they may fail to consider a diagnosis of diphtheria as a cause of pharyngitis in adults with waning immunity levels (National Center for Infectious Diseases, 1997).

Health system factors may also contribute more actively to childhood diseases and their effects. For example, nosocomial infection in hospitals and physicians' offices is a significant factor in the spread of varicella (Holmes, et al., 1996). Similarly, medical treatment for conditions such as asthma and autoimmune diseases that require immunosuppressive therapy place individuals at greater risk for complications of varicella (Choo, et al., 1995). In some instances, immunization itself may contribute to disease. For example, from 1980 to 1994, administration of oral polio vaccine led to 125 cases of vaccine-associated paralytic poliomyelitis (94% of all reported cases) (Childhood Vaccine Preventable Disease Bureau, 1997a). These findings have led to recent recommendations for use of inactivated poliovirus vaccine (IPV) for the first two doses followed by two doses of oral poliovirus vaccine (OPV) (Prevots, Sutter, Strebel, Wharton, & Hadler, 1997).

Finally, failure to mount intensive immunization campaigns directed toward populations at risk has resulted in the continuing incidence of many childhood diseases. Inattention to booster immunization for persons beyond childhood and lack of initiation of tetanus immunization for older persons, for example, have both resulted in a pool of susceptible adults. Similarly, failure to target immunization campaigns to members of minority groups and those of lower socioeconomic levels and to design an intensive campaign for HiB immunization for children in day care

centers have contributed to the extent of preventable morbidity and mortality related to childhood diseases.

Factors related to the biophysical, physical, social, behavioral, and health system dimensions influence the incidence and consequences of childhood diseases. These epidemiologic factors are summarized in Table 30–4. Additional information related to each of the diseases discussed here is presented in Appendix S, Information on Selected Communicable Diseases.

Diagnostic Reasoning and Care of Clients with Childhood Diseases

The community health nurse may derive a variety of nursing diagnoses related to childhood diseases. These diagnoses may reflect the health needs of individuals, families, or population groups. For example, the nurse working with a family may diagnose "inadequate immunization status due to poor knowledge of children's immunization needs." A nursing diagnosis related to an individual client is "potential for infection with tetanus due to increased risk of occupational injury," or "failure to obtain routine immunizations due to lack of transportation."

Other nursing diagnoses may reflect the health needs of groups of people. For example, the community health nurse might diagnose "poor immunization levels among minority children due to limited access to immunization services." Other community-related diagnoses are "potential for measles outbreak due to large number of unimmunized children and young adults with declining immunity levels" and "increased incidence of congenital rubella syndrome due to low rubella immunity levels among women of childbearing age."

Planning and Implementing the Dimensions of Health Care in Childhood Diseases

Efforts to control childhood illnesses and their effects can occur at the primary, secondary, or tertiary levels of prevention. Planning of control strategies at each level is based on the general principles of program planning discussed in Chapter 19.

TABLE 30–4. EPIDEMIOLOGIC FACTORS IN CHILDHOOD DISEASES

BIOPHYSICAL DIMENSION

Genetic inheritance
- Many women of childbearing age are unimmunized for rubella.
- Complications of mumps are more frequent in males.

Maturation and aging
- Measles may occur in children too young for immunization.
- Children under 2 years of age are at a greater risk for HiB infection and complications of measles.
- Complications of mumps are more frequent in adults than in children.
- Polio occurs in young children and adolescents in developed nations and in infants and young children in developing nations.
- Many young adults lack immunity to measles, mumps, and varicella.
- Older adults may be at high risk for tetanus.
- Neonates are at high risk for death and complications from varicella.

PHYSIOLOGIC FUNCTION

- Presence of asplenia, sickle cell disease, or immunodeficiency increases susceptibility to HiB infection.
- Immunodeficiency may inhibit immunization response.
- Tonsillectomy may predispose one to bulbar involvement and paralysis in polio.
- Malnutrition increases the risk of complications in measles.

PHYSICAL DIMENSION

- Overcrowding increases spread of airborne diseases.
- Incidence of measles, mumps, rubella, pertussis, polio, and HiB infection is high in inner-city areas.
- Poor sanitation leads to fecal–oral polio spread in developing nations.

SOCIAL DIMENSION

- Poverty impedes access to immunization services for all age groups and to prenatal care for pregnant women.
- Media coverage of adverse reactions to immunization results in fear of immunization.
- Increased incidence of pertussis occurs in the homeless.
- Social factors necessitating employment of both parents and day care for children increases risk of HiB infection.
- Poverty impedes access to care when disease occurs.
- School attendance enhances the potential for the spread of disease.
- Homelessness decreases resistance and increases the potential for exposure to childhood illnesses.
- Social upheaval and migration may tax health system abilities to control childhood diseases.

BEHAVIORAL DIMENSION

- Poor nutrition is a contributing factor.
- Lack of attention to immunization needs contributes to disease.
- Lack of rest may increase susceptibility to polio.

HEALTH SYSTEM DIMENSION

- Inaccurate knowledge of immunization needs has led to (1) giving immunizations at inappropriate times and (2) assuming adequate immunity to measles following initial immunization.
- Access to immunization services has been impeded by (1) fees for immunization services and (2) refusal of some agencies to immunize women of childbearing age against rubella.
- Failure to educate public about need for immunization and failure to mount intensive immunization campaigns have lowered immunity levels.
- Missed opportunities for immunization have increased risks for childhood diseases.
- Failure to accurately diagnose childhood diseases has increased the potential for spread of diseases.
- Nosocomial exposure to childhood diseases enhances their transmission.
- Medical treatment for some conditions increases the risk of complications of some childhood diseases.
- Use of trivalent oral poliovirus vaccine (OPV) results in occasional cases of poliomyelitis.

Primary Prevention

Primary prevention for childhood disease includes immunization, chemoprophylaxis, and other measures as appropriate.

Immunization.   The major primary preventive measure for reducing the incidence of childhood diseases is, of course, immunization. The community health nurse should ensure that all susceptible individuals, particularly children, receive immunizations as appropriate.

The usual recommended schedule for measles immunization is an initial dose at 15 months of age, with a booster at either school entry or entry into junior high, or, for adults, college entry or employment in a health care setting. The initial dose of measles vaccine may be given earlier (at a few months of age) in areas of high incidence, but should be repeated after the child's first birthday. Measles immunization can also be given to susceptible adults, but should not be given to pregnant women because of the theoretical risk of harm to the fetus (Advisory Committee on Immunization Practices, 1994). Immunization should be given to unimmunized persons with HIV infection (Advisory Committee, 1993).

Immunization for rubella should be planned for all susceptible persons except pregnant women (Advisory Committee, 1994), particularly women of childbearing age. Planned immunization sites targeting women of childbearing age might include postpartum and family planning clinics, and college health services.

All youngsters over the age of 1 and susceptible adults, especially males, should receive mumps immunization. Immunization is contraindicated in immunosuppressed clients, except as mumps/measles/rubella (MMR) vaccine for children with HIV infection, and live-virus vaccines should not be given to pregnant women (Advisory Committee, 1993).

Immunization with diphtheria-tetanus-pertussis (DTP) vaccine in childhood with continued boosters for tetanus and diphtheria (TD) every 10 years throughout life is the major primary preventive strategy for these diseases. Immunizations for diphtheria and pertussis are particularly recommended for health care personnel, whereas tetanus should be of particular concern in occupational groups prone to injury. Older persons should be evaluated for their diphtheria and tetanus immunization status, and an initial series of immunizations should be planned and initiated as needed. Immunization of unimmunized travelers to areas with high incidence rates for these diseases is also recommended, especially for young children.

Inactivated poliovirus vaccine (IPV) should be given to infants at 2 and 4 months of age followed by oral poliovirus vaccine (OPV) at 18 months and school entry. Persons who are immunodeficient, their family members, and nursing personnel caring for them should be given inactivated polio vaccine (IPV) rather than OPV (Prevots, et al., 1997). Immunization is not generally recommended for adults unless they are working with infectious clients during a polio outbreak, in which case IPV should be given.

Primary prevention for HiB-caused illnesses involves immunizing children under 6 years of age. Immunization may consist of three doses at 2, 4, and 6 months of age with a booster at 12 to 15 months. When possible, the same brand of HiB vaccine should be used for the primary series of three doses, but vaccines may be interchanged if necessary (Advisory Committee, 1994).

Varicella virus vaccine (VZV) is recommended for routine immunization in a single dose at 12 to 18 months of age. Children under 13 years of age who have not yet been immunized and who do not have demonstrated immunity should receive one dose of VZV. Susceptible persons 13 years of age or older should be given two doses of vaccine 4 to 8 weeks apart. Those at high risk of exposure, such as health care workers, should be a priority for immunization services. The vaccine may be given during mild illness without diminution of effectiveness, but is not recommended for persons with immunosuppression or untreated tuberculosis. Household contacts of immunocompromised persons, however, should be immunized (Holmes, et al., 1996).

At the community level, efforts are needed to increase immunization levels within the population. By the end of 1996, 81% of children aged 19 to 35 months had completed the primary series of four DTP injections, 91% had received three doses of polio vaccine, and 92% had received three doses of HiB vaccine. In addition, 91% of children in this age group had received some form of measles-containing vaccine (usually MMR) and 82% had received three doses of hepatitis B vaccine (National Center for Health Statistics, 1997b). These figures suggest a need for continued community efforts to boost immunization levels. The National Association of County Health Officials (1993) has suggested several strategies that communities might use to achieve this goal. Some of these strategies are expanding immunization service hours and the availability of more convenient sites, providing transportation to immunization clinic sites, public education, special outreach programs targeted to specific populations (eg, migrants, day care enrollees, homeless), and using culturally and linguistically appropriate staff. These and other recommended strategies are summarized here:

- Establish links between health departments and other community agencies (eg, community clinics).
- Mobilize community resources (eg, churches, schools).
- Use volunteers for such responsibilities as clerical tasks, transportation, crowd control, and child care.
- Provide nurses with medical standing orders for immunization.
- Expand service hours.
- Establish new immunization sites.
- Provide transportation.
- Educate health care providers to prevent missed immunization opportunities.
- Provide linguistically and culturally appropriate services.
- Develop outreach programs for special target groups.

- Provide "walk-in" immunization services.
- Conduct public education on the need for immunization.
- Develop data systems for surveillance/tracking.
- Collaborate with other agencies to contain costs.
- Develop funding alternatives.
- Pursue legislative mandates related to immunization (including funding authorization).

Chemoprophylaxis. Chemoprophylaxis may be used as a primary preventive measure for those childhood diseases for which prophylactic medications are available. Chemoprophylaxis is given when an unimmunized person has already been exposed to the infectious agent causing a particular disease. In most cases, routine immunization for the disease should be initiated once the immediate danger has been averted. The community health nurse would use the following guidelines in planning chemoprophylaxis.

MEASLES. Live vaccine given within 72 hours of exposure may provide protection. Measles immune serum globulin may be given to household contacts and those with symptomatic HIV infection or other severely immunocompromised persons within 6 days of exposure (Benenson, 1995).

RUBELLA. Chemoprophylaxis is not recommended. Large doses of immunoglobulin have been given to pregnant women exposed to disease who refuse to consider abortion, but the effectiveness of this practice has not been evaluated (Benenson, 1995).

MUMPS. It is not known whether postexposure immunization for mumps is effective, but it is not contraindicated. Immunoglobulin is not effective following mumps exposure (Benenson, 1995).

DIPHTHERIA. Previously immunized contacts should receive a booster and a primary immunization series begun for other contacts. Antibiotic prophylaxis should be given to all contacts whether previously immunized or not. Those with positive cultures should receive extended treatment (Benenson, 1995).

PERTUSSIS. Close contacts under age 7 who have not received four doses of DTP or one dose in the last 3 years should be given a booster. Immunization has also been shown to protect against disease in previously unimmunized contacts when acellular pertussis vaccine is used (Schmitt, et al., 1996). All close contacts should be given a 14-day course of erythromycin regardless of immunization status (Division of Epidemiology and Surveillance, 1995).

TETANUS. Previously immunized persons should be given a booster dose of TD vaccine if 10 years or more has elapsed since the last dose (5 years for major or contaminated wounds). Unimmunized persons should receive a dose of tetanus toxoid. If the wound is major or contaminated, unimmunized persons should receive tetanus immunoglobulin (TIG) (Benenson, 1995). TIG should also be given to immunocompromised persons (Advisory Committee on Immunization Practices, 1993).

POLIOMYELITIS. Close contacts may be immunized, but may not be protected against disease unless previously immunized. No specific chemoprophylaxis is recommended (Benenson, 1995).

HiB INFECTION. Chemoprophylaxis using rifampin, an antituberculin drug, may be given to all household contacts in homes with children under age 4 who are unimmunized. Staff and young unimmunized children exposed in day care settings may also receive chemoprophylaxis (Benenson, 1995).

VARICELLA. Zoster immunoglobulin (ZIG) should be given to exposed neonates and severely immunocompromised individuals within 96 hours of exposure. ZIG may also be given to healthy children within 72 hours of exposure. Prophylaxis with acyclovir may also limit the number and severity of cases in household contacts (Holmes, et al., 1996).

Other Primary Prevention Measures. In some cases, other primary prevention measures may be planned and implemented to prevent childhood diseases. These measures include public education regarding control of these diseases and advocacy.

Education of clients includes the use of protective clothing in certain occupational groups to prevent injuries and the need for adequate cleansing of wounds with soap and water to prevent tetanus when injuries do occur. Education of individual clients and the general public regarding the need for immunization is another community health nursing activity directed toward primary prevention. At present there is also a need to inform previously immunized persons of the need for a booster dose of measles vaccine and periodic boosters for tetanus and diphtheria after school entry.

Interventions related to advocacy might entail ensuring access to immunization services for those most in need of them. Eliminating fees for primary immunization of children would be one means of ensuring access to services. The community health nurse might also advocate the enactment and enforcement of immunization policies designed to protect the general public. For example, community health nurses might advocate requirements that college entrants provide evidence of measles immunity. Community health nurses can also advocate HiB immunization prior to day care admission, and may be involved in efforts to promote legislation to this effect.

Secondary Prevention

Generally speaking, secondary preventive measures usually include screening efforts and activities designed to diagnose and treat existing illness. With the exceptions of screening pregnant women for susceptibility to rubella and screening contacts to diphtheria for carrier status, however, screening is not an effective control measure for childhood illnesses because of the relatively short incubation periods involved. Consequently, this discussion focuses on planning other categories of secondary prevention: diagnosis and treatment.

Diagnosis.   Secondary prevention of childhood diseases, as well as other communicable diseases, involves prompt identification and care of persons with the disease. Diagnosis of childhood diseases is usually made on the basis of the clinical symptomatology and immunization history, but may be confirmed by laboratory procedures in some instances. The community health nurse refers suspected cases of childhood diseases for diagnostic confirmation. The nurse also informs clients of the types of diagnostic procedures likely to be used, based on the following guidelines developed by the Centers for Disease Control (1997a).

MEASLES.   Diagnosis may be confirmed by isolation of the virus from blood, conjunctivae, nasopharynx, or urine by a rise in measles antibody titer.

RUBELLA.   Presumptive diagnosis made on the basis of history and physical findings should be confirmed by rising rubella antibody titers. Diagnosis may also be made on the basis of viral cultures of the pharynx, blood, urine, or stool within 1 to 2 weeks of the onset of rash.

MUMPS.   Diagnosis is usually made on the basis of physical findings but may be confirmed by serologic tests or isolation of the virus from saliva, blood, urine, or cerebrospinal fluid.

DIPHTHERIA.   Diagnosis is made on the basis of the characteristic lesion in the throat and is confirmed by bacteriologic examination of lesions.

PERTUSSIS.   Diagnosis is based on identifying the causative organism in clinical specimens or positive

polymerase chain reactions to *Bordatella pertussis*. A paroxysmal cough, an inspiratory whoop, or posttussive vomiting in contacts to laboratory-confirmed cases is also diagnostic.

TETANUS.   Diagnosis is made on the basis of clinical symptoms including acute onset of hypertonia, severe and painful contractions of neck and jaw muscles, and generalized muscle spasms without other cause.

POLIO.   Diagnosis is based on clinical signs of acute onset flaccid paralysis and diminished deep tendon reflexes without sensory or cognitive loss and with no other apparent cause. Diagnosis must be confirmed by review of an expert panel.

HiB INFECTIONS.   Diagnosis is based on isolating the virus from a normally sterile site (eg, blood or cerebrospinal fluid).

VARICELLA.   Diagnosis is based on clinical signs and symptoms. Laboratory confirmation is not usually required but may be made by isolating the virus in cell cultures or by a rise in serum antibody levels.

Treatment.   Community health nursing involvement in the treatment of childhood diseases includes referring clients with suspected diseases for diagnosis and for medical supervision. The community health nurse also educates parents or clients regarding the disease and its treatment. Community health nurses can educate parents or clients on measures to reduce fever and promote comfort for all childhood diseases, until the particular disease runs its course. Nurses also should educate caretakers on the symptoms of potential complications. Families whose members have rubella should be specifically cautioned by the community health nurse about the risks of exposing pregnant women. In the event exposure does occur during pregnancy, the nurse can counsel the family on options available and aid them in decisions about the pregnancy. Specific education about treatment measures for childhood illnesses should be planned to include the following information.

MEASLES, RUBELLA, MUMPS, AND POLIO.   Treatment is symptomatic and focuses on controlling fever and maintaining hydration and nutrition. In the case of polio, treatment may also entail maintenance of respiration through mechanical assistance.

DIPHTHERIA.   Diphtheria antitoxin and antibiotics such as penicillin and erythromycin are administered. Diphtheria antitoxin is no longer commercially available in the United States, but may be obtained from the Centers for Disease Control (National Center for Infectious Diseases, 1997).

PERTUSSIS.   Antibiotics such as erythromycin limit the period of communicability although they do little to speed recovery (Benenson, 1995). Attention to rest is important. Rest may be facilitated by the use of cough suppressants.

TETANUS.   Tetanus immune globulin (TIG) or tetanus antitoxin accompanied by intravenous metronidazole is administered. Excision of the wound, airway maintenance, sedation or muscle relaxants, or use of ventilators may be necessary (Benenson, 1995).

HiB INFECTIONS.   Usually ampicillin is administered. Ampicillin-resistant strains of HiB may be treated with ceftriaxone, cefotaxime, or chloramphenicol. Initial treatment is followed by a course of rifampin to ensure elimination of the organism (Benenson, 1995).

VARICELLA.   Treatment in most instances is symptomatic, consisting of control of fever and itching and maintenance of hydration. Acyclovir can be given within 24 hours of the onset of lesions to decrease duration and severity of illness (Holmes, et al., 1996).

Tertiary Prevention

Tertiary prevention for the individual client with a childhood disease involves preventing complications and long-term sequelae. For population groups, tertiary prevention is aimed at curtailing the spread of infection and preventing a recurrence of an outbreak. Preventing recurrent infection is not relevant for individual clients with most childhood diseases because infection usually confers lifelong immunity. In planning tertiary prevention of childhood illnesses, the community health nurse considers the following interventions.

MEASLES.   People who have suffered complications of measles may need help in adjusting to handicaps such as blindness and mental retardation. Families can be referred to sources of assistance and can be given emotional support in caring for handicapped members.

Recurrent outbreaks of measles can be prevented by immunizing children as young as 6 months, with repeated MMR immunization at 15 months of age. Using door-to-door immunization teams and giving immunizations in emergency rooms can also curtail the spread of an epidemic.

RUBELLA, MUMPS, DIPHTHERIA, AND PERTUSSIS.   Tertiary prevention is not usually required for individuals who recover

from these diseases. In the case of congenital rubella syndrome, however, families of affected children may require support and assistance in dealing with a variety of handicapping conditions. Recurrent outbreaks of disease in the community can be prevented by immunizing susceptible individuals.

TETANUS.   Tertiary prevention is not usually required for individuals who recover from tetanus. Control of animal feces in the environment can prevent the spread of disease. Hygienic midwifery practices in developing countries and immunization of susceptible persons can prevent recurrent epidemics.

POLIO.   Rehabilitation may be required to strengthen affected muscles or to promote individual and family adjustment to permanent disabilities. Active and passive range of motion may help restore muscle strength and prevent contractures. Maintaining skin integrity for clients with braces or those confined to bed or wheelchair is also important. Observation for recurrent disease (even many years later) is also needed. Families may also require assistance in financing rehabilitative care and procuring needed equipment and appliances. Mass immunization campaigns can curtail the spread of polio in the community and prevent recurrent epidemics.

HiB INFECTIONS.   Rehabilitation may be required for lasting consequences of HiB infections in individuals. Developmental levels should be carefully monitored and referrals made for assistance as needed. Parents should also be discouraged from becoming overprotective.

Immunization of household contacts and children in day care centers can curtail the spread of infection; immunization of all children under the age of 5 can prevent recurrent epidemics in the community.

VARICELLA.   Minimizing scratching can prevent secondary infection of lesions. Observation for complications such as encephalitis and pneumonia is important. Parents should be particularly cautioned not to use aspirin for fever control due to the risk of Reye syndrome. Persons experiencing congenital varicella syndrome or other long-term complications of varicella infection will need referral for assistance in a variety of areas. Those who develop later cases of shingles, a relatively common consequence of chickenpox, will also need referral for treatment.

Primary, secondary, and tertiary preventive activities are very similar for all of the diseases discussed thus far. Interventions at each level of prevention are summarized in Table 30–5.

TABLE 30–5. PRIMARY, SECONDARY, AND TERTIARY PREVENTION MEASURES AND COMMUNITY HEALTH NURSE FUNCTIONS IN CONTROL OF CHILDHOOD DISEASES

Level of Prevention	Community Health Nurse Function
PRIMARY PREVENTION	
Immunization	Identify persons in need and refer for immunization; provide immunizations
Prophylaxis (diphtheria, pertussis, measles, rubella, polio, HiB infection), varicella	Identifiy person in need and refer for prophylaxis; monitor use of prophylactics
SECONDARY PREVENTION	
Diagnosis and symptomatic treatment for most diseases	Employ case finding and refer for diagnosis and treatment
	Assist with supportive measures
	Observe for complications
Antibiotics/antitoxins/antivirals (pertussis, diphtheria, tetanus, HiB infection, varicella)	Educate regarding medications
TERTIARY PREVENTION	
Prevention of complications	Observe for complications, prevent use of aspirin, prevent scratching (varicella)
Mass immunization to prevent spread of disease	Plan and implement immunization programs
Rehabilitation (poliomyelitis, HiB infection, complications of measles and varicella, congenital rubella and varicella syndromes)	Monitor and promote development; promote client and family adjustment

TABLE 30–6. STATUS OF SELECTED NATIONAL OBJECTIVES RELATED TO CHILDHOOD DISEASES

	Objective	1988	1995	Target
20.1	Reduce number of cases of			
	a. Diphtheria	1	0	0
	b. Tetanus	3	5	0
	c. Wild polio	0	0	0
	d. Measles	3396	309	0
	e. Rubella	225	128	0
	f. Congenital rubella syndrome	6	6	0
	g. Mumps	4866	906	500
	h. Pertussis	3450	5137	1000
20.7	Reduce bacterial meningitis (per 100,000)	6.5	NDA[a]	4.7
20.11	Basic immunization in 2-year-olds	54–64%	75%	90%
20.13	States with immunization laws covering all recommended antigens	10	34	50
20.16	Health department provision of recommended adult immunizations	13%	48%	90%

[a]NDA, no data available.

(Source: U.S. Department of Health and Human Services, 1996.)

secondary and tertiary prevention is the incidence of complications resulting from these conditions. For example, if there are fewer instances of measles encephalitis among persons who get measles, secondary and tertiary preventive measures are probably effective.

Evaluating Control Strategies for Childhood Diseases

A number of the health-related statistics discussed in Chapter 8 can be used to evaluate the effects of primary prevention of childhood illnesses at the community level. Incidence rates for each of the childhood diseases provide information on the efficacy of primary preventive measures. Immunization levels in the population also indicate whether immunization programs, a primary preventive measure, are reaching high-risk populations. Evidence of primary prevention for the individual client is reflected in whether the client is immunized or develops a particular disease.

Another approach in evaluating control measures is examining the extent to which the national objectives for childhood diseases have been met. Table 30–6 presents information on the current status of many of these objectives.

Rates of death due to childhood illnesses are indicators of the success or failure of secondary and tertiary interventions. Another evaluative criterion for

Human Immunodeficiency Virus Infection and AIDS

Human immunodeficiency virus (HIV) infection, which results in AIDS in its most extreme manifestation, may well go down in the history of the 20th century as a disease comparable in terms of human devastation to the plagues of the Middle Ages. HIV is also an anomaly in that, with increasing survival time, it is both a communicable and a chronic disease. The growing concern about HIV infection and AIDS prompted the inclusion of several objectives related to control of this disease in the national health objectives for the year 2000 (U.S. Department of Health and Human Services, 1991) (see Appendix A).

HIV infection occurs on a continuum of related conditions characterized by inadequate immune system function. Within weeks of exposure to the virus, the new host may develop an acute primary HIV infection with mild symptoms similar to those of infectious mononucleosis or influenza (Carpenter, et al., 1996). Symptoms generally subside to be followed by a variable period of asymptomatic HIV infection.

In 1993, the Centers for Disease Control revised the classification system for the progression of HIV infection based on the presence or absence of clinical symptomatology and clients' CD4+ T-lymphocyte counts (Castro, Ward, Slutsker, Buehler, Jaffe, & Berkelman, 1992). This system uses the nine categories of HIV infection presented in Table 30–7. Symptoms in categories B1, B2, and B3 are those attributable to HIV infection, but not related to the AIDS indicator diseases included in categories C1, C2, and C3. Examples of B-category symptoms include persistent fever or diarrhea (lasting longer than 1 month), oral thrush, persistent or frequent vulvovaginal candidiasis, cervical dysplasia or carcinoma in situ, and recurrent shingles. Categories A3, B3, C1, C2, and C3 are included in the current surveillance case definition of AIDS, and clients in these categories are considered to have AIDS. The following AIDS indicator diseases are known as opportunistic infections:

- Candidiasis of bronchi, trachea, lungs, or esophagus
- Invasive cervical cancer
- Disseminated or extrapulmonary coccidioidomycosis
- Extrapulmonary cryptosporidiosis
- Intestinal cryptosporidiosis (longer than 1 month)
- Cytomegalovirus disease (except of liver, spleen, nodes)
- Cytomegalovirus retinitis
- HIV-related encephalopathy
- Herpes simplex bronchitis, pneumonitis, esophagitis, or chronic ulcers (longer than 1 month)
- Disseminated or extrapulmonary histoplasmosis
- Intestinal isosporiasis (longer than 1 month)
- Kaposi's sarcoma
- Burkitt's lymphoma
- Immunoblastic lymphoma
- Primary lymphoma of the brain
- Disseminated or extrapulmonary *Mycobacterium avium* complex or *Mycobacterium kansasii*
- *Mycobacterium tuberculosis*

- Disseminated or extrapulmonary *Mycobacterium*, other
- *Pneumocystis carinii* pneumonia
- Recurrent pneumonia
- Progressive multifocal leukoencephalopathy
- Recurrent *Salmonella* septicemia
- Toxoplasmosis, brain
- HIV-related wasting syndrome (Castro, et al., 1992)

Opportunistic infections are diseases caused by organisms that either do not usually cause illness in humans or that usually cause only mild disease.

Additional data presently known about AIDS, such as incubation period, transmission, and communicability, are presented in Appendix S. It should be particularly noted that the modes of transmission for HIV infection are relatively limited. Despite widespread fear of casual transmission, most actual transmission of HIV infection occurs via sexual contact; inoculation by contaminated needles and syringes; exposure to infected blood, blood products, or tissue; and transplacental or perinatal transmission from mother to infant. Specific behaviors that contribute to transmission of the disease include injection drug use (particularly using contaminated needles and syringes) and anal intercourse as practiced by male homosexuals and bisexuals and by some heterosexuals.

Trends in HIV Infection and AIDS

The incidence of AIDS rose sharply in the late 1980s and early 1990s from 5.36 per 100,000 population in 1986 to 40.2 in 1993. Incidence has since declined somewhat to 27.2 per 100,000 population in 1995 (Kao, et al., 1996).

The prevalence of HIV infection, of course, greatly exceeds the number of persons with actual cases of AIDS. Worldwide, an estimated 18 million adults and 1.5 million children are infected with HIV

TABLE 30–7. CLASSIFICATION CATEGORIES FOR HIV INFECTION

A1 HIV SEROPOSITIVE	B1 HIV SEROPOSITIVE	C1 HIV SEROPOSITIVE
Asymptomatic, primary HIV or PGL[a] and CD4+ T-cell count >500/µL	Symptomatic, not A or C conditions, and CD4+ T-cell count >500/µL	AIDS indicator conditions and CD4+ T-cell count >500/µL
A2 HIV SEROPOSITIVE	**B2 HIV SEROPOSITIVE**	**C2 HIV SEROPOSITIVE**
Asymptomatic, primary HIV or PGL and CD4+ T-cell count 200–499/µL	Symptomatic, not A or C conditions, and CD4+ T-cell count 200–499/µL	AIDS indicator conditions and CD4+ T-cell count 200–499/µL
A3 HIV SEROPOSITIVE	**B3 HIV SEROPOSITIVE**	**C3 HIV SEROPOSITIVE**
Asymptomatic, primary HIV or PGL and CD4+ T-cell count <200/µL	Symptomatic, not A or C conditions, and CD4+ T-cell count <200/µL	AIDS indicator conditions and CD4+ T-cell count <200/µL

[a]PGL, persistent generalized lymphadenopathy.
(*Source: Castro, et al., 1992.*)

(Division of HIV/AIDS Prevention, 1995b). Incidences of both HIV infection and AIDS are expected to continue at high levels in the next few years. AIDS was formerly believed to be uniformly fatal with a *case fatality rate* (number of persons who have a disease who will die as a result of it) approaching 100%. Antiviral therapy and primary prevention of opportunistic infections are increasing survival time for people with AIDS. For example, the number of deaths due to AIDS decreased by 23% from 1995 to 1996. Increased survival has led to an increase in AIDS prevalence, and in late 1997 there were more than 235,000 people in the United States living with AIDS (Division of HIV/AIDS Prevention—Surveillance and Epidemiology, 1997).

Assessing the Dimensions of Health in HIV Infection and AIDS

Factors in several dimensions of health influence the development and effects of HIV infection and AIDS.

The Biophysical Dimension

Knowledge of the epidemiology of HIV infection has been growing ever since the condition was first identified. Human biological factors, particularly age and health status, are known to influence the incidence of HIV infection and AIDS. An individual's race and

sex also influence the disease's incidence, probably through differential risk of exposure. In conducting an assessment related to AIDS and HIV infection, the community health nurse identifies factors related to the community or to individuals that foster the spread of disease. The nurse also assesses the effects of the disease on the individual, his or her family, and the community.

Maturation and Aging. The nurse begins by assessing the client or community for factors related to age that may increase susceptibility to HIV infection. AIDS is currently primarily a disease of young adults because of behaviors that put them at risk. There is, however, a growing number of young children who have developed AIDS. By September 1996, more than 7000 cases of AIDS had been diagnosed in children under age 13 (Division of HIV/AIDS Prevention, 1996a). The relative age distribution of all cases of AIDS diagnosed through October 1995 is presented in Figure 30–1. Infants appear to be more susceptible to HIV infection, and up to 30% of infants born to HIV-infected mothers are themselves infected. In the United States, perinatal transmission accounted for 92% of pediatric AIDS reported in 1994 (Davis, Byers, Lindegren, Caldwell, Karon, & Gwinn, 1995).

Twenty percent of infants who are actually infected with HIV perinatally develop AIDS within the first year of life. AIDS mortality is higher among those who develop symptoms within the first year, and in 1992, HIV infection became the seventh leading cause

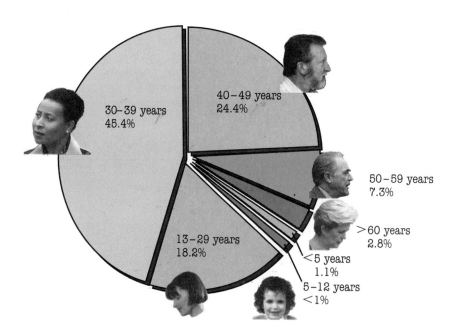

Figure 30–1. Age distribution of AIDS cases diagnosed prior to October 1995. (Source: Division of HIV/AIDS Prevention, 1995b)

of death in children aged 1 to 4 years. In 1994, there were more than 12,000 children under 13 years of age with AIDS in the United States (Davis, et al., 1995).

Adolescents are at high risk of HIV infection because of prevalent risk behaviors. Despite education related to HIV prevention, adolescents are more sexually active today than ever before. Incidence of AIDS among older people is increasing. More than 10% of all diagnosed cases of AIDS up to October 1995 occurred in people over 50 years of age (Division of HIV/AIDS Prevention, 1995b). Older persons have shorter periods of time between exposure and development of symptomatic AIDS. In addition, survival time, even after adjusting for normal mortality, is less for persons diagnosed with AIDS at age 55 or older than for younger persons (Darby, Ewart, Giangrande, Spooner, & Rizza, 1996).

Sex and Race.   Far more men than women have AIDS, again probably because men are more likely to engage in high-risk behaviors such as anal intercourse and injection drug use. More and more women are becoming infected, however, either through these risk behaviors or through sexual intercourse with someone who engages in high-risk behaviors (National Center for HIV, STD, and TB Prevention, 1996a). In 1992,

AIDS became the fourth leading cause of death for women aged 25 to 44 years (Davis, et al., 1995). Because the majority of females with AIDS are of childbearing age, there is increased potential for pediatric infection.

Racial and ethnic group differences are noted as well in the incidence of AIDS. Rather than contributing to HIV infection or AIDS, race and ethnicity are considered *markers* for groups at higher risk of disease due to other contributing factors (Division of HIV/AIDS, 1994). Although the majority of cases to date have occurred among whites, the incidence of AIDS is disproportionately high for African Americans and Latinos. Relative incidence rates for AIDS among whites, African Americans, Latinos, Asians and Pacific Islanders, and Native Americans are depicted in Figure 30–2. Racial and ethnic group differences in the incidence of pediatric AIDS are even more marked, as indicated in Figure 30–3.

Significant differences are noted for HIV-related mortality among racial and ethnic groups. In 1991, HIV infection was the leading cause of death among African American and Latino men aged 25 to 44 years and the sixth leading cause of death in Asian Americans and Native Americans. Mortality differences are even greater for women. For example, the 1991 AIDS

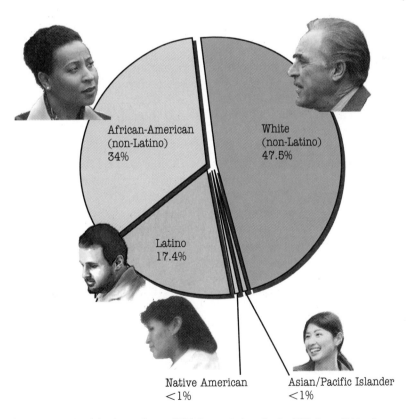

Figure 30–2.   Racial distribution of cases of AIDS diagnosed prior to October 1995. (Source: Division of HIV/AIDS Prevention, 1995b)

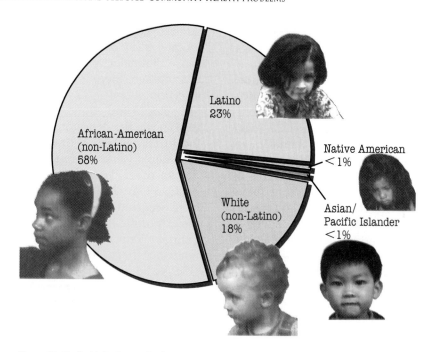

Figure 30–3. Racial distribution of pediatric AIDS cases diagnosed prior to September 1996. (Source: Division of HIV/AIDS Prevention, 1996a)

mortality rate for black women was ten times that of white women (Division of HIV/AIDS, 1994).

Physiologic Function. The presence or absence of other health conditions can influence the transmission of HIV infection as well as the development of AIDS. In assessing the potential for AIDS in the community, the community health nurse determines the prevalence of these conditions and their relationship to other risk factors. To determine an individual client's risk of AIDS, the nurse assesses the presence or absence of these conditions in the client.

Health conditions requiring transfusion or organ transplantation provide the potential for HIV transmission. The potential for transfusion-related HIV transmission has been greatly reduced by screening of potential donors for HIV antibodies. Only a few transfusion-related cases of AIDS have been diagnosed since 1985, when donor screening and blood testing began; at present, the risk of HIV infection is estimated at one in every 450,000 to 660,000 donations (Lackritz, et al., 1995).

Pregnancy is a risk factor in the development of AIDS for both mother and baby. As noted earlier, the majority of pediatric AIDS cases are due to perinatal transmission. The potential for infection of the infant appears to increase if the mother is actually symptomatic for AIDS. Transmission can also occur, however, if the mother is asymptomatic. Perinatal transmission may occur in utero with transplacental

transfer of the virus, by contact with maternal blood and vaginal secretions during delivery, or through breastfeeding (Langston, et al., 1995). Mothers are also at risk during pregnancy. Pregnant women with HIV infection have a greater probability of developing AIDS than those who are not pregnant.

Several other physical conditions appear to increase an individual's susceptibility to HIV infection. For both men and women, the presence of genital ulcers from diseases such as syphilis and genital herpes also increases the potential for HIV infection (Benenson, 1995).

Prior to the development of AIDS indicator conditions, some HIV-infected individuals display nonspecific symptoms that increase in frequency or duration with progression toward AIDS. Some of these conditions were addressed earlier. Other common findings include thrush, rashes, persistent fatigue, fever, and anemia, and the community health nurse should be alert to these findings in HIV-infected clients.

Because HIV compromises and eventually destroys the immune system, persons with AIDS are highly susceptible to a variety of other infections, and the community health nurse assesses the person with AIDS or HIV infection for signs and symptoms of opportunistic infections. Persons with AIDS, for example, have approximately 100 times the risk of developing tuberculosis as healthy individuals, or even those with other chronic conditions. The physiologic effects of AIDS can also be seen in the increased levels of mortality from pneumonia and influenza among individuals with AIDS. It is important for the nurse to remember that HIV-infected individuals may not always exhibit signs and symptoms of these conditions typical among non-HIV-infected individuals. Symptoms of common opportunistic infections for which the community health nurse should assess the client with AIDS are listed in Table 30–8.

The Psychological Dimension

Elements of the psychological dimension can also present problems related to AIDS that should be assessed by the community health nurse. Psychological factors such as poor self-esteem and poor interpersonal skills may lead individuals to engage in behaviors such as sexual promiscuity and injection drug use, thus increasing their risk of exposure to HIV infection. In addition, fear of a diagnosis of AIDS may cause individuals to delay seeking treatment for suspected illness.

For clients who have been diagnosed as having HIV infection or AIDS, there are tremendous psychological implications. These clients may face guilt related to past high-risk behaviors that contributed to their diagnoses and to possibly infecting loved ones with HIV. In addition, they face the possibility of rejection by significant others and of their own untimely death. Severe depression occurs in 5 to 10% of people with HIV infection but may be ignored as a common response to diagnosis. In addition, symptoms of depression such as fatigue, change in appetite, and sleep disturbance occur in many other conditions experienced by clients with AIDS and may make the diagnosis of depression difficult (McEnany, Hughes, & Lee, 1996). Suicide is a serious problem among persons with HIV infection and AIDS, and the community health nurse should assess these clients for depression, withdrawal, and suicidal ideation or gestures. The nurse should also assess family members for signs of emotional stress, fear and anxiety, or grief regarding the client's possible death. Because of the social stigma attached to AIDS, many bereaved families hide their loss and are denied the comfort usually afforded by friends.

Another consideration in the psychological dimension is that of boundaries between client and health care provider. Because of the intense nature of client–provider relationships in conditions like AIDS, providers may overidentify with clients and impair the therapeutic nature of their interaction (Rosica, 1995).

The final psychological factor to be assessed is confusion or disorientation in the client with AIDS. HIV infection has central nervous system effects that may result in loss of memory and confusion or in aggressive or combative behavior. Approximately 6% of people with AIDS display some level of dementia (Monastersky, 1992). The community health nurse assesses the client's level of orientation and the presence or absence of confusion.

The Social Dimension

The primary social dimension factors related to becoming infected with HIV are the prevalence of HIV infection within a particular population and the extent to which individuals within that population engage in high-risk practices. The prevalence of HIV seropositivity varies across the country as does the incidence of full-blown cases of AIDS. AIDS has been diagnosed

---

TABLE 30–8. SYMPTOMS OF SELECTED OPPORTUNISTIC INFECTIONS IN HIV-INFECTED INDIVIDUALS

Opportunistic Infection	Typical Symptoms in HIV-infected Individuals
Candidiasis	Thrush, dysphagia with esophageal infection, redness, itching, and burning in skin folds, inflammation of tissue around nails, vaginitis
Coccidioidomycosis	Malaise, fever, weight loss, cough, fatigue
Cryptosporidiosis	Profuse watery diarrhea, abdominal cramps, flatulence, weight loss, anorexia, malaise, fever, nausea and vomiting, muscle pain
Cytomegalovirus (CMV)	Retinal or choroidal inflammation, pneumonitis, encephalitis, colitis, esophagitis, hepatitis, impaired vision (disseminated)
Herpes simplex virus	Painful lesions on lips, tongue, or buccal mucosa; fever; cervical lymphadenopathy; genital lesions (with proctitis: pain, difficult urination or defecation, rectal discharge)
Histoplasmosis	Fever, weight loss, enlarged liver, spleen, lymph nodes, anemia
Isosporiasis	Profuse, watery, fatty, nonbloody diarrhea; abdominal pain; nausea; anorexia; weight loss; low-grade fever
Mycobacterium avium–intracellulare	Fever, fatigue, weight loss, anorexia, night sweats, abdominal pain, cough, diarrhea
Pneumocystis carinii pneumonia	Fever, fatigue, shortness of breath, cough (6–7% may be asymptomatic)
Salmonellosis	Diarrhea, weight loss, anorexia, fever, chills, sweats
Toxoplasmosis (CNS)	Headache, altered mental status, hemiparesis, aphasia, ataxia, visual impairment, motor disorders
Tuberculosis	Fever, weight loss, night sweats, fatigue, dyspnea, productive cough, hemoptysis, chills, lymphadenopathy, chest pain

(Source: Ungvarsky & Schmidt, 1992.)

in all 50 states, Washington, DC, and U.S. territories. Figure 30–4 presents AIDS incidence rates by state for the period from July 1995 through June 1996.

Specific risk behaviors prevalent in areas with high AIDS incidence rates account for those high rates. In New York City, for example, the highest incidence of HIV infection occurs among injection drug users and their sexual partners. The nurse in a particular community assesses the prevalence of these risk behaviors in the population to determine community risk for problems related to AIDS.

Prison inmates constitute another institutionalized group with high incidence rates because of the high proportion of injection drug use and needle sharing and high-risk sexual behaviors in correction settings (Koehler, 1994). Incidence of AIDS among inmates is seven times that of the general population (Mahon, 1996). Homeless individuals may also be at high risk for infection due to drug abuse, mental illness, and use of sex for monetary gain.

Some of the differences between racial and ethnic groups in the incidence of AIDS and the prevalence of HIV infection may be due to the social dimension factor of lack of knowledge regarding the transmission of AIDS. Knowledge differences related to AIDS and HIV infection have been noted among members of different racial and ethnic groups, with African Americans and Latinos being less knowledgeable than the white population.

Community attitudes toward AIDS can often influence the effect of having AIDS on individual clients. The social stigma attached to a diagnosis of AIDS may deter people with possible infection from being tested or from seeking treatment. The social stigma and fear attendant on a diagnosis of HIV infection may also prevent those who know that they are infected with HIV from notifying their contacts or limiting their sexual or needle-sharing drug use behaviors. Some authors note that the overwhelming psychological effects of massive mortality in the gay community of San Francisco have led some HIV-infected individuals to attempt to rebuild their lives in small Midwestern communities. The conservatism typical of these communities necessitates a "closet" existence, movement to bisexuality, and consequent spread of infection in the heterosexual population (Joseph, 1992).

Negative attitudes toward HIV-infected individuals are displayed in attempts at mass isolation as called for in California's Proposition 64 (which was

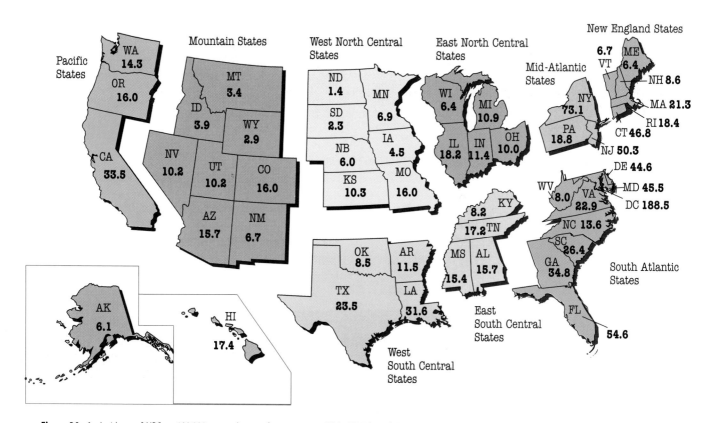

Figure 30–4. Incidence of AIDS per 100,000 persons by state for cases reported July 1995 through June 1996. (Source: Centers for Disease Control. (1996). AIDS rates. *MMWR, 45,* 316.)

defeated in 1987). Although we would like to believe that the social stigma attached to HIV/AIDS has diminished, that does not appear to be the case. In findings reported in 1993, respondents still voiced desires to isolate and avoid infected individuals and a willingness to blame them for their condition (Herek & Capitano, 1993).

In communities with high anxiety levels and fear of casual exposure to HIV infection, individuals with AIDS are unlikely to seek assistance until they are desperate. Such attitudes by community members may also limit the availability of services for persons with AIDS. In addition, fear of contagion has led to difficulty in finding foster placement for babies born to HIV-infected women and has resulted in the "boarder baby" phenomenon of infants left in hospital nurseries indefinitely. In assessing individual and community risk of health problems related to AIDS, the community health nurse explores community members' knowledge, beliefs, and attitudes toward AIDS, as well as the sources of their knowledge, beliefs, and attitudes. Community attitudes are frequently influenced by social role models as in the case of celebrity disclosures of HIV infection.

Social norms that contribute to high-risk behaviors also foster the spread of HIV infection. For example, relaxed sexual mores have led to greater sexual promiscuity and increased risk of exposure to HIV infection. Similarly, a social environment in which it is relatively easy to obtain drugs for injection drug use promotes the spread of infection.

One aspect of the social and physical environment is *not* considered to influence the transmission of HIV infection. Casual social or physical contact with persons who have AIDS or who are infected with HIV has not been implicated in transmission of the infection. In studies of families with AIDS, household contact with infected persons has not led to seroconversion in other members of the household. This has also been true of health care workers caring for clients with AIDS; casual contact has not been a source of infection. Beliefs by community residents that casual contact does transmit infection, however, can impede efforts to provide care for people with AIDS and should be identified by the community health nurse.

The nurse working with individuals with AIDS should assess the extent of their social support networks. Clients with AIDS may have diminished social networks due to social isolation resulting from other people's reactions to their diagnosis or to the death of significant others from AIDS. In addition, abstinence from sexual contact to prevent the spread of disease may limit the client's social contacts. Loss of occupation and financial resources may also occur as a result of reaction to the diagnosis or as a result of diminish-

ing health. The nurse should determine the people who constitute the client's social support network and the types of support available from each. Gaps in social support available and additional avenues for obtaining support from the social network can also be determined.

Occupation is another social dimension factor that may contribute to HIV infection and AIDS. Health care workers are one of the occupational groups at increased risk for infection. HIV infection occurs in approximately 0.3% of percutaneous injuries among health care workers (Division of HIV/AIDS Prevention, 1995a). There is also some potential for infection of other persons exposed to blood and body fluids such as paramedics and laboratory personnel. Prostitutes are another occupational group that are at extremely high risk for HIV infection as well as other sexually transmitted diseases.

Although the risk of transmission of HIV infection to health care workers is small, the possibility exists. For this reason, the Centers for Disease Control recommends the application of universal blood and body fluid precautions by all health care workers with clients with AIDS and other bloodborne diseases. Under these recommendations, blood and other body fluids of all patients are to be treated as though HIV infection were present. Potentially infectious bodily fluids include blood, semen, vaginal secretions, cerebrospinal fluid, pleural fluid, pericardial fluid, and amniotic fluid. Universal precautions *do not* apply to feces, nasal secretions, sputum, sweat, tears, urine, or vomitus. Special precautions for dental professionals are suggested for contact with saliva, more because of the likelihood of transmission of hepatitis B than concern for HIV infection. Observance of universal precautions provides protection against hepatitis and other bloodborne diseases, as well as AIDS. Universal precautions for bloodborne pathogens are summarized here:

- Wash hands before and after client contact and immediately after contamination with blood or other body fluids.
- Wear gloves when contamination with blood or body fluids is likely.
- Wear masks when splashing of blood or body fluids is likely.
- Wear protective eyewear when splashing of fluids is likely.
- Wear a gown if soiling of exposed skin or clothing is likely.
- No special precautions are needed for dishes.
- Do not bend, clip, or recap contaminated needles. Dispose of contaminated sharps in puncture-resistant containers.

- Contaminated reusable equipment should be appropriately cleaned.
- Have mechanical ventilation devices available for resuscitation.
- Use gloves to clean spilled blood or body fluids. Wipe up excess with disposable towels; clean area first with soap and water, then with dilute solution of household bleach (1:100, smooth surfaces; 1:10, porous surfaces).
- Health care workers with open lesions and dermatitis should not engage in direct client care or handle contaminated equipment.
- Health care workers should be thoroughly acquainted with these precautions by their employers and compliance should be enforced.

Two additional elements of the social dimension that may influence the health of HIV-infected clients are violence and pet ownership. Because of the social attitudes toward AIDS discussed earlier, some people who are fearful of infection may resort to violence against those who are infected. A group that may be at particular risk of violence are HIV-infected women whose partners become aware of their exposure for infection (Rothenberg & Paskey, 1995). Pet ownership is another area of concern because of the potential for *zoonoses,* diseases transmitted to humans by animals. In one study of people with AIDS who had pets, only 10% had been informed of the risk of zoonoses (Conti, Lieb, Liberti, Wiley-Bayless, Hepburn, & Diaz, 1995).

The Behavioral Dimension

Behavioral factors play a greater role in the development of AIDS than any other epidemiologic factor. The primary behavioral dimension factors involved in the development of HIV infection and AIDS are sexual activity and injection drug use. In assessing the risk of HIV infection and its effects in a community or for an individual client, the community health nurse determines the presence of factors in each of these areas.

Sexual Activity.   In the United States, approximately 90% of all AIDS cases are related to sexual transmission (Division of HIV/AIDS Prevention, 1995b). Most cases of sexually transmitted AIDS early in the epidemic (approximately 95%) occurred among homosexual men. More recently, however, heterosexual transmission of AIDS has increased. As of October 1995, nearly 8% of AIDS cases among adults were the result of heterosexual transmission (Division of HIV/AIDS Prevention, 1995b). Among women, heterosexual exposure accounts for 37% of cases of AIDS (Division of HIV/AIDS, 1994). The people most at risk for heterosexually transmitted HIV infection are those with multiple partners, those with other sexually transmitted diseases (STDs), and those living in areas with high prevalence rates for HIV seropositivity.

Several factors increase one's risk for heterosexual disease transmission. Male-to-female HIV transmission is facilitated when the infected male has advanced HIV disease, the woman is over 45 years of age or has another STD, and the couple engages in anal intercourse. The risk of female-to-male transmission increases when the infected woman is in an advanced stage of disease or is menstruating at the time of intercourse. Homosexual (male-to-male) transmission increases with receptive anal intercourse. Lesbians and bisexual women are also at risk of HIV infection, and female-to-female transmission has been documented (Guly, 1994). Prostitution by both males and females also enhances disease transmission.

An individual's risk of HIV infection increases as the number of his or her sexual partners increases. This is true whether one engages in homosexual or heterosexual activities. A significant number of adults and adolescents engage in sexual activity with multiple partners, thus increasing their risk of AIDS and other STDs.

One final factor related to sexual activity that influences the incidence of HIV infection and AIDS is the use of condoms. Latex condoms have been shown to be about 90% effective in preventing HIV infection. Despite this fact, only 14% of sexually active single women reported condom use in a 1995 national survey (National Center for Health Statistics, 1997a). The use of a spermicide in conjunction with a condom may provide additional protection, but this has not yet been satisfactorily demonstrated in clinical practice.

Injection Drug Use.   Injection drug use is another behavioral factor implicated in the transmission of HIV infection. Injection drug use in the United States accounted for 35% of AIDS cases diagnosed in the United States in 1995 (Division of HIV/AIDS Prevention, 1996b).

The prevalence of HIV infection among injection drug users (IDUs) varies widely across the country. From 10 to 70% of IDUs in a given locale may be HIV positive. *Seroprevalence rates,* or the proportion of people with positive blood tests, among IDUs also vary geographically. The low prevalence of HIV infection among drug users in Los Angeles, as compared with New York City, may be due to environmental factors that limit the potential for spread of the infection. These include the widespread nature of metropolitan Los Angeles and the absence of large "shooting galleries," where multiple patrons share needles and syringes, common on the East Coast. Because of relatively great distances between small groups of IDUs in the Los Angeles area and the lack of a mass transportation system, there is little interaction between groups of drug users. Hence, HIV infection is confined to the small local group of IDUs rather than being spread to drug users throughout the city.

Some of the differences in AIDS incidence and prevalence of HIV infection among racial and ethnic groups may be explained by differences in the prevalence of injection drug use within groups. African American clients are significantly more likely to develop AIDS as a consequence of injection drug use than their white counterparts, among whom homosexuality is the more common risk factor (Division of HIV/AIDS Prevention—Surveillance and Epidemiology, 1997).

Specific behaviors among drug users increase the risk of HIV infection. The primary risk behavior in this group is needle sharing (this includes sharing any drug-related paraphernalia such as needles and syringes that may be contaminated with blood). Several studies have indicated widespread needle sharing among IDUs.

In assessing the risk of AIDS in the community and for the individual client, the community health nurse explores the extent of injection drug use (if any). The nurse determines the extent to which unsafe practices such as needle sharing are prevalent. The nurse also assesses the extent to which sexual and drug use behaviors are combined by members of the community, because the combination of risk behaviors associated with injection drug use and sexual activity is particularly significant in the transmission of HIV infection. HIV seropositivity for heterosexuals is higher for those whose partners are IDUs than for those whose partners are not. Other findings that link combined sexual and drug use behaviors with HIV infection include the fact that many prostitutes who are seropositive for HIV antibodies are IDUs. Moreover, an increased incidence of AIDS is linked to sexual contact with multiple partners from urban areas with high rates of injection drug use, prostitution, and other STDs.

Condom use by IDUs engaging in sexual activity could significantly reduce the risk of HIV infection; however, several studies indicate that condoms are rather infrequently used by IDUs.

The Health System Dimension

As noted earlier, blood transfusions were a source of HIV infection prior to the institution of donor screening. HIV transmission has also occurred in organ transplants from infected donors (Rogers, Simonds,

Lawton, Moseley, & Jones, 1994). HIV transmission via infected semen used in artificial insemination (Araneta, et al., 1995), nuclear medicine procedures, and spring-loaded finger-stick devices has also been documented. At present, no known mechanism exists for processing human semen that can prevent transmission of HIV infection. The Centers for Disease Control also recently released a report that, in a few cases, HIV infection was transmitted from infected health care workers to their patients; however, the risk of becoming infected is extremely low.

The health care system has influenced the HIV epidemic in other ways as well. Steven Joseph, former Commissioner of Health for New York City, notes that the failure of New York and other states to permit private laboratories to conduct early HIV screening tests made screening inaccessible to large numbers of people at a time when control of the epidemic would have been much easier. On the other hand, he credits the medical and scientific communities with the rapid growth in understanding of HIV infection and its management, a feat that would not have been possible with technology 20 years earlier (Joseph, 1992).

Expertise in managing HIV-infected clients also influences the course of disease. For example, an inverse relationship has been found between hospital experience with AIDS clients and AIDS mortality. Hospitals that saw fewer AIDS clients had higher AIDS mortality despite more intensive resource use (Stone, Seage, & Epstein, 1992).

Health care providers may also contribute to the spread of HIV infection by omission. Despite a national objective that 75% of health care providers engage in age-appropriate HIV prevention counseling, many providers do not counsel clients at all in this area. In one study, for example, fewer than half of primary care physicians routinely obtained a sexual history from their clients, and only 40% reported that they were likely to encourage HIV testing for sexually active adolescents (National AIDS Information and Education Program, 1994).

Refusal of some health care workers to provide care to persons with AIDS is another health care system factor influencing the impact of this disease. Both the American Medical Association and the American Nurses Association have issued statements relative to the responsibility of health care professionals to care for those with communicable diseases, including AIDS. The ethical implications of refusal to care for clients with AIDS are addressed in Chapter 15.

Finally, the lack of facilities for the care of persons with AIDS may lead to an increased burden of suffering for the individual and his or her family. This is particularly true for clients with central nervous system effects of the disease that cause aggressive behavior. In many instances, these clients are not able to be placed in nursing homes, hospices, or other facilities for the terminally ill because of their combativeness. This may either place the burden of care for the client on significant others or create a situation in which the person with AIDS becomes part of the homeless population discussed in Chapter 24.

Biophysical, psychological, social, behavioral, and health system factors contributing to HIV infection are summarized in Table 30–9.

Diagnostic Reasoning and Care of Clients with HIV Infection and AIDS

Nursing diagnoses related to HIV infection and AIDS may be derived for population groups and individual clients and their families. Diagnoses at the community level may reflect the current incidence of disease or the potential for spread of infection. Examples of such diagnoses are "increased incidence of AIDS due to injection drug use" and "potential for increased transmission of HIV infection due to widespread use of unsafe sexual practices by a large adolescent population."

Diagnoses related to individual clients and families may also reflect potential for infection or active disease. A possible diagnosis for a sexually active adolescent is "potential for HIV infection due to multiple sexual partners and failure to use condoms." Nursing diagnoses for a client who has AIDS and his or her significant others may be many and varied.

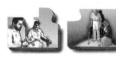

Planning and Implementing the Dimensions of Health Care for HIV Infection and AIDS

Planning and implementation of control strategies for HIV infection and AIDS occur at the primary, secondary, and tertiary levels of prevention.

Primary Prevention

Efforts to control the incidence of HIV infection and AIDS are hampered by several factors. The first of these is the disease's prolonged incubation period, during which infected persons are communicable but asymptomatic and thus difficult to identify. Second, based on current knowledge the potential for reduced

TABLE 30–9. EPIDEMIOLOGIC FACTORS IN HIV INFECTION

BIOPHYSICAL DIMENSION

Maturation and aging	• Infants in utero are particularly susceptible.
	• Incidence is highest in young adults.
Physiologic function	• Conditions requiring transfusion or organ transplantation slightly increase risk of HIV infection.
	• Pregnancy increases maternal susceptibility and potential for infant exposure in utero.
	• Cervicitis, vaginitis, or menstruation increases susceptibility.
	• Genital ulcer disease increases susceptibility.

PSYCHOLOGICAL DIMENSION

- Psychological factors that increase high-risk behaviors increase the potential for exposure.
- Fear associated with diagnosis of HIV infection may prevent infected individuals from seeking screening.
- Persons with HIV infection may experience fear, guilt, and anxiety.

SOCIAL DIMENSION

- Prevalence of HIV infection in population affects risk of exposure.
- Increased prevalence is noted in large metropolitan areas.
- Potential for spread is increased in institutions for mentally disabled.
- Casual contact *does not* transmit HIV infection
- Social stigma attached to HIV infection impedes control efforts.
- Social norms that contribute to high-risk behaviors lead to increased incidence.
- Lack of knowledge about HIV transmission may lead to high-risk behaviors.
- Social support networks of persons with AIDS may be diminished.
- Use of universal precautions for blood and body fluids limits chances of health care worker exposure.

BEHAVIORAL DIMENSION

Sexual activity	• Increased number of sexual partners increases risk of exposure.
	• Receptive anal intercourse increases risk of infection.
	• Homosexual and bisexual behavior increases risk of exposure.
	• Use of condoms decreases risk of infection.
Injection drug use	• Drug use and needle-sharing practices increase risk of exposure.
	• Prostitution to support a drug habit increases risk of exposure.

HEALTH SYSTEM DIMENSION

- Screening of blood and organ donors limits potential for exposure.
- Failure to provide health insurance for persons with HIV infection leads to decreased access to care.
- Refusal of health care workers to care for infected persons leads to poor care.
- Lack of facilities for care leads to increased suffering and societal burden.
- Infected providers may spread HIV infection to clients.
- Lack of expertise in managing clients with AIDS leads to increased mortality.

communicability with treatment is uncertain. Finally, AIDS is largely spread by private behaviors that are associated with some degree of social stigma, making it difficult to identify individuals at greatest risk for the disease.

Currently, there is no vaccine for AIDS, although human testing of potential vaccines has been initiated.

> ## POTENTIAL NURSING DIAGNOSES FOR THE INDIVIDUAL CLIENT WITH AIDS
>
> *Physical Health*
> - Fever due to opportunistic infection
> - Cough due to opportunistic infections of the respiratory system
> - Dyspnea due to lung congestion related to opportunistic pulmonary infection
> - Skin lesions related to opportunistic infection
> - Weakness due to debilitation from recurrent opportunistic infections
> - Fluid and electrolyte loss due to diarrhea from opportunistic gastrointestinal infection
> - Poor nutritional status due to loss of appetite, nausea, and vomiting related to opportunistic infections
> - Increased susceptibility to infection due to immune deficiency
>
> *Psychological Health*
> - Confusion/disorientation due to central nervous system effects of AIDS
> - Fear of impending death due to diagnosis of AIDS
> - Grief of individual and/or family due to impending death
> - Impaired self-image due to diagnosis of AIDS
> - Guilt related to past high-risk behavior and possible exposure of loved ones
>
> *Socioeconomic Health*
> - Potential for spread of disease due to communicability of HIV infection
> - Social isolation due to stigma of AIDS diagnosis
> - Financial problems resulting from loss of job and medical bills
> - Lack of source of care due to inadequacy of facilities for caring for clients with AIDS

Progress in developing an AIDS vaccine has been hampered by the ease with which the virus mutates, creating new strains. Zidovudine (AZT) has proven effective in slowing the course of infection among many individuals, but whether it will render these individuals noncommunicable is not known. The U.S. Public Health Service recommended zidovudine for pregnant HIV-infected women to prevent perinatal disease transmission (Mofenson, Balsley, Simonds, Rogers, & Moseley, 1994).

At present the most effective method of decreasing the incidence of HIV infection and AIDS is eliminating high-risk behaviors. Two approaches can be taken to achieve this end. The first is to change behaviors among those who are uninfected so as to prevent or minimize exposure to HIV infection. The second is to promote behavioral changes in those who are infected to prevent transmission to others.

Several approaches have been suggested for decreasing the risk of exposure for persons who are currently uninfected. These include avoiding unsafe sexual practices and high-risk drug behaviors, continued screening of blood and organ donors, using universal precautions in the handling of blood and body fluids, and offering premarital/preconceptual HIV testing and counseling.

Optimal risk reduction relative to sexually transmitted HIV infection would result from abstinence or lifelong monogamy. Serial monogamy (only one partner at a time) is less effective than lifelong monogamy, but less risky than having multiple partners. It has been suggested that legitimizing same-sex relationships in terms of the rights and privileges accorded to married people might contribute to greater lifelong monogamy among these individuals, thus reducing the incidence of AIDS among gay men. Community health nurses can educate the public on the advantages of monogamous relationships, or they can use political activity to legitimize same-sex unions.

In the absence of monogamy or abstinence, the use of barrier methods such as condoms and spermicidal preparations limits exposure to HIV infection and other STDs, as well as pregnancy. Education about condom use alone does not seem to affect use appreciably (Catania, et al., 1995); however, education coupled with easy access to condoms does seem to increase use of this barrier method. The development of barrier methods that are female controlled has also been advocated as has assertiveness training regarding condom use among prostitutes (Karim, Karim, Soldan, & Zondi, 1995). Limiting the number of sexual partners and refraining from anogenital intercourse are other ways to limit sexual transmission of HIV infection. Community health nurses can educate individual clients and the general public about safe sexual practices and use advocacy to ensure easy availability of condoms. For example, community health nurses might participate in programs to provide free condoms to sexually active young people.

For drug users, preventive measures might include increased availability of drug treatment centers and methadone programs. Failing elimination of drug use, clients can be educated regarding "safe shooting" practices such as not sharing needles and disinfecting them after use. Again, education along with ready access to bleach as a disinfectant has resulted in some behavioral changes among injection drug users (Division of HIV/AIDS Prevention, 1995c). Advocacy is also needed to change laws that make possession of injection equipment a criminal offense, creating a need to share drug paraphernalia.

It has also been suggested that drug users be provided assertiveness training and support groups that might improve users' abilities to resist peer pressure to share needles or avoid condom use during intercourse. Community health nurses can refer willing drug users to drug treatment centers. They might also be involved in advocating access to drug treatment centers and in planning education programs for IDUs related to safe shooting practices, avoiding needle sharing, and using bleach to disinfect equipment. Nurses might also plan and implement needle exchange programs for IDUs to reduce needle-sharing behaviors.

Another approach to reducing high-risk sexual activity and drug use is to provide alternatives to prostitution and drug abuse. This might be accomplished in part by providing employment and other social needs. Other approaches to the primary prevention of drug abuse are discussed in Chapter 33.

Education is one approach to bring about some of the behavioral changes suggested. First, there is a need to educate health care providers about risks for HIV infection and the kinds of interventions that can prevent transmission of disease. When health care professionals are knowledgeable, they can more effectively educate clients on safe and unsafe behaviors. As noted earlier, community health nurses may play a role in education programs for health care professionals related to AIDS and other sexually transmitted diseases. They may be involved in planning and implementing formal education programs for other health care providers, or they may educate other providers more informally on a one-to-one basis.

Educating the general public and members of high-risk groups about AIDS has had some impact, and community health nurses can be actively involved in educational endeavors. Increases in knowledge of AIDS and its transmission have been noted both among adolescents and adults. In neither group, however, did knowledge of the risk of transmission lead to greater use of condoms. In addition to providing information about HIV infection and its transmission, community health nurses should plan educational campaigns that motivate clients to change their behavior. Motivational techniques were reviewed in Chapter 9.

Among high-risk groups, education and counseling have been somewhat more effective. Homosexuals have demonstrated rather profound decreases in numbers of sexual partners and unsafe sexual practices. Among some groups of drug users there has also been evidence of a decrease in high-risk behaviors as a result of education and counseling. Community health nurses should reinforce positive behavior changes among clients that diminish potential for exposure to HIV infection.

Measures can also be taken to prevent the spread of HIV infection from infected individuals to others in the community. By and large, these should be voluntary measures. Research indicates that voluntary changes in behavior to reduce the risk of transmission to others have occurred in groups of homosexual men.

Some people, however, have called for isolation of those with AIDS and HIV carriers as a means of preventing the spread of the epidemic. Because casual contact is not a means of transmission for HIV infection, isolation measures would be unwarranted. There may occasionally be a need to restrict persons who knowingly continue to infect others. Authority to do so should be provided to the states as is the case in other communicable diseases, but this should be exercised only as a last resort and only in instances in which the individual is definitely infected, continues to put others at risk, and refuses to control his or her behavior. Control in such cases should be exercised using the least restrictive method possible. Community health nurses should be active in ensuring that punitive measures not be enacted against persons with AIDS. They might also need to plan and implement political campaigns to promote legislation against broad-based measures to isolate individuals with AIDS and to monitor isolation proceedings when they occur to be sure that they are warranted.

Prenatal or even preconceptual screening for HIV infection in high-risk groups could serve as a primary prevention measure in the control of pediatric AIDS. In addition, use of zidovudine during pregnancy has been shown to decrease the risk of fetal infection (Mofenson, et al., 1994). Refraining from breastfeeding may also prevent postpartum transmission (Bertolli, et al., 1996). Community health nurses could be active in planning and implementing screening programs for high-risk women in STD and family planning clinics and drug treatment centers so as to facilitate counseling those with seropositive results regarding the risks of pregnancy. Any counseling should be coupled with opportunities to receive contraceptive services. Women who are HIV-positive and who are already pregnant can be counseled regarding the potential for infection of the infant and options available to them. Community health nurses can also refer women of childbearing age in high-risk groups for HIV infection to screening and counseling services.

Community health nurses may also engage in primary prevention for persons with HIV infection and/or AIDS. In this case, intervention focuses on preventing opportunistic infections (Kaplan, Masur, & Holmes, 1997) and psychosocial problems stemming from infection. For example, the community health nurse might refer clients for *Pneumocystis carinii* pneumonia prophylaxis (Grubman, Oleske, Simonds, Rogers, & Moseley, 1995) or provide immunization against influenza, pneumonia, measles, and other diseases for susceptible persons. Because of the HIV-infected individual's reduced immune response, immunization schedules may need to be altered, with inactivated polio virus vaccine used instead of live vaccine. Zoster immunoglobulin (ZIG) may also be warranted after chickenpox exposure or measles immunoglobulin for measles exposure. The community health nurse might also educate HIV-infected clients regarding nutrition and other avenues for health promotion.

Secondary Prevention

Secondary prevention involves identifying HIV-infected persons and those with AIDS and appropriately treating their infection. The first step is screening those at risk. Other secondary prevention measures involve diagnosis and treatment of AIDS and related opportunistic infections.

Screening. For screening programs to be effective in controlling the incidence of AIDS, health care professionals should be adequately educated regarding those who need screening, interpretation of screening tests, and need for counseling after testing. Community health nurses can be active in planning and implementing this education. Initial screening is done using enzyme immunoassays (EIAs), the most common of which is the enzyme-linked immunosorbent assay (ELISA). Reactive (positive) tests should be repeated until there have been more than two reactive tests on the same sample. They should then be confirmed by means of the Western blot (WB) test. Screening tests for viral RNA or DNA, such as the polymerase chain reaction (PCR), are also being used on a limited basis due to lack of availability.

Screening results are reported as positive, indeterminate, or negative. A positive test is one in which more than two positive reactions were obtained on an EIA subsequently confirmed with a Western blot or immunofluorescence assay (IFA) (Rogers, et al., 1995). Indeterminate tests necessitate further observation of the client and retesting, as he or she may be in the process of *seroconversion,* or changing from a negative to a positive test. Generally, seroconversion occurs within 30 to 50 days of exposure (Carpenter, et al., 1996). Health care providers, including community health nurses, who are interpreting screening tests for HIV should be aware that false-positive results may be obtained due to pregnancy, immunoglobulin derived from infected persons, and circulating maternal antibodies in young infants. Test results should be assessed in the light of client history and questionable results confirmed with subsequent blood tests before clients are informed that they are infected with HIV. Infants who are actually uninfected experience a process of *seroreversion* in which their blood test results revert back to negative after a transient seropositivity due to circulating maternal antibodies. This usually occurs at about 9 months of age (Caldwell, Oxtoby, Simonds, Lindegren, & Rogers, 1994).

HIV screening has been suggested for a number of groups, including blood and tissue donors, persons with other STDs, prisoners, hospitalized persons, injection drug users, women of childbearing age, pregnant women, men and women contemplating impregnation, children of infected women, those who have been transfused, those with tuberculosis and other signs of opportunistic infection, prostitutes, persons applying for marriage licenses, military recruits, and the general public.

Screening of the general public is unwarranted at this time. Because of the slow spread of HIV infection in populations without identified risk factors, the cost of screening and posttest counseling would outweigh the benefits in terms of cases of HIV infection identified. Although premarital screening for HIV infection in the general population has also been suggested, the incidence of HIV seropositivity among those without identified risk factors is relatively low, limiting the cost-effectiveness of screening. Premarital screening for HIV infection has been mandated in two states, Louisiana and Illinois. Screening was never implemented in Louisiana, and the Illinois law mandating screening was repealed. Studies during its implementation indicated that the law, rather than promoting HIV screening, caused increasing numbers of couples to be married in adjoining states rather than be tested for HIV infection (McKillip, 1991).

Mandatory testing of prisoners has been advocated by some because of the increased prevalence of both drug abuse and homosexual activity within correctional settings. Current recommendations are for the provision of voluntary testing for inmates (Koehler, 1994), with emphasis on those in high-risk groups or who have symptoms suggestive of AIDS. Federal prisons have received directives to test all inmates on admission and at release. Screening for HIV infection is mandatory for sex offenders, prostitutes, and drug users arrested in some states.

Routine HIV screening is advisable among some population groups. HIV screening for clients seen in STD clinics and drug treatment centers, for example, is warranted because of the prevalence of risk behaviors among these groups. Routine screening of all pregnant women is now recommended by the U.S. Public Health Service (Rogers, et al., 1995). Because of the devastating effect of learning that one is HIV-infected after one is already pregnant, more intensive screening of women of childbearing age is also recommended (U.S. Department of Health and Human Services, 1995b). Screening is also warranted for individuals in high-risk groups who are contemplating pregnancy or those who feel themselves to be at risk for AIDS. In addition, screening is recommended for all people who were transfused between 1978 and 1985.

It has been suggested that all hospital admissions be screened for HIV infection. In populations with HIV seroprevalence of less than 1%, however, routine screening of all hospital admissions could cost as much as $753 million per infection prevented in health care workers. There is also a high probability of many people being labeled as seropositive due to false-positive results in populations with low HIV prevalence (Lurie, Avins, Phillips, Kahn, Lowe, & Ciccarone, 1994). Public Health Service recommendations are for screening of hospital admissions for high-risk behaviors and offering of voluntary testing as well as the use of universal precautions with all admissions (Ward, Janssen, Jaffe, & Curran, 1993).

Screening for HIV, even in groups in which screening is recommended, should be a voluntary activity, with adequate provision for the protection of confidentiality. Reporting of positive test results to state or local health authorities facilitates determination of the incidence of HIV infection, allows for follow up of infected individuals for medical care, and permits contact notification. Screening also permits earlier diagnosis and promotes better medical management and efforts to prevent opportunistic infections.

The only generally accepted exception to voluntary HIV screening is screening of blood and tissue donors. The cost of screening in these instances are outweighed by the benefits of identifying infected donors. Also, calculations of the relative costs and benefits per case of AIDS prevented are comparable to those for other screening programs.

In spite of efforts to promote screening among high-risk groups, many people at risk for HIV infection do not avail themselves of screening opportunities. According to the National AIDS Behavior Survey, there was virtually no change in the proportion of the population screened for HIV infection from 1990 to 1992 (Catania, et al., 1995). Similarly, in 1993, only 32% of U.S. women of childbearing age had been screened for infection (Division of Health Interview Statistics, 1996). Among adolescents, another high-risk group, rates of HIV screening have been shown to increase when parental consent requirements are eliminated (Meehan, Hansen, & Klein, 1997).

Community health nurses are often actively involved in planning and implementing HIV screening programs. They educate clients at risk for HIV infection of the need for testing and may either refer them to screening clinics or conduct screening tests in those clinics. Community health nurses working in HIV screening clinics also interpret test results for clients and counsel them on avoiding high-risk behaviors that may lead to HIV exposure. Nurses refer clients with positive tests for further diagnosis and treatment as needed and provide counseling to prevent the spread of disease to others. Community health nurses may also refer clients for counseling related to the psychological effects of positive test results.

Diagnosis. Community health nurses refer clients with positive HIV screening results and others with conditions suggestive of AIDS for further diagnostic evaluation. Diagnosis of AIDS is based on diagnostic classifications addressed earlier in the chapter. A diagnosis of AIDS is a reportable condition in every state.

Treatment. At present, treatment for AIDS and HIV infection is in transition. Zidovudine (AZT) is currently being used to treat many people with symptomatic AIDS and those with asymptomatic HIV infection. Zidovudine has been shown to decrease the rate of HIV infection in infants born to HIV-infected mothers by two thirds (Mofenson, et al., 1994). New therapies for AIDS include protease inhibitors such as saquinavir, ritonavir, and indinavir. Some authorities recommend use of these drugs with persons at risk for rapid progression of AIDS (Carpenter, et al., 1996), whereas others suggest their use in combination with older antiretrovirals for initial treatment of HIV infection (Collier, Coombs, Schoenfeld, et al., 1996).

Additional treatment of clients with AIDS is primarily supportive. Treatment for current opportunistic infections is provided as necessary as a secondary prevention measure. Community health nurses working with clients with AIDS can educate them regarding treatment with zidovudine or other primary drugs for AIDS and treatment for opportunistic infections. Areas to be addressed in planning include the client's need to know the effects and side effects of the medications and how to take medications as prescribed. Community health nurses should also plan interventions related to maintaining nutritional status, oral and personal hygiene, observation for effects and side effects of medications, and advocacy. At the community level, secondary prevention by community health nurses may include political action to ensure the availability of funding and adequate diagnostic and treatment facilities for those with HIV infection and AIDS.

Tertiary Prevention

Teritiary prevention in AIDS may be directed toward the individual client or population groups.

The Individual Client.   Tertiary prevention measures for HIV-infected clients are aimed at limiting the debilitating effects of infection, preventing the occurrence of opportunistic infections, and normalizing the client's life as much as possible. Prophylaxis may be given to prevent certain opportunistic infections such as *Pneumocystis carinii* pneumonia (PCP) and tuberculosis. Tuberculosis chemoprophylaxis is given to persons with HIV infection who have a reactive tuberculin skin test and no evidence of active disease. Isoniazid (INH) is the drug most often used. In the presence of HIV infection, INH is given for at least a year, compared with the usual prophylactic regimen of 6 months (Kaplan, et al., 1997).

Trimethoprim–sulfamethoxazole is most often used for prophylaxis of PCP (Kaplan, et al., 1997), especially in clients with multiple episodes. PCP prophylaxis may also be achieved with aerosolized pentamidine, which ensures delivery of drug to the alveolar site of infection. Trimethoprim–sulfamethoxazole may also be used for PCP prophylaxis in children (Grubman, et al., 1995). Recently, PCP prophylaxis has been recommended for all HIV-infected persons with CD4+ T-cell counts below 200/µL (Kaplan, et al., 1997).

The community health nurse working with HIV-infected clients receiving prophylaxis for tuberculosis, PCP, or other opportunistic infections educates clients regarding the medication used, its therapeutic effects, and its side effects. In addition, the nurse monitors the effectiveness of medication and the occurrence of side effects.

Community health nurses can plan referral for clients with AIDS and HIV infection to health care sources that provide both prevention for opportunistic infection and routine health care. Nurses may also be involved in educating health care providers regarding the special health needs of those with AIDS or HIV infection.

The community health nurse working with clients with AIDS and HIV infection should monitor them closely for signs of opportunistic infection. When signs or symptoms of opportunistic infections are noted, the nurse makes a referral for treatment. The nurse also monitors the effectiveness of treatment for opportunistic infections.

Community health nurses may also need to function as advocates to prevent AIDS-related discrimination and to foster a client's integration into the community to the extent permitted by the client's health status. To achieve this, the nurse may need to educate those who interact with the client about how HIV infection is and is not transmitted. When working with children with AIDS, advocacy by the community health nurse may necessitate planning activities that foster normal growth and development in each child. Owing to fear of infection, for example, teachers and schoolmates and their parents may be reluctant to let the child with AIDS participate in group activities. Or, parents of the child with AIDS may become overprotective and prevent the child from engaging in activities that would promote growth and development.

Another role for the community health nurse in tertiary prevention to limit the impact of AIDS on the individual client and his or her family lies in providing emotional support. Clients will probably need assistance in working through their feelings about having the disease and their guilt at possibly having infected others (especially their children). Clients and family members may need the help of the community health nurse in adjusting to the debilitating effects of the disease and in dealing with the possibility of death. If referral is needed for additional counseling, the community health nurse should be prepared to make such referrals and to act as a liaison in linking the client and family with appropriate resources.

Assistance may also be needed in dealing with the financial impact of AIDS. The community health nurse can help in this respect by referring the client and his or her family to sources of financial assistance. Advocacy by community health nurses may be required to ensure client eligibility for financial assistance programs. At the level of public policy, community health nurses may need to plan political activity to ensure necessary funding for AIDS-related assistance programs.

The Community Client.   Tertiary prevention with population groups is directed primarily toward preventing the spread of infection. In the absence of a cure for AIDS, the most significant approach to tertiary prevention at the community level is contact notification.

Contact notification for AIDS and HIV infection has been a controversial issue because of fear about loss of confidentiality and discrimination against HIV-infected individuals. Other arguments against contact notification for HIV are based on concerns over cost and the lack of a definitive treatment. These concerns are largely unfounded. The history of contact notification in other STDs and the precautions taken against loss of confidentiality have been very effective, and similar precautions would be taken in notifying contacts to HIV infection.

Some argue that contact notification is of no benefit in the absence of a cure for HIV infection. It is argued that knowledge of exposure only creates anxiety on the part of contacts. With the advent of zidovudine, protease inhibitors, and drugs used to prevent opportunistic infections, however, HIV infection is closer today to becoming a manageable chronic illness than it ever was before.

Even in the absence of effective treatment for HIV infection, contact notification can help control the spread of this disease, particularly in view of the fact that about 14% of contacts tested prove seropositive and are in danger of infecting others (Pavia, Benyo, Niler, & Risk, 1993). Contact notification and subsequent testing for HIV infection counteract the tendency of many high-risk individuals to avoid testing. Contact notification also permits several avenues for action that would be unavailable without this measure. If contacts are seronegative on examination, they can be counseled regarding measures that may limit their chances of subsequent exposure (eg, condom use, not sharing needles, discontinuing receptive anogenital intercourse). If contacts are seropositive, they can be encouraged to take precautions to avoid infecting others. Studies have shown that contacts tend to change high-risk behaviors whether they test positive or negative for HIV infection.

Furthermore, earlier identification of HIV-infected persons through contact notification and testing permits preventive measures for opportunistic infections. For example, seropositive contacts can be screened for tuberculosis and given chemoprophylaxis to prevent development of active disease. Female contacts who are HIV-positive can be assisted to make informed decisions regarding pregnancy. Contact notification also provides opportunities to offer other needed services, such as treatment for other STDs, immunization, contraceptive services, and psychological support services.

In some jurisdictions community health nurses are involved in notifying contacts of HIV-infected persons. In carrying out contact notification, community health nurses need to keep in mind that individuals might be emotionally devastated by news of possible HIV infection. Fear of AIDS can cause contacts to react with anger, depression, or anxiety. Consequently, the nurse should plan interventions to assist the contact to deal with his or her emotional reaction. The nurse can be an effective support person in helping the contact deal with these feelings. The nurse can be an effective support person in helping the contact deal with these feelings. The nurse can explain that not everyone becomes seropositive after exposure to HIV and that testing can help determine whether the contact is indeed infected. The nurse can also use the opportunity to educate the client regarding high-risk practices and can suggest changes in behavior to minimize risk of disease transmission. Nurses who are engaged in contact notification also have the opportunity to refer contacts for other needed services. For example, an injection drug user can be referred to a treatment program if desired. Or, the nurse may discuss the potential effects of HIV infection in pregnancy with a female contact of childbearing age and refer her for contraceptive services (or high-risk prenatal services if she is already pregnant).

Contacts should be reassured as to the confidential nature of screening. The nurse should emphasize that information about the need for screening and test results will not be shared with others (eg, employers). Reassurance should also be provided that illegal behaviors will not be reported to the authorities and that, although information about high-risk behaviors is requested at the time of screening, this information is strictly confidential and will not be used in criminal proceedings.

When contacts arrive for screening tests, they might encounter the same nurse or other community health nurses. These nurses reinforce information about the screening test and about high-risk behaviors and how these behaviors can be modified. When the client returns to obtain test results, the community health nurse has another opportunity to inform the client about measures to prevent the transmission of AIDS. Clients who have positive test results need a great deal of emotional support from the nurse. They may need assistance in dealing with feelings and fears regarding AIDS and HIV infection. The nurse can provide information about the need for medical supervision and make referrals for these services as well as for psychological counseling. Referrals may also be needed for other services such as drug abuse treatment, prenatal or contraceptive services, and financial aid.

Numerous primary, secondary, and tertiary prevention measures can be employed to control HIV infection. Community health nurses are actively involved in controlling this disease at all three levels. Table 30–10 summarizes primary, secondary, and tertiary prevention activities for HIV infection and AIDS.

TABLE 30–10. PRIMARY, SECONDARY, AND TERTIARY PREVENTION MEASURES TO CONTROL HIV INFECTION

Level of Prevention	Community Health Nurse Function	Goal
Primary prevention	• Educate clients and public on preventive measures. • Educate on "safe sex." • Refer drug abusers for treatment. • Educate drug users on "safe shooting" practices. • Engage in political activity.	• Decrease number of sex partners. • Increase use of condoms. • Decrease receptive anal intercourse. • Decrease injection drug use. • Decrease needle sharing. • Ensure funding for education and prevention.
Secondary prevention	• Identify and refer those in need of screening. • Provide screening and counseling. • Monitor treatment for HIV infection. • Monitor treatment for opportunistic infections. • Engage in political activity.	• Increase screening of members of high-risk groups. • Increase compliance with treatment. • Provide adequate treatment of opportunistic infections. • Ensure funding for facilities and treatment.
Tertiary prevention	• Counsel HIV-infected women. • Counsel and screen blood and tissue donors. • Educate infected persons on means of preventing transmission. • Interview cases and notify contacts. • Provide prophylaxis for opportunistic infections. • Assist clients and families with grieving. • Engage in political activity.	• Prevent fetal HIV infection. • Ensure safe blood and tissue supply. • Prevent spread of infection. • Prevent spread of infection. • Prevent opportunistic infection. • Help clients and families accept death. • Ensure funds to care for terminally ill (including hospice care).

Evaluating Control Strategies for HIV Infection and AIDS

The effects of control strategies for HIV infection and AIDS for various population groups can be evaluated in terms of trends in HIV incidence and HIV-related mortality as well as indicators of the extent of risk behaviors in the population. For example, the nurse could examine the extent to which members of a community or target group engage in unsafe sexual practices or needle sharing during drug use. At the national level, the objectives for the year 2000 provide criteria for future evaluation of the effectiveness of control measures in preventing HIV infection. The current status of selected HIV-related objectives is presented in Table 30–11.

Evaluation of care for individuals with HIV infection and AIDS focuses on the extent of disruption of clients' lives caused by their condition. How effective is antiretroviral therapy in preventing the development of AIDS? Has the person with HIV infection refrained from practices that enhance the spread of infection? Have further opportunistic infections been prevented or resolved in the client with AIDS? Have the social and economic effects of his or her condition been minimized?

Hepatitis

Hepatitis, or inflammation of the liver caused by viral agents, occurs with alarming frequency, and because of the ease of transmission of most forms of viral hepatitis, it has become a public health problem of major concern. To date, five specific hepatitis-causing viruses have been identified: hepatitis A virus (HAV), hepatitis B virus (HBV), hepatitis C virus (HCV), hepatitis D virus (HDV), and hepatitis E virus (HEV). One additional virus, hepatitis G (HGV), has also been identified, but its role in human hepatitis is unclear at present (Alter, et al., 1997). Prior to identification of the specific viruses involved, hepatitis, C, D, and E were collectively known as non-A, non-B hepatitis.

Trends in Hepatitis

Various forms of hepatitis are found throughout the world, and hepatitis contributes to significant morbidity and mortality.

Approximately 33% of the U.S. population has antibodies to hepatitis A, indicating infection at some point in their lives (Shapiro, Bell, & Margolis, 1996). The annual cost of HAV infection is estimated at $200 million (Smith, Kline Beecham, 1995a). In 1995, the incidence rate for HAV was 12.13 per 100,000 persons (Centers for Disease Control, 1996). Worldwide, an estimated 350 million people are chronically infected with hepatitis B (Marchou, et al., 1995). More than one million people in the United States are chronic carriers of HBV and up to 300,000 new infections occur each year (Marsano, et al., 1996). In 1995, the incidence rate for HBV in the United States was 4.19 per 100,000 population (Centers for Disease Control, 1996).

Hepatitis C occurs in approximately 150,000 persons each year in the United States (Bryan, Pinner,

TABLE 30–11. STATUS OF SELECTED NATIONAL OBJECTIVES FOR HIV INFECTION

Objective	Base	Current Status	Target
18.1 Decrease annual incidence (per 100,000)	17 (1989)	28.6	43
18.2 Decrease prevalence of HIV infection (per 100,000)	400 (1989)	NDA[a]	≤400
18.4 Increase condom use among sexually active unmarried persons aged 15–44 years	19% (1988)	25% (1995)	50%
18.5 Increase proportion of injection drug users in treatment	11% (1989)	34% (1995)	50%
18.6 Increase use of uncontaminated injection equipment	31% (1991)	60% (1992–1996)	75%
18.7 Decrease risk of transfusion-transmitted HIV infection (per unit of blood)	1 per 40,000–150,000 (1989)	1 per 225,000 (1991)	1 per 250,000
18.8 Increase testing for HIV infection in those infected	72.5% (1990)	NDA	80%
18.9 Increase counseling for HIV infection	10% (1987)	83% (1995)	80%
18.10 Increase proportion of schools with HIV education curricula	66%	86% (1995)	95%

[a]NDA, no data available.

(Sources: U.S. Department of Health and Human Services, 1995a; 1997.)

Gaynes, Peters, Aguilar, & Berkelman, 1994) and is the cause of approximately 90% of transfusion-related hepatitis cases in the United States (Tong, El-Farra, Reikes, & Co, 1995). The 1995 incidence rate for HCV was 1.78 per 100,000 people (Centers for Disease Control, 1996). Hepatitis D was previously known as delta hepatitis. Because it requires hepatitis B virus for replication, HDV disease can exist only in clients with HBV disease. Enteric hepatitis or hepatitis E infection is seen more frequently in developing countries than in the United States. Outbreaks have occurred in Africa, Asia, and Mexico (Crowe, 1994). As many as 29,000 people have been affected in some HEV outbreaks (Hepatitis Bureau, 1993).

Assessing the Dimensions of Health in Hepatitis

Factors related to biophysical, physical, psychological, social, behavioral, and health system dimensions influence the incidence of hepatitis in its various forms. The community health nurse assesses for the factors present in each area to determine the risk of these diseases for an individual client or for a community.

The Biophysical Dimension

Elements of the biophysical dimension to be addressed include the influence of age, race and ethnicity, and health status on the development of disease as well as the physiologic effects of hepatitis. Although hepatitis A occurs in all age groups, it is most commonly seen in children and young adults. For example, 30% of all cases of HAV infection occurs in children under 15 years of age (Shapiro, et al., 1996), and in some communities with periodic outbreaks 30 to 40% of children are infected before age 5 (Hematologic Diseases Bureau, 1997). Although the incidence

of disease is higher in the young, the severity of the disease seems to increase with age, and children often have subclinical cases without noticeable symptoms.

Hepatitis B can be transmitted from mother to fetus, and an estimated 20,000 babies are born each year to American women with chronic hepatitis B infection (Epidemiology and Surveillance Division, 1996). Despite the availability of an effective vaccine, only 82% of U.S. children aged 19 to 35 months had received three or more doses of hepatitis B vaccine in 1996 (National Center for Health Statistics, 1997b). Although the initial infection in neonates tends to be mild, these children tend to develop persistent chronic infection and have a high incidence of later cirrhosis and liver cancer (Hepatitis Bureau, 1997b). Adolescents are also at high risk for HBV infection because of risk behaviors such as sexual promiscuity and drug use.

All age groups are susceptible to hepatitis C and D, but HDV infection tends to be quite severe in children. HEV tends to occur most often in young adults. During disease outbreaks, those between 15 and 40 years of age are most frequently affected.

Hepatitis tends to occur with equal frequency in both males and females. Among racial and ethnic groups, Native Americans and Mexican Americans are at higher risk of hepatitis A infection than other ethnic groups. Up to 67% of Mexican Americans and 80% of people in some Native American communities have HAV antibodies (Hepatitis Bureau, 1997a; Shapiro, et al., 1996).

Two aspects of physiologic function must be considered in assessing individuals or communities for problems related to viral hepatitis: physiologic factors that may increase one's susceptibility to disease and the physiologic effects of disease. With respect to physiologic precursors to disease, conditions requiring transfusion may contribute to infection with hepatitis B, C, and D, all of which can be transmitted parenterally. The likelihood of transmission of HBV and HCV has declined dramatically with the advent of donor testing for antibodies to these two viruses. For example, since the initiation of donor testing for HCV, the current risk of posttransfusion hepatitis is less than 0.8% (National Institutes of Health, 1995).

As noted earlier, pregnancy in a woman with HBV infection may result in perinatal exposure of the infant. Hepatitis C may be transmitted to the infant by an infected mother who is coinfected with HIV (Crowe, 1994). Other conditions that increase risk for HBV infection include hemodialysis and immunosuppression. Hemodialysis patients and those with hemophilia are likewise at higher risk for HCV than the general population, as are those who are immunocompromised. Immunodeficiency may also result in a longer period between infection and seroconversion in HCV infection. Hepatitis D occurs only in the presence of HBV, and pregnant women are at higher risk for mortality due to HEV.

The various forms of viral hepatitis differ in their consequences as well. Generally speaking, hepatitis A is a relatively mild disease, as are most cases of hepatitis C and E (except in pregnant women) (Benenson, 1995). Hepatitis B and D, on the other hand, may cause more severe disease, and the severity of HBV increases with HDV coinfection (Smith Kline Beecham, 1992). Chronic disease and a carrier state are highly characteristic of hepatitis B and C and occur in some cases of hepatitis D, but rarely in hepatitis A or E. Hepatitis D is more likely than other viral forms of the disease to result in fulminant hepatitis, a particularly severe manifestation of disease (Farci, et al., 1994). Chronic hepatitis B, C, and D are implicated in the development of cirrhosis and liver cancer, and HBV may be a causal factor in 80% of hepatocellular carcinoma worldwide (Benenson, 1995).

Hepatitis mortality rates also vary with different forms of hepatitis. For HAV, for example, overall mortality is less than 1 per 1000 cases. Death is slightly more likely in children under age 5 (1.5 per 1000 cases), and people 50 years of age and older are 27 times more likely than younger people to die of HAV (Benenson, 1995). Persons with underlying chronic liver disease are more likely than others to experience fulminant HAV and death (Shapiro, et al., 1996). Fulminant HBV, on the other hand, occurs in approximately 1% of cases (Crowe, 1994) and the case fatality rate is also 1% overall, with more frequent deaths in persons over age 40. HCV rarely causes fulminant disease and death but 30 to 60% of infected persons develop chronic disease and 5 to 20% develop cirrhosis (Benenson, 1995). Mortality due to HDV is much higher and ranges from 2 to 20% in some outbreaks. HEV mortality is generally low except for pregnant

women among whom mortality can be as high as 20% (Crowe, 1994), particularly if infection occurs in the third trimester (Benenson, 1995).

The Physical, Psychological, and Social Dimensions

Poor sanitation, inadequate plumbing, and overcrowding are physical dimension conditions that contribute to the incidence of both hepatitis A and E, which involve fecal–oral transmission. Travel to developing countries where HAV and HEV are endemic also increases one's risk of disease. Factors in the psychological dimension that contribute to intravenous drug use may also lead to infection with HBV, HCV, and HDV. Within the social dimension, institutional care and enrollment in day care have been associated with hepatitis A infection, and social factors that contribute to drug abuse also influence the incidence of parenterally transmitted forms of hepatitis.

Occupation is another aspect of the social dimension that can influence one's risk of developing hepatitis. Because of the potential for sexual transmission of HBV, HCV, and HDV, prostitutes are extermely high risk for infection. Other occupational groups at risk for hepatitis include health care providers and military personnel. Military personnel may be at increased risk for HAV with overseas assignments in developing countries. Health care providers are at risk for most forms of hepatitis. With HBV, HCV, and HDV the risk comes primarily from potential for needle sticks and other exposures to bloodborne pathogens, with HBV being the most common exposure reported. In fact, occupational exposure to HBV accounts for approximately 12,000 cases annually (Smith Kline Beecham, 1995b). The seroconversion rate following needle-stick injuries is approximately 6% (Hepatitis Bureau, 1997c). Providers are also at risk for hepatitis A and C. One study indicated that increased hepatitis A incidence was associated with 12-hour shifts. The explanation given was the increased propensity for eating on the unit during a longer shift (Mosley, 1993). Other occupational groups at risk for hepatitis include staff caring for mentally disabled clients and clients receiving dialysis, law-enforcement and correctional facilities personnel, and laboratory personnel. Environmental factors in each of these three dimensions contribute to geographic differences in the incidence of hepatitis A and B as seen in Figures 30–5 and 30–6, respectively.

The Behavioral Dimension

Poor personal hygiene, particularly lack of handwashing after toileting, is a lifestyle factor associated with both hepatitis A and E. Consumption of unwashed foods and contaminated shellfish or water is also a

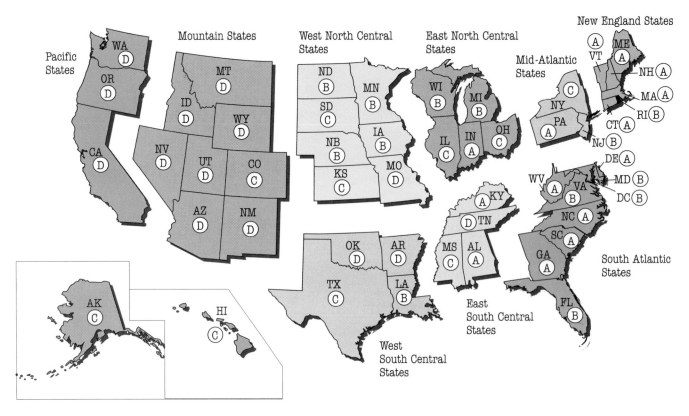

Figure 30–5. Incidence of hepatitis A per 100,000 population, by state, 1995. A = 0–3.26 cases per 100,000 population; B = 3.27–4.74 cases per 100,000 population; C = 4.75–17.24 cases per 100,000 population; D = >17.25 cases per 100,000 population. (Source: Centers for Disease Control, 1996.)

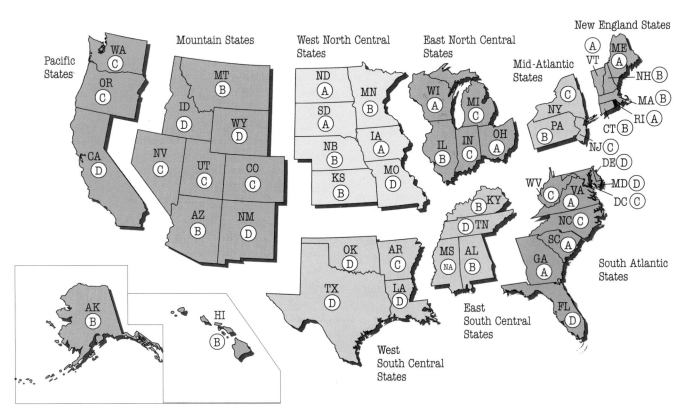

Figure 30–6. Incidence of hepatitis B per 100,000 population, by state, 1995. A = 0–1.78 cases per 100,000 population; B = 1.79–2.89 cases per 100,000 population; C = 2.90–4.69 cases per 100,000 population; D = >4.70 cases per 100,000 population. (Source: Centers for Disease Control, 1996.)

risk factor in these diseases. Anogenital intercourse has also been shown to be associated with HAV transmission, probably because of the fecal–oral nature of the disease (Smith Kline Beecham, 1995a). Injection drug use is highly correlated with infection with HBV, HCV, and HDV. Sexual activity has also been associated with all forms of viral hepatitis except HEV (Benenson, 1995; Kao, et al., 1996).

The Health System Dimension

Health system factors also contribute to the incidence of hepatitis, particularly hepatitis B and C. For HBV, failure to mount effective motivational campaigns to foster immunization has led to a large reservoir of susceptible individuals. Similarly, reluctance of employers to provide immunizations to health care providers at risk for infection has contributed to increased incidence. Lack of routine screening of pregnant women for HBV has also led to increased disease in neonates. Although transmission via blood transfusion is now rare, persons receiving clotting factor concentrate have developed both hepatitis A and C, sometimes in conjunction with home infusion by family members (Hematologic Diseases Bureau, 1996; 1997). On occasion, hepatitis B and C have been transmitted to patients during invasive procedures (Esteban, et al., 1996; Harpaz, et al., 1996). Hepatitis C transmission has also been associated with administration of some brands of intravenous immunoglobulin (Bresee, et al., 1996). Finally there have been several accounts of hepatitis infection transmitted by contaminated medical equipment such as finger-stick devices (Division of Cancer Prevention and Control, 1997). Health system factors, as well as other factors contributing to morbidity and mortality related to hepatitis, are summarized in Table 30–12.

Diagnostic Reasoning and Care of Clients with Hepatitis

Nursing diagnoses related to hepatitis in the individual may reflect either the potential for infection or health problems associated with acute or chronic hepatitis. Typical nursing diagnoses are "potential for exposure to hepatitis B due to injection drug use" and "nausea and vomiting due to inability to digest fatty foods." Nursing diagnoses for population groups might reflect increased incidence of viral hepatitis or the existence of conditions contributing to infection. Examples of community nursing diagnoses are "increased incidence of hepatitis B due to unprotected sexual intercourse among adolescents" and "potential for outbreak of hepatitis A due to broken sewer lines following earthquake."

TABLE 30–12. EPIDEMIOLOGIC FACTORS IN HEPATITIS

BIOPHYSICAL DIMENSION
- Hepatitis A severity increases with age.
- Children often have asymptomatic hepatitis A.
- Hepatitis B is generally mild in children.
- Neonates with hepatitis B often develop persistent chronic infection and later cirrhosis or liver cancer.
- Adolescents are at high risk for hepatitis B due to risk behaviors.
- Hepatitis D infection is usually severe in children.
- Hepatitis E occurs most often in young adults.
- Native Americans are at higher risk for hepatitis A than other ethnic groups.
- Hepatitis B is endemic in Alaskan Natives.
- Hepatitis C is seen more often among Japanese than other groups.
- Conditions requiring transfusion increase risk of hepatitis B, C, and D, especially in developing countries.
- Pregnancy may result in hepatitis B infection in the infant.
- Pregnancy increases mortality risk in hepatitis E.
- Hemodialysis and immunosuppression increase one's risk of hepatitis B and C.
- Chronic hepatitis occurs with hepatitis B, C, and occasionally D.
- Hepatitis D is more likely than the other forms to result in fulminant hepatitis.

PSYCHOLOGICAL DIMENSION
- Poor self-esteem may lead to sexual activity or substance abuse resulting in increased risk for hepatitis A, B, C, and D.

PHYSICAL DIMENSION
- Poor sanitation and crowding increase risk for hepatitis A and E.
- Contaminated water supplies transmit hepatitis A and E infection.

SOCIAL DIMENSION
- Institutional care and day care are associated with hepatitis A transmission.
- Lack of mandate for hepatitis B immunization in most states hampers control.
- Prostitutes are at increased risk for hepatitis B, C, and D, and health care workers are at increased risk for all forms of viral hepatitis.

BEHAVIORAL DIMENSION
- Poor personal hygiene and lack of handwashing contribute to hepatitis A and E.
- Consumption of contaminated shellfish, food, and water increases the risk of hepatitis A.
- Anogenital intercourse increases risk for hepatitis A and B.
- Unprotected sexual intercourse contributes to hepatitis B, C, and D, and occasionally A.
- Injection drug use contributes to hepatitis B, C, and D.

HEALTH SYSTEM DIMENSION
- Failure to promote immunization for hepatitis B contributes to incidence of both hepatitis B and D.
- Reluctance of employers to immunize health care workers against hepatitis B has contributed to disease.
- Lack of hepatitis B screening for pregnant women has contributed to neonatal infection.
- Contaminated medical equipment has been implicated in hepatitis B transmission.
- Infected health care providers have transmitted hepatitis B and C to clients.

Planning and Implementing the Dimensions of Health Care for Hepatitis

Primary, secondary, and tertiary prevention measures may be planned to control the incidence and consequences of hepatitis.

Primary Prevention

Primary prevention of hepatitis focuses on immunization or chemoprophylaxis when available and control measures related to the modes of disease transmission.

Immunization and Chemoprophylaxis. Immunization is currently available only for hepatitis A and B. Hepatitis B immunization is recommended for all infants (including premature infants), health care workers, persons on hemodialysis, immunosuppressed clients, injection drug users, and any others who engage in high-risk behaviors including adolescents as well as adults. Exposed infants should also be given hepatitis B immunoglobulin (HBIG) (Benenson, 1995). Hepatitis A immunization is suggested for travelers to endemic areas, military personnel, children in communities with periodic outbreaks, IDUs, men engaging in homosexual activity, persons working with nonhuman primates, laboratory personnel, food handlers in high-prevalence areas, and persons with chronic liver disease or clotting disorders (Shapiro, et al., 1996).

Preexposure chemoprophylaxis for HAV is recommended for international travel to developing countries. Chemoprophylaxis with immunoglobulin, in conjunction with hepatitis A vaccine, may be warranted for travelers who live in or visit rural areas, eat or drink in areas with poor sanitation, or engage in close contact with persons (especially children) in areas with poor sanitation (Atkinson, 1997).

Primary prevention of hepatitis A can also involve prophylaxis following exposure to HAV. Immunoglobulin should be given within 2 weeks of exposure. Prophylaxis can also be given to household and sexual contacts of cases, day care staff and children exposed to the disease, and staff and residents of institutions for the developmentally disabled. Routine prophylaxis is no longer recommended for health care personnel or persons exposed at work (Benenson, 1995).

Chemoprophylaxis with hepatitis B immunoglobulin (HBIG) is also used following potential exposures to HBV in sexual and household contacts of acute cases, neonates born to infected mothers, exposed health care workers, homosexual men, high-risk populations (eg, Alaskan Natives), and travelers who will be spending more than 6 months in endemic areas. HBIG is accompanied by a three-dose series of hepatitis B vaccine (Benenson, 1995). Prevention of hepatitis B also prevents HDV infection. Community health nurses are frequently involved in identifying contacts of those with hepatitis and in educating them regarding the need for prophylaxis. Nurses may then either plan to refer contacts to appropriate health care services or administer chemoprophylaxis directly under appropriate protocols.

Other Control Measures. Other primary preventive measures for hepatitis are dependent on interrupting the mode of transmission of a particular virus. For hepatitis A and E, control measures are aimed at improving sanitation, protecting food and water from contamination, and promoting adequate handwashing. Washing fruits and vegetables before eating, boiling contaminated water, and discouraging use of human waste as fertilizer may also serve to prevent both diseases in developing countries.

Primary prevention for hepatitis B, C, and D involves screening blood donors for disease, educating drug users regarding the risks of needle sharing, and the use of universal precautions for blood and body fluids by health care workers and other occupational groups that may experience blood exposures (eg, firefighters, law enforcement, emergency personnel).

Secondary Prevention

Secondary preventive measures for hepatitis include diagnostic and treatment measures. Diagnosis of most forms of viral hepatitis depends on the presence of identifiable antibodies to the viruses involved. In hepatitis A, during and shortly after symptom manifestation, clients exhibit elevated serum immunoglobulin M (IgM) anti-HAV antibody, which is replaced by elevations in IgG anti-HAV antibody levels during and after convalescence. Elevated serum hepatitis B surface antigen levels late in the incubation period and afterward are diagnostic for HBV. In addition, high levels of HBe antigen indicate greater communicability of disease. Diagnosis may also be made on the basis of antibody to core or surface HBV (anti-HBc or anti-HBs) antigens. Anti-HCV antibody is found in chronic infection with HCV, but may be difficult to detect early in the disease process. Polymerase chain reaction (PCR) for HCV RNA may be used in clients with negative anti-HCV antibody tests and symptomatic disease. Viral antigen tests are also used to diagnose HDV (eg, anti-HDV). Although antibody tests have been developed for HEV, they are not widely available in the United States, and diagnosis is based primarily on clinical features and negative tests for other forms of hepatitis (Benenson, 1995).

In recent years, antiviral therapy has been shown to be somewhat effective in treating both hepatitis B and C infection. Interferon alfa has been used with moderate results in chronic forms of both diseases (Crowe, 1994; Niederau, et al., 1996; Poynard, et al., 1995). In HBV, interferon alfa is successful in approximately 40% of cases of chronic infection. Some clients who have not responded to interferon have obtained favorable results with lamivudine (Dienstag, Perrillo, Schiff, Bartholomew, Vicary, & Rubin, 1995). The effectiveness of interferon alfa in chronic HCV is approximately 25% (Benenson, 1995). Ribavirin has been used with poor results in the treatment of chronic HCV infection (Di Bisceglie, et al., 1995). Neither acyclovir nor corticosteroids have been shown to have any effect in treating HCV (Benenson, 1995). Additional treatment for hepatitis B and C, as well as other forms of viral hepatitis, includes adequate diet and rest and treatment of symptoms such as pruritis and nausea.

Tertiary Prevention

Tertiary prevention of hepatitis reinfection in individual clients is generally unnecessary, because antibodies developed confer immunity after infection with a specific virus. Immunity to one virus does not, however, confer immunity to other hepatitis viruses. Tertiary preventive efforts are geared toward preventing complications of disease and preventing infection of others. Changes in drug use and sexual behaviors (eg, using condoms) and use of universal precautions can prevent the spread of hepatitis B, C, and D, whereas handwashing, improved sanitation, and other similar measures can prevent transmission of hepatitis A and E. Refraining from drinking alcohol is one way of preventing complications of hepatitis whatever the causative agent. Primary, secondary, and tertiary prevention strategies for hepatitis are summarized in Table 30–13.

Evaluating Control Strategies for Hepatitis

Evaluating control strategies for hepatitis involves monitoring the incidence and prevalence of disease in the population. Other indicators of successful control include declining mortality figures for these diseases. National objectives for the year 2000 can also be used to evaluate the effectiveness of efforts to prevent hepatitis. The status of selected national objectives related to hepatitis A, B, and C is presented in Table 30–14. The current set of national health objectives do not address either hepatitis D or E.

Other Sexually Transmitted Diseases

Several other diseases are also transmitted via sexual intercourse. This section examines trends, epidemiologic factors, nursing diagnoses, control strategies, and evaluation related to syphilis, gonorrhea, herpes simplex virus (HSV) infection, and chlamydia. Epidemiologic and treatment information about each of these diseases is summarized in Appendix S.

Trends in Sexually Transmitted Diseases

Overall, the incidence of most sexually transmitted diseases (STDs) has risen in recent years. Because of the sometimes devastating consequences of these diseases (eg, blindness in infants exposed to syphilis, gonorrhea, or herpes), their increasing incidence is of concern to community health practitioners and the general public. Evidence of this concern can be seen in the fact that 15 of the national health objectives for the

---

TABLE 30–13. PRIMARY, SECONDARY, AND TERTIARY PREVENTION MEASURES TO CONTROL HEPATITIS

Level of Prevention	Community Health Nurse Function	Goal
Primary prevention	• Monitor community sanitation. • Monitor food and water supplies. • Discourage use of human waste as fertilizer. • Educate clients and public. • Notify contacts and refer for chemoprophylaxis. • Refer drug users for treatment. • Educate drug users on "safe shooting" practices. • Engage in political activity. • Encourage immunization with hepatitis A and B vaccines.	• Prevent spread of disease. • Ensure safe food and water supplies. • Prevent contamination of food and water supplies. • Increase handwashing and hygiene to prevent the spread of infection. • Provide prophylactic treatment for contacts. • Decrease drug use and potential for exposure. • Decrease needle sharing. • Ensure adequate sanitation and safe food and water supplies. • Promote immunity to disease.
Secondary prevention	• Educate clients about relief of symptoms. • Refer for diagnosis and treatment as needed.	• Relieve symptoms. • Effective treatment of disease.
Tertiary prevention	• Educate infected persons to prevent spread to others. • Interview individuals and notify contacts. • Educate clients about alcohol effects on inflamed liver.	• Change behavior to prevent the spread of infection. • Provide chemoprophylaxis for exposed persons. • Prevent complications.

TABLE 30–14. STATUS OF SELECTED NATIONAL OBJECTIVES FOR HEPATITIS

	Objective	Base	Most Recent	Target
19.7	Reduce the number of cases of sexually transmitted hepatitis B	47,593 (1987)	58,393 (1991)	30,500
20.3	Reduce incidence per 100,000 population for			
	a. Hepatitis A	33 (1987)	12.13 (1995)	16
	b. Hepatitis B	63.5 (1987)	4.19 (1995)	40
	c. Hepatitis C	18.3 (1987)	1.78 (1995)	13.7
20.11	Increase hepatitis B immunization among			
	a. Infants of antigen-positive mothers	40% (1987)	78% (1994)	90%
	b. Occupationally exposed workers	37% (1989)	67% (1994)	90%

(Sources: Centers for Disease Control, 1996; U. S. Department of Health and Human Services, 1993; 1995a; 1996.)

year 2000 are specifically related to sexually transmitted diseases other than AIDS (U.S. Department of Health and Human Services, 1991).

Syphilis.   Through the use of antibiotics and the contact notification strategies discussed earlier, the incidence of syphilis seemed to be well controlled for several years. In the late 1980s and early 1990s, however, there was an increase in both early syphilis among adults and congenital syphilis in young children. In 1990, for example, the incidence of primary and secondary syphilis was the highest it has been since the advent of antibiotics (20.3 per 100,000 population) (Epidemiology and Surveillance Bureau, 1996). In 1990, approximately 110 of every 100,000 infants in the United States had congenital syphilis (Centers for Disease Control, 1993). By 1995, the incidence of primary and secondary syphilis had declined to 6.3 per 100,000 population, and the incidence of congenital syphilis had dropped to 39 cases per 100,000 live births (National Center for HIV, STD, and TB Prevention, 1996b).

Gonorrhea.   Adequate treatment for gonorrhea has been available since the 1940s, and incidence rates decreased 65% from 1975 to 1993 (Epidemiology Research Bureau, 1995). Nevertheless, attempts to control gonorrhea have not been as successful as attempts to control syphilis and incidence remains high. Approximately 700 million cases of gonorrhea occur worldwide each year (Castro, Sara, & Wyrwinski, 1997). Gonorrhea incidence in the United States was 149.5 cases per 100,000 population in 1995 (Centers for Disease Control, 1996). This translates to more than 392,000 cases of disease (National Center for HIV, STD, and TB Prevention, 1996b).

Further complicating the situation, the incidence of antibiotic-resistant strains of *Neisseria gonorrhoeae*, the causative organism in gonorrhea, has risen steadily in the last few years. Most antibiotic resistance is related to penicillinase-producing *N. gonorrhoeae* (PPNG); however, other strains such as chromosomally mediated resistant *N. gonorrhoeae* (CMRNG) and tetracycline-resistant *N. gonorrhoeae* (TRNG) have been reported. CMRNG is resistant not only to penicillin therapy, but also to treatment with tetracycline, spectinomycin, cephalosporin, and, more recently, the fluoroquinolones. In 1995, nearly one third of gonococcal isolates tested were resistant to one or more antibiotics (National Center for HIV, STD, and TB Prevention, 1996b).

Herpes Simplex Virus Infection.   Unlike the STDs discussed so far, reporting of herpes simplex virus (HSV) infection, or genital herpes, is not required by law. Consequently, precise incidence figures are not available. HSV infection is caused by one of two distinct strains of the virus, HSV-1 or HSV-2. In the past, HSV-1 was most often associated with herpes stomatitis and subsequent "cold sores," whereas HSV-2 infection was primarily genital in nature. Today, although HSV-2 is still the causative agent in most cases of genital herpes, either type may be involved. An estimated 50 to 90% of U.S. adults have circulating HSV-1 antibodies (prevalence increases with declining socioeconomic status), whereas 20% of people over age 15 have experienced HSV-2 infection (Wald, Zeh, Barnum, Davis, & Corey, 1996). This amounts to 55 million people, up to 25% of whom may be unaware of infection (Sacks, Aoki, Diaz-Mitoma, Sellors, & Shafran, 1996).

Chlamydia.   Chlamydia, caused by infection with the organism *Chlamydia* trachomatis, is the most prevalent of all STDs, with a possible incidence of 4 million cases annually (Surveillance and Information Systems Bureau, 1994). From 1987 to 1995, the incidence of chlamydia infection increased 281%, and 5 to 15% of sexually active adolescents are infected (Division of Sexually Transmitted Disease Prevention, 1997a; 1997b). An additional 7 to 20% of pregnant women are also affected (Anderson, 1995). In 1995, there were 182.2 cases of chlamydia per 100,000 population in the United States (Centers for Disease Control, 1996).

 ## Assessing the Dimensions of Health in Sexually Transmitted Diseases

Factors in the biophysical, psychological, social, behavioral, and health system dimensions contribute to the growing problem of STDs.

The Biophysical Dimension

Biophysical dimension factors to be assessed in relation to STDs are age, race, sex, and physiologic function.

Age. The incidence of all STDs is higher among adolescents and young adults than in other age groups. This is primarily a function of lifestyle factors rather than biological susceptibility because of one's age. Infants are, however, more susceptible to the effects of STD exposure, particularly in utero or during birth.

Women of childbearing age constitute the majority of women with syphilis, increasing the potential for congenital syphilis in babies born to these women. Syphilis contracted early in pregnancy results in fetal demise in up to 40% of cases if untreated. Untreated maternal infection in the 4 years prior to pregnancy causes congenital syphilis in 70% of infants (National Center for HIV, STD, and TB Prevention, 1996b). Congenital syphilis may result in fetal death, blindness, mental retardation, or cardiovascular disease. There is also an increased incidence of syphilis among the elderly in some areas.

Children exposed to other STDs are also at higher risk of complications than are adults. Infants exposed to gonorrhea during passage through the birth canal, for example, may develop a gonorrheal conjunctivitis called ophthalmia neonatorum. In addition, as many as 400 to 1000 babies with neonatal HSV infection are born each year in the United States. Transmission of HSV infection to infants rarely occurs transplacentally, but is usually due to perinatal exposure as the infant passes through the birth canal of an infected mother (Benenson, 1995). HSV-infected infants have a high incidence of visceral and central nervous system complications.

As many as 20% of pregnant women may have chlamydia, placing their infants at risk for neonatal conjunctivitis and chlamydial pneumonia (Division of Sexually Transmitted Disease Prevention, 1997b). As is true with gonorrhea, exposure to chlamydia occurs during passage through the birth canal. Approximately two thirds of infants exposed in this manner become infected. Even with chemoprophylaxis, 15 to 25% of infected infants develop conjunctivitis, compared with 50 to 75% without prophylactic treatment (Berman, et al., 1993). Occurrence of STDs in children beyond the neonatal period is a potential indication of sexual abuse (Anderson, 1995).

Community health nurses should assess both the extent of these pediatric effects of STDs in the community and the factors contributing to them. The extent of disease in other age groups should also be assessed.

Sex. Sex also plays a part in the incidence and effects of some STDs, and the nurse assessing the potential for cases of STDs in the community determines the community's sex composition and the relative incidence of STDs in males and females in the community. For example, chlamydia is more often diagnosed in women than in men, primarily because men are not routinely screened for chlamydial infection (National Center for HIV, STD, and TB Prevention, 1996b). Risk of chlamydial infection, however, appears to be similar for male-to-female and female-to-male transmission (Quinn, et al., 1996). In addition, women are more likely to experience complications of chlamydial infection than men. For example, chlamydia is believed to contribute to infertility in 20% of women infected (Johnson, Grun, & Haines, 1996), but only rarely in men (Tagg, 1996).

Males and females may also differ somewhat in the symptoms associated with STDs. Males with gonorrhea, for example, may experience a penile discharge with burning on urination, whereas females may have an increased vaginal discharge that may have a foul odor. In addition, females are more likely than males to be asymptomatic with gonococcal infection, creating a large reservoir of untreated persons capable of spreading disease. Both men and women are frequently asymptomatic in chlamydial infection (Tagg, 1996).

Race. Generally speaking, in the United States, members of various minority groups have higher incidence rates for STD diagnoses than whites. This is primarily a function of socioeconomic factors rather than innate racial susceptibility, making racial or ethnic group membership a marker for STDs rather than a risk factor (National Center for HIV, STD, and TB Prevention, 1996b).

Physiologic Function. Physiologic factors also influence the incidence and course of several STDs, and the community health nurse assesses for the presence of specific factors in an individual client as well as their prevalence in the community in assessing the risk of STDs. As noted earlier, the presence of syphilitic lesions facilitates HIV transmission (Kilmarx & St. Louis, 1995). Concurrent HIV infection influences the diagnosis, treatment, and consequences of syphilis. The presence of HIV infection may cause false-negative results on screening and confirmatory tests for syphilis. HIV-infected individuals also have a greater risk of developing neurosyphilis (deterioration of the central nervous system in the late stages of syphilis). In addition, treatment for syphilis may be less effective when HIV infection is present (Yinnon, Coury-Doniger, Polito, & Reichman, 1996). In men, lack of circumcision is a physiologic factor that has been linked to syphilis, as well as to gonorrhea and herpetic infection (Cook, Koutsky, & Holmes, 1994). Gonorrhea and chlamydia also facilitate HIV transmission (National Center for HIV, STD, and TB Prevention, 1996b).

In terms of the physiologic consequences of STDS, gonorrheal infection has been associated with later prostatitis in men and with pelvic inflammatory disease (PID) and tubal pregnancy in women. The risk of ectopic pregnancy increases with each episode of chlamydia (Hillis, Owens, Marchbanks, Amsterdam, & MacKenzie, 1997). Chlamydia is responsible for significant epididymitis in men and is the causative agent in 5 to 50% of cases of PID in women. Approximately 17% of women treated for PID will have later fertility problems with increased risk of tubal pregnancy. Chronic pelvic pain is another possible outcome of chlamydial infection in women (Berman, et al., 1993).

Chlamydia is suspected as the causative agent in 25 to 70% of cases of nongonococcal urethritis (NGU) (Greendale, Haas, Holbrook, Walsh, Schacter, & Phillips, 1993) and epididymitis, and is implicated as well in the development of PID, ectopic pregnancy and infertility, increased perinatal mortality, postpartum endometritis, ophthalmia neonatorum, and pneumonia in the neonate. It is estimated that direct and indirect costs of chlamydial infection amount to $2 billion a year (Division of Sexually Transmitted Disease Prevention, 1997b).

Absence of symptoms is a relatively common feature of HSV, chlamydial, and gonococcal infection, contributing to the spread of infection by those who do not realize they are infected. Approximately 25% of men and 75% of women with chlamydial infection are asymptomatic (Benenson, 1995; Tagg, 1996).

The Psychological Dimension

The psychological dimension contributes to the incidence of STDs to the extent that it creates an emo-

tional climate conductive to exposure to infection, usually through sexual activity or injection drug use. Individuals with low self-esteem or poor interpersonal skills may use sexual activity as a means of interacting with others. In a similar vein, those with poor coping skills or those confronting feelings of hopelessness may turn to illicit drug use as an escape.

Among teenagers, the sense of invulnerability characteristic of this age group may lead to experimentation with sex or drugs in the belief that adverse consequences are unlikely. In addition, the need for peer acceptance and for conformity to peer group norms may lead the adolescent to engage in sexual activity or drug use in an effort to be accepted by peers.

The Social Dimension

One of the major social factors to be assessed relative to the incidence of STDs is the prevalence of the disease in the community. In areas where the incidence of disease is high, large reservoirs of infected individuals increase the risk of exposure to disease. Generally speaking, the incidence of STDs is higher in urban than in rural areas. Variations in incidence rates for gonorrhea by state for 1995 are depicted in Figure 30–7. Incidence of syphilis and chlamydia also vary from place to place. State-by-state variations in annual incidence rates for syphilis and chlamydia are shown in Figures 30–8 and 30–9, respectively.

Incidence rates for gonorrhea and syphilis also seem to rise during the summer and at certain holidays (particularly Labor Day and Memorial Day). It is unclear whether this increase is due to increased sexual activity at these times or because antibiotics used to treat wintertime infections may also treat incubating gonorrhea and syphilis, thus reducing their incidence during the winter months.

Other social environmental factors that contribute to STDs include poverty, lack of access to health care, and social attitudes condoning behaviors that foster exposure to these diseases. For example, higher incidence rates for congenital syphilis among African Americans may be a function of lack of prenatal care and associated opportunities for early diagnosis and treatment of pregnant women with syphilis. Similar factors may be operating in outbreaks of syphilis among Native Americans.

Changes in behavioral norms in the society at large, with greater acceptance of sexual activity outside of marriage, have led to increases in sexual activity and subsequent increases in the incidence of STDs. At the same time, social constraints on discussing

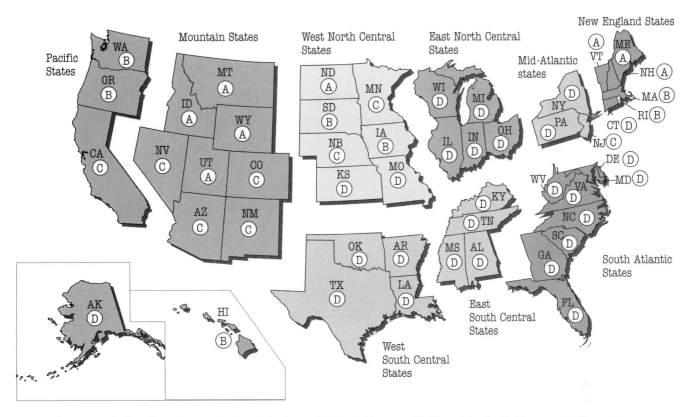

Figure 30–7. Incidence of gonorrhea per 100,000 population, by state, 1995. A = 0–16 cases per 100,000 population; B = 17–61 cases per 100,000 population; C = 62–100 cases per 100,000 population; D = >100 cases per 100,000 population. (Source: Centers for Disease Control, 1996.)

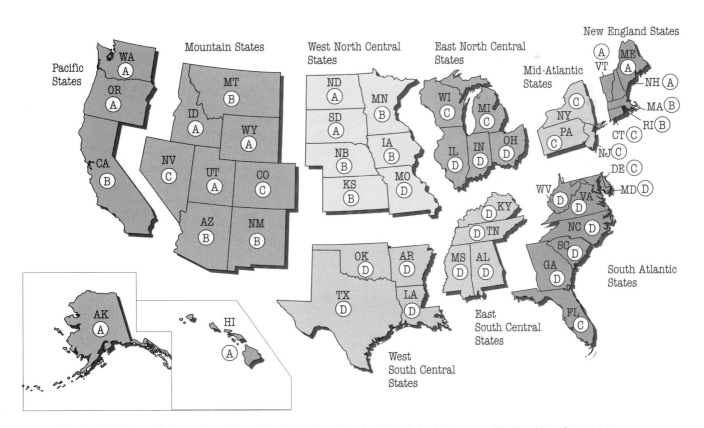

Figure 30–8. Incidence of primary and secondary syphilis per 100,000 population, by state, 1995. A = 0–0.3 cases per 100,000 population; B = 0.4–2.0 cases per 100,000 population; C = 2.1–4.0 cases per 100,000 population; D = > 4.0 cases per 100,000 population. (Source: Centers for Disease Control, 1996.)

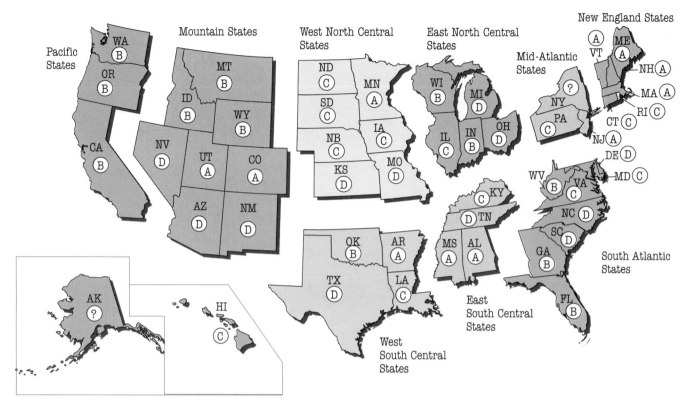

Figure 30–9. Incidence of reported chlamydia per 100,000 women, by state, 1995. A = 0–199.9 per cases per 100,000 women; B = 200–279.9 cases per 100,000 women; C = 280–339.9 cases per 100,000 women; D = > 340 cases per 100,000 women. (Source: Centers for Disease Control, 1996.)

sexuality have limited the ability of public health officials and school personnel to provide sex education to young people at high-risk for STDs.

Media presentations of sexual activity as desirable behavior have also contributed to the incidence of STDs. Portrayals of popular heroes and heroines as "sexy" and sexually active have fostered imitative behavior, particularly among adolescents.

The Behavioral Dimension

Behavioral factors to be assessed by the nurse in determining the risk of STDs in the community or for the individual client include sexual activity and injection drug use.

Sexual Activity. The primary behavioral factor associated with STDs is, of course, sexual activity itself. Increased sexual activity, failure to use protective devices, and male homosexual activity are some of the specific factors that contribute to STDs.

As noted earlier, changes in social mores have led to increased sexual activity by large numbers of Americans. Increased sexual activity, particularly with multiple partners, increases one's risk of expo-

sure to STDs (Quinn, et al., 1996). Widespread use of oral contraceptives over the last few decades led to more sexual activity among women as fear of pregnancy diminished. Another effect of increased use of oral contraceptives is a concomitant decline in the use of barrier methods of contraception that also provided protection against STDs.

Male homosexual activity has also been associated with increased incidence of some STDs. Both gonorrhea and syphilis have been more prevalent among homosexual men than among the general population. The incidence of both these diseases declined in the 1980s during the first wave of the AIDS epidemic, but may be on the increase due to reinstitution of high-risk behavior such as anogenital intercourse (Gonorrhea, Chlamydia and Chancroid Bureau, 1997). Male homosexuals are more likely to develop chlamydial proctitis or proctocolitis than other forms of the disease (Berman, et al., 1993).

Injection Drug Use. Injection drug use is a lifestyle factor implicated in the development of syphilis. Drug-related prostitution is another lifestyle factor that increases the incidence of STDs. Some drug users, particularly those who use crack cocaine, trade sex directly for drugs or engage in prostitution to obtain money to support their drug habits (Epidemiology and Surveillance Bureau, 1996; Gourevitch, et al., 1996).

The Health System Dimension

Health care system factors have also contributed to the rise of STDs. Health care system factors that influence the occurrence of STDs include lack of adequate attention to the problem on the part of many health care providers, failure of health care providers to educate individuals and the general public about STDs, inappropriate use of antibiotics, and failure to provide diagnostic and treatment facilities. Community health nurses assess the extent to which factors in each of these areas contribute to problems related to STDs in the community.

Unless clients specifically request services for signs and symptoms that may be related to STDs, many health care providers do not address sexuality issues with their clients. Despite recommendations for obtaining a sexual history on all adolescent and adult clients, few primary care providers regularly do so. Health care providers have also failed to routinely screen clients at risk for STDs (Division of Sexually Transmitted Disease Prevention, 1997a).

Health care providers often use antibiotics inappropriately both in treating STDs and in treating other conditions. For example, a sizable proportion of primary care providers do not prescribe the appropriate drugs for treating STDs. In addition, many providers fail to recognize the fact that clients with one STD may have been exposed to others and thus fail to provide treatment with broad-spectrum antimicrobial agents that treat both incubating and symptomatic disease. Finally, health care professionals may prescribe antibiotics inappropriately for other conditions (eg, a viral respiratory infection). If the client is exposed to a STD, the amount of antibiotic prescribed may not be sufficient to treat the STD, but may present the infecting organism with an opportunity to develop resistance to the antibiotic, creating antibiotic-resistant strains of microorganisms.

Failure to provide adequate preventive, diagnostic, and treatment services to clients with STDs is another way in which the health care system has contributed to the rising incidence of these diseases. Lack of affordable prenatal care for pregnant women at risk for STDs, for example, has added to an increased incidence of gonorrhea, syphilis, and HSV infection in newborns. In addition, concern for the rising incidence of AIDS has led to diversion of funds

from control programs for other STDs and has resulted in a shortage of diagnostic and treatment services for these diseases.

Factors related to the biophysical, psychological, social, behavioral, and the health system dimensions influence the development of STDs in communities and in individual clients. Factors in each of these areas are summarized in Table 30–15.

TABLE 30–15. EPIDEMIOLOGIC FACTORS IN OTHER SEXUALLY TRANSMITTED DISEASES

BIOPHYSICAL DIMENSION

Genetic inheritance	• Increased incidence of syphilis in women of childbearing age leads to increased congenital syphilis. • More women than men are asymptomatic for gonorrhea. • More women than men are diagnosed with chlamydia.
Maturation and aging	• Incidence of STDs is highest among adolescents and young adults. • Infants in utero are at risk for infection with syphilis and chlamydia. • Infants are at risk of ophthalmia neonatorum due to gonorrhea and chlamydia infection.
Physiologic function	• Concurrent HIV infection may invalidate tests for syphilis. • Syphilitic, gonorrheal, and chlamydial infections are associated with HIV risk. • Passage through birth canal may infect infant with HSV, gonorrhea, or chlamydia. • Presence of one STD increases potential for others.

PSYCHOLOGICAL DIMENSION

• Psychological factors that lead to increased sexual activity increase risk of exposure.
• Psychological factors that contribute to drug use increase risk of exposure to syphilis and hepatitis B.

SOCIAL DIMENSION

• Incidence of STDs is higher in large urban areas.
• Changes in social norms and increased use of contraceptives have led to greater sexual activity and risk of exposure.
• Media presentations of sexual activity as desirable have led to increases in risk behaviors.
• Peer pressure for injection drug use increases the risk of exposure to syphilis.

BEHAVIORAL DIMENSION

• Sexual activity with multiple partners increases risk of infection.
• Homosexual activity increases risk of exposure to some STDs.
• Failure to use condoms or other barrier methods increases risk of exposure to STDs.
• Injection drug use and needle sharing increase risk of exposure to syphilis.

HEALTH SYSTEM DIMENSION

• Failure to educate public regarding STDs impedes control.
• Inappropriate use of antibiotics leads to ineffective control of STDs.
• Reduced funding impedes adequate control of STDs.
• Lack of access to prenatal care contributes to congenital infections.

Diagnostic Reasoning and Care of Clients with Sexually Transmitted Diseases

Nursing diagnoses related to other STDs, like those for HIV infection or infection with hepatitis B, C, or D, may be related to individual clients or population groups. Examples of diagnoses for the individual are "potential for exposure to syphilis due to intravenous drug use and needle sharing" and "pain on urination due to gonococcal urethritis." At the group level, nursing diagnoses might reflect an "increased incidence of chlamydia in adolescent girls due to sexual activity with multiple partners" or "potential for increased incidence of congenital syphilis due to lack of prenatal care for women in high-risk groups."

Planning and Implementing the Dimensions of Health Care for Sexually Transmitted Diseases

Planning control strategies for STDs may occur at the primary, secondary, or tertiary levels of prevention.

Primary Prevention

Primary prevention strategies for STDs consist of prophylaxis and other general prevention measures. No immunizations are currently available for STD prevention; however, a vaccine against chlamydia has been shown to be effective in mice (Whittum-Hudson, An, Saltzman, Prendergast, & MacDonald, 1996).

Chemoprophylaxis. Prophylactic treatment of those exposed to an STD can prevent not only the spread of STDs to others but also development in the exposed individual. Prophylaxis is available for several STDs including syphilis, gonorrhea, and chlamydia. Community health nurses can notify contacts who are candidates for chemoprophylaxis of their exposure to one of these diseases and inform them of the availability of prophylactic treatment. Community health nurses might refer clients to other sources of prophylactic services or provide prophylactic treatment themselves on the basis of medically approved protocols. In either case, the nurse educates the client about the medications used, how to take them, and potential side effects.

Prophylactic treatment of those exposed to syphilis is usually accomplished with a long-acting form of penicillin in a dose similar to that used for treatment of confirmed cases of early syphilis. Early treatment of pregnant women with syphilis is also prophylactic for congenital syphilis in the infant.

Prophylaxis is also available for ophthalmia neonatorum due to gonorrhea or chlamydia in the newborn. Prophylaxis for gonorrhea is accomplished with the instillation of a 1% silver nitrate solution or tetracycline or erythromycin ointment in both eyes immediately after birth. Prevention of ophthalmia neonatorum due to chlamydia involves the application of erythromycin ointment in the eyes of the newborn immediately after delivery. Tetracycline can also be an effective prophylactic for this condition. Silver nitrate solution has not been found to be effective in preventing chlamydial conjunctivitis in the newborn, and antibiotic ointments are not 100% effective but do prevent most chlamydial conjunctivitis. Treatment of pregnant women who have chlamydial infection provides primary prevention for other forms of the disease in the neonate.

Cesarean section can be performed on pregnant women with active HSV infection at the time of delivery to prevent transmission of infection to the newborn. Another alternative is prophylactic use of acyclovir in infected mothers. This is not routine, however, due to lack of knowledge regarding the effects of acyclovir on the fetus. Community health nurses refer pregnant women with possible HSV infection for appropriate diagnostic and treatment services to prevent infection of their infants.

Other Measures. Several other measures may also be used in the primary prevention of STDs. Primary prevention of all STDs relies heavily on achieving change in high-risk behaviors such as limiting the number of sexual partners (preferably to a monogamous relationship), using barrier forms of contraception such as condoms and spermicides that may also prevent exposure to STDs, and refraining from drug use. Some authors recommend substituting "outercourse" or heavy petting and mutual mastubation without vaginal penetration as an alternative to intercourse among adolescents (Cobb, 1997).

Primary prevention for congenital syphilis, neonatal herpes infection, and ophthalmia neonatorum involves early identification and treatment of pregnant women with early syphilis, HSV infection, gonorrhea, and chlamydia. This may be accomplished by screening pregnant women in the first trimester of pregnancy and again early in the third trimester. It has been suggested that male partners of pregnant women also be screened to identify risk for infection during pregnancy. An alternative approach is to screen women for pregnancy if they have STDs or are sexual contacts of men who have STDs. Pregnant women living in neighborhoods with a high incidence of STDs also can be screened for these conditions as well as referred for prenatal care and treatment if necessary. Women diagnosed as having an STD might also need counseling regarding the risks associated with pregnancy and the need for prenatal care for current or future pregnancies.

Women who are injection drug users are at high risk for pregnancy and syphilis and should be asked about their menstrual history and referred for pregnancy testing as needed. Screening for STDs in family planning clinics and drug treatment centers and among female prisoners can also identify pregnant women for whom treatment would constitute primary prevention of STDs in their babies.

Pregnant women with genital lesions can be tested for HSV infection. Those with positive tests or those who have a history of prior episodes of symptomatic herpes or contact with an infected person can be closely monitored for symptoms near term. If lesions are present at delivery, a cesarean section can be performed.

Community health nurses may also educate and motivate clients to modify lifestyle factors that contribute to STDs. Limiting sexual activity and using condoms are primary preventive measures aimed at the population of sexually active individuals at risk for infection. Limiting needle sharing and treating drug abuse may reduce transmission of STDs in intravenous drug users.

Community health nurses are actively involved in primary prevention of STDs. They are frequently involved in educating the public, particularly young people, regarding the risks of indiscriminate sexual activity and the use of preventive measures such as condoms to reduce the risk of infection.

Nurses also make frequent referrals for prenatal care and follow women throughout their pregnancy. During this prenatal period they can continue to educate clients regarding the risks of STDs and identify women whose babies are at risk for congenital syphilis or other STDs. Women with identified risk factors can then be referred for diagnosis and treatment to prevent disease in their babies.

At the aggregate level, primary prevention of STDs entails the allocation of adequate funds for STD control efforts. Community health nurses can influence policy makers, using the processes described in Chapter 13, to ensure that monies will be made available for education regarding STDs and for prenatal care for women at risk.

Nurses can also campaign for adequate sex education for young people that includes information on the prevention of STDs. In addition, they can educate injection drug users regarding "safe shooting practices" or refer clients desiring assistance with drug abuse problems.

Secondary Prevention

Several strategies are used in secondary prevention of STDs. These include screening, diagnosis, and treatment, each of which is discussed briefly.

Screening. Screening procedures are available for syphilis, gonorrhea, HSV infection, and chlamydia. Community health nurses educate individual clients and the public about the need for and availability of screening for STDs. Areas to be addressed in education programs include groups at high risk for disease who should be screened and the signs and symptoms of these STDs that indicate a need for screening. Information about symptoms of the STDs discussed here is presented in Appendix S. Nurses can also refer clients for screening or actually conduct screening programs. In addition, they explain screening results to those tested and educate them regarding the meaning of the tests. When screening tests are positive, they refer clients for further diagnosis or treatment as needed.

Screening for STDs should be routinely performed on persons seen for STDs, those in family planning clinics who are at risk because of multiple sexual partners, prostitutes, males engaging in homosexual activity, and injection drug users. Screening for selected STDs may also be done on a routine basis for arrestees, hospital admissions in high-risk groups such as young adults or drug users, and persons with identified high-risk behaviors or sexually active persons who live in areas with a high incidence of STDs. Premarital screening for syphilis is required to obtain a marriage license in most states; however, this approach to screening has not been shown to be cost-effective because of the low prevalence of the disease in the general population.

Screening for reactive serology is usually the initial step in identifying persons with syphilis. Screening for syphilis is generally done with a nontreponemal test, such as that developed by the Venereal Disease Research Laboratory (VDRL), or with the Rapid Plasma Reagin test (RPR). These tests are relatively inexpensive and easy to perform. They are not, however, specific for syphilis because they react to a variety of conditions other than syphilis. For example, pregnancy and injection drug use, as well as several diseases, may cause a biological false-positive (BFP) reaction. Positive screening tests are followed by specific diagnostic tests discussed later in this chapter.

Screening for gonorrhea is accomplished by culture of vaginal secretions in women or of urine in men. Vaginal cultures are not foolproof in women, and a negative test should not be interpreted as conclusive evidence of the absence of infection.

Screening for HSV infection using Pap smears, immunoperoxidase tests, immunofluorescence, or enzyme assay has been suggested. The sensitivity of such tests is too low, however, and the yield of positive cases too few to warrant routine screening except in the case of pregnant women at high risk as noted earlier.

Since the advent of reliable nonculture screening tests for *Chlamydia trachomatis,* such as enzyme immunoassays and polymerase chain reaction assay, screening for chlamydia is more feasible. Rapid office screening tests are also available. Screening samples obtained by women at home and mailed for analysis have also been shown to be accurate (Ostergaard, Moller, Andersen, & Olesen, 1996). High-risk groups that should be targeted for screening are pregnant women; women with mucopurulent cervicitis (MPC); sexually active adolescents; women with multiple sexual partners; women who use barrier contraceptives inconsistently; women attending prenatal, family planning, or STD clinics; and female prisoners. Positive screening tests should be confirmed by culture or a second nonculture test (Berman, et al., 1993).

Diagnosis.   Sexually transmitted diseases are diagnosed using a variety of laboratory procedures as well as physical signs and symptoms and history of risk behaviors or actual exposure to disease. Community health nurses might plan to refer clients with suspected STDs for diagnostic evaluation or obtain specimens for diagnostic tests themselves based on medically approved protocols.

Laboratory diagnosis of syphilis is made on the basis of confirmatory treponemal antibody tests such as the Fluorescent Treponemal Antibody (FTA) test and the *Treponema pallidum* Immobilizing (TPI) test or actual identification of treponemes on dark-field examination of material taken from primary or secondary lesions. Diagnosis of gonorrhea and chlamydia may be confirmed through urine, vaginal, or rectal cultures.

Symptomatic HSV infection is diagnosed on the basis of clinical findings and the result of viral cultures of lesions; however, it is estimated that as many as two thirds of infected persons are asymptomatic. The typical lesion in genital herpes is vesicular in nature and very painful. Lesions tend to occur in anogenital and oral–facial areas depending on the site of exposure. Viral culture of lesions is an effective method of identifying HSV infection in an initial episode of symptomatic genital herpes. Cultures of lesions are less sensitive during recurrent episodes. Immunofluorescent and enzyme assay tests for HSV antibodies indicate the presence of infection, but they do not predict the likelihood of infecting others.

Treatment.   Antibiotic therapy is available for syphilis, gonorrhea, and chlamydia and antiviral therapy has been used with variable success in HSV infection. Acyclovir has been shown to reduce viral shedding in both symptomatic and asymptomatic recurrences of HSV in about 50% of cases; famcyclovir also suppresses HSV recurrence (Mertz, et al., 1997). Medications used to treat these diseases are presented in Appendix S. Community health nurses can refer clients with suspected STDs for medical management or provide treatment themselves when there are established protocols for doing so. Community health nurses are also responsible for educating clients about medications used, how to take them if they are self-administered, and potential side effects. Nurses also monitor the effectiveness of treatment. To prevent the spread of infection, community health nurses should also plan to caution clients to refrain from sexual activity until they have returned for follow-up testing and cure has been demonstrated.

At the community level, community health nurses can be active in educating the public, especially those at risk, regarding the signs and symptoms of STDs and the availability of treatment. Nurses may also need to educate health care professionals, particularly those in the private sector, regarding the appropriate diagnostic and treatment measures for STDs. Political activity by nurses might also be needed to ensure the adequacy of facilities for the diagnosis and treatment of STDs.

The treatment of choice for syphilis is still penicillin. Gonorrhea can be treated with a variety of antibiotics, although ceftriaxone or another cephalosporin is the therapy of choice because of its effectiveness in treating strains of gonorrhea resistant to other antibiotics (Benenson, 1995).

Treatment for chlamydia may be provided routinely in conjunction with gonococcal therapy because the two infections often occur together. Doxycycline, tetracycline, and azithromycin have been found to be effective in treating chlamydia (Benenson, 1995; Johnson, et al., 1996).

Tertiary Prevention

Tertiary prevention of STDs in the individual client involves a follow-up visit to determine the efficacy of treatment and education to prevent reinfection. Community health nurses should emphasize to all clients the necessity for returning for follow-up to determine the effectiveness of treatment. This is particularly true of syphilis, in which the VDRL is used to monitor treatment effects.

Community health nurses should also inform clients with syphilis that blood tests for syphilis usually continue to be positive even after adequate treatment. These clients, therefore, should be encouraged to inform subsequent health care providers that they have been treated for syphilis in the past. Records of initial and posttreatment VDRLs can then be obtained from the Centers for Disease Control and Prevention and compared with current test results to determine whether reinfection has occurred and treatment is required.

Babies with STDs may have a variety of subsequent health problems, even though they have been adequately treated and the progression of the disease has been halted. For this reason, community health nurses continue to monitor these children over extended periods to provide for early identification of developmental delays and other problems.

Preventing reinfection, another aspect of tertiary prevention with the individual client, requires limiting exposure to the causative organism. Community health nurses can educate clients on the need to limit their sexual activity and the number of sexual partners and on the efficacy of condoms and other barrier methods in preventing STDs.

Another means of preventing reinfection with syphilis among drug users is discontinuing needle sharing. When an infected person shares equipment contaminated with his or her blood, the infection is transmitted to the new host. Community health nurses should educate injection drug users regarding the risks of needle sharing and refer those who desire treatment to available treatment centers.

Tertiary prevention at the community level involves preventing the spread of STDs. The primary mode of preventing the spread of many STDs is contact notification. Contacts of persons with syphilis, gonorrhea, and chlamydia, if identified and treated soon after exposure, can be prevented from developing the disease and transmitting it to others.

When STDs in children are the result of child abuse, the nurse will be involved in referrals and counseling to prevent subsequent abuse and reinfection. The involvement of community health nurses in cases of child abuse is dealt with in more detail in Chapter 34.

Tertiary prevention may also require planning for political activity on the part of nurses. As noted earlier, monies previously allocated to contact notification and STD prevention programs have been shifted to HIV infection control. Community health nurses can help acquaint policy makers with the need to continue to fund control programs for syphilis as well as for other communicable diseases. Primary, secondary, and tertiary control measures for STDs are summarized in Table 30–16.

TABLE 30–16. PRIMARY, SECONDARY, AND TERTIARY PREVENTION MEASURES TO CONTROL OTHER SEXUALLY TRANSMITTED DISEASES

Level of Prevention	Community Health Nurse Function	Goal
Primary prevention	• Refer for chemoprophylaxis. • Use antibiotics that not only treat gonorrhea but also treat incubating syphilis and chlamydia. • Educate on condom use. • Educate persons at risk. • Refer pregnant women for prenatal care and STD screening. • Refer intravenous drug users for treatment. • Educate on "safe shooting" practices.	• Provide prophylaxis for persons exposed to STDs. • Prevent developing infection. • Increase condom use. • Decrease number of sexual partners. • Identify and treat women with STDs to prevent fetal infection. • Decrease drug use and potential for exposure. • Decrease needle sharing.
Secondary prevention	• Refer for screening persons at risk for STDs. • Refer persons with symptoms for diagnosis and treatment. • Educate clients on relief of symptoms of STDs. • Educate clients on use of medications. • Engage in political activity.	• Screen groups at risk. • Adequately diagnose and effectively treat STDs. • Relieve symptoms of STDs. • Treat STDs adequately. • Ensure funds and facilities for treatment.
Tertiary prevention	• Monitor effects of treatment. • Educate clients about risk behaviors. • Educate drug abusers on "safe shooting" practices. • Interview cases and notify contacts. • Observe for signs of complications and refer for care as needed. • Refer children with STDs for child protective services.	• Client compliance and effective treatment of STDs. • Prevent reinfection. • Prevent reinfection. • Prevent communicability and spread of infection. • Prevent long-term consequences of infection. • Investigate possible sexual abuse and prevent recurrence.

Evaluating Control Strategies for Sexually Transmitted Diseases

For individual clients, evaluation of the effectiveness of control strategies focuses on whether clients develop STDs (evaluation of primary prevention), whether they are adequately treated for existing STDs (secondary prevention), and whether they develop complications or become reinfected (tertiary prevention). At the aggregate level, criteria for evaluation can be derived from the objectives for control of communicable diseases developed for the year 2000. Evaluative data and the status of STD objectives are presented in Table 30–17.

Tuberculosis

Tuberculosis (TB) in the United States is primarily a disease of the lungs in immunocompetent persons. In developing countries and in persons with immunodeficiencies, however, tuberculosis occurs in a variety of extrapulmonary sites including bone, kidneys, pericardium, joints, and the lymphatic system. There is also a disseminated form of the disease that manifests in multiple organ systems. Tuberculosis is transmitted by the airborne route as ***droplet nuclei*** (small droplets of respiratory secretions propelled into the air by coughing, sneezing, or talking) that are inhaled by the host. Several strains of related bacteria produce tuberculosis, but the primary cause of pulmonary tuberculosis is *Mycobacterium tuberculosis* in immunocompetent persons. Atypical strains of mycobacteria also cause disease in persons who are immunocompromised and constitute a serious threat to HIV-infected individuals (U.S. Public Health Services Task Force on Prophylaxis and Therapy for *Mycobacterium avium*

Complex, 1993). Basic information about tuberculosis is presented in Appendix S.

Trends in Tuberculosis Incidence

With the advent of antituberculin drugs, both morbidity and mortality due to TB declined precipitously. In fact, from the early 1950s to 1985, TB incidence declined 5 to 6% per year (National Center for HIV, STD and TB Prevention, 1996c). Prior to the availability of treatment, approximately half of those with TB died.

Despite the remarkable decline in morbidity and mortality, new cases of TB continue to occur, and incidence rates increased 20% between 1985 and 1992 (National Center for HIV, STD and TB Prevention, 1996c). The 1996 incidence was 8 cases per 100,000 population (Division of Tuberculosis Elimination, 1997c). Worldwide, there are 1 billion people infected with *Mycobacterium tuberculosis* (Johnson, et al., 1992). Approximately 10% of these people will develop active disease at some point in their lives (National Center for HIV, STD and TB Prevention, 1996c). Approximately 7.5 million cases of active TB and 2.5 million deaths occur each year throughout the world (Wilkinson, Davies, & Connolly, 1996). Expectations for the last decade of the millenium include 90 million new cases and as many as 30 million TB-related deaths (Division of Tuberculosis Elimination, 1996). These alarming morbidity and mortality estimates reflect the increasing incidence of HIV infection as well as deteriorating socioeconomic conditions in much of the world.

In 1989, the Advisory Committee for the Elimination of Tuberculosis (ACET) develop a *Strategic Plan for the Elimination of Tuberculosis in the United States*. The goal of this plan, reduction of overall TB incidence to less than one case per 100,000 population by 2010, has been further refined in national objectives for the year 2000 related to tuberculosis in several

---

TABLE 30–17. STATUS OF SELECTED NATIONAL OBJECTIVES FOR SEXUALLY TRANSMITTED DISEASES

	Objective	Base	Most Recent	Target
19.1	Reduce gonorrhea incidence (per 100,000)	300 (1989)	149.5 (1995)	225
19.3	Reduce incidence of primary and secondary syphilis (per 100,000)	18.1 (1989)	6.3 (1995)	10
19.4	Reduce incidence of congential syphilis (per 100,000 live births)	91 (1991)	39 (1995)	40
19.5	Reduce annual number of first visits for genital herpes infection	163,000 (1988)	285,000 (1991)	142,000
19.12	Increase STD education in schools	95% (1988)	NDA[a]	100%
19.13	Increase correct management of STDs by providers	70% (1988)	NDA	90%
19.14	Increase provider counseling regarding STDs	10% (1987)	50% (1995)	75%
19.15	Increase partner notification of STD exposure	20% (1988)	NDA	50%

[a]NDA, no data available.

(Sources: Centers for Disease Control, 1996; U.S. Department of Health and Human Services. 1993; 1995a.)

high-risk groups (U.S. Department of Health and Human Services, 1991).

 ## Assessing the Dimensions of Health in Tuberculosis

The incidence and consequences of TB are influenced by factors in each of the six dimensions of health. The community health nurse assesses factors related to biophysical, psychological, physical, social, behavioral, and health system dimensions that may place individual clients or communities at risk for TB. Factors that may affect the course of the disease for the individual or the community are also identified.

The Biophysical Dimension

Both the very young and the very old are at particular risk for TB (Colditz, et al., 1995; Division of Tuberculosis Elimination, 1997c). From 1985 to 1995, TB incidence among children under 14 years of age increased nearly 24% when overall TB incidence increased only 3% (National Center for HIV, STD and TB Prevention, 1996c). Worldwide, 170,000 children died of tuberculosis in 1995 (Division of Tuberculosis Elimination, 1997b). Children may be less likely than adults to transmit infection to others, but should be considered communicable if they have a forceful cough, cavitation on x-ray, or other signs of infectiousness, or are involved in procedures that induce coughing or aerosolization (Bozzi, et al., 1994). Currently, incidence rates for tuberculosis are highest for persons over 65 years of age (22.3 cases per 100,000 population in 1996) (Division of Tuberculosis Elimination, 1997c).

Members of ethnic minority groups are vastly overrepresented among persons with active tuberculous disease. In 1996, for example, Asians and Pacific Islanders were nearly 14 times more likely than non-Latino whites to develop TB, and non-Latino blacks were 7 times as likely as whites to have active disease. Incidence rates for Latinos were slightly more than 6 times higher, and those for Native Americans 5 times higher, than those of their white counterparts (National Center for HIV, STD and TB Prevention, 1996c). Overall, two thirds of TB cases in the United States occur in minority group members (Boutotte, 1993). These findings reflect socioeconomic factors rather than innate susceptibility to tuberculous disease.

The presence of other physiologic conditions can also contribute to the incidence of TB, and the community health nurse identifies physical conditions that increase the susceptibility of an individual to disease. The nurse also assesses the prevalence of these conditions in the population to determine the aggregate risk for TB. Leanness, diabetes, silicosis, steroid therapy, renal disease, and chronic malabsorption syndromes are all risk factors for TB, as is immunosuppression due to any cause (Graham & Cruise, 1996). Persons with HIV infection have an 8 to 10% annual risk of developing active TB compared to a 10% lifetime risk for the general population (National Center for HIV, STD and TB Prevention, 1996c). Among Latinos, the presence of diabetes seems to increase the risk of TB to a level commensurate with the risk in HIV-infected persons (Pablos-Mendez, Blustein, & Knirsch, 1997). Other conditions that increase the risk of tuberculosis include some hematologic disorders (eg, leukemia), gastrectomy, and jejunoileal bypass (Bloch, 1995).

In addition to being more susceptible to TB due to reduced immune system capabilities, HIV-infected individuals progress more rapidly to active disease than immunocompetent individuals (National Center for HIV, STD and TB Prevention, 1996c). Finally, many HIV-infected individuals develop *anergy,* a condition in which one is incapable of reacting to antigens commonly used in tuberculosis skin testing due to suppression of cellular immunity (Bozzi, et al., 1994). Malnutrition is another factor which may cause false-negative TB tests (Division of Tuberculosis Elimination, 1997b). Failure to react appreciably to the primary screening tool for TB means increased difficulty in identifying a population group at high risk for TB and for severe complications of the disease.

Another aspect of the physiologic dimension of tuberculosis of interest to the community health nurse is the course of the disease process itself. Tuberculosis begins with a primary infection in which the causative agent invades the host, leading to an antigen–antibody response. In most people, the body's immune system succeeds in isolating the infecting organisms within a small area of tissue (usually in the lungs), creating an asymptomatic period of latent infection that may last years or even for life. Under conditions of physiologic stress, the infection "reactivates," with resumed replication of bacteria resulting in active tuberculosis (Grimes & Grimes, 1995). As noted earlier, the progression to active disease occurs in a shorter time among HIV-infected individuals than in the general population.

Pregnancy or any other condition that puts undue stress on the body may also increase susceptibility to tuberculosis. In addition, tubercular symptoms, such as fatigue and increased respiratory rate, may be mistaken for normal physiologic changes of pregnancy. Poor nutrition, particularly that experienced by alcohol and drug abusers, also increases the risk of TB. The presence of these conditions also heightens the severity of TB.

The Psychological Dimension

Factors in the psychological dimension may also contribute to reactivation of tuberculous infection. Psychological stress may lead to reactivation. Psychological factors may also contribute to behavioral dimension elements such as substance abuse that increase susceptibility to tuberculosis. Finally, substance abuse, as well as other forms of psychopathology, may reduce compliance with treatment for TB, increasing the potential for relapse and for the development of drug-resistant organisms.

The Physical Dimension

Exposure to infected individuals in one's environment increases the risk of disease. This is particularly true in conditions of overcrowding. The more crowded the living conditions and the more frequent and prolonged the contact with an infected person, the greater the risk of infection. Areas of the country in which exposure to TB is most likely to occur owing to the

widespread nature of the disease are presented in Figure 30–10. Seven nations of the world—Mexico, the Philippines, Vietnam, India, the Republic of Korea, the People's Republic of China, and Haiti—accounted for 66% of foreign-born people with tuberculosis in the United States in 1996 (Division of Tuberculosis Elimination, 1997c).

Poor ventilation and recirculated air contribute to the spread of droplet nuclei that contain *M. tuberculosis*. Negative air pressure ventilation that prevents the escape of bacteria into corridors and other areas is recommended for hospital rooms and other institutional settings where clients with active TB may be housed. Exposure to ultraviolet light kills *M. tuberculosis*, so the presence of ultraviolet light in an area can limit the spread of disease; however, care must be taken to avoid retinal damage where ultraviolet light is strong (Bozzi, et al., 1994).

The Social Dimension

Social dimension factors can contribute to increases in cases of TB. War and social upheaval cause TB rates to rise. The recent influx of refugees from parts of the

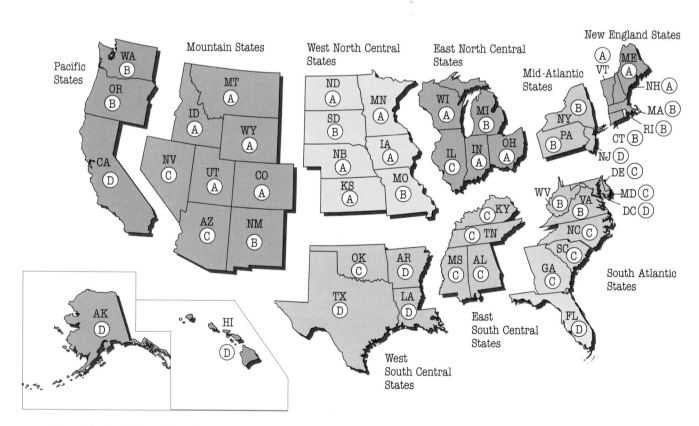

Figure 30–10. Incidence of tuberculosis per 100,000 population, by state, 1995. A = 0–3.5 cases per 100,000 population; B = 3.6–5.9 cases per 100,000 population; C = 6.0–10.5 cases per 100,000 population; D = >10.5 cases per 100,000 population. (Source: Centers for Disease Control, 1996.)

world with high incidence rates for TB has contributed to the rising incidence in the United States (National Center for Infectious Diseases, 1995). Undocumented immigrants from countries with high TB incidence rates, such as Mexico, also facilitate the spread of TB in the United States. In 1996, 37% of TB cases diagnosed in the United States occurred in foreign-born individuals (Division of Tuberculosis Elimination, 1997c).

Other population groups at high risk for TB include the homeless and institutionalized individuals. Physical debilitation, street living, and crowded shelters contribute to TB incidence among the homeless. In one New York City shelter, for example, 79% of homeless men had positive tuberculin skin tests (Paul, Lebowitz, Moore, Hoven, Bennett, & Chen, 1993). Persons in hospitals (especially hospitalized clients with immunodeficiency), nursing homes, residential facilities for the mentally disabled, and correctional institutions are also at high risk for TB than the general public. For example, as many as 14 to 25% of inmates may be infected (Graham & Cruise, 1996). Institutional settings, including prisons and hospitals, tend to favor the spread of multidrug-resistant tuberculosis (MDR-TB), and several outbreaks of MDR-TB in such institutions have been reported. These outbreaks have been characterized by case fatality rates of 72 to 89% with extremely short intervals between diagnosis and death (National Center for HIV, STD and TB Prevention, 1996c).

Social concerns for confidentiality related to HIV infection have hampered efforts to control TB in coinfected populations (Division of Tuberculosis Elimination, 1994a). The problems of TB and HIV coinfection have also led to a nationwide review of state laws related to TB control. In many instances, existing laws have been found to be inadequate to deal with the ever-increasing incidence of TB, and the Advisory Council for the Elimination of Tuberculosis has developed a set of comprehensive recommendations to address these inadequacies (Willis, Schwartz, & Knowlton, 1993). Selected recommendations from the resulting document will be addressed in later sections of this chapter.

Occupation is another social dimension factor that poses a risk for health care providers caring for persons with communicable TB. The risk of infection is probably less, however, in working with persons diagnosed as having TB than in working with those in high-risk groups who are undiagnosed. This is so because, when a definitive diagnosis of TB has been made, precautions can be taken to prevent transmission to health care providers. Any person providing services to people in high-risk groups is at increased risk for infection. These include persons working with immigrants and refugees, persons who work in shelters for the homeless, and those working with hospitalized clients with active TB.

Migrant farm workers are another occupational group at high risk for tuberculosis. Poor living conditions, crowding, and malnutrition are all factors that contribute to increased TB incidence among migrant workers. Workers exposed to silica are also at increased risk for tuberculosis (National Institute for Occupational Safety and Health, 1995).

Active TB infection may lead to legal restrictions on certain employment categories. In 1993, 22 states restricted persons with active TB from engaging in one or more occupations while they were considered contagious. Occupations affected included food handling, work with schoolchildren, day care, and work in nursing homes and home health care (Willis, et al., 1993).

The Behavioral Dimension

Poor nutrition and consumption patterns related to substance abuse and smoking increase susceptibility to TB. Substance abuse in particular may lead to debilitation, making one susceptible to active disease. In 1993, 2.4% of active tuberculosis was associated with injection drug use and 13% with excessive alcohol use (Division of Tuberculosis Elimination, 1994a). Drug abuse, particularly opiate use, may also result in anergy, reducing the validity of tuberculin tests as a screening tool in this high-risk population. In some studies, as many as 25% of injection drug users display anergy (Bellin, Fletcher, & Safyer, 1993; Zoloth, et al., 1993). As noted earlier, substance abuse may interfere with compliance in the treatment of tuberculosis. For example, in one study, 40% of injection drug users with positive skin tests did not understand the importance of medication compliance (Wolfe, et al., 1995).

The Health System Dimension

Many authors have blamed a variety of health system factors for the overwhelming upsurge of TB incidence in the United States. Four particular errors in judgment have been identified as major contributing factors: inadequate initial treatment regimens, improper modification of treatment regimens, insufficient drug susceptibility testing, and failure to promote treatment adherence. These factors are particularly strong contributors to increased MDR-TB (National Center for HIV, STD and TB Prevention, 1996c). A fifth factor is a significant reduction in funding for TB control programs (Chaulk, Moore-Rice, Rizzo, & Chaisson, 1995).

Health care system factors also contribute to the incidence of TB in that many health care providers are not aware of the growing magnitude of the problem and fail to consider TB as a potential diagnosis. In addition, based on the number of cases of TB occurring in people under 35 years of age who should have received chemoprophylaxis, prophylactic services are not being provided to those in need of them. Another health care system factor contributing to tuberculosis incidence is lack of access to diagnostic and treatment services for large segments of high-risk populations. Lack of adherence to infection control measures also contributes to the spread of disease in institutional settings.

Long waits in crowded emergency facilities that promote disease transmission is another possible health system factor contributing to disease in both staff and clients (Redd & Susser, 1997). In addition, inaccurate diagnosis may lead to inappropriate treatment of individuals who are uninfected and misdiagnosis of those who are. For example, laboratory errors leading to false-positive cultures for *M. tuberculosis* led to unnecessary treatment of several persons in 1996 (Division of Tuberculosis Elimination, 1997a). On the other hand, failure to distinguish between tuberculosis infection and an immune response due to BCG vaccine in young children entering the United States from countries where BCG is routinely given also leads to misdiagnosis (Division of Tuberculosis Elimination, 1997b). Finally, medical treatment for other conditions may interfere with effective treatment of tuberculosis. For example, use of protease inhibitors, the most promising therapy for HIV infection, interacts with rifamycin derivatives diminishing their effectiveness in treating TB (Center for Drug Evaluation and Research, 1996). Factors in the epidemiology of tuberculosis are summarized in Table 30–18.

Diagnostic Reasoning and Care of Clients with Tuberculosis

Nursing diagnoses related to TB in the individual may reflect the potential for exposure to disease or problems arising from existing disease. Examples of individual diagnoses are "need for chemoprophylaxis due to close contact with family member with TB" and "visual disturbances due to ethambutol therapy for TB." At the aggregate level, nursing diagnoses may reflect increased incidence of TB or the existence of conditions that increase the risk of infection. Typical diagnoses at this level are "increased incidence of TB among homeless persons" and "increased incidence of TB due to recent settlement of Southeast Asian refugees."

TABLE 30–18. EPIDEMIOLOGIC FACTORS IN TUBERCULOSIS

BIOPHYSICAL DIMENSION

Genetic inheritance	• Men are more often affected than women.
Maturation and aging	• The very young and elderly are at greater risk of infection than other age groups. • Risk of death is greater for the elderly than other age groups.
Physiologic function	• Presence of leanness or diabetes increases susceptibility to infection. • Pregnancy increases susceptibility. • Immunosuppression or immunodeficiency increases susceptibility. • Other existing conditions such as diabetes, leukemia, and gastrectomy increase susceptibility.

PSYCHOLOGICAL DIMENSION

• Increased psychological stress heightens potential for developing active disease.

PHYSICAL DIMENSION

• Overcrowding increases risk of exposure.

SOCIAL DIMENSION

• Times of social disruption such as war and famine increase incidence.
• Homelessness contributes to increased risk of disease.
• Immigration from countries with a high incidence of TB contributes to increased prevalence and incidence of disease in the United States.
• Members of minority groups account for a large portion of TB incidence in the United States.
• Institutionalization increases risk of TB.
• Persons caring for those with active TB are at increased risk of exposure.

BEHAVIORAL DIMENSION

• Substance abuse contributes to physical debilitation, leading to increased susceptibility to disease.
• Poor nutrition increases susceptibility to TB.
• Smoking increases susceptibility to TB.

HEALTH SYSTEM DIMENSION

• Failure to diagnose and adequately treat TB contributes to spread of infection and recurrence of active disease.
• Relaxation of tuberculin screening requirements for certain groups of people has contributed to the spread of disease.
• Failure to provide chemoprophylaxis to persons under age 35 with positive TB skin tests contributes to the incidence of active TB.
• Use of protease inhibitors to treat HIV infection reduces the effectiveness of some TB drugs.
• Prolonged exposure to infectious cases of TB in crowded emergency departments increases risk of infection for staff and clients.

Planning and
Implementing
the Dimensions of Health Care
for Tuberculosis

Planning control strategies for tuberculosis is based on general principles of program planning presented in Chapter 19. Control efforts may be planned and implemented at primary, secondary, and tertiary levels of prevention.

Primary Prevention

Primary prevention for tuberculosis includes basic health promotion to limit susceptibility to disease. Prevention of HIV infection by measures described earlier in this chapter can also limit susceptibility to tuberculosis in the population. Improvement in living conditions, promotion of good nutrition, and efforts to relieve conditions of poverty increase the resistance of the population to developing TB.

Immunization. There is a vaccine available for tuberculosis—bacille Calmette–Guérin (BCG) vaccine—developed from an attenuated strain of *Mycobacterium bovis*. *Attenuated organisms* are those rendered incapable of causing disease. The efficacy of BCG is somewhat unpredictable, but has been shown to reduce risk of infection by an average of 50 to 80% of children and infants in developing countries (Colditz, et al., 1995; Villarino, Huebner, Lanner, & Geiter, 1996). Because it causes conversion of tuberculin skin tests to positive, BCG is not widely used in the United States, where the prevalence of tuberculosis has been relatively low and tuberculin screening is widely used as a control measure. BCG is recommended for children who experience continuous exposure to persons with active TB but who cannot be given routine chemoprophylaxis. The vaccine should also be administered to those individuals exposed to persons who have TB that is resistant to the usual forms of therapy. Additionally, BCG should not be given to individuals who are immunocompromised and should be administered only with caution to those at risk for HIV infection (Villarino, et al., 1996). BCG may also be appropriate for health care workers in settings where MDR-TB is prevalent and in which infection control strategies have proven ineffective.

Chemoprophylaxis. Chemoprophylaxis is used for primary prevention of tuberculosis in the United States. Persons who are at risk for TB or who have reactive tuberculin skin tests without evidence of current disease are offered antibiotic treatment to prevent its development. The most frequently used form of prophylaxis is administration of isoniazid (INH), an antituberculin medication. Chemoprophylaxis is recommended for individuals of any age who have reactive skin tests and who are in close contact with a diagnosed case of active TB, have recently converted from a negative to a positive skin test, have medical conditions that increase their risk of disease, are HIV-infected, have previously untreated or inadequately treated infection, who are injection drug users, or who have demonstrated anergy. Other candidates for preventive therapy include persons under 35 years of age who were born in high-prevalence countries, who are part of a high-risk minority group, or who are residents of institutional facilities (including prisons) (Graham & Cruise, 1996).

Other Measures. Other primary prevention measures include the use of adequate ventilation and ultraviolet light in areas that increase the risk of TB transmission. For example, areas in which aerosol sputum specimens are collected provide an environment conducive to the spread of disease that can be modified using these measures. Providing appropriate facilities for isolating infectious clients in hospitals also minimizes the risk of transmission to health care personnel.

Community health nurses are often involved in primary preventive efforts for control of tuberculosis. In a few cases, they may identify persons in need of BCG vaccine and assist them to obtain needed services. It is more likely, however, that they will supervise chemoprophylaxis for clients at risk for developing TB. Prophylaxis has been shown to be 90% effective in preventing the development of TB if the regimen is completed. For this reason, community health nurses should carefully educate clients regarding the need for preventive therapy and should monitor their compliance. When clients are judged to be unreliable, it is suggested that they be given directly observed therapy twice a week. (In *directly observed therapy,* the nurse actually watches the client take the medication). Another means of assessing compliance is periodic spot-testing of urine for INH metabolites.

Community health nurses should educate clients regarding medication dosage and potential side effects. They also monitor clients on chemoprophylaxis for evidence of side effects.

Nurses are also involved in efforts to alleviate social conditions that contribute to tuberculosis incidence. They can help influence policy makers to provide for the needs of the homeless and to improve the conditions of others in poverty. They can also intervene directly with these clients to refer them to sources of housing and financial assistance.

Secondary Prevention

Secondary prevention efforts for tuberculosis center around screening, diagnosis, and treatment of existing disease.

Screening. Secondary prevention of TB begins with screening members of high-risk groups. Persons who should be screened include those in contact with someone with active TB (especially household contacts) and others at risk for close contact with infected persons such as staff in tuberculosis clinics, shelters for the homeless, nursing homes, substance abuse programs, and prisons. Other high-risk groups that should be screened are recent immigrants from areas of high TB incidence, migrant workers, prisoners, nursing home residents, the homeless, and persons with HIV infection and other debilitating conditions.

The screening test of choice is the Mantoux skin test, an intradermal injection of tuberculin purified protein derivative (PPD). Health care providers evaluating HIV-infected persons or injection drug users for evidence of TB should bear in mind that these clients may have anergy, resulting in a false-negative PPD and that a negative test should not exclude a diagnosis of TB.

A positive tuberculin skin test indicates that the person has at some time been exposed to TB and has developed circulating antibodies to infection. It does not, however, indicate whether the person has active disease. Unlike HIV infection, TB infection is not *necessarily* communicable. Individuals with what is termed a *primary infection* have been exposed to the causative agent, but bodily defense mechanisms have successfully combatted the invading organism. Usually the organism is walled off in an encapsulated area within the lung. During this process, antibody formation is stimulated and the tuberculin skin test becomes reactive.

Persons with primary infection cannot transmit the disease to others; however, when any of a variety of physical or psychological stressors undermine the body's ability to confine the invading organism, active disease can occur. Clients with active disease can transmit the disease to others. Preventing the development of active disease is the aim of chemoprophylactic therapy discussed earlier.

Community health nurses are frequently involved in referring clients for screening. They may also give and interpret the TB test. The nurse should be sure to inform clients of the need to return to have the TB skin test read in 48 to 72 hours. When the test results are positive, the nurse refers the client for further diagnostic studies and treatment as needed. A positive skin test in an immunocompetent individual is indicated by an area of *induration,* or swelling, of more than 10 mm at the test site. For individuals with possible HIV coinfection or other reason for anergy, a reaction greater than 5 mm is considered positive (Bloch, 1995). Individuals with known or suspected HIV infection or injection drug users can be tested for anergy prior to tuberculin skin testing with a panel of skin test antigens to which most people would normally react (eg, mumps or candida antigens or tetanus toxoid). Community health nurses may be involved in anergy testing as well as TB screening.

Diagnosis. When a person has a reactive TB skin test, there is a need for further diagnostic testing to determine whether the individual does or does not have active tuberculosis. Diagnosis of active pulmonary disease is based on sputum smears or cultures positive for acid-fast bacilli. In the absence of positive cultures, diagnosis is made in the presence of any two of the following: symptoms suggestive of TB (see Appendix S), x-ray findings consistent with TB, and a positive PPD (Centers for Disease Control, 1997a). Diagnosis of TB in persons with HIV infection may be complicated by the fact that symptoms may not reflect the typical clinical picture of TB and by differences from characteristic x-ray findings. In addition, a large proportion of TB in those with concurrent HIV infection is extrapulmonary in nature.

Treatment. Treatment with antituberculin drugs is highly effective in most clients, resulting in return to negative sputum cultures in most clients within 6 months when the infecting organism is sensitive to the drugs of choice and the client is consistent in taking the medication. Given the prevalence of multidrug-resistant TB, recommended initial therapy consists of a four-drug regimen including INH, rifampin (RIF), pyrazinamide (PZA), and either streptomycin (SM) or ethambutol (EMB). In institutional outbreaks of MDR-TB, a six-drug initial regimen may be needed (Division of Tuberculosis Elimination, 1994b). Duration of treatment for immunocompetent clients is a minimum of 6 months, whereas therapy for those who are immunocompromised should continue at least 9 months. Directly observed therapy (DOT) is recommended for all persons with tuberculosis (El-Sadr, Medard, & Barthaud, 1996). DOT has been associated with treatment completion rates of 78 to 90% even when volunteers supervise therapy (Wilkinson, et al., 1996).

Community health nurses working with clients with active TB will most likely be monitoring clients' compliance with the treatment regimen and observing them for side effects. It is important that the nurse emphasize to clients the need to complete therapy and to take the medications as directed because sporadic therapy frequently results in the development of drug-resistant bacteria.

Community health nurses should educate clients on antituberculin therapy regarding potential side effects of medications and measures that can be taken to minimize them. They should also ensure that vision, liver function, hearing, and kidney function are periodically tested to identify adverse effects of chemotherapy.

Tertiary Prevention

Tertiary preventive efforts for tuberculosis focus on three areas: preventing recurrence of the disease in the individual, notifying and treating contacts of cases of tuberculosis, and isolating infected persons as needed.

Prevention of Recurrence. Tertiary prevention of TB takes place at both the individual client level and the community level. With the individual client, there is the potential for reactivation of disease following treatment, particularly if treatment has been inadequate. Most inadequate treatment is related to client failure to comply with treatment recommendations.

Community health nurses can prevent recurrence of TB. Case finding and referral of clients for treatment can eliminate lack of therapy as a cause of recurrent disease. Community health nurses are frequently involved in educating other health care providers regarding the appropriate treatment for tuberculosis as well as other communicable diseases. Community health nurses can also help to ensure that clients take their medications as directed and complete their therapy.

Some of the actions that can be taken to achieve this have already been discussed and include directly observed therapy, periodic spot-testing of urine, and, most important, education to promote client understanding of the need to complete an adequate course of therapy. In addition, community health nurses can monitor clients after treatment for signs of recurrent disease and may be involved in obtaining follow-up sputum cultures or arranging for follow-up x-rays to determine the adequacy of treatment.

Contact Notification. At the community level, tertiary prevention of TB focuses on preventing the spread of disease within the community. Contact notification is the major activity in this area. The strategic plan for tuberculosis control developed by the Centers for Disease Control calls for interviews of clients with diagnosed cases of TB within 3 days of diagnosis and examina-

tion of close contacts within 7 days, at which time contacts would be offered prophylactic chemotherapy (Advisory Committee for the Elimination of Tuberculosis, 1989).

Isolation. A final tertiary preventive measure for TB is involuntary isolation of persons with active disease; this is designed to prevent the spread of disease. This intervention has the potential for use in the control of several communicable diseases, but is most frequently invoked in TB control. What is involved is the involuntary isolation or quarantine of an infected person who refuses to discontinue behaviors that expose others to infection. Such measures are a last resort and are used only when all other efforts to control the spread of infection fail (Bayer, Dubler, & Landesman, 1993). In 1993, 44 states had legal procedures in place permitting involuntary commitment as a potential control measure for TB (Willis, et al., 1993). Rapid screening of emergency department clients to identify those in need of immediate isolation has also been suggested. Criteria for isolation in this setting include an abnormal chest x-ray, temperature over 101°F, homelessness or shelter dwelling, and history of positive skin test, exposure, or active TB (Redd & Susser, 1997). Similar criteria could be used in isolation decisions in correctional settings. A summary of primary, secondary, and tertiary preventive measures for TB is presented in Table 30–19.

Evaluating Control Strategies for Tuberculosis

Evaluating primary preventive measures for TB control involves monitoring the incidence and prevalence of the disease as well as the effectiveness of measures to prevent active disease. Secondary and tertiary prevention can be evaluated on the basis of mortality rates for TB and adequacy of therapy in individual cases. The status of the national objectives related to TB control is summarized in Table 30–20.

Influenza

Between 1972 and 1992, nine influenza epidemics occurred in the United States, each accounting for more than 20,000 deaths and four of them causing more than 40,000 deaths each (Arden, Cox, & Schonberger, 1997). Influenza is a viral disease caused by three types of viruses (influenza, A, B, and C.) Type A influenza virus has three subtypes, and both type A and type B viruses undergo frequent genetic mutations that cause periodic development of variant strains for

TABLE 30–19. PRIMARY, SECONDARY, AND TERTIARY PREVENTION MEASURES TO CONTROL TUBERCULOSIS

Level of Prevention	Community Health Nurse Function	Goal
Primary prevention	• Educate public regarding health promotion and good nutrition. • Identify and refer those in need of BCG immunization. • Identify and refer those in need of chemoprophylaxis.	• Increase resistance to disease. • Increase resistance to disease. • Prevent developing active disease.
Secondary Prevention	• Provide screening and counseling services. • Engage in case finding and refer for treatment. • Educate regarding medications. • Monitor and treat medication side effects.	• Screen persons at risk. • Diagnose and treat with appropriate antituberculin agents. • Ensure client compliance and effective treatment of disease. • Prevent adverse reactions.
Tertiary prevention	• Interview cases and notify contacts. • Monitor effects of treatment. • Educate health care providers on appropriate treatment. • Identify need for and initiate isolation procedures for noncompliant clients with active disease or in high-transmission settings.	• Prevent spread of infection. • Ensure effective treatment. • Prevent inadequate treatment. • Prevent spread of infection.

which prior immunization is ineffective. Thus, despite the development of vaccines for influenza, the disease continues to occur throughout the world. It is usually type A and type B viruses that cause major epidemics of influenza, whereas type C influenza appears only sporadically throughout the world (Benenson, 1995). For most people, influenza is a short-lived illness producing moderate discomfort. For others, however, influenza is a far more serious illness.

Trends in Influenza Incidence

Thousands of people are exposed to influenza and develop active disease each year. Influenza outbreaks often result in excessive school absenteeism and have occasionally led to school closures to prevent spread of the infection. Hospitalization rates may increase two- to fivefold among persons in high-risk groups

who develop influenza (Arden, et al., 1997), and annual costs for influenza are estimated at $1 billion for hospitalization under Medicare alone (Health Care Financing Administration, 1997).

 ## Assessing the Dimensions of Health in Influenza

Biophysical, psychological, physical, social, behavioral, and health system factors contribute to the development of influenza and affect its outcome.

The Biophysical Dimension

Human biological factors influence susceptibility to and consequences of influenza infection, and the nurse should identify factors present in individual clients or in communities that may place them at risk for influenza or its complications. Influenza occurs in all age groups, but mortality is highest among the young and the very old. Generally, influenza B outbreaks occur most often among school-age children, with low mortality associated with infection. Influenza A, on the other hand, frequently affects both children and the elderly, particularly in nursing home outbreaks. Approximately 90% of influenza-related deaths occur among those over 65 years of age (Adult Vaccine Preventable Diseases Bureau, 1997). Males are more often affected than females, and all racial groups are susceptible, but African Americans have mortality rates nearly one and one-half times those of the white population (Mortality Statistics Bureau, 1996).

Persons with other debilitating physical conditions, particularly chronic pulmonary diseases, diabetes, stroke, heart disease, and malnutrition are at higher risk for death due to influenza (Potter, et al., 1997). Other illnesses that increase susceptibility in-

TABLE 30–20. STATUS OF SELECTED NATIONAL OBJECTIVES FOR TUBERCULOSIS

	Objective	Base	Current Status	Target
20.4	Reduce tuberculosis incidence (per 100,000)			
	Overall	9.1 (1988)	8.0 (1996)	3.5
	Among Asians/Pacific Islanders	36.3 (1988)	41.6 (1996)	15.0
	Among African Americans	28.3 (1988)	22.3 (1996)	10.0
	Among Latinos	18.3 (1988)	16.0 (1996)	5.0
	Among Native Americans	18.1 (1988)	14.5 (1996)	5.0
20.18	Increase proportion of infected persons completing TB therapy	66.3% (1987)	65.3% (1993)	85%

(Sources: U.S. Department of Health and Human Services, 1993; 1996; Division of Tuberculosis Elimination, 1997c.)

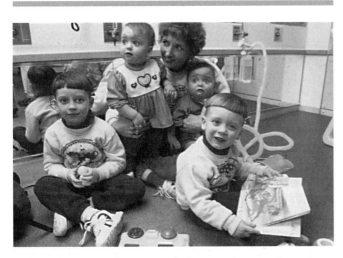

Influenza is easily transmitted in settings such as day care centers, where children handle common objects.
From: Ball, J., & Bindler, R. (1999). Pediatric nursing: Caring for children (2nd ed.). Stamford, CT: Appleton & Lange.

clude renal dysfunction, hemoglobinopathies, and diseases or treatment regimens that result in immuno-suppression. Persons with HIV infection are at particular risk for influenza, and the death rate among persons with both diseases is much higher than that for the rest of the population. Children who are on long-term aspirin therapy are of particular concern because of the potential for developing Reye syndrome following viral infections such as influenza. Pregnancy may also present significant risk of complications of influenza, particularly in the second and third trimesters (Arden, et al., 1997).

In working with clients with influenza, the nurse also assesses the extent of the disease. Clients' complaints generally include fever, headache, muscle aches, coryza, sore throat, and cough. The cough, in particular, may linger for some time after other symptoms have resolved. Gastrointestinal symptoms such as nausea, vomiting, and diarrhea can also occur, particularly in children, so the nurse should assess clients for signs of dehydration resulting from these symptoms. The nurse also assesses clients for signs of croup, pneumonia, and other respiratory complications of influenza, as well as pericarditis and central nervous system disease.

The Psychological and Physical Dimensions

Psychological stress can lower one's resistance to influenza, but the psychological dimension, otherwise, has little effect on influenza incidence or conse-quences. Like other diseases spread by airborne transmission, influenza occurs more frequently when people congregate in close quarters. This would explain the increased incidence of influenza in temperate areas in the winter months because people are gathered indoors, making the spread of disease from an infected individual to others more likely. Low temperatures and low humidity promote viral viability and have been associated with summer outbreaks of influenza in highly air conditioned areas (Kohn, Farley, Sundin, Tapia, McFarland, & Arden, 1995). Epidemics occur throughout the year in tropical areas, and from April to September in the Southern Hemisphere. Transmission of influenza is particularly likely in conditions of overcrowding. On rare occasions, animal strains of influenza virus may be transmitted to humans. Animals that can serve as reservoirs for disease include pigs, horses, mink, and seals, as well as many domestic and wild birds (Benenson, 1995).

The Social Dimension

A variety of social factors also contribute to the spread of influenza and to the severity of its effects. For example, poverty can prevent people at risk for influenza from obtaining immunizations or prevent infected persons from seeking medical assistance, thereby increasing their chances for complications from the disease.

Occupation presents opportunity for exposure to influenza as well as the potential for exposing others. Health care personnel and staff in residential settings, including correctional settings, are at increased risk of exposure. Occupational factors also play a part in increased susceptibility to infection or increased exposure to influenza virus. Occupations that result in exposure to high levels of dust and other particulate matter or chemical vapors that may damage lung tissue can increase susceptibility to disease. School teachers are another occupational group with an increased risk, as they are frequently exposed to infected children in their classrooms.

Homelessness may also contribute to the onset of influenza. Exposure to cold, poor nutrition, and other conditions related to homelessness can increase the homeless individual's susceptibility to disease. In addition, crowded conditions in shelters or in other areas where the homeless sleep can increase the spread of disease from infected individuals. Institutionalization can also contribute to the spread of disease (Arden, et al., 1997).

The Behavioral Dimension

Any behavioral factor that contributes to a generally poor state of health increases susceptibility to influenza, so the community health nurse should be alert to lifestyle factors that may contribute to the development of influenza. Consumption patterns such as poor nutrition and substance abuse lower one's general state of health; smoking impairs respiratory function and increases susceptibility to infection. Overexertion and fatigue can decrease resistance to disease in general, including influenza.

The Health System Dimension

The nurse assesses health care system factors that may influence the risk of influenza in an individual or in a community. For example, the nurse might explore the extent to which immunization programs are targeted to members of high-risk groups. In some areas, influenza vaccine is available primarily to those who can pay for it, so many who are in need of protection do not obtain it. Health care providers may miss significant opportunities to immunize those at greatest risk for influenza. During a 1-year period, opportunities for influenza immunization were missed in 65% of Medicare hospitalizations for pneumonia (Health Care Financing Administration, 1997). In addition, health care providers may not recognize the need for supportive services for persons with influenza who are at greatest risk for complications such as pneumonia.

Influenza surveillance by designated segments of the health care system also influences the progress of disease in any given influenza season. Because of frequent antigenic mutations in viral strains, it is important that annual influenza vaccines target strains of influenza virus likely to occur in the population. Using national and international surveillance systems to identify early cases of disease, viral strains can be identified and the appropriate vaccine developed for the coming season. In recent years, vaccine developers have been quite successful in providing immunity to viral strains actually experienced within the population. Health care system and other factors in the epidemiology of influenza are summarized in Table 30–21.

Diagnostic Reasoning and Care of Clients with Influenza

Nursing diagnoses for the individual client will probably relate to the potential for exposure to, or problems resulting from, influenza. Examples of individual diagnoses are "need for influenza immunization due to chronic respiratory disease"; "impaired oxygen exchange due to respiratory effects of influenza";

TABLE 30–21. EPIDEMIOLOGIC FACTORS IN INFLUENZA

BIOPHYSICAL DIMENSION

Maturation and aging	• The elderly are at increased risk for influenza and death due to complications of influenza.
Physiologic function	• Conditions such as chronic obstructive pulmonary disease, diabetes, stroke, and heart disease increase susceptibility to disease.
	• Renal dysfunction, hemoglobinopathies, and immunosuppression increase susceptibility and risk of complications.
	• Children on long-term aspirin therapy are at risk for Reye syndrome as an influenza-related complication.
	• Persons with HIV infection are more susceptible to influenza infection and complications.
	• Pregnancy increases the risk of complications due to influenza.

PSYCHOLOGICAL DIMENSION

• Psychological stress increases susceptibility.

PHYSICAL DIMENSION

• Overcrowding contributes to spread of disease.
• Influenza incidence increases during weather that keeps people indoors.
• Animal strains of influenza may occasionally be transmitted to humans.

SOCIAL DIMENSION

• Poverty may prevent people at risk from seeking immunization or disease treatment services.
• Conditions associated with homelessness can contribute to increased susceptibility to influenza.
• Institutionalization contributes to the spread of disease.
• Care providers in residential and health care facilities are at increased risk of exposure.
• Persons with occupational exposure to dust, fumes, etc., may be at increased risk of influenza infection.

BEHAVIORAL DIMENSION

• Poor nutrition increases susceptibility to influenza.
• Substance abuse increases susceptibility to influenza.
• Failure to get adequate rest increases susceptibility to influenza.
• Smoking increases susceptibility to influenza infection.

HEALTH SYSTEM DIMENSION

• Failure to provide immunization to persons at risk impedes control of influenza.
• Surveillance permits development of strain-appropriate vaccines each year.

"electrolyte imbalance from diarrhea due to influenza"; and "dehydration due to vomiting and diarrhea."

Nursing diagnoses at the community level may reflect the incidence or consequences of influenza or the potential for an outbreak in the population. Examples of population-oriented diagnoses are "increased mortality from influenza in minority group members due to lack of access to medical care" and "potential for increased influenza incidence due to poor immunization levels in high-risk groups."

Planning and
Implementing the
Dimensions of Health Care for Influenza

Primary, secondary, and tertiary preventive efforts are warranted in the control of influenza. Primary measures are geared toward preventing outbreaks or individual cases of disease, whereas secondary measures focus on resolving existing problems. Tertiary prevention is directed toward preventing complications or recurrence of disease.

Primary Prevention

Primary prevention measures center on immunizing susceptible individuals. Other primary strategies include chemoprophylaxis and general hygiene and health promotion.

Immunization. The major emphasis in primary prevention of influenza is immunization. Because of the tendency of the influenza virus to produce new strains, a vaccine is developed each year to provide protection against the viral strains identified in early cases of the disease and expected to cause most of that year's cases of influenza. For this reason, community health nurses should educate those persons at greatest risk (eg, the elderly or those with debilitating illnesses) about the need to be reimmunized annually. Routine yearly influenza immunization is recommended for heath care workers, the elderly, and persons with chronic diseases including chronic pulmonary or cardiovascular diseases, asthma, chronic metabolic diseases such as diabetes, renal dysfunction, hemoglobinopathies, or immunosuppression.

Immunization should also be provided to household contacts of persons in high-risk groups to minimize the risk of exposing high-risk individuals to influenza. Other candidates for immunization include travelers to areas of high incidence, children 6 months to 18 years of age who are on long-term aspirin therapy (immunization is to prevent the development of Reye syndrome), and persons with HIV infection. Influenza vaccine is made from inactivated viruses and cannot cause influenza in the person immunized. For this reason, it is safe to administer influenza vaccine to persons with immunosuppression due to AIDS, and immunization is recommended; however, these individuals may not develop adequate immunity in response to the vaccine and should be protected from exposure to the virus whenever possible. Immunization can also be safely given to pregnant women who demonstrate risk factors for influenza. Immunization is most effective in preventing disease when it is administered before the onset of the influenza season in late fall. Immunization is not recommended for those who have experienced an anaphylactic reaction to egg protein.

Failure to adequately immunize groups at risk for influenza results in unnecessary infection, disease, and death. For example, in one study only 48% of persons over 65 years of age with cardiac conditions received influenza immunization, and only 52% of those with pulmonary conditions were immunized (Advisory Committee on Immunization Practices, 1995). In 1995, roughly 59% of persons over age 65 were immunized against influenza (Powell-Griner, Anderson, & Murphy, 1997). Immunization of health care workers in long-term care facilities protects them as well as the frail elderly residents who may not respond well to immunization (Potter, et al., 1997). In addition, influenza A vaccine appears to play a protective role in preventing otitis media in young children (Clements, Langdon, Bland, & Walter, 1995).

Community health nurses identify persons at risk for influenza and plan to refer them for immunization services. Nurses may also plan and implement immunization programs, targeting groups at high risk for influenza. In addition to referring clients for or providing immunizations, the community health nurse educates clients about potential side effects of immunization (soreness at injection site, fever, and myalgia) and their control.

Chemoprophylaxis. Chemoprophylaxis is not routinely used as a primary preventive measure for persons exposed to influenza except for those at high risk of complication and their caretakers (Arden, et al., 1997). Prophylaxis with an antiviral agent such as amantadine, however, is recommended for individuals involved in outbreaks of influenza A in closed populations (Kohn, et al., 1995). For example, if an outbreak of influenza has taken place in a nursing home or institution for the developmentally disabled, all residents and staff who do not already have the disease might be given amantadine to prevent illness. Chemoprophylaxis is also recommended for persons at high risk for influenza who cannot be immunized (eg, those having severe allergic reactions to eggs). Amantadine is not effective in the prevention of influenza B.

Other Measures. Public education regarding personal hygiene, particularly respiratory hygiene, is another primary prevention measure for influenza. Community health nurses can be instrumental in such education as well as in identifying persons at risk for influenza. The nurse can then acquaint those at risk with the need for immunization and refer them to the appro-

TABLE 30–22. PRIMARY, SECONDARY, AND TERTIARY PREVENTION MEASURES TO CONTROL INFLUENZA

Level of Prevention	Community Health Nurse Function	Goal
Primary prevention	• Educate clients on nutrition and health promotion. • Identify and refer persons at risk; provide immunizations.	• Promote general health. • Immunize persons at risk.
Secondary prevention	• Educate clients in symptom control.	• Relieve symptoms.
Tertiary prevention	• Educate clients for self-care and about signs of complications. • Monitor for signs of complications and refer for treatment. • Plan and implement mass immunization campaigns.	• Prevent complications. • Prevent long-term consequences. • Prevent spread of disease through immunization.

priate source of care. Oftentimes community health nurses are also involved in the implementation of influenza immunization programs.

Secondary Prevention

No routine screening test exists for influenza. Even if a test were available, it would not be widely used because the incubation period for influenza is not long enough for action to be taken to prevent development of symptomatic disease in those infected. Persons who had reactive tests would more than likely already be exhibiting symptoms of the disease.

Diagnosis of influenza is based on the presence of characteristic respiratory or gastrointestinal symptoms and the absence of indicators that these symptoms are due to some other cause. Diagnosis also depends on the potential for exposure at any given time. Because influenza in temperate zones is a cold-weather disease, influenza-like symptoms experienced in the summer months are probably not due to influenza but to some other disease process. Likewise, if jaundice accompanies gastrointestinal upset, a more likely cause is hepatitis rather than influenza. If necessary, clinical diagnosis can be confirmed with a viral culture or increase in antibody titer during convalescence (Benenson, 1995).

Treatment for influenza is generally symptomatic, although early administration of amantadine in influenza A infection may reduce symptoms. Unimmunized clients who are at particular risk for influenza or its complications may be referred for amantadine therapy in areas where viral cultures of infected persons demonstrate the presence of influenza A strains.

The community health nurse working with individuals with influenza should give particular attention to maintaining hydration and conserving energy. If gastrointestinal symptoms are severe, antiemetics or antidiarrheal agents may be given. Antipyretics can be given for fever and analgesics for the headache and myalgia frequently associated with influenza. Nonsalicylate analgesics and antipyretics (for example, acetaminophen) are recommended for influenza-related fever and discomfort in children because of the risk of Reye syndrome.

Community health nurses are frequently involved in educating the public regarding the symptoms of influenza and elements of self-care. They may also be instrumental in identifying clients who need professional care for severe infection. In such cases, community health nurses make referrals for medical care. If clients are seriously ill or markedly dehydrated, hospitalization may be necessary, and the nurse may need to plan an emergency referral.

Tertiary Prevention

Tertiary prevention for the individual client involves preventing complications due to influenza. Clients who are infected should be cautioned by community health nurses not to overexert themselves. Particularly debilitating strains of influenza may require a relatively prolonged period of convalescence before the client is able to return to normal activity levels. Community health nurses may need to help clients

TABLE 30–23. STATUS OF SELECTED NATIONAL OBJECTIVES FOR INFLUENZA

	Objective	Base	Most Recent	Target
20.2	Reduce epidemic-related pneumonia and influenza deaths among older adults (per 100,000)	19.9 (1979–1987)	15.7 (1993)	15.9
20.11	Increase immunization among noninstitutionalized high-risk populations	33% (1989)	55% (1994)	60%
20.16	Increase proportion of health departments providing influenza immunization	70% (1991)	91% (1992–1993)	90%

(Sources: U.S. Department of Health and Human Services, 1995a; 1996.)

give priority to their activities until they are fully recovered. For example, a mother with influenza may need to continue feeding her children if no other help is available, but she can suspend other activities until she is recuperated. Resuming one's former activity level before fully recuperating from influenza frequently leads to relapse or the onset of complications.

Another aspect of tertiary prevention with the individual is dealing with complications that do arise. Antibiotic therapy is warranted for persons with bacterial infections secondary to influenza. Again, community health nurses monitor the health status of persons with influenza, identifying those who have developed disease complications and referring them for appropriate treatment.

Tertiary prevention measures used to prevent the spread of other diseases are not routinely employed for influenza. Contact notification is not useful because of the short incubation period of the disease. Contacts at high risk for fatality may be provided with chemoprophylaxis, and immunization may be provided for those not yet exposed. Both of these measures may limit the spread of disease within the population. Community health nurses are likely to be involved in immunization as a tertiary as well as a primary preventive measure. Isolating persons with influenza is usually not practical because of the short incubation of the disease. Occasionally, schools and other institutions may be closed in major epidemics to limit the spread of disease to any persons who are not already infected, but more often because too few

teachers, students, or employees are well enough to make it practical to keep the institution operating. Primary, secondary, and tertiary measures for control of influenza are presented in Table 30–22.

Evaluating Control Strategies for Influenza

Evaluating the extent to which the year 2000 objectives for influenza immunization have been achieved is one way of assessing the effectiveness of primary prevention strategies in the control of influenza in a community. The community health nurse examines the extent to which immunization coverage had been achieved in his or her community. The status of objective accomplishment at the national

Critical Thinking in Practice: A Case in Point

Jasmine is an 18-year-old college student. She lives in the dorm with her roommate, Sarah. Shortly after Jasmine returned from Christmas vacation, she developed a fever and a rash. She didn't feel too bad, but Sarah persuaded her to see a doctor. Because it was Saturday, Jasmine went to the emergency room of the local hospital. The physician there made a diagnosis of rubella. Later that night he and the nurses in the ER became very busy with victims of a multicar accident. As a result no one completed the health department form reporting Jasmine's rubella until 2 days later.

By the time a community health nurse contacted Jasmine to complete a rubella case report, Sarah and several other girls in Jasmine's dorm also developed rubella. Sarah gave it to her boyfriend, who exposed those in his classes. One of the women in his English class is pregnant.

1. What primary preventive measures could have been employed to prevent this situation? What primary prevention measures are appropriate at this point?
2. What secondary and tertiary measures by the community health nurse are appropriate at this time?
3. What roles will the community health nurse perform in dealing with this situation?

level is presented in Table 30–23. Other criteria for evaluating the effectiveness of control measures for influenza include the annual incidence of the disease and complications and mortality attributable to influenza.

TESTING YOUR UNDERSTANDING

1. Describe the trends in at least five major communicable diseases. Identify at least one factor contributing to each of these trends. (pp. 744–745, 755–756, 771–772, 777–779, 788–789, 796)
2. What are the six major modes of transmission for communicable diseases? Describe a preventive strategy appropriate to each mode of transmission. (pp. 738–739)
3. Identify at least four roles for community health nurses in controlling communicable diseases. Give an example of a nursing activity that might be performed by a nurse in fulfilling each role. (pp. 742–744)
4. Name the two major approaches to the control of communicable diseases. Give an example of how each approach might be implemented. (pp. 740–742)
5. Discuss the influences of at least two factors in each dimension of health dealing with childhood diseases. (pp. 745–748)
6. Describe at least two nursing interventions for controlling childhood diseases at each level of prevention. (pp. 749–753)
7. Compare and contrast the epidemiologic factors contributing to HIV infection and other STDs. (pp. 756–759, 779–783)
8. Describe at least two nursing interventions for controlling HIV infection and other STDs related to each level of prevention. (pp. 764–771, 784–787)
9. Discuss the influence of at least two factors in each of the dimensions of health related to hepatitis. (pp. 772–775)
10. Describe at least two nursing interventions for controlling hepatitis related to each level of prevention. (pp. 776–777)
11. Discuss the influence of at least two factors in each of the dimensions of health related to TB. (pp. 789–792)
12. Describe at least two nursing interventions for controlling TB related to each level of prevention. (pp. 793–795)
13. Discuss the influence of at least two factors in each of the dimensions of health related to influenza. (pp. 796–798)
14. Describe at least two nursing interventions for

controlling influenza related to each level of prevention. (pp. 799–801)

WHAT DO YOU THINK?
Questions for Critical Thinking

1. What effect does the length of the incubation period have on efforts to control a specific communicable disease?
2. What would your response be if you were told that you had been in contact with someone with TB? HIV? Would your response differ based on the form that contact took? If so, why?
3. What are the advantages and disadvantages of contact notification regarding STD exposure by a health professional versus your sexual contact?
4. Does the role of the community health nurse in controlling communicable diseases differ with the disease to be controlled? If so, how does it differ?
5. Should mandatory HIV screening be required for all hospital admissions? For prisoners? Why or why not?
6. Should people who knowingly infect others with communicable diseases be confined involuntarily? Does your response differ depending on the disease involved? If so, why?

REFERENCES

Adult Vaccine Preventable Diseases Bureau. (1997). Pneumococcal and influenza vaccination levels among adults aged > 65 years—United States, 1995. *MMWR, 46,* 913–919.

Advisory Committee for the Elimination of Tuberculosis. (1989). A strategic plan for the elimination of tuberculosis in the United States. *MMWR, 38*(S-3), 1–25.

Advisory Committee on Immunization Practices. (1993). Use of vaccines and immune globulins in persons with altered immunocompetence. *MMWR, 42*(RR-4), 1–18.

Advisory Committee on Immunization Practices. (1994). General recommendations on immunization. *MMWR, 43*(RR-1), 1–38.

Advisory Committee on Immunization Practices. (1995). Assessing adult vaccination status at age 50 years. *MMWR, 44,* 561–563.

Alter, H., Nakatsuji, Y., Melpolder, J., et al. (1997). The incidence of transfusion-associated hepatitis G virus infection and its relation to liver disease. *New England Journal of Medicine, 336,* 747–754.

Anderson, C. (1995). Childhood sexually transmitted diseases: One consequence of sexual abuse. *Public Health Nursing, 12,* 41–46.

Arden, N. H., Cox, N. J., & Schonberger, L. B. (1997). Prevention and control of influenza: Recommendations of the Advisory Committee on Immunization Practices (ACIP). *MMWR, 46*(RR-9), 1–25.

Araneta, M. R. G., Mascola, L., Eller, A., et al. (1995). HIV transmission through donor artificial insemination. *JAMA, 273,* 854–858.

Atkinson, W. L. (1997). Ask the experts. *Needle Tips and the Hepatitis B Coalition News, 7*(1), 1, 6–8.

Bayer, R., Dubler, N. N., & Landesman, S. (1993). The dual epidemics of tuberculosis and AIDS: Ethical and policy issues in screening and treatment. *American Journal of Public Health, 83,* 649–653.

Bellin, E., Fletcher, D., & Safyer, S. (1993). Abnormal chest x-rays in intravenous drug users: Implications for tuberculosis screening programs. *American Journal of Public Health, 83,* 698–700.

Benenson, A. S. (Ed.). (1995). *Control of communicable diseases manual* (16th ed.). Washington, DC: American Public Health Association.

Berman, S. M., Campbell, C. H., Geisman, K., et al. (1993). Recommendations for the prevention and management of *Chlamydia trachomatis* infections, 1993. *MMWR, 42*(RR-12), 1–39.

Bertolli, J., St. Louis, M. E., Simonds, R. J., et al. (1996). Estimating the timing of mother-to-child transmission of human immunodeficiency virus in a breast-feeding population in Kinshasa, Zaire. *Journal of Infectious Diseases, 174,* 722–726.

Bloch, A. B. (1995). Screening for tuberculosis infection in high-risk populations: Recommendations of the Advisory Council for the Elimination of Tuberculosis. *MMWR, 44*(RR-11), 18–34.

Boutotte, J. (1993, May). TB the second time around. *Nursing 93,* 42–49.

Bozzi, C. J., Burwen, D. R., Dooley, S. W., et al. (1994). Guidelines for preventing the transmission of *Mycobacterium tuberculosis* in health care facilities, 1994. *MMWR, 43*(RR-13), 1–132.

Bresee, J. S., Mast, E. E., Coleman, P. J., et al. (1996). Hepatitis C virus infection associated with administration of intravenous immune globulin. *JAMA, 276,* 1563–1567.

Bryan, R. T., Pinner, R. W., Gaynes, R. P., Peters, C. J., Aguilar, J. R., & Berkelman, R. L. (1994). Addressing emerging infectious disease threats: A prevention strategy for the United States. Executive summary. *MMWR, 43*(RR-15), 1–18.

Caldwell, M. B., Oxtoby, M. J., Simonds, R. J., Lindegren, M. L., & Rogers, M. F. (1994). 1994 revised classification system for human immunodeficiency syndrome virus infection in children less than 13 years of age. *MMWR, 43*(RR-12), 1–10.

Carpenter, C. C. J., Fischl, M. A., Hammer, S. M., et al. (1996). Antiretroviral therapy for HIV infection in 1996. *JAMA, 276,* 146–154.

Castro, K. G., Ward, J. W., Slutsker, L., Buehler, J. W., Jaffe, H. W., & Berkelman, R. L. (1992). 1993 revised classification system for HIV infection and expanded surveillance case definition for AIDS among adolescents and adults. *MMWR, 41*(RR-17), 1–19.

Castro, V. J., Sara, M., & Wyrwinski, P. (1997). Gonococcal endocarditis: An unusual deadly complication. *Resident & Staff Physician, 43*(8), 31–34.

Catania, J. A., Binson, D., Dolcini, M. M., et al. (1995). Risk factors for HIV and other sexually transmitted diseases and prevention practices among US heterosexual adults: Changes from 1990 to 1992. *American Journal of Public Health, 85,* 1492–1499.

Center for Drug Evaluation and Research. (1996). Clinical update: Impact of HIV protease inhibitors on the treatment of HIV-infected tuberculosis patients with rifampin. *MMWR, 45,* 921–925.

Centers for Disease Control. (1993). Summary of notifiable diseases, United States, 1992. *MMWR, 41*(55), 1–73.

Centers for Disease Control. (1994). *Addressing emerging infectious disease threats: A prevention strategy for the United States.* Atlanta: Centers for Disease Control and Prevention.

Centers for Disease Control. (1996). Summary of notifiable diseases, United States, 1995. *MMWR, 44*(53), 1–87.

Centers for Disease Control. (1997a). Case definitions of infectious conditions under public health surveillance. *MMWR, 46*(RR-10), 1–55.

Centers for Disease Control. (1997b). Measles eradication: Recommendations from a meeting cosponsored by the World Health Organization, the Pan American Health Organization, and CDC. *MMWR, 46*(RR-11), 1–20.

Centers for Disease Control. (1997c). Pertussis vaccination: Use of acellular pertussis vaccines among infants and young children. *MMWR, 46*(RR-7), 1–25.

Chaulk, C. P., Moore-Rice, K., Rizzo, R., & Chaisson, R. E. (1995). Eleven years of community-based directly observed therapy for tuberculosis. *JAMA, 274,* 945–951.

Childhood and Respiratory Diseases Bureau. (1996). Progress toward the elimination of *Haemophilus influenza* type b disease among infants and children—United States, 1987–1995. *MMWR, 45,* 901–906.

Childhood Vaccine Preventable Diseases Bureau. (1995). Pertussis—United States, January 1992–June 1995. *MMWR, 44,* 525–529.

Childhood Vaccine Preventable Diseases Bureau. (1996). Update: Diphtheria epidemic—New Independent States of the former Soviet Union, January 1995–March 1996. *MMWR, 45,* 693–697.

Childhood Vaccine Preventable Diseases Bureau. (1997a). Paralytic poliomyelitis—United States, 1980–1994. *MMWR, 46,* 79–83.

Childhood Vaccine Preventable Diseases Bureau. (1997b). Pertussis outbreak—Vermont, 1996. *MMWR, 46,* 822–826.

Childhood Vaccine Preventable Diseases Bureau. (1997c). Rubella and congenital rubella syndrome—United States, 1994–1997. *MMWR, 46,* 350–354.

Choo, P. W., Donahue, J. G., Manson, J. E., & Platt, R. (1995). The epidemiology of varicella and its complications. *Journal of Infectious Diseases, 172,* 706–712.

Clements, D. A., Langdon, L., Bland, C., & Walter, E. (1995). Influenza A vaccine decreases the incidence of otitis media in 6- to 30-month-old children in day care. *Archives of Pediatric and Adolescent Medicine, 149,* 1113–1117.

Cobb, J. C. (1997). Outercourse as a safe and sensible alternative to contraceptives. *American Journal of Public Health, 87,* 1380–1381.

Colditz, G. A., Berkey, C. S., Mosteller, F., et al. (1995). The efficacy of Bacillus Calmette–Guerin vaccination of newborns and infants in the prevention of tuberculosis: Meta-analyses of the published data. *Pediatrics, 96*(1), 29–35.

Collier, A. C., Coombs, R. W., Schoenfeld, D. A., et al. (1996). Treatment of human immunodeficiency virus infection with saquinavir, zidovudine, and zalcitabine. *New England Journal of Medicine, 334,* 1011–1017.

Committee on Infectious Diseases. (1995). Recommendations for the use of live attenuated varicella vaccine. *Pediatrics, 95,* 791–795.

Conti, L., Lieb, S., Liberti, T., Wiley-Bayless, M., Hepburn, K., & Diaz, T. (1995). Pet ownership among persons with AIDS in three Florida counties. *American Journal of Public Health, 85,* 1559–1561.

Cook, S. L., Koutsky, L. A., & Holmes, K. K. (1994). Circumcision and sexually transmitted diseases. *American Journal of Public Health, 84,* 197–201.

Crowe, H. M. (1994). Hepatitis A, B, C, D, E: Infection prevention issues. *Asepsis: The Infection Prevention Forum, 16*(2), 13–17.

Darby, S. C., Ewart, D. W., Giangrande, P. L. F., Spooner, R. J. D., & Rizza, C. R. (1996). Importance of age at infection with HIV-1 for survival and development of AIDS in UK haemophilia population. *Lancet, 347,* 1573–1579.

Davis, S. F., Byers, R. H., Lindegren, M. L., Caldwell, M. B., Karon, J. M., & Gwinn, M. (1995). Prevalence and incidence of vertically acquired HIV infection in the United States. *JAMA, 274,* 952–955.

Di Bisceglie, A. M., Conjeevaram, H. S., Fried, M. W., et al. (1995). Ribavirin as therapy for chronic hepatitis C: A randomized, double-blind, placebo-controlled study. *Annals of Internal Medicine, 123,* 897–903.

Dienstag, J. L., Perrillo, R. P., Schiff, E. R., Bartholomew, M., Vicary, C., & Rubin, M. (1995). A preliminary trial of lamivudine for chronic hepatitis B infection. *New England Journal of Medicine, 333,* 1657–1661.

Division of Cancer Prevention and Control. (1997). Nosocomial hepatitis B infection associated with reusable fingerstick blood sampling devices—Ohio and New York City, 1996. *MMWR, 46,* 217–221.

Division of Epidemiology and Surveillance. (1995). Transmission of pertussis from adult to infant—Michigan, 1993. *MMWR, 44,* 74–76.

Division of Health Interview Statistics. (1996). HIV testing among women aged 18–44 years—United States, 1991 and 1993. *MMWR, 43,* 733–737.

Division of HIV/AIDS. (1994). AIDS among racial/ethnic minorities—United States, 1993. *MMWR, 43,* 644–647, 653–655.

Division of HIV/AIDS Prevention. (1995a). Case-control study of HIV seroconversion in health-care workers after percutaneous exposure to HIV-infected blood—France, United Kingdom, and United States, January 1988–August 1994. *MMWR, 44,* 929–933.

Division of HIV/AIDS Prevention. (1995b). First 500,000 AIDS cases—United States, 1995. *MMWR, 44,* 849–853.

Division of HIV/AIDS Prevention. (1995c). Syringe exchange programs—United States, 1994–1995. *MMWR, 44,* 684–685, 691.

Division of HIV/AIDS Prevention. (1996a). AIDS among children—United States, 1996. *MMWR, 45,* 1005–1010.

Division of HIV/AIDS Prevention. (1996b). AIDS associated with injecting drug use—United States, 1995. *MMWR, 453,* 392–398.

Division of HIV/AIDS Prevention—Surveillance and Epidemiology. (1997). Update: Trends in AIDS incidence—United States, 1996. *MMWR, 46,* 861–867.

Division of Sexually Transmitted Disease Prevention. (1997a). Chlamydia screening practices of primary-care providers—Wake County, North Carolina, 1996. *MMWR, 46,* 819–822.

Division of Sexually Transmitted Disease Prevention. (1997b). *Chlamydia trachomatis* genital infections—United States, 1995. *MMWR, 46,* 193–198.

Division of Tuberculosis Elimination. (1994a). Expanded tuberculosis surveillance and tuberculosis mortality—United States, 1993. *MMWR, 43,* 361–366.

Division of Tuberculosis Elimination. (1994b). Multidrug-resistant tuberculosis in a hospital—Jersey City, New Jersey, 1990–1992. *MMWR, 43,* 417–419.

Division of Tuberculosis Elimination. (1996). Characteristics of foreign-born Hispanic patients with tuberculosis—eight U.S. counties bordering Mexico, 1995. *MMWR, 45,* 1032–1036.

Division of Tuberculosis Elimination. (1997a). Multiple

misdiagnosis of tuberculosis resulting from laboratory error—Wisconsin, 1996. *MMWR, 46,* 797–801.

Division of Tuberculosis Elimination. (1997b). Tuberculin skin test survey in a pediatric population with high BCG vaccine coverage——Botswana, 1996. *MMWR, 46,* 846–851.

Division of Tuberculosis Elimination. (1997c). Tuberculosis morbidity—United States, 1996. *MMWR, 46,* 695–700.

El-Sadr, W., Medard, F., & Barthaud, V. (1996). Directly observed therapy for tuberculosis: The Harlem Hospital experience. *American Journal of Public Health, 86,* 1146–1149.

Epidemiology and Surveillance Bureau. (1996). Outbreak of primary and secondary syphilis—Baltimore City, Maryland, 1995. *MMWR, 45,* 166–169.

Epidemiology Research Bureau. (1995). Increasing incidence of gonorrhea—Minnesota, 1994. *MMWR, 44,* 282–287.

Esteban, J. I., Gomez, J., Martell, M., et al. (1996). Transmission of hepatitis C virus by a cardiac surgeon. *New England Journal of Medicine, 334,* 555–560.

Farci, P., Mandas, A., Coiana, A., et al. (1994). Treatment of chronic hepatitis D with interferon alpha-2a. *New England Journal of Medicine, 330,* 88–94.

Global Program on Vaccines and Immunization. (1996). Poliomyelitis outbreak—Albania, 1996. *MMWR, 45,* 819–820.

Gonorrhea, Chlamydia, and Chancroid Bureau. (1997). Gonorrhea among men who have sex with men—Sexually transmitted disease clinics, 1993–1996. *MMWR, 46,* 889–892.

Gourevitch, M. A., Hartel, D., Schoenbaum, E., et al. (1996). A prospective study of syphilis and HIV infection among injection drug users receiving methadone in Bronx, New York. *American Journal of Public Health, 86,* 1112–1115.

Graham, S. M., & Cruise, P. E. (1996). Prevention and control of tuberculosis in correctional facilities: Recommendations of the Advisory Council for the Elimination of Tuberculosis. *MMWR, 45*(RR-8), 1–27.

Greendale, G. A., Haas, S. T., Holbrook, K., Walsh, B., Schachter, J., & Phillips, R. S. (1993). The relationship of *Chlamydia trachomatis* to male infertility. *American Journal of Public Health, 83,* 996–1001.

Grimes, D. E., & Grimes, R. M. (1995). Tuberculosis: What nurses need to know to help control the epidemic. *Nursing Outlook, 43,* 164–173.

Grubman, S., Oleske, J. M., Simonds, R. J., Rogers, M. F., & Moseley, R. R. (1995). 1995 revised guidelines for prophylaxis against *Pneumocystis carinii* pneumonia for children infected with or perinatally exposed to human immunodeficiency virus. *MMWR, 44*(RR-4), 1–11.

Guly, C. (1994, September 6). The invisible lesbian face of AIDS. *The Advocate,* 45.

Harpaz, R., Von Seidlein, L., Averhoff, F. M., et al. (1996). Transmission of hepatitis B virus to multiple patients from a surgeon without evidence of inadequate infection control. *New England Journal of Medicine, 334,* 549–554.

Health Care Financing Administration. (1997). Missed opportunities for pneumococcal and influenza immunization of Medicare pneumonia patients—12 western states, 1995. *MMWR, 46,* 919–923.

Hematologic Diseases Bureau. (1996). Hepatitis A among persons with hemophilia who received clotting factor concentrate—United States, September–December 1995. *MMWR, 45,* 29–32.

Hematologic Diseases Bureau. (1997). Transmission of hepatitis C virus infection associated with home infusion therapy for hemophilia. *MMWR, 46,* 597–599.

Hepatitis Bureau. (1993). Hepatitis E among U.S. travelers, 1989–1992. *MMWR, 42,* 1–4.

Hepatitis Bureau. (1997a). Hepatitis A vaccination programs in communities with high rates of hepatitis A. *MMWR, 46,* 600–603.

Hepatitis Bureau. (1997b). Program to prevent perinatal hepatitis B virus transmission in a health-maintenance organization——Northern California, 1990–1995. *MMWR, 46,* 378–380.

Hepatitis Bureau. (1997c). Recommendations for follow-up of health-care workers after occupational exposure to hepatitis C virus. *MMWR, 46,* 603–606.

Herek, G. M., & Capitano, J. P. (1993). Public reactions to AIDS in the United States: A second decade of stigma. *American Journal of Public Health, 83,* 574–577.

Hillis, S. D., Owens, L. M., Marchbanks, P. A., Amsterdam, L. E., & MacKenzie, W. R. (1997). Recurrent chlamydial infections increase the risks of hospitalization for ectopic pregnancy and pelvic inflammatory disease. *American Journal of Obstetrics and Gynecology, 176,* 103–107.

HIV Laboratory Investigations Bureau. (1997). Transmission of HIV possibly associated with exposure of mucous membrane to contaminated blood. *MMWR, 46,* 620–623.

Holmes, S. J., Reef, S., Hadler, S. C., Williams, W. W., & Wharton, M. (1996). Prevention of varicella: Recommendations of the Advisory Committee on Immunization Practices. *MMWR, 45*(RR-11), 1–36.

International Task Force for Disease Eradication. (1993). Recommendations of the International Task Force for Disease Eradication. *MMWR, 42*(RR-16), 1–38.

Izurieta, H. S., Sutter, R. W., Strebel, P. M., et al. (1997). Tetanus surveillance—United States, 1991–1994. *MMWR, 46*(SS-2), 15–25.

Johnson, A. M., Grun, L., & Haines, A. (1996). Controlling genital chlamydial infection. *British Medical Journal, 313,* 1160–1161.

Johnson, M. P., Coberly, J. S., Clermont, H. C., et al.

(1992). Tuberculin skin test reactivity among adults infected with human immunodeficiency virus. *Journal of Infectious Diseases, 166,* 194–198.

Joseph, S. C. (1992). *Dragon within the gates: The once and future AIDS epidemic.* New York: Carroll & Graf.

Kao, J., Hwang, Y., Chen, P., et al. (1996). Transmission of hepatitis C virus between spouses: The important role of exposure duration. *American Journal of Gastroenterology, 91,* 2087–2090.

Kaplan, J. E., Masur, H., & Holmes, K. K. (1997). 1997 USPHS/ISDA guidelines for the prevention of opportunistic infections in persons infected with human immunodeficiency virus. *MMWR, 46*(RR-12), 1–46.

Karim, Q. A., Karim, S. S. A., Soldan, K., & Zondi, M. (1995). Reducing the risk of HIV infection among South African sex workers: Socioeconomic and gender barriers. *American Journal of Public Health, 85,* 1521–1525.

Kilmarx, P. H., & St. Louis, M. E. (1995). The evolving epidemiology of syphilis. *American Journal of Public Health, 85,* 1053–1054.

King, G. E., Markowitz, L. E., Health, J., et al. (1996). Antibody response to measles-mumps-rubella vaccine of children with mild illness at the time of vaccination. *JAMA, 275,* 704–707.

Koehler, R. J. (1994). HIV infection, TB, and health crisis in corrections. *Public Administration Review, 54*(1), 31–35.

Kohn, M. A., Farley, T. A., Sundin, D., Tapia, R., McFarland, L. M., & Arden, N. H. (1995). Three summertime outbreaks of influenza type A. *Journal of Infectious Diseases, 175,* 246–249.

Lackritz, E. M., Satten, G. A., Aberle-Grasse, J., et al. (1995). Estimated risk of transmission of the human immunodeficiency virus by screened blood in the United States. *New England Journal of Medicine, 333,* 1721–1725.

Langston, C., Lewis, D. E., Hammill, H. A., et al. (1995). Excess intrauterine fetal demise associated with maternal human immunodeficiency virus infection. *Journal of Infectious Diseases, 172,* 1451–1460.

Lurie, P., Avins, A. L., Phillips, K. A., Kahn, J. G., Lowe, R. A., & Ciccarone, D. (1994). The cost-effectiveness of voluntary counseling and testing of hospital inpatients for HIV infection. *JAMA, 272,* 1832–1838.

Mahon, N. (1996). New York inmate's HIV risk behaviors: The implications for prevention policy and programs. *American Journal of Public Health, 86,* 1211–1215.

Marchou, B., Excler, J., Bourderioux, C., et al. (1995). A 3-week hepatitis B vaccination schedule provides rapid and persistent protective immunity: A multicenter, randomized trial comparing accelerated and classic vaccination schedules. *Journal of Infectious Diseases, 172,* 258–260.

Marsano, L. S., Greenberg, R. N., Kirkpatrick, R. B., et al.

(1996). Comparison of a rapid hepatitis B immunization schedule to the standard schedule for adults. *American Journal of Gastroenterology, 91,* 111–115.

McEnany, G. W., Hughes, A. M., & Lee, K. A. (1996). Depression and HIV: A nursing perspective on a complex relationship. *Nursing Clinics of North America, 31,* 57–80.

McKillip, J. (1991). Public health and the law: The effects of mandatory premarital testing on marriage: The case of Illinois. *American Journal of Public Health, 81,* 650–653.

Measles Virus Section, Respiratory and Enteric Viruses Bureau. (1996). Measles——United States, 1995. *MMWR, 45,* 305–307.

Meehan, T. M., Hansen, H., & Klein, W. C. (1997). The impact of parental consent on the HIV testing of minors. *American Journal of Public Health, 87,* 1338–1341.

Mertz, G. J., Loveless, M. O., Levin, M. J., et al. (1997). Oral famcyclovir for suppression of recurrent genital herpes simplex virus infection in women. *Archives of Internal Medicine, 157,* 343–349.

Mofenson, L., Balsley, J., Simonds, R. J., Rogers, M. F., & Moseley, R. R. (1994). Recommendations of the U.S. Public Health Service Task Force on the use of zidovudine to reduce perinatal transmission of human immunodeficiency virus. *MMWR, 43*(RR-11), 1–20.

Monastersky, R. (1992). Pentamidine may have dementia payoff. *Science News, 141,* 191.

Mortality Statistics Bureau. (1996). Mortality patterns—United States, 1993. *MMWR, 456,* 161–164.

Mortimer, E. A. (1994). Communicable diseases. In I. B. Pless (Ed.), *The epidemiology of childhood disorders* (pp. 229–274). New York: Oxford University Press.

Mosley, J. W. (1993). Virus transmission in health care settings: Precautions, epidemiologic experience, and common sense. *American Journal of Public Health, 83,* 1164–1165.

National AIDS Information and Education Program. (1994). HIV prevention practices of primary-care physicians—United States, 1992. *MMWR, 42,* 988–992.

National Association of County Health Officials. (1993). *Local health department strategies for improving childhood immunization rates.* Washington, DC: National Association of County Health Officials.

National Center for Health Statistics. (1997a). *Fertility, family planning and women's health: New data from the 1995 National Survey of Family Growth.* Washington, DC: Centers for Disease Control and Prevention.

National Center for Health Statistics. (1997b). Status report on the Childhood Immunization Initiative: National, state, and urban area vaccination coverage levels among children aged 19–35 months—United States, 1996. *MMWR, 46,* 657–664.

National Center for HIV, STD, and TB Prevention. (1996a, November). The Scope of the HIV/AIDS epidemic. *Focus on HIV/AIDS Prevention,* 1–3.

National Center for HIV, STD, and TB Prevention. (1996b, November). STDs in the United States. *Focus on STD Prevention,* 1–4.

National Center for HIV, STD, and TB Prevention. (1996c, November). Trends in TB cases in the United States. *Focus on TB Elimination,* 1–3.

National Center for Infectious Diseases. (1995). Tuberculosis among foreign-born persons who had recently arrived in the United States—Hawaii, 1992–1993, and Los Angeles County, 1993. *MMWR, 44,* 703–707.

National Center for Infectious Diseases. (1996). Progress toward global eradication of poliomyelitis, 1995. *MMWR, 45,* 565–568.

National Center for Infectious Diseases. (1997). Toxigenic *Corynebacterium diphtheriae*—Northern Plains Indian community, August–October 1996. *MMWR, 46,* 506–510.

National Immunization Program. (1994a). Outbreak of measles among Christian Science students—Missouri and Illinois, 1994. *MMWR, 43,* 463–465.

National Immunization Program. (1994b). Rubella and congenital rubella syndrome—United States, January 1, 1991–May 7, 1994. *MMWR, 43,* 397–401.

National Immunization Program. (1994c). Update: Childhood vaccine-preventable diseases—United States, 1994. *MMWR, 43,* 718–720.

National Institutes of Health. (1995). *NIH consensus statement: Infectious disease testing for blood transfusions.* Bethesda, MD: National Institutes of Health.

National Institute for Occupational Safety and Health. (1995). Proportionate mortality from pulmonary tuberculosis associated with occupations—28 states, 1979–1990. *MMWR, 44,* 14–19.

Niederau, C., Heintges, T., Lange, S., et al. (1996). Long-term follow-up of HBeAg-positive patients treated with interferon alfa for chronic hepatitis B. *New England Journal of Medicine, 334,* 1422–1427.

Nennig, M. E., Shinefield, H. R., Edwards, K. M., Black, S. B., & Fireman, B. H. (1996). Prevalence and incidence of adult pertussis in an urban population. *JAMA, 275,* 1672–1674.

Ostergaard, L., Moller, J. K., Anderson, B., & Olesen, F. (1996). Diagnosis of urogenital *Chlamydia trachomatis* infection in women based on mailed samples obtained at home: Multipractice comparative study. *British Medical Journal, 313,* 1186–1189.

Pablos-Mendez, A., Blustein, J., & Knirsch, C. A. (1997). The role of diabetes mellitus in the higher prevalence of tuberculosis among Hispanics. *American Journal of Public Health, 87,* 574–579.

Paul, E. A., Lebowitz, S. M., Moore, R. E., Hoven, C. W., Bennett, B. A., & Chen, A. (1993). Nemesis revisited: Tuberculosis in a New York City men's shelter. *American Journal of Public Health, 83,* 1743–1745.

Pavia, A. T., Benyo, M., Niler, L., & Risk, I. (1993). Partner notification for control of HIV: Results after 2 years of a statewide program in Utah. *American Journal of Public Health, 83,* 1418–1424.

Potter, J., Stott, D. J., Roberts, M. A., et al. (1997). Influenza vaccination of health care workers in long-term-care hospitals reduces the mortality in elderly patients. *Journal of Infectious Diseases, 175,* 1–6.

Powell-Griner, E., Anderson, J. E., & Murphy, W. (1997). State- and sex-specific prevalence of selected characteristics—Behavioral Risk Factor Surveillance System, 1994 and 1995. *MMWR, 46*(SS-3), 1–31.

Poynard, T., Bedossa, P., Chevallier, M., et al. (1995). A comparison of three interferon alfa-2b regimens for the long-term treatment of chronic non-A, non-B hepatitis. *New England Journal of Medicine, 334,* 1457–1462.

Prevots, D. R., Sutter, R. W., Strebel, P. M., Wharton, M., & Hadler, S. C. (1997). Poliomyelitis prevention in the United States: Introduction of a sequential vaccination schedule of inactivated poliovirus vaccine followed by oral poliovirus vaccine. *MMWR, 46*(RR-3), 1–25.

Quinn, T. C., Gaydos, C., Shepherd, M., et al. (1996). Epidemiologic and microbiologic correlates of *Chlamydia trachomatis* infection in sexual partnerships. *JAMA, 276,* 1737–1742.

Redd, J. T., & Susser, E. (1997). Controlling tuberculosis in an urban emergency department: A rapid decision instrument for patient isolation. *American Journal of Public Health, 87,* 1543–1547.

Rogers, M. F., Moseley, R. R., Simonds, R. J., et al. (1995). U.S. Public Health Service recommendations for human immunodeficiency virus counseling and voluntary testing for pregnant women. *MMWR, 44*(RR-7), 1–15.

Rogers, M. F., Simonds, R. J., Lawton, K. E., Moseley, R. R., & Jones, W. K. (1994). Guidelines for preventing transmission of human immunodeficiency virus through transplantation of human tissue and organs. *MMWR, 43*(RR-8), 1–17.

Rosica, T. C. (1995). AIDS and boundaries: Instinct versus empathy. *Focus: A Guide to AIDS Research and Counseling, 10*(2), 1–4.

Rothenberg, K. H., & Paskey, S. J. (1995). The risk of domestic violence and women with HIV infection: Implications for partner notification, public policy, and the law. *American Journal of Public Health, 85,* 1569–1576.

Sacks, S. L., Aoki, F. Y., Diaz-Mitoma, F., Sellors, J., & Shafran, S. D. (1996). Patient-initiated, twice daily oral famcyclovir for early recurrent genital herpes. *JAMA, 276,* 44–49.

Schmitt, H. J., von Konig, W., Neiss, A., et al. (1996). Efficacy of acellular pertussis vaccine in early childhood after household exposure. *JAMA, 275,* 37–41.

Schulman, S. T., McKendrick, W. P., & Atamos, J. K.

(1993). *Handbook of pediatric infectious disease and antimicrobial therapy.* St. Louis: Mosby Year Book.

Shapiro, C. N., Bell, B. P., & Margolis, H. S. (1996). Prevention of hepatitis A through active or passive immunization: Recommendations of the Advisory Committee on Immunization Practices (ACIP). *MMWR, 45*(RR-15), 1–30.

Smith Kline Beecham Pharmaceuticals. (1992). *Chronic viral hepatitis backgrounder.* Philadelphia: Smith Kline Beecham.

Smith Kline Beecham Pharmaceuticals. (1995a). *Havrix: Hepatitis A vaccine, inactivated.* Philadelphia: Smith Kline Beecham.

Smith Kline Beecham Pharmaceuticals. (1995b). *Hepatitis B prevention.* Philadelphia: Smith Kline Beecham.

Stone, V. E., Seage, G. R., & Epstein, A. M. (1992). The relations between hospital experience and mortality for patients with AIDS. *JAMA, 268*, 2655–2661.

Stutman, H. R. (1996, Winter). Varicella vaccine. *Perinatal Care Matters, 1*, 4.

Surveillance and Information Systems Bureau. (1994). Chlamydia prevalence and screening practices—San Diego County, California, 1993. *MMWR, 43*, 366–369, 375.

Tagg, P. I. (1996). Chlamydia: What you should know. *Nurse Practitioner, 21*, 133–134.

Tong, M. J., El-Farra, N. S., Reikes, A. R., & Co, R. L. (1995). Clinical outcomes after transfusion-associated hepatitis C. *New England Journal of Medicine, 332*, 1463–1466.

Ungvarsky, P. J., & Schmidt, J. (1992). The most common opportunistic infections. *RN, 55*(11), 37–45.

U.S. Department of Health and Human Services. (1991). *Healthy people 2000: National health promotion and disease prevention objectives.* Washington, DC: Government Printing Office.

U.S. Department of Health and Human Services. (1993). *Health United States, 1992, and healthy people 2000 review.* Washington, DC: Government Printing Office.

U.S. Department of Health and Human Services. (1995a). *Healthy people 2000: Midcourse review and 1995 revisions.* Washington, DC: Government Printing Office.

U.S. Department of Health and Human Services. (1995b). *Untitled communication.* Washington, DC: U.S. Public Health Service.

U.S. Department of Health and Human Services. (1996, October 31). *Healthy people 2000: Progress review—Immunization and infectious diseases.* Washington, DC: Government Printing Office.

U.S. Department of Health and Human Services. (1997, July 8). *Healthy people 2000: Progress review: HIV infection.* Washington, DC: Government Printing Office.

U.S. Public Health Service Task Force on Prophylaxis and Therapy for *Mycobacterium avium* complex.

(1993). Recommendations on prophylaxis and therapy for disseminated *Mycobacterium avium* complex for adults and adolescents with human immunodeficiency virus. *MMWR, 42*(RR-9), 13–19.

Villarino, M. E., Huebner, R. E., Lanner, A. H., & Geiter, L. J. (1996). The role of BCG vaccine in the prevention and control of tuberculosis in the United States: A joint statement by the Advisory Council for the Elimination of Tuberculosis and the Advisory Committee on Immunization Practices. *MMWR, 44*(RR-4), 1–18.

van Loon, F. P. L., Holmes, S. J., Sirotkin, B. I., et al. (1995). Mumps surveillance—United States, 1988–1993. *MMWR, 44*(SS-3), 1–14.

Wald, A., Zeh, J., Barnum G., Davis, L. G., & Corey, L. (1996). Suppression of subclinical shedding of herpes simplex virus type 2 with acyclovir. *Annals of Internal Medicine, 1241*, (pt. 1), 8–15.

Ward, J. S., Janssen, R. S., Jaffe, H. W., & Curran, J. W. (1993). Recommendations for HIV testing services for inpatients and outpatients in acute-care hospital settings. *MMWR, 42*(RR-2), 1–6.

Whittum-Hudson, J. A., An, L., Saltzman, W. M., Prendergast, R. A., & MacDonald, A. B. (1996). Oral immunization with an anti-idiotypic antibody to the exoglycolipid antigen protects against experimental *Chlamydia trachomatis* infection. *Nature Medicine, 2*, 1116–1121.

Wilkinson, D., Davies, G. R., & Connolly, F. (1996). Directly observed therapy for tuberculosis in rural South Africa, 1991 through 1994. *American Journal of Public Health, 86*, 1094–1097.

Willis, B. M., Schwartz, L. P., & Knowlton, S. B. (1993). Tuberculosis control laws—United States, 1993. *MMWR, 42*(RR-15), 1–28.

Wolfe, H., Marmor, M., Maslansky, R., et al. (1995). Tuberculosis knowledge among New York City injection drug users. *American Journal of Public Health, 85*, 985–988.

Yinnon, A. M., Coury-Doniger, P., Polito, R., & Reichman, R. C. (1996). Serologic response to treatment of syphilis in patients with HIV infection. *Archives of Internal Medicine, 156*, 321–325.

Zoloth, S. R., Safyer, S., Rosen, J., et. al. (1993). Anergy compromises screening for tuberculosis in high-risk populations. *American Journal of Public Health, 83*, 749–751.

RESOURCES FOR COMMUNICABLE DISEASE CONTROL

American Council for Healthful Living
c/o Jane Westlake
Elite Graphics
285 Changebridge Road
Pine Brook, NJ 07058
(201) 808–9769

American Foundation for AIDS Research
733 Third Avenue, 12th Floor
New York, NY
(212) 682–7440

American Foundation for Prevention of Venereal
    Disease, Inc.
799 Broadway, Ste. 638
New York, NY 10003
(212) 759–2069

American Medical Association
515 N. State Street
Chicago, IL 60610–0174
(312) 464–4470

American Social Health Association
PO Box 13827
Research Triangle Park, NC 27709
(919) 361–8400

CDC National AIDS Clearinghouse (NAC)
Centers for Disease Control
PO Box 6003
Rockville, MD 20849–6003
(800) 458–5231

Centers for Disease Control
Center for Infectious Diseases
1600 Clifton Road
Atlanta, GA 30333
(404) 639–3401

Citizens' Alliance for VD Awareness
PO Box 31915
Chicago, IL 60631–0915
(847) 398–3378

Hepatitis B Coalition
1573 Selby Avenue, Ste. 229
St. Paul, MN 55104
(612) 647–9009

Herpes Resource Center/American Social Health
    Association
PO Box 13827
Research Triangle Park, NC 27709
(919) 361–8488

March of Dimes Birth Defects Foundation
1275 Mamaroneck Avenue
White Plains, NY 10605
(914) 428–7100

National Institute of Allergy and Infectious Diseases
Office of Communications
Building 31, Room 7A32
9000 Rockville Pike
Bethesda, MD 20892
(301) 496–5717

Operation Venus
1213 Clover Street
Philadelphia, PA 19107
(215) 567–6969

People with AIDS Coalition
50 West 17th Street, 8th Floor
New York, NY 10011–1607
(212) 647–1415

Shanti Project
1546 Market Street
San Francisco, CA 94102
(415) 864–2273

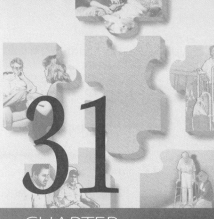

CHRONIC PHYSICAL HEALTH PROBLEMS

► KEY TERMS

chronic health problems
disability
impairment
handicap
risk markers

Because of the effectiveness of control measures developed for many previously fatal communicable diseases, chronic health problems have largely replaced communicable diseases as the leading causes of death and disability in the United States. Each year millions of people experience the suffering and the economic costs associated with chronic problems, and many die as a result. Diabetes, for example, caused more than 61,000 deaths in 1996 (Mortality Statistics Bureau, 1997) and costs the U.S. economy $92 billion annually (Division of Diabetes Translation, 1994a).

Chronic health problems are those that are present for extended periods and that are characterized by one or more distinctive features. These features may include nonreversible pathological changes, a need for lifestyle adjustment, or a prolonged period of supervision and care by health professionals. Chronic conditions include disease entities, injuries with lasting consequences, or other enduring abnormalities (Verbrugge & Patrick, 1995).

Chronic health problems may be either physical or emotional, and both types of chronic conditions are addressed in the national health objectives developed for the year 2000 (U.S. Department of Health and Human Services, 1991) (see Appendix A). The focus of this chapter, however, is chronic physical health problems. Chronic emotional conditions are addressed in Chapter 32.

▶ Chapter Objectives

After reading this chapter, you should be able to:

- Describe at least three personal effects and four population effects of chronic physical health problems.
- Identify at least three factors in the biophysical dimension that influence the development of chronic physical health problems.
- Describe at least two factors related to each of the psychological, physical, and social dimensions that influence chronic physical health problems and their consequences.
- Identify at least five behavioral dimension factors that contribute to the development of chronic physical health problems.
- Describe three health system factors that impede efforts to control chronic physical health problems.
- Describe at least four approaches to primary prevention of chronic physical health problems.
- Identify at least three aspects to the treatment of chronic physical health problems.
- Describe five considerations in tertiary prevention of chronic physical health problems.

▶ THE EFFECTS OF CHRONIC HEALTH PROBLEMS

Chronic health problems can arise from a variety of sources. For example, a person might develop a chronic disability as a result of a serious accident or because of arthritis. Other chronic conditions arise out of other disease processes such as cardiovascular disease, chronic respiratory diseases, and cancer. Some chronic conditions, such as some cancers, may result in death. Others, although not fatal, cause persistent pain and disability.

The effects of chronic health conditions are experienced not only by individuals. Population groups and society at large are also affected by the consequences of chronic health problems.

Personal Effects

The advent of a chronic condition has many personal effects for individual clients. The consequences of disease and injury include impairment, disability, and handicap (Disabilities Prevention Program, 1994). A fourth consequence is economic burden. *Impairment* refers to the loss of psychological, physiological, or anatomical structure or function. *Disability*, on the other hand, is a limitation in functional ability resulting from impairment (Disabilities Prevention Program, 1994). In 1994, approximately 14% of the U.S. population experienced some form of activity limitation due to a chronic condition (U.S. Department of Health and Human Services, 1996).

Activity restrictions often require a change in lifestyle. Individuals with arthritis, for example, may need to adjust to their inability to do some things that they have done in the past or may need to learn to use special implements to accomplish everyday tasks like closing a zipper or buttoning a shirt. Similarly, clients with chronic respiratory conditions may find that they are less able to engage in vigorous activity than in the past and may require more frequent rest periods, and the client seriously injured in an automobile accident may need to adjust to using a wheelchair. Frequently, such physical limitations make it necessary to rely on others to perform routine tasks of daily living. This enforced dependence on others may, in turn, adversely affect an individual's self-image.

Even when activities are not restricted, the presence of a chronic health problem usually requires lifestyle adjustments. For the person with diabetes or a heart condition, for example, changes in diet are required. The person with diabetes may also need to make changes in eating patterns. This might mean not skipping meals or not eating on the run.

Pain also accompanies a number of chronic conditions and is often unremitting. The client with arthritis or cancer, for example, may have to endure a long period of pain despite the continued use of analgesics. The constant battle with chronic pain can be disheartening and can lead to depression and possible suicide.

The third consequence of chronic conditions is *handicap* which is the disadvantage one experiences in interaction with the environment as a result of impairment or disability (Disabilities Prevention Program, 1994). The pain, lifestyle changes, decreased activity levels, and impaired mobility associated with chronic conditions can contribute to social isolation. The chronically ill individual may be less able to interact with others in familiar patterns or be unable to engage in activities that friends and family enjoy. Consequently, this person may feel left out unless concerted efforts are made to incorporate him or her into family and community life.

Finally, chronic health problems often entail considerable financial burden. Most chronic conditions require the individual to take prescribed medications for the rest of his or her life. For those taking medications for several chronic conditions, the cost can escalate rapidly. Add to this the cost of frequent visits to health care providers to monitor the condition and the effects of therapy. Moreover, many individuals with chronic conditions require expensive special equipment or services.

Population Effects

Chronic conditions also affect the general population. These effects are reflected in financial costs, mortality, and morbidity.

Societal Costs

Chronic health problems cost society millions of dollars each year. Societal costs of chronic health conditions include the direct monetary costs of health care as well as the indirect costs of lost productivity and use of limited resources. The overall cost of disabling conditions is estimated to be almost $170 billion per year (Disabilities Prevention Program, 1994). In 1990, health care costs for asthma amounted to $6.2 billion, or 1% of all U.S. health care expenditures (Air Pollution and Respiratory Health Bureau, 1996b), and, in 1993, accounted for 198,000 hospitalizations (Air Pollution and Respiratory Health Bureau, 1996a). Diabetes accounts for almost 15% of total U.S. health care spending (Division of Diabetes Translation, 1997a). Arthritis, which is the leading cause of disability in the United States, was associated with nearly $65 million in direct and indirect costs in 1992 (Division of Adult and Community Health, 1996).

Accidental injuries account for a major portion of societal costs related to chronic conditions. In 1994, for example, unintentional injuries in the United States cost $440 billion, with motor vehicle accidents accounting for $176.5 billion of these costs (U.S. Department of Commerce, 1996). Alcohol-related traffic accidents in 1990 cost more than $46 billion, only $5.1 billion of which was for medical care (Division of Unintentional Injury Prevention, 1994). Near drownings are another expensive form of accidental injury. Initial hospitalizations for near drownings in California children in 1991 cost more than $11 million, more than a third of which were paid by Medicaid (Ellis & Trent, 1995). It would seem clear from these cost figures alone that the United States can no longer bear the burden of chronic disease and must take steps to control the cost of these and other chronic conditions.

Morbidity

Societal costs of chronic health conditions are measured not only in dollars but also in terms of the ex-tent of morbidity resulting from these conditions. Although some progress has been made in preventing mortality due to chronic conditions, their prevalence has been increasing over the years. Because the reporting of chronic health conditions is not mandatory, however, prevalence figures probably grossly underrepresent the extent of these conditions in the population.

For example, hypertension affects approximately 50 million people in the United States (Lenfante, 1996). Cancer incidence has risen for most forms of cancer. In fact, it is estimated that 30% of the U.S. population will have some form of cancer during their lifetimes. From 1973 to 1992, annual incidence rates increased for cancers of the esophagus, colon and rectum, lungs, prostate, and bladder among men. For women, annual incidence increased for pancreatic, lung, breast, and ovarian cancers (U.S. Department of Health and Human Services, 1996). Each year approximately 182,000 women develop breast cancer (Ferris, Golden, Petry, Litaker, Nachenson, & Woodward, 1996), and roughly 30,000 people develop oral cancers (Division of Cancer Prevention and Control, 1994). In 1996, 1 million new diagnoses of malignant melanoma (Centers for Disease Control, 1996c) and more than 133,000 cases of colorectal cancer were expected (Division of Cancer Prevention and Control, 1996a).

Various forms of heart disease affect major segments of the U.S. population as well. Approximately 22 million Americans reported heart conditions in 1994 (U.S. Department of Commerce, 1996).

Approximately 16 million individuals in the United States have diabetes mellitus, a third of whom are not aware of their diagnosis (Centers for Disease Control, 1997). Each year, roughly 625,000 new diagnoses of diabetes are made (Centers for Disease Control, 1996b), and from 1980 to 1994 the prevalence of diabetes in the U.S. population increased 17% to 29.8 cases per 100,000 persons (Division of Diabetes Translation, 1997b).

Asthma affects about 14 million Americans (Air Pollution and Respiratory Health Bureau, 1996b), and its prevalence has increased steadily since 1982 to a rate of 49.4 per 1000 people in 1992, a 42% increase (Air Pollution and Respiratory Health Bureau, 1995). As noted in Chapter 20, asthma accounts for more school absences than any other condition. Asthma is also a significant problem in the workplace, where hypersensitive individuals may be exposed to small but significant amounts of respiratory irritants (Reilly, et al., 1994).

Arthritis is another chronic condition with significant health effects experienced by 40 million people in the United States. By 2020, arthritis may affect 60 million people (Centers for Disease Control, 1996a). Arthritic conditions include osteoarthritis, rheumatoid arthritis, gout, ankylosing spondylitis, and juvenile rheumatoid arthritis.

Accidental injuries also result in a significant proportion of chronic disability. Approximately one fourth of the entire U.S. population is injured each year (U.S. Department of Commerce, 1996). For example, bicycle accidents contribute to more than 180,000 head injuries each year, 76% of which occur in children under 15 years of age (Macknin & Mendendorp, 1994). Add to these the morbidity related to falls, poisonings, near drownings, and fires, and it becomes obvious that accident prevention should be a major health priority in the United States.

Obesity, itself a chronic condition as well as a contributor to other chronic health problems, is also highly prevalent in the U.S. population. More than 30% of Americans are 20% or more in excess of their ideal body weight (Zhang, Proenca, Maffei, Barone, Leopold, & Friedman, 1994). From 1987 to 1993, the prevalence of overweight in the United States increased by 5% (Galuska, Serdula, Pamuk, Siegel, & Byers, 1996).

Some of the increase in incidence and prevalence figures for chronic health problems is attributable to better diagnosis as well as to the ability to prevent deaths due to these conditions. These and similar figures for other chronic conditions, however, indicate that Americans are making little progress in the primary prevention of chronic health problems.

Mortality

Many chronic health conditions contribute to increased mortality and loss of productive years of life among the population. As with morbidity figures, mortality figures also provide only a partial picture of the extent of chronic health problems within the population; however, they can provide information on patterns and trends in chronic conditions over time.

Despite a marked decline in mortality, cardiovascular disease remains the leading cause of death in industrialized nations. The 1996 data indicated an age-adjusted mortality rate for heart disease in the United States of 134.6 deaths per 100,000 population, a 3% decline from the 1995 rate (Mortality Statistics Bureau, 1997). Age-adjusted cardiovascular mortality has shown a progressive decline with a 56% decrease in deaths from 1950 to 1996 (Mortality Statistics Bureau, 1977; U.S. Department of Health and Human Services, 1996).

Mortality due to stroke is also declining. The crude cerebrovascular disease mortality rate in 1996 was 60.5 deaths per 100,000 population, a considerable decline from 134 per 100,000 at the turn of the century (Mortality Statistics Bureau, 1997). Much of this progress, however, has been in preventing deaths due to stroke rather than in preventing the occurrence of stroke.

Mortality figures for malignant neoplasms are less favorable. Age-adjusted death rates for all forms of malignancy increased from 125.3 per 100,000 population in 1950 to 132.6 in 1993 (U.S. Department of Health and Human Services, 1996), then declined slightly to 129.1 per 100,000 in 1996 (Mortality Statistics Bureau, 1997). Some forms of cancer are greater contributors to increased mortality than others. Mortality due to lung cancer, for example, more than tripled from 1950 to 1993, whereas breast cancer deaths decreased by about 3% (U.S. Department of Health and Human Services, 1996). The greatest increase in mortality rates for malignancies occurred for malignant melanomas, which increased 34% from 1973 to 1992 (Centers for Disease Control, 1996c). In 1996, melanoma was expected to result in over 7000 deaths (Division of Cancer Prevention and Control, 1996b), and deaths due to colorectal cancer were expected to approach 55,000 (Division of Cancer Prevention and Control, 1996a).

Other chronic conditions also contribute to mortality figures for the nation. Diabetes mellitus, for example, accounted for more than 13 deaths per 100,000 population in 1996 (Mortality Statistics Bureau, 1997). This figure somewhat underrepresents the extent of the problem, as diabetes may contribute to death without being reported on death certificates. Chronic obstructive pulmonary disease (COPD) and allied conditions have also shown marked increases in mortality rates in recent years and were the fourth leading cause of death in the United States in 1996 (Mortality Statistics Bureau, 1997). For the general population, age-adjusted COPD mortality has increased from 4.4 deaths per 100,000 population in 1950 to 21.4 in 1993 (U.S. Department of Health and Human Services, 1996). Each year, 4000 to 5500 asthma-related deaths occur in the United States (Epidemiology Program Office, 1997), many of them among people under 25 years of age (Air Pollution and Respiratory Health Bureau, 1996a). Finally, chronic liver disease and cirrhosis caused 7.5 deaths per 100,000 people in 1996, and constituted the tenth highest cause of death. Accidents were the fifth leading cause of death at 30 deaths per 100,000 population (Mortality Statistics Bureau, 1997).

► THE DIMENSIONS MODEL AND CONTROL OF CHRONIC PHYSICAL HEALTH PROBLEMS

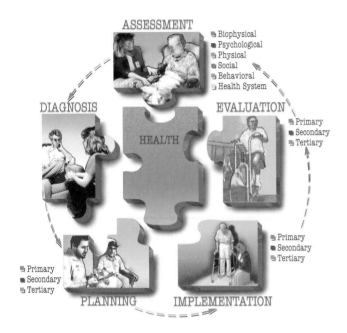

The Dimensions Model can be used to direct community health nursing actions to control chronic physical health problems experienced by individual clients or by population groups.

Critical Dimensions of Nursing in the Control of Chronic Physical Health Problems

Elements of each of the dimensions of nursing are employed in the control of chronic physical health problems, but elements of some dimensions are more critical to those efforts than others. For example, motivation to change unhealthful behaviors to prevent chronic diseases or to adhere to treatment regimens for existing chronic conditions may be difficult to achieve given the relatively low priority the American public assigns to health. Interpersonal skills by community health nurses will be critical in educating clients and the general public regarding the need for behavior changes and in motivating them to make those changes.

Nursing action may also be required in both the process and ethical dimensions to address the need for health promotion. In the process dimension, community health nurses will need to be actively involved in effecting a change in health care policy to reflect a greater focus on prevention, rather than cure, of chronic health problems. For example, nurses may engage in the political process to work for legislation in-

tended to foster health-promoting behaviors such as helmet use and smoking cessation. At the same time, community health nurses need to direct attention to the need to change environmental conditions that contribute to chronic disease. In the ethical dimension, nurses must make sure that the emphasis on personal responsibility for healthful behavior does not result in blaming the victims of chronic disease and withdrawal of needed assistance for those with existing health problems.

In the reflective dimension, there is a growing need for nursing research to identify interventions that motivate health-promoting behaviors. Research is also needed to develop strategies for assisting clients with existing chronic health problems to achieve the greatest possible quality of life in spite of their condition.

 Assessing the Dimensions of Health in Chronic Physical Health Problems

Community health nurses use their assessment skills to assess for risk factors that contribute to chronic health problems and for existing chronic conditions and their effects. Factors related to the biophysical, psychological, physical, social, behavioral, and health system dimensions can increase the risk of the individual or a population group with respect to a particular chronic condition. Conversely, the presence of a chronic health problem might affect factors in each of these areas.

The Biophysical Dimension

Human biological factors related to age, sex, race, specific genetic inheritance, and physiologic function can increase one's risk of developing several chronic health problems.

Maturation and Aging. Many people think of chronic health problems as occurring primarily among the elderly, despite the fact that nearly 4 million U.S. children experience some form of disability related to a variety of chronic conditions (Disabilities Prevention Program, 1995), many of which were discussed in Chapter 20. Both the young and the elderly are at higher risk for accidental injuries and resulting disabilities. In part, this increased risk is due to maturational events of childhood and aging. The inability of a young infant to roll over or support his or her head contributes to suffocation as the leading cause of accidental death and disability in this age group. Similarly, normal toddler development involves a great

ASSESSMENT TIPS: Assessing Risk for Chronic Health Problems

Biophysical Dimension

What age groups are most likely to develop the problem? What age groups will be most seriously affected by the problem?

Are there racial or gender differences in disease incidence?

Is there a genetic predisposition to the problem?

Are there other physiologic conditions that increase the risk of developing the problem? If so, what are they?

What are the signs and symptoms of the problem?

What are the physiologic effects of the problem?

Does the problem limit functional abilities?

Psychological Dimension

Does exposure to stress increase risk of the problem?

What are the psychological effects of the problem?

What is the extent of adaptation to the problem?

Physical Dimension

Do environmental pollutants contribute to the problem?

What effect, if any, do weather conditions have on the problem?

Does the problem necessitate environmental changes (eg, installation of ramps for a wheelchair)?

Social Dimension

Do social norms support behaviors that increase the risk of developing the problem (eg, smoking)?

What are societal attitudes to the problem? Do they hamper control efforts?

Is there social stigma attached to having the problem?

Do occupational factors influence the incidence of the problem? In what way?

Does socioeconomic status influence the effects of the problem?

What effect, if any, do cultural beliefs and behaviors have on incidence of the problem?

What effect, if any, does legislation have on risk factors for the problem?

What social support systems are available to people with the problem?

Behavioral Dimension

Do dietary factors influence the incidence of the problem? In what way?

Does having the problem necessitate dietary changes? If so, what changes are required?

Does alcohol or drug use contribute to the incidence of the problem?

What effect does alcohol or drug use have on the course of the problem?

What effect does physical activity have on the incidence of the problem?

Does smoking contribute to the incidence of the problem?

What effects do self-care behaviors (eg, breast self-examination) have on the course of the problem?

Health System Dimension

Do health system factors contribute to the development of the problem? If so, how?

What primary preventive measures are available for the problem? Are they widely used?

To what extent do health care providers educate the public on primary prevention of the problem?

Is there a screening test for the problem? If so, are persons at risk for the problem adequately screened?

How is the problem diagnosed?

Can the problem be controlled with conventional medical therapy? Are there alternative therapies that may contribute to the control of the problem? If so, what are they?

Are diagnostic and treatment services for the problem available and accessible to persons with the problem?

What is the attitude of health care providers to persons with the problem?

---

deal of experimentation that may lead to accidental injury and disability if close supervision and safety precautions are not employed. The risk taking and feelings of invulnerability characteristic of preadolescent and adolescent development places young people at risk for motor vehicle and firearms accidents.

Among the elderly, death and disabilities due to fires and falls are of the greatest concern. Typical causes of accidental injury and disability for selected age groups are presented in Table 31–1.

Some chronic conditions and their effects are more prevalent in adults. For example, despite the

TABLE 31–1. TYPICAL CAUSES OF INJURY AND DISABILITY

Age Group	Typical Causes of Injury and Disability
Infants (birth–1 year)	Suffocation, aspiration of food and other objects, fire, drowning
1–9 years	Motor vehicle accidents, drowning, poisoning, fires
10–14 years	Motor vehicle accidents, drowning, firearms, fires
15–64 years	Motor vehicle accidents, occupational injury, falls, fires
Over 65 years	Falls, fires

popular belief that people with arthritis are elderly, most cases of arthritis have their onset in the fourth decade of life. For women over age 45, for example, arthritis is the major cause of activity limitation (Division of Chronic Disease Control and Community Intervention, 1995). Older persons do, however, tend to experience greater disability as a result of this condition. The prevalence of COPD tends to increase dramatically in the fifth through the seventh decades of life. The incidence of malignant neoplasms, in general, also increases with advancing age, particularly after midlife, as does the prevalence of diabetes (Division of Diabetes Translation, 1997b).

Sex. One's sex can also influence the risk of developing a variety of chronic health conditions. Women, for example, have lower incidence rates for hypertension, and those who do have hypertension are more likely than men to have their blood pressure under control. Men are almost twice as likely as women to die of heart disease and one and one-half times more likely to die of malignant neoplasms than women. Similarly, men have higher risks for death from stroke, COPD, diabetes, and unintentional injuries (Mortality Statistics Bureau, 1996).

Arthritis incidence by gender tends to depend on the type of arthritis involved. For all types of arthritis combined, women tend to have higher incidence rates than men, and these differences persist with increasing age (U.S. Department of Commerce, 1996). Looking at specific types of arthritis, osteoarthritis is more common in younger men and then becomes more common in women after age 55, whereas rheumatoid arthritis is more common in women than men of all ages. The opposite is true for ankylosing spondylitis and gout, but girls have a higher risk of juvenile rheumatoid arthritis than boys.

Race. Differences exist in the incidence and prevalence of some chronic conditions among different racial and ethnic groups. These may, in part, be due to environmental factors and access to health care, but some differences may be the result of genetic factors. For example, there are differences in cancer survival rates among racial and ethnic groups that are not totally explained by stage of the neoplasm at diagnosis and quality of care received. Persons of Japanese ancestry have the highest cancer survival rates followed by Latinos, Chinese, and the dominant white population. Survival rates for blacks and Filipinos are less encouraging, and Native Americans experience the worst survival rates for cancer in general.

The incidence and prevalence of other chronic health problems also differ among racial and ethnic groups. African Americans, for example, tend to have higher diabetes and hypertension prevalence rates than do whites (Kingston & Smith, 1997). Among some Native American tribes, the prevalence of diabetes is as high as 50% of the adult population (Stuart, Smith, Gilkison, Shaheb, & Stahn, 1994). Race may also play a part in the propensity to develop arthritis, as the incidence of this disease is low in Asian populations, and African Americans and Native Americans are more likely to report being affected by arthritis than Asian Americans or Caucasians (National Arthritis Data Workgroup, 1996). Latinos experience higher prevalence rates of hypertension and diabetes and fewer heart conditions than Anglos (Kingston & Smith, 1997).

For many chronic conditions, ethnic or racial factors function as risk markers rather than risk factors. *Risk markers* are factors that help to identify persons who may have an elevated risk of developing a specific condition, but that do not themselves contribute to its development. For many chronic diseases, race and ethnicity are probably markers for differences in health behaviors, access to health care, and other factors that contribute to the development of disease. For example, when socioeconomic status is controlled, there is very little difference in mortality rates for cardiovascular disease between black Americans and their white counterparts. Socioeconomic status and access to health care are also believed to explain significant differences in asthma mortality between blacks and whites (Targonsky, Persky, Orris, & Addington, 1994).

Genetic Inheritance. Some chronic diseases seem to be associated with genetic predisposition. Thus, community health nurses should obtain a family history of chronic diseases to help determine the individual client's risk for these conditions. Genetic inheritance is thought to be a major contributing factor for some cancers, for diabetes, and for cardiovascular disease.

Breast, ovarian, and colon cancers, in particular, seem to have a hereditary component. In one study, women with a first-degree relative with ovarian cancer had more than four times the risk of ovarian cancer as those without a family history. Family histories of breast, uterine, and pancreatic cancers also increased women's risk of ovarian cancer (Kerber & Slattery, 1995). Both colorectal cancer and malignant melanoma also exhibit tendencies to occur in some families more often than others (Fuchs, Giovannucci, Colditz, Hunter, Speizer, & Willett, 1994; Division of Cancer Prevention and Control, 1996b). The genetic component of coronary disease is supported by findings that about 5% of the families in the general U.S. population account for approximately 50% of early coronary deaths (those occurring before age 55). A family history of diabetes is also a strong indicator that an individual client may be at risk for diabetes, and a possible genetic disposition to rheumatoid arthritis is suggested by the presence of a specific histocompatibility antigen in persons with rheumatoid arthritis compared with the general population. There is also some evidence that morbid obesity has a genetic component (Clement, et al., 1995).

In assessing the potential for chronic health problems in individual clients, the nurse obtains a family history and constructs a genogram as described in Chapter 20. Positive findings related to chronic conditions with a genetic component direct the assessment to possible signs and symptoms of existing chronic health problems discussed later in this chapter.

Physiologic Function.   Assessment of physiologic factors related to chronic conditions focuses on three areas: presence of physiologic risk factors, physiologic evidence of existing chronic health problems, and evidence of physiologic consequences of chronic conditions.

Certain physiologic conditions may predispose one to develop some chronic health problems. Activity limitations and impaired balance and mobility, for example, may contribute to injuries with long-term consequences, particularly in elderly individuals, whereas hypertension, elevated serum cholesterol, and diabetes are all physiologic factors in the development of cardiovascular disease. Diabetes also tends to increase the risk of stroke.

Obesity is a physiologic factor that can contribute to diabetes, and coexistent hypertension may increase the risk of diabetic complications such as blindness. Obesity also places greater strain on joints and may exacerbate the effects of arthritis on affected joints. Other conditions in which obesity is a contributing factor include gallbladder disease, hypercholesterolemia, and some cancers (Galuska, et al., 1996).

Past infection may also be implicated in the development of some chronic conditions. For example, viral infection is suspected as a contributing factor in both cancer and diabetes (Helfand, Gary, Freeman, & Anderson, 1995), particularly in children. As noted in Chapter 30, genital herpes simplex virus may contribute to later development of cervical cancer. A history of recurrent respiratory infections, particularly a history of severe viral pneumonias early in life, has been found to be associated with COPD. Respiratory allergy and asthma may also be predisposing physiologic factors in COPD; whereas viral infection may be a predisposing factor in childhood asthma (Buchdahl, Parker, Stebbings, & Babiker, 1996). There is also some evidence to suggest that chronic *Chlamydia pneumoniae* may be a risk factor for coronary heart disease (Muhlestein, et al. 1996). Other physiologic conditions may be complicated by the existence of chronic illnesses. For example, diabetes places both the pregnant woman and her child at increased risk of adverse outcomes (Division of Diabetes Translation, 1994b). Conversely, pregnancy complicates diabetes control.

In addition to assessing individual clients for the presence of physiologic risk factors for chronic health problems, the community health nurse examines the incidence and prevalence of these risk factors in the general population to determine the potential for chronic health problems in the community. The nurse also assesses individual clients and groups of people for indications of existing chronic health problems. Finally, the nurse assesses clients with existing chronic conditions for evidence of related physical effects. Assessment considerations related to physiologic risk factors, signs and symptoms of existing chronic conditions, and evidence of physical problems related to selected conditions are summarized in Table 31–2.

The Psychological Dimension

The major psychological dimension factor contributing to chronic health problems is stress. Stress can result in carelessness and contribute to accidents that lead to chronic disability. Similarly, stress has been implicated as a contributing factor in the development of cancer and cardiovascular disease. Stress may also lead to poor compliance with control measures in persons with diabetes, resulting in diabetic complications. In one study, persons with a history of a major depressive episode had more than four times the risk of heart attack of those without depression (Pratt, Ford, Crum, Armenian, Gallo, & Eaton, 1996). Anger and anxiety have also been associated with myocardial infarction and hypertension (Kubzansky, Hawachi, Spiro, Weiss, Vokonas, & Sparrow, 1997; Markovitz, Matthews, Kannel, Cobb, & D'Agostino, 1993; Mittleman, et al., 1995).

In addition to assessing individual clients for levels and sources of stress and the adequacy of their

TABLE 31–2. ASSESSMENT CONSIDERATIONS RELATED TO SELECTED CHRONIC PHYSICAL HEALTH PROBLEMS

Condition	Physiologic Risk Factors	Signs and Symptoms	Potential Effects
Arthritis	Previous injury, obesity	Painful, swollen joints, limited range of motion	Contractures, limited mobility, inability to perform ADL
Cancer	Cervical dysplasia, viral infection	Weight loss, change in bowel or bladder habits, changes in voice quality, pain, skin changes, palpable lumps or growths, persistent cough, rectal bleeding or blood in stool	Debility
Cardiovascular disease	Hypertension, hypercholesterolemia, diabetes, atherosclerosis, obesity, infection	Chest pain, shortness of breath on exertion, fatigue, arrhythmias, elevated blood pressure, cardiac enlargement, edema	Debility, myocardial infarction
Cerebrovascular disease	Hypertension, atherosclerosis, congenital anomaly, heart disease, diabetes, polycythemia	Headaches, confusion, vertigo, diplopia, parasthesia of extremities, transient ischemic attacks, slurred speech, weakness	Paralysis, aphasia, incontinence
Chronic obstructive pulmonary disease	Asthma, respiratory allergy, frequent respiratory infections	Shortness of breath on exertion, cough, weakness, weight loss, diminished libido	Debility, inability to perform ADL, heart failure
Diabetes mellitus	Obesity, viral infection	Polyuria, polydipsia, polyphagia, weight loss, frequent infections (especially monilia)	Ketoacidosis with nausea, anorexia, vomiting, air hunger, and coma; diabetic retinopathy; poor wound healing and infection; sensory loss; postural hypotension; male impotence; nocturnal diarrhea
Hypertension	Atherosclerosis	Headache, blurred vision, dizziness, flushed face, fatigue, epistaxis, elevated blood pressure	Heart disease, stroke

coping mechanisms, the community health nurse assesses the psychological effects of chronic health problems on persons experiencing them. Psychological effects of chronic and debilitating conditions occur in response to three aspects of loss: physical loss, social loss, and psychological loss. Physical loss may reflect the loss of physical abilities to function or changes in one's physical appearance. Social loss may result from the immobilizing and isolating features of chronic conditions. Psychological loss involves movement through the stages typical of grieving in other similar loss situations (Fraley, 1992).

Adaptation to psychological loss typically occurs in stages. These stages include initial disbelief or denial followed by awareness of the loss and anger that it has occurred. Other feelings that may occur during the awareness stage include guilt, anxiety, and depression. This stage is followed by a period of information seeking that may be accompanied by feelings of being overwhelmed or helpless. The final stage is one of conditional acceptance, when those affected begin to view the chronic condition as a part of life and accommodate to its presence in their lives. In assessing the psychological consequences of a chronic health problem, the nurse explores with the client and family their progression through these four stages. The nurse also assesses the client's emotional response to his or her condition and its treatment, the effects of the condition on the client's self-image, and

any effects of the condition on the client's ability to interact effectively with others. The psychological consequences of pain should also be assessed and evidence of depression and potential for suicide sought. Depression may result from diminished functional ability, and may, in turn, cause further disability creating a downward spiral effect on health (Bruce, Seeman, Merrill, & Blazer, 1994). Considerations in assessing clients for depression are addressed in Chapter 32.

The Physical Dimension

Physical dimension factors contribute to chronic health problems such as long-term sequelae of accidents, cancer, and COPD. Road conditions, weather, dangerous conditions for swimming, and other physical safety hazards can contribute to accidents that result in permanent physical disability, and the nurse assesses the existence of these types of hazardous conditions in the community.

The community health nurse also assesses the environment for pollutants that may be carcinogenic. Air pollution, in particular, contributes to COPD and asthma (Buchdahl, et al., 1996). In 1991, it was estimated that 63% of persons in the United States with asthma lived in areas that have not attained National Ambient Air Quality Standards for one or more pollutants (Air Pollution and Respiratory Health

Bureau, 1995). Other environmental factors that may influence chronic respiratory conditions, particularly those with an allergic basis, include house dust, mites, molds, tobacco smoke, and occupational exposures to respiratory irritants. Long-term lead exposure, on the other hand, has been linked to hypertension (Hu, et al., 1996). The effects of environmental pollution on health were addressed in more detail in Chapter 17.

The other aspect of the physical environment related to chronic health problems is its effect on the functional abilities of persons with existing chronic conditions. From this perspective, the nurse assesses the need to adapt the environment to accommodate the needs of the client with a chronic condition. For example, does the home have a shower to make personal hygiene easier for the person with arthritis who may have difficulty getting in and out of a bathtub? Or does the home of the person with cardiovascular disease or COPD have numerous stairs that cause the individual to become short of breath? Similarly, the nurse assesses for potential barriers that limit community services for persons with chronic disabilities.

The Social Dimension

The social dimension contributes to the development of chronic health problems primarily in terms of social support for unhealthful behaviors and factors that enhance or impede access to health care. Social norms that condone or promote behaviors such as smoking, drinking alcohol, and a sedentary lifestyle contribute to the development of a variety of chronic health problems.

Social factors also include role modeling of healthful behaviors. Social dimension factors may also promote health and healthy behaviors and impede the development of chronic health problems. For example, social pressures to quit smoking may motivate many smokers to abandon their habit. Similarly, no-smoking policies in work settings have led to an overall decrease in smoking in many instances (Stephens, Pederson, Koval, & Kim, 1997). The existence of strong social support networks has also been shown to reduce the risk of cardiovascular disease.

Social environmental factors such as low income, low education levels, and unemployment may prevent access to health care for persons who have existing chronic conditions. Lack of care leads to the development of complications that might be averted if adequate treatment and monitoring are available. These types of socioeconomic factors explain some of the differences in survival rates for members of different ethnic groups who have cancer, and par-

ticularly explain the poor survival rates of African Americans with cancer. Income may also affect health behaviors. For example, sedentary lifestyle has been shown to be inversely related to income levels, with those at lower levels engaging in less physical activity.

Legislative factors can also influence health behaviors and consequent chronic health problems. For example, smoking has been shown to decrease when cigarette prices or taxes increase (Office on Smoking and Health, 1996a; Stephens, et al., 1997). Similarly, bicycle helmet use increases when use legislation is enforced (Kraus, Peek, & Williams, 1995).

Occupational factors are another element of the social dimension that can contribute to the development of chronic health problems. As noted in Chapter 26, safety hazards in the work environment can result in accidents that lead to chronic disability. Clients' occupations may also increase their potential for exposure to various carcinogens found in the workplace. Repetitive movements involved in some jobs can lead to joint injuries and subsequent arthritis. Occupations involving exposure to organic and inorganic dusts or noxious gases increase the probability of COPD. Employment in plastics factories and in cotton mills is particularly associated with increased incidence of COPD.

The community health nurse assesses the jobs performed by individual clients and identifies any risk factors for chronic health problems posed by the work environment or the work performed. The nurse also assesses the community for potential occupational risk factors related to chronic health problems by determining the major employers and occupations present in the community and the types of products, services, and processes involved.

The community health nurse also assesses the social effects of chronic health problems on those clients experiencing them. For example, the nurse might note that the physical effects of arthritis or COPD may prevent clients from engaging in activities that provided them with opportunities for social interaction in the past, thus resulting in social isolation.

In addition, the nurse should assess the adequacy of the client's social support network for dealing with the problems posed by chronic health problems. Areas to be considered include those who make up a client's social support network, the assistance provided by each, the adequacy of the network for meeting the client's needs, and the extent to which the network is appropriately used. For example, the nurse might note that the client's support network is not sufficiently broad to meet his or her needs or that the client is not using the existing network as fully as possible.

The Behavioral Dimension

Behavioral factors are the major contributors to the development of most chronic health problems. Behavioral considerations to be assessed by the nurse include consumption patterns, exercise, and other behaviors.

Consumption Patterns.   Consumption patterns that play a role in the development and course of chronic health problems include diet and the use of tobacco and alcohol. Poor dietary patterns contribute to chronic diseases such as diabetes and cardiovascular disease and to obesity, which is a risk factor for both of these conditions.

Cholesterol consumption patterns are well-known correlates of cardiovascular disease, and excess blood cholesterol is a prevalent problem throughout the United States. A large percentage of the fat consumed by Americans comes from animal sources known to be high in cholesterol. In 1995, a median of 19% of people in states participating in the Behavioral Risk Factor Surveillance Survey (BRFSS) reported being told they had elevated cholesterol levels (Powell-Griner, Anderson, & Murphy, 1997). In addition, as the percentage of calories derived from fat increases, intake of more healthful foods such as fruits, vegetables, and dietary sources of vitamins A and C, folates, and fiber decreases. As a result, not only does increased fat intake contribute to obesity and thereby to chronic disease, it may also contribute to a variety of dietary deficiencies.

Diet has also been implicated in the development of some forms of cancer. For example, rates of colon cancer have been shown to increase with diets high in fat (Division of Cancer Prevention and Control, 1996a). Baseline data for the national health objectives indicate that American women aged 20 to 50 years eat less than half the recommended daily amounts of vegetables and fruits or grain products (U.S. Department of Health and Human Services, 1993). Selenium, a trace element, has been associated with decreased risk of lung, colorectal, and prostate cancers (Clark, et al., 1996).

Use of tobacco is another consumption pattern highly correlated with the development of a variety of chronic health problems. In fact, smoking is estimated to be the underlying cause of 400,000 deaths annually in the United States. These smoking-related deaths are due to heart disease, various forms of cancer, COPD, stroke, and other conditions caused by smoking.

Tobacco use remains one of the primary behavioral factors contributing to cancer of the lungs, bladder, mouth, pharynx, larynx, and esophagus. In fact, tobacco consumption patterns are thought to explain some of the regional variation in cancer incidence. For example, higher rates of oral cancer in the rural South are related to the use of snuff, whereas cigarette smoking is associated with high lung cancer rates in other areas. Pipe smoking, on the other hand, is associated with cancers of the oral cavity and lips. Smoking mentholated tobacco appears to increase the risks of lung cancer even more than nonmentholated cigarette smoking (Sidney, Tekawa, Friedman, Sadler, & Tashkin, 1995).

Smoking has also been found to influence the incidence of cardiovascular disease and complications of diabetes and COPD. The association between smoking and cardiovascular disease is supported by findings that people who quit smoking reduce their risk of coronary heart disease by about half after a year of abstinence from tobacco. Smoking cessation also markedly reduces the risk of premature death in persons with existing cardiovascular disease. Smoking has been found to interact with diabetes to result in greater risk of complications. There is also some evidence that smoking is an independent risk factor in the development of diabetes (Rimm, Chan, Stampfer, Colditz, & Willett, 1995). Smoking is also the primary contributing factor in the development of COPD. In addition to being the single most significant factor in the development of this disease, smoking interacts with all other contributing factors to increase the potential for COPD.

Despite a significant decline in the number of smokers in the United States, the 1995 BRFSS indicated that a median of 22% of the population in participating states were current smokers (Office on Smoking and Health, 1996b). These figures indicate that smoking will continue to be a contributing factor in the incidence of cancer, cardiovascular disease, chronic liver disease and cirrhosis, and complications of diabetes and COPD.

Alcohol use also contributes to the development of certain chronic health problems and their consequences. For example, alcohol is implicated in motor vehicle accidents, bicycling accidents, fires, falls, and boating accidents, many of which result in chronic disability. For example, alcohol was involved in 44% of all traffic fatalities in 1993 (Division of Unintentional Injury Prevention, 1994). Alcohol abuse also contributes to asthma (Epidemiology Program Office, 1997), but moderate alcohol use appears to have a protective effect for diabetes (Perry, Wannamethee, Walker, Thomson, Whincup, & Shaper, 1995).

In assessing the influence of consumption patterns on chronic health problems, the community health nurse identifies consumption patterns that place individuals at risk for chronic conditions. The nurse also determines the prevalence of high-risk consumption patterns in the community. In addition, the nurse explores unhealthful consumption patterns with clients who have existing chronic diseases and determines their effects on the course of the condition. For example, the nurse would determine whether a client with diabetes is adhering to a diabetic diet. The nurse also assesses for factors related to food preferences and modes of preparation that may impede adherence to special diets.

Exercise and Leisure Activity. Exercise, or the lack of it, can influence the development and course of some chronic conditions. Exercise may enhance the control of diabetes or contribute to hypoglycemic reactions. The community health nurse should assess the extent of the diabetic client's exercise in relation to his or her dietary intake and the amount of insulin used to determine the potential for hypoglycemic reaction related to exercise.

Physical activity has also been shown to be directly related to the incidence of heart disease. Several studies have documented that adults with active lifestyles have significantly lower risk of developing heart disease than their less active contemporaries. A sedentary lifestyle, on the other hand, is closely associated with obesity, a risk factor for cardiovascular disease. In the 1995 BRFSS, more than one fourth of the U.S. adult population continued to report no leisure time physical activity (Powell-Griner, et al., 1997). The association of lack of exercise, obesity, and cardiovascular risk holds true for children as well as for adults.

Television viewing is frequently a component of a sedentary lifestyle and has been shown to be associated with obesity. Watching television is the third most time-consuming activity in the United States, and the typical adult watches TV an average of 4 hours each day. As viewing time increases, physical fitness declines. The nurse assessing an individual client or a community for risk factors related to exercise or its lack would determine the extent of regular exercise obtained by the individual or the proportion of sedentary individuals who make up the population.

Other Behaviors. Other lifestyle behaviors that might influence the development and course of chronic diseases include the practice of self-assessment behaviors for breast and testicular cancers and the use of safety devices and precautions.

Despite the advantages of early detection of breast cancer through breast self-examination, few women engage in this practice on a regular basis, and even fewer men engage in regular testicular examinations. In assessing this aspect of lifestyle and its effects on chronic health problems, the nurse would ascertain how often individual clients engage in breast or testicular self-examination. The nurse would also assess the extent to which these practices are employed within the community to determine the community's potential for increased mortality due to breast and testicular cancer.

The use of safety devices and safety precautions can prevent accidents that may result in chronic disability, and the nurse should determine the extent to which individual clients and their families practice safety measures. Are there smoke detectors in the home? Are hazardous items, such as sharp objects and poisons, stored appropriately? Is there potential for falls owing to multiple obstacles in the homes of elderly persons? Do family members consistently use seat belts? Seat belt use is an important behavioral factor in preventing motor vehicle fatalities. In the 1995 BRFSS, roughly two thirds of respondents reported consistent seat belt use (Powell-Griner, et al., 1997).

The community health nurse also appraises the extent to which these and similar safety conditions and practices are found in the general population or in the work setting. Are smoke detectors and sprinkler systems present in public buildings or in business and industries? Is seat belt use mandatory in the jurisdiction and, if so, is it enforced? Are appropriate safety equipment and safety precautions employed in work settings?

Other behaviors can contribute to or prevent skin cancer. For example, reducing direct exposure to sunlight (particularly from 10 A.M. to 4 P.M.), using sunscreen protection, and wearing a broad-brimmed hat can minimize the risk of malignant melanoma. In the 1992 National Health Interview Survey, however, less than one third of U.S. adults indicated routinely engaging in these behaviors (Division of Cancer Prevention and Control, 1996b).

The Health System Dimension

Health care system factors may contribute to the development of chronic health problems or influence their course and consequences. The failure of health care professionals to educate their clients and the general public on the effects of diet, exercise, smoking, alcohol, and other factors in the development of chronic health problems contributes to the increased incidence of these conditions.

The extent of screening services for existing chronic conditions may influence their course and effects. It is estimated that diabetic screening programs, for example, detect only about half of the population affected by this disease (Centers for Disease Control, 1996b).

The extent to which low-cost screening procedures for various forms of cancer are available varies considerably throughout the country. Although screening services may often be obtained from private health care providers, they are often costly and many low-income people are prevented from taking advantage of them.

Even in those states where screening services are provided, they may not be used effectively. In 1996, for example, a median of 74% of adult women included in the BRFSS reported ever having had a clinical breast examination by a health care professional, and 69% reported having had a mammogram (Powell-Griner, et al., 1997). Research also indicates that persons with existing chronic diseases may be less likely to receive cancer screening services (Fontana, Baumann, Helberg, & Love, 1997).

Health care system factors influence the availability and quality of treatment obtainable for persons with chronic conditions. The aggressiveness of treatment received also affects the outcome of chronic health conditions. Some studies, for example, suggest that poorer cancer survival rates among low-income populations may be related to reduced access to care (Gorey, et al., 1997). The quality of treatment received for diabetes may also vary widely and affect the consequences of this disease. Medical technology, on the other hand, has greatly reduced mortality from cardiovascular and cerebrovascular diseases. This is largely due to a concerted effort to control hypertension, smoking, and diet. Medical therapy has also been shown to increase one's risk for chronic health conditions. Asthma mortality, for example, has been linked to overuse of inhaled β-agonists and underuse of corticosteroids (Epidemiology Program Office, 1997), as well as failure of clinicians to recognize the severity of disease (Targonski, et al., 1994). Similarly, there is growing evidence that some approaches to antihypertensive therapy, particularly the use of β-blockers, increases the risk of myocardial infarction (Merlo, et al., 1996).

In assessing individual and community risk for chronic health problems, the community health nurse determines the extent of preventive, diagnostic, and treatment services offered to community residents as well as their cost and accessibility. The nurse also assesses the extent to which available services are used and possible reasons for nonuse if appropriate.

Risk factors related to the biophysical, psychological, physical, social, behavioral, and health system dimensions all influence the development and outcomes of chronic physical health problems. Risk factors for selected chronic conditions are summarized in Appendix T, Factors in the Epidemiology of Selected Chronic Physical Health Problems.

 ## Diagnostic Reasoning and Care of Clients with Chronic Physical Health Problems

Nursing diagnoses are derived from information collected relative to the incidence and prevalence of chronic health problems in the population and the factors contributing to these conditions. These diagnoses may relate to individual clients or to the general population. Examples of nursing diagnoses related to an individual client are "potential for cardiovascular disease due to smoking and sedentary lifestyle" and "uncontrolled diabetes due to failure to adhere to diabetic diet." At the group level, the nurse might derive diagnoses such as "increased prevalence of lung cancer due to smoking and occupational exposure to carcinogens." In each case, the nursing diagnosis contains a statement of the probable cause or etiology of the problem that directs interventions designed to resolve it.

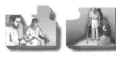 ## Planning and Implementing the Dimensions of Health Care in the Control of Chronic Physical Health Problems

Planning interventions related to chronic health problems is based on the understanding of contributing factors derived from the assessment. It is particularly important to involve the client and his or her family in planning solutions to chronic health problems because the client or a significant other will probably be responsible for implementing the plan. By involving the client and members of the client's family, the nurse can tailor the plan of care to the client's circumstances. It is important to remember that the presence of a chronic health problem affects many facets of life for the client and his or her family. Effective planning accounts for these effects and minimizes the consequences of chronic illness for client and family alike.

When chronic health problems exist at the community or group level, the nurse collaborates with other members of the community to plan health programs that address the problems identified. For example, if the prevalence of cardiovascular disease is particularly high in the community, programs to prevent and control cardiovascular disease might be developed. In planning these programs, the nurse and other health planners employ the general principles of health programming discussed in Chapter 19.

Control strategies for chronic health problems can be undertaken at the primary, secondary, or tertiary level of prevention. To date, the major emphasis has been on secondary prevention, with only recent attention to primary and tertiary levels.

Primary Prevention

Nursing strategies for primary prevention of chronic conditions focus on two major areas: health promotion and risk factor modification. Both aspects of primary prevention can be applied to individual clients or to population groups.

Health Promotion.

General health promotion is aimed at making people healthier and reducing their chances of developing a variety of health problems including chronic conditions. Health promotion at both the individual and group levels involves education for a healthier lifestyle, political activity to create conditions that promote health, and immunization for selected conditions.

HEALTH EDUCATION. Health education efforts in primary prevention of chronic health problems focus on diet, exercise, and coping skills. The nurse employs the principles of health education discussed in Chapter 9 to educate both individual clients and the general public on basic nutrition and specific nutritional requirements based on a person's age and activity level. For example, to prevent obesity the nurse would teach parents about the nutritional needs of infants and young children and encourage a well-balanced diet with minimal amounts of junk food. Similarly, the nurse would teach a pregnant woman, a nursing mother, or a physically active person about their specific nutritional needs. The nurse would also try to inform the general public about proper nutrition.

Exercise is another area in which health education may be required, and nurses would plan to inform both individual clients and the general public about the need for regular exercise. The nurse might also assist clients to plan ways of incorporating exercise into their daily routine or develop plans for exercise programs in the community or for employees of local businesses.

Teaching general coping skills is another way for community health nurses to promote health and prevent chronic health problems that are influenced by stress. In this respect, the nurse might assist a harried mother of several small children to develop ways of coping with stress, or the nurse might assist school personnel to develop a program to teach basic coping skills as part of elementary and secondary school curricula. Another approach might be to plan a program to foster adequate coping among employees of local businesses.

POLITICAL ACTIVITY. Political activity related to primary prevention focuses on measures to promote access to preventive health services and to create a healthful environment. Nursing involvement in efforts at this level include planning strategies to influence health policy making discussed in Chapter 13. For example, community health nurses might campaign for better access to prenatal care for pregnant women or legislation to prevent or reduce pollution so as to prevent its contribution to chronic respiratory conditions and other chronic health problems.

Political activity by community health nurses might also be required to establish and enforce policies and legislation that foster healthful behaviors. For example, failure to enforce laws related to sale of tobacco products to minors has enabled youngsters to purchase tobacco. Conversely, bicycle helmet laws meet with compliance in about 85% riders when enforced and coupled with community education (Macknin & Mendendorp, 1994).

IMMUNIZATION. Although immunization is generally considered a primary preventive measure for communicable diseases, it can also serve to prevent some chronic conditions and their effects. For example, immunization of persons at risk for hepatitis B can serve to eliminate this risk factor for chronic liver disease and cirrhosis. Those clients with existing liver disease should receive pneumococcal vaccine and annual immunizations for influenza as should persons with diabetes.

Risk Factor Modification.

Activities designed to eliminate or modify risk factors include quitting smoking, reducing weight, controlling hypertension, using safety and protective devices, and creating environments free of safety hazards. Again, educational efforts by community health nurses are an important aspect of risk factor modification, and nurses would plan to educate both individual clients and the general public about the elimination or modification of identified risk factors for chronic health problems.

SMOKING. Some progress has been made in eliminating smoking as a risk factor for chronic health problems. Two general approaches have been used in this area: personal efforts and public activity. Personal efforts are designed to keep people from ever starting to smoke and encouraging smokers to quit. Among adults, these efforts have been relatively successful, and as of 1996, less than 23% of the adult population in the United States were smokers (Powell-Griner, et al., 1997). Unfortunately, smoking is on the rise among young people.

Community health nurses can educate smokers regarding the hazards of smoking and direct them to sources of assistance to quit smoking. In addition, the community health nurse can provide support and encourage family members to support the smoker's efforts to quit. Nurses can also educate young people regarding the hazards of smoking and develop programs that discourage them from initiating the habit. Finally, nurses can educate individual clients and groups of people to eliminate other forms of tobacco use such as snuff and chewing tobacco.

Community health nurses may also be involved in political activity to limit smoking. Legislative and regulatory activities to control smoking can be of two types: legislation controlling smoking in public places and taxation of tobacco sales. In Great Britain, for example, prohibitively high taxes on cigarettes and other forms of tobacco have greatly reduced tobacco use. Legislation has also been effective in controlling smoking behavior by limiting smoking in public places.

Another area of the public effort to reduce smoking lies in workplace restrictions, and community health nurses can be active in promoting no-smoking policies in business and industry.

OBESITY.   Control efforts for obesity have been less extensive than those for smoking. Health education related to caloric intake and fat consumption, particularly saturated fats, is required, and community health nurses should educate individual clients about the need to consume fewer calories and to reduce fat consumption. Dietary recommendations related to the year 2000 health objectives include reducing fat intake to less than 30% and saturated fat to less than 10% of total caloric intake (U.S. Department of Health and Human Services, 1991). Community health nurses can educate clients about reading package labels to determine the fat and caloric content of various foods. They can also inform clients about foods that are low in saturated fats and about food preparation methods that minimize fat consumption.

Development of modified food products also assists in controlling fat intake. Community health nurses can encourage the food industry to pursue research on food modification. They can also campaign for legislation to require accurate labeling of food packages and disclosure of food contents.

Regular exercise can also be emphasized as a control strategy for obesity, as well as a means of counteracting the effects of a sedentary lifestyle, itself a risk factor in many chronic conditions. Community health nurses can encourage overweight or sedentary clients to incorporate more exercise into their daily routine. Nurses may also be involved in planning exercise programs for groups of overweight or sedentary clients in the community or in work settings.

HYPERTENSION.   In addition to being a chronic condition itself, hypertension is a risk factor for several other chronic health problems and their complications. For example, hypertensive men have a twofold risk of congestive heart failure compared to normotensive men. Among women there is a threefold increase in risk (Levy, Larson, Vasan, Kannel, & Ho, 1996). For this reason, efforts to control hypertension constitute primary prevention for cardiovascular and cerebrovascular diseases as well as for complications of diabetes.

Community health nurses should educate individual clients and the general public regarding the effects and signs and symptoms of hypertension. They can also identify people with hypertension and be involved in planning hypertension screening programs or in referring clients with elevated blood pressures for further evaluation and treatment.

The second aspect of hypertension control is encouraging behaviors that promote control of existing hypertension. Community health nurses can educate hypertensive clients on the appropriate use of antihypertensive medications and potential side effects. In addition, nurses should convey to clients the need to continue with therapy and to report any adverse effects of treatment to their primary care providers.

SAFETY PRECAUTIONS.   The use of safety devices and other safety precautions can modify risk factors for accidents that may lead to chronic disability. Community health nurses can encourage clients to install smoke detectors in residences, provide adequate supervision for small children, store hazardous items appropriately, and remove hazards that promote falls for the elderly. They can also promote the use of seat belts in vehicles and campaign for legislation that makes seat belt use mandatory in all vehicles. Community health nurses can promote safety devices and safety precautions in the work setting to prevent accidental injury. Finally, community health nurses can motivate clients to use sunscreen and protective clothing to prevent melanoma. Primary prevention goals in the control of chronic physical health problems and related community health nursing activities are summarized in Table 31–3.

TABLE 31–3. GOALS FOR PRIMARY PREVENTION AND RELATED COMMUNITY HEALTH NURSING INTERVENTIONS IN THE CONTROL OF CHRONIC PHYSICAL HEALTH PROBLEMS

Primary Prevention Goal	Nursing Intervention
1. Health promotion. a. Provide prenatal care.	1. Promote client health. a. Educate clients and public about the need for prenatal care. Refer to or provide prenatal care.

b. Maintain appropriate body weight through adequate nutrition.
  i. Breastfeed infants.
  ii. Delay introduction of solid foods.
  iii. Avoid use of food as pacifier or reward.
  iv. Establish healthy food habits from childhood.
	b. Educate clients and public about adequate nutrition.
	  i. Obtain diet history and identify poor food habits.
	  ii. Assist with breastfeeding.
	  iii. Assist with menu planning and budgeting.
	  iv. Refer for food-supplement plans as needed.
	  v. Encourage use of nonfood reward systems.

c. Engage in graduated program of exercise.	c. Educate public about need for exercise. Assist clients to plan appropriate exercise program.
d. Develop coping skills.	d. Teach coping skills.

2. Risk factor modification.
 a. Quit smoking and prevent initiation of smoking.
	2. Screen for risk factors. Educate public regarding risk factors.
	 a. Foster self-help groups for smokers and overeaters.
	  i. Educate nonsmokers about the hazards of smoking.
	  ii. Promote no-smoking policies in public places and in the workplace.

b. Decrease dietary intake of saturated fats, cholesterol, sodium, and alcohol.	b. Educate and help clients plan adequate nutritional intake.

c. Identify and treat existing health problems that are risk factors for chronic illness (hypertension, obesity).	c. Screen for and refer clients with existing conditions.
	  i. Educate clients regarding therapy for existing conditions.
	  ii. Adjust therapy to client's situation when possible.
	  iii. Monitor for compliance, therapeutic effects, and side effects.

d. Eliminate environmental pollutants contributing to chronic disease.	d. Educate public about pollution. Become politically active on environmental legislation.

e. Decrease exposure to sources of radiation (x-ray, sunlight).	e. Educate public about risks of radiation.
	  i. Discourage sunbathing.
	  ii. Encourage use of sunscreen and protective clothing.

f. Eliminate occupational exposure to hazardous substances.	f. Monitor occupational safety conditions.
g. Eliminate or modify effects of emotional stress. Avoid stressful situations when possible.	g. Assist clients to identify stressful situations. Explore with clients ways of decreasing stress.

Secondary Prevention

Secondary prevention activities in the control of chronic illness are aimed at dealing with chronic health problems once they have occurred. The three major foci at this level of prevention are screening for existing chronic conditions, early diagnosis, and prompt treatment of these conditions.

Screening. Screening tests are available for several chronic health problems. Pap smears, for example, are used to screen women for cervical cancer, and breast self-examination and mammography assist in early detection of breast cancer. Testicular self-examination is an equally important screening procedure for men. Early detection of colorectal cancers is assisted with regular stool examination for occult blood and an annual rectal exam. Dermatologic screening for skin cancers and hypertension and diabetes screenings are readily available and easily accessible in most areas.

Community health nurses play an important role in screening for chronic illness. They are conversant with the prevalence of various risk factors in the community and can plan screening programs needed to detect conditions related to the most prevalent risk

factors. They may also plan to motivate client participation in screening by educating the public regarding the need for screening. Interpretation of test results and referrals for further diagnosis and treatment of suspected conditions are also functions of community health nurses in secondary prevention of chronic health problems. Recommendations for routine screening tests for men and women are included in Table 31–4. In addition to routine screening recommendations, persons with specific risk factors for chronic conditions should be screened as needed (U.S. Preventive Health Services Task Force, 1996).

Early Diagnosis. The effects of many chronic health conditions can be minimized when they are diagnosed and treated early in the course of the disease. As noted earlier, positive screening test results are always an indication of a need for further diagnostic testing. Persons with obvious symptoms associated with chronic diseases should also be referred for diagnostic evaluation.

Community health nurses frequently engage in case finding with respect to chronic diseases, identifying community members with possible symptoms of

TABLE 31–4. RECOMMENDATIONS FOR ROUTINE SCREENING FOR CHRONIC CONDITIONS IN ADULT MEN AND WOMEN

Screening Test	Recommendations for Men	Recommendations for Women
Blood cholesterol	Periodically from age 35–65 years	Periodically from age 45–65 years
Fecal occult blood	Periodically for all children and adults	Periodically for all children and adults
Gross hearing	Elderly	Elderly
Hypertension	Periodically for all children and adults	Periodically for all children and adults
Iron-deficiency anemia		Pregnant women
Mammography and clinical breast examination		Every 1–2 years from age 50–69 years
Obesity	Periodic height and weight for all adults and children	Periodic height and weight for all adults and children
Papanicolau smear		At least every 3 years after onset of sexual activity
Problem drinking (by history)	All adolescents and adults	All adolescents and adults
Visual acuity (Snellen chart)	Elderly	Elderly

(Source: U.S. Preventive Health Services Task Force, 1996.)

disease and referring them for diagnosis and treatment as appropriate. Community health nurses are also active in educating clients and the general public regarding signs and symptoms of chronic diseases and the need for medical intervention. Community health nurses who are nurse practitioners may also be involved in making medical diagnoses of chronic illnesses.

Prompt Treatment. The third aspect of secondary prevention in the control of chronic health problems is the treatment of existing conditions. Treatment considerations in chronic conditions include stabilizing the client's condition as rapidly as possible, establishing a medical treatment regimen, and preventing progression of the disease by monitoring treatment effectiveness.

STABILIZING THE CLIENT'S CONDITION.   Community health nurses may need to provide emergency care to stabilize clients who are experiencing some chronic conditions. For example, the client having a heart attack may need CPR; emergency care is also required for the client in diabetic coma. Community health nurses may actually provide emergency care in situations of this type or may educate clients and the public in emergency care procedures. Once the client has been stabilized, the nurse would refer the client to an appropriate source of medical care.

ESTABLISHING A TREATMENT REGIMEN.   The medical treatment regimen for a chronic health problem may involve medication, radiation, chemotherapy, surgery, or other types of therapy. Although nurse practitioners may be involved in providing some of these forms of care, most community health nurses are not. They are, however, involved in preparing clients for treatments both physically and psychologically, and they provide supportive measures as needed during therapy. For example, the nurse may administer intravenous pain

medication to clients in the terminal stages of cancer or help clients deal with the side effects of radiation or chemotherapy.

Nurses also educate clients about their treatment and motivate them to comply with treatment recommendations. For example, community health nurses can educate clients with hypertension about antihypertensive medications and their effects and side effects as well as about diet, weight loss, and the need for continued medical supervision.

At the community level, community health nurses may be politically involved in efforts to ensure the presence and accessibility of prompt treatment for chronic conditions. They may also be involved in planning health care programs for the treatment of a variety of chronic health problems using the principles of health program planning discussed in Chapter 19.

MOTIVATING COMPLIANCE.   Many persons with chronic conditions are noncompliant in following prescribed recommendations. Reasons for noncompliance include inability to understand recommendations, inconvenience of required actions, disruption of lifestyle, financial or situational constraints, and lack of belief in the severity of the problem or the efficacy of treatment.

Monitoring client compliance with therapy for chronic conditions is an important community health nursing function. Identifying and eliminating factors in a client situation that promote noncompliance may foster compliance instead. Clients may be physically or mentally unable to comply with recommendations. Clients who cannot remove the childproof cap, cannot get into the tub for a sitz bath, or cannot remember to take their medication will not be compliant because of sheer inability. These are some of the considerations the nurse must make when planning to enhance client compliance with the recommended treatment plan. This is also further reason for incorporating the client and/or family members in the design of the treatment plan.

Other clients may be noncompliant because treatment requires too great an alteration in lifestyle. In this case the nurse can plan adjustments in the treatment plan to more closely fit the client's lifestyle. For example, the nurse can assist the client who has diabetes to incorporate culturally preferred foods into a diabetic diet.

Situational constraints can also lead to noncompliance. Clients who cannot afford to purchase their medication will not take it. Lack of running water may make warm soaks difficult for the arthritic client. The effort of bringing water from a well and heating it on the stove may be more detrimental to inflamed joints than doing nothing. The nurse plans measures to eliminate situational barriers to clients' compliance with treatment plans. For example, the nurse may plan a referral to assist a client to obtain Medicaid coverage to help pay for medical expenses, or help the client plan for other ways to provide moist heat to arthritic joints.

Noncompliance may also result when the client has a vested interest in being ill. Clients who use illness to get attention or qualify for disability benefits are unlikely to comply fully with a treatment program. In such cases, community health nurses must identify the goal of the client's noncompliance. They may then be able to help the client plan other means of achieving that goal and motivate greater compliance.

Finally, lack of motivation can contribute to noncompliance. Clients may lack motivation owing to a poor self-concept or because of discouragement. The nurse, family members, and friends can help improve the client's self-concept by encouraging independence, helping the client accomplish short-term goals, and positively reinforcing accomplishments. Above all, the client must be accepted by family and friends as a unique individual worthy of respect.

Discouragement can be abated through realistic goal setting and achievement of short-term goals. Emotional support by the nurse, provided through opportunities on the part of the client to express feelings of fear and frustration, as well as positive reinforcement of accomplishments, can help to alleviate discouragement and foster compliance. Another way to deal with this type of noncompliance is referral to an appropriate self-help group.

MONITORING TREATMENT EFFECTS. The nurse involved in secondary prevention for chronic health problems also monitors clients for the presence of side effects related to treatment. For example, the nurse may note that a client is experiencing postural hypotension due to an-

tihypertensives and will then educate the client about the need to change position gradually and will continue to monitor blood pressure levels to be sure that they do not drop too low.

At the same time, the nurse monitors the therapeutic effects of treatment. For instance, the nurse may obtain periodic blood pressure measurements for the client with hypertension. In the event the nurse determines that antihypertensive therapy has not noticeably affected the client's blood pressure, the nurse would make sure that the client is taking the medication appropriately and refer the client to his or her physician for further follow-up. Goals for secondary prevention of chronic physical health problems and related community health nursing interventions are summarized in Table 31–5.

Tertiary Prevention

In tertiary prevention the aim is to promote the client's optimal level of function despite the presence

TABLE 31–5. **GOALS FOR SECONDARY PREVENTION AND RELATED COMMUNITY HEALTH NURSING INTERVENTIONS IN THE CONTROL OF CHRONIC PHYSICAL HEALTH PROBLEMS**

Secondary Prevention Goal	Nursing Intervention
1. Screening. a. Perform periodic health examinations. b. Periodically screen for chronic disease.	1. Screen for existing chronic diseases. a. Educate public about need for health examinations. Provide periodic examinations. b. Educate public about need for periodic screening. Plan and implement screening programs for high-risk groups.
2. Early diagnosis.	2. Educate public about warning signs and symptoms of chronic disease. a. Engage in case finding and refer for diagnosis as appropriate. b. Prepare client for diagnostic procedures (physically and emotionally). c. Conduct diagnostic tests as appropriate.

3. Prompt treatment.
 a. Stabilize condition as soon as possible.
 	
 b. Establish treatment regimen.
  i. Medication
  ii. Radiation
  iii. Chemotherapy
  iv. Surgery
 	
c. Prevent disease progression.
	3. Assist with management of chronic disease.
	 a. Provide emergency care as needed.
	  i Educate public to provide emergency care (CPR).
	  ii. Refer for further treatment.
	 b. Prepare client for treatment procedures (physically and emotionally).
	  i. Carry out treatment regimen.
	  ii. Provide supportive measures during treatment (relief of pain).
	  iii. Educate clients about medications: dosage, side effects, etc.
	  iv. Encourage client compliance with treatment.
	 c. Monitor therapeutic effects of treatment.
	  i. Monitor side effects.
	  ii. Refer for follow-up as needed.

of a chronic health problem. This entails preventing further loss of function in affected and unaffected systems, restoring function, monitoring health status, and assisting the client to adjust to the presence of a chronic condition.

Preventing Loss of Function in Affected Systems.   Chronic health problems frequently result in some loss of function in organ systems affected by the condition, and tertiary prevention activities should be planned to prevent further loss of function in these systems. Activities may be planned to minimize losses or to eliminate risk factors that might lead to adverse consequences of the condition. Such activities on the part of the community health nurse might include motivating client compliance with treatment recommendations and assisting clients to identify and change risk factors that may lead to further loss of function. For example, the client with arthritis may be assisted to identify safety factors in the home that might contribute to falls, leading to further mobility limitation. Or, the client who has had a myocardial infarction may be assisted to plan a regimen of diet and exercise that will prevent future infarcts.

Preventing Loss of Function in Unaffected Systems.   Chronic health problems may also result in loss of function in other physical and nonphysical systems not directly affected by the condition. For example, the client with arthritis may develop skin lesions due to limited mobility, or the client with COPD may become malnourished because meal preparation is too exhausting.

Nursing interventions will be directed toward preventing both physical and social disability. Physical complications of chronic conditions may be prevented by activities such as teaching breathing exercises to clients with COPD, providing good skin care for the client with arthritis, and teaching foot care for clients with diabetes.

Nurses can also help prevent social disability by encouraging the client to interact with others, assisting clients to maintain their independence as much as possible, assisting with necessary role changes within the family, and referring the client to appropriate self-help groups. At the group level, community health nurses can work to prevent social isolation of those with chronic illnesses by advocacy and political activities to ensure access to services. They can also work to educate the public and to develop positive attitudes to persons with chronic or disabling conditions.

Restoring Function.   The restoration aspect of tertiary prevention focuses on regaining as much lost function as is possible given the client's situation. Particular areas of function to be considered include bed activities, po-

Critical Thinking in Research

Wagner and colleagues (1994) conducted a study of a nursing intervention to prevent falls and diminished functional status in older adults. They randomly assigned more than 1500 health maintenance organization (HMO) enrollees over age 65 to one of three treatment conditions: (1) a nursing assessment visit to review risk factors for falls and development of a tailored intervention plan to address risk factors exhibited; (2) a general health promotion nursing visit; and (3) usual HMO care. The assessment/risk factor modification group had significantly fewer falls and less decline in functional status than the usual care group, while the general health promotion group had outcomes intermediate between the other two groups. The differences between groups narrowed 2 years after the interventions. The authors interpreted the results to indicate that "a modest, one-time prevention program appeared to confer short-term health benefits on ambulatory HMO enrollees."

1. What features of the intervention might have contributed to the differences in group outcomes?
2. If you were going to replicate this study, how would you obtain data on the two outcome measures used?
3. Do you think the intervention used in the study would be cost-effective? How would you design a study to answer this question?

sitioning, range of motion, transfer abilities, dressing, bowel and bladder control, hygiene, locomotion, and eating. Other functional considerations include vision, hearing, speech, mental ability, and capacity for social interaction. The nurse, together with the client and his or her significant others, can foster renewed abilities to perform these functions. For example, the nurse may develop a plan and teach the client and family how to reestablish bowel control following a stroke, or the nurse might assist the client with passive and active range-of-motion exercises to restore function after a broken arm has healed.

Monitoring Health Status.   Another aspect of tertiary prevention in the control of chronic health problems is monitoring the client's health status. The nurse would be actively involved in periodic reassessment of a client's situation, being particularly alert to changes in circumstances that may affect health. For example, the nurse may note that cessation of unemployment benefits will limit the client's capacity to pay for health care. In this case, a referral might be made for additional financial assistance.

The nurse monitors the client's overall health status as well as the status of the chronic condition. When warranted, the nurse refers the client for medical follow-up. For example, the nurse may note that a client disabled by a serious accident is developing pressure sores due to long periods in a wheelchair. In this case, the nurse would suggest interventions to heal the pressure sores and prevent their recurrence or refer the client for medical assistance for severe lesions.

Promoting Adjustment.   Adjustments to the presence of a chronic disease need to be both functional and psychological. Functional adjustments reflect changes in lifestyle necessitated by the illness. Such changes may involve diet, activity patterns, restrictions (eg, limiting alcohol use or caloric intake), and the need to take medications. Some diseases necessitate learning special skills. For example, insulin-dependent diabetic clients need to learn to give themselves insulin injections, and hypertensive clients may need to learn how to take their blood pressure. In other chronic conditions, such as arthritis, there may be a need for special apparatus to assist in performing routine activities. The need for medication may also necessitate budgetary changes that the client must adjust to.

Psychological adjustments are also necessary. Psychological adjustment to a chronic condition may be required in a number of areas. Self-esteem is one of these areas. A chronic disease may make a client more dependent on others and less able to engage in activities that promote a positive self-image. For example, the client may need to stop working or begin to rely on others for assistance with basic functions such as eating and toileting. This dependence may be demeaning to one who has been self-reliant. The nurse should encourage the client to maintain as many functions as possible and help families to see the client's need for independence.

Loss of independence also necessitates adjustments in one's sense of control. Clients may feel they are not in control of events when the food they eat or the activities they perform are dictated in part by the chronic health problem. For some clients, noncompliance with recommendations might be an attempt to regain control over their own lives. Nurses can help prevent noncompliance by providing the client with other avenues for exercising control. Ways of doing this include involving the client in planning interventions and providing, whenever possible, choices in which the client can exercise control over actions and outcomes.

Guilt may also require adjustments in the way clients think about themselves. Because behavioral factors are widely known to make a significant contribution to the majority of chronic conditions, clients may feel guilty about behaviors that may have contributed to their current health problems. The nurse

can help clients explore their feelings and assist them to turn from an irredeemable past to present behaviors that minimize the effects of health problems.

The final area that may require adjustment for clients with chronic conditions is that of intimacy. Among men, for example, some chronic conditions or their treatments may result in impotence. In other cases, pain or changes in self-image may limit a client's ability to maintain intimate relationships with others. Another potential problem may be the withdrawal of significant others. Clients and their families can be encouraged to discuss intimacy issues openly, and significant others can be assisted to find ways of fulfilling intimacy needs that are congruent with the presence of a chronic health problem.

In dealing with clients who have chronic illnesses, the nurse must plan to assist them to return to a normal level of functioning as far as this is possible. In addition to the assistance of the nurse, it may be appropriate to refer the client to a relevant self-help group. Self-help groups can be particularly helpful in dealing with the psychosocial adjustments required by a chronic condition. Clients may be able to relate better to persons experiencing similar problems than to the authority figures represented by health care professionals.

Self-help groups have been shown to be quite effective in dealing with many health problems. The effectiveness of these groups stems from several assumptions. First, the emotional support of others with similar problems reduces the social isolation experienced by many clients with chronic conditions. Second, a collective self-identity emerges through group participation, allowing group members to develop new personal self-concepts. Third, group participation permits sharing of experiential knowledge and practical suggestions for coping with problems encountered. Finally, group participation fosters a more active orientation to health, greater reliance on individual and group support systems, and less dependence on health care providers.

Community health nurses may be involved in the initiation of self-help groups or in subsequent support of such groups. Nurses also refer individual clients to groups as appropriate. Nurses should function as facilitators of the group process, not as "leaders" or active participants in the group unless they also experience the chronic condition involved.

Community health nurses can facilitate the work of self-help groups in several ways. These include monitoring and directing active involvement by group members, encouraging the sharing of experiences and solutions to common problems, encouraging provision of mutual aid, and encouraging utilization of professional assistance as needed. Other facilitative measures include emphasizing personal responsibility for and control over events, maintaining positive pressure for behavior change, and emphasizing the need for positive coping strategies. Finally, the nurse should facilitate group interaction by providing the least amount of personal input possible.

Community health nurses can refer clients to self-help groups or other community agencies that provide assistance in dealing with problems arising from chronic health conditions. Community health nurses should determine the availability of such agencies within their own communities and identify the services provided and eligibility requirements for each type of service so as to make appropriate referrals.

Tertiary prevention related to individuals with chronic health problems focuses on assisting clients to adjust to their condition and on preventing additional problems. Tertiary prevention at the community level might involve planning and implementing programs to assist with client adjustment or political activity to ensure the availability of tertiary prevention programs. Tertiary prevention goals and related nursing interventions are summarized in Table 31–6.

Evaluating Care of Clients with Chronic Physical Health Problems

Evaluating care related to chronic health problems is done in terms of care outcomes. Care may be evaluated in relation to the individual client or to a population group. In the case of the individual client, the nurse evaluates the status of the chronic condition as well as the client's adjustment to having a chronic health problem. If interventions, both medical and nursing, have been effective, the condition will be controlled or may even be improving or will provide the least disruption possible to the life of the client and his or her significant others. Evaluative criteria re-

---

TABLE 31–6. GOALS FOR TERTIARY PREVENTION AND RELATED COMMUNITY HEALTH NURSING INTERVENTIONS IN THE CONTROL OF CHRONIC PHYSICAL HEALTH PROBLEMS

Tertiary Prevention Goal	Nursing Intervention
1. Preventing further loss of function in affected systems. Decrease risk factors for recurrence, exacerbation, or development of crises.	1. Motivate client to comply with treatment regimen. Assist client to identify risk factors amenable to change. Assist client to identify ways of decreasing risk factors.

2. Preventing loss of function in unaffected systems.
  a. Prevent physical disability.
	2. Assist client to maintain function in unaffected systems.
	  a. Prevent physical complications of illness through:
	    i. Breathing exercises
	    ii. Skin care
	    iii. Range-of-motion exercises
	    iv. Adequate nutrition and fluids
	  Provide physical care as required. Refer for assistance with physical care as needed.

b. Prevent social disability.	b. Accept client as a unique person. Encourage interaction with others. Assist significant others to deal with feelings about client's illness. Assist client to maintain independence as much as possible. Assist with identification of need for changes in family roles. Work to change public attitudes toward the disabled. Promote legislation to aid chronically ill to maintain their independence.
3. Restoring function.	3. Assist with planning and implementation of programs to regain function (bowel training, physical therapy). Teach client and others to carry out program and evaluate effects.
4. Monitoring health status.	4. Monitor client health status. Identify changes in client situation that affect health. Refer for follow-up as appropriate.

5. Promoting adjustment.
  a. Deal with feelings about disease.
	5. Assist client to adjust to presence of chronic disease.
	  a. Accept client at his or her level of development and acceptance of disease. Encourage client to discuss fears and apprehensions. Refer to self-help groups as appropriate.

b. Adjust lifestyle to accommodate chronic disease and its effects.	b. Assist client to identify needed changes in lifestyle. Assist client to plan and carry out lifestyle changes.
c. Adjust environment to meet changed needs.	c. Identify need for self-help devices and help client obtain them. Identify environmental changes needed to foster independence. Assist client to make necessary environmental changes.
d. Adjust self-image.	d. Assist client to adjust to change in self-image. Refer for counseling as needed.
e. Adjust to expense of chronic care.	e. Refer for financial aid as needed.

TABLE 31–7. **STATUS OF SELECTED NATIONAL OBJECTIVES FOR PHYSICAL HEALTH PROBLEMS**

Objective		Base	Most Recent	Target
1.3	Proportion of people engaged in regular exercise	22% (1985)	71% (1995)	30%
2.3	Reduce overweight prevalence	26% (1976–1980)	28% (1995)	20%
2.5	Reduce percentage of calories from fat	36% (1976–1980)	34% (1988–1991)	10%
3.4	Reduce smoking prevalence	29% (1987)	22% (1995)	15%
3.11	Increase worksite smoking policies	27% (1985)	59% (1992)	75%
3.16	Increase providers who counsel about smoking	52% (1986)	75% (1992)	75%
8.1	Increase years of healthy life	64 (1990)	NDA[a]	65
9.2	Reduce accidental injury hospitalizations (per 100,000 population)	887 (1988)	699 (1993)	754
9.9	Reduce nonfatal head injury (per 100,000)	118 (1988)	90 (1993)	106
9.10	Reduce nonfatal spinal cord injury (per 100,000)	5.3 (1988)	4.7 (1993)	5
9.12	Increase use of motor vehicle occupant protection systems	42% (1988)	66% (1995)	85%
9.13	Increase use of			
	Motorcycle helmets	60% (1988)	62% (1994)	80%
	Bicycle helmets	8% (1984)	5–10% (1994)	50%
9.14	Increase the number of states with laws regarding			
	Seat belt use	33 (1989)	48 (1994)	50
	Helmet use	22 (1989)	25 (1994)	50
10.2	Reduce work-related injuries (per 100 workers)	7.7 (1983–87)	8.4 (1994)	6
11.1	Reduce asthma hospitalizations (per 100,000)	188 (1987)	179 (1992)	160
15.1	Reduce coronary heart disease (CHD) deaths (per 100,000)	135 (1987)	122 (1991)	100
15.2	Reduce stroke deaths (per 100,000)	30.4 (1987)	26.5 (1996)	20
15.4	Increase control of blood pressure	11% (1976–1980)	21% (1991)	50%
15.6	Reduce mean serum cholesterol	213 (1976–1980)	NDA	200
16.1	Reduce cancer deaths (per 100,000)	134 (1987)	129 (1996)	130
16.2	Reduce lung cancer deaths (per 100,000)	38.5 (1987)	39.6 (1991)	42
16.3	Reduce breast cancer deaths (per 100,000)	23 (1987)	13.2 (1992)	20.6
16.4	Reduce cervical cancer deaths (per 100,000)	2.8 (1987)	2.7 (1992)	1.3
16.5	Reduce colorectal cancer deaths (per 100,000)	14.4 (1987)	21.9 (1992)	13.2
16.11	Increase clinical breast examination and mammography	36% (1987)	77% (1995)	80%
16.12	Increase Pap smear	88% (1987)	94% (1995)	95%
17.2	Reduce major activity limitation due to chronic conditions	9.4% (1988)	9.6% (1991)	8%
17.9	Reduce diabetes deaths (per 100,000)	38 (1986)	13.6 (1996)	34
17.11	Reduce diabetes incidence (per 1000)	2.9 (1987)	3.7 (1994)	2.5

[a]NDA, no data available.

flect both the client's physiologic status and his or her quality of life.

When the recipient of care is a community or population group, evidence of success in controlling chronic health problems lies primarily in changes in morbidity and mortality figures. Are there fewer cases of hypertension or cardiovascular disease in the population now than before the initiation of control efforts? Are there fewer disabilities due to accidental injuries? Do those with diabetes live longer or have fewer hospitalizations for diabetic complications? Based on the evaluative data, decisions can be made regarding the need to attempt other control strategies or to continue with current measures.

Evaluation of control strategies for chronic conditions in the population may focus on the extent to which chronic disease objectives for the year 2000 have been achieved. Table 31–7 provides information on selected objectives related to control of chronic health problems.

TESTING YOUR UNDERSTANDING

1. Describe at least three personal effects and four population effects of chronic physical health problems. (pp. 812–814)
2. Identify at least three biophysical factors that influence the development of chronic physical health problems. (pp. 815–818)
3. Describe at least two factors related to the physical, psychological, and social dimensions that influence chronic physical health problems and their consequences. (pp. 818–820)
4. Identify at least five behavioral dimension factors

Critical Thinking in Practice: A Case in Point

You have just started working as a community health nurse for the Wachita County Health Department in Mississippi. During your employment interview the nursing supervisor mentioned that one of your responsibilities would be to participate in developing plans for dealing with the high rate of hypertension in the county. The incidence rate for hypertension here is three times that of the state and twice that of the nation.

The population of the county is largely African American with high unemployment rates and little health insurance. Folk health practices are quite common, one of them being drinking pickle brine for a condition called "high blood." Although this condition is not related to high blood pressure, the two terms are frequently confused by both lay members of the community and professionals alike. Dietary intake is typical of the rural South, consisting of a variety of fried foods, beans and other boiled vegetables, and corn bread.

Few health services are available in the county itself, although there is a major hospital 50 miles away. There are two general practitioners in the area and one pediatrician. The health department holds well-child, immunization, tuberculosis, and family planning clinics regularly and all are well attended. Transportation is a problem for many community residents.

1. What are the biophysical, psychological, physical, social, behavioral, and health system factors influencing the incidence and prevalence of hypertension?
2. Write two objectives for your efforts to resolve the community's problem with hypertension.
3. What primary, secondary, and tertiary activities might be appropriate in dealing with the problem of hypertension? Which of these activities might you carry out yourself? Which would require collaboration with other community members?
4. How would you evaluate the outcome of your interventions?

---

that contribute to the development of chronic physical health problems. (pp. 821–822)
5. Describe three health care system factors that impede efforts to control chronic physical health problems. (pp. 822–823)
6. Describe at least four general approaches to primary prevention of chronic physical health problems. Give an example of an activity that a community health nurse might perform in relation to each. (pp. 824–825)
7. Identify at least three aspects of the treatment of chronic physical health problems. What is the role of the community health nurse with respect to each? (pp. 827–828)
8. Describe five considerations in tertiary prevention of chronic physical health problems. How might a community health nurse be involved in each? (pp. 828–831)

WHAT DO YOU THINK?
Questions for Critical Thinking

1. What are some of the reasons for the increased prevalence of chronic physical health problems in the United States? Could the same be said of developing countries in the world?

2. Given the limited resources available for health care services, do you think priority should be given to dealing with problems of communicable diseases or chronic diseases?
3. Should healthful behavior be legislated (eg, helmet-use laws, smoking prohibitions)? Why or why not?
4. What chronic physical condition would be most devastating for you personally? Why? What effects do you think this condition would have on your life?
5. If you could only choose one target population, what would be the "ideal" group for interventions designed to prevent chronic conditions? Why?

REFERENCES

Air Pollution and Respiratory Health Bureau. (1995). Asthma—United States, 1982–1992. *MMWR, 43,* 952–955.

Air Pollution and Respiratory Health Bureau. (1996a). Asthma mortality and hospitalization among children and young adults—United States, 1980–1993. *MMWR, 45,* 350–353.

Air Pollution and Respiratory Health Bureau. (1996b). Asthma surveillance programs in public health departments—United States. *MMWR, 45,* 802–804.

Bruce, M. L., Seeman, T. E., Merrill, S. S., & Blazer, D. G.

(1994). The impact of depressive symptomatology on physical disability: MacArthur studies of successful aging. *American Journal of Public Health, 84,* 1796–1799.

Buchdahl, R., Parker, A., Stebbings, T., & Babiker, A. (1996). Association between air pollution and acute childhood wheezy episodes: Prospective observational study. *British Medical Journal, 312,* 661–665.

Centers for Disease Control. (1996a). National arthritis month—May 1996. *MMWR, 45,* 373.

Centers for Disease Control. (1996b). National diabetes awareness month—November 1996. *MMWR, 45,* 937.

Centers for Disease Control. (1996c). National melanoma/skin cancer detection and prevention month, May 1996. *MMWR, 45,* 345.

Centers for Disease Control. (1997). National diabetes awareness month—November 1997. *MMWR, 46,* 1013.

Clark, L. C., Combs, G. F., Turnbull, B. W., et al. (1996). Effects of selenium supplementation for cancer prevention in patients with carcinoma of the skin. *JAMA, 276,* 1957–1963.

Clement, K., Vaisse, C., Manning, B. S. J., et al. (1995). Genetic variation in the β-adrenergic receptor and an increased capacity to gain weight in patients with morbid obesity. *New England Journal of Medicine, 333,* 352–354.

Disabilities Prevention Program. (1994). Prevalence of diabetes and associated health conditions—United States, 1991–1992. *MMWR, 43,* 730–731, 737–739.

Diabilities Prevention Program. (1995). Disabilities among children aged < 17 years—United States, 1991–1992. *MMWR, 44,* 609–613.

Division of Adult and Community Health. (1996). Factors associated with prevalent self-reported arthritis and other rheumatic conditions—United States, 1989–1991. *MMWR, 45,* 487–491.

Division of Cancer Prevention and Control. (1994). Examinations for oral cancer—United States, 1992. *MMWR, 43,* 198–200.

Division of Cancer Prevention and Control. (1996a). Screening for colorectal cancer—United States, 1992–1993, and new guidelines. *MMWR, 45,* 107–110.

Division of Cancer Prevention and Control. (1996b). Survey of knowledge of and awareness about melanoma—United States, 1995. *MMWR, 45,* 346–349.

Division of Chronic Disease Control and Community Intervention. (1995). Prevalence and impact of arthritis among women—United States, 1989–1991. *MMWR, 44,* 329–334.

Division of Diabetes Translation. (1994a). Continuing diabetes care—Rhode Island, 1991. *MMWR, 43,* 798–800.

Division of Diabetes Translation. (1994b). Pregnancies complicated by diabetes—North Dakota, 1980–1992. *MMWR, 43,* 837–839.

Division of Diabetes Translation. (1997a). Diabetes-specific preventive-care practices among adults in a managed-care population—Colorado, Behavioral Risk Factor Surveillance System, 1995. *MMWR, 46,* 1018–1023.

Division of Diabetes Translation. (1997b). Trends in the prevalence and incidence of self-reported diabetes mellitus—United States, 1980–1994. *MMWR, 46,* 1014–1018.

Division of Unintentional Injury Prevention. (1994). Update: Alcohol-related traffic fatalities—United States, 1982–1993. *MMWR, 43,* 861–867.

Ellis, A. A., & Trent, R. B. (1995). Hospitalizations for near drowning in California: Incidence and costs. *American Journal of Public Health, 85,* 1115–1118.

Epidemiology Program Office. (1997). Asthma mortality—Illinois, 1979–1994. *MMWR, 46,* 877–880.

Ferris, D. G., Golden, N. H., Petry, J., Litaker, M. S., Nackenson, M., & Woodward, L. D. (1996). Effectiveness of breast self-examination prompts on oral contraceptive packaging. *Journal of Family Practice, 42,* 43–48.

Fontana, S. A., Baumann, L. C., Helberg, C., & Love, R. R. (1997). The delivery of preventive services in primary care practices according to chronic disease status. *American Journal of Public Health, 87,* 1190–1196.

Fraley, A. M. (1992). *Nursing and the disabled across the life span.* Boston: Jones and Bartlett.

Fuchs, C. S., Giovannucci, E. L., Colditz, G. A., Hunter, D. J., Speizer, F. E., & Willett, W. C. (1994). A prospective study of family history and the risk of colorectal cancer. *New England Journal of Medicine, 331,* 1669–1674.

Galuska, D. A., Serdula, M., Pamuk, E., Siegel, P. Z., & Byers, T. (1996). Trends in overweight among US adults from 1987 to 1993: A multistate telephone survey. *American Journal of Public Health, 86,* 1729–1735.

Gorey, K. M., Holowaty, E. J., Fehringer, G., et al. (1997). An international comparison of cancer survival: Toronto, Ontario, and Detroit, Michigan, metropolitan areas. *American Journal of Public Health, 87,* 1156–1163.

Helfand, R. F., Gary, H. E., Freeman, C. Y., & Anderson, L. J. (1995). Serologic evidence of an association between enteroviruses and the onset of Type I diabetes mellitus. *Journal of Infectious Diseases, 172,* 1206–1211.

Hu, H., Aro, A., Payton, M., et al. (1996). The relationship of bone and blood lead to hypertension: The normative aging study. *JAMA, 275,* 1171–1176.

Kerber, R. A., & Slattery, M. L. (1995). The impact of family history on ovarian cancer risk. *Archives of Internal Medicine, 155,* 905–912.

Kington, R. S., & Smith, J. P. (1997). Socioeconomic status and racial and ethnic differences in functional status associated with chronic diseases. *American Journal of Public Health, 87,* 805–810.

Kraus, J. F., Peek, C., & Williams, A. (1995). Compliance with the 1992 California motorcycle helmet use law. *American Journal of Public Health, 85,* 96–99.

Kubzansky, L. D., Kawachi, I., Spiro, A., Weiss, S. T., Vokonas, P. S., & Sparrow, D. (1997). Is worrying bad for your heart? A prospective study of worry and coronary heart disease in the normative aging study. *Circulation, 95,* 818–824.

Lenfante, C. (1996). High blood pressure: Some answers, new questions, continuing challenges. *JAMA, 275,* 1604–1606.

Levy, D., Larson, M. G., Vasan, R. S., Kannel, W. B., & Ho, K. K. L. (1996). The progression from hypertension to congestive heart failure. *JAMA, 275,* 1557–1562.

Macknin, M. L., & Mendendorp, S. V. (1994). Association between bicycle helmet legislation, bicycle safety education, and use of bicycle helmets in children. *Archives of Pediatric and Adolescent Medicine, 148,* 255–259.

Markovitz, J. H., Matthews, K. A., Kannel, W. B., Cobb, J. L., & D'Agostino, R. B. (1993). Psychological predictors of hypertension in the Framingham study: Is there tension in hypertension? *JAMA, 270,* 2439–2443.

Merlo, J., Ranstam, J., Liedholm, H., et al. (1996). Incidence of myocardial infarction in elderly men being treated with antihypertensive drugs: Population based cohort study. *British Medical Journal, 313,* 457–461.

Mittleman, M. A., MacClure, M., Sherwood, J. B., et al. (1995). Triggering of acute myocardial infarction onset by episodes of anger. *Circulation, 92,* 1720–1725.

Mortality Statistics Bureau. (1996). Mortality patterns—United States, 1993. *MMWR, 45,* 161–164.

Mortality Statistics Bureau. (1997). Mortality patterns—Preliminary data, United States, 1996. *MMWR, 46,* 941–944.

Muhlestein, J. B., Hammond, E. H., Carlquist, J. F., et al. (1996). Increased incidence of *Chlamydia* species within the coronary arteries of patients with symptomatic atherosclerotic versus other forms of cardiovascular disease. *Journal of the American College of Cardiology, 27,* 1555–1561.

National Arthritis Data Workgroup. (1996). Prevalence and impact of arthritis by race and ethnicity—United States, 1989–1991. *MMWR, 45,* 373–378.

Office on Smoking and Health. (1996a). Cigarette smoking before and after an excise tax increase and an antismoking campaign—Massachusetts, 1990–1996. *MMWR, 45,* 966–970.

Office on Smoking and Health. (1996b). State-specific prevalence of cigarette smoking—United States, 1995. *MMWR, 45,* 962–966.

Perry, I. J., Wannamethee, S. G., Walker, M. K., Thomson, A. G., Whincup, P. H., & Shaper, A. G. (1995). Prospective study of risk factors for development of non-insulin dependent diabetes in middle aged British men. *British Medical Journal, 310,* 560–564.

Powell-Griner, E., Anderson, J. E., & Murphy, W. (1997). State- and sex-specific prevalence of selected characteristics—Behavioral Risk Factor Surveillance System, 1994 and 1995. *MMWR, 45*(SS-3), 1–31.

Pratt, L. A., Ford, D. E., Crum, R. M., Armenian, H. K., Gallo, J. J., & Eaton, W. W. (1996). Depression, psychotropic medication, and risk of myocardial infarction. *Circulation, 94,* 3123–3129.

Reilly, M. J., Rosenman, K. D., Watt, F. C., et al. (1994). Surveillance for occupational asthma—Michigan and New Jersey, 1988–1992. *MMWR, 43*(SS-1), 9–17.

Rimm, E. B., Chan, J., Stampfer, M. J., Colditz, G. A., & Willett, W. C. (1995). Prospective study of cigarette smoking, alcohol use, and the risk of diabetes in men. *British Medical Journal, 310,* 555–559.

Sidney, S., Tekawa, I. S., Friedman, G. D., Sadler, M. C., & Tashkin, D. P. (1995). Mentholated cigarette use and lung cancer. *Archives of Internal Medicine, 155,* 727–732.

Stephens, T., Pederson, L. L., Koval, J. J., & Kim, C. (1997). The relationship of cigarette prices and no-smoking bylaws to the prevalence of smoking in Canada. *American Journal of Public Health, 87,* 1519–1521.

Stuart, C. A., Smith, M. M., Gilkison, C. R., Shaheb, S., & Stahn, R. M. (1994). Acanthosis Nigricans among Native Americans: An indicator of high diabetes risk. *American Journal of Public Health, 84,* 1839–1842.

Targonski, P. V., Persky, V. W., Orris, P., & Addington, W. (1994). Trends in asthma mortality among African Americans and whites in Chicago, 1968 through 1991. *American Journal of Public Health, 84,* 1830–1833.

U.S. Department of Commerce. (1996). *Statistical abstract of the United States, 1996.* Washington, DC: Government Printing Office.

U.S. Department of Health and Human Services. (1991). *Healthy people 2000: National health promotion and disease prevention objectives.* Washington, DC: Government Printing Office.

U.S. Department of Health and Human Services (1993). *Health United States, 1992, and healthy people 2000 review.* Washington, DC: Government Printing Office.

U.S. Department of Health and Human Services. (1996). *Health United States, 1995.* Washington, DC: Government Printing Office.

U.S. Preventive Health Services Task Force. (1996). *Guide*

to clinical preventive services (2nd ed.). Alexandria, VA: International Medical.

Verbrugge, L. M., & Patrick, D. L. (1995). Seven chronic conditions: Their impact on US adults' activity levels and use of medical services. *American Journal of Public Health, 85,* 173–182.

Wagner, E. H., LaCroix, A. Z., Grothaus, L., et al. (1994). Preventing disability and falls in older adults: A population-based randomized trial. *American Journal of Public Health, 84,* 1800–1806.

Zhang, Y., Proenca, R., Maffei, M., Barone, M., Leopold, L., & Friedman, J. M. (1994). Positional cloning of the mouse obese gene and its human homologue. *Nature, 372,* 425–432.

RESOURCES FOR NURSES DEALING WITH CHRONIC PHYSICAL HEALTH PROBLEMS

Accident Prevention

American Association of Poison Control Centers
3201 New Mexico Avenue, NW, Ste. 310
Washington, DC 20016
(202) 362–7271

American Red Cross National Headquarters
431 18th Street, NW
Washington, DC 20006
(202) 737–8300

American Trauma Society
8903 Presidential Pkwy, Ste. 512
Upper Marlboro, MD 20772
(301) 420–4189

National Safety Council
1121 Spring Lake Drive
Itasca, IL 60143–3201
(708) 285–1121

National Spinal Cord Injury Association
545 Concord Avenue, No. 29
Cambridge, MA 02138–1122
(617) 441–8500

Airway Disease

American Lung Association
1740 Broadway
New York, NY 10019–4374
(212) 315–8700

Asthma and Allergy Foundation of America
1125 15th Street, NW, Ste. 502
Washington, DC 20005
(202) 466–7643

Emphysema Anonymous
PO Box 3224
Clearwater, FL 34617
(813) 391–9977

National Jewish Center for Immunology and Respiratory Medicine
1400 Jackson Street
Denver, CO 80206
(303) 388–4461

Arthritis

Arthritis Foundation
1314 Spring Street, NW
Atlanta, GA 30309
(404) 872–7100

Cancer

American Cancer Society
1599 Clifton Road, NE
Atlanta, GA 30329
(404) 320–3333

R. A. Bloch Cancer Foundation
H & R Block Bldg.
4410 Main
Kansas City, MO 64111
(816) 932–8453

Cancer Care, Inc. and The National Cancer Foundation, Inc.
1180 Avenue of the Americas
New York, NY 10036
(212) 221–3300

National Cancer Center
88 Sunnyside Blvd.
Plainview, NY 11803
(516) 349–0610

Oncology Nursing Society
501 Holiday Drive
Pittsburgh, PA 15220
(412) 921–7373

Reach to Recovery
c/o American Cancer Society
1599 Clifton Road, NE
Atlanta, GA 30329
(800) ACS–2345

United Ostomy Association
36 Executive Park, Ste. 120
Irvine, CA 92714
(714) 660–8624

Diabetes

American Diabetes Association
National Service Center
PO Box 25757
1660 Duke Street
Alexandria, VA 22314
(703) 549–1500

Joslin Diabetes Center
One Joslin Place
Boston, MA 02215
(617) 732–2400

Juvenile Diabetes Foundation
120 Wall Street
New York, NY 10005–3904
(212) 889–7575

Heart Disease

American Heart Association
7272 Greenville Avenue
Dallas, TX 75231–4596
(214) 373–6300

Council on Arteriosclerosis of American Heart
  Association
7320 Greenville Avenue
Dallas, TX 75231
(214) 706–1293

Mended Hearts, Inc.
7272 Greenville Avenue
Dallas, TX 75231–4596
(214) 706–1442

Hypertension

National High Blood Pressure Education Program
National Heart, Lung, and Blood Institute
National Institutes of Health, Bldg. 31
9000 Rockville Pike
Bethesda, MD 20892
(301) 496–0554

National Hypertension Association
324 East 30th Street
New York, NY 10016
(212) 889–3557

Obesity

Overeaters Anonymous
6075 Zenith Court, NE
Rio Rancho, NM 87124–6424
(505) 891–2664

TOPS Club
PO Box 07360
4575 South 5th Street

Milwaukee, WI 53207
(414) 482–4620

Weight Watchers International
500 North Broadway, Ste. 200
Jericho, NY 11753–2196
(516) 949–0400

Pain

National Chronic Pain Outreach Association
7979 Old Georgetown Road, Ste. 100
Bethesda, MD 20814–2429
(301) 652–4948

National Committee on the Treatment of Intractable
  Pain
c/o Wayne Coy, Jr.
Cohn and Marks
1333 New Hampshire, NW
Washington, DC 20036
(202) 452–4836

Smoking

Action on Smoking and Health
2013 H Street, NW
Washington, DC 20006
(202) 659–4310

American Cancer Society
(see entry under Cancer)

American Heart Association
(see entry under Heart Disease)

American Lung Association
(see entry under Airway Disease)

Other

Medic Alert Foundation International
1735 N Lynn Street, Ste. 950
Arlington, VA 22209–2022
(703) 524–7710

National Center for Chronic Disease Prevention
  and Health Promotion
4770 Buford Hwy., NE
Mailstop K 13
Atlanta, GA 30333
(770) 488–5080

U.S. Senate Committee on Labor and Human
  Resources
Subcommittee on the Handicapped
SH-639 Hart
Washington, DC 20510
(202) 224–5630

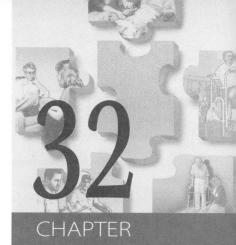

CHRONIC MENTAL HEALTH PROBLEMS: SCHIZOPHRENIA AND MOOD DISORDERS

Working with individual clients who have chronic mental illness and with their families is an increasingly important dimension of community health nursing. Community health nurses may be called on to follow clients after they are discharged from a psychiatric facility, often with little or no ongoing support from psychiatrists or mental health specialists. Nurses may also discover that a client they are following for some other reason has signs and symptoms of chronic mental illness. In such situations, community health nurses understandably feel uncertain about the nature and scope of their responsibility. Those who have limited experience with psychiatric disorders beyond basic education are likely to feel unprepared to assess, evaluate, and intervene effectively with chronically mentally ill clients and their families.

Schizophrenia and mood disorders—bipolar disorder and major depressive disorder—are discussed in this chapter. In dealing with these conditions, community health nurses function primarily in a supportive role. They may assess clients' responses to medication and their adjustment to home, work, and social life. Community health nurses work most effectively as part of a treatment team of health care providers who cooperate to develop treatment plans, establish clearly defined roles and expectations commensurate with educational preparation, and communicate regularly to coordinate care.

▶ ## Chapter Objectives

After reading this chapter, you should be able to:

- Identify at least five symptoms characteristic of schizophrenia.
- Identify three common forms of disorganized speech associated with schizophrenia.
- Discuss the major thrust of secondary prevention in the control of schizophrenia.
- Discuss at least three areas of emphasis in tertiary prevention for schizophrenia.
- Identify at least three biophysical factors that may influence the development of mood disorders.
- Describe at least five social dimension factors that may contribute to the development of schizophrenia or mood disorders.
- Identify three approaches to primary prevention of mood disorders.
- Describe at least three community health nursing activities related to secondary prevention of mood disorders.
- Identify at least two considerations in tertiary prevention of mood disorders.

▶ ## THE IMPACT OF CHRONIC MENTAL HEALTH PROBLEMS

A *chronic mental illness* is a syndrome with specific symptoms that impairs an individual's cognition, perceptions, emotions, and/or behavior and that recurs over an extended period. Schizophrenia is the most disabling of severe mental illnesses (Andreasen & Carpenter, 1993b), and new cases occur at an annual rate of one for every 10,000 people in the United States. The lifetime prevalence of schizophrenia is 0.5 to 1% (American Psychiatric Association, 1994). Depression is even more common, affecting 25 million Americans (Badger, 1996) and 340 million people worldwide (*The Nation's Health*, 1996). Approximately 17% of the U.S. population will experience major depression during their lifetimes (Badger, 1996).

Chronic mental illness not only takes a toll on an individual's quality of life but can also tax a family's emotional, physical, and financial resources. These family problems frequently become society's problems. For example, the monetary costs of schizophrenia exceed those for cancer (Andreasen & Carpenter, 1993a). Health care costs associated with major depression amount to nearly 44 billion each year in the United States (Shao, et al., 1997). Depressed persons also incur higher costs for health care unrelated to their depression. In one study, for example, annual health care costs for clients with diagnosed depression exceeded those for nondepressed clients by an average of nearly $2000 (Simon, Von Korff, & Barlow, 1995).

As noted in Chapter 24, chronic mental illness is a major contributing factor in the growing problem of homelessness. In fact, it is believed as many as 150,000 people with severe mental illness may be among the homeless (Flynn, 1993). Mental illness also places many other stresses on individuals, families, and society as a whole. The importance of chronic mental health problems in the United States is highlighted by the number of objectives related to these disorders in the national health objectives for the year 2000 (U.S. Department of Health and Human Services, 1991). These objectives are summarized in Appendix A.

▶ ## CRITICAL DIMENSIONS OF NURSING IN THE CARE OF CLIENTS WITH CHRONIC MENTAL HEALTH PROBLEMS

Like chronic physical illness, dealing with chronic mental health problems is a lifelong undertaking. This means that motivation is a critical feature of controlling the effects of mental illness. For this reason, the interpersonal dimension of community health nursing is particularly crucial to working effectively with clients with chronic mental health problems. Assisting clients with motivational issues may be even more difficult in these conditions than in the case of chronic physical health problems because of the cognitive deficits that frequently characterize diseases such as schizophrenia. Clients may often be unaware of the effects of their own behavior on their health and, thus, are unmotivated to change.

The cognitive dimension is also particularly important in community health nurse's care of clients with chronic mental health problems. Community health nurses frequently express concerns regarding the adequacy of their knowledge and skills for working with this population (Reutter & Ford, 1996). Discomfort in caring for clients with chronic mental illness may also stem from the social stigma associated with these diseases. Social stigma may prevent clients with problems from seeking help and makes the case finding and referral functions of the community health nurse particularly important. Social stigma also gives rise to a need to engage in the advocacy element of the ethical dimension of nursing. Crucial to advocacy are the process dimension elements of political activity and change. Community health nurses must work to change societal attitudes toward mental illness and to incorporate these changed attitudes into effective health care policy that assures access to care for those with chronic mental health problems.

▶ THE DIMENSIONS MODEL AND CONTROL OF SCHIZOPHRENIA

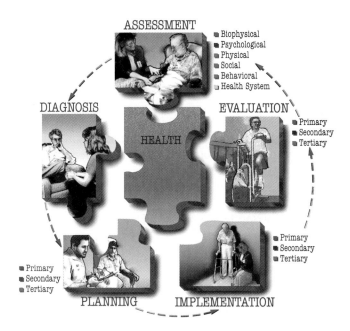

The disorder called schizophrenia was described in Sanskrit writings as early as 1400 BC. *Schizophrenia* is a psychotic condition that manifests itself in massive disruptions in perception, cognition, emotion, and behavior (American Psychiatric Association, 1994). For many clients this illness results in lifetime psychological disability and disrupted family relationships.

The term *schizophrenia* is derived from the Greek, meaning "split mind." Although the term itself has existed since 1912, its definition has changed over time and is different in various parts of the world. A common misconception is that a person who has schizophrenia has dual personalities, a Dr. Jekyll and Mr. Hyde. Rather than a dual personality, schizophrenia involves a disassociation of thinking from feeling and from actions. Schizophrenia may be defined as a severe emotional disorder marked by disturbances of thinking, mood, and behavior, with thought disorder (confused or bizarre thinking) as the primary feature. According to the DSM-VI (American Psychiatric Association, 1994), schizophrenia is characterized by the presence of at least two of the following symptoms for a significant portion of the month: delusions, hallucinations, disorganized speech, grossly disorganized or catatonic behavior, and "negative" symptoms such as flattened affect and avolition (inability to make deci-

sions). Schizophrenia is also characterized by significant social or occupational dysfunction.

People with chronic schizophrenia who are in remission often appear "normal." It is only during exacerbations that they exhibit symptoms. Other clients may never be totally without some residual symptomatology even with treatment (Kane & Marder, 1993).

Diagnosis of schizophrenia is difficult. Because it encompasses such a nonspecific cluster of symptoms, some experts believe that schizophrenia is not a distinct disorder. Diagnosis is further complicated by the fact that people with schizophrenia are a heterogeneous group whose illness is marked by the presence of various symptoms and whose course of recovery differs.

Misunderstanding about schizophrenia and the wide variation in its course have led to its being understood by some physicians, including psychiatrists, and lay people as equivalent to a diagnosis of cancer in that it is incurable. Although it is true that there is no cure for schizophrenia, comparing it with diabetes is more appropriate because both diseases are chronic, marked by exacerbations, and can be controlled. In fact, schizophrenia has been referred to as "cerebral diabetes" because of the similarities between the two conditions (Holden, 1995).

Assessing the Dimensions of Health in Schizophrenia

Factors in each of the dimensions of health have been associated with schizophrenia.

The Biophysical Dimension

Biological findings suggest a variety of explanations of schizophrenia including genetics and physiologic dysfunctions in the neurotransmitter systems of the brain.

Genetics. Various studies of families, twins, and adopted children provide strong evidence that some people have a genetic predisposition to develop schizophrenia. First-degree relatives of persons with schizophrenia are ten times more likely to develop the illness than those without a family history of the disease (American Psychiatric Association, 1994). Only 1% of the general population develops schizophrenia, but 10% of the parents, siblings, and children of people with schizophrenia also are diagnosed with the illness.

Studies of twins show that both heredity and environment play a role in schizophrenia. The potential for schizophrenia developing in both members of identical twins is 48%, and the risk of schizophrenia in both members of fraternal twins is 4%. In addition, any family members who do not have schizophrenia may exhibit schizophrenia-like symptoms (Kendler & Diehl, 1993). Because the chance of identical twins both developing schizophrenia is not 100%, environmental influences apparently play a significant part in the emergence of the disease.

How much of a role either heredity or environment plays in the etiology of schizophrenia remains unknown. There is no single biological marker consistently found in schizophrenic people that is not also found in people without, and no single biological change is consistently found in all those with schizophrenia (Bogerts, 1993).

Physiologic Function.   Researchers have investigated the action of the drugs that control the symptoms of schizophrenia in an attempt to understand the biochemical basis of the disease. It is known that the two classes of drugs used in the treatment of schizophrenia, phenothiazines (chlorpromazine [Thorazine]) and butyrophenones (haloperidol [Haldol]), both block dopamine receptors. On this basis, researchers suspect that schizophrenia may be related to excessive levels of dopamine linked to overactive neuronal activity (Lieberman & Koreen, 1993). Both genetics and environmental factors like stress, nutrition, and exposure to viruses can influence biochemical states. The dopamine hypothesis—that the amount of dopamine available at particular synapses is altered in people with schizophrenia—is the most promising explanation of schizophrenia. The monoamine oxidase (MAO) explanation of schizophrenia, on the other hand, postulates that levels of a type of MAO (an enzyme that oxidizes monoamines such as epinephrine) are lower in people with schizophrenia than in the general population.

Other physiologic phenomena have also been associated with schizophrenia. Brain ventricular size is significantly larger in chronic schizophrenic clients than in members of control groups, and other anatomical brain abnormalities have been noted in persons with schizophrenia (Bogerts, 1993; Selemon, Rajkowska, & Goldman-Rakic, 1995). Research has also suggested that schizophrenia may be an autoimmune disease (Kirch, 1993).

Another aspect of assessing factors related to physiologic function in clients with schizophrenia is identification of physical illness. In general, psychiatric clients have higher rates of undiagnosed physical illness, particularly cardiovascular diseases and diabetes, than the general population. Assessing the individual with schizophrenia for physical symptoms may be difficult because nonspecific behavior and

mood changes may be the only signs of physical illness exhibited. Or, physical illness may manifest through psychological symptoms, leading the nurse to focus on the psychological aspects of disease. Finally, symptoms of physical illness may mimic symptoms of an earlier schizophrenic episode. In one study, more than 46% of individuals with serious mental illness reported unmet physical health needs (Flynn, 1993).

Maturation and Aging.   The onset of schizophrenia typically occurs from late adolescence to the middle of the fourth decade and cases among children are rare (American Psychiatric Association, 1994). In fact, a diagnosis of schizophrenia is 50 times more likely after 15 years of age than before (Kronenberger & Meyer, 1996). Diagnosis of schizophrenia in children is complicated by the number of other conditions in these age groups with similar characteristics (eg, attention deficit hyperactivity disorder [ADHD] and pervasive developmental disorders) (American Psychiatric Association, 1994).

The Psychological Dimension

Elements of the psychological dimension to be considered in schizophrenia include the characteristic manifestations of the disease, psychological risk factors, other psychiatric comorbidity, coping skills used by clients with schizophrenia, and the potential for suicide.

Characteristic Psychological Manifestations of Schizophrenia.   The characteristic features of schizophrenia are manifested in cognitive and affective abnormalities that fall into two categories, positive symptoms and negative symptoms. Positive symptoms reflect an excess or distortion of normal thought patterns, whereas negative symptoms reflect a decrease or loss of normal function (American Psychiatric Association, 1994). Positive symptoms include delusions, hallucinations, disorganized speech, and grossly disorganized or catatonic behavior.

Delusions are distortions of inferential thinking that lead to misperceptions of experiences and erroneous beliefs. Delusions differ in type and may include perceptions of being persecuted or of being capable of amazing feats (grandiose delusions). In referential delusions, the client believes that unrelated gestures or messages are directed at him or her. Delusions are misperceptions of phenomena in the real world. Hallucinations, on the other hand, occur in the absence of external stimuli (Silbersweig, et al., 1995). **Hallucinations** are sensory experiences that occur without any sensory input and may be noted in any sensory modality (taste, smell, hearing, sight, or touch). Auditory hallucinations, in which the client hears sounds or voices that do not exist, are the most common (American Psychiatric Association, 1994). Visual hallucinations involve seeing objects that are not visible to others, while tactile, olfactory, and gustatory hallucinations reflect inappropriate sensations of touch, smell, and taste, respectively.

Disorganized thinking is inferred in clients whose speech is disorganized. This disorganization may be reflected in loose associations (wandering from one topic to another), *tangentiality* (oblique relationships between topics), or incoherence in which words are strung together without producing any coherent meaning. Typical forms of disorganized thinking are summarized in Table 32–1. Grossly disorganized behavior, the fourth positive symptom of schizophrenia, may be manifested in a variety of ways as unusual modes of dress, inappropriate sexual behavior, unpredictable agitation, and so on.

Negative symptoms of schizophrenia include flattened affect, alogia, and avolition. *Flattened affect* is characterized by lack of emotional response, facial inexpressiveness, and diminished body language. *Alogia* is an inability to express oneself verbally, and *avolition* is the inability to make decisions.

The community health nurse would assess clients for evidence of both positive and negative symptoms of schizophrenia and make referrals for further evaluation as needed. The nurse should also assess clients with schizophrenia for prodromal symptoms suggesting imminent relapse. These may be unique to the individual client and should be elicited from the client or family members. Such symptoms may include difficulty sleeping, changes in thought patterns, social withdrawal, deteriorating physical appearance due to lack of self-care, and impaired verbal communication reflected in changes in thought patterns. Behavioral changes and changes in self-concept and body image may also be prodromal symptoms of relapse.

Psychological Risk Factors.   Although schizophrenia seems to have a significant biological basis, psychological

stress appears to play an important part in development of the disease (Holden, 1995). Stress and an emotionally charged environment are also implicated in symptomatic relapses in clients with diagnosed disease. Conversely, decreasing stress and increasing personal and interpersonal competencies appears to contribute to better control of the disease and its manifestations (Bellack & Meuser, 1993).

Psychiatric Comorbidity.   Many clients with schizophrenia also experience manifestations of other psychiatric illnesses such as depression, obsessive-compulsive disorder, panic disorder, and substance abuse. In addition, depression may be part of the relapse prodrome in schizophrenia (Kane & Marder, 1993). Schizophrenia is also associated with increased risk of delusional disorder and atypical psychosis (Kendler & Diehl, 1993). Because of this marked comorbidity, it may be difficult to make diagnoses of schizophrenia. Comorbidity also makes treatment decisions more complicated and will be addressed later in this chapter.

Coping Skills in Clients with Schizophrenia.   Clients with severe mental illness are often believed to be deficient in coping abilities. Research has indicated, however, that clients with schizophrenia have fairly well-developed coping skills used to control their symptoms. Some of these coping strategies are healthier than others and can be encouraged by community health nurses working with clients with schizophrenia and their families. One category of coping skill displayed by schizophrenic clients dealt with behavior control by means of passive or active distraction (eg, listening to music

 QUESTIONS FOR ASSESSING INDIVIDUALS FOR SIGNS OF SCHIZOPHRENIA

- Have you noticed any change in your sleeping patterns?
- Have you noticed that you are spending more time by yourself lately?
- Have you noticed any change in the way you think? Have you had nagging thoughts that will not go away?
- Have you noticed that you have less energy for keeping up your appearance, for example, putting on your make-up, taking showers or baths?
- Have you been feeling more nervous lately? More anxious?
- Have you noticed any change in your eating patterns? Have you suddenly gained weight? Lost weight?
- Have you noticed people reacting differently to you at home? At work?
- How are you liking yourself these days?

TABLE 32–1. COMMON FORMS OF DISORGANIZED SPEECH

Type of Disorganized Speech	Manifestation
Loose associations	Barely connects one thought to the next thought
Tangentiality	Begins with one thought and leads "round the mulberry bush" before answering the question
Incoherence	Makes no logical connection between words, "word salad"

or reading vs. playing an instrument or writing poetry), rest or physical activity (eg, running), or indulgence (eg, eating, drinking, or smoking). Other coping strategies included socializing with and talking to others, avoiding thinking about or ignoring misperceptions, shifting one's attention to other thoughts, engaging in future planning or problem solving, seeking medical care, prayer, and acceptance of symptoms. One final strategy, symptomatic behavior (eg, telling voices to "shut up" or doing as told by voices) is a less healthy approach to dealing with symptoms of schizophrenia (Kingdon & Turkington, 1994).

Suicide Potential.   Another aspect of psychological assessment related to schizophrenia is the potential for suicide in the schizophrenic client. Suicide is the most devastating potential outcome of schizophrenia, and studies indicate that there is a 10% probability of suicide among clients with schizophrenia (American Psychiatric Association, 1994). Community health nurses need to be particularly attentive to the potential for suicide when clients with schizophrenia experience depressive episodes.

The Physical Dimension

There is little evidence, as yet, that elements of the physical environment influence the development of schizophrenia. Some authors, however, have postulated a link between urban environments, with their increased stress levels and intensity of environmental pollution, and schizophrenia. Support for these hypotheses lie in the increased prevalence of schizophrenia in urban versus rural areas and in developed versus developing countries as well as the fact that schizophrenia was not recognized as a disease entity until the early 1800s at the beginning of the Industrial Revolution. It is hypothesized that heterocyclic amines (HCAs) present in some foods, cigarette smoke, and associated with some air pollutants, may play a role in the development of schizophrenia (Holden, 1995).

The Social Dimension

In the past, schizophrenia was thought to be largely a result of impaired family interactions. More recent evidence refutes this attribution of causality. Although there do appear to be familial tendencies toward schizophrenia, these are now thought to be more genetic in origin than the product of family interaction. The community health nurse working with clients with schizophrenia, however, should be aware of the profound influence this disease has on family members as well as on the individual involved. With the closure of many institutions for the mentally ill in the early 1960s, families became the "institution of

choice" for the care of mentally ill clients (Parker, cited in Loukissa, 1995). In approximately 60% of cases, clients with mental illness are cared for by parents, many of whom are aging and do not have other relatives nearby to share the burden of care (Flynn, 1993). Like clients themselves, families of persons with schizophrenia have been found to engage in several types of behavior to minimize the impact of the client's symptoms on the family. Again, some of these are healthy and others are not. Relatively positive coping behaviors displayed by families include positive actions to minimize symptoms (eg, distracting the client), ignoring or accepting bizarre behavior, becoming resigned to the client's behavior, and reassuring the client. Negative responses include avoiding interaction with the client, use of coercion or threats, condoning or supporting symptomatic behavior, and becoming hopeless and disorganized (Kingdon & Turkington, 1994). The community health nurse should assess the effect of schizophrenia on the family and on family interactions with the client, paying particular attention to factors that may increase stress and potential for symptomatic relapse.

Culture is another feature of the social dimension that has implications for schizophrenia, particularly for diagnosis of the disease. What appear to be delusions in one cultural context are perfectly accepted and understandable in another. For example, in some cultures religious experiences of hearing God speak are considered normal. Culture may also influence the expression of affect, and differences between client and health care providers may lead to inappropriate diagnostic inferences.

Homelessness among the chronically mentally ill is a serious social dimension problem. As noted earlier, the severely mentally ill make up a significant portion of the homeless population in the United States due to a number of factors discussed in Chapter 24. Early in the 1980s, Judge Robert Coates wrote in *A Street is not a Home,* "severely mentally ill people have never before been permitted to roam the nation's streets unassisted, bringing their private (treatable) hells out in the open to haunt us and our cities" (cited in White, 1993). Unfortunately, too often the problem of the mentally ill among the homeless population has been addressed with inappropriate incarceration, and an estimated 37,500 to 150,000 mentally ill persons may be inappropriately placed in correctional settings (White, 1993). It is also estimated that 5 to 10% of the correctional population is in need of care for severe mental illness including schizophrenia (Flynn, 1993).

The Behavioral Dimension

Behavioral choices can precipitate the onset of an episode of schizophrenia. People who have had one or more episodes of schizophrenia do best when they minimize stress and live balanced lives. The community health nurse needs to assess leisure activities to ensure that the person exercises in a regular and balanced way.

With regard to consumption patterns, there is a growing awareness among health care providers that many of the same people who abuse substances have underlying chronic mental disorders that they are attempting to mask with the use of mind-altering drugs. This becomes evident when the person is weaned from the substance and the symptoms of schizophrenia become more prominent. It is also known that abuse of alcohol, marijuana, or hallucinogens can cause hallucinations in persons vulnerable to schizophrenia. As noted earlier, HCAs created by some modes of cooking food (eg, frying and broiling) and contained in azo food dyes used in some soft drinks and hard candies may also contribute to schizophrenia. Smoking also creates HCAs and may have a similar effect (Holden, 1995). Smoking also increases the risk of tardive dyskinesia, a serious side effect of the use of neuroleptics to treat schizophrenia (Jeste & Caligiuri, 1993).

The Health System Dimension

In most cases, the current public mental health care delivery system is unable to provide more than custodial care to people suffering from chronic disorders like schizophrenia. The trend toward reimbursement systems favoring prospective payment means that hospital stays will be shorter and coverage for outpatient services will be decreased. As treatment for psychiatric problems is increasingly focused on short-term therapy for acute problems, clients with chronic mental health problems suffer. Health insurance, if it covers mental illness treatment at all, does so only to a limited extent and discriminates against those with chronic disorders (Carter, 1993). Access to needed services is even less for children, and less than 20% of children with mental illness, including schizophrenia, receive care (Gore, 1993).

While federal and state funding of mental health services is decreasing, treatment of chronic mental illness is becoming increasingly complex. At the same time, fewer persons are now trained or interested in dealing with the chronically mentally ill. In the face of fewer treatment options for the chronically mentally ill, community health nurses are more likely to see clients with chronic mental illness in their caseloads. This is particularly true as many people suffering from chronic mental illness are living with their families.

Most of the mentally ill can live normally in the community if they receive outpatient care, rehabilitative services, and decent housing. Research findings indicate that a system of halfway houses and day treatment facilities is needed to provide ongoing care, support, and treatment for the chronically mentally ill. At present, too few of these facilities are available, and although they are much less costly than inpatient facilities, their services are covered by few insurance companies.

Diagnostic Reasoning and Care of Clients with Schizophrenia

Community health nurses may make a variety of nursing diagnoses related to schizophrenia. These diagnoses can reflect the health needs of an individual client, the client's family, or a population group. For example, the nurse might diagnose "impaired reality orientation due to schizophrenic episode" in an individual client or an "exacerbation of psychotic symptoms due to family stress" in a client with diagnosed schizophrenia. Another nursing diagnosis at this level might reflect "disruption of family function due to exhibition of symptoms of schizophrenia" on the part of one member.

Nursing diagnoses may also be made that reflect problems related to schizophrenia affecting population groups. For example, the community health nurse might diagnose an "increased incidence of schizophrenia in the homeless population," or "inadequate treatment facilities for persons with chronic mental health problems due to reduced program funds."

Planning and Implementing the Dimensions of Health Care in the Control of Schizophrenia

Planning control of schizophrenia may occur at primary, secondary, and tertiary levels of prevention. Primary prevention involves identifying families at risk and providing support and education around topics such as parent effectiveness. Secondary prevention includes the diagnosis and treatment of clients with schizophrenia. Preventing further episodes by monitoring compliance with medication and other treatment regimens falls under tertiary prevention.

Primary Prevention

The role of primary prevention in reducing risks for schizophrenia among the general population and among those at high risk for the disease is reflected in the Institute of Medicine's (*The Nation's Health,* 1994) call for federal funding of research on preventive interventions in the field of mental health. The community health nurse's role lends itself to primary prevention in the area of stress or risk factor reduction. To plan effectively for primary prevention, the nurse needs to keep in mind the current understanding of the major factors contributing to schizophrenia discussed earlier.

The major aspect of primary prevention in the control of schizophrenia is eliminating or reducing stress or risk factors for the disease. Families who are at risk for schizophrenia may need anticipatory guidance to cope with major changes and major life transitions. Some family therapists believe that schizophrenia is one of the symptoms that can emerge when families have difficulty moving from one stage of family development to another. Basing primary prevention efforts on this psychological developmental theory, the community health nurse can plan to give anticipatory guidance when the family is making the transition to a new stage of development that may be stressful, for example, when families with preadolescent children move into the stage of adolescence or when young adult children begin to leave home. Nurses can encourage families at risk to seek family counseling before or early in the process of undergoing disruptive transitions in their lives, including major geographic moves or divorce. If research confirms the links hypothesized between HCAs in food, smoke, and environmental pollution and schizophrenia, community health nurses may encourage avoidance of HCAs. For example, nurses can promote abstinence from smoking or advocate antipollution legislation (Holden, 1995).

Secondary Prevention

Secondary prevention may entail referring for diagnosis and treatment; educating both client and family about the disease and about medications and other aspects of treatment. Secondary prevention of schizophrenia focuses on the control of psychotic symptoms through the use of medication. Any of several different classes of antipsychotic drugs may be used in the initial treatment of clients with schizophrenia. Some clients will not respond to initial drug therapy or may experience adverse effects or annoying side effects that may limit compliance with the therapeutic regimen. In such cases, alternative drugs may be tried until the desired effect is achieved. A newer drug, clozapine, is frequently reserved for use with clients whose symptoms fail to respond to other medications (Kane & Marder, 1993). Community health nursing

during this phase of treatment consists of monitoring treatment compliance, treatment effects, and adverse or side effects of medications.

Tertiary Prevention

Once relief of symptoms is achieved, the emphasis in treatment shifts to tertiary prevention which focuses on rehabilitating the client and preventing relapse. Maintenance treatment with medications can take one of two alternative paths (Kane & Marker, 1993). The first is continuous low-dose administration of medications with increases in dosage with the advent of symptoms, and the second is "targetted or intermittent" use of medication initiated with the first appearance of symptoms suggestive of relapse. Both of these approaches are intended to minimize the risk of tardive dyskinesia and extrapyramidal side effects and to maximize client compliance.

Tertiary prevention also includes a variety of other interventions in addition to medication. As noted by one author, "Medication may be a cornerstone of treatment, but treatment cannot be successful unless all dimensions of an affected individual's life are addressed and supported" (Wingerson, 1996). Community health nurses may be asked to follow clients with diagnoses of schizophrenia to provide support, encourage compliance, and monitor the effects of treatment. Community health nurses can assist clients to plan a regular lifestyle that includes sufficient sleep, regular patterns of waking and sleeping (not rotating shifts), and limited-to-no-use of stimulants such as coffee, tobacco, and stimulant-containing decongestant medications that may trigger schizophrenic episodes. Hallucinogens, amphetamines, and even marijuana can trigger episodes, and the nurse should educate the client about the risks involved in their use. Moderate alcohol use does not appear to trigger symptomatic episodes, but clients should be cautioned about use, particularly in conjunction with medication.

Nurses should also assist clients to limit exposure to stressful situations. Some stressors occur without warning, but clients can plan to minimize the aggregation of stressors over which they have control. For example, the client would be wise not to plan to buy a new house and change employment at the same time. The nurse can also help clients and their families to identify prodromal symptoms that signal a symptomatic relapse and to seek professional assistance when these symptoms are noted.

In addition, community health nurses can educate clients and their families regarding medication side effects and ways to deal with them as well as educating them about serious adverse effects that should be reported to their health care provider. Potentially harmful effects include liver disturbances and bone marrow suppression as well as tardive dyskinesia. Tardive dyskinesia occurs in approximately one fourth of clients taking neuroleptics and the risk of this condition increases with age, length of medication use, smoking, diabetes, and the presence of mood disorder and extrapyramidal side effects of antipsychotic drugs (Jeste & Caligiuri, 1993). Clients experience involuntary muscle movements of the face, tongue, limbs, or trunk that may contribute to dental ulcers and infection, falls, and shortness of breath, as well as social stigmatization and isolation. The effects of tardive dyskinesia are reversible, to a point, and the nurse should monitor the client closely so medications can be changed or the condition treated if symptoms occur.

Clients and families need to know that depression often occurs sometime during or following a schizophrenic episode. Several types of depression are associated with schizophrenia. Stress can trigger depression, which can trigger a schizophrenic episode. In addition, some people experience recovery depression, normal feelings during recovery from what some people have called a "living hell." A third type of depression arises in response to knowledge of an incurable disease. Again, this is a normal response. Depression may also result from medication. Finally, there is a chronic depression that sometimes accompanies schizophrenia. The remarkable reversal of schizophrenic symptoms that sometimes occurs with the use of clozapine may lead to depression when clients "awaken" to reality to find themselves without social or job skills and little to live for (Kopelowicz, 1996). As noted by one author, "Lifting the veil of delusion can bring a reactive depression so legitimate and so powerful it may lead to immobilization or even thoughts of suicide" (Lefley, 1996). When nurses observe depression in clients, they need to alert the treatment team and monitor clients for suicidal behaviors.

Persons with chronic mental illness often have a high incidence of physical health problems and sometimes lack the capacity to seek health care in today's complex delivery systems. In some areas, nurse practitioners are being employed by community mental health centers to assess and meet the physical health needs of these clients. The community health nurse may be in the situation of following a person for a physical health problem who suddenly begins to show signs of schizophrenia discussed earlier in this chapter. The nurse's role in this case is to refer the client for further diagnosis and treatment. The community health nurse also refers the client who is exhibiting signs of exacerbation of the disease.

 Evaluating Control Strategies for Schizophrenia

Evaluating the treatment plan for schizophrenia includes assessing clients and families for their understanding of schizophrenia and their ability to monitor client status and behaviors in response to the nursing interventions discussed above. The nurse's role often includes evaluating interventions to ensure that they focus on the behavioral, perceptual, cognitive, and emotional aspects of the client's functioning as evidenced by improved communication, self-care, and judgment. These interventions and plans need to be realistic, reflecting the client's level of functioning and the course of the disorder.

Evaluation at the group or population level focuses on the incidence and prevalence of schizophrenia in the population. If primary prevention efforts are effective, these rates should decline. Other foci for evaluation at the group level include the adequacy of treatment facilities and the extent of *recidivism*, or rehospitalization, as a result of recurrent episodes of schizophrenia. When secondary and tertiary interventions are effective, evaluation should indicate that hospitalization occurs less frequently.

▶ THE DIMENSIONS MODEL AND CONTROL OF MOOD DISORDERS

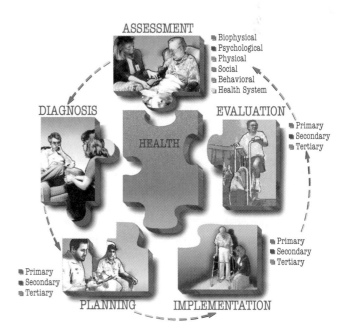

A *mood disorder* is a disturbance in mood that manifests mainly as depression but can also involve elation or mania. In the DSM-IV, mood disorders include major depressive disorder and bipolar disorder, as well as other forms of depression such as dysthymic disorder (American Psychiatric Association, 1994).

Affect refers to emotional tone. Affect includes verbal descriptions of emotional states and nonverbal behaviors like facial expression, motor activity, and physiologic responses. Another way to think of affect is on a continuum from depression through "normal" to manic. People diagnosed as having major depression experience loss of interest in life and an unresponsive mood lasting at least 2 weeks. Bipolar episodes include times when the person is depressed and periods where the person experiences elation, needs less sleep, and exhibits an enormous capacity for activity. The manic phase begins suddenly and the depressive phase is briefer than in major depressive disorder.

Although an estimated 13% of men and 21% of women in the general population experience depressive episodes at some time in their lives (Hagerty, 1995), only a minority seek psychiatric or mental health care. Given this, community health nurses are likely to encounter many individuals suffering from various forms of mood disorders that have never been treated.

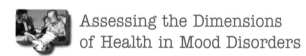

Assessing the Dimensions of Health in Mood Disorders

A variety of factors are associated with the development of mood disorders. These factors occur in each of the dimensions of health.

The Biophysical Dimension

Human biological factors related to age and sex, genetic inheritance, and physiologic function have been associated with the incidence and course of mood disorders.

Age and Sex. Approximately 25 million Americans suffer from depression. Women have approximately twice the risk of depression of men (Hagerty, 1995). The prevalence of depression among children ranges from 1.7 to 6% (Anderson & Werry, 1994), and incidence in children of depressed parents has been as high as 45% in some reports (Badger, 1996). These children continue to experience difficulties even when their parents are in remission. Among the elderly, depression may be seen as a normal effect of losses occurring with age. Conversely, depression may be di-

agnosed in elderly clients experiencing delirium due to physical illness (Farrell & Ganzini, 1995).

Genetic Inheritance. Strong evidence exists for the role of genetic factors in mood disorders. It is highly possible that genetic factors make some individuals more susceptible to environmental stressors or styles of parenting that may contribute to depression. Evidence suggests that genetic etiologies play a role in both major depression and bipolar disorder.

Genetic factors have been linked to the development of mood disorders. Close relatives of people with mood disorders face a 1.5 to 3 times higher risk of developing these disorders than the general population. In addition, studies of twins suggest a strong genetic component to bipolar disorder (American Psychiatric Association, 1994).

In assessing the potential for depression in individuals and families, the community health nurse can use a genogram to describe familial patterns of mood disorder. Evidence of a family history of depression would direct the nurse's attention to a more in-depth assessment for signs of depression in current family members. These signs and symptoms of mood disorder are discussed later in this chapter.

Physiologic Function. Other physiologic theories have been advanced to explain depression. The endocrine model holds that endocrine changes that occur after exposure to stress result in the biophysical changes known as the "vegetative signs of depression." Hormones, particularly cortisol, growth hormone, thyroid-stimulating hormone, thyroid-releasing hormone, leutenizing hormone, and prolactin, have all been found in abnormal levels in depressed clients, supporting belief in a psychoendocrinologic mechanism for depression. Community health nurses can assess clients at risk for depression for vegetative signs including psychomotor slowing, sleeping disorders, appetite disturbances, diminished libido (sexual desire), difficulty concentrating, and constipation.

One test used to diagnose endogenous depression (chronic depression not caused by external factors like grief or loss) is related to the psychobiological theory of depression. The dexamethasone suppression test (DST) involves administering a single dose of dexamethasone followed by blood or urine monitoring of cortisol levels. In depressed people, dexamethasone does not suppress adrenocortical functioning because of a failure of the normal inhibitory influence of the brain in release of adrenocorticotropic hormone (ACTH) and cortisol. This suggests that this limbic system dysfunction is not simply a response to stress. Rather, it is associated with disturbances in mood, affect, appetite, sleep, and autonomic nervous system

> ## VEGETATIVE SIGNS OF DEPRESSION
>
> *Disturbances in sleep patterns*
> Difficulty falling asleep
> Early morning awakening
> Difficulty waking up
>
> *Alterations in eating habits*
> Significant weight gain
> Significant weight loss
>
> *Diminished energy level*
>
> *Decreased interest in sex*
>
> *Difficulty concentrating*
>
> *The presence of one or more of these symptoms can indicate that a client is experiencing depression.*

activity. A related theory suggests that depressed people suffer from a failure of the central nervous system circadian inhibitory mechanism. Seasonal affective disorders (SADs) are being studied in people who live in the Northern Hemisphere and who suffer increased depressions during winter when there is less sunlight.

Community health nurses should assess clients with possible depression for changes in biorhythms, mood, affect, and appetite. The nurse may also assess seasonal patterns to depressive episodes that suggest SADs.

In assessing individual clients with mood disorders, the nurse should conduct a head-to-toe physical examination. Organically caused depression is due to a person's changed biochemical condition and should not be confused with normal reactions to illness. Organically caused depression may result from hormonal or chemical imbalances and even from some physical diseases. Postpartum depression is a fairly common depressive response thought to be physiologically induced by changes in hormone levels and relationships as the body readjusts to a nonpregnant state. Although most postpartum depression lasts a few days to a week, a small percentage of postpartum women may experience depression lasting months and requiring treatment.

Because depression often precedes or results from physical illnesses, the nurse needs to be particularly sensitive to the powerful connections between mind and body when people with depression experience exacerbations of conditions such as eczema or psoriasis, asthma, ulcerative colitis, and Crohn's disease. AIDS, multiple sclerosis, systemic lupus erythematosus, thyroid and parathyroid disorders, adrenal

insufficiency, carcinoid syndrome, and central nervous system tumors are among the disorders associated with depression. As an example, 20 to 25% of people with cancer may experience diagnosable depression (Valente & Saunders, 1997). In addition to the potential for depression in the face of physical illness, depression increases the risk of death in conditions such as cardiovascular disease (Shao, et al., 1997). Management of physical illness is also complicated by the presence of depression (American Psychiatric Association, 1994).

Some clients experience "iatrogenic depression" as a side effect of some medications taken for physical illnesses. Medications implicated in iatrogenic depression include opiates, antineoplastics, phenothiazines, digitalis, guanethidine, hydralazine, methyldopa, propranolol, reserpine, levodopa, sedatives, and steroids. Community health nurses caring for clients who are on any of these medications should assess clients carefully for evidence of depression.

Clients who exhibit symptoms mimicking depressive or bipolar disorders may be experiencing serum electrolyte imbalance instead, and the community health nurse should assess the client for other signs of electrolyte imbalance and refer the client for further diagnosis and treatment of imbalance.

The Psychological Dimension

In addition to assessing clients for actual signs of psychological depression, two other elements of the psychological dimension should be assessed. The first is the existence of psychiatric comorbidity, and the second is the potential for suicide in the depressed client. Several other major psychiatric disorders tend to occur concurrently with depressive disorders. These include substance abuse disorders, panic disorder, obsessive-compulsive disorder, eating disorders, and borderline personality disorder (American Psychiatric Association, 1994). The lifetime incidence of psychiatric comorbidity with major depression is estimated to be as high as 43% (Hagerty, 1995). The presence of these conditions may mask depression, contribute to depression, or occur independently of the depressive disorder, and the community health nurse should be alert to signs of these conditions and their implications for control of depression. There is also some evidence that children of persons with major depressive disorders may be at increased risk for attention deficit hyperactivity disorder (ADHD) (American Psychiatric Association, 1994).

Another aspect of assessing the client with a mood disorder is to determine the potential for suicide. Depression and suicide are highly correlated, with up to 15% of those with severe major depressive disorder dying from suicide (American Psychiatric Association, 1994). The nurse should explore with the client any suicidal tendencies or thoughts of suicide. Suicide tends to occur most frequently when clients are recovering from an episode of depression; this is because the severely depressed client probably does not have the energy to commit suicide.

The Physical Dimension

As noted earlier, it is believed that lack of exposure to sunlight may be a contributing factor in seasonal depression, indicating that the physical environment may influence the occurrence of mood disorders. Seasonal affective disorder is diagnosed when there is an established relationship between seasonal variations and development of depressive symptoms for at least 3 years (Hagerty, 1995). Seasonal affective disorder most often occurs in the winter months with clients experiencing symptom relief with the advent of spring. It is estimated that 5 to 10% of the general population may experience this form of depression at clinically significant levels with prevalence increasing with more northerly latitude (Lam, et al., 1995).

The Social Dimension

Elements of the social dimension to be addressed include the contribution of social factors to the development of depression and the effects of depression on family interactions. Hypothesized social risk factors for depression include increased urbanization, geographic mobility with consequent loss of family support systems, social anomie, changes in family structures, and changes in the role of women in society. Lower socioeconomic status may also contribute to major depression, whereas higher socioeconomic status has been associated with bipolar disorder (Hagerty, 1995). Lack of social support systems has also been associated with depression, particularly in elderly widows and widowers (Kanacki, Jones, & Galbraith, 1996).

Culture may influence expression of symptoms in depressive disorders. Asian clients, for example, may exhibit more somatic complaints. Caucasians, on the other hand, may have more complaints of altered mood and cognition (Hagerty, 1995). The social stigma attached to depression, which also varies from culture to culture, may prevent many clients from seeking assistance when symptoms are experienced (American Psychiatric Association, 1994).

The social effects of depression on families with depressed members are many and varied and may be quite severe. For example, marital adjustment is often poor and dissatisfaction high. In addition, these families often have difficulties communicating and are characterized by high levels of tension and low levels of mutual support. These effects have been found to be more severe than in families with problems of alcohol dependence, adjustment disorder, or schizophrenia and create a risk of divorce nine times that of the general population. Family difficulties tend to continue even when the depressed family member is in remission and these families often exhibit diminished levels of social support resources (Badger, 1996).

The Behavioral Dimension

Behavioral factors related to consumption patterns and leisure activities may also influence mood disorders.

Consumption Patterns.   Consumption patterns in the form of substance abuse can mask the symptoms of affective illness. Substance abuse can be an attempt at self-medication to relieve the symptoms of mood disorders. For individuals with mood disorders, alcohol, barbiturates, and tranquilizers are the substances most often abused. Some experts estimate that as many as 70% of alcoholics, for example, may have a bipolar disorder.

The community health nurse should assess a client's consumption of alcohol and other substances that may mask or exacerbate mood disorders. The nurse should pay particular attention to tendencies to

---

Critical Thinking in Research

Kanacki, Jones, and Galbraith (1996) studied the relationship of social support to depression in older people who had lost a spouse. They found that widows and widowers experienced similar incidence of depression and that there was a significant negative relationship between social support as perceived by participants and the amount of depression experienced. Social support was measured using the Personal Resource Questionnaire and depression was assessed using the Beck Depression Inventory. Nearly half of the participants had at least a moderate level of depression and those with lower levels of perceived social support had higher levels of depression.

1. What are the implications of the findings of this study for preventing depression in widows and widowers?
2. Would you expect to obtain similar findings if you studied the relationship of social support to depression in middle-aged women whose children are leaving home? Why or why not?
3. How would you go about determining whether or not your hypothesis is accurate?
4. How might you identify potential subjects for your study?

ASSESSMENT TIPS: Assessing Risk for Chronic Mental Health Problems

Biophysical Dimension

What age groups are most likely to develop the chronic mental health problem?

Are there racial or gender differences in the incidence of the problem?

Is there a genetic contribution to the problem?

What effect does existing physical illness have on the chronic mental health problem?

How does the chronic mental health problem affect control of physical health problems?

Do physical health problems or their treatment cause signs and symptoms suggestive of the chronic mental health problem?

Psychological Dimension

What life stresses contribute to the chronic mental health problem?

Does stress exacerbate the chronic mental health problem?

What are the psychological manifestations of the problem?

What is the extent of adaptation to the chronic mental health problem? How does the client cope with the problem?

Is there existing psychiatric comorbidity? If so, what form does it take?

Is the client at risk for suicide as a result of the chronic mental health problem?

Physical Dimension

What effect, if any, do weather conditions have on the chronic mental health problem?

Do environmental pollutants contribute to the incidence of the problem?

Social Dimension

What are the effects of the chronic mental health problem on social interactions (with family and others)?

What are societal attitudes to the problem? Do they hamper control efforts?

Is there social stigma attached to having the chronic mental health problem?

What effect, if any, do cultural beliefs and behaviors have on incidence of the problem?

Does the chronic mental health problem contribute to homelessness?

What social support systems are available to people with the problem?

How do social factors (eg, unemployment) influence the problem?

How does the mental health problem affect the client's ability to work?

Behavioral Dimension

Does alcohol or drug use contribute to the incidence of the chronic mental health problem or its effects?

Are alcohol or drugs used in an effort to control the problem?

What effect, if any, does exercise have on the problem?

Does smoking influence the chronic mental health problem? In what way?

What effect does the problem have on self-care behaviors?

Health System Dimension

What is the attitude of health care providers to persons with the chronic mental health problem?

Are health care providers alert to signs and symptoms of the problem?

What treatment facilities are available to persons with the problem? How adequate are they?

What types of therapy are available for the problem? How effective are they?

Are diagnostic and treatment services available and accessible to persons with the chronic mental health problem?

Does the client exhibit treatment side effects or adverse effects?

Does treatment for other health problems cause or exacerbate the mental health problem?

---

mix alcohol and medications as these may be lethal combinations.

Leisure Activity.   As was the case with schizophrenia, balance is the key in assessing leisure activity. In the case of depression, nurses need to determine whether the individual is including leisure activities into his or her schedule. Most people suffering from depression have very little energy, and they often lose their ability to enjoy life. Leisure activities for the person in the manic stage of bipolar disorder may pose safety hazards if excessive risks are taken during periods of grandiose thinking. Evidence of the effects of physical exercise in preventing mental health problems is somewhat mixed. Some authors, for example, extol the beneficial effects of exercise for mental health (Brill & Cooper, 1993). Others have found no association between exercise and risk of depression or other psychiatric conditions (Cooper-Patrick, Ford, Mead, Chang, & Klag, 1997).

The Health System Dimension

The major issue in mood disorders related to the health care system is reaching those persons suffering from depression—many individuals do not seek treatment. Lack of attention to symptoms of depression by health care providers may further decrease the opportunity to treat people with mood disorders (Lyness, Noel, Cox, King, Conwell, & Caine, 1997). Primary care providers are often inclined to ignore signs and symptoms of depression or attribute them to physical illnesses, and as many as 35 to 50% of persons with depression may be undiagnosed or inadequately treated (Shao, et al., 1997). Providers may also fail to warn clients of the potential for depression caused by many medications and to monitor them for evidence of depression.

Lack of access to care is another health care system factor that may impede diagnosis and treatment of mood disorders. For example, some health insurance policies may not cover care for emotional disorders, particularly if they are not yet severe enough to warrant hospitalization. The nurse should assess clients' ability to pay for care as well as the availability and accessibility of resources for care of mood disorders in the community.

 Diagnostic Reasoning and Care of Clients with Mood Disorders

Nursing diagnoses related to mood disorders might reflect the presence or consequences of these diseases for individual clients or the existence of a high incidence of mood disorders or lack of care facilities in the community. Possible nursing diagnoses for an individual are "depression due to recent divorce and financial stress" and "potential for loss of job due to manic manifestations of bipolar disorder." At the community level, the nurse might diagnose "increased incidence of depressive disorder due to economic instability" or "lack of facilities for care of mood disorders due to diminished tax revenues."

 Planning and Implementing the Dimensions of Health Care in the Control of Mood Disorders

As was the case with schizophrenia, it is important that both client and family be actively involved in planning and implementing control strategies for mood disorders. Effective strategies can involve primary, secondary, and tertiary prevention measures depending on whether the disorder has already manifested itself in a particular client.

Primary Prevention

Because depression is the most prevalent mental disorder identified in primary health care settings, the community health nurse is in an excellent position to engage in primary prevention of mood disorders. Because the number of people suffering from mood disorders far exceeds the number of those who seek treatment, the nurse is likely to encounter individuals with active disorders who are either unaware they are depressed or do not want to face it.

Primary preventive measures may include family teaching, referral, and risk factor reduction. Awareness of the pivotal role of community health nurses in preventing depression has led to the development of training programs to increase knowledge and skills related to assessment and intervention with those at risk for depression. Prevention measures can be developed for individuals and families who are at risk for mood disorders owing to family history or situational stressors. Teaching them about the prevalence of depression in society, the genetic factors involved, and the potential for stressful life events that can cause depression can help clients and their families deal with feelings about the disorder. Teaching how to handle stress is another way of preventing depression in people who are at risk for mood disorders.

Because many chronically depressed people are socially isolated and do not seek help, community health nurses need to increase the level of support available to clients. Community support groups exist for those who are adjusting to separation, divorce, or the death of a loved one, and nurses can make referrals to these and similar support groups for clients who are undergoing stressful life events. The nurse can also refer parents to parenting groups that can provide them with opportunities for social interaction as well as parenting support.

Reducing or eliminating stressors and risk factors for depression is another way to lessen the feelings of helplessness and hopelessness that can lead to depression. Working to improve the social conditions of persons at risk for depression may effectively reduce their exposure or vulnerability to socioeconomic stressors and associated higher risks of physical and mental illness.

Secondary Prevention

When the community health nurse suspects that an individual is suffering from a major depressive or bipolar disorder, the nurse can refer the client for further diagnosis and treatment. Again, the nurse would want to consider the type of referral that will be most appropriate to the client's circumstances. Areas to be considered include the client's financial resources, the acceptability of a particular source of services to the client, and any other circumstances that might influence the client's ability to follow through on the referral (eg, lack of transportation). Because depressed clients frequently do not have the energy to seek care, the nurse may make an appointment for the client and help the client plan the logistics of getting there.

In caring for the client with a diagnosis of a mood disorder, the nurse may plan to obtain a "mood history." Particularly useful in bipolar disorder, the *mood history* is a picture obtained from the client and family about the cyclical ups and downs of the client's moods over the last several years. When this picture is completed, the nurse, client, and family can often identify particular times of the year or particularly stressful events that precipitated either manic or depressive episodes. This knowledge can then be used to design strategies or minimize stress at expected periods of exacerbation, thus limiting response. In addition, the nurse and the family can plan intensive observation of the client at these times to identify early signs of depression or manic behavior so treatment can be initiated or reinforced.

Antidepressant medications are effective in all forms of depressive disorders and may be used alone or in conjunction with other therapies. Because depression and anxiety often go hand in hand, both symptoms can be treated pharmacologically. Several categories of antidepressant and antianxiety agents are commonly prescribed. Two classes of antidepressants have been prescribed since 1960, tricyclics like amitriptyline (Elavil) and imipramine hydrochloride (Tofranil), and monoamine oxidase (MAO) inhibitors like phenelzine sulfate (Nardil) and tranylcypromine sulfate (Parnate).

Although the reason for their effectiveness is not known, both types of antidepressants share one property: the ability to boost the action of serotonin and norepinephrine. While the tricyclics block reabsorp-

tion of these neurotransmitters, MAO inhibitors interfere with enzymes that break them down. When a client is started on a traditional tricyclic, he or she spends several weeks taking progressively larger doses. The provider uses blood tests to determine the effective serum concentration, which is different for each individual. Because an overdose of tricyclics can be extremely toxic, resulting in low blood pressure, heart disturbances, blurred vision, constipation, dizziness, sluggishness, and weight gain, many doctors often prescribe too little. Because the therapeutic range is so narrow, too little medication is often ineffective. The MAO inhibitors can cause a hypertensive response to foods containing retsin (eg, chocolate, cheese, wines). Many people choose depression over these side effects.

The community health nurse caring for clients on antidepressant medications educates them about the medication and its therapeutic and toxic effects as well as potential side effects. Fluoxetine (Prozac), a new classification of antidepressant introduced in 1987, is now the most commonly prescribed antidepressant in the United States. Prozac works like a tricyclic that focuses on serotonin. Although Prozac takes 3 weeks to become effective, there is no blood monitoring, because a dose of 20 to 40 mg is usually effective. There is less risk of overdose, and the most common side effects are nuisance effects such as headaches, nausea, insomnia, nervousness, weight loss, decreased sexual interest and loss or delay of orgasm, and a slight risk of seizures. In rare cases, suicidal thoughts and overtly violent behavior have been traced to Prozac. A small number of clients develop a "caffeine syndrome" in which they become restless and sometimes experience tremors. Because it is a new drug, the long-term effects of Prozac are unknown. There is concern that because administration of Prozac is so simple, the drug may be indiscriminately prescribed like Valium was in the 1970s. Psychiatrists are cautioned that Prozac may not be as effective as the tricyclics. Clients may not be helped if they are suffering depression associated with a hidden illness like cancer, hypothyroidism, or AIDS. Finally, because trials have been done exclusively on young, healthy adults, the effects on the less robust and the elderly remain unknown.

Antianxiety agents, sedatives, and hypnotics are often prescribed when symptoms of anxiety are related to depression. These classes of drugs share similar pharmacologic properties, and they can be effective in small doses to relieve anxiety and in larger doses to induce sleep. Meprobamate (Miltown, Equanil) was the first antianxiety agent released in the 1960s. Both its questionable level of effectiveness and its addictive and fatal overdose potential resulted in its obsolescence. The benzodiazepines are the most commonly used antianxiety agents today. These include chlordiazepoxide hydrochloride (Librium) and diazepam (Valium), both of which are widely prescribed and widely abused. Newer drugs in the benzodiazepine family include lorazepam (Ativan), alprazolam (Xanax), clonazepam (Klonopin), and triflupromazine (Vesprin). Drugs in the benzodiazepine family offer rapid, effective, and safe treatment for anxiety states. They have a low addiction potential and do not affect the metabolism of medications taken concurrently, although caffeine interferes with their effectiveness. The major side effect of the benzodiazepines is drowsiness, and community health nurses should warn clients not to drive when they feel drowsy.

The barbiturates (secobarbital [Seconol]) are a group of sedative–hypnotic drugs. These are often contraindicated in treating anxiety states because they are very addictive, used in suicide attempts, depress the central nervous and respiratory systems, and depress REM sleep, possibly resulting in the insomnia these drugs are intended to control.

Many well-controlled clinical studies have found lithium to be the most effective agent for treating acute manic and hypomanic states. Tegretol and valproic acid amide are being used to treat clients who cannot tolerate lithium; however, lithium continues to be the drug of choice for treating bipolar and cyclic unipolar depression as well as "rapid cyclers," persons who have bipolar episodes spaced unusually close together. Lithium is a salt whose ion can be detected in the blood. Lithium is given in divided doses with increases in the daily dose until, in the acute phase of an affective episode, the blood level is between 1.0 and 1.5 mEq/L, the effective level. After a week to 10 days, as the symptoms subside, the blood level should be maintained in the range 1.0 to 1.2 mEq/L.

Because the gap between the therapeutic level and the toxic level of lithium is the narrowest of any psychopharmacologic drug, blood levels must be monitored after each change. When lithium is first prescribed, daily blood tests may be necessary, decreasing to weekly and, finally, to monthly checks during maintenance. Kidney function must be tested before putting a person on lithium. Significant side effects are correlated with blood levels above 1.5 mEq/L.

Community health nurses educate clients who are on lithium about the need to drink eight glasses of water a day, eat foods high in potassium (lithium can deplete potassium levels), and watch for early signs of toxicity. The nurse also monitors the client closely for signs of lithium toxicity. The nurse refers the client

▶ SIGNS OF LITHIUM TOXICITY

Confusion	Seizures
Dizziness	Slurred speech
Hyperactive reflexes	Somnolence
Incontinence	Stupor
Nausea	Thirst
Polyuria	Tremor
Restlessness	Vertigo

back to the psychiatrist if signs of toxicity are evident. The nurse also reinforces the need for periodic checks of blood levels of lithium to ensure early identification of toxic levels.

Tertiary Prevention

When a person has suffered repeated bouts of major depression or bipolar disorder, tertiary prevention is an issue. As in schizophrenia, the entire family should be included in the treatment of both major depression and bipolar disorder. Both depression and bipolar disorder are cyclical, and there are exacerbations and remissions. Seasonal patterns have been noted in both disorders. In the first session with a client, it is enlightening to the family and helpful to the clinician to draw a time line that reflects the client's history of mood swings over several years. Trends might begin to appear. For example, for the last 5 years a client has experienced mood alterations in late summer or early fall. The nurse, client, and family would then be alerted that late September or early October is a time when the client and family will need to pay special attention to the client's affective state. Nurses must rely heavily on family members' monitoring of the prodromal signs of mania because clients who have bipolar disorder are notoriously poor at identifying these signs in themselves. For this reason, the nurse should make family members thoroughly conversant with prodromal signs of mania. Not sleeping is often the first sign of a person moving toward mania. If the client has difficulty sleeping more than two nights, the nurse and the psychiatrist should be notified.

It is important that community health nurses learn to assess levels of depression and suicide risk and refer clients at risk to a mental health provider immediately if they are not already involved in some ongoing therapy. Community health nurses are also using approaches such as diary writing and physical exercise to help individuals deal more effectively with depressive symptoms. Open lines of communication are imperative among nurse, mental health provider,

TABLE 32–2. STATUS OF SELECTED NATIONAL OBJECTIVES RELATED TO CHRONIC MENTAL HEALTH PROBLEMS

Objective		Base	Most Recent	Target
6.3	Prevalence of mental disorders in children and adolescents	20% (1988)	NDA[a]	17%
6.4	Prevalence of mental disorders in adults	20.4% (1983)	16% (1992)	10.7%
6.5	Adverse health effects due to stress	44.2% (1985)	39.2% (1993)	35%
6.6	Use of community support programs by persons with severe mental disorders	15% (1986)	NDA	30%
6.7	Treatment for depressive disorders	34.7% (1983)	34.2% (1992)	54%
6.8	Proportion of people who seek help in coping with personal and emotional problems	11.1% (1985)	14.3% (1993)	20%

[a]NDA, no data available.

(Sources: U.S. Department of Health and Human Services, 1995; 1996.)

family, and client at times when the client is deeply depressed or actively suicidal.

Evaluating Control Strategies for Mood Disorders

Evaluating the effectiveness of care for clients with mood disorders demands constant vigilance, given the changeable nature of mood disorders. For the in-dividual client, functional ability and family interactions are good indicators of the success of treatment for depression.

At the aggregate level, community health nurses can use the national objectives for the year 2000 to gauge progress in controlling chronic mental health problems, including both schizophrenia and depression. The nurse might be involved in collecting data to evaluate achievement of these objectives in the local community. Information on the status of mental health objectives at the national level is presented in Table 32–2.

Critical Thinking in Practice: A Case in Point

You are the community health nurse assigned to see Donna for a well-baby visit several weeks after she delivered a healthy son. Donna is 39 and has been married to Jack, 48, for a year. Stephen is their first child. When you arrive at Donna's house, you note that she and her family live in a comfortable home in an upper-middle-class neighborhood. Donna answers the door, and you see that her eyes and nose are red as though she has been crying. You explain the purpose of your visit and examine the baby, who is in a freshly painted nursery with a bright mobile over the crib and plenty of stuffed animals and toys around. Stephen is neat, clean, and appears to be well-fed, happy, and healthy.

When you finish with the baby, you ask how Donna is doing. Donna bursts into tears. She tells you that she has been feeling desperately unhappy since her pregnancy began. She has been feeling so depressed, she reports, that she is not sure she will be able to get out of bed anymore to take care of her son. You say, "Tell me about this past year." Donna tells you that this is a first marriage for her and for Jack, and neither of them has children from previous relationships. In their discussions prior to marriage, she and Jack had never resolved their differences about having children. Donna was ambivalent about having a child; her husband was sure he did not want one. Because they are devout Roman Catholics, they used the rhythm method of birth control. When Donna told Jack she was pregnant after 2 months of marriage, he became very angry and blamed Donna for tricking him into having a baby. Although she had not tricked him, Donna felt guilty and blamed herself for becoming pregnant. Terrified that Jack would leave her if she told him how she felt, she kept all her own feelings of sadness, anger, and depression inside. She did not want to be a single parent. Abortion was never considered because of their religious beliefs.

During the pregnancy, Jack was emotionally withdrawn, depressed, and refused to take part in any activity related to the up-coming birth. Donna's sister attended Lamaze classes with her and coached her during the birth because Jack would not attend. Donna felt jealous of the women whose husbands were so attentive during these classes. Ever since her son's birth, Donna says that she has had "postpartum depression." She has told no one how depressed she feels because she is afraid she will have to be hospitalized as she was several times in her late twenties and early thirties for episodes of clinical depression.

(continued)

Critical Thinking in Practice: A Case in Point (cont.)

When you do a genogram with her, you discover a family history of depression. Both her grandmother and mother suffered bouts of deep depression, and her grandmother had been hospitalized for a year in a psychiatric institution following menopause. Donna's father is an emotionally withdrawn man whose only sister committed suicide when she was 40. Donna's sister has an eating disorder; she is bulimic.

Now that Donna has been home for 3 weeks with her son, she sees her sister twice a week. Jack is pleased that they have a son and he is beginning to spend time after he comes home from work playing with Stephen. Donna cannot understand why it makes her angry instead of happy that Jack is becoming involved with their child. Because Jack has refused to support them in a manner that would allow Donna to stay home with Stephen, Donna must return to work after her 6-week maternity leave. She is afraid she will be unable to function at work and has yet to find a day-care facility for Stephen. Donna worries about these things and has difficulty both in falling asleep and in getting up during the night to feed her son. She cries for "no reason" several times a day and has lost weight. She weighs less now than before she was pregnant. She has little interest in anything, including her baby, and she says that life does not really seem worth living anymore.

1. Does Donna have any vegetative signs of depression? If so, describe them.
2. How would you assess her potential for suicide?
3. How would you determine whether Donna's depression is "normal" postpartum depression or clinical depression requiring psychiatric assessment and treatment?
4. Based on your assessment, will you follow Donna yourself or refer her to a psychiatrist or mental health worker?
5. How will you involve Donna's husband and sister in the plan of care?

TESTING YOUR UNDERSTANDING

1. Identify at least five symptoms of schizophrenia for which the community health nurse might assess an individual client. (pp. 842–843)
2. Identify three common forms of disorganized speech associated with schizophrenia. Give an example of each. (p. 843)
3. Discuss the major thrust of secondary prevention in the control of schizophrenia and the related role of the community health nurse. (p. 846)
4. Discuss at least three areas of emphasis in tertiary prevention for schizophrenia. Give an example of community health nursing involvement in each. (pp. 846–847)
5. Identify at least three biophysical factors that may influence the development of mood disorders. (pp. 848–849)
6. Describe at least five social dimension factors that may contribute to the development of schizophrenia or mood disorders. (pp. 844, 850)
7. Identify three approaches to primary prevention of mood disorders. Give an example of community health nursing involvement in each. (pp. 852–853)
8. Describe at least three community health nursing activities related to secondary prevention of mood disorders. (pp. 853–854)
9. Identify at least two considerations in tertiary pre-

vention of mood disorders. Give an example of a community health nursing action related to each. (pp. 854–855)

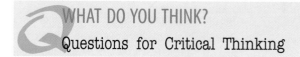

WHAT DO YOU THINK?
Questions for Critical Thinking

1. What is your personal risk of developing a depressive disorder? What factors are contributing to that risk? What could you do about them?
2. How would you differentiate a mood disorder characterized by depression from other causes of apparent depression in an elderly client?
3. Discuss the possible relationship between homelessness and schizophrenia and between homelessness and depression. What similarities and differences are there in the relationships?
4. What effect does dysfunctional family communication have on schizophrenia?

REFERENCES

American Psychiatric Association. (1994). *Diagnostic and statistical manual of mental disorders* (4th ed.). (DSM-IV). Washington, DC: American Psychiatric Association.

Anderson, J., & Werry, J. S. (1994). Emotional and behavioral problems. In I. B. Pless (Ed.), *The epidemiology of childhood disorders* (pp. 304–338). New York: Oxford University Press.

Andreasen, N. C., & Carpenter, W. T. Jr. (1993a). Diagnosis and classification of schizophrenia. In D. Shore (Ed.), *Special report: Schizophrenia* (pp. 25–40). Rockville, MD: National Institute of Mental Health.

Andreasen, N. C., & Carpenter, W. T. Jr. (1993b). General overview. In D. Shore (Ed.), *Special report: Schizophrenia* (pp. 1–4). Rockville, MD: National Institute of Mental Health.

Badger, T. A. (1996). Family members' experiences living with members with depression. *Western Journal of Nursing Research, 18,* 149–171.

Bellack, A. S., & Meuser, K. T. (1993). Psychosocial treatment. In D. Shore (Ed.), *Special report: Schizophrenia* (pp. 12–13). Rockville, MD: National Institute of Mental Health.

Bogerts, B. (1993). In D. Shore (Ed.), *Special report: Schizophrenia* (pp. 22–25). Rockville, MD: National Institute of Mental Health.

Brill, P. A., & Cooper, K. H. (1993). Physical exercise and mental health. *National Forum, LXXIII*(1), 44–45.

Carter, R. (1993). Mental health policy and health care reform. *National Forum, LXXIII*(1), 13–15.

Cooper-Patrick, L., Ford, D. E., Mead, L. A., Chang, P. P., & Klag, M. J. (1997). Exercise and depression in midlife: A prospective study. *American Journal of Public Health, 87,* 670–673.

Farrell, K. R., & Ganzini, L. (1995). Misdiagnosing delirium as depression in medically ill elderly patients. *Archives of Internal Medicine, 155,* 2459–2464.

Flynn, L. M. (1993). Political impact of the family-consumer movement. *National Forum, LXXIII*(1), 8–12.

Gore, T. (1993). Children and mental illness. *National Forum, LXXIII*(1), 16–17.

Hagerty, B. M. (1995). Advances in understanding major depressive disorder. *Journal of Psychosocial Nursing, 33*(11), 27–34.

Holden, R. J. (1995). Schizophrenia, smoking, and smog. *Holistic Nursing Practice, 9*(2), 74–82.

Jeste, D. V., & Caligiuri, M. P. (1993). Tardive dyskinesia. In D. Shore (Ed.), *Special report: Schizophrenia* (pp. 129–141). Rockville, MD: National Institute of Mental Health.

Kanacki, L. S., Jones, P. S., & Galbraith, M. E. (1996). Social support and depression in widows and widowers. *Journal of Gerontological Nursing, 22*(2), 39–45.

Kane, J. M., & Marder, S. R. (1993). Pharmacologic treatment of schizophrenia. In D. Shore (Ed.), *Special report: Schizophrenia* (pp. 113–128). Rockville, MD: National Institute of Mental Health.

Kendler, K. S., & Diehl, S. R. (1993). Genetics. In D. Shore (Ed.), *Special report: Schizophrenia* (pp. 8–10). Rockville, MD: National Institute of Mental Health.

Kingdon, D. C., & Turkington, D. (1994). *Cognitive-behavioral therapy of schizophrenia.* New York: Guilford Press.

Kirch, D. G. (1993). Infection and autoimmunity. In D. Shore (Ed.), *Special report: Schizophrenia* (pp. 16–18). Rockville, MD: National Institute of Mental Health.

Kopelowicz, A. (1996). And when they awaken what will they find? *The Journal of the California Alliance for the Mentally Ill, 7*(2), 15–16.

Kronenberger, W. G., & Meyer, R. G. (1996). *The child clinician's handbook.* Boston: Allyn and Bacon.

Lam, R. W., Gorman, C. P., Michalon, M., et al. (1995). Multicenter, placebo-controlled study of fluoxetine in seasonal affective disorder. *American Journal of Psychiatry, 152,* 1765–1770.

Lefley, H., P. (1996). Awakenings and recovery: Learning the beat of a different drummer. *The Journal of the California Alliance for the Mentally Ill, 7*(2), 4–6.

Lieberman, J. A., & Koreen, A. P. (1993). Neurochemistry and neuroendocrinology. In D. Shore (Ed.), *Special report: Schizophrenia* (pp. 19–22). Rockville, MD: National Institute of Mental Health.

Loukissa, D. A. (1995). Family burden in chronic mental illness: A review of research studies. *Journal of Advanced Nursing, 21,* 241–255.

Lyness, J. M., Noel, T. K., Cox, C., King, D. A., Conwell, Y., & Caine, E. D. (1997). Screening for depression in elderly primary care patients. *Archives of Internal Medicine, 157,* 449–454.

The Nation's Health. (1994, March). *IOM report says prevention is key to mental health crisis,* p. 11.

The Nation's Health. (1996, September). *WHO releases figures on mental health,* p. 30.

Reutter, L. I., & Ford, J. S. (1996). Perceptions of public health nursing: Views from the field. *Journal of Advanced Nursing, 24,* 7–15.

Selemon, L. D., Rajkowska, G., & Goldman-Rakic, P. S. (1995). Abnormally high neuronal density in the schizophrenic cortex. *Archives of General Psychiatry, 52,* 805–818.

Shao, W., Williams, J. W., Lee, S., et al. (1997). Knowledge and attitudes about depression among non-generalists and generalists. *The Journal of Family Practice, 44,* 161–168.

Silbersweig, D. A., Stern, E., Frith, C., et al. (1995). A functional neuroanatomy of hallucinations in schizophrenia. *Nature, 378,* 176–179.

Simon, G. E., Von Korff, M., & Barlow, W. (1995). Health care costs of primary care patients with recognized depression. *Archives of General Psychiatry, 52,* 850–856.

U.S. Department of Health and Human Services. (1991). *Healthy people 2000: National health promotion and disease prevention objectives.* Washington, DC: Government Printing Office.

U.S. Department of Health and Human Services. (1995). *Healthy people 2000: Midcourse review and 1995 revi-*

sions. Washington, DC: Government Printing Office.

U.S. Department of Health and Human Services. (1996, July 9). *Healthy people 2000: Progress review—Mental health and mental disorders.* Washington, DC: Government Printing Office.

Valente, S. M., & Saunders, J. M. (1997). Diagnosis and treatment of major depression among people with cancer. *Cancer Nursing, 20,* 168–177.

White, S. W. (1993). Mental illness and national policy. *National Forum, LXXIII*(1), 2–3.

Wingerson, D. (1996). Awakenings—To what? *The Journal of the California Alliance for the Mentally Ill, 7*(2), 12–14.

....

RESOURCES FOR NURSES DEALING WITH CHRONIC MENTAL HEALTH PROBLEMS

American Psychiatric Association
1400 K Street NW
Washington, DC 20005
(202) 682–6000

American Psychiatric Nurses Association
1200 19th Street NW, Ste. 300
Washington, DC 20036
(202) 857–1133

Depression and Related Affective Disorders
  Association
Johns Hopkins Hospital, Meyer 3-181
600 North Wolfe Street
Baltimore, MD 21287–7381
(410) 955–4647

Depressives Anonymous, Recovery from Depression
329 East 62nd Street
New York, NY 10021
(212) 689–2600

Emotional Health Anonymous
PO Box 63236
Los Angeles, CA 90063–0236
(213) 268–7220

National Alliance for the Mentally Ill (NAMI)
200 N. Glebe Road, No. 1015
Arlington, VA 22203–3728
(703) 524–7600

National Depressive and Manic Depressive
  Association
730 North Franklin, Ste. 501
Chicago, IL 60610
(312) 642–0049

National Foundation for Depressive Illness
PO Box 2257
New York, NY 10116
(212) 268–4260

National Institute of Mental Health
5600 Fishers Lane
Rockville, MD 20857
(301) 443–4513

National Mental Health Association
Information Center
1021 Prince Street
Alexandria, VA 22314–2971
(703) 684–7722

Project Overcome
50 4th Avenue
Minneapolis, MN 55401
(612) 340–0165

SUBSTANCE ABUSE

Most drugs are used appropriately for medicinal purposes, but substance abuse is a growing world problem. The illegal drug trade is big business, and the fact that many substances with the potential for abuse also have legitimate use has made control of substance abuse difficult. *Drug use* is the taking of a drug in the correct amount, frequency, and strength for its medically intended purpose. *Drug abuse,* on the other hand, is the deliberate use of a drug for other than medicinal purposes in a manner that can adversely affect one's health or ability to function.

In the United States, the abuse of alcohol and other drugs and the use of tobacco products are of particular concern. The magnitude of these concerns is seen in the development of more than 30 national health promotion and disease prevention objectives for the year 2000 related to tobacco use and the abuse of alcohol and other drugs (see Appendix A).

In this chapter, theoretical perspectives on abuse and trends in substance use and abuse are examined. Risk factors contributing to all forms of substance abuse, signs and symptoms of specific types of abuse, and community health nursing interventions in the control of substance abuse are addressed. The focus of the chapter is the abuse of psychoactive substances addressed by the *Diagnostic and Statistical Manual of Mental Disorders, Fourth Edition,* of the American Psychiatric Association (DSM-IV) (1994).

▶ Chapter Objectives

After reading this chapter, you should be able to:

- Describe at least two theories of substance abuse.
- Identify at least three criteria for diagnosing psychoactive substance dependence.
- Distinguish between psychoactive substance dependence and abuse.
- Identify at least five substances that lead to dependence and abuse.
- Describe at least two personal effects, two family effects, and two societal effects of substance abuse.
- Describe the five aspects of community health nursing assessment in relation to substance abuse.
- Identify two major approaches to primary prevention of substance abuse.
- Describe the components of the intervention process in secondary prevention of substance abuse.
- Identify at least four general principles in the treatment of substance abuse.
- Describe at least three treatment modalities in secondary prevention of substance abuse.
- Identify three major goals of harm reduction.

▶ PSYCHOACTIVE SUBSTANCES: DEPENDENCE AND ABUSE

Substance abuse involves the inappropriate use of psychoactive substances. *Psychoactive substances* are drugs or chemicals that alter ordinary states of consciousness including mood, cognition, or behavior (Insel & Roth, 1998). The DSM-IV recognizes abuse of several substances under umbrella diagnoses of psychoactive substance dependence and psychoactive substance abuse. The *psychoactive substance dependence syndrome* is a cluster of cognitive, behavioral, and physiologic symptoms that indicate impaired control over the use of a psychoactive substance and continued use despite adverse consequences (American Psychiatric Association, 1994). Diagnosis of psychoactive substance dependence is based on the following signs:

- Increasing amounts of substance used, or use extending over a longer period than intended
- Persistent desire for the substance or one or more unsuccessful attempts to control its use
- Increased time spent in obtaining, using, or recovering from the effects of the substance

- Frequent symptoms of intoxication or withdrawal interfering with obligations
- Elimination or reduction of important occupational, social, or recreational activities as a result of substance use
- Continued use of the substance despite recurrent problems caused
- Increased tolerance to the substance
- Experience of characteristic withdrawal symptoms
- Increased substance use to decrease withdrawal symptoms

Psychoactive substance abuse involves maladaptive patterns of substance use that do not meet the criteria for dependence. Criteria for a diagnosis of abuse include continued use of a substance (or substances) despite persistent or recurrent physical, psychological, or social problems related to its use or recurrent use of the substance in physically dangerous situations (eg, driving while intoxicated). Because substance abuse is a precursor to dependence, the term *substance abuse* is used throughout this chapter in discussing the role of the community health nurse in its prevention and control.

▶ THEORIES OF SUBSTANCE ABUSE

Inappropriate drug use behavior usually proceeds through three phases: initial use, habitual use, and relapse. During the initial use phase, the user engages in experimental, occasional or light irregular use of the psychoactive substance. The habitual phase involves regular use of the drug over time and includes both dependence and abuse diagnoses described above. Relapse involves a return to habitual use after a period of abstinence longer than the usual time between doses (Akers, 1992). Not every user, however, progresses from the initial to the habitual phase of use. What explains progression to abuse and dependence in some people and not in others?

At present there is no definitive answer to this question. Several theories have been advanced, however, to explain this selective development of substance abuse. The anomie or *social strain theory* suggests that abusers are not fully integrated into society because of rapid social changes and the strain of attempting to conform to high social expectations of material success without access to socially acceptable means of achieving that success (Akers, 1992). This state of affairs leads to decreased affiliation with society and its norms and deviant behavior in the form of drug use, either as a means to material success or as an escape from one's lack of success.

In the *selective interaction theory,* abusers are socialized into a drug subculture through attraction to and selective interaction with people who hold values similar to their own. Examples of values that may characterize this subculture include religious alienation, extremist politics, and sexual promiscuity. Drug abuse, from this perspective, may represent an attempt to gain acceptance or status within the group.

Social learning theory explains drug abuse in terms of behavior learned by observation of social models and perceptions of positive or negative consequences of that behavior for the model. *Social control theory,* or bonding theory, on the other hand, suggests that drug abuse results from weak socialization to conformity with social norms of behavior and inadequate development of internal and external controls on behavior. The bonding aspect of this type of theory suggests that attachment to others and commitment to and involvement in activities incompatible with drug use lead to internalization of societal norms and values that promote self-control (Akers, 1992). This theory is exemplified in efforts to involve inner-city minority boys in Boy Scouting to deter drug use.

The basic premise of *labeling theory* is that individuals are labeled as deviant by significant others and so engage in deviant behavior as a form of self-fulfilling prophesy (Witters, Venturelli, & Hanson, 1992). The basic theme here might be, "If you think I'm deviant now, wait 'til you see what I do next." The final theory of substance abuse, the self-esteem or *derogation theory,* is closely related, but the negative perceptions of self arise from one's own low self-esteem rather than from labeling by others. In this theory, drug abuse is seen as an attempt to increase self-esteem or to minimize negative self-attitudes (Akers, 1992).

▶ PSYCHOACTIVE SUBSTANCES AND THEIR USE

Whatever the theoretical reasoning involved, it is estimated that approximately 6% of the adult population of the United States uses some type of illicit nonprescription psychoactive drug (Gfroerer, 1995). Psychoactive substances are abused because of their desirable initial effects. Some of these effects and the drugs associated with them are presented in Table 33–1. Unfortunately, many psychoactive drugs with potential for abuse have rebound effects that are usually the opposite of their initial effects and that lead to repeated use to eliminate the undesirable symptoms created by the rebound. These adverse effects are discussed later in this chapter. Because of the phenomenon of tolerance, the user requires larger and larger

doses of many drugs to combat rebound effects and to achieve the desired pleasurable effect. *Drug tolerance* is an adaptation of the body to a substance such that previous doses do not have the desired effect. The following psychoactive substances may be involved in either dependence or abuse:

- Alcohol
- Sedatives, hypnotics, and anxiolytics
- Opioids
- Cocaine
- Amphetamines
- Hallucinogens
- Cannabis
- Inhalants
- Nicotine

Alcohol

The alcohol contained in alcoholic beverages is ethyl alcohol created by the fermentation of grain mixtures or the juice of fruits and berries. After ingestion, alcohol is rapidly absorbed into the bloodstream through the gastrointestinal tract and functions as a central nervous system depressant.

Alcohol abuse is a serious problem in the United States and elsewhere in the world. The prevalence of alcohol abuse in the United States is estimated at 15 to 22 million people (Robertson, 1993). In 1993, the median percentage of binge drinkers in states participating in the Behavioral Risk Factor Surveillance System (BRFSS) was slightly over 14%. The percentage of drinkers in this category varied from state to state and ranged from just over 4% of adults in Tennessee to almost 29% in Wisconsin. Chronic drinking was reported by a median of 3% of adults and ranged from 1.4% in Tennessee to 6.1% in Nevada (Frazier, Okoro, Smith, & McQueen, 1996). In 1994, more than half of all persons (53%) in the United States over 12 years of age reported alcohol use in the previous month (U.S. Department of Health and Human Services, 1996). Although figures on the extent of alcohol abuse are alarming, the fact that an estimated 75% of abusers do not receive treatment for their disorder (*The Nation's Health,* 1994) is even more disconcerting. Another alcohol-related tragedy is that 40,000 babies born each year in the United States suffer from alcohol-related defects (Robertson, 1993), and 4 of every 10,000 babies experience full fetal alcohol syndrome (FAS) (Fetal Alcohol Syndrome Prevention Section, 1997).

Sedatives, Hypnotics, and Anxiolytics

A second group of drugs frequently abused are the sedatives, hypnotics, and anxiolytics. Sedatives are

TABLE 33–1. SELECTED PSYCHOACTIVE SUBSTANCES, STREET NAMES, TYPICAL ROUTES OF ADMINISTRATION, AND EFFECTS PROMOTING ABUSE

Substance	Street Names	Typical Route of Administration	Effects Promoting Abuse
Alcohol	Beer, wine, spirits, booze, various brand names	Orally ingested	Relaxation, decreased inhibitions, increased confidence, euphoria
Sedatives, hypnotics, and anxiolytics		Orally ingested, injected	Calming effect, decreased nervousness and anxiety, ability to sleep, relaxation, mild intoxication, loss of inhibition
Barbiturates			
Amytal	Blues, downers		
Nembutal	Yellows, yellow jackets		
Phenobarbital	Phennie, purple hearts		
Seconal	Reds, F-40s, Redbirds		
Tuinal	Rainbows, tooies		
Quaalude	Ludes, 714s, Q's, Quay, Quad, mandrex		
Tranquilizers (minor)	Tranks, downs, downers, goof balls, sleeping pills, candy		
Dalmane			
Equanil/Miltown	Muscle relaxants, sleeping pills		
Librium			
Valium			
Serax			
Opioids			
Codeine	Schoolboy	Orally ingested	Relief of pain, euphoria
Demerol	Demies, dolls, dollies, Amidone	injected	
Dilaudid	Little D, Lords	Injected	
Heroin	Smack, junk, downtown, H, black tar, horse, stuff	Injected, smoked, sniffed	
Methadone	Meth, dollies	Injected	
Morphine	M, Miss Emma, morph, morpho, tab, white, stuff, monkey	Injected	
Opium	Blue velvet, black stuff, Dover's powder, paregoric	Orally ingested, smoked, injected	
Percodan	Perkies	Orally ingested	
Cocaine	Coke, snow, uptown, flake, crack, bump, toot, c, candy	Snorted, injected, smoked	Increased alertness and confidence, euphoria, reduced fatigue
Amphetamines		Orally ingested	Increased alertness and confidence, decreased fatigue, euphoria
Benzedrine	Bennies, pep pills, uppers, truck drivers		
Biphetamine	Black beauties		
Desoxyn	Co-pilots		
Dexedrine	Dex, speed, dexies		
Methedrine	Meth, crank, speed, crystal, go fast		
MDMA	Ecstasy		
Hallucinogens		Orally ingested, smoked, injected	Altered perceptions, mystical experience
Phencyclidine	Angel dust, krystal, DOA, hog, PCP, peace pill	Smoked, orally ingested, injected	Dream-like state producing hallucinations
LSD	Acid, microdot, cubes		
MDA	The love drug		
Mescaline	Cactus, mesc		
Peyote	Buttons		
Psilocybin	Magic mushrooms, shrooms, sacred mushrooms		
Cannabis		Smoked, orally ingested	Relaxation, euphoria, altered perceptions
Hashish	Kif, herb, hash		
Hashish oil	Honey, hash oil		
Marijuana	Grass, ganja, weed, dope, reefer, Thai sticks, pot, Acapulco gold, roach, loco weed, Maui wowie, joint, Mary Jane		
Inhalants		Inhaled	Relaxation, euphoria, intoxication
Amyl nitrate	Poppers		
Butyl nitrate	Locker room, rush		
Nitrous oxide	Laughing gas		
Nicotine	Various brand names of tobacco products	Smoked, chewed	Relaxation, mild stimulation

used to calm nervousness, irritability, and excitement, whereas hypnotics induce sleep. Many drugs have sedative effects in lower doses and hypnotic effects in higher doses. Anxiolytics (also known as antianxiety agents or minor tranquilizers) are used to reduce anxiety and tension and promote sleep. All three types of drugs are central nervous system (CNS) depressants.

These drugs are frequently prescribed for symptoms of nervousness, anxiety, or difficulty sleeping. Unfortunately, their prescription for legitimate use often creates a dependence. In low doses, these drugs produce a mild state of euphoria, reduce inhibitions, and create feelings of relaxation and decreased tension. Their major pharmacologic action is CNS depression. Drugs involved in this category of substance abuse include tranquilizers such as chlordiazepoxide hydrochloride (Librium) and diazepam (Valium); barbiturate sedatives; nonbarbiturates such as hydroxyzine hydrochloride (Atarax) and meprobamate (Equanil); and hypnotics such as methaqualone hydrochloride (Quaalude) and diphenhydramine hydrochloride (Nytol, Sleep-eze, Sominex). Because of their widespread use for both legitimate and illegitimate reasons and their easy availability, precise figures on the abuse of these drugs are difficult to obtain. In national surveys, however, 1.2% of the U.S. population engaged in inappropriate use of prescription drugs in 1994 (Gfroerer, 1995).

Opioids

Opioids are also CNS depressants and are derived naturally from the opium poppy or created synthetically. Opioids bind to CNS cell receptors to mimic the action of naturally produced endorphins that relieve pain. In addition to relief of pain, opioids create a psychological euphoria that prompts continued use.

Opioid dependence (along with barbiturate dependence) was once a primary concern in relation to substance abuse, and continued use of opioids is still of concern to health care professionals. In 1994, the prevalence of current heroin use among persons aged 18 to 25 years was less than 1% (U.S. Department of Commerce, 1996), but health care providers in many areas of the country are reporting increased use (Brown, 1995b).

Cocaine

Cocaine is a stimulant derived from the leaves of the coca plant. Its use produces euphoria and a sense of competence. Other desired effects include increased energy and clarity of thought. Unlike many of the other drugs presented here, the pleasurable effects of cocaine are extremely short-acting (approximately 30 minutes) and are followed by an intense letdown and craving for another dose. Use of cocaine may be accompanied by the practice of "freebasing." Normally, to maintain its stability, cocaine is combined with a hydrochloride base, creating a substance that is usually only about 25% cocaine. *Freebasing* involves the use of heat and ether to free the cocaine from its hydrochloride base, thus creating a purer product that produces a more intense effect. Because of the combination of heat and the highly volatile and explosive ether, freebasing is an extremely dangerous practice. To eliminate the need for freebasing, drug dealers created *crack*, a stable form of cocaine without the hydrochloride base that can be smoked rather than inhaled, for a more rapid and more intense effect (National Institute on Drug Abuse, 1995).

Next to alcohol, cocaine is the abusive substance of greatest concern because of the rapid escalation in its use and its severe adverse effects. Although current use of cocaine declined from 4.2 million persons in 1979 to 1.3 million in 1993 (Brown, 1995a), the number of current users subsequently increased to 1.4 million in 1994 (National Institute on Drug Abuse, 1994).

Amphetamines

Amphetamines are CNS stimulants manufactured chemically. Amphetamines have, on occasion, been prescribed to assist weight loss and relative fatigue, but they are not recommended for either condition. Amphetamines and similar drugs produce feelings of euphoria, energy, confidence, increased ability to concentrate, and improved physical performance. They are often used by truck drivers and students who wish to stay awake to study or by athletes desiring to improve their performance.

An estimated 4 million people in the United States have abused amphetamines at least once, and related morbidity and mortality nearly tripled from 1991 to 1994 (Sajo, 1996). Regular use of amphetamines and related drugs is higher in some areas than in others. Methamphetamine use, for example, is particularly prevalent in Southern California.

Amphetamines lend themselves to chemical modifications to create "designer drugs." *Designer drugs* are legal modifications of drugs whose use in their original form is restricted. One of the most widely known designer drugs is 3,4-methylenedionymethamphetamine (MDMA), better known as "ectasy." Originally developed as an appetite suppressant, MDMA no longer has any legitimate medical use because of its neurotoxicity and contributions to cardiac arrhythmias. Recently, MDMA has also been implicated in acute renal failure and hepatotoxicity (Henry, Jeffreys, & Dawling, 1992).

Hallucinogens

Phencyclidine (PCP) was originally developed as an anesthetic, but its use was discontinued because of its many adverse side effects. The effects of PCP are variable and may include stimulation or depression of the CNS or hallucinations. Its more desirable effects include heightened sensitivity to stimuli, mood elevation, a sense of omnipotence, and relaxation. Unfortunately, PCP has some serious adverse effects. PCP-induced psychosis constitutes a psychiatric emergency, and PCP use may lead to seizures, coma, and death (Akers, 1992).

Other hallucinogens or psychedelic drugs such as *d*-lysergic acid diethylamide (LSD), mescaline, peyote, and psilocybin mushrooms alter experience to create hallucinations. They also distort the distinction between self and the environment to make the user extremely vulnerable to environmental stimuli. Common effects of these drugs include changes in mood (euphoria or terror and despair), heightened sensation or synesthesia (merging of the senses so colors, eg, are experienced as odors or vice versa), changes in perceptions of time and objects, and changes in relations leading to depersonalization and feelings of merging with other people and objects.

In 1993, 18 million people reported ever having used hallucinogens (Brown, 1995a). Just over 1% of 12 to 17 year olds and 1.5% of people aged 18 to 25 years reported current use of hallucinogens in 1994 (U.S. Department of Commerce, 1996).

Cannabis

Cannabis species of plants are the source of marijuana and hashish. The primary psychoactive substance in these drugs is delta-9-tetrahydrocannabinol (THC). THC may be inhaled by smoking marijuana or hashish or ingested and produces relaxation, euphoria, and occasionally altered perceptions of time and space. Marijuana use may contribute to exacerbation of other mental health problems such as schizophrenia and depression. *Sensemilla,* a form of marijuana consisting of dried flowers of female plants without seeds, may be as much as 10 times more potent than regular marijuana mixtures that also contain leaves and seeds (National Institute on Drug Abuse, 1996).

Marijuana is used by 80% of people who use illicit drugs (Gfroerer, 1995). Approximately 10 million Americans over the age of 12 use marijuana in any given month (National Institute on Drug Abuse, 1996). Overall, marijuana use in the general population has declined from a high of 13% in 1979 to 5% in 1994 (U.S. Department of Commerce, 1996).

Inhalants

Inhalants are abused by sniffing products such as airplane model glue, nail polish remover, gasoline, aerosols, and anesthetics such as nitrous oxide. They usually produce a sense of euphoria, loss of inhibition, and excitement. Inhalants are often used by people who do not have the financial resources to support more expensive drug habits. In addition to a variety of adverse physical effects such as kidney and heart damage, there is the potential for suffocation while inhaling these substances from a plastic bag. Because of their volatile nature, explosion is another hazard presented by inhalants.

Approximately 17% of adolescents report ever having used inhalants (National Institute on Drug Abuse, 1994). In 1994, 2% of those aged 12 to 17 years reported current inhalant use compared to less than 1% of persons aged 18 to 25 years and 26 years of age and older. Inhalant use in all age groups declined significantly from 1979 to 1994 (U.S. Department of Commerce, 1996).

Nicotine

Nicotine, the last of the abusive substances included in the DSM-IV categories of psychoactive substance dependence and abuse, is the psychoactive substance present in tobacco smoke. Nicotine produces feelings of well-being, increases mental acuity and ability to concentrate, and heightens one's sense of purpose. Nicotine may also exert a calming effect on the smoker. Unfortunately, nicotine also contributes to a host of adverse physical effects including heart disease, several forms of cancer, and chronic respiratory diseases. Although a great deal of progress has been made in efforts to limit tobacco use in the United States, its use among young people continues to be relatively prevalent.

Because of the highly addictive nature of nicotine and its adverse health effects, all forms of tobacco use should be discouraged. Unlike moderate alcohol use, even moderate smoking produces negative effects on health. Nicotine, unlike many other abused substances, has no medical applications.

Efforts to eliminate smoking in the U.S. population have been somewhat successful. For example, in 1993, 25% of people over 18 years of age smoked compared with 42% in 1965. Results of efforts to eliminate smoking among young people have also been effective, resulting in an 81% decrease in the proportion of smokers aged 12 to 17 between 1974 and 1994, and a 61% decrease in 18 to 25 year olds during the same time period (U.S. Department of Commerce, 1996).

► EFFECTS OF SUBSTANCE ABUSE

Substance abuse contributes to adverse effects for the abusing individual, for his or her family, and for society at large.

Personal Effects

The effects of substance abuse on the individual are physical, psychological, and social. Physical effects include increased morbidity directly related to the effects of the drug or drugs abused, as well as increased potential for exposure to diseases such as AIDS and hepatitis when abuse involves use of contaminated needles or results in sexual promiscuity as a means of financing a drug habit or because of lowered inhibitions. Other physical effects of substance abuse include physical deterioration due to malnutrition and poor hygiene. Some drugs such as alcohol, nicotine, and barbiturates also result in withdrawal symptoms when the drug is removed from the client's system. The *withdrawal syndrome* caused by these and other drugs is a complex of symptoms usually including severe discomfort, pain, nausea, vomiting, and, possibly, convulsions. Some drugs also produce chromosomal changes that cause congenital malformations in children as well as increased potential for spontaneous abortion. Death is the ultimate adverse effect of drug use and may result from a drug overdose, from withdrawal, or from the long-term effects of drug use such as cirrhosis, cancer, and cardiovascular disease. Assessment for both short-term and long-term physical effects of specific substances is discussed later in this chapter.

In addition to the desired effects that promote drug use and abuse, psychological effects of drug abuse can include personality disturbances, anxiety, and depression. Organic mental disorders characterized by hallucinations, delusions, dementia, delirium, and disorders of mood or perception may also be caused by substance abuse. In addition, substance abuse may trigger exacerbations of existing schizophrenic or mood disorders.

Preoccupation with the abused substance can lead to a variety of social problems for the substance abuser. Relationships with family and friends may be impaired, or abusers may become incapable of or disinterested in performing their jobs and may be fired. Unemployment can lead to difficulties in obtaining housing and can contribute to homelessness. The need to obtain money to support a drug habit or to obtain necessities may lead to criminal activity. Table 33–2 lists the possible legal penalties for the manufacture and distribution of drugs regulated by the Narcotics Penal-

TABLE 33–2. MAXIMUM PENALTIES FOR ILLEGAL DRUG MANUFACTURE OR SALE

Drug		Penalty for Sale or Manufacture
Cocaine		
500–4999 g	First offense	5–40 years in prison
	Second offense	10 years to life in prison
5 kg or more	First offense	10 years to life in prison
	Second offense	20 years to life in prison
Cocaine base		
5 g or more	First offense	If death or serious injury, 20 years to life in prison
	Second offense	If death or serious injury, life in prison
Fentanyl		
40–399 g	First offense	Fine up to $2 million
	Second offense	Fine up to $4 million
400 g or more	First offense	Fine up to $4 million
	Second offense	Fine up to $8 million
Fentanyl analog		
10–99 g	First offense	Fine up to $2 million
	Second offense	Fine up to $4 million
100 g or more	First offense	Fine up to $4 million
	Second offense	Fine up to $8 million
Heroin		
100–999 g	First offense	5 to 40 years in prison
	Second offense	10 years to life in prison
1 kg or more	First offense	10 years to life in prison
	Second offense	20 years to life in prison
LSD		
1–10 g	First offense	Fine up to $2 million
	Second offense	Fine up to $4 million
10 g or more	First offense	Fine up to $4 million
	Second offense	Fine up to $8 million
Marijuana		
100–999 kg	First offense	Fine up to $2 million, 5 to 40 years in prison; if death or serious injury, 20 years to life in prison
	Second offense	Fine up to $4 million, 10 years to life in prison; if death or serious injury, life in prison
1000 kg or more	First offense	Fine up to $4 million, 10 years to life in prison; if death or serious injury, 20 years to life in prison
	Second offense	Fine up to $8 million, 20 years to life in prison; if death or serious injury, life in prison
Phencylidine (PCP)		
10 g or more	First offense	If death or serious injury, 20 years to life in prison
	Second offense	If death or serious injury, life in prison

(Source: Akers, 1992.)

ties and Enforcement Act of 1986. The drugs are classified as Schedule I through V based on their abuse potential, with Schedule I drugs having the highest potential for abuse and Schedule V the lowest. Legal penalties are also warranted for theft, violence, or prostitution committed in efforts to support a drug habit.

Family Effects

The effects of substance abuse on the family of the abuser can be many and severe. These families are characterized by frequent conflict, anger, ambivalence, fear, guilt, confusion, mistrust, and violence as a mode of conflict resolution. The family frequently becomes socially isolated in efforts to cover up the problem of abuse and so are not able to make use of sources of assistance that might be available to them. Substance abuse may also be a factor in family violence.

In families in which one parent or the other is a substance abuser, the husband–wife coalition present in most families is frequently absent. Often it is replaced by a strong dyad of the nonabusing parent and a child. Such coalitions may require children to assume adult responsibilities, either as a "little mother" or as a parental confidant. The pressure caused by these responsibilities may be one of the contributing factors in later substance abuse by children of abusers.

The effects of parental alcoholism on children has been widely studied. More than 28 million people in the United States were raised in homes where alcohol abuse was evident. These individuals tend to exhibit both physical and psychological effects of parental alcoholism both as children and as adults. They may experience feelings of guilt, premature responsibility, and a sense of being trapped by the situation. As adults, children of alcohol abusers tend to have frequent marital problems and psychosomatic illnesses, and experience high levels of guilt and anxiety.

Some researchers have described stages of family response to alcohol abuse that are similar to responses to abuse of other substances by family members (Finley, 1991). The first stage is usually characterized by denial of the problem and attempts to mitigate the social effects of abuse. For example, a spouse may call to explain the abuser's absence from work as illness when it is actually due to a drug hangover. In this stage, family members exhibit the phenomenon of "codependency." A *codependent* is a person in a continuing relationship with the substance abuser, whose behavior enables the abuser to continue his or her drug-dependent existence (Insel & Roth, 1998). Codependents practice maladaptive behaviors to cope with the problem of abuse. Characteristics of codependents are summarized here:

- Assumption of responsibility for others' feelings or behaviors
- Difficulty in identifying and expressing feelings
- Excessive worry over the response of others to one's feelings
- Difficulty in forming or maintaining close relationships

- Fear of rejection
- Unrealistic expectations of self and others
- Difficulty making decisions
- Tendency to minimize or deny personal feelings or needs
- Emotional dependence on others
- Reluctance to ask for help
- Reluctance to share problems with others
- Though misplaced, steadfast loyalty to others
- Need to be needed
- Perfectionism
- Depression
- A need to control
- Anxiety

The second state of family response to substance abuse involves unsuccessful attempts to eliminate the problem. For example, the family may conspire to prevent the alcohol abuser from having access to alcohol. In the third stage, the family becomes disorganized, control attempts are abandoned, and there is diminished support for the abuser in his or her family roles. The fourth stage of response is characterized by the attempt of the other spouse (or a child) to control the family and to function without the input of the abusing member. This is usually followed by an escape stage in which a separation may occur. In the sixth stage, the family reorganizes and redistributes family roles in the absence of the abuser. With effective treatment, families may also experience a seventh stage in which the family is again reorganized to reintegrate the recovered abuser into his or her previous family roles. The stages of family response to substance abuse are summarized here:

1. Denial of the problem and attempts to mitigate the social effects of substance abuse
2. Unsuccessful attempts by family members to control or eliminate the problem
3. Disorganization, abandonment of control efforts, diminished support for substance abuser in prior family roles
4. Attempts by one or more family members to control the family and to function without the input of the abusing member
5. Separation or other attempts to escape the problem
6. Reorganization and redistribution of family roles without the abuser
7. Reintegration of the recovered substance abuser into the family and into prior family roles

Direct exposure of children to psychoactive substances has a variety of adverse physical and psychological effects. Children with perinatal exposure to alcohol, nicotine, or other drugs may be lower in birth weight, be particularly irritable and difficult to comfort, and experience poor school performance later in life. Drug use during pregnancy may also contribute to premature labor.

Home exposure to tobacco smoke also affects the health status of children and may contribute to a variety of respiratory conditions as well as childhood cancers. The health effects of drug exposures for children are discussed in more detail later in this chapter.

Societal Effects

Societal effects of substance abuse include increased morbidity and mortality, higher economic costs, and increased crime. Physical morbidity related to psychoactive substance abuse was addressed in relation to personal effects of substance abuse. At the societal level, abuse leads to increased incidence and prevalence of these conditions.

Mortality

As noted earlier, substance abuse also leads to increased mortality, either directly as a result of drug overdose or withdrawal or indirectly due to other conditions related to abuse. The contribution of smoking to increased mortality was discussed in Chapter 31. The 1993 age-adjusted mortality rates for drug-induced and alcohol-induced causes were 4.8 and 6.7 per 100,000 population, respectively (U.S. Department of Health and Human Services, 1996).

Mortality related to alcohol abuse is of particular concern. Each year, alcohol is a contributing factor in 100,000 deaths (Addiction Research Center, 1995). In spite of decreases in the number of alcohol-related motor vehicle fatalities, more than 17,000 people died in alcohol-related crashes in 1996 (Centers for Disease Control, 1997). Alcohol use is also implicated in other injury fatalities (Li, Smith, & Baker, 1994). In addition to accident fatalities, alcohol is a factor in other deaths, including homicide; suicide; deaths due to cancers of the lip, oral cavity, pharynx, esophagus, stomach, liver, and larynx; cardiovascular deaths; and deaths due to respiratory diseases, digestive diseases, and diabetes mellitus. Morbidity and mortality due to amphetamine use are also significant societal problems. For example, the number of amphetamine-related deaths in the United States tripled from 1991 to 1994, and a similar increase was noted in emergency room visits due to amphetamines (Substance Abuse and Mental Health Services Administration, 1995).

Cost

Substance abuse also affects society in terms of its economic costs. Alcohol abuse, for example, is considered the most expensive health problem in the United States. Alcohol in the workplace costs employers nearly $55 million a year, and the total 1995 societal costs related to alcohol abuse were expected to be $150 billion (Robertson, 1993). Emergency room costs for alcohol-related injuries are more than twice those for other injuries (Waller, Skelley, & Davis, 1997). In 1991, 20% of all hospital days charged to Medicaid were for substance-abuse-related conditions (Fox, Merrill, Chang, & Califano, 1995).

Crime

One final social effect associated with the abuse of many substances (excluding nicotine) is increased crime (Brown, 1995c). For example, drugs have been implicated in the commission of many crimes that are not strictly related to drugs (selling or possessing drugs, driving while intoxicated). In 1993, drugs were involved in more than 5% of all murders (Brown, 1995a), and drug abuse violations figured in 1.1 million arrests in 1994 (U.S. Department of Commerce, 1996).

▶ THE DIMENSIONS MODEL AND CONTROL OF SUBSTANCE ABUSE

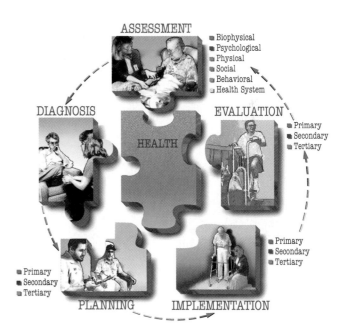

To control problems of substance abuse, community health nurses must identify those persons and groups at risk for substance abuse and its adverse effects, as well as those who are actually experiencing problems of abuse. The Dimensions Model provides a framework for identifying these people and for planning, implementing, and evaluating interventions to assist them in controlling substance abuse.

ASSESSMENT TIPS: Assessing Risk for Substance Abuse

Biophysical Dimension

Are there existing physical health problems contributing to substance abuse?

Is there a family history of substance abuse?

Does the client exhibit signs of intoxication? Or withdrawal?

What influence, if any, does age have on the effects of substance abuse?

What effects does substance abuse have on efforts to control existing physical health problems (eg, diabetes)?

Is the client pregnant? What effects will substance abuse have on the fetus?

Does the client exhibit long-term effects of substance use or abuse? If so, what are these effects?

Psychological Dimension

Does the client have a poor self-image?

What are the client's life goals? Are they realistic?

Does the client exhibit poor impulse control? What is the client's level of frustration tolerance?

What is the extent of the client's coping abilities? What defense mechanisms does the client display?

What life stresses is the client experiencing? How does he or she deal with stress?

Is there underlying psychopathology contributing to substance abuse?

Social Dimension

To what extent do social mores contribute to substance abuse?

What effect does legislative activity have on substance abuse?

Does the client's peer network support substance use and abuse?

Is substance use a regular part of social interaction?

What cultural or religious values or practices influence substance abuse?

Has the client been a victim or perpetrator of family violence?

What social factors (eg, unemployment) contribute to substance abuse?

How readily available are abused substances?

What contribution, if any, does occupation make to substance abuse?

What is the effect of substance abuse on the client's ability to work?

What is the contribution of substance abuse to criminal activity? To homelessness?

What is the extent of substance abuse among homeless individuals?

Behavioral Dimension

What substances are abused? Is there evidence of multisubstance abuse?

Are abused substances used recreationally?

Is substance use associated with leisure activities?

To what extent does the client engage in other high-risk behaviors (eg, driving while intoxicated, high-risk sexual activity)?

Health System Dimension

What is the attitude of health care providers to clients with substance abuse problems?

Are health care providers alert to signs and symptoms of substance abuse?

To what extent do health care providers educate clients about substance abuse?

What health system factors contribute to substance abuse (eg, inappropriate prescription of psychoactive drugs)?

What treatment facilities are available to substance abusers? To special populations of substance abusers (eg, pregnant women, adolescents)?

Does the client have financial access to substance abuse treatment?

Critical Dimensions of Nursing and Substance Abuse

Substance abuse disorders are pervasive phenomena that influence multiple facets of clients' lives and the lives of their families. As was the case with chronic physical and mental health problems, resolution of substance abuse problems requires significant levels of motivation on the part of clients and their families. One critical element of the dimensions of nursing in working with these clients is the interpersonal skill of motivation. Dealing with substance abuse requires changes in behavior on the part of the affected family member and, frequently, on the part of other family members. Because community health nurses often interact with people in their homes where most substance abuse occurs, they are in a unique position to identify persons with substance abuse problems. Community health nurses assess individuals and families for signs of problems related to substance abuse and work with them to create the motivation for change. They also use their interpersonal skills to support individuals and families in dealing with problems of substance abuse.

Like diagnoses of chronic mental illness, substance abuse is associated with social stigma that may be applied to both the person involved and his or her family. This stigma may prevent clients or family members from seeking the help that they need. Nursing advocacy may be required within the ethical dimension to assure sensitive treatment of persons with substance abuse by other health care providers and to prevent or ameliorate discrimination against them in the general society.

At the community level, the nurse employs the process dimension skills of change, leadership, and political activity to create societal changes that modify risk factors contributing to substance abuse. For example, they might campaign for stricter laws related to substance use by, and sales to, minors or driving while intoxicated. Or, they might work to promote increased taxes on tobacco and alcohol as a means of decreasing sales. In addition, community health nurses may promote access to treatment services for persons with substance abuse disorders.

 Assessing the Dimensions of Health in Substance Abuse

Several aspects of community health nursing assessment relate to problems of substance abuse. These include assessing for risk factors, for signs of abuse and dependence, for intoxication, for signs of withdrawal, and for long-term physical and psychological effects of substance abuse. Because of the negative connotations associated with substance abuse, the nursing assessment must be conducted with tact and with an accepting and a nonjudgmental, nonthreatening approach. Nurses must first examine their own attitudes toward substance abuse and work through any negative feelings that may interfere with nurse–client interactions. If clients sense a disparaging or judgmental attitude on the part of the nurse, they are less likely to respond truthfully to questions about their use of psychoactive substances.

Assessing for Risk Factors

The epidemiology of substance abuse indicates that there are contributing factors in five of the six dimensions of health. Community health nurses should keep in mind that the interplay of biological, psychological, and social factors that lead to substance abuse are unique to each individual, and all areas of clients' lives should be assessed in relation to the potential for substance abuse.

The Biophysical Dimension. Human biological factors influencing substance abuse and its effects include genetic inheritance, maturation and aging, and physiologic function.

GENETIC INHERITANCE. A growing body of evidence suggests that substance abuse may be associated with some form of genetic predisposition. Studies of adopted children, for example, indicate that alcohol abuse by one or both of the biological parents is associated with alcohol abuse by the child, even if the adoptive parents are nonabusers. Further support for a genetic predisposition for alcoholism comes from the increased risk of alcohol abuse in the second twin if the first of monozygotic twins in alcohol-dependent when compared with dizygotic twins (Kendler, Heath, Neale, Kesales, & Eaves, 1992).

Research indicating similar ways of processing alcohol and other drugs (eg, opioids) in the brain suggests that there may also be a genetic component in the abuse of drugs other than alcohol. In assessing individuals and families for the level of risk for substance abuse, the community health nurse prepares a detailed genogram that includes information about the family history of substance abuse as well as the presence of physical and emotional illnesses with a genetic component.

Gender, race, and ethnicity are other factors that may influence substance abuse. Male abusers of illicit drugs usually begin with early alcohol use, whereas female abusers are more likely to have been early smokers (Kandel & Yamaguchi, 1993). Gender differences also occur in drug effects. For example, women experience faster progression and more alcohol-related consequences in a shorter period of time than men (Boyd & Hauenstein, 1997). In addition, women alcohol abusers have a greater risk of cardiomyopathy than men (Urbano-Marquez, Estruch, Fernandez-Sola, Nicolas, Pare, & Rubin, 1995). Finally, men and women differ in terms of the incidence of substance abuse disorders, with men, in general, more often affected than women, although these differences are diminishing.

With respect to racial or ethnic factors, Asians

and African Americans are the ethnic groups most likely to abstain from alcohol use altogether. Marijuana, hallucinogen, and amphetamine abuse tends to be more common among whites than blacks, whereas the reverse is true for heroin and cocaine (Akers, 1992). Risk factors for substance abuse have also been shown to vary substantially among ethnic groups.

MATURATION AND AGING.   Age influences one's risk for exposure to drugs and alcohol through social factors. For example, young people are more likely to be exposed to peer influence for drug use or smoking than older people. Adolescents and preadolescents are particularly vulnerable to this type of influence because of their developmental need to conform to peer expectations and to be part of a group. Often, being part of the group depends on engaging in behaviors that place the individual at risk, such as sexual activity, smoking, and drug and alcohol use. For example, illicit drug use was reported by nearly 36% of high school seniors in 1994 compared to 27% in 1992 (Office of National Drug Control Policy, 1995). In 1995, more than a quarter of high school students participating in the Youth Risk Behavior Surveillance System (YRBSS) reported current marijuana use and more than 3% reported current cocaine use (Kann, et al., 1996). Community health nurses working with young people should assess their level of maturity and their ability to resist pressure to conform.

One's age also influences the effects of drug exposure, and perinatal exposures to drugs and alcohol have a variety of adverse effects on the fetus. As many as 7 to 15% of neonates may be exposed to drugs in utero (Robins & Mills, 1993). Some psychoactive substances, such as alcohol, amphetamines, and cocaine,

have teratogenic effects when taken during pregnancy. *Teratogenic substances* are those that cause physical defects in the developing embryo. Other drugs do not affect fetal development per se, but have other adverse health effects for the neonate or long-term effects for the child. For example, fetal alcohol exposure may result in prenatal and postnatal growth deficits, CNS abnormality, and delayed psychomotor development (Larroque, Kaminski, Dehaene, Subtil, Delfosse, & Querleu, 1995; Sampson, Bookstein, Barr, & Streissguth, 1994). Amphetamine use during pregnancy also causes growth retardation, low birth weight, and cerebral injury, and may result in preterm labor or abruptio placenta (Sajo, 1996). Similar effects are noted with perinatal exposure to cocaine (Division of Reproductive Health, 1996). Other fetal, neonatal, and developmental effects of selected psychoactive substances are presented in Table 33–3.

The elderly may also be at increased risk for substance abuse. It is estimated, for example, that 20 to 30% of older persons in the United States abuse alcohol. Factors contributing to abuse in this age group include pain, lack of family support, loneliness, difficulty sleeping, prescription of drugs with abuse potential for pain or sleep, and misuse of prescribed medications due to confusion (Witters, et al., 1992).

The elderly are also at risk for adverse effects of drugs because of decreased ability to metabolize drugs, a condition that occurs with advancing age. In addition, aging itself results in cell loss in target organs, thus increasing their sensitivity to the effects of alcohol and other drugs.

Two general types of substance abuse have been noted among the elderly: early-onset abuse and late-onset abuse. In early-onset abuse, the abuser has de-

TABLE 33–3.   FETAL, NEONATAL, AND DEVELOPMENTAL EFFECTS OF PERINATAL PSYCHOACTIVE SUBSTANCE EXPOSURE

Substance	Fetal Effects	Neonatal Effects	Developmental Effects
Alcohol	Growth deficiency, microcephaly, stillbirth, low birth weight (LBW), joint and facial anomalies, cardiac and kidney anomalies	Acute withdrawal with sedation, seizures, poor feeding	Developmental delay, low IQ, hyperactivity
Sedatives, hypnotics	Sedation at delivery	Tremors, hypertonicity, poor suck, high-pitched cry	Unknown
Opioids	Intrauterine growth retardation, prematurity, microcephaly, hyperactivity	Withdrawal with tremors, hypertonicity, poor feeding, diarrhea, seizures, irritability	Increased rate of sudden infant death syndrome (SIDS)
Cocaine	Spontaneous abortion	Tremors, hypertonicity, muscle weakness, seizures	Developmental delay, increased rate of SIDS
Amphetamines	Intrauterine growth retardation, biliary atresia, transposition of great vessels	Stillbirth, LBW, cardiac anomalies, withdrawal	Poor school performance
Hallucinogens	Agitation at delivery, microcephaly	Irritability, poor fine-motor coordination, sensory input problems	Unknown
Cannabis	Bleeding problems in delivery	Sedation, tremors, excessive response to light	Unknown
Inhalants	Unknown	Unknown	Unknown
Nicotine	Intrauterine growth retardation, microcephaly	Jitteriness, poor feeding	Poor school performance, increased rate of SIDS

veloped a pattern of substance abuse over a lifetime and continues abuse in old age. The late-onset abuser begins to abuse alcohol or other drugs in response to the stresses that occur as a result of aging.

In working with newborns and young children the community health nurse is alert to signs of perinatal drug exposure. He or she also assesses for risk factors that would make the child or older person particularly vulnerable to substance abuse and its effects.

PHYSIOLOGIC FUNCTION.   Deterioration in physiologic function as the result of physical disability may be a contributing factor in substance abuse. For example, in one study, younger people with disabilities were more likely to report use of heroin or crack cocaine than those without disabilities. In older people, sedatives and tranquilizers were used more often by disabled than nondisabled subjects (Gilson, Chilcoat, & Stapleton, 1996). In another study, however, chronic back pain sufferers were no more likely to engage in substance abuse than the comparison group (Brown, Patterson, Rounds, & Papasouliotis, 1996).

In many instances, disability is due to injuries caused by substance abuse (eg, in motor vehicle accidents that occur while one is intoxicated). Cocaine use, for example, has been implicated in more than a quarter of fatal injuries in New York City (Marzuk, et al., 1995). At other times, the person with a disability may abuse drugs or alcohol as an escape from pain, depression, or stress related to the disability. Or, substance abuse may stem from a desire for gratification when other avenues are denied or as a method of regaining control over one's choices and actions. In working with disabled clients, community health nurses assess clients' responses to disability and their vulnerability to substance abuse as a means of coping with disability.

The Psychological Dimension.   Both personality traits and the presence of psychopathology may contribute to problems of substance abuse. There seem to be some commonalities in the personalities of substance abusers regardless of the type of substance abused. Personality traits that may place one at risk for substance abuse include rebelliousness and nonconformity that may lead to substance abuse as an expression of defiance or as an escape from the constraints and expectations of the adult world. Other common traits in abusers are a greater tolerance of deviant behavior, a poor self-concept, and passive surrender to their belief of their own inevitable failure in life. Abusers of psychoactive substances also tend to be impulsive, unable to value themselves, and have poor tolerance for frustration and anxiety. They may also have difficulty in acknowledging their feelings and in developing inter-

ests and deriving pleasure from them. In addition, people who abuse psychoactive substances frequently feel alienated from those around them and are socially isolated. They may also feel powerless, and they usually have poor coping skills. Many of these same personality traits are also exhibited by codependents (Yates & McDaniel, 1994).

Substance abusers also tend to display a common set of defense mechanisms that include denial, projection, rationalization, and conflict minimization and avoidance. Abusers frequently deny that they have a problem with substance abuse and assert that they can change their behavior. They may exhibit inability to accept responsibility for their own behavior in other areas as well, and they frequently project or transfer the blame for their own behavior onto others. They also rationalize their behavior without developing true insights into the reason for that behavior. They tend to try to avoid conflict, and may turn to substance abuse as a means of escaping from the stress generated by conflict rather than engaging in positive modes of conflict resolution. Their thinking is characterized by an all-or-nothing quality, and they often make decisions that are inflexible and narrow in scope.

The presence of definite psychopathology also places many people at increased risk of substance abuse, and substance abuse is frequently an attempt to relieve or mask the symptoms of underlying psychiatric disorders (Sajo, 1996). Women alcohol abusers may be particularly likely to have other psychiatric di-

Critical Thinking in Research

Yates and McDaniel (1994) suggested that nurses as a general group exhibit many of the symptoms of codependence, including the following:

- minimizing one's own problems
- being out of touch with one's feelings
- needing to control the outcomes of events
- perfectionism
- low self-esteem
- being unable to distinguish responsibilities of others
- emotional dependency
- going to extremes with coworkers

1. If this is true, do codependent people gravitate to nursing or does nursing create codependency? How would you design a study to answer this question?
2. How would you go about determining if similar traits are present in members of other helping professions (eg, teachers)?
3. How would you determine why some nurses exhibit codependency and others do not?

agnoses, most commonly major depressive disorder (Boyd & Hauenstein, 1997).

Psychological factors involved in smoking initiation are somewhat different from those involved in the abuse of other substances, although there are some commonalities. Approximately one third of smokers report that they smoke as a means of dealing with stress, fear, anxiety, or pressure, indicating an absence of other effective coping skills. Smokers do not tend to display the psychopathology, alienation, or defense mechanisms typical of other substance abusers; however, young people who begin smoking in the face of current social pressures not to smoke may be exhibiting the defiance that is typical of those who abuse other substances.

The Social Dimension. Factors in the social dimension may also contribute to problems of substance abuse. These factors can exist within the family unit, one's peer group, or society at large. Within the family, research indicates that favorable parental attitudes toward marijuana use are associated with the use of marijuana by children. Similarly, the use of alcohol or drugs by parents or older siblings may influence drug use by children. Families with low cohesion, high levels of conflict, few shared interests and activities, poor coping strategies, and marital dissatisfaction increase the risk of substance abuse in their members. Families encountering multiple stressors and who have inadequate resources are also at risk. Episodes of violence within the family can also lead family members to abuse substances as a means of escape from family tensions (Fendrich, Mackesy-Amiti, Wislar, & Goldstein, 1997). Community health nurses should assess families for conditions that may contribute to substance abuse by family members.

Peer influence is another factor in the social environment that may contribute to substance abuse. In adolescents and preadolescents in particular, pressure from peers to smoke, drink, or use other psychoactive drugs is a powerful motivator for initiating these behaviors. For example, socialization with people who use or abuse psychoactive substances has been shown to contribute to cocaine use as well as the use of other drugs (Witters, et al., 1992). In working with young people, in particular, the nurse carefully assesses peer attitudes toward substance use and abuse as well as the degree to which the individual feels a need to conform to peer dictated norms.

Social factors such as poverty, unemployment, and discrimination may create a sense of hopelessness and powerlessness that leads to substance abuse as an escape or to enhance one's own feelings of competence. These factors might explain the higher prevalence of some forms of substance abuse among members of minority groups and the poor. Societal

attitudes to drug use and abuse also influence the extent of substance abuse in the population. For example, attitudes that promote building jails rather than providing treatment are not only ineffective but more costly than substance abuse treatment (Leshner, 1996). Societal action to restrict access to drugs, on the other hand, may be more effective. In one study, for example, prohibiting alcohol possession in Alaskan Native communities has significantly decreased the consumption of alcohol during pregnancy (Bowerman, 1997).

Culture also seems to play a part in the development of alcohol abuse. Cultural attitudes and modes of introducing alcohol use to young people can either contribute to or impede the development of alcohol abuse. Religion is an aspect of culture that may strongly influence drug use. Strong religious affiliation, whatever the denomination, is associated with reduced risk of drug and alcohol abuse. Religious denomination, however, does have some influence on alcohol use, with generally higher rates of use among Roman Catholics, Episcopalians, and Lutherans, and less use by Baptists, Mormons, and Christian Fundamentalists groups (Akers, 1992).

In assessing individuals, families, and communities for potential for substance abuse, the community health nurse investigates both the influence of cultural norms and sources of stress on the use of psychoactive substances. In addition, the nurse looks for risk factors such as poverty and unemployment that increase stress and prompt substance abuse.

Other societal factors that contribute to substance abuse should also be assessed, including general norms for abusive behaviors and the availability of psychoactive substances. Media portrayals of drinking and smoking as desirable behaviors influence use of these substances. Ready availability of amphetamines in Southern California, where methamphetamine labs abound, make this a drug of choice in the area and increase its abuse relative to other psychoactive substances.

Occupation is another social dimension factor that may contribute to substance abuse. Some occupational groups are at increased risk for substance abuse. People whose work involves travel outside the United States may have access to illicit drugs that promote abuse. Similarly, there is a relatively high incidence of substance abuse among health care providers because of easy access to controlled drugs.

Athletes are another occupational group with relatively high rates of drug abuse. Drugs of choice for this group tend to be *ergogenic agents,* drugs used to enhance athletic performance (Witters, et al., 1992). Increased prevalence of substance abuse has occurred among both professional and amateur athletes. In the 1995 YBRSS survey, nearly 4% of high school students reported steroid use without a physician's prescription (Kann, et al., 1996).

Use and abuse of psychoactive substances in other occupational settings is also of concern. Approximately two thirds of substance abusers and most casual users of psychoactive substances are employed, and it is estimated that 12% of the U.S. work force suffers from drug and alcohol problems (Robertson, 1993). Further, an estimated one fourth of U.S. workers have come to work under the influence of psychoactive substances at some time (Akers, 1992). Users are more likely than nonusers to be injured on the job and are less productive and have more work absences than nonusers.

Employer sanctions against substance use and abuse have been shown to decrease these practices. For example, policies related to drug use in the U.S. military have led to reduced rates of drug abuse in this occupational group compared with the civilian population. On the other hand, lack of attention to alcohol use and smoking by military personnel has led to increased prevalence of these behaviors. Employer policies related to smoking in the workplace have also been shown to decrease smoking behaviors both on and off the job.

Mandatory screening of employees, although controversial, is believed by many to contribute to control of drug use in occupational settings. Federal regulations require drug testing of workers employed in the rail, trucking, airline, and nuclear power industries. Many private concerns are also using drug tests to screen employees. More and more companies are instituting employee assistance programs (EAPs) to help drug- and alcohol-impaired employees.

Easy access to alcohol and cigarettes has also contributed to abuse of these substances. On the other hand, laws controlling access to alcohol through higher taxes on alcohol sales and by raising the minimum age of purchase have decreased both the use and misuse of alcohol. Recent reductions in alcohol-related traffic fatalities in the United States have also been attributed to changes in social environmental factors such as enactment and enforcement of minimum drinking age laws and penalties for driving while intoxicated.

The Behavioral Dimension.   Behavioral factors that influence substance abuse are related to consumption patterns and leisure activities. The community health nurse assesses individual and family consumption patterns related to tobacco, alcohol, and medications. The nurse should ascertain the frequency and amount of substance use as well as the appropriateness of its use. For example, the nurse might determine whether sedatives are in fact being used as prescribed, whether they are kept away from young people in the home,

and whether they are ever used in conjunction with alcohol. Nurses should also determine the extent of alcohol use by families. Many people, for example, do not consider taking medications with an alcohol base as drinking, but may be receiving a hefty dose of alcohol through repeated use. Similarly, Mexican American families might return to Mexico to obtain medications such as paregoric (an opioid preparation) for use for diarrhea without even knowing about their potential for abuse. The nurse also asks about medicinal uses of alcohol, particularly with children, such as giving alcohol for teething pain or to quiet a fretful child.

Recreational activities can contribute to the use of psychoactive substances in that alcohol and tobacco use are frequent adjuncts of such activities. People tend to drink and smoke when they socialize with others. In fact, 80 to 95% of alcohol abusers are also smokers (Robertson, 1993). Friday or Saturday night binges are a relatively common phenomenon, when people can "let go" and drink because they know they will have time to recover before returning to work on Monday. Next to alcohol, marijuana is the most widely used recreational drug, but cocaine is also used recreationally and has the connotation of high status, glamour, and excitement. PCP is also used for recreational purposes.

Substance abuse has also been shown to be related to other high-risk lifestyle behaviors. The relationship of alcohol use to motor vehicle fatalities has already been discussed, but it is also believed that 60 to 80% of marijuana users drive under the influence (Witters, et al., 1992). The relationship of drugs to violent crime has also been addressed. One other behavior associated with substance abuse is high-risk sexual activity. Crack smoking, particularly in conjunction with injection drug use, has been shown to be associated with prostitution and unprotected intercourse (Booth, Watters, & Chitwood, 1993). Male amphetamine users are also likely to engage in high-risk sexual behaviors (Sajo, 1996). Similarly, use of alcohol, tobacco, marijuana, cocaine, and other illicit drugs was associated with increased sexual activity, multiple sexual partners, and lack of condom use among adolescents (Lowry, Holtzman, Truman, Kann, Collins, & Kolbe, 1994).

The Health System Dimension.   Many of the psychoactive substances with abuse potential originated within the health care system. Opioids were widely used for pain control even during the American Civil War (Akers, 1992), and are still the drug of choice for relief of severe pain. Cocaine and PCP were first used as surgical anesthetics (Witters, et al., 1992), and marijuana may have some medical use in the treatment of glaucoma. Sedatives and hypnotics are widely used for controlling anxiety, and amphetamines were originally developed as diet aids, although they no longer have any accepted medical use.

Several aspects of the U.S. health care system have contributed to the growing problem of substance abuse. Lack of attention to educating clients and the public about the hazards of substance abuse and failure to identify clients with substance abuse problems have impeded efforts to control abuse. Practitioners have been particularly slow to identify pregnant women and older clients with problems of abuse, and until recently it was difficult for pregnant abusers to find accessible treatment facilities (Breitbart, Chavkin, & Wise, 1994). At the same time, some health care providers have actively fostered drug abuse by prescribing psychoactive drugs inappropriately or by not monitoring the extent of clients' use of these drugs.

The health care system also impedes control of substance abuse by failing to provide adequate treatment for persons affected. For example, health insurance coverage for treatment for substance abuse is minimal at best. Provision of adequate treatment of substance abuse may be further impeded by negative feelings on the part of health care providers toward those who abuse psychoactive substances. Many clients in need may not have access to services. For instance, many shelters for the homeless refuse abusers despite the fact that a large proportion of homeless individuals abuse alcohol and other drugs.

The health care system may pose additional barriers to care that are particularly burdensome for some population groups. For example, most treatment programs are geared toward the needs of younger people and may not recognize the unique needs of the elderly substance abuser. Certainly Medicare, in the implementation of the DRG (diagnosis-related group) system, does not take note of the extended time needed to safely detoxify the elderly substance abuser. In addition, because older people are often considered nonproductive members of society, priority for placement in treatment facilities may be given to younger people.

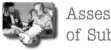 Assessing for Signs of Substance Abuse

In addition to assessing individuals, families, and communities for risk factors that may contribute to substance abuse, the nurse should assess individual clients for general indications of existing abuse. General indicators that a person has a problem with abuse of a psychoactive substance include frequent intoxication, preoccupation with obtaining and using the sub-

stance, binge use, changes in personality or mood, withdrawal, problems with family members related to use of the substance, problems with friends or neighbors, problems on the job (absenteeism, poor performance, interpersonal difficulties), and conflicts with law enforcement officials. Additional indicators include belligerence, financial problems, inability to discontinue substance use despite attempts, continued use of the substance despite related health conditions and other problems, and increasing tolerance to the substance.

Assessing for Intoxication

Another aspect of the community health nurse's assessment related to substance abuse is assessing individuals for signs of intoxication. **Intoxication** is a state of diminished physical or mental control that occurs as a result of the current use of psychoactive drugs. Intoxication with different drugs may be reflected in differing symptoms. For example, cocaine intoxication is characterized by disinhibition, impaired judgment and impulsivity, grandiosity, and compulsively repeated actions. Other common symptoms include hy-

TABLE 33–4. SIGNS OF INTOXICATION WITH SELECTED PSYCHOACTIVE SUBSTANCES

Substance	Typical Indications of Intoxication
Alcohol	Decreased alertness, impaired judgment, slurred speech, nausea, double vision, vertigo, staggering, unpredictable emotional changes, stupor, unconsciousness, increased reaction time
Sedative, hypnotics, anxiolytics	Slurred speech; slow, shallow respiration; cold and clammy skin; nystagmus; weak and rapid pulse; drowsiness, blurred vision, unconsciousness; disorientation; depression; poor judgment; motor impairment
Opioids	Sedation, hypertension, respiratory depression, impaired intellectual function, constipation, pupillary constriction, watery eyes, increased pulse and blood pressure
Cocaine	Irritability, anxiety, slow weak pulse, slow shallow breathing, sweating, dilated pupils, increased blood pressure, insomnia, seizures, dysinhibition, impulsivity, compulsive actions, hypersexuality, hypervigilance, hyperactivity
Amphetamines	Sweating, dilated pupils, increased blood pressure, agitation, fever, irritability, headache, chills, insomnia, agitation, tremors, seizures, wakefulness, hyperactivity, confusion, paranoia
Hallucinogens	Dilated pupils, mood swings, elevated blood pressure, paranoia, bizarre behavior, nausea and vomiting, tremors, panic, flushing, fever, sweating, agitation, aggression, nystagmus (PCP)
Cannabis	Reddened eyes; increased pulse, respirations, and blood pressure; laughter; confusion, panic; drowsiness
Inhalants	Giddiness, drowsiness, increased vital signs, headache, nausea, fainting, stupor, fatigue, slurred speech, disorientation, delirium
Nicotine	Headache, loss of appetite, nausea, increased pulse, blood pressure, and muscle tone

persexuality, hypervigilance, and hyperactivity. Nicotine intoxication, on the other hand, is characterized by increased blood pressure, heart rate, and muscle tone. Signs of intoxication with selected psychoactive substances are presented in Table 33–4.

Assessing for Withdrawal

The physiologic dependence engendered by some psychoactive substances leads to withdrawal or abstinence syndrome when the substance is withheld. A withdrawal syndrome is a complex of symptoms that accompany abstinence from a psychoactive substance, usually characterized by severe discomfort, pain, nausea, vomiting, and, possibly, convulsions. The severity of withdrawal may vary with the abusive substance and the degree of dependence experienced by the client. The community health nurse working with clients who may abuse psychoactive substances assesses the client for signs of withdrawal. Typical withdrawal symptoms for selected psychoactive substances are presented in Table 33–5.

Withdrawal can be extremely dangerous and may even be life-threatening, especially for vulnerable clients. Withdrawal is a particularly serious event for pregnant women, when both mother and fetus are at risk, and for the elderly, and the community health nurse should be alert in assessing these clients for signs of withdrawal. Interventions during the withdrawal phase are addressed later in this chapter.

The physical and psychological discomfort and the deep depression that may occur with withdrawal from psychoactive drug use may lead to suicide. The community health nurse assessing clients for withdrawal symptoms should also carefully assess them for potential suicide. Clients should be monitored carefully and asked about suicidal thoughts.

Because of the duration and unique features of cocaine abstinence, the cocaine withdrawal syndrome merits specific discussion here. Cocaine abstinence occurs in three phases: crash, withdrawal, and extinction (Witters, et al., 1992). The crash occurs anywhere from 1 hour to 4 days after discontinuing use of the drug and is characterized by agitation, depression, anorexia, and intense craving. This phase is also characterized by feelings of extreme exhaustion following a cocaine binge. During the withdrawal phase, the client first experiences normal sleep patterns, low anxiety levels, and low cravings for cocaine. Later in this phase, which may last up to 10 weeks, the client experiences *anhedonia* (an inability to experience pleasure), high anxiety, and high levels of craving. Cravings are exacerbated by conditioned cues associated with prior drug use such as seeing people with whom one used drugs or re-

TABLE 33–5. INDICATIONS OF WITHDRAWAL FROM SELECTED PSYCHOACTIVE SUBSTANCES

Substance	Indications of Withdrawal
Alcohol	Anxiety, insomnia, tremors, delirium, convulsions
Sedatives, hypnotics, anxiolytics	Anxiety, insomnia, tremors, delirium, convulsions (may occur up to 2 weeks after stopping use of anxiolytics)
Opioids	Restlessness, irritability, tremors, loss of appetite, panic, chills, sweating, cramps, watery eyes, runny nose, nausea, vomiting, muscle spasms, impaired coordination, depressed reflexes dilated pupils, yawning
Cocaine	*Early crash:* agitation depression, anorexia, high level of craving suicidal ideation *Middle crash:* fatigue, depression, no craving, insomnia *Late crash:* exhaustion, hypersomnolence, hyperphagia, no craving *Early withdrawal:* normal sleep and mood, low craving, low anxiety *Middle and late withdrawal:* anhedonia, anxiety, anergy, high level of craving exacerbated by conditioned cues *Extinction:* normal hedonic response and mood, episodic craving triggered by conditioned cues
Amphetamines	Fatigue, hunger, long periods of sleep, disorientation, severe depression
Hallucinogens	Slight irritability, restlessness, insomnia, reduced energy level, depression
Cannabis	Insomnia, hyperactivity, decreased appetite
Inhalants	None reported
Nicotine	Nervousness, increased appetite, sleep disturbances, anxiety, irritability

turning to places where drugs have been used. The extinction phase, which lasts an indefinite period, is characterized by normal hedonic experience, normal moods, and episodic cravings triggered by conditioned cues. Cravings occurring in both the withdrawal and extinction phases may lead to resumed drug use.

Assessing for Long-term Effects of Substance Abuse

In addition to assessing clients for signs and symptoms of intoxication and withdrawal, community health nurses should also assess individual clients for symptoms of long-term effects of substance abuse. These effects can be physical or psychological and vary with the psychoactive substance. For example, long-term effects of alcohol abuse include malnutrition, cirrhosis, and liver cancer, and typical effects of phencyclidine abuse are psychoses and insomnia. Typical long-term effects that should be considered with specific substances are presented in Table 33–6. The community health nurse assessing the health of population groups assesses morbidity and mortality related to these long-term effects of substance abuse in the population.

TABLE 33–6. LONG-TERM EFFECTS ASSOCIATED WITH ABUSE OF SELECTED PSYCHOACTIVE SUBSTANCES

Substance	Long-term Effects of Abuse
Alcohol	Malnutrition; impotence, ulcers; cirrhosis; esophageal, stomach, and liver cancers; organic brain syndrome; deafness
Sedatives, hypnotics, anxiolytics	Potential for death due to overdose from increasing doses due to tolerance, impaired sexual function
Opioids	Lethargy, weight loss, sexual disinterest and dysfunction, increased susceptibility to infection and accidents, constipation
Cocaine	Damage to nasal tissue, high blood pressure, weight loss, muscle twitching, paranoia, hallucinations, disrupted sleeping and eating patterns, irritability, liver damage
Amphetamines	Depression, paranoia, hallucinations, weight loss, impotence
Hallucinogens	Memory loss, inability to concentrate, insomnia, chronic or recurrent psychosis, flashbacks
Cannabis	Chromosome changes, reduced sperm count, impaired concentration, poor memory, reduced alertness, inability to perform complex tasks
Inhalants	Organic brain syndrome, liver and kidney damage, bone marrow damage, anemia, hearing loss, nerve damage
Nicotine	Cardiovascular disease, lung cancer, bladder cancer, chronic disease, diabetic complications

Diagnostic Reasoning and Control of Substance Abuse

Community health nurses make nursing diagnoses related to substance abuse at two levels. The first level is diagnoses related to individuals who have problems of substance abuse and their families. For example, the nurse might make a diagnosis for the individual client of "increased risk of substance abuse due to family history of alcohol abuse" or "abuse of sedatives due to increased life stress and poor coping skills." Nursing diagnoses related to the family of a substance abuser might include "codependency due to family feelings of guilt related to daughter's cocaine abuse" and "school behavior problems due to children's anxiety over mother's alcoholism."

At the second level, the community health nurse might make diagnoses of community problems related to substance abuse. For example, the nurse might diagnose an "increased incidence of motor vehicle fatalities due to driving under the influence of psychoactive drugs," or "increased prevalence of drug abuse among minority group members due to discrimination and feelings of powerlessness." Another community-based diagnosis is "increased prevalence of fetal alcohol syndrome due to alcohol abuse among pregnant women."

Planning and Implementing the Dimensions of Health Care in Controlling Substance Abuse

Strategies for controlling problems of substance abuse can involve primary, secondary, or tertiary prevention.

Primary Prevention

There are three major goals for primary prevention of substance abuse. The first goal is to prevent nonusers from initiating use of psychoactive substances. The second goal is to prevent progression from experimentation to chronic use. And the third goal is to prevent expansion to the use of other substances. Using smoking as an example, primary prevention may be aimed at preventing the initiation of smoking in the first place, preventing movement from occasional smoking to regular use of tobacco, and preventing movement from tobacco use to the use of other drugs such as marijuana.

Primary prevention efforts to control substance abuse usually focus on two approaches: education and risk factor modification. In addition, there has been some preliminary success in immunizing laboratory rats against the effects of cocaine that may have implications for preventing substance abuse in humans (Rocio, et al., 1995; Swan, 1996).

Education. Education usually focuses on acquainting the public with the hazards of substance abuse. Both general public education campaigns and school-based educational programs have shown moderate success in limiting the use of psychoactive substances; however, they tend to be more effective in moderating the effects of substance abuse such as preventing drug-related motor vehicle fatalities. One of the criticisms of school-based programs is that they may not be reaching groups at greatest risk for substance abuse, those with a family history of abuse or who display characteristics associated with potential abusers.

Community health nurses may be involved in educating individual clients and families or in providing substance abuse education for groups of people. In either case, the nurse would employ the principles of teaching and learning discussed in Chapter 9.

Risk Factor Modification. Risk factor modification can occur with individuals, families, or society at large. Community health nurses may assist individuals to modify factors that put them at increased risk for substance abuse. For example, the nurse might assist clients experiencing stress to eliminate or modify sources of stress in their lives. Or, the nurse can assist clients to develop more effective coping skills.

Community health nurses might also assist families to develop more effective coping skills. In addition, the nurse may make referrals for social services to eliminate financial difficulties and other sources of stress. Or, the nurse might assist a harried single parent to obtain respite care. Nurses can also assist families to plan means of enhancing family communication and cohesion to minimize the risk of substance abuse among children.

At the societal level, community health nurses can engage in political activity to control access to and limit the availability of psychoactive substances as well as to modify societal factors that contribute to abuse. For example, the nurse might work to see that laws restricting the sale of alcohol and tobacco to minors are enforced. Or, the nurse might work to reduce discrimination against members of minority groups or to ensure a minimal income for all families.

Secondary Prevention

Secondary prevention is employed when there is an existing problem with substance abuse. The goal in secondary prevention is early intervention aimed at those who have not yet developed irreversible pathological changes due to substance abuse. Planning secondary prevention necessitates mutual goal setting by the nurse and the family of the person experiencing a substance abuse problem. Goals relate to "intervention" and to treatment for substance abuse.

Intervention. **Intervention,** in terms of substance abuse, is the act of confronting the substance abuser with the intent of making a referral for assistance in dealing with the abuse (Sajo, 1996). The goal of the intervention is to elicit an agreement from the individual involved to be evaluated for a possible problem with substance abuse.

Community health nurses may facilitate intervention by families of individual abusers but are not usually the interveners themselves. In this respect, the family, rather than the abuser, is the community health nurse's client.

Many families may not see themselves as clients, and the community health nurse may need to reinforce the idea that substance abuse is a family disorder to motivate family members to engage in intervention. To this end, the first step in preparing for intervention is providing the family or significant others with basic information about substance abuse and the defense mechanisms used by both the abuser and his or her significant others. In this way, family members can be helped to see their role as codependents or enablers of the abusive behavior. The nurse also educates family members about the intervention process, their responsibility for that process, and some of the feelings that they may experience during intervention.

In assisting family members to prepare for intervention, the nurse aids them to determine who should be involved. It may be that some members will not be able to follow through with confronting the individual with his or her behavior and should be asked not to participate in the intervention. Individuals who should be involved in the intervention include those who are close to and concerned for the abuser, those who may be able to influence the abuser's behavior in a positive way, and those who are able to engage in the intervention.

Next the nurse assists those who will be involved in the intervention to identify in writing the causes for their concern and to describe how they felt when significant events related to substance abuse occurred. Areas that the group should plan to address during the intervention are the problem as they perceive it, statements about the individual's behavior that indicate a problem of substance abuse, effects of the abuse problem, and their concern for the individual.

Prior to the intervention, the group should arrange an appointment for an evaluation for substance abuse to take place immediately after the intervention session, as it is wise to follow through on the referral as soon as possible while the individual is motivated to seek help. It is suggested that appointments be made in more than one facility so the individual can exercise some choice in the matter and will feel less coerced.

The group planning the intervention should also consider potential roadblocks to the success of the effort. For example, the individual might be concerned about the cost of care or about the need for child care while he or she is in treatment. If anticipated, these difficulties can be circumvented.

The nurse can also assist family members to plan their response to the individual's possible refusal to comply with a request for evaluation for substance abuse. If the wife plans to threaten divorce if the husband does not seek help, will she be able to carry through this threat in the face of his refusal? The nurse can help the family plan for these contingencies and work through feelings created by the proposed intervention by helping group members practice the intervention (who will say what, when, and so on). Practice should also include who will sit nearest the individual (those with the greatest influence) and between the abuser and the door and who will initiate the intervention.

Once the group is ready for the intervention, the individual should be brought to the place selected and the intervention initiated. Just prior to the intervention, while waiting for the individual to arrive, the nurse may remind family members why they are there and what is planned. The nurse is present to keep the intervention moving, but is not otherwise an active participant.

If the individual agrees to be evaluated, one or more of the group members should accompany him or her to the evaluation appointment to prevent a potential suicide attempt. While this is occurring, the nurse may meet with the other members of the group to discuss their feelings about the process and its outcome. If the intervention has not been successful, the nurse can reassure group members and assist them to plan a subsequent intervention.

Treatment

GENERAL PRINCIPLES OF TREATMENT FOR SUBSTANCE ABUSE.   Treatment for problems of substance abuse vary somewhat depending on the type of substance involved. There are, however, some general principles that guide treatment for substance abuse. First, a combination of modalities of treatment is usually more effective than a single mode. Second, treatment should be geared to individual problems, responses, and resources. For example, issues of aging related to retirement, physical loss, and loss of significant others leading to social isolation are issues that may need to be addressed with the elderly person but may not be factors in substance abuse by others. Similarly, the effects of physical disability must be dealt with in the handicapped person who abuses psychoactive substances, whereas this is not likely to be an issue with most other clients.

The third principle is that treatment should be administered by both professionals and laypersons. For example, a combination of professional psychotherapy and participation in a self-help group such as Alcoholics Anonymous may be far more effective in dealing with alcohol abuse than either mode by itself. Family members or significant others should also be actively involved in treatment to refrain from enabling behaviors that allowed the individual to continue his or her substance abuse.

Fourth, detoxification is necessary before any further treatment can be undertaken. Fifth, associated psychopathology requires psychiatric treatment, not just the assistance of a self-help group. Finally, social and vocational rehabilitation may be needed to reintegrate the person into the family and into society at large.

► GENERAL PRINCIPLES OF TREATMENT FOR SUBSTANCE ABUSE

- A combination of modalities is usually more effective than a single treatment modality.
- Treatment should be tailored to the problems, responses, and resources of the individual abuser.
- Treatment should be provided by both professionals and laypersons.
- Detoxification and achievement of sobriety constitute the first step in treatment.
- Associated psychopathology requires psychiatric treatment.
- Social and vocational rehabilitation may be required to reintegrate the substance-abusing individual into the family and society.

TREATMENT MODALITIES FOR SUBSTANCE ABUSE.   Treatment modalities that may be employed include pharmacologic methods, psychosocial methods, sociotherapies, and self-help groups. Pharmacologic methods use medication to help the abuser deal with the symptoms of withdrawal or to handle cravings for the substance involved. For example, Librium and Valium may be used to help the alcohol abuser relieve the anxiety caused by alcohol withdrawal, while disulfiram (Antabuse) may be given to modify the craving for alcohol. Similarly, methadone may be used to control cravings for heroin. Psychosocial methods of treatment include individual, group, and family therapy; behavior modification; contracting; and aversion or relaxation therapies. Sociotherapy involves participation in therapeutic communities and residential programs where clients learn new lifestyles consistent with sobriety. Finally, self-help groups consist of people who are abusers of the same substance and who provide for each other understanding and support in conquering their substance abuse habit. For example, Alcoholics Anonymous is a self-help group for alcohol abusers, and Potsmokers Anonymous is a self-help group for marijuana abusers. Treatment modalities typically used for specific types of substance abuse are indicated in Table 33–7.

Community health nurses may plan involvement in treatment for substance abuse in a number of ways. First, nurses might identify cases of substance abuse and plan to refer clients and their families to treatment resources in the community. Nurses may also educate the general public on the signs and symptoms of substance abuse as well as the availability of treatment facilities. In addition, community health nurses can monitor the use of medications dur-

TABLE 33–7. TREATMENT MODALITIES TYPICALLY USED FOR SELECTED FORMS OF PSYCHOACTIVE SUBSTANCE ABUSE

Substance	Typical Treatment Modalities
Alcohol	Detoxification; psychotherapy; group therapy; family therapy; self-help groups (Alcoholics Anonymous, Al-Anon); pharmacologic therapy (disulfiram, short-term use of tranquilizers or antidepressants); residential programs; referral for vocational rehabilitation and social services as needed
Sedatives, hypnotics, anxiolytics	Detoxification; psychotherapy and group therapy (for underlying psychiatric disorders)
Opioids	Pharmacologic therapy (methadone, opioid antagonists); therapeutic communities (Synanon, Odyssey House, Daytop, Phoenix House); group therapy; assistance with social skills, vocational training and job placement; family therapy; self-help groups (Narcotics Anonymous, Chemical Dependency Anonymous); psychotherapy
Cocaine	Hospitalization; self-help groups; contingency contracting (client agreement to urinary monitoring and acceptance of aversive contingencies for positive results); pharmacologic therapy (tricyclic antidepressants)
Amphetamines	No established treatment guidelines; may be similar to treatment for cocaine abuse
Hallucinogens	Detoxification; psychotherapy (for underlying psychiatric disorders); group therapy; residential programs
Cannabis	Same as for Hallucinogens; self-help groups
Inhalants	Psychosocial interventions; psychotherapy (for underlying psychiatric disorder); sociodrama; vocational rehabilitation; family therapy; social support services
Nicotine	Aversive conditioning; desensitization; substitution; hypnotherapy; group therapy; relaxation training; supportive therapy; abrupt abstinence

ing withdrawal (if this is done on a outpatient basis) or on a long-term basis.

Community health nurses might also be involved in psychosocial therapies in referring clients to sources of group, individual, or family therapy, or the nurse might reinforce contracts made for reducing the use of substances. This is particularly true in measures to help clients stop smoking. In this instance, community health nurses may initiate behavioral contracts with clients to enable them gradually to cut down on tobacco consumption or to quit smoking for gradually lengthened periods.

Community health nurses' involvement with therapeutic communities and self-help groups usually occurs in the form of referrals for these types of services. In some instances, however, community health nurses are actively involved in initiating support groups.

At the community level, nursing efforts to control substance abuse might include political activity to support the development of adequate treatment facilities, especially those geared to the needs of currently underserved population groups such as pregnant women, the homeless, and the elderly. Community health nurses might also be involved in political activity and advocacy to encourage insurance coverage of treatment for substance abuse.

The goals of treatment for substance abuse include intervening early for persons who have not yet become abusers but who use psychoactive substances; managing withdrawal and reducing cravings for the substance involved; and building a foundation for recovery. Successful treatment efforts are usually characterized by patience, perseverance, and commitment by the helper; realistic goals; abstinence during treatment and as the ultimate goal; some degree of coercion involving the setting of limits, contracts, or substance control measures; breaking through the abuser's denial to acceptance of the problem; bolstering his or her motivation to maintain abstinence; and development of alternate coping styles and enhanced self-esteem.

EARLY TREATMENT. For some psychoactive substances, such as cocaine, use at any level frequently leads to abuse because of the vicious rebound cycle that occurs. For other substances like alcohol, sedatives, and tranquilizers, moderate use may be acceptable when these substances are used appropriately. Some authors suggest early intervention with people using these substances to allow them to use the substance in moderation. To this end, brief treatment is undertaken to stabilize and to moderate use of the substance in question so that it does not reach the level of abuse. Programs of this type involve teaching clients self-control skills and skills for decision making about responsible behavioral choices.

MANAGING WITHDRAWAL AND CRAVINGS. For clients who have already reached a level of substance abuse that does not admit to moderate use or with substances for which there is no level of moderate use, the goal of treatment is abstinence and long-term sobriety. The first step to abstinence is detoxification, which often involves supporting the client through withdrawal. Community health nurses may be involved in referring clients to detoxification facilities and in supporting them during detoxification.

Persons who are at risk for serious consequences of withdrawal should always go through detoxification under medical supervision. Of particular concern are pregnant women and the elderly. Many of the drugs used to mitigate the adverse symptomatology of withdrawal from psychoactive substances are contraindicated in pregnancy. For example, Valium and

Librium, both of which may be used to combat the anxiety and sleeplessness that may accompany withdrawal, may be teratogenic and should not be given to the pregnant substance abuser. Similarly, detoxification procedures may need to be modified for older adults because of their tendency to be overmedicated by relatively small doses of medication.

Community health nurses may monitor medication use during withdrawal or on a long-term basis, and they should be alert to the potential for use of medications for suicide purposes and to the potential for abuse of some of the substances used (eg, Valium). The nurse should assess clients on medications for suicide potential and should monitor mood changes closely. The nurse should also educate clients and their families as to the adverse effects of combining medications with alcohol or other psychoactive drugs. Because disulfiram (Antabuse), in particular, is contraindicated in both pregnant women and clients with cardiac arrhythmias and pulmonary disease, the nurse should monitor clients for evidence of these conditions.

Other nursing considerations related to withdrawal and craving include maintaining levels of hydration and nutrition. Hydration is particularly important for the client who abuses alcohol because of the diuretic effects of alcohol. Nutrition is important for most drug abusers because substance abuse frequently leads to a disinterest in food in favor of consumption of the abusive substance. Decreased intake of stimulants such as caffeine is also advisable. Treatment can also be enhanced by a regular program of exercise that will improve self-esteem, prevent excessive weight gain, and stimulate the release of endorphins. Community health nurses can educate clients on the need for hydration and nutrition and suggest exercise. Vigorous aerobic exercise should not be undertaken before a thorough medical assessment of cardiovascular status has been conducted. In the interim, however, the nurse can suggest a program of stretching exercises.

BUILDING A FOUNDATION FOR RECOVERY.   Treatment for substance abuse is more than a matter of detoxification and modification of cravings for the drug in question. It is usually a total program of modification that results in changes in modes of thinking and acting. This may be achieved through professional therapy, participation in self-help groups, changes in environment and lifestyle, self-image enhancement, and development of new coping skills and new patterns of family interaction.

Community health nursing involvement in therapy and in self-help groups was addressed earlier. Nurses can also assist clients to plan changes in their environment to minimize stresses that may contribute to substance abuse. For example, the nurse can refer a client for help with financial difficulties or for respite from the care of a handicapped child or elderly parent. Socially isolated older persons who abuse substances can be linked to sources of social support, and unemployed persons can be assisted to find employment or to learn skills that enhance their employability.

Community health nurses can also help clients develop stronger self-images by reinforcing their successes and helping them realistically examine their failures and their expectations for themselves. In addition, nurses can help clients who abuse psychoactive substances to develop alternative ways of coping with stress by taking action to modify stressors or changing their perceptions of and responses to stressors.

Treatment efforts are also needed for members of the abuser's family to enable them to recover from codependency. Goals in the care of families of substance abusers include stabilizing the family system, making changes in family interactions, and developing mechanisms for maintaining those changes. Family stabilization may be achieved by linking families to needed support services and engaging in the crisis intervention strategies described in Chapter 18. The nurse can also make referrals for marital or family therapy as needed and can assist families to identify their use of defense mechanisms similar to those used by the substance abuser.

The community health nurse might also provide families with anticipatory guidance about the negative effects of life change events and help them deal with these events without resorting to substance abuse. Family members may also need help in working through resentment related to substance abuse and subsequent behaviors by the abuser.

Building positive experiences in the life of the family also fosters cohesion and helps to stabilize the family. The community health nurse can assist the family to plan activities in which all members can participate. It is particularly important to integrate the substance-abusing member into these occasions to prevent further alienation.

The community health nurse can also assist families to develop new patterns of interaction. For example, the nurse might help the family realign members into the more usual husband–wife coalition rather than parent–child coalitions by improving family communication and developing joint problem-solving skills. The nurse can also assist family members to identify and express feelings and learn negotiating strategies.

Harm Reduction.   An alternative approach to the control of substance abuse is based on the philosophy of harm reduction. Traditionally, the goal of policy development and implementation related to substance abuse has been a reduction in drug use. It has been suggested that a more appropriate focus would be to reduce the harm to society resulting from drug abuse (Reuter & Caulkins, 1995). *Harm reduction* is an approach to drug use that focuses on moderation of substance use and minimization of its harmful effects (Tatarsky, 1995). Harm reduction is based on the premises that (1) nonmedical use of drugs is inevitable given the ease of drug accessibility in society, (2) use inevitably produces personal and social harm, but that harm can be minimized, (3) drug policies must be realistic, (4) drug users must be integrated into, rather than isolated from, the larger community, and (5) it is not always necessary to eliminate use to minimize harm (Des Jarlais, 1995). Suggested goals for harm reduction include providing adequate treatment for abusers, reducing HIV and other disease transmission through drug use (eg, by way of needle-exchange programs), and creating new legal, but inconvenient and expensive mechanisms for distribution of some drugs among adults to minimize the criminal aspects of drug abuse. Many of these strategies remain controversial, but there is growing recognition of the potential for harm reduction (Des Jarlais, 1995), and some of these strategies are reflected in the 1995 National Drug Control Strategy (Brown, 1995a).

Tertiary Prevention

Tertiary prevention is aimed at preventing a relapse into prior substance-abusing behaviors by the individual or into enabling behaviors by family members and significant others. Community health nurses can contribute to these efforts by providing emotional support to recovering abusers and their families and by linking them with other support groups. Other tertiary prevention measures might include efforts to eliminate or modify stressors that contribute to relapse. For example, assisting the recovering abuser to find work can alleviate the stress of unemployment and financial worries.

The nurse can also reinforce the individual's motivation to abstain from drug use by commending and highlighting successes and periods of sobriety. Development of positive coping skills may also prevent relapse. Other tertiary prevention needs may involve providing information on resources, providing respite from onerous burdens of care, or helping individuals plan time for themselves. Table 33–8 lists primary, secondary, and tertiary prevention goals in the control of substance abuse.

TABLE 33–8. PRIMARY, SECONDARY, AND TERTIARY PREVENTION GOALS AND RELATED COMMUNITY HEALTH NURSING INTERVENTIONS IN THE CONTROL OF SUBSTANCE ABUSE

Goal of Prevention	Nursing Intervention
Primary Prevention	
1. Positive coping skills	1. Teach coping skills
2. Strong self image	2. Foster and reinforce development of strong self-image
3. Public education on the hazards of substance abuse	3. Educate clients and public
4. Policies and programs to prevent abuse	4. Engage in political activity and advocacy
Secondary Prevention	
1. Early detection of persons with substance abuse problems	1. Engage in case finding
2. Early intervention for persons with problems related to substance abuse	2. Assist families to plan and carry out intervention
3. Treatment of substance abuse	3. Refer client for treatment; monitor client during treatment
4. Public education on signs of abuse and resources available	4. Educate clients and public
5. Treatment facilities	5. Engage in political activity to support treatment facilities and programs
6. Insurance coverage for treatment	6. Engage in political activity and advocacy
Tertiary Prevention	
1. Support for abusers	1. Provide emotional support and encouragement; refer to support groups
2. Lifestyle changes that discourage abusive behavior	2. Assist with lifestyle changes
3. Modification of stressors that contribute to substance abuse	3. Assist with modification of stressors

Evaluating Control Strategies for Substance Abuse

Evaluating interventions with individual substance abusers and their families focuses on the extent to which problems of substance abuse have been resolved. Has the abuser been able to remain sober for extended periods? Have stresses contributing to substance abuse been modified?

At the level of the community, the nurse could evaluate the effects of intervention programs on the incidence and prevalence of substance abuse as well as indicators of morbidity and mortality related to abuse. The nurse evaluating the effects of programs directed at substance abuse might examine the extent to which national health promotion and disease prevention objectives have been met in the community. Table 33–9 presents evaluative information on national efforts to meet the year 2000 objectives, and similar information could be obtained by the nurse relative to the local community.

TABLE 33–9. STATUS OF SELECTED NATIONAL OBJECTIVES RELATED TO SUBSTANCE ABUSE

Objective		Base	Most Recent	Target
4.1	Reduce alcohol-related motor vehicle deaths (per 100,000)	9.8 (1987)	6.7 (1993)	8.5
4.2	Reduce cirrhosis deaths (per 100,000)	9.2 (1987)	7.5 (1996)	6.0
4.3	Reduce drug-related deaths (per 100,000)	3.8 (1987)	4.8 (1993)	3.0
4.4	Reduce drug abuse-related emergency room visits (per 100,000)	175.8 (1991)	NDA[a]	131.9
4.5	Increase average age of first use of			
	Cigarettes	11.6 (1988)	11.7 (1993)	12.6
	Alcohol	13.1 (1988)	12.9 (1993)	14.1
	Marijuana	13.4 (1988)	13.9 (1993)	14.4
4.6	Reduce youth use in the past month			
	a. Alcohol			
	12–17 years	25.2% (1988)	16% (1994)	12.6%
	18–25 years	57.9% (1988)	64% (1994)	29.0%
	b. Marijuana			
	12–17 years	6.4% (1988)	7% (1994)	3.2%
	18–25 years	15.5% (1988)	12% (1994)	7.8%
	c. Cocaine			
	12–17 years	1.1% (1988)	0.4% (1994)	0.6%
	18–25 years	4.5% (1988)	1% (1994)	2.3%
4.7	Reduce heavy drinking last 2 months			
	High school seniors	33.0% (1989)	29.8% (1991)	28.0%
	College students	41.7% (1989)	42.8% (1991)	32.0%
4.8	Reduce gallons per capita alcohol consumption	2.54 (1987)	2.31 (1991)	2.0
4.14	Increase worksite policies for			
	Alcohol	88% (1992)	88% (1992)	60%
	Other drugs	89% (1992)	89% (1992)	60%
3.4	Decrease cigarette smoking (age 20 and over)	29% (1987)	22% (1995)	15%
3.5	Reduce smoking initiation by youth	30% (1987)	27% (1993)	15%
3.7	Increase smoking cessation during pregnancy	39% (1985)	31% (1991)	60%
3.13	Increase states with laws prohibiting tobacco sales to minors	44 (1990)	50 (1994)	50
3.16	Increase tobacco use counseling by health care providers	52% (1986)	75% (1992)	75%

[a]NDA, no data available.

(Sources: U.S. Department of Commerce, 1996; U.S. Department of Health and Human Services, 1993; 1995; 1996.)

TESTING YOUR UNDERSTANDING

1. Identify at least three criteria for diagnosing psychoactive substance dependence. Give examples of behaviors that might be performed by clients who meet these criteria. (p. 860)
2. Distinguish between psychoactive substance dependence and abuse. (p. 860)
3. Identify at least five psychoactive substances that lead to dependence and abuse. (pp. 861–864)
4. Describe at least two personal effects, two family effects, and two societal effects of substance abuse. (pp. 865–867)
5. What are the five aspects of community health nursing assessment in relation to substance abuse? (pp. 868–876)
6. Identify two major approaches to primary prevention of substance abuse. How might community health nurses be involved in each? (pp. 876–877)
7. Describe the components of the intervention process in secondary prevention of substance abuse. What might be the role of the community health nurse in the intervention process? (pp. 877–878)
8. Identify at least four general principles in the treatment of substance abuse. (p. 878)
9. Describe at least three treatment modalities in secondary prevention of substance abuse. What is the role of the community health nurse with respect to each? (pp. 878–879)
10. Identify three major goals of harm reduction. (pp. 880–881)

WHAT DO YOU THINK?
Questions for Critical Thinking

1. Should marijuana use be legalized? If so, for whom?
2. What factors make control of substance abuse so difficult? How could these factors be modified or eliminated?

Critical Thinking in Practice: A Case in Point

You have been working with the Schumacher family for the last several months. The youngest child, who is 18 months old, has multiple physical handicaps and has been in and out of the hospital numerous times for surgery. He is currently enrolled in physical and occupational therapy programs to promote his development. You have been following this child and working with the family to meet his needs. On your most recent home visit, Mrs. Schumacher voiced concern about her husband's drinking.

Since the birth of the baby, Mr. Schumacher has gone on periodic drinking binges. Initially, these occurred about once a month, but lately he has been getting drunk almost every weekend. This week Mrs. Schumacher had to call her husband's office, where he is employed as a civil engineer, to tell his employer that her husband was ill. Actually, he was too hung over to go to work. She has tried to talk to her husband about his drinking, but he becomes angry and storms out of the house. When he returns, he is drunk. Each time, after he sobers up, he is repentant and promises not to imbibe again. Mrs. Schumacher thinks her husband's drinking is the result of his worry about financial problems.

Since Mr. Schumacher's drinking problem has escalated, the older children have been reluctant to bring friends home because they are embarrassed by their father's drunken behavior. They have begun to ask Mrs. Schumacher rather pointed questions about their father, such as "Is daddy an alcoholic?" They know that their grandfather, Mr. Schumacher's father, died of cirrhosis stemming from alcoholism. Mrs. Schumacher says she has told the children their father is not an alcoholic but is just tired and has been under a lot of stress at work.

Mr. Schumacher has always been a successful provider for the family and did not drink much before the baby was born. He did well in school, completing a master's degree in engineering, and was promoted to a new position with his engineering firm about 2 years ago. His job pays relatively well, but because their health insurance did not cover the baby when he was born, they have had to pay all of the new infant's medical expenses out-of-pocket. Mrs. Schumacher says they have exhausted their savings and indicates that they are having some difficulty meeting mortgage payments on their house. She would like to work but would have trouble finding someone to care for the baby, who has a tracheostomy and requires periodic suctioning. She has discussed her willingness to work with her husband, but he insists that he is not going to have his wife working when the children need her at home and that he will take care of things.

1. What are the biophysical, psychological, social, behavioral, and health system factors influencing these problems?
2. What are the health problems evident in this situation? Develop several nursing diagnostic statements related to these problems.
3. What evidence of codependence is present in this family situation?
4. What client care objectives would you set in working with this family?
5. What primary, secondary, and tertiary intervention strategies should be employed with this family? Why?
6. How would you evaluate the effectiveness of your interventions with the Schumacher family? What evaluative criteria would you use? How would you obtain the evaluative data needed?

---

3. What risk factors for substance abuse are present in your own life? What are you doing, or what can you do to eliminate or minimize your risks of substance abuse?
4. Would you be willing to be a foster parent for a drug-exposed infant? Why or why not?

REFERENCES

Addiction Research Center. (1995). Symptoms of substance dependence associated with use of cigarettes, alcohol, and illicit drugs—United States, 1991–1992. *MMWR, 44*, 830–831, 837–839.

Akers, R. L. (1992). *Drugs, alcohol, and society: Social structure, process, and policy.* Belmont, CA: Wadsworth.

American Psychiatric Association. (1994). *Diagnostic and statistical manual of mental disorders* (4th ed.) (DSM-IV). Washington, DC: American Psychiatric Association.

Booth, R. E., Watters, J. K., & Chitwood, D. D. (1993). HIV risk-related sex behaviors among injection drug users, crack smokers, and injection drug users who smoke crack. *American Journal of Public Health, 83*, 1144–1148.

Bowerman, R. J. (1997). The effect of a community-supported alcohol ban on prenatal alcohol and other substance abuse. *American Journal of Public Health, 87*, 1378–1379.

Boyd, M. R., & Hauenstein, E. J. (1997). Psychiatric assessment and confirmation of dual disorders in rural substance abusing women. *Archives of Psychiatric Nursing, XI*(2), 74–81.

Breitbart, V., Chavkin, W., & Wise, P. H. (1994). The accessibility of drug treatment for pregnant women: A survey of programs in five cities. *American Journal of Public Health, 84*, 1658–1661.

Brown, L. P. (1995a). *National drug control strategy: Executive summary.* Washington, DC: Office of National Drug Control Policy.

Brown, L. P. (1995b). *Pulse check: National trends in drug abuse.* Washington, DC: Office of National Drug Control Policy.

Brown, L. P. (1995c). *What America's users spend on illegal drugs, 1988–1993.* Washington, DC: Office of National Drug Control Policy.

Brown, R. L., Patterson, J. J., Rounds, L. A., & Papasouliotis, O. (1996). Substance abuse among patients with chronic back pain. *Journal of Family Practice, 43*, 152–160.

Centers for Disease Control. (1997). National drunk and drugged driving prevention month—December 1997. *MMWR, 46*, 1129.

Des Jarlais, D. C. (1995). Editorial: Harm reduction—A framework for incorporating science into drug policy. *American Journal of Public Health, 85*, 10–12.

Division of Reproductive Health. (1996). Population-based prevalence of perinatal exposure to cocaine—Georgia, 1994. *MMWR, 45*, 887–891.

Fendrich, M., Mackesy-Amiti, M. E., Wislar, J. S., & Goldstein, P. J. (1997). Childhood abuse and the use of inhalants: Differences by degree of use. *American Journal of Public Health, 87*, 765–769.

Fetal Alcohol Syndrome Prevention Section. (1997). Surveillance for fetal alcohol syndrome using multiple sources—Atlanta, Georgia, 1981–1989. *MMWR, 46*, 1118–1120.

Finley, B. G. (1991). The family and substance abuse. In G. A. Bennet (Ed.), *Substance abuse: Pharmacologic, developmental, and clinical perspectives* (2nd ed.). New York: Wiley.

Fox, K., Merrill, J. C., Chang, H.-h., & Califano, J. A., Jr. (1995). Estimating the costs of substance abuse to the Medicaid hospital care program. *American Journal of Public Health, 85*, 48–54.

Frazier, E. L., Okoro, C. A., Smith, C., & McQueen, D. V. (1996). State- and sex-specific prevalence of selected characteristics—Behavioral Risk Factor Surveillance System, 1992 and 1993. *MMWR, 45*(SS-6), 1–36.

Gilson, S. F., Chilcoat, H. D., & Stapleton, J. M. (1996). Illicit drug use by persons with disabilities: Insights from the National Household Survey on Drug Abuse. *American Journal of Public Health, 86*, 1613–1615.

Gfroerer, J. (1995). *Preliminary estimates from the 1994 national household survey on drug abuse.* Rockville, MD: Substance Abuse and Mental Health Services Administration.

Henry, J. A., Jeffreys, K. J., & Dawling, S. (1992). Toxicity and deaths from 3,4-methylenedioxymethamphetamine ("ecstasy"). *Lancet, 340*(1), 384–387.

Insel, P., & Roth, W. T. (1998). *Core concepts in health* (8th ed.). Mountain View, CA: Mayfield.

Kandel, D., & Yamaguchi, K. (1993). From beer to crack: Developmental patterns of drug involvement. *American Journal of Public Health, 83*, 851–855.

Kann, L., Warren, C. W., Harris, W. A., et al. (1996). Youth Risk Behavior Surveillance—United States, 1995. *MMWR, 45*(SS-4), 1–84.

Kendler, K. S., Heath, A. C., Neale, M. C., Kesales, R. C., & Eaves, L. J. (1992). A population-based twin study of alcoholism in women. *JAMA, 268*, 1877–1882.

Larroque, B., Kaminski, M., Dehaene, P., Subtil, D., Delfosse, M., & Querleu, D. (1995). Moderate prenatal alcohol exposure and psychomotor development at preschool age. *American Journal of Public Health, 85*, 1654–1661.

Leshner, A. I. (1996). Bridging the "great disconnect." *NIDA Notes, 11*(2), 3, 4.

Li, G., Smith, G. S., & Baker, S. P. (1994). Drinking behavior in relation to cause of death among US adults. *American Journal of Public Health, 84*, 1402–1406.

Lowry, R., Holtzman, D., Truman, B. I., Kann, L., Collins, J. L., & Kolbe, L. J. (1994). Substance abuse and HIV-related sexual behaviors among US high school students: Are they related? *American Journal of Public Health, 84*, 1116–1120.

Marzuk, P. M., Tardiff, K., Leon, A. C., et al. (1995). Fatal injuries after cocaine use as a leading cause of death among young adults in New York City. *New England Journal of Medicine, 332*, 1753–1757.

National Institute on Drug Abuse. (1994). *Inhalant abuse: Its dangers are nothing to sniff at.* Washington, DC: National Institute on Drug Abuse.

National Institute on Drug Abuse. (1995). Facts about cocaine abuse and treatment. *NIDA Notes, 10*(5), 15.

National Institute on Drug Abuse. (1996). Facts about marijuana and marijuana abuse. *NIDA Notes, 11*(2), 15.

The Nation's Health. (1994, January). *Substance abuse costs society millions*, p. 18.

Office of National Drug Control Policy. (1995, June). *Fact sheet: Drug use trends.* Rockville, MD: National Criminal Justice Reference Service.

Reuter, P., & Caulkins, J. P. (1995). Redefining the goals of national drug policy: Recommendations from a working group. *American Journal of Public Health, 85*, 1059–1063.

Robertson, B. (1993). *Alcohol disabilities primer: A guide to physical and psychosocial disabilities caused by alcohol use.* Boca Raton, LA: CRC.

Robins, L. N., & Mills, J. L. (Eds.). (1993, December). Effects of in utero exposure to street drugs. *American Journal of Public Health, 83*(Suppl.), 1–23.

Rocio, M., Carrera, A., Ashley, J. A., et al. (1995). Suppression of psychoactive effects of cocaine by active immunization. *Nature, 378,* 727–730.

Sampson, P. D., Bookstein, F. L., Barr, H. M., & Streissguth, A. P. (1994). Prenatal alcohol exposure, birthweight, and measures of child size from birth to age 14 years. *American Journal of Public Health, 84,* 1421–1428.

Sajo, E. (1996). Nurses can intervene to stop abuse of methamphetamine. *NURSEweek, 9*(17), 8–9.

Substance Abuse and Mental Health Services Administration. (1995). Increasing morbidity and mortality associated with abuse of methamphetamine—United States, 1991–1994. *MMWR, 44,* 882–886.

Swan, N. (1996). Rats immunized against effects of cocaine. *NIDA Notes, 11*(2), 1, 4.

Tatarsky, A. (1995, Fall). Clinical psychology and harm reduction are a good match. *Harm Reduction Communication, 7,* 17.

Urbano-Marquez, A., Estruch, R., Fernandez-Sola, J., Nicholas, J. M., Pare, J. C., & Rubin, E. (1995). The greater risk of alcoholic cardiomyopathy and myopathy in women compared with men. *JAMA, 274,* 149–154.

U.S. Department of Commerce. (1996). *Statistical abstract of the United States, 1996.* Washington, DC: Government Printing Office.

U.S. Department of Health and Human Services. (1993). *Health United States, 1992, and healthy people 2000 review.* Washington, DC: Government Printing Office.

U.S. Department of Health and Human Services. (1995). *Healthy People 2000: Midcourse review and 1995 revisions.* Washington, DC: Government Printing Office.

U.S. Department of Health and Human Services. (1996). *Health United States, 1995.* Washington, DC: Government Printing Office.

Waller, J. A., Skelly, J., & Davis, J. H. (1997). Substance abuse: Medicaid disproportionately burdened by trauma care related to alcohol. *The Medicaid Letter, 3*(3), 5–6.

Witters, W., Venturelli, P., & Hanson, G. (1992). *Drugs and society* (3rd ed.). Boston: Jones and Bartlett.

Yates, J. G., & McDaniel, J. L. (1994). Are you losing yourself in codependency? *American Journal of Nursing, 94*(4), 32–36.

RESOURCES FOR NURSES DEALING WITH SUBSTANCE ABUSE

Alcohol Abuse

Al-Anon
Family Group Headquarters, Inc.
PO Box 862
Midtown Station
New York, NY 10018
(212) 302–7240

Alcohol Research Information Service
1106 East Oakland
Lansing, MI 48906
(517) 485–9900

Alcoholics Anonymous World Services
475 Riverside Drive
New York, NY 10163
(212) 870–3400

American Council on Alcohol Problems
3426 Bridgeland Drive
Bridgeton, MO 63044
(314) 739–5944

Calix Society
7601 Wayzata Blvd.
St. Louis Park, MN 55426
(612) 546–0544

Children of Alcoholics Foundation
PO Box 4185
Grand Central Station
New York, NY 10163
(212) 754–0656

National Association for Children of Alcoholics
11426 Rockville Pike, Ste. 100
Rockville, MD 20852
(301) 468–0985

National Institute on Alcohol Abuse and Alcoholism
6000 Executive Blvd., Ste. 514
Bethesda, MD 20892–7003
(301) 443–4897

The Other Victims of Alcoholism
PO Box 1528
Radio City Station
New York, NY 10101
(212) 247–8087

Drug Abuse

American Council for Drug Education
164 W. 74th Street
New York, NY 10023
(800) 488–DRUG

Ethos Foundation
5201 Leesburg Pike, Ste. 100
Falls Church, VA 22041
(703) 671–5335

Families Anonymous
PO Box 3475
Culver City, CA 90231–3475
(310) 313–5800

Narcotics Anonymous
PO Box 9999
Van Nuys, CA 91409
(818) 773–9999

National Association on Drug Abuse Problems
355 Lexington Avenue
New York, NY 10017
(212) 986–1170

National Families in Action
National Drug Information Center
2296 Henderson Mill Road, Ste. 300
Atlanta, GA 30345
(770) 934–6364

National Institute on Drug Abuse
5600 Fishers Lane
Rockville, MD 20857
(301) 443–6480

National Parents Resource Institute for Drug
   Education
3610 DeKalb Technology Parkway, Ste. 105
Atlanta, GA 30340
(770) 458–9900

Potsmokers Anonymous
208 West 23rd Street, Apt. 1414
New York, NY 10011–2139
(212) 254–1777

U.S. House of Representatives
Select Committee on Narcotics Abuse and Control
H2-234 House Office Bldg., Annex II
Washington, DC 20515
(202) 226–3040

Dual Agencies

Alcohol and Drug Problems Association
   of North America
1555 Wilson Blvd., Ste. 300
Arlington, VA 22209
(703) 875–8684

"Just Say No" International
2101 Webster Street, Ste. 1300
Oakland, CA 94612
(510) 451–6666

Substance Abuse, and Mental Health Administration
5600 Fishers Lane
Rockville, MD 20857
(301) 443–4111

U.S. Senate Committee on Labor
   and Human Relations
Subcommittee on Children, Family, Drugs,
   and Alcoholism
SH-639 Hart Bldg.
Washington, DC 20510
(202) 224–5630

Nursing

Drug and Alcohol Nursing Association
66 Lonely Cottage Drive
Upper Black Eddy, PA 18972–9313
(610) 847–5396

National Consortium of Chemical
   Dependency Nurses
1720 Willow Creek Circle, Ste. 519
Eugene, OR 97402
(503) 485–4421

National Nurses Society on Addictions
4101 Lake Boone Trail, Ste. 201
Raleigh, NC 27607
(919) 783–5871

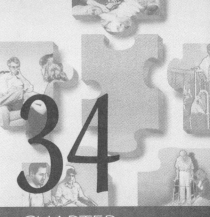

VIOLENCE

► KEY TERMS

child abuse
durable power of attorney
elder abuse
emotional abuse
expressive homicides
expressive violence
family violence
homicide
incest
instrumental homicides
instrumental violence
neglect
organized sadistic abuse
physical abuse
psychological
  maltreatment
sexual abuse
spouse abuse
suicidal ideation
suicide
suicide cluster
suicide prevention
  contract
victim-precipitated
  homicide

34

CHAPTER

Violence is a pervasive phenomenon in our society. In part, this is a function of the American heritage and the activities required to carve a nation from a wild and uncivilized land. Violence has historically been seen as a mode of resolving conflict and even of ensuring support of law and order. The vigilante approach to justice on the Western frontier is one example of the use of violence to protect society.

In societies in which survival is subjected to physical threats that must be countered by physical force, violent behavior may be more or less of a necessity. Some authorities, however, contend that humankind has failed to adapt to changes in survival needs and has continued to exercise proclivities to violence that are not warranted in today's society. Societal violence has become a global concern, and in 1996 the World Health Organization (WHO) declared violence a worldwide public health problem (Division of Violence Prevention, 1996b).

Societal violence costs millions of dollars in hospital care alone and results in millions of days of lost work productivity. Add to this the personal costs of victimization as well as the mounting cost of police and other protective services and related court costs, and it becomes apparent that the United States cannot afford the current level of violence and must do something to contain it.

Family violence, homicide, and suicide are forms of violence that are of particular concern to society and, hence, to community health nurses who are charged with promoting the health of the population. Violence contributes to a variety of physical and psychological health problems that can be prevented by community health nursing efforts to modify factors that contribute to violence against self or others.

▶ Chapter Objectives

After reading this chapter, you should be able to :

- Describe at least three theories of assaultive violence.
- Describe four types of child abuse.
- Describe the three stages of spouse abuse.
- Identify at least five forms of elder abuse.
- Describe the influence of at least three biophysical factors in family violence.
- Identify at least four social dimension and four psychological dimension factors that influence family violence.
- Describe at least three areas of focus in primary prevention of family violence.
- Identify at least two approaches to the secondary prevention of family violence.
- Describe at least two factors in the biophysical, psychological, social, behavioral, and health system dimensions related to homicide.
- Describe at least two factors in the biophysical, psychological, social, behavioral, and health system dimensions related to suicide.
- Identify at least three primary prevention measures for homicide and suicide.

▶ THEORIES OF ASSAULTIVE VIOLENCE

Why does violence occur? Several theoretical perspectives have been advanced in an effort to answer this question; none has been completely successful. Generally, theories that explain violence are categorized as biological, psychological, sociological, anthropological, and multifactorial theories. Biological theories attribute violence to an innate, instinctual drive for aggression, genetics, head injury, or a variety of neurochemical imbalances such as an imbalance in levels of serotonin, dopamine, norepinephrine, or other neurotransmitters (Sigler, 1995).

Psychological theories may take one of several approaches: developmental; interpersonal dynamics; dependency; or psychoanalytic. In the developmental approach, it is believed that early life experiences, particularly relationships with parents (or lack of them), that foster the development of personal behavioral control mediate propensities for violence (Rosenberg & Mercy, 1991). According to the interpersonal violence or intraindividual dynamics model, violence is the result of some form of psychopathology, for example, mental illness or substance abuse. From this perspective, the violent person lacks the ability to communicate effectively with others and to use nonviolent strategies to reduce stress or deal with conflict (Stark & Flitcraft, 1991).

The dependency and exchange theory of violence has been advanced specifically in relation to elder abuse (Pillemer & Frankel, 1991) but may also be applicable to other forms of violence. In this theory, violence is believed to result from dependence of the abused on the abuser, which leads to excessive caregiver stress, or, conversely, from dependence of the abuser on the abused, resulting in feelings of powerlessness and frustration.

In psychoanalytic theory, human beings have an internal need to discharge hostility. When one's ego has insufficient strength to channel this hostility into acceptable forms of expression, violence may result. From this perspective, we all have "tendencies" toward violence that can be triggered by internal and external events, but that are controlled by the ego in most of us (Sigler, 1995).

Some authors also consider social learning theory a psychological explanation for violence, whereas others would classify it as a sociological theory. Social learning theory was discussed in relation to substance abuse in Chapter 33, and posits that violence is learned from behavior modeled by others and perceptions of the rewards or sanctions awarded that behavior. The family violence model, or generational theory, is essentially an application of social learning theory to family violence in which violence is learned from family role models in a society that provides normative support for physical punishment and views family interactions as highly private (Jackson, 1996).

Other sociological explanations of violence include the subculture model, structural model, interactionist model, and economic or deterrence model, as well as the gender-politics model and social isolation model. In the subculture model, it is believed that violence, like substance abuse, arises from a subculture in which violence is the accepted mode of conflict resolution and results in status within the subcultural group (Sigler, 1995). The primary thesis of structural explanations of violence is that the structure of society (eg, poverty, discrimination, lack of opportunity) prevents members of some groups from achieving material success, creating frustrations that may be expressed in violence.

The interactionist model suggests that violence is the outcome of an interactive sequence of events in which one person "moves" in response to the "moves" of another, escalating conflict to the point of violence. From this perspective, the moves of the other person are seen as a threat to one's personal identity and self-esteem that must be countered

(Rosenberg & Mercy, 1991). This kind of interplay might be viewed as an extreme of "one-upsmanship."

In the economic or deterrence model, violence is seen as a rational choice based on perceptions of risks and benefits of one's actions. Violence is "reasonable" when it results in a perceived gain (eg, monetary in robbery or personal gratification in the abuse of one's spouse or child) and is deterred when the risks are perceived to outweigh potential gains. The gender-politics model is basically a power model, in which violence is used to exert power over others—men over women, children, and others in the gender application of the concept. This model may also be labeled a feminist model (Letellier, 1996).

The final sociological approach to explaining violence is the social isolation model. In this model, violence is possible because the victim is isolated and violent behavior and its effects are unlikely to come to light (Pillemer & Frankel, 1991). This model is the basis for insistence on the concept of "two-deep leadership" advocated by youth organizations such as the Boy Scouts of America. The two-deep policy requires that a minimum of two adults be present during all activities to minimize the potential for clandestine abuse (Boy Scouts of America, 1993).

Anthropological explanations for violence involve social organization and cultural patterning, particularly with respect to the place of women in the society. In the sexual inequality model, women within the society are perceived as property and, thus, subject to the control of male family members (Hanrahan, Campbell, & Ulrich, 1993).

This control is exercised in terms of cultural patterns of accepted behavior, which may, in some societies, include abuse. Violence may also result from cultural norms regarding the discharge of innate hostilities, something of an amalgam of biological and anthropological theory. Finally, it is believed that the complexity of social and family organization may influence societal levels of violence (American Psychological Association, 1996). Increasingly complex societies, for example, have been shown to have higher rates of violence. Similarly, family complexity in the form of polygamy or single parenthood may also contribute to family violence (Hanrahan, et al., 1993).

Finally, multifactorial theories explain violence in terms of multiple contributing factors (Humphreys & Ramsey, 1993) that may interact in different ways in different situations. Theoretical perspectives that acknowledge the interplay of a variety of factors in the development of violent behaviors are probably the most useful in directing nursing intervention. Later in this chapter, we examine the application of the multifactorial Dimensions Model to various facets of societal violence.

► TYPES OF SOCIETAL VIOLENCE

Societal violence occurs in a variety of forms. Three of these are of particular concern in community health nursing practice: family violence, homicide, and suicide. General information regarding each of these forms of violence will be presented and then discussed in the context of the Dimensions Model.

Family Violence

Family violence involves action by one family member with the intent to inflict harm on or control another member (American Psychological Association, 1996). For the most part, violence occurring within family constellations is a hidden phenomenon, so the actual frequency of family violence is unknown. Cases that come to light are probably only a small proportion of what actually occurs. Targets of family violence may be children, spouses, or the elderly.

Child Abuse

As defined by the Child Abuse Prevention and Treatment Act, *child abuse* is any physical or mental injury, sexual abuse or exploitation, negligent treatment, or maltreatment of a child by someone responsible for the child's welfare that poses a threat to that child's welfare (Humphreys & Ramsey, 1993). Child abuse is manifested at the level of individual abusive families. It is potentiated, however, by institutional policies that permit children to be abused and by social mores and policies that foster circumstances leading to abuse.

Four categories of child abuse are recognized: physical abuse, psychological maltreatment, sexual abuse, and organized sadistic abuse (American Psychological Association, 1996). *Physical abuse* occurs when a child is subjected to intentional use of force by a parent or caregiver that results in pain, physical injury, or death. *Psychological maltreatment* encompasses both neglect and psychological or emotional abuse. *Neglect* occurs when the physical, emotional, or educational resources necessary to the child's health and development are withheld. In instances of physical neglect, for example, the child might be deprived of food, clothing, housing, or health care, or be exposed to hazardous environmental conditions. Emotional neglect occurs when the child is denied the emotional nurturance and support that would foster normal psychosocial development. Educational neglect occurs when inadequate attention is given to the child's educational needs. This might involve permitting truancy as well as failure to make arrangements to meet routine or special education needs. *Emotional abuse* involves subjecting the child to psychological harm or anguish and may include attempts to erode the child's self-esteem and sense of self-worth as well as forcing the child to witness abuse of others.

Sexual abuse consists of deliberate involvement of a child in involuntary sexual activity for which the child is developmentally unprepared. This may include fondling, exposure, or exploitation, in addition to actual sexual intercourse (U.S. Department of Health and Human Services, 1992). *Incest* is a subtype of child sexual abuse in which the child is subjected to sexual contact by relatives such as parents, stepparents, or siblings. *Organized sadistic abuse* is extreme abusive behavior including torture, severe psychological coercion, or sadistic sexual or physical abuse. Other manifestations of organized sadistic abuse include ritualistic abuse, pornography, and forced prostitution as well as forcing children to commit violent acts against others (American Psychological Association, 1996).

The problem of child abuse seems to be escalating in the United States. From 1990 to 1994, the total number of substantiated reports of child abuse increased by 57% to nearly 1.2 million cases. Most of these cases (45%) involved neglect. Physical abuse accounted for 22% of cases, sexual abuse for 12%, emotional abuse for 4%, and medical neglect for 2%. The remaining cases were of other or unknown types. Actual numbers of cases in each category represent an increase over 1990 figures (U.S. Department of Commerce, 1996). In part, these increases are attributable to better recognition and reporting of the problem, but there is also a definite increase in the actual number of instances of abuse.

The effects of abuse on children are many and varied. Abused youngsters are more likely than their agemates to have problems with discipline and fighting at home and at school. They are also more likely to engage in vandalism or theft, develop problems related to drug or alcohol abuse, and get arrested than are children who are not abused. In addition, childhood abuse predisposes these youngsters to become abusive parents in later years.

Spouse Abuse

Spouse abuse is also a problem in this country. Family violence may be either expressive or instrumental in nature. *Expressive violence* involves aggressive behavior by both parties in a conflict that escalates to violence. *Spouse abuse,* on the other hand, involves instrumental violence between partners in an intimate relationship, who may or may not be legally married. In spouse abuse situations, *instrumental violence* involves the expression of feelings, the goal of which is

to force or control the partner's behavior, or to achieve some other goal (National Commission on Correctional Health Care, 1993). Instrumental violence may involve face-to-face confrontation in which fear is the motivating force that influences the behavior of the victim, or it can involve instilling feelings of guilt to manipulate the behavior of the other person as well as actual physical mistreatment.

Spouse abuse involving overt physical violence is a cyclical phenomenon that occurs in three stages (American Psychological Association, 1996). The first stage is one of rising tension in which the abuser is irritated by minor events or behavior on the part of the abused spouse. The second stage is the acute battering episode, in which the tension explodes in anger manifested in physical violence. The third phase is a period of calm and loving reconciliation in which the abuser expresses contrition, tries to make amends, and vows to change.

The New York State Office for the Prevention of Domestic Violence has developed a typography of spousal violence similar to those developed for child and elder abuse. Types of spouse abuse include physical, sexual, psychological, emotional, and economic abuse (Chez, 1994). Physical abuse includes actual or attempted infliction of physical injury or illness, as well as withholding access to resources necessary to maintain health or forcing one to use alcohol or other drugs. Sexual abuse involves the use of physical or psychological coercion to force sexual contact with the abuser or with others (eg, forced prostitution) or attempts to undermine the victim's sexual identity. Attempting to control the victim through fear and threats or isolating the victim from social interaction with others constitutes psychological abuse, while economic abuse consists of attempts to make the victim financially dependent. In any given spousal abuse situation, several types of abuse may occur simultaneously. For example, an abuser might prevent his or her victim from working (economic abuse) and threaten physical harm or loss of children if the victim attempts to leave the abusive situation (psychological abuse).

It is estimated that 1 in every 26 American women is physically abused each year. This estimate rises to 1 in 10 women involved in heterosexual relationships (Campbell & Fishwick, 1993). Intimate violence is the leading cause of injuries to women. Approximately 22 to 35% of female trauma seen in emergency rooms is attributable to abuse, and half of female homicides involve domestic abuse (Eilenberg & Fullilove, 1996). Violence does not always occur between marital or intimate partners during the relationship. In fact, approximately three fourths of abuse victims (3 to 4 million) are divorced, separated, or single. Frequently, the abuse occurs precisely because the victim has attempted to terminate the relationship (Campbell, 1992; Hammers, 1993; Sugg & Inui, 1992). Nor is abuse usually a single incident within relationship.

Spouse abuse can result in a variety of both physical and psychological effects. Abused women, for example, have been found to experience poor health and symptoms of psychological distress such as headaches, nervousness, depression, and feelings of worthlessness and hopelessness. They are also more likely than women who are not abused to contemplate or attempt suicide.

Elder Abuse

Elder abuse is purposeful physical or psychological harm directed toward elderly persons. Elder abuse can occur within families or in institutional settings such as nursing homes and other residential facilities for the elderly. The focus of this chapter, however, is on abuse of older persons by family members.

As is the case with child abuse and spouse abuse, elder abuse takes several forms including physical abuse, emotional abuse, financial abuse, active and passive neglect, denial of civil rights, and self-abuse and neglect (American Psychological Association, 1996). Physical abuse can involve inflicting physical pain or injury, sexual molestation, or involuntary and inappropriate restraint of the individual. Overmedicating older people to keep them quiescent is another form of physical abuse. Emotional abuse is intended to cause mental suffering and may consist of name calling, insults, humiliation, intimidation, or threats directed at the older person. Intentional, illegal, or unethical confiscation or use of money or personal property belonging to an older person constitutes financial abuse. Active and passive neglect may be either physical or emotional. Passive neglect usually involves unintentional failure to engage in needed care or leaving the older person alone and socially isolated. In active neglect, items necessary for daily life such as food, medication, and assistance are deliberately withheld. Older people may also be abused by intentional denial of their personal rights, particularly their right to self-determination. Overprotection, denial of the older person's need for independence, and removal from active participation in personal decisions also constitute denial of the individual's civil rights. Finally, older people may engage in self-injurious behaviors or neglect, either by self-inflicted injury, failure to eat, or failure to take reasonable safety precautions. Self-abuse can be either intentional or unintentional.

The extent of elder abuse in the United States is largely unknown. It is estimated that approximately 3% of elderly Americans are victims of abuse (Pillemer & Frankel, 1991). From 1986 to 1994, the number or reported cases in the United States increased by 106% to more that 240,000 cases. More than half of the cases (58%) involved neglect; 16% of cases involved physical abuse; and 12% involved financial abuse (American Psychological Association, 1996).

The figures cited here represent only a small portion of the actual cases of elder abuse. It is estimated that only 1 of 14 cases of elder abuse are actually reported (American Psychological Association, 1996). Reasons for this failure to report instances of abuse may include the reluctance of older persons to admit that they raised a child who could abuse them (because most abusers are family members), love of the abuser, dependence on the abuser and fear of further injury, and a lack of alternatives.

The physical effects of neglect and abuse in elderly persons can lead to malnutrition, mobility limitations due to injuries, or skin breakdown due to poor hygiene. Psychological effects can include fear, anxiety, and depression, as well as feelings of hopelessness and helplessness that may lead to substance abuse or suicide as attempts to escape the situation.

Societal consequences of all forms of family violence are also of concern. Naturally, there are the economic costs of medical care for physical injury. Family violence results in more hospitalizations each year than heart attacks, and the annual cost of related medical care is estimated at $44 million. There are also other costs, including the cost of counseling, legal, and social services and the cost of imprisoning convicted abusers all of which amount to more that $41 million a year (Mellman & Bell, 1996). In addition there is the pain and suffering experienced by the victims of abuse. When abuse leads to substance abuse, there are additional costs related to these problems, which were discussed in Chapter 33.

Homicide

There are an average of 65 homicides each day in the United States. Homicide is the second leading cause of death among people aged 15 to 34 years and one of the top five causes of death in children under the age of 15 (Goetting, 1994). In 1993, more than 26,000 homicides occurred in the United States. The rate of homicides increased by 4% per year from 1985 to 1991, then declined by 1% per year from 1992 to 1994 (Division of Violence Prevention, 1996b). The homicide rate for 1993 was 10.7 per 100,000 population (U.S. Department of Health and Human Services, 1996a) compared to a 1994 rate of 9.6 per 100,000 (Cummings, Koepsell, Grossman, Savarino, & Thompson, 1997).

Suicide

In 1994, suicide was the ninth leading cause of death in the general population with a rate of 12 suicides per 100,000 population (Division of Violence Prevention, 1997b). Among adolescents 15 to 19 years of age, suicide is the third leading cause of death, and for every successful suicide, there are approximately 31 nonfatal attempts (National Center for Injury Prevention and Control, 1995). In the 1995 Youth Risk Behavior Surveillance System (YRBSS) survey, fully one fourth of students surveyed had considered suicide in the past year (Kann, et al., 1996). All of these figures underscore the magnitude of violence in American society and the need for public health interventions to control violence.

▶ THE DIMENSIONS MODEL AND CONTROL OF VIOLENCE

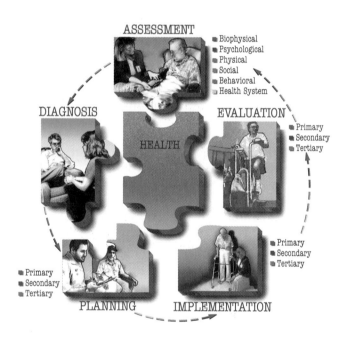

Critical Dimensions of Nursing in the Control of Violence

Perhaps the most critical of the dimensions of nursing related to control of societal violence is the ethical dimension. Advocacy, which is an important element of this dimension, is needed in a variety of areas related to violence. For example, community health nurses advocate for changes in social forces such as discrimination and unemployment that may contribute to all forms of violence. Likewise, nurses advocate for access to treatment facilities to deal with substance abuse and psychiatric illness, both associated with violence. In the case of family violence, the nurse has a multifaceted advocacy role advocating for victims,

perpetrators, and observers of family violence to receive the necessary treatment services to minimize the effects of violence and to stop the intergenerational cycle of family violence.

Elements of the process dimension are also important to community health nurses in controlling societal violence. The political process may be one means of engaging in advocacy as described above. In addition, community health nurses use the health education process to educate persons at risk for violence, either as perpetrators or victims, to develop coping strategies and modes of conflict resolution that avoid violence. Finally, in the cognitive dimension, the community health nurse must have a thorough knowledge of the risk factors and signs of incipient or actual violence as well as the resources available in the community to deal with problems of societal violence.

Within the reflective dimension, well-designed research into the causes of and solutions to societal violence is imperative. There is a critical need for a sound research base for public policy related to violence control. Some authors make the association between flawed research studies and ineffective, or even harmful, policies on weapons availability (Webster, Vernick, Ludwig, & Lester, 1997). In addition, many violence control strategies have not been adequately evaluated.

 Assessing the Dimensions of Health in Family Violence

Nursing assessment related to family violence focuses on two major areas. First, the nurse assesses families for risk factors that may contribute to violence. The second aspect of the community health nurse's assessment is related to indicators of abuse actually occurring within families. Both aspects of assessment would also be applied to population groups. Nurses could assess communities for risk factors for family violence as well as for the actual incidence of cases of abuse.

Prior to engaging in either aspect of assessment for family violence, community health nurses should examine their own feelings with respect to violence and their commitment to nursing intervention related to family violence. There is a need for early identification of families with potential for violence or in which actual abuse is occurring. To intervene effectively, community health nurses need to be able to deal with their own emotional responses to the fact of abuse.

Assessing Risk Factors

For family violence of any kind to occur, three conditions must exist. There must be motivation for

---

ASSESSMENT TIPS: Assessing Risk for Family Violence

Biophysical Dimension

Does the family include persons in age groups at particular risk for abuse?

Are there existing physical health problems in potential abusers or victims?

Does physical or mental disability increase the risk of abuse?

Is there physical evidence of injury due to abuse? If so, what form does that evidence take?

Is there physical evidence of neglect or sexual abuse?

Is pregnancy an issue in the family?

Psychological Dimension

What psychological stressors impinge on the family?

What is the extent of coping skills exhibited by the potential abuser? By potential victims?

What is the level of self-esteem of the potential abuser? Of potential victims?

Is depression a factor in family violence or neglect?

Does underlying psychopathology contribute to family violence?

Does the potential victim exhibit annoying psychological traits?

Does the emotional climate in the family foster abuse?

Are there unrealistic expectations of others within the family?

What is the distribution of power within the family? Does it influence the potential for abuse?

What are the psychological effects of abuse for the victim? For the perpetrator? For other family members?

Is the victim of family violence willing to accept help?

Is the perpetrator of family violence willing to accept help?

Social Dimension

What is the character of interactions among family members?

What contribution do social definitions of and attitudes toward family violence make to abuse?

Have family members been previously socialized to family violence?

What socioeconomic factors influence the potential for violence (eg, unemployment)?

Is the family socially isolated? What is the extent of social support available to the potential abuser? To potential victims?

What cultural or religious values or practices influence violence in the family?

What social factors pose barriers to escape from an abusive situation?

Is agism a contributing factor in family violence?

What is the attitude of protective services personnel to family violence?

What facilities are available to protect victims of family violence (eg, safe shelter)? What legal services are available?

Behavioral Dimension

Is substance abuse a contributing factor in family violence?

Do victims of the abuse use alcohol or drugs as an escape?

Is cohabitation a factor in the family violence?

Health System Dimension

Are health care providers alert to evidence of family violence?

What are the attitudes of health care providers to victims of family violence? To perpetrators?

What health care services are available to meet the needs of victims of family violence? What is available to perpetrators of violence?

What is the extent of health care services used by victims of abuse?

Do health care providers report suspected cases of family violence and abuse?

---

abuse on the part of the abuser, acquiescence on the part of the victim, and a situation conducive to abuse. Various factors related to the biophysical, psychological, social, behavioral, and health system dimensions contribute to the existence of these conditions.

The Biophysical Dimension

MATURATION AND AGING.   Generally speaking, both physical abuse and sexual abuse rates among children vary with age. For example, approximately two thirds of physical abuse occurs among children under 6 years of age (one third are under 1 year of age). Younger children are more likely than their older peers to sustain serious physical injury. The age differential for sexual abuse is essentially reversed with one third of cases occurring in children under 6 and two thirds of cases in older children (American Psychological Association, 1996).

The age of the abuser can also influence the incidence of child abuse. It has often been purported that adolescent parents are more likely than older parents to engage in child abuse because of their emotional immaturity. However, it may be that adolescent parents are under closer surveillance than other potential child abusers and that cases of child abuse are more readily identified in this group, thus accounting for associations of adolescent parenthood with child abuse.

Age may also be a factor in the type of long-term consequences of abuse experienced by victims. With respect to sexual abuse, for example, preschool children most often exhibit anxiety, nightmares, posttraumatic stress disorder (PTSD), fearfulness, aggression, and inappropriate sexual behavior such as public masturbation or requests for sexual stimulation from adults. School-age children also display fearfulness, aggression, and nightmares, but may also demonstrate poor school performance, hyperactivity, or regression. Common sequelae for adolescents include depression, withdrawal, attempted suicide, somatic complaints, delinquency, running away, and substance abuse (Bower, 1993).

Age is also a factor in elder abuse. Abuse of older people most often occurs in the "old elderly," those over 75 years of age. Increasing age may increase a victim's dependence on others beyond levels able to be tolerated by family members. Because of increased longevity, this burden of dependence may be prolonged over many years. The age and developmental level of the abuser can also be a contributing factor in elder abuse. At the point when many older persons become dependent, family members are frequently engaged in significant developmental life changes that engender considerable stress. This stress is compounded by the dependent needs of the elder at a point when family members may be looking forward to children leaving home, retirement, and a chance to live their own lives in relative freedom (Sengstock & Barrett, 1993). Spouse abuse tends to occur more frequently in younger than in older couples (Family and Intimate Violence Prevention Team, 1996).

SEX. Girls are at higher risk than boys for physical, emotional, and sexual abuse, but both boys and girls are at equal risk for neglect. The relative risk ratio for sexual abuse for girls is more than three times that for boys (Cappelleri, Eckenrode, & Powers, 1993).

Spouse abuse is usually directed toward women; however, men are also occasionally subjected to violence perpetrated by females. Approximately one sixth of U.S. couples employ violence by both parties at some point in a given year, underscoring the prevalence of physical aggression (Fullilove, 1996). In one national study, 8% of women described being victims of domestic abuse (Bell, et al., 1996). In another study in New York State, nearly 6% of women and 7% of men reported abuse by their partners. Men are generally subjected to more severe forms of violence, but, because of their limited strength and ability to defend themselves, women are more likely than men to be physically injured during domestic disputes (Family and Intimate Violence Prevention Team, 1996). Battering does not occur exclusively in heterosexual couples and is reported in 25 to 48% of lesbian couples and 38% of gay couples (Coleman, 1996).

Victims of elder abuse are more likely to be female than male. Gender differences in the incidence of abuse among older persons may be a function of age; women typically live longer than men and are therefore older and more vulnerable. Abusers of older victims may also differ by gender and type of abuse, with male abusers more often engaging in physical abuse and females in psychological abuse and neglect (American Psychological Association, 1996).

PHYSIOLOGIC FUNCTION. The health of both the victim and the abuser, as well as the health of other family members, can be influencing factors in child abuse. Children who are born prematurely, who are the result of a multiple pregnancy, who have physical or mental handicaps, who are hyperactive, or who experience feeding or sleep problems have been found to be at somewhat higher risk of abuse than other children.

Diminished health of the perpetrator has also been associated with child abuse and other forms of violence. For example, victims of head injury frequently display behavior changes that increase aggression. This has been referred to as "episodic discontrol syndrome" and is thought to result from damage to centers of self-regulation in the brain (Warnken, Rosenbaum, Fletcher, Hoge, & Adelman, 1996).

Pregnancy is a physiologic state that may precipitate spouse abuse. The incidence of abuse among pregnant women is estimated to be about 23% (Eilenberg & Fullilove, 1996). Abused women are more likely to experience spontaneous abortion and are more likely to not begin prenatal care until the third trimester of pregnancy.

There is some question of the role of physical

disability in the abuse of older persons. Several authors have suggested that abused elders are likely to suffer from a variety of physical impairments or be physically dependent on the abuser. Other research, however, suggests that abused older persons are no less healthy or more debilitated than their nonabused counterparts. In fact, in some areas, abused elders have been found to be more self-sufficient than those not abused. Physiologic function may also influence the detection of elder abuse when physical effects of abuse are mistaken for normal consequences of aging (Pillemer & Frankel, 1991).

The Psychological Dimension.   Factors in the psychological dimension that may contribute to family violence include poor coping skills, the emotional climate in the family, personality traits of the abuser or the victim, and the presence of psychopathology. Families with poor coping skills have difficulty dealing with situational stressors that create tension, resulting in violence. Constant family crises or upheavals indicative of poor coping abilities are frequently characteristic of abusive families.

The emotional climate in the family can also contribute to abuse. Families that exhibit increased emotional tension and anxiety, with little display of visible affection or emotional support, are considered emotionally impoverished and are at risk for violence. Similarly, family communication patterns that are nonnurturing, destructive, or ambiguous may also indicate risk for family violence.

The distribution of power within the family is another element of the emotional climate that may lead to abuse. Abusive families are characterized by autocratic decision making and power struggles between members. Abusers tend to abuse the power they have over other family members when they feel their power is threatened. Various studies of elder abuse, for example, have indicated that some abusers are economically dependent on the victims of abuse, and abuse may be an indication of frustration over their helplessness.

Personality traits of either the abuser or the victim can influence the incidence of family violence. Abusers and victims alike tend to have poor self-esteem. Abusers may also be emotionally immature, hostile, and unable to cope with problems in a healthy manner. They frequently feel personally insecure and inadequate, although they often appear successful to others.

Child abusers tend to have unrealistic expectations of children, particularly as sources of warmth and love. When they are disappointed in these expectations, abuse may occur. For example, children who are irritable, who cry often, or who do not care to be cuddled may be perceived as rejecting the parent. For parents with low self-esteem, this perceived rejection can set the stage for abuse.

Abused women tend to be dependent, passive, and reluctant to make changes. Grief and guilt are other frequent feelings exhibited by victims of spouse abuse. Furthermore, an abused woman may respond to abuse by adopting what is termed a *hostage response.* This adaptive behavior is characterized by feelings of responsibility for the abuse, feeling unworthy of help, fearing one will be disbelieved, and wariness of the motivation of others.

Depression is also frequently encountered in abused females. Women with a history of sexual abuse constitute up to 75% of women in some substance abuse treatment programs (Eilenberg & Fullilove, 1996). In addition, abused women are more than four times more likely to attempt suicide than women in general (McCauley, et al., 1995). Childhood sexual abuse is also associated with increased incidence of bulimia (Wonderlick, Wilsnack, Wilsnack, & Harris, 1996).

Psychological traits can also lead to decisions to care for older individuals in the family home, resulting in the potential for abuse. Feelings of obligation or responsibility or even of personal satisfaction may be involved in these decisions.

Psychological traits exhibited by the older person might also contribute to abuse. For example, the older person may have difficulty adjusting not only to physical and emotional losses but also to the loss of autonomy associated with age and the need to move in with family members. This difficulty in adjusting can make people querulous and difficult to live with, adding to the stress experienced by family caregivers and, possibly, leading to abuse.

The presence of psychopathology can also contribute to family violence. In one study, for example, 88% of male spouse abusers exhibited demonstrable psychopathology (Maiuro & Avery, 1996). Antisocial personality and other psychopathology have been asociated with child abuse as well (Kelleher, Chaffin, Hollenberg, & Fischer, 1994). Mental illness on the part of the abuser has also been found to be associated with elder abuse. Mental retardation on the part of the caregiver can also be a factor in abuse.

In assessing families for potential for violence, the nurse explores family coping methods and observes for evidence of an emotional climate that might contribute to violence. Families experiencing stress and who demonstrate poor coping skills, poor communication patterns, or lack of affection and cohesion are at risk for abusive behaviors. The nurse is also alert to evidence of personality traits that might place some family members at greater risk for victimization (eg, passivity or whining and complaining). The nurse may also note personality traits such as immaturity and feelings of insecurity and personal inadequacy on the part of family members who might become abusive.

The Social Dimension.   Clinical interventions in family violence must address the social forces that foster violence. As noted by one author, "To the extent that violence is accepted as a legitimate tool for goal achievement, the ability of society to control violence will be limited" (Sigler, 1995, p. 126). Social dimension factors can influence family violence in four primary ways. First, social definitions of abuse and violence influence societal responses to abusive behaviors. Second, myths regarding family violence impede efforts to control it. Third, the socialization of individuals may contribute to the use of violence as a mode of conflict resolution. Finally, the social environment may create stressors that contribute to violence in families.

The concept of abuse presumes that one individual is acting toward another in a manner that violates societal norms. In this respect, then, family violence is socially defined. A permissive societal attitude toward family violence contributes to abuse within families. Several researchers have noted that in societies where family life is a relatively public matter and where neighbors and friends actively interfere with abusive behavior, the incidence of family violence is limited. Until fairly recently, however, violence within families was an accepted way of life in the United States and few people, including health care providers and law enforcement officials, intervened to curtail violent episodes.

Societal attitudes toward and definitions of violence influence legal sanctions that are employed to prevent or curtail family violence. In the United States, legal action to protect children and the elderly from abuse are more extensive than those designed to protect spouses. Most states have some form of legislation related to spouse abuse, but legal sanctions vary from arrest to mandated treatment for the abuser. Even when protective social systems exist, they may not function effectively. For example, the American Psychological Association (1996, p. 47) noted that "the child protective system in this country is in an emergency state because it can neither provide adequate protection for children nor provide adequate treatment and prevention efforts to stop child abuse and maltreatment."

Community health nurses assessing community responses to the problems of family abuse should familiarize themselves with relevant legislation in their own jurisdictions. They should also assess the extent to which legislation is enforced in their communities. This type of information might be obtained from domestic court personnel, from law enforcement officials, or from protective services personnel in the area.

In the past, physical and emotional mistreatment of children was perceived by some people as in the best interests of the child and as an appropriate form of socialization. Mistreatment has occasionally been defended on religious grounds of teaching children right from wrong. More recently, however, such behavior is perceived as abuse, and reporting of suspected child abuse is mandated in all 50 states and the District of Columbia.

Some cultural groups define child abuse somewhat differently from the legal system. In some cultures, behaviors that would be defined as abusive by the majority culture are perceived as beneficial to the child. These culturally prescribed behaviors were described in Chapter 16, and include practices such as pinching to release harmful gases, coining (abrasion of the skin with a coin), and burning with a lighted cigarette or a wisp of burning cotton to treat diarrhea. The community health nurse should assess the prevalence of these and similar practices, particularly among Asian clients.

Although physical abuse of spouses is a criminal offense, enforcement of legislation is frequently predicated on the victim pressing charges, which many abused women are reluctant to do for fear of repercussions for themselves, their children, or the abuser. In some jurisdictions, for example, both victims and perpetrators of family violence have been arrested (Hamberger & Potente, 1996).

States vary greatly in their approach to protecting the abused spouse. In some states, courts may order eviction of the abuser or counseling for the abuser, the victim, or both. Even when legislation does exist protecting potentially abused spouses, it is not always enforced. Or, if the abuser is arrested, he or she is often released in a short period to return to exact retribution.

All 50 states have laws mandating reporting of abuse of older persons and have penalties for the failure of health care professionals to report suspected abuse. State statutes differ greatly in their definitions of elder abuse and the types of abuse covered.

Strongly held myths about family violence are another social environmental factor influencing abusive behavior within families. These myths may dissuade members of society, including health care professionals, from interfering in abusive situations. Some common myths and related realities in family violence are presented in Table 34–1. Community health nurses can assess the extent to which these myths prevail in their communities by talking with

TABLE 34–1. COMMON MYTHS AND REALITIES REGARDING FAMILY VIOLENCE

Myth	Reality
Family violence is rare.	Family violence is a common occurrence and its incidence is increasing.
Family violence is confined to families in which there is mental illness.	Family violence occurs in many families without psychopathology.
Family violence occurs more frequently in certain racial and cultural groups.	Family violence occurs among all racial and ethnic groups.
Violence occurs only between heterosexual couples.	Homosexuals are also at risk for abuse by spousal partners.
Social factors do not influence family violence because it occurs in all societies.	Social factors that tax family coping abilities do contribute to family violence.
Abused spouses can end the abuse by leaving the situation.	Without protection, divorced or separated women are frequently at higher risk of abuse if they attempt to terminate the relationship.
Abused children invariably become abusers.	Abused children may become abusive adults if the cycle of violence is not broken.
Substance abuse is the real cause of family violence.	Substance abuse may trigger an abusive episode or may be used as an excuse for abusive behavior, but does not *cause* abuse.
Violence and love do not coexist in abusing families.	Abusive family members frequently love each other, but may have difficulty expressing that love or controlling other emotions.
Family violence is classless.	Both spouse abuse and child abuse occur more often among the poor.
Abused women must like being abused or they would leave.	Abused women do not like being abused, but may feel like they deserve abuse. They may also be unable to leave an abusive situation because of economic, cultural, or religious constraints or because they fear for the safety of themselves or their children.
Violence among family members is a private matter, and they have a right to privacy.	No one has a right to abuse another. Early intervention by family, friends, or outsiders can prevent family violence.
Abused women deliberately provoke attacks.	Abused women go to great lengths to avoid confrontation with the abuser.
Abusers are uneducated people who are unable to cope with the world.	Abusers are frequently successful and respected citizens.
Children need their parents even if they are abusive.	Child abuse or witnessing other family violence can have lasting effects on young children, and removal of victims from an abusive situation may be necessary.
Once an abused wife, always an abused wife.	Violent families can be rehabilitated, and many women who escape abusive situations are careful not to enter others.
Once an abuser, always an abuser.	Abusive family members can be helped and families can be reconstructed with assistance.

health care providers, social services personnel, and other members of the community. The nurse should also assess for belief in these myths among potential perpetrators or victims of abuse. Victims, in particular, may internalize societal beliefs that they are somehow to blame for or deserving of abuse.

Socialization to violence as an acceptable means of resolving conflict is the third type of social dimension factor influencing family violence. Violence as a way of resolving conflict is a learned behavior that tends to be communicated from one generation to the next. Child abusers, for example, have frequently been found to have been abused children themselves (Jackson, 1996). It is believed, in these instances, that abusive parenting roles enacted by the abuser's parents are interpreted as normal parenting behavior. Children who witness violence in the home come to view violence as an acceptable means for conflict resolution that may lead to abuse of their own children, their spouses, or their parents in later life.

Abused spouses, particularly women, have also frequently been socialized to violence in their own families. It has also been suggested that elder abuse is a function of prior socialization to violence in one's family of origin. Media exposure to violence is another way in which people are socialized to violent behavior. This occurs in three ways: (1) increased fear of victimization and use of violence as a protective measure, (2) desensitization to violence and apathy in the face of violent behavior, and (3) an increased affinity for violent behaviors (American Psychological Association, 1996).

In assessing families for risk factors contributing to family violence, the community health nurse asks about family patterns of conflict resolution and observes for evidence of verbal aggression, threats of violence, or inability to resolve conflicts successfully without resorting to violence. The nurse also assesses forms of discipline used to socialize children, their appropriateness, and who administers disciplinary action. In addition, the nurse should inquire about conflict resolution strategies and modes of discipline used when adult family members were growing up. Construction of a genogram detailing a family history of violence may be helpful in identifying families at risk.

The last way in which the social environment may contribute to family violence is through stressful circumstances that tax family members' coping abilities. Stress-producing factors are similar for all forms of family violence and include restricted family resources related to unemployment, poverty, and poor social support systems. Low income and the resultant stress have been linked to both spouse abuse and child abuse. Overall, child maltreatment is seven times more likely to occur in families with annual incomes under $15,000 than in those with higher incomes (American Psychological Association, 1996). Other social factors that may create stress within the family include intolerance of differences of opinion and rigid or unsatisfactory role allocation. The existence of a strong social support system can act as a protective buffer against family violence. The absence of support, on the other hand, is a risk factor for family violence of all types. The extent of support available also influences the outcomes for victims and perpetrators after family violence occurs (Duncan, 1996). The nurse explores with family members their economic status and the existence and use of support systems that can provide emotional as well as material support. In addition, the nurse examines the appropriateness of role allocation and family members' satisfaction with roles allocated. Patterns of decision making within the family can also be assessed because family violence tends to occur more often in families where one partner is the exclusive decision maker.

One social factor that may contribute to abuse of older persons is "ageism." *Ageism* is a generally negative attitude toward the elderly held by members of a society. Ageism promotes stereotypes of older persons as senile, demanding, or debilitated, thus increasing their vulnerability to exploitation.

Social, cultural, and economic factors may also result in decisions to care for elderly family members in the home when this may not be in the best interests of either the older person or the caregiver. For example, the family may not be able to afford nursing home care or may perceive social expectations that they will care for their elderly members at home. The increase in the average age of the American population is also a factor in that, as a greater proportion of the population becomes elderly, the responsibility for their care falls to a diminishing number of younger people, thus increasing the burden of caregiving for these younger people.

Social factors not only influence the potential for abuse within families, but may also pose barriers to escaping an abusive situation for the victim of abuse. Victims of family violence may be economically dependent on the abuser or have no other alternative. Culture and religious beliefs may also make it difficult for abused women to leave an abusive relationship. In addition, the woman may fear loss of her children if she leaves an abusive situation. Abused elders may be

the economic support of the abuser and may be reluctant to abandon that individual or any grandchildren in the home.

The Behavioral Dimension.   Behavioral factors may be associated with all forms of family violence. For example, lifestyles experienced by single parents produce stressors not encountered by two-parent families. Single parents must assume the roles of both mother and father and function as the family's primary wage earner. Because single-parent families more often experience economic difficulties, the single parent is typically under considerably more stress than parents in the average two-parent household. Single parents may also have little outside emotional or material support and may have little or no respite from the responsibilities of parenthood.

The use of both alcohol and drugs has received mixed reviews in terms of contributing to family violence. Some studies indicate that alcohol and drug use plays a significant role in abusive families. Other researchers contend that alcohol and drugs are used as a justification or rationalization for abusive behavior (Raistick, 1994). Psychoactive substances such as alcohol and other drugs do diminish inhibitions against violence; however, sober abusers often inflict more damage than their intoxicated counterparts.

Research has established a link between spouse abuse and abuse of alcohol and other drugs by the victim (McCauley, et al., 1995), however it may be that alcohol use by the abused woman may be an attempt to escape from the realities of her situation. Whatever the causal relationship between substance abuse and family violence, substance abuse is an indication of a family that may be at risk for violence. For this reason, the nurse should be alert to indications of substance abuse, discussed in Chapter 33, as a possible risk factor for, or an effect of, family violence.

For abused women, a lifestyle that involves cohabitation, frequently with a substance-abusing male, may contribute to abuse. Cohabiting women are more likely to be abused than married women. Possible explanations may be the loss of social support that accompanies the social stigma of cohabitation or greater acceptability of violence against someone who is not officially part of one's family (Jackson, 1996).

The Health System Dimension.   The nation's health care system tends to ignore the problem of family violence. Victims of abuse are seen in a variety of health care settings such as well-child and prenatal clinics, schools, and emergency rooms, yet the diagnosis of abuse is frequently overlooked because of provider inattention to significant cues. In one study of abused women seen in emergency rooms, physicians failed to identify abuse in seven out of eight cases. In another study, 43% of women had sought care for violence-related injury more than six times without being identified by providers as battered (Innes & Mellman, 1996).

The average health care provider's index of suspicion for abuse due to family violence is relatively low. One study demonstrated that physicians were more likely to recognize child abuse than other forms of family violence. In this same study, a third of the physicians reported no training about family violence during their medical education (Tilden, Schmidt, Limandri, Chiodo, Garland, & Loveless, 1994). Lack of attention to the possibility of family violence is also demonstrated by other studies indicating that few physicians routinely make direct inquiries regarding possible abuse. Mandatory screening for abuse in emergency departments has been initiated in many jurisdictions to promote identification of victims and perpetrators (Schiavone, 1996).

Even when providers do identify potential cases of abuse, they may not take action to deal with the abuse. Reasons given for this inaction in one study included fear of offending clients by intruding, close identification with the victim (particularly among female physicians), feelings of powerlessness to do anything about the situation, and time needed to address issues of abuse in a busy practice (Sugg & Inui, 1992). In addition, many physicians do not see themselves as responsible for addressing family violence. Ethical considerations can also surface relative to the potential for damage to the abuser, further injury to the victim, or violation of a client's confidence (Limandri & Tilden, 1996). The potential for depression and suicide for the victim of abuse is another ethical concern. With adult clients there may be the additional issue of countering the victim's wishes in reporting an instance of abuse. For example, a community health nurse may need to decide whether to report an instance of abuse when the victim prefers, for whatever reasons, that it not be reported. Finally, the health care provider may fear that he or she will not be able to intervene successfully, that dealing with abusive situations will evoke painful memories, that the provider's concern and efforts will be rejected, or that the provider might be in danger from the abuser.

Health care providers may also impede efforts to control family violence by exhibiting attitudes and values that can prevent victims of abuse from seeking help. For example, failure to believe clients or intimating that they are exaggerating the problem might be interpreted as rejection. Clinical procedures that force victims to relive traumatic events also contribute to injury by providers. Similarly, expressing value judg-

ments that the person is weak or could have prevented the abuse are not helpful. Abused adults may be reluctant to make changes or to initiate legal proceedings, and their feelings and decisions should be respected.

Health care providers who address the problem of violence in the families with whom they work typically take a militant attitude toward intervention. Militancy may involve recommendations for the arrest of the abuser, legal protection of the victim, or removal of the victim from the situation. Although actions might protect the victim from further abuse, they might also serve to increase the danger to the victim. In fact, as many as three fourths of instances of spouse abuse may involve partners from a relationship that has been terminated. Militancy may also violate the victim's desires or needs and may further impair the health care professional's ability to assist the client. In addition, militancy merely treats the symptoms of family violence rather than getting at the underlying causes of the problem and rehabilitating both the abuser and the family.

Assessing for Evidence of Family Violence

The second aspect of community health nursing assessment related to family violence is observing for actual evidence of abuse. To this end, the nurse should routinely include questions related to possible abuse in taking health histories from all clients. In addition, the nurse should check for physical signs and symptoms of abuse and observe for behaviors on the part of either the client or significant others that might indicate abuse.

The behavior of both parents and children should be observed on each encounter with the community health nurse. Children who are withdrawn, fearful, or particularly clinging may be victims of abuse, and parents who give vague or conflicting histories for child injuries may be perpetrators of abuse. Abusive parents may exhibit excessive concern given the nature of the child's injuries or display little or no concern.

Physical examination of a child can provide a variety of indicators of abuse. Of particular concern are bruises in unlikely locations for the child's age or in various stages of resolution, indicating multiple injury incidents, fractures sustained in suspicious circumstances, burns in unusual places or with characteristic outlines (eg, of a cigarette touched to the skin; burns in the shape of an iron or heater grill; immersion burns), and abdominal injuries in the absence of a history of major trauma. Evidence of sexually transmitted disease in young children is highly suggestive of sexual abuse (Anderson, 1995). Additional physical

TABLE 34–2. PHYSICAL AND PSYCHOLOGICAL INDICATIONS OF CHILD ABUSE

Type of Abuse	Physical Indications	Psychological Indications
Neglect	• Persistent hunger • Poor hygiene • Inappropriate dress for the weather • Constant fatigue • Unattended physical health problems • Poor growth patterns	• Delinquency due to lack of supervision • School truancy • Begging or stealing food
Physical abuse	• Bruises or welts in unusual places or in several stages of healing; distinctive shapes • Burns (especially cigarette burns; immersion burns of hands, feet, or buttocks; rope burns; or distinctively shaped burns) • Fractures (multiple or in various stages of healing, inconsistent with explanations of injury) • Joint swelling or limited mobility • Long-bone deformities • Lacerations and abrasions to the mouth, lip, gums, eye, genitalia • Human bite marks • Signs of intracranial trauma • Deformed or displaced nasal septum • Bleeding or fluid drainage from the ears or ruptured eardrums • Broken, loose, or missing teeth • Difficulty in respirations, tenderness or crepitus over ribs • Abdominal pain or tenderness • Recurrent urinary tract infection	• Wary of physical contact with adults • Apprehensive when other children cry • Behavioral extremes of withdrawal or aggression • Appears frightened of parents • Inappropriate response to pain
Emotional abuse	• Nothing specific	• Overly compliant, passive, and undemanding • Extremely aggressive, demanding, or angry • Behavior inappropriate for age (either overly adult or overly infantile) • Developmental delay • Attempted suicide
Sexual abuse	• Torn, stained, or bloody underwear • Pain or itching in genital areas • Bruises or bleeding from external genitalia, vagina, rectum • Sexually transmitted disease • Swollen or red cervix, vulva, or perineum • Semen around the mouth or genitalia or on clothing • Pregnancy	• Withdrawn • Engages in fantasy behavior or infantile behavior • Poor peer relationships • Unwilling to participate in physical activities • Wears long sleeves and several layers of clothes even in hot weather • Delinquency or running away • Inappropriate sexual behavior or mannerisms

and psychological signs of child abuse are included in Table 34–2.

The nurse should also assess children exposed to abuse of other family members for adverse effects. Generally speaking, children from homes where violence is a frequent occurrence respond with withdrawal, anxiety, or aggression. These effects seem to be most pronounced in boys under the age of 10, although they are also seen in girls. There may also be a difference in the types of responses exhibited by boys and girls. Boys are more prone to externalize symptoms. Girls, on the other hand, more often display internalizing behaviors.

In a similar fashion, the nurse assesses spouses, especially women, for physical and psychological evidence of abuse. A history of nonspecific complaints, frequent hospitalizations, and frequent emergency room visits for injuries are suggestive of abuse. Abused women may also exhibit anxiety, substance abuse, or eating disorders, or attempt suicide in response to abuse. Similarly, women who respond overly casually to serious injuries or are overly emotional regarding relatively minor injuries may be victims of abuse.

Again, injuries that are inconsistent with the explanation given are possible indicators of abuse. Particularly suspicious injuries include lacerations of the face; injuries to the chest, breasts, back, abdomen, and genitalia; symmetrical injuries; and distinctive burn patterns. Frequent illness is another indicator of possible abuse because abused women seek medical care nearly twice as often as nonabused women (McCauley, et al., 1995). Typical signs and symptoms of spouse abuse are presented in Table 34–3.

Assessment of the older adult for possible abuse should focus on a general assessment, physical assessment, behavioral patterns, social interaction, and medical assessment. The general assessment includes

TABLE 34–3. PHYSICAL AND PSYCHOLOGICAL INDICATIONS OF SPOUSE ABUSE

Physical Indications	Psychological Indications
• Chronic fatigue	• Casual response to a serious injury or excessively emotional response to a relatively minor injury
• Vague complaints, aches, and pains	
• Frequent injuries	
• Recurrent sexually transmitted diseases	• Frequent ambulatory or emergency room visits
• Muscle tension	
• Facial lacerations	• Nightmares
• Injuries to chest, breasts, back, abdomen, or genitalia	• Depression
	• Anxiety
• Bilateral injuries of arms or legs	• Anorexia or other eating disorder
• Symmetric injuries	• Drug or alcohol abuse
• Obvious patterns of belt buckles, bite marks, fist, or hand marks	• Poor self-esteem
	• Suicide attempts
• Burns of hands, feet, buttocks, or with distinctive patterns	
• Headaches	
• Ulcers	

TABLE 34–4. PHYSICAL AND PSYCHOLOGICAL INDICATIONS OF ELDER ABUSE

Type of Abuse	Physical Indications	Psychological Indications
Neglect	• Constant hunger or malnutrition • Poor hygiene • Inappropriate dress for the weather • Chronic fatigue • Unattended medical needs • Poor skin integrity or decubiti • Contractures • Urine burns/excoriation • Dehydration • Fecal impaction	• Listlessness • Social isolation
Emotional abuse	• Hypochondria	• Habit disorder (biting, sucking, rocking) • Destructive or antisocial conduct • Neurotic traits (sleep or speech disorder, inhibition of play) • Hysteria • Obsessions or compulsions • Phobias
Physical abuse	• Bruises and welts • Burns • Fractures • Sprains or dislocations • Lacerations or abrasions • Evidence of oversedation	• Withdrawal • Confusion • Fear of caregiver or other family members • Listlessness
Sexual abuse	• Difficulty walking • Torn, stained, or bloody underwear • Pain or itching in genital area • Bruises or bleeding on external genitalia or in vaginal or anal areas • Sexually transmitted diseases	• Withdrawal
Financial abuse	• Inappropriate clothing • Unmet medical needs	• Failure to meet financial obligations • Anxiety over expenses
Denial of rights	• Nothing specific	• Hesitancy in making decisions • Listlessness and apathy

observation of hygiene, confusion that may be due to over medication or to anxiety, emotional state, and appropriateness of dress for the weather. Physical manifestations of abuse in older people can include bruises and other injuries. Behavioral patterns reflect the client's nutritional level and possible substance abuse or self-neglect. Information on lifestyle might also indicate a lack of assistance with necessary functions. The extent and quality of the client's social interaction might indicate passive neglect or suggest depression or withdrawal due to abuse or neglect. Finally, the medical assessment, focusing on signs and symptoms of existing disease, might disclose unattended medical needs indicative of neglect or sexually transmitted diseases suggesting sexual abuse. Specific signs and symptoms of elder abuse for which the community health nurse should assess older clients are presented in Table 34–4. The nurse should be particularly careful in assessing the older client to differentiate signs of abuse from signs and symptoms that accompany aging or that reflect existing chronic conditions. Assessment for the effects of aging and chronic disease in the elderly was discussed in Chapter 23.

Diagnostic Reasoning and Control of Family Violence

Community health nurses use the information obtained during client assessments to derive nursing diagnoses related to family violence for individual families or population groups. At the group level, nursing diagnoses would most likely reflect the prevalence of or potential for family violence in the community. For example, the nurse might diagnose "potential for increased child abuse due to an increase in single-parent families," or "increased incidence of elder abuse due to lack of residential facilities for the elderly and increased stress on family caregivers."

Nursing diagnoses may also be made relative to violence in families with whom the nurse is working. Examples of diagnoses at this level are "potential for emotional neglect due to lack of parental recognition of affective needs of children" and "excessive physical punishment due to unrealistic parental expectations of children."

Planning and Implementing the Dimensions of Health Care in Family Violence

Control of violence may be undertaken with communities or target groups or with individuals and their families. Control efforts may be employed at the primary, secondary, or tertiary level of prevention.

Planning to resolve problems of family violence is based on three general principles. First, the nurse and the family should establish mutually acceptable goals that are put in writing. When the goals of individual family members are contradictory or inconsistent with those of the nurse, discrepancies should be discussed and compromises achieved. Second, the nurse and family members should set concrete achievable objectives that lead to accomplishment of identified goals. Finally, the nurse should refrain from imposing solutions on the family.

Primary Prevention

Primary prevention for family violence can be aimed at potential abusers, potential victims of abuse, or society in general.

Interventions Directed Toward Potential Abusers.
When the nurse identifies a family in which factors that may lead to violence are present, the nurse can plan efforts to modify those factors. Areas of emphasis include increasing the potential abuser's coping skills, improving his or her self-esteem and sense of competence and decreasing dependence, treating existing psychopathology or substance abuse, discussing development issues and expectations, providing emotional support and relief from stress, and changing attitudes toward violence.

IMPROVING COPING SKILLS. The community health nurse can plan to assist a potential abuser to improve his or her coping abilities by exploring with the client currently used coping strategies and their effectiveness. The nurse can then assist the client to develop more effective and more appropriate coping strategies. For example, the nurse might assist the client to change his or her perceptions of circumstances that create stress and that lead to abuse. Or, the client might be assisted to change his or her response to stressors. The nurse can also assist clients to learn how to modify or eliminate stress by teaching them the process of problem solving. In teaching this process, the nurse assists the client to identify desired outcomes of action, to determine and evaluate alternative means of achieving out-

comes, and to implement selected alternatives and evaluate their effectiveness in achieving the desired outcomes.

ENHANCING SELF-ESTEEM. Community health nurses can also assist potential abusers to create a more positive self-image. To this end, the community health nurse might plan to praise and reinforce positive qualities displayed by the client, foster self-reliance, and use problem-solving skills to help the client decrease his or her dependence on others. For example, if the client is economically dependent on an older person living in the home, the nurse might assist the client to obtain employment or show the person how to budget for his or her own needs. The client could also be encouraged to contribute to the support of the household either monetarily or through activities in the home, such as making repairs around the house.

TREATING PSYCHOPATHOLOGY AND SUBSTANCE ABUSE. If treatment is required for existing psychopathology or for substance abuse by a potentially violent family member, the nurse can make referrals for a variety of treatment services. For example, the nurse might assist the potential abuser to enter a program of psychotherapy or might refer the person to a self-help group. Community health nursing involvement in treatment for psychiatric disorders and substance abuse was discussed in Chapters 32 and 33.

CREATING REALISTIC DEVELOPMENTAL EXPECTATIONS. Another aspect of primary prevention of family violence is educating potential abusers about developmental expectations at various stages of life. For example, the potentially abusive parent can be acquainted with expected behavior as children mature and can be given anticipatory guidance in dealing with these behaviors. Anticipatory guidance and information about parenting skills may even be given before couples have children. In this way they can make decisions about starting a family with a clear idea of the expectations of parenthood. In families that already have children, the nurse can refer potentially abusive parents to parenting programs that focus on skills needed to deal effectively with the expectations and stresses of parenthood.

Similarly, family members may need to be acquainted with the difficulties that older persons might experience in adjusting to aging and changed circumstances and that may make them querulous and difficult to live with. The nurse can also suggest to family members ways in which the older person's adjustment can be made easier. For example, the nurse can suggest that the older person be afforded as much privacy as possible, given the home situation, and that he or she be allowed to keep cherished possessions, even if it means that the home becomes somewhat crowded.

The nurse might also educate the potential abuser about personal developmental changes that he or she can expect. For example, if the primary caregiver of an older adult is a woman entering menopause, the nurse can discuss with her the psychological effects of menopause and strategies for minimizing them. The nurse can also refer the client for assistance as needed.

PROVIDING EMOTIONAL AND MATERIAL SUPPORT. Nurses can also plan to provide emotional support to clients who are under stress, which may cause them to engage in violence. In addition, the nurse can help the client modify or eliminate sources of stress that contribute to family tension and, potentially, to violence. For example, the nurse might refer the family for financial assistance or help them obtain respite care for a handicapped child or an older member.

CHANGING ATTITUDES TOWARD VIOLENCE. The final aspect of primary prevention directed toward the potential abuser is changing his or her perceptions of violence as an acceptable mode of conflict resolution. This is particularly needed for clients who come from a family in which violence was common. In working with these families, the nurse might discuss with parents the purpose of disciplining children and help them to develop appropriate forms of discipline to accomplish those purposes without the risk of physical or psychological damage to the child. (See Chap. 20 for a discussion of considerations related to discipline.) Similarly, the nurse can assist families to develop positive conflict resolution strategies similar to those presented in Chapter 12.

Interventions Directed Toward Potential Victims. Many of the primary prevention strategies directed toward potential victims of abuse are similar to those for potential abusers. For example, the nurse might work with women who grew up in violent families to change their perceptions of violence as an acceptable form of family interaction. To this end, the nurse might educate children, spouses, and older persons about abuse and some of the factors that contribute to family violence.

Similarly, community health nurses can help family members develop strong self-images that prevent them from accepting abusive situations. The nurse might also assist potential victims to develop good coping, problem-solving, and conflict resolution skills so that they can look for ways of circumventing potential violence. In addition, the nurse can plan to assist family members to develop effective communication skills that are assertive but do not prompt others to perceive them as whining or demanding.

Another primary prevention strategy directed toward potential victims of abuse is empowerment. *Empowerment* is the process of creating within the individual the ability to care for and protect oneself from imposition by others. Children can be empowered by being educated about abuse and what constitutes abuse. They can also be taught, in health care settings or in schools, what to do if they are being abused. Similarly, adults at risk for abuse can be educated about their options and ways of protecting themselves. Teaching both children and adults that no one has a right to abuse them, no matter what, is another form of empowerment.

Empowerment can also come from encouraging potential victims of abuse to maintain relationships with people outside of the family situation who could spot signs of possible abuse. It is particularly important to encourage family members to invite outside friends into the home. Family members who may be at risk for abuse should also be encouraged to participate in groups and activities outside the home and to ask for help when needed.

One final primary prevention measure that is particularly relevant to older persons in potentially abusive situations is to make arrangements to prevent financial abuse. Four financial arrangements can be made to safeguard the funds and property of older people: a financial representative trust, durable power of attorney, designation of a representative payee, and joint tenancy (Weiler, 1989).

In a *financial representative trust,* the older person transfers to a trustee, selected by him- or herself, responsibility for managing his or her property. In this type of arrangement the trustee is required to manage the older person's assets in a particular manner for the benefit of the older person or others designated (eg, grandchildren).

A *durable power of attorney* is a written document in which the older person grants another person the authority to act in his or her stead. The durable power of attorney comes into force only when the older person (the "principal") chooses to relinquish control of his or her affairs to the designated person or when the principal becomes incapacitated.

A *representative payee* is a person or organization that receives payments as a substitute for the beneficiary. For example, an older person may make arrangements for his or her Social Security benefits to be paid to a specific family member who uses that money to meet the beneficiary's financial obligations. This type of arrangement is restricted to payments to veterans, recipients of Social Security and supplemental security income, and retirees from railroad companies or state agencies. The agreement covers only that one source of the older person's income. The person receiving the money is required by law to use the funds for the care of the beneficiary, and the agency remitting the checks may demand an accounting of expenditures.

In *joint tenancy,* the person is coowner of the assets covered with one or more designated others. All parties involved have the use of funds or property covered under joint tenancy. In the event of the death of one party, ownership automatically devolves on other members of the joint tenancy agreement. Advantages and disadvantages of these four methods of preventing financial abuse of older people are summarized in Table 34–5. The community health nurse can assist older clients at risk for financial abuse to evaluate these financial management options and select those best suited to their needs. If the older person needs help in implementing the alternative suggested, the nurse could refer the individual to a source of assistance.

Interventions Directed Toward Society. Community health nurses may also be involved in primary prevention measures at the community or societal level. For the most part, these measures involve advocacy and political activity. For example, nurses might be active in promoting nonviolence at a societal level by teaching people more effective strategies for conflict resolution, or they might work to decrease the level of violence portrayed on television and in films. Nurses might also be involved in teaching positive conflict resolution strategies and effective coping skills to school populations.

Critical Thinking in Research

Dorfman, Woodruff, Chavez, & Wallack (1997) examined local television news stories related to young people or violence or both to determine whether or not the stories were framed episodically or thematically. Episodically framed stories focused on the events that had occurred without addressing the context in which they occurred. Thematic stories, on the other hand, included material on trends and conditions related to the events covered. They contended that thematically framed stories help to define violence as a public health issue, whereas episodic stories address violence as a criminal justice issue and that the approach taken influences policy makers to assume either a preventive public health approach or a punitive criminal justice approach to the control of societal violence. Their findings included the following:

- violence dominated news coverage
- crime details dominated coverage of violence
- more than half of the stories about youth related to violence
- more than two thirds of stories on violence related to youth
- most of the coverage reflected an episodic framework rather than a thematic framework

1. What are the implications of the findings of this study for public policy related to violence? Do you think the direction policy making is likely to take is an appropriate one? Why or why not?
2. What would the effects be if news coverage related to young people were more positive in nature? Why do you think news coverage focuses on the negative side of youth behavior?
3. Do you think news media coverage of youth behaviors has changed over time? How would you find out if your assumption was true or false?
4. Do you think a study of print news media would result in similar findings? How would you go about doing such a study? What types of print news media would you examine?

TABLE 34–5. ADVANTAGES AND DISADVANTAGES OF FINANCIAL ARRANGEMENTS TO PREVENT FINANCIAL ABUSE OF THE ELDERLY

Type of Financial Arrangement	Advantages	Disadvantages
Financial representative trust	• Legal accountability for use of funds • Ability to specify use of funds and beneficiaries	• Cost of establishing and administering trust
Durable power of attorney	• Financial needs met if older person becomes incapacitated • Ability to designate person to control funds • Retention of control of funds by older person until he or she chooses to relinquish it or becomes incapacitated	• Limited measures to safeguard older person if designee does not use funds as intended
Representative payee	• Limited control of funds by designated payee • Legal responsibility to use funds for the benefit of the stated beneficiary • Mechanism for demanding accounting of use of funds	• Restrictions on types of funds covered
Joint tenancy	• Ability of older person to designate recipient of funds • Automatic right of survivorship eliminates inheritance taxes	• Both parties have access to and use of property, and the joint tenant may use them for his or her own benefit and not that of the older person

Activity is also warranted to promote positive attitudes toward the elderly and to reduce the effects of ageism in society. Community health nurses might be involved in advocacy efforts that encourage older people to remain involved in the community and to become politically active.

Community health nurses may also be involved in political activity to promote legal sanctions for family violence that serve as deterrents to abuse. Nurses may also need to engage in community organization activities to ensure that law enforcement officials and judges enforce legislation.

Political activity may also be needed to eliminate societal conditions that contribute to family violence. Nurses may campaign, for example, for access to alternative forms of care for older adults for families already experiencing high levels of stress, or they might advocate respite care for family members caring for handicapped children or debilitated elders. Action may also be warranted to ensure adequate income for families in need.

Finally, community health nurses can engage in research related to family violence and its contributing factors. They can then convey their findings to policy makers to promote efforts aimed at preventing family violence.

Secondary Prevention

Secondary prevention takes place when violence and abuse are identified within a family. Two major goals in secondary prevention of family violence are protecting the victim from further abuse and breaking the cycle of violence. Protecting the victim may require treatment for serious injuries, reporting the abuse (or suspected abuse) to the proper authorities, and/or removing the victim from the abusive situation. Breaking the cycle of violence involves treatment of the abuser, the victim, and the family.

Reporting Confirmed or Suspected Abuse.   Health care providers and some other personnel (eg, teachers or child caregivers) are required by law in all 50 states and the District of Columbia to report all confirmed or suspected instances of child abuse. Usually the report is made immediately by telephone to the local child protection agency or similar government bureau, followed by a written report within 24 hours. If a provider encounters a suspected or confirmed case of child abuse during nonbusiness hours, he or she should report the incident to the local law enforcement agency at that time and follow with a report to the child protection agency on the next business day. The nurse should ascertain the agency designated to receive reports of po-

tential cases of abuse in his or her jurisdiction and obtain copies of the forms to be used in submitting reports. Examples of reporting forms used in one jurisdiction are included in Appendix U, Suspected Abuse Report Forms.

Health care providers are also required to report suspected abuse of older individuals, and community health nurse's should determine the status of reporting laws in their state as well as the procedures to be followed. The nurse should also determine the agency to which cases of abuse should be reported. Requirements for reporting spouse abuse vary from place to place. The community health nurse can, however, report instances of spouse abuse to law enforcement agencies, family courts, or other agencies that may be concerned with family violence. Although these agencies may not be required to take any action, they will at least be alert to the possibility of violence in the particular family. Another possible resource to which the nurse may report cases of abuse are ombudsman organizations that function as advocates for abused women (or occasionally men).

In addition to making the report, the nurse should inform the abuser that he or she will be reporting the incident to the appropriate authorities. Even if the agencies involved take no action, the fact of having been reported may deter future abuse in some situations.

The question of reporting possible abuse of adults or even older children may pose some ethical dilemmas for the nurse. These include the possibility that reporting instances of abuse may place the victim at greater risk for subsequent abuse, questions of violating client confidentiality, and questions of violating a client's autonomy and right of self-determination. Victims may not want the abuse reported for fear of the consequences for themselves or for the abuser. Reporting of self-neglect or self-abuse by elderly clients may violate their right of self-determination, as can decisions to report abuse when the victim does not want it reported. The nurse needs to determine what is really in the client's best interest based on the ethical principles discussed in Chapter 15.

Removing the Victim from an Abusive Situation.   Promoting the safety of the victim may necessitate his or her removal from the abusive situation. This may mean placement of an abused child in foster care or arranging for an abused spouse or older person to go to a temporary shelter until more permanent arrangements can be made.

Forcibly removing a child from his or her home may pose ethical questions for health care providers and social services personnel. Although community health nurses are not usually directly responsible for the decision for foster placement, their assessments of family situations often figure prominently in decisions by child protection services personnel. In removing a child from the home, there is the possibility that removal from familiar surroundings and people that the youngster loves may cause more trauma for the child than leaving him or her in the abusive situation.

Adults cannot be removed involuntarily from an abusive situation unless they are mentally incompetent to make their own decisions. The nurse, however, can encourage the spouse or older person who seems to be in danger to go to a shelter or other source of care. In general, three guidelines can assist the nurse and client to determine whether removal is warranted. First, the person should be encouraged to leave if he or she is experiencing a life-threatening medical condition that is not being treated. Second, removal may be warranted by hazards within the environment (eg, lack of heat, food, or water). Third, the client should be encouraged to leave if there is unimpeded access to the client by an individual who has previously harmed them.

It may be very difficult for abused women or older clients to leave an abusive situation. For the woman, she is leaving a home and a relationship into which she has put considerable time and energy. In addition, the woman may not have any source of economic support should she leave. Or she may fear the loss of her children. Older clients may be reluctant to leave a familiar place or fear going to a nursing home as the only alternative to remaining in an abusive situation. Moreover, the older client may fear complete isolation from family members or the effects of their removal on others in the family (eg, grandchildren).

The nurse should help the client explore the advantages and disadvantages of leaving the situation. If the client decides to leave, he or she should be encouraged to take along personal valuables or place them for safekeeping with a responsible friend or family member. Important personal documents (eg, children's birth certificates and health records, wills) should also be taken. If the woman has young children, she should take the children and a small amount of clothing (as well as important toys) with her. Once the client has been placed in a shelter there may be a need to assist in planning further action such as permanent housing, employment, or legal action. The community health nurse can either help the client with these matters or make referrals for appropriate services.

The client may also require assistance in helping children cope with the upheaval created in their lives. The community health nurse can help the client understand that children are apt to act out their fear and frustration in the situation by being disobedient or quarrelsome with the parent or at school. The nurse can help the client deal with frustrations stemming from these behaviors by children and can also make referrals for counseling for both client and children as needed.

If either abused women or older clients decide not to leave an abusive situation, the community health nurse must accept that decision without conveying disgust for the client or abandoning the person. The nurse can also provide the client with shelter information and suggest contingency plans that the client might make for reaching the shelter should this become necessary later.

Treating the Abuser. The abusive family member usually also requires assistance from the community health nurse. As noted earlier, the militant approach to family violence taken by some health care providers may (or may not) result in the accomplishment of short-term goals but does nothing to restore the "personhood" of the abuser or the victim. Treatment of the abuser should focus not only on strategies to cope or to manage anger but also on reconstructing a whole person who has dealt with the psychological factors that may have contributed to the abuse. The goals of treatment for the abuser are cessation of violence, expanding the abuser's emotional repertoire beyond anger to acknowledge other positive and negative feelings, and providing an environment in which violence is *not* reinforced and nonviolence *is* reinforced. To achieve these goals, the community health nurse should make referrals for counseling, for psychotherapy for underlying psychopathology, and for treatment for problems of substance abuse if these exist. The nurse may also make referrals to residential programs in which families can learn new patterns of interaction in a nonviolent environment. In addition, the community health nurse provides emotional support while the abuser learns a new way of thinking and acting and new attitudes toward interpersonal interactions.

The nurse can also help bolster the abuser's self-esteem and sense of personal competency and assist the client to eliminate or modify situational stresses that contributed to abuse. For example, the nurse might assist the abuser to find employment or obtain assistance. Assistance in developing intimacy skills and decreasing loneliness has also been shown to be effective in treating child sexual abusers (Marshall, Bryce, Hudson, Ward, & Moth, 1996). Medication has also been recommended as an adjunct to psychotherapy and social interventions. Medication may be particularly important to modify biological factors that may interfere with motivation to accept other forms of therapy (Maiuro & Avery, 1996).

Treating the Victim.   Victims of abuse also require treatment. Treatment may be needed for both the physical and psychological effects of abuse, and the community health nurse may make referrals for both types of services. When extensive medical care is needed for severe injuries, the nurse may also need to make referrals for financial assistance. In addition, the nurse can also make referrals for counseling to deal with the emotional effects of abuse.

The nurse should also support the victim emotionally through the treatment of physical defects resulting from abuse. Clients may need assistance adjusting to the long-term consequences of abuse (eg, permanent deformity or other disability). Victims of abuse should be encouraged to ventilate and work through their fears and anxieties about future abuse and to develop strategies for coping with their changed life circumstances. Clients may also need assistance in obtaining financial support, housing, and other necessities.

Treating the Family.   Family members other than the direct victim of abuse also suffer the effects of family violence. As noted earlier, children exposed to family violence, even when they are not the target of that violence, tend to accept violence as an appropriate way of resolving differences. In addition, these children may exhibit symptoms related to the increased tension caused by family violence. Community health nurses should assist these youngsters and other family members to deal with their feelings about violence and its effects on their lives. They should be encouraged to develop adaptive responses toward previous abuse and to learn effective strategies for resolving interpersonal conflict without resorting to violence. Community health nurses can assist family members in developing these skills and refer them to sources of additional help as needed.

Families may also need to be assisted to reconstruct themselves along lines that do not include violence. It is particularly important for families that maintain their structure (including the abuser) to plan activities that enhance family cohesion. To this end, the community health nurse might help the family plan social activities in which all can engage.

Tertiary Prevention

Many of the activities discussed as primary prevention measures can also be used in tertiary prevention, preventing the recurrence of abuse once an abusive situation unfolds. For example, abusive parents can be assisted to develop parenting skills and more realistic expectations of their children. Abusers of all types can be helped to develop more appropriate ways of dealing with stress. Both abusers and victims can be assisted to develop more positive self-concepts. This is particularly important for victims of child abuse if the intergenerational cycle of abusive behavior is to be broken.

Elimination of social and behavioral dimension factors contributing to abuse may also prevent recurrence. Community health nurses can work to reduce long-term vulnerability factors such as poor social support networks, historical patterns of abuse, and poor coping abilities. Nurses can also plan to reduce short-term stresses, such as unemployment, and increase long-term and short-term protective factors. Furthermore, nurses need to increase the independence of abusers of older persons as a means of minimizing elder abuse. Other potential tertiary strategies for elder abuse include providing alternatives to home care of the elderly and increasing community support services for persons who are caring for older family members. For example, respite services or adult day care centers might reduce the burden on caregivers and prevent recurring incidents of abuse. Intervention goals for family violence and related community health nursing actions at the primary, secondary, and tertiary levels of prevention are summarized in Table 34–6.

....

► HOMICIDE AND SUICIDE

Family violence is not the only form of violence evident in today's society. Homicide and suicide are two other forms of violence that are of particular concern. Community health nurses may be involved in assessing risk factors that contribute to homicide and suicide both for individuals and for communities. Factors related to biophysical, psychological, social, behavioral, and health system dimensions are associated with both homicide and suicide. Because factors associated with each of these conditions may differ somewhat, each is addressed separately before interventions related to both are discussed.

 Assessing the Dimensions of Health in Homicide

The Biophysical Dimension

Differences exist in the incidence of homicide in different age and ethnic groups. From 1950 to 1993,

TABLE 34–6. GOALS FOR PRIMARY, SECONDARY, AND TERTIARY PREVENTION OF FAMILY VIOLENCE AND RELATED COMMUNITY HEALTH NURSING INTERVENTIONS

Goal of Prevention	Nursing Intervention
PRIMARY PREVENTION	
1. Development of effective coping skills	1. Teach coping skills.
2. Development of strong self-image	2. Foster and reinforce development of strong self-image. Foster independence of potential abusers.
3. Treatment of psychopathology or substance abuse	3. Refer abusers for counseling or therapy. Refer to self-help groups.
4. Development of realistic expectations of self and others	4. Educate parents on child development. Educate caregivers on developmental needs of the elderly. Assist clients to recognize own limitations.
5. Development of parenting skills	5. Teach parenting skills.
6. Provision of emotional and material support	6. Assist clients to modify sources of stress. Refer to outside assistance. Provide emotional support. Engage in political activity to change conditions conducive to abuse.
7. Change in attitudes toward violence	7. Teach nonviolent modes of conflict resolution. Teach problem-solving and decision-making skills. Discuss attitudes and approaches to discipline. Discourage societal glorification of violence.
8. Development of policies that discourage violence and protect potential victims	8. Engage in political activity and advocacy.
9. Empowerment of potential victims	9. Foster self-esteem. Teach coping, communication, and problem-solving skills. Educate clients about abuse. Encourage clients to maintain relationships outside the family. Assist older clients to make appropriate financial arrangements.
10. Elimination of negative attitudes toward potential victims of abuse	10. Engage in advocacy. Convey a positive attitude toward the elderly. Educate the public on abuse and dispel myths.
SECONDARY PREVENTION	
1. Reporting of confirmed and suspected cases of abuse	1. Engage in case finding. Report potential cases of abuse.
2. Removal of victims from abusive situations	2. Refer to shelters. Arrange for foster home placement of abused children.
3. Treatment of abusers	3. Refer for counseling. Foster self-esteem. Provide emotional support. Engage in political activity to ensure availability of treatment services.
4. Treatment of victims	4. Refer for physical care. Refer for counseling. Provide emotional and material support.
5. Treatment of families	5. Refer for counseling. Provide emotional support. Encourage activities that foster family cohesion. Assist family members to deal with feelings about abuse.
TERTIARY PREVENTION	
1. Provision of support to abusers	1. Provide emotional support. Teach parenting skills. Assist with the development of realistic expectations. Foster self-esteem.
2. Provision of support to victims	2. Foster self-esteem. Foster independence.
3. Reduction of sources of stress	3. Refer for financial help and other material support. Assist in obtaining respite care. Increase social support networks.

childhood homicide rates tripled to become the fourth leading cause of death among children aged 1 to 4 years and the third leading cause of death in those 5 to 14 years of age (Division of Violence Prevention, 1997a). Homicide rates increase still further among young adults with one third of all 1993 homicides occurring in people aged 15 to 24 years (Division of Violence Prevention, 1996b). The age distribution of U.S. homicide victims in 1994 is presented in Table 34–7. Homicide victims are nearly equally distributed between blacks and whites in terms of actual numbers, but homicide rates are eight times higher for black males than for white males and more than four times higher for black females (U.S. Department of Commerce, 1996). Gender differences in homicide are the result of differential exposure to social factors that contribute to homicide and favor women four to one. Women are also less likely than men to perpetrate homicide (Dawson & Langan, 1994).

Physiologic health status does not seem to play a significant role in homicide. One exception, however, is the small number of combined murder–suicide incidents in which elderly persons with seriously ill spouses may kill their spouse and then kill themselves.

The Psychological Dimension

Psychological dimension factors associated with homicide are similar to those discussed in relation to family violence and include poor coping strategies and perceptions of violence as an acceptable means of resolving conflict. Other psychological factors associated with homicide include poor impulse control and, on occasion, psychopathology. The feelings of hopelessness and powerlessness that may occur with poverty and discrimination may also lead to defiance that erupts in the form of violence and homicide.

One other aspect of the psychological environment is the state of mind of the victim at the time of the homicide. Homicides often occur as a result of arguments (frequently when both parties have been drinking). In fact, in 1994, nearly one third of all homicides were preceded by an argument (U.S. Depart-

TABLE 34–7. AGE DISTRIBUTION OF HOMICIDE VICTIMS, 1994

Age	Number	Percent
< 1 year	257	1%
1–4 years	470	2%
5–9 years	138	0.6%
10–14 years	317	1.4%
15–19 years	3021	14%
20–39 years	12,492	57%
40–59 years	3698	17%
60–74 years	871	4%
> 75 years	436	1%
age unknown		1%

(Source: U.S. Department of Commerce, 1996.)

ment of Commerce, 1996). It has been suggested that a fair number of these altercations are provoked by the victims in an effort to motivate another person to kill them. This phenomenon is referred to as *victim-precipitated homicide* and occurred in nearly 20% of murders committed in 1988 (Dawson & Langan, 1994). In other studies, victim-precipitated homicide may be involved in 22 to 38% of cases (Goetting, 1994).

The Social Dimension

Social dimension factors that contribute to homicide include societal acceptance of personal violence, stress due to a variety of underlying factors, crime and gang membership, and availability of weapons. Many of the societal factors that influence family violence also contribute to homicide. The use of force to settle conflicts and the failure of members of society to interfere in the face of escalating violence contribute to homicide as well as to other forms of violence. In addition, media portrayal of violence without elucidating its consequences glamorizes violence.

Stress due to social conditions appears to be a contributing factor in homicide although its contribution is somewhat unclear. Poverty, poor job opportunity, education, movement from rural to urban settings, changes in family structure, increased population mobility, drug trafficking, and racial discrimination have all been cited as sources of stress that may influence the risk of homicide.

Levels of stress experienced and the poverty and other social factors that contribute to stress may partially explain the difference in homicide rates noted between urban and rural areas. Significant differences in urban and rural homicide rates are seen even

---

ASSESSMENT TIPS: Assessing Risk for Homicide

Biophysical Dimension

Is the client in an age group at increased risk for homicide?

Is the client in an ethnic group with a high incidence of homicide?

Psychological Dimension

Does the client have a wish for death that may precipitate homicide?

What is the extent of coping skills exhibited by persons in a potential homicide situation?

Does the client perceive violence as a means of conflict resolution?

Is there a history of family violence or exposure to other forms of violence?

What is the effect of homicide on surviving family members?

Social Dimension

To what extent does society accept violent behavior?

What socioeconomic factors influence the potential for homicide (eg, poverty, social unrest)?

How easy is it to obtain weapons?

Behavioral Dimension

Does the client use alcohol or other drugs?

Does the client frequent high crime areas? Places where drug and alcohol use are common?

Does the client work in a high crime area or occupation?

Does the client work with the public or handle money?

Is the client involved in criminal activity?

Is the client a member of a gang?

Health System Dimension

Do health care providers promote nonviolent means of conflict resolution?

Do health care providers report cases of assault?

Are there services available to family members of homicide victims to help them deal with the death?

among segments of the population already at risk. Urban areas are frequently characterized by poverty, high population density, and poor housing, which create stress that may lead to violence. Homicide rates tend to be particularly high in cities where economic status contributes to interpersonal confrontations.

Crime and gang activity in urban areas also place residents at greater risk of homicide. Homicides may be committed in the process of other criminal activity, particularly robbery and the sale of illegal drugs. For example, cities with high rates of crime related to robbery and drug trafficking also tend to have high homicide rates. Although much attention is given in the media to homicide connected with criminal behavior, the proportion of total homicides related to crime is less than one might expect. In 1994, for example, less than 20% of homicides occurred during the commission of a felony (U.S. Department of Commerce, 1996). Unfortunately, many of the victims of crime-related homicides are innocent bystanders.

The availability of weapons is a significant social environmental contribution to homicide. Weapons used to commit homicide vary, but in the majority of cases the weapon used is some type of firearm. This choice of weapon is probably influenced by the lethality of the method as well as the ease of access to guns. In some studies, for example, 20 to 22% of high school students had brought guns to school (Arria, Wood, & Anthony, 1995; Kann, et al., 1996). Weapon carrying appears to be associated with peers who engage in similar behaviors (Myers, McGrady, Marrow, & Mueller, 1997). Homicide rates have been shown to be positively correlated with household gun ownership (Cummings, et al., 1997). Other weapons used include cutting implements and bludgeons.

A person's occupation is another social factor that can increase his or her risk of being homicide victim. In 1992, the U.S. occupational homicide rate was 0.64 per 100,000 workers. American women seem to be at greater risk of occupational homicide than men. Homicide accounted for 42% of occupational fatalities for women and only 11% of fatalities for men. Jobs that require frequent contact with the public or the exchange of money increase one's risk for homicide. Driving a taxicab, working in a liquor store, gas station, or jewelry store, and working as a detective or security personnel are the occupations with the greatest risk of homicide. Most occupational homicides occur in the context of robbery, and, media portrayals to the contrary, only 4 to 6% of occupational homicides are perpetrated by coworkers (National Institute for Occupational Safety and Health, 1996). Working at night in a high-crime area is another occupational risk factor for homicide. The risk of homicide can be reduced, however, by factors within the work setting itself. Examples of risk reduction strategies include train-

ing employees in conflict management, limiting the amount of money available or access to that money by employees, increasing employee visibility to the general public, and controlling access to the premises.

The Behavioral Dimension

Drug and alcohol use may contribute to one's propensity to commit homicide as well as the probability of being a victim of homicide. Use of psychoactive substances frequently decreases a person's inhibitions against violent behavior and may lead to homicide, particularly as the culmination of an argument. Studies of alcohol and drug intake among perpetrators are understandably few; this is because the arrest of a murder suspect frequently does not occur until some time after the crime, when blood and urine levels of psychoactive substances are likely to be quite different from those that might be obtained earlier. It is estimated, however, that more than half of the homicides committed in the United States involve drug or alcohol use by perpetrators or victims (Dawson & Langan, 1994).

Use of alcohol and drugs can also contribute to a person's likelihood of becoming a victim of homicide. The relationship of alcohol use to homicide tends to be stronger for homicides that occur as a result of arguments than for those that do not. It has even been suggested that just being present in places where alcohol use occurs may increase one's risk of being a homicide victim. Homicide has been described as a "leisure-related activity" because it occurs at times and places where leisure activities generally take place (Goetting, 1994).

Drug use and abuse may also contribute to homicides both while one is under the influence of the drug and during activities performed to support a drug habit (eg, robbery). Drug traffickers are at particular risk for homicide.

The Health System Dimension

The major contribution of the health care system to homicide lies in failure to engage in primary preventive efforts to control the problem. Other health care system factors may also contribute to homicide. Emergency facilities in many cities with high homicide rates are sometimes ill equipped to deal with the sheer numbers of people seriously injured in assaults, and many of these people become part of the statistical picture of homicide. In addition, a significant number of nonfatal assault cases seen in emergency rooms are not reported to police. If health care providers were more consistent in reporting cases of nonfatal assault, more of the perpetrators of these assaults might be apprehended by law enforcement authorities before they eventually kill someone.

ASSESSMENT TIPS: Assessing Risk for Suicide

Biophysical Dimension

Is the client in an age group at increased risk for suicide?

Is the client in an ethnic or gender group with a high incidence of suicide?

Does the client have a physical health problem that might contribute to suicide?

Is the client experiencing a maturational crisis (eg, adolescence)?

Psychological Dimension

Is the client depressed?

Does the client express suicidal thoughts? How well developed are plans for suicide?

Does the client exhibit other underlying psychopathology?

Does the client express feelings of hopelessness or despair?

Has the client been exposed to suicide by others?

Has the client previously attempted suicide?

What sources of stress are present in the client's life?

Social Dimension

Is the client experiencing family or interpersonal difficulties? Have there been recent changes in interpersonal relationships (eg, divorce)?

Is there a history of family violence?

Does the client exhibit poor school performance? Lack of goals for the future?

Has the client been exposed to media coverage of suicide?

How accessible are lethal methods of suicide?

Are there social factors contributing to the potential for suicide (eg, unemployment)?

Has the client recently experienced some kind of failure?

Behavioral Dimension

Does the client use alcohol or other drugs?

Is there evidence of substance abuse?

Does the client engage in regular exercise?

Does the client have difficulty sleeping?

Does the client have any outside interests?

Health System Dimension

Do health care providers promote effective coping skills among clients?

Are health care providers alert to signs and symptoms of potential suicide?

What is the attitude of health care providers to suicidal individuals?

Does the client have a regular source of health care who might identify suicide potential?

 ## Assessing the Dimensions of Health in Suicide

The Biophysical Dimension

Human biological factors that may be related to suicide include effects of maturation and aging, gender, racial group membership, and physiologic function. Some age groups have higher suicide rates than others. Suicide rates among children quadrupled from 1950 to 1993 (Division of Violence Prevention, 1997a), but remain highest among persons over 75 years of age? Differences in suicide rates for different age groups vary with gender and race. For white women, the incidence of suicide peaks in midlife and then declines. For example, the highest incidence of suicide among white women in 1993 occurred among those who were 45 to 54 years of age (7.8 per 100,000 women). For men, on the other hand, the incidence of suicide rises with increasing age, with the highest rates experienced by white men 85 years of age and older (over 70 cases per 100,000 men in 1993). Among blacks, the peak incidence of suicide occurs in the 20- to 24-year-old age group for both men and women. White males over the age of 85 continue to have the highest rate of suicide for any age group (U.S. Department of Commerce, 1996).

Age–gender differences in suicide may be explained, in part, by maturational events. Women at midlife usually experience menopause accompanied by hormonal changes that may lead to severe depression and consequent suicide. At the same time, women may be experiencing social factors, such as children leaving home, that may contribute to depression. Men, on the other hand, may be responding to the effects of age on physical and mental abilities and social interaction, again leading to depression and, possibly, to suicide.

Although objectively not as high as rates for older people, suicide rates for young people are also of concern because of their rapid escalation in recent years. For example, from 1980 to 1992, suicide rates increased for only two age groups, children aged 5 to 19 years and the elderly (Division of Violence Prevention, 1996a). During this time, suicide rates for 10- to 14-year olds increased by 120%, with a 28% increase among adolescents aged 15 to 19 years (Division of Violence Prevention, 1995). Again, this is a period in one's life characterized by rapid hormonal and social changes with which the individual may have difficulty coping, thus leading to increased potential for suicide. When working with people in age groups at particular risk for suicide, the community health nurse is careful to assess for other suicidal risk factors as well as specific indicators of suicidal intent.

There is also some evidence that physiologic function may contribute to suicide. Pregnancy was the reason given in 2.4% of adolescent suicide attempts in one study (National Center for Injury Prevention and Control, 1995), and wounded Vietnam veterans, particularly those wounded more than once, have a higher risk of suicide than unwounded veterans (Bullman & Kang, 1996). Research has indicated rather consistently that lower levels of the biochemical neurotransmitter serotonin, also linked to depressive illness, are associated with suicide. Less consistent associations have also been demonstrated between suicide and other neurotransmitters such as norepinephrine, dopamine, and acetylcholine. Suicide may also be associated with depression due to severe illness or intractable pain (Fishbain, 1996). Symptomatic HIV disease is also strongly associated with increased risk of suicide (Dannenberg, McNeil, Brundage, & Brookmeyer, 1996).

The Psychological Dimension

Some authors assert the most victims of suicide suffer from some type of mental disorder (Shaffer & Hicks, 1994). As noted in Chapter 32, both schizophrenics and persons with depressive disorders have higher incidence rates for suicide than the general population. In some cases of suicide associated with mental illness, it is unclear whether the suicide is a result of the illness or the effects of psychotropic drugs used in treatment of mental illness. Antidepressants, in particular, can reverse depression sufficiently to give severely depressed clients the energy they lacked to commit suicide.

The hopelessness that may accompany severe debilitating or terminal illness is another psychological factor that may lead to suicide. Clients with terminal cancers or AIDS, for example, may see suicide as an escape from a painful and lingering illness for which there is no cure. Community health nurses working with clients with either mental or serious physical illness or disability should carefully assess them for suicide potential, focusing particularly on inability to cope with the effects of the illness or its treatment and on the presence of signs of depression discussed in Chapter 32.

Exposure to suicide by others may create a psychological climate that encourages suicide in vulnerable individuals. Both direct knowledge of someone who has committed suicide and indirect knowledge via media presentations of suicide have been found to be associated with subsequent suicide (National Center for Injury Prevention and Control, 1995; Shaffer & Hicks, 1994). Community health nurses obtain information related to suicide and attempted suicide as well as other conditions in constructing family genograms early in their interactions with individuals and families. This information might help to identify people exposed to prior suicides. The nurse then explores with the client the client's resolution of grief related to the prior suicide.

Other psychological signs of suicide potential for which the nurse should assess clients include a sudden change in mood, particularly from agitation and depression to calm, and expression of suicidal thoughts. Generally speaking, the more persistent the thoughts of suicide, the more likely the event. Also, the more detailed the plan for suicide and the more lethal the method described in the plan, the more likely the person is to attempt suicide. Finally, clients who make few references to the future in terms of plans or goals are at risk for suicide. *Suicidal ideation,* or thoughts of committing suicide, is a relatively common phenomenon among adolescents. In the 1995 Youth Risk Behavior Surveillance Survey (YRBSS), 24% of high school students reported having considered suicide, nearly 18% had formulated a specific suicide plan, and almost 9% had actually attempted suicide in the previous year (Kann, et al., 1996).

The nurse should ask the clients if they have ever thought about committing suicide. If the response is yes, the nurse should ask the client about the frequency and persistence of these thoughts and also inquire as to what plans, if any, have been made for a potential suicide. The nurse should assess for the following indicators of potential suicide:

- Family history of suicide
- History of prior suicide attempt(s)
- Recent loss (particularly in the last 6 months)
- Signs of depression
- Feelings of hopelessness and helplessness expressed
- Feelings of anxiety, irritability, or panic exhibited
- Lack of references to future goals or activities

- Frequent or persistent thoughts of committing suicide
- Carefully thought-out plan for suicide
- Lethal method planned for suicide
- Reduced likelihood of rescue, given method planned and other aspects of suicide plan
- Specific time frame planned for suicide
- Suicide planned for near future
- Behaviors designed to "put one's house in order" (making a will, giving away prized possessions, making a final contact with significant others)

The Social Dimension

Social dimension factors that influence the incidence of suicide may arise from the personal social environment or from the larger environment. Within the personal social environment, poor interpersonal relationships, particularly family relationships, have been associated with suicide.

Suicide among adults has also been linked to changes in interpersonal relationships, particularly to divorce or death of a spouse, whereas marriage appears to be a protective factor against suicide for men and, to a lesser extent, for women as well. Widowed and divorced men have suicide rates nearly three times higher than those for married men, whereas rates for single men are nearly twice as high as for their married counterparts. Divorced women commit suicide nearly twice as often as married women, and single women have suicide rates 30% higher than those of married women (Division of Violence Prevention, 1996a).

Societal factors that have been associated with increased incidence of suicide include the easy availability of firearms and drugs, joblessness, and media coverage of suicide. Firearms are the most frequently used mode of committing suicide. In 1993, for example, nearly two thirds of suicides by males and 39% of female suicides were committed using firearms; poisoning accounted for another 14% of suicides by males and 35% by females. Hanging or strangulation and suffocation were less frequently used methods of suicide by women (13%) but were used in 15% of male suicides (U.S. Department of Commerce, 1996).

The relationship of joblessness to suicide is not completely clear, however, it is a reasonable conjecture that joblessness contributes to hopelessness and depression, which may culminate in suicide as a means of escape from an unbearable situation. It may also be that people with psychiatric disorders that can culminate in suicide are unemployed as a result of their disease rather than depressed because of their unemployment. Suicide victims do exhibit more frequent job changes and periods of unemployment than do the general population, which may be evidence of general mental instability.

Prominent coverage of suicides in the news media is another societal factor that has been shown to be associated with suicide, particularly among young people (O'Carroll & Potter, 1994). This is particularly true of "cluster suicides." A *suicide cluster* is a group of suicides or suicide attempts that occur closer together in time and space than would otherwise be expected. Suicide clusters account for only 1 to 5% of all suicides, but they are especially traumatizing to communities in which they occur. There is some evidence that such events arise from imitative behavior due to exposure to suicide by knowing the victim or through media coverage of the event.

The Behavioral Dimension

The major behavioral factors associated with suicide are drug and alcohol abuse. Psychoactive substance abuse may lead to depression that culminates in suicide. In addition, the use of both alcohol and drugs results in disinhibition and may minimize the effects of religious and ethical strictures against suicide. In several studies, suicidal ideation among adolescents has been linked to a variety of high-risk behaviors including sexual activity, smoking, psychoactive substance use and abuse, and aggressive behavior. Community health nurses should be alert to evidence of suicide potential among persons who abuse alcohol or other psychoactive substances or engage in other high-risk activities. Another study, however, indicated that coffee intake had a strong inverse relationship with suicide. Women who consumed two to three cups of coffee per day had about one third the risk of suicide of noncoffee drinkers (Kawachi, Willett, Colditz, Stampfer, & Speizer, 1996).

The Health System Dimension

Health care system factors that contribute to suicide include lack of attention to persons at high risk and failure to identify potential suicide victims. This failure to identify persons at risk for suicide is highlighted by findings that many suicide victims are seen by health care providers in the month prior to death (Division of Violence Prevention, 1996a). Lack of access to a regular source of health care may also be a contributing factor because it limits the opportunity of health care professionals to identify persons at risk. Another potential health system influence on suicide is the possibility of physician-assisted suicide. Studies in Oregon (Lee, et al., 1996) and Michigan (Bachman, et al., 1996) indicated that the majority of physicians would support assisted-suicide legislation, and 35 to 46% would be willing to participate in assisted suicide.

Diagnostic Reasoning and Control of Homicide and Suicide

Nursing diagnoses related to homicide and suicide may reflect existing or potential health problems for individuals, families, or population groups. For example, a nursing diagnosis for an individual client might be "potential for homicide due to night work in a high-crime area" or "potential for suicide due to depression following father's death." The nurse working with a family might diagnose "unresolved grief due to suicide of eldest child."

Similar diagnoses at the community level might also reflect either existing problems related to homicide and suicide or potential for increased incidence of either. For example, the nurse might diagnose a "potential for increased incidence of teenage suicide due to media coverage of a group suicide pact" or "increased incidence of homicide due to relaxation of gun control laws."

Planning and Implementing the Dimensions of Health Care in Homicide and Suicide

Control of homicide and suicide may require primary, secondary, or tertiary prevention measures. At each of these levels, intervention may be directed toward the individual or family experiencing the problem or the population as a group.

Primary Prevention

Primary prevention for homicide and suicide is similar to that for family violence and substance abuse and involves promoting a positive self-image and developing adequate coping abilities among clients, particularly those at high risk for suicide or homicide. Educating individual clients and the public with respect to stress management and coping is one means of limiting the incidence of both homicide and suicide. In addition, teaching conflict management strategies can help to prevent homicide. Community health nurses can also encourage clients not to frequent places where homicides commonly occur (eg, a bar in a high-crime area) and not to use alcohol or drugs in circumstances where interpersonal conflict is likely to take place. Another approach to primary prevention of suicide in individuals is treatment of existing psychopathology or substance abuse.

At the aggregate level, limiting access to firearms and other weapons employed in suicide and homicide can contribute to prevention, and community health nurses can plan political activity related to control of guns and other weapons. Nurses can also advocate control of alcohol and drugs that contribute to suicide and homicide or that may be used as a method of suicide.

School-based education about suicide has been suggested as a means of decreasing the incidence of violence among young people (Farrell & Meyer, 1997). It is, however, possible that discussion of suicide may lead to imitative behavior on the part of vulnerable individuals within the group. For this reason, caution is suggested in the implementation of such programs. Any programs that are instituted should make provision for counseling of those students who seem unduly disturbed by discussion of suicide.

Secondary Prevention

Secondary prevention involves the early identification of persons who are contemplating suicide or homicide and intervention to prevent the act or limit the consequences. Nurses, teachers, and counselors may recognize the signs of impending suicide or escalating aggression and should take immediate action. Such action might include counseling, referral, or hospitalization if the danger appears imminent. Community health nurses may also be involved in educating individuals who work with young people, the elderly, and others at risk for suicide to recognize indicators of a potential suicide attempt.

There is at present no evidence to suggest that providing suicide "hotlines" decreases the incidence of suicide. There is also no evidence that such services are harmful, so they may at least be worth a try as a secondary prevention strategy.

Community health nurses and other health care providers can employ a suicide prevention contract with an individual client who has expressed thoughts of committing suicide. A *suicide prevention contract* is a mutual agreement between the nurse and the client that specifies the contributions of each party in preventing the client's self-destruction. The exact nature of what is or is not to be done should be spelled out clearly and simply. For example, the nurse might get the client to agree not to kill himself or herself without first talking to the nurse.

Because clients are reluctant to commit themselves to giving up the notion of suicide permanently, the contract may need to be time-limited at first. For example, the nurse might be able to get the client to agree not to kill oneself until after completing at least

▶ RECOMMENDATIONS FOR A COMMUNITY PLAN TO PREVENT SUICIDE CLUSTERS

1. The community should develop a response plan before the onset of a suicide cluster.
2. The response should involve all concerned segments of the community and should be planned by representatives of all concerned agencies.
3. One agency should be designated to coordinate response planning and be responsible for:
   a. Calling the initial meeting of the planning committee
   b. Establishing a mechanism for notification of a potential suicide cluster
   c. Convening the group when a suicide cluster appears to be occurring
   d. Maintaining the response plan and seeing that the planning group reviews and updates it periodically
4. Relevant community resources should be identified, including hospitals and emergency services, local academic resources, clergy, parent groups, suicide crisis centers or hotlines, survivor groups, students, police, media personnel, and representatives of local government.
5. The plan should be implemented when a suicide cluster occurs or when one or more trauma-related deaths occur that may influence others to commit suicide.
6. Plan implementation should include:
   a. Contacting agencies involved
   b. A review of responsibilities and tasks to be accomplished
   c. Preparation for dealing with the problems and stresses encountered by those responding to the crisis
7. The response should be conducted in a manner that avoids glorifying the victims and minimizes sensationalism by:
   a. Having the spokesperson present as accurate a picture of the victim as possible to students, parents, family, media, and others
   b. Announcing suicides among persons of school age in a manner that maximizes support and minimizes hysteria
8. Persons at risk for suicide should be identified and have at least one screening with a trained counselor. These individuals include relatives of victims, boyfriends or girlfriends, close friends, fellow employees, or students. Identification may be accomplished by:
   a. Identifying people present at funerals who seem particularly upset
   b. Asking teachers to identify students who seem to be at risk
   c. Identifying those associated with the victim who themselves have attempted suicide
   d. Identifying and referring depressed persons
   e. Identifying those with poor social support systems
9. The community may establish a suicide hotline or a walk-in crisis center.
10. Counselors should be provided at a particular site and their availability made known to community residents.
11. The assistance of local media should be sought to disseminate information on sources of help.
12. Counseling services should also be made available to those responding to the crisis.
13. Plans should be made for a timely flow of accurate and appropriate information to the media, including:
    a. Designating a single spokesperson or one spokesperson from each agency involved in the response
    b. Providing accurate information without whitewashing or sensationalism
    c. Providing information on positive steps being taken
    d. Not disclosing the precise mode of suicide employed
    e. Enlisting the help of the community in referring all requests for information to the spokespersons
14. Elements in the initial suicide that might increase the likelihood of other suicides should be identified and changed (eg, erecting barriers along a cliff where suicide has occurred).
15. Long-term issues suggested by the nature of a suicide cluster should be addressed (eg, if all those committing suicide were unemployed, action can be taken to reduce unemployment levels).

(Source: Centers for Disease Control, 1988.)

a month of therapy. Whatever agreement is reached, the nurse witnesses the client's verbal statement of the terms of the contract. This verbalization seems to increase the reality of the contract for the client and strengthens the contract's chances for success. Contracts made in a group setting appear to have even more influence than those made only in the presence of the nurse. Care should be taken not to initiate a suicide prevention contract, particularly with manipulative adolescents, until rapport has been established between nurse and client. Clients with poor impulse control or those who have difficulty forming interpersonal relationships are also poor candidates for suicide prevention contract (Valente, 1992).

Tertiary Prevention

Tertiary prevention is particularly relevant in the prevention of cluster suicides. Because of the traumatic nature of such occurrences, a working group has developed specific guidelines for preventing and controlling cluster suicides. These guidelines include community development of a response plan in the event of the onset of a suicide cluster, involvement of all concerned segments of the community (especially the media to prevent overdramatization of instances of suicide), and coordination of the planned response by one designated agency (Centers for Disease Control, 1988).

Tertiary prevention of suicide and homicide may also involve working with families of victims. The community health nurse can assist family members to work through their grief over the death of a loved one. They can also assist families to deal with any feelings of guilt that they may be suffering. In addition, the nurse can assist violence-prone families to find ways of coping with their loss that prevent further suicide or homicide. Primary, secondary, and tertiary control measures for suicide and homicide are summarized in Table 34–8.

Evaluating Control Strategies for Societal Violence

Whether intervention takes place at the primary, secondary, or tertiary level of prevention, there is a need to evaluate its effectiveness in solving problems of violence. Evaluation of interventions directed toward individuals and their families is assessed in terms of whether the factors underlying a problem have been

TABLE 34–8. GOALS FOR PRIMARY, SECONDARY, AND TERTIARY PREVENTION OF HOMICIDE AND SUICIDE AND RELATED COMMUNITY HEALTH NURSING INTERVENTIONS

Goal of Prevention	Nursing Intervention
PRIMARY PREVENTION	
1. Development of effective coping skills	1. Teach coping skills and stress management skills.
2. Development of self-esteem	2. Foster self-image. Advocate school programs to foster self-esteem in young people.
3. Promotion of nonviolent conflict resolution	3. Teach nonviolent conflict management strategies.
4. Reduction of risk behaviors	4. Encourage clients not to frequent places where homicides occur and not to use drugs and alcohol in circumstances in which interpersonal conflict is likely.
5. Decreased availability of weapons, drugs, and alcohol	5. Engage in political activity to promote control of weapons and limit access to drugs and alcohol.
SECONDARY PREVENTION	
1. Identification of persons contemplating suicide	1. Engage in case finding. Teach teachers and counselors to recognize signs of possible suicide.
2. Provision of counseling for persons at risk for suicide or who express suicidal thoughts	2. Refer for counseling. Use a suicide prevention contract to motivate the client not to commit suicide.
3. Provision of treatment for homicide and suicide victims	3. Engage in political activity and advocacy to ensure adequate treatment facilities.
TERTIARY PREVENTION	
1. Prevention of suicide clusters	1. Assist in the development of community response plans.
2. Provision of care to families of homicide and suicide victims	2. Assist family members to work through feelings of grief and guilt. Assist families to find positive ways to cope with loss.

modified in such a way that the problem is controlled. If the individual is suicidal, have interventions contributed to better abilities to cope with stress? Has recurrent child abuse been prevented? Or, has family communication improved?

TABLE 34–9. STATUS OF SELECTED NATIONAL OBJECTIVES RELATED TO VIOLENCE

	Objective	Base	Most Recent	Target
7.1	Reduce homicide incidence (per 100,000)	10.8 (1991)	9.4 (1995)	7.2
7.2	Reduce suicide incidence (per 100,000)	11.7 (1987)	11 (1995)	10.5
7.3	Reduce weapon-related violent deaths (per 100,000)	14.6 (1990)	13.5 (1995)	11.6
7.4	Reduce the incidence of maltreatment of children (per 1000)	22.6 (1986)	41.9 (1993)	22.6
7.5	Reduce abuse of women by partners (per 1000)	30 (1985)	NDA[a]	27.0
7.8	Reduce adolescent suicide attempts	2.1% (1991)	2.8% (1995)	1.8%
7.10	Reduce weapon carrying by adolescents (incidents per 100 per month)	107 (1991)	81 (1995)	86
7.13	Increase states with child death review systems	33 (1991)	48 (1995)	45
7.15	Reduce proportion of women turned away from shelters	40% (1987)	NDA[a]	10%

[a]NDA, no data available.

(Sources: U.S. Department of Health and Human Services, 1995; 1996b.)

Programs designed to resolve problems of violence at the community or group level are also evaluated in terms of their outcomes; however, the outcome is measured in terms of the extent of the problem in the population. Several national objectives deal with societal violence and can be used as a basis for evaluating control strategies for family violence, homicide, and suicide. The current status of selected objectives related to violence are presented in Table 34–9.

Critical Thinking in Practice: A Case in Point

On a routine postpartum visit, your client, Mrs. Montañez, mentions that she is very concerned about her next-door neighbor, Mrs. Abood, who is pregnant. Mrs. Montañez tells you that she thinks Mr. Abood beat his wife last night. She heard shouting during the night, and this morning she noticed that Mrs. Abood had a black eye that she said she got when she ran into the bedroom door in the dark. Before leaving the apartment complex, you knock on the Aboods' door, but no one answers. You leave your card asking Mrs. Abood to call you.

When Mrs. Abood phones the next day, you explain that you were responding to the concern of a friend for her safety and ask if she is in need of assistance. Mrs. Abood tells you that there is nothing wrong. When you mention that Mrs. Montañez described some injuries, she denies that her husband is abusive. She states that she is receiving prenatal care from a private physician, will contact him if she has any problems with the pregnancy, and is not in need of your services. You accept her refusal of help, but you inform her that you are available and can be reached by phone if she needs assistance at some time in the future.

A month later you receive a call from Mrs. Abood, who asks to see you. She indicates that she is afraid to have you come to her home lest her husband return while you are there. She agrees to meet you at the health department when she comes to get a copy of her daughter's immunization record for school entry.

When you see Mrs. Abood, she admits that her husband beat her the previous day. This is the second time he has assaulted her since she became pregnant. She has several bruises on her face and one particularly large bruise on her abdomen where her husband hit her. Mrs. Abood says that her husband is very jealous and does not believe the baby is his. She insists that she has been faithful to her husband and has tried to convince him of this. She says her husband gets angry because she "shows herself off to other men and gives them a come-on." She comments, "I guess he's right. I do wear shorts a lot, because they're comfortable in this hot weather. I really should try to respect his wishes more."

Mrs. Abood has tried to convince her husband that the baby is his. She has stopped going out with female friends and even tries to avoid talking to the mailman and other males who come to the house. She has not even been to see her family because her husband refuses to go with her and accuses her of meeting her lover on these excursions.

Since the beating yesterday, Mrs. Abood says she is afraid for her own safety as well as that of her unborn child. She says that her husband loves their daughter and would not hurt her. Mrs. Abood has never worked although she completed nursing school before she got married. She feels as though she should get away from her husband even though she still loves him; however, she has no money to support herself and her daughter. She does not feel she can go to relatives because her husband would be able to find her there and bring her back home. She is also afraid that if she leaves him, her husband will attempt to get custody of their daughter.

1. What are the health problems evident in this situation? What are the biophysical, psychological, social, behavioral, and health systems factors influencing these problems?
2. What considerations are important in planning care for Mrs. Abood?
3. What secondary prevention measures would be warranted to deal with existing health problems? Describe specific actions that you would take to resolve these problems.
4. What could be done in terms of tertiary prevention to prevent further consequences or recurrence of health problems in this situation?
5. What primary prevention measures might have prevented the development of the health problems in this situation? How might you, as a community health nurse, be involved in such measures?

TESTING YOUR UNDERSTANDING

1. Describe the four types of child abuse. (pp. 889–890)
2. Describe the three stages of spouse abuse. (p. 890)
3. Identify at least five forms of elder abuse. (p. 891)
4. Describe the influence of at least three biophysical factors in family violence. (pp. 893–895)
5. Identify at least four social dimension and four psychological dimension factors that influence family violence. (pp. 895–898)
6. Describe at least three areas of focus in primary prevention of family violence. How might the community health nurse be involved in each? (pp. 902–905)
7. Identify at least two approaches to the secondary prevention of family violence. What community health nursing activities might be related to each? (pp. 905–907)
8. Describe at least two factors in each of the biophysical, psychological, social, behavioral, and health system dimensions related to homicide. (pp. 907–910)
9. Describe at least two factors in each of the biophysical, psychological, social, behavioral, and health system dimensions related to suicide. (pp. 911–913)
10. Identify at least three primary prevention measures for homicide and suicide. How might the community health nurse be involved in each? (p. 914)

WHAT DO YOU THINK?
Questions for Critical Thinking

1. How would you feel about providing services to a woman who abuses her children? Would you be able to work effectively with this type of client? Why or why not?
2. What considerations would lead you to decide to remove a victim of abuse from an abusive situation? Under what circumstances would you recommend leaving the victim in the home?
3. What recommendations would you have for reducing violence in school settings?
4. You encounter a situation in which an Asian refugee mother has inflicted several round lesions on her 3-year-old daughter's abdomen in the process of "coining" her to cure a stomach ache. One of the lesions has become infected. Would you report the mother to child protective services? Why or why not?

REFERENCES

American Psychological Association. (1996). *Violence and the family: Report of the American Psychological Association Presidential Task Force on Violence and the Family.* Washington, DC: American Psychological Association.

Anderson, C. (1995). Childhood sexually transmitted diseases: One consequence of sexual abuse. *Public Health Nursing, 12,* 41–46.

Arria, A. M., Wood, N. P., & Anthony, J. C. (1995). Prevalence of carrying a weapon and related behaviors in urban school children, 1989 to 1993. *Archives of Pediatric and Adolescent Medicine, 149,* 1345–1350.

Bachman, J. G., Alcser, K. H., Doukas, D. J., et al. (1996). Attitudes of Michigan physicians and the public toward legalizing physician-assisted suicide and voluntary euthanasia. *New England Journal of Medicine, 334,* 303–309.

Bell, R., Duncan, M., Eilenberg, J., et al. (1996). Executive summary. In R. Bell, M. Duncan, & J. Eilenberg, et al. (Eds.), *Violence against women in the United States: A comprehensive background paper* (2nd ed.) (pp. xi–xv). New York: Commonwealth Fund.

Bower, B. (1993). The survivor syndrome. *Science News, 144,* 202–204.

Boy Scouts of America. (1993). *Youth protection guidelines.* Irving, TX: Boy Scouts of America.

Bullman, T. A., & Kang, H. K. (1996). The risk of suicide among wounded Vietnam veterans. *American Journal of Public Health, 86,* 662–667.

Campbell, J. C. (1992). Violence against women. *Nursing & Health Care, 13,* 464–470.

Campbell, J., & Fishwick, N. (1993). Abuse of female partners. In J. Campbell & J. Humphreys (Eds.), *Nursing care of survivors of family violence* (pp. 68–104). St. Louis: Mosby Year Book.

Cappelleri, J. C., Eckenrode, J., & Powers, J. L. (1993). The epidemic of child abuse: Findings from the second national incidence and prevalence study of child abuse and neglect. *American Journal of Public Health, 83,* 1622–1624.

Centers for Disease Control. (1988). CDC recommendations for a community plan for the prevention and containment of suicide clusters. *MMWR, 37*(SS-6), 1–12.

Chez, N. (1994). Helping the victim of domestic violence. *American Journal of Nursing, 94*(7), 33–37.

Coleman, V. E. (1996). Lesbian battering: The relationship between personality and the perpetration of violence. In L. K. Hamberger & C. M. Renzetti (Eds.), *Domestic partner abuse* (pp. 77–102). New York: Springer.

Cummings, P., Koepsell, T. D., Grossman, D. C., Savarino, J., & Thompson, R. S. (1997). The association between purchase of a handgun and homicide or suicide. *American Journal of Public Health, 87,* 974–978.

Dannenberg, A. L., McNeil, J. G., Brundage, J. F., & Brookmeyer, R. (1996). Suicide and HIV infection. *JAMA, 276,* 1743–1746.

Dawson, J. M., & Langan, P. A. (1994). Murder in families. *Bureau of Justice Special Report.* Washington, DC: U.S. Department of Justice.

Division of Violence Prevention. (1995). Suicide among children, adolescents, and young adults—United States, 1980–1992. *MMWR, 44,* 289–291.

Division of Violence Prevention. (1996a). Suicide among older persons—United States, 1980–1992. *MMWR, 45,* 3–6.

Division of Violence Prevention. (1996b). Trends in rates of homicide—United States, 1985–1994. *MMWR, 45,* 460–464.

Division of Violence Prevention. (1997a). Rates of homicide, suicide, and firearm-related death among children—26 industrialized countries. *MMWR, 46,* 101–105.

Division of Violence Prevention. (1997b). Regional variation in suicide rates—United States, 1990–1994. *MMWR, 46,* 789–793.

Dorfman, L., Woodruff, K., Chavez, V., & Wallack, L. (1997). Youth and violence on local television news in California. *American Journal of Public Health, 87,* 1311–1316.

Duncan, M. (1996). Help-seeking and social support. In R. Bell, M. Duncan, & J. Eilenberg, et al. (Eds.), *Violence against women in the United States: A comprehensive background paper* (2nd ed.) (pp. 53–79). New York: Commonwealth Fund.

Eilenberg, J., & Fullilove, M. (1996). Introduction. In R. Bell, M. Duncan, & J. Eilenberg, et al. (Eds.), *Violence against women in the United States: A comprehensive background paper* (2nd ed.) (pp. 1–5). New York: Commonwealth Fund.

Family and Intimate Violence Prevention Team. (1996). Physical violence and injuries in intimate relationships—New York, Behavioral Risk Factor Surveillance System, 1994. *MMWR, 45,* 765–767.

Farrell, A. D., & Meyer, A. L. (1997). The effectiveness of a school-based curriculum for reducing violence among urban sixth-grade students. *American Journal of Public Health, 87,* 979–984.

Fishbain, D. A. (1996). Current research on chronic pain and suicide. *American Journal of Public Health, 86,* 1320–1321.

Fullilove, M. (1996). Patterns of violence. In R. Bell, M. Duncan, & J. Eilenberg, et al. (Eds.), *Violence against women in the United States: A comprehensive background paper* (2nd ed.) (pp. 7–23). New York: Commonwealth Fund.

Goetting, A. (1994). *Homicide in families and other special populations.* New York: Springer.

Hamberger, L. K., & Potente, T. (1996). Counseling het-erosexual women arrested for domestic violence: Implications for theory and practice. In L. K. Hamberger & C. M. Renzetti (Eds.), *Domestic partner abuse* (pp. 53–75). New York: Springer.

Hammers, M. (1993). Domestic violence: Facing the epidemic. *NURSEweek, 6*(1), 6–8.

Hanrahan, P., Campbell, J., & Ulrich, Y. (1993). Theories of violence. In J. Campbell & J. Humphreys (Eds.), *Nursing care of survivors of family violence* (pp. 3–35). St. Louis: Mosby Year Book.

Humphreys, J., & Ramsey, A. M. (1993). Child abuse. In J. Campbell & J. Humphreys (Eds.), *Nursing care of survivors of family violence* (pp. 36–67). St Louis: Mosby Year Book.

Innes, L., & Mellman, L. (1996). Treatment for victims of violence. In R. Bell, M. Duncan, & J. Eilenberg, et al. (Eds.), *Violence against women in the United States: A comprehensive background paper* (2nd ed.) (pp. 39–51). New York: Commonwealth Fund.

Jackson, N. A. (1996). Observational experiences of intrapersonal conflict and teenage victimization: A comparative study among spouses and cohabitors. *Journal of Family Violence, 11,* 191–203.

Kann, L., Warren, C. W., Harris, W. A., et al. (1996). Youth Risk Behavior Surveillance—United States, 1995. *MMWR, 45*(SS-4), 1–84.

Kawachi, I., Willett, W. C., Colditz, G. A., Stampfer, M. J., & Speizer, F. E. (1996). A prospective study of coffee drinking and suicide in women. *Archives of Internal Medicine, 156,* 521–525.

Kelleher, K., Chaffin, M., Hollenberg, J., & Fischer, E. (1994). Alcohol and drug disorders among physically abusive and neglectful parents in a community-based sample. *American Journal of Public Health, 84,* 1586–1590.

Lee, M. A., Nelson, H. D., Tilden, V. P., et al. (1996). Legalizing assisted suicide—Views of physicians in Oregon. *New England Journal of Medicine, 334,* 310–315.

Letellier, P. (1996). Gay and bisexual male domestic violence victimization: Challenges to feminist theory and responses to violence. In L. K. Hamberger & C. M. Renzetti (Eds.), *Domestic partner abuse* (pp. 1–21). New York: Springer.

Limandri, B. J., & Tilden, V. P. (1996). Nurses' reasoning in the assessment of family violence. *Image: Journal of Nursing Scholarship, 28,* 247–252.

Maiuro, R. D., & Avery, D. H. (1996). Psychopharmacological treatment of aggressive behavior: Implications for domestically violent men. In L. K. Hamberger & C. M. Renzetti (Eds.), *Domestic partner abuse* (pp. 153–190). New York: Springer.

Marshall, W. L., Bryce, P., Hudson, S. M., Ward, T., & Moth, B. (1996). The enhancement of intimacy and the reduction of loneliness among child molesters. *Journal of Family Violence, 11,* 219–235.

McCauley, J., Kern, D. E., Kolodner, K., et al. (1995). The

"battering syndrome:" Prevalence and clinical characteristics of domestic violence in primary care internal medicine practices. *Annals of Internal Medicine, 123,* 737–746.

Mellman, L., & Bell, R. (1996). Consequences of violence against women. In R. Bell, M. Duncan, & J. Eilenberg, et al. (Eds.), *Violence against women in the United States: A comprehensive background paper* (2nd ed.) (pp. 31–37). New York: Commonwealth Fund.

Myers, G. P., McGrady, G. A., Marrow, C., & Mueller, C. W. (1997). Weapon carrying among black adolescents: A social network perspective. *American Journal of Public Health, 87,* 1038–1040.

National Center for Injury Prevention and Control. (1995). Fatal and nonfatal suicide attempts among adolescents—Oregon, 1988–1993. *MMWR, 44,* 312–315, 321–323.

National Commission on Correctional Health Care. (1993). *Correctional health care and the prevention of violence.* Chicago: National Commission on Correctional Health Care.

National Institute for Occupational Safety and Health. (1996). *Violence in the workplace: Risk factors and prevention strategies.* Cincinnati: National Institute for Occupational Safety and Health.

O'Carroll, P. W., & Potter, L. B. (1994). Suicide contagion and the reporting of suicide: Recommendations from a national workshop. *MMWR, 43*(RR–6), 9–18.

Pillemer, K., & Frankel, S. (1991). Domestic violence against the elderly. In M. L. Rosenberg & M. A. Fenton (Eds.), *Violence in America: A public health approach* (pp. 158–183). New York: Oxford University Press.

Raistick, D. (1994). Alcohol, other drugs, and violence. In J. Shepherd (Ed.), *Violence in health care: A practical guide to coping with violence and caring for victims* (pp. 43–62). Oxford: Oxford University Press.

Rosenberg, M. L., & Mercy, J. A. (1991). Assaultive violence. In M. L. Rosenberg & M. A. Fenton (Eds.), *Violence in America: A public health approach* (pp. 15–50). New York: Oxford University Press.

Schiavone, F. M. (1996). Routine screening is good health policy. *Health Alert, 4*(1), 1–2, 4.

Senstock, M. C., & Barrett, S. A. (1993). Abuse and neglect of the elderly in family settings. In J. Campbell & J. Humphreys (Eds.), *Nursing care of survivors of family violence* (pp. 173–208). St. Louis: Mosby Year Book.

Shaffer, D., & Hicks, R. (1994). Suicide. In I. B. Pless (Ed.), *The epidemiology of childhood disorders* (pp. 339–365). New York: Oxford University Press.

Sigler, R. T. (1995). The cost of tolerance for violence. *Journal of Health Care for the Poor and Underserved, 6,* 124–134.

Stark, E., & Flitcraft, A. H. (1991). Spouse abuse. In M. L. Rosenberg & M. A. Fenton (Eds.), *Violence in Amer-*ica: A public health approach* (pp. 123–157). New York: Oxford University Press.

Sugg, N.K., & Inui, T. (1992). Primary care physicians' response to domestic violence: Opening Pandora's box. *JAMA, 267,* 3157–3160.

Tilden, V. P., Schmidt, T. A., Limandri, B. J., Chiodo, G. T., Garland, M. J., & Loveless, P. A. (1994). Factors that influence clinicians' assessment and management of family violence. *American Journal of Nursing, 84,* 628–633.

U.S. Department of Commerce. (1996). *Statistical abstract of the United States, 1996.* Washington, DC: Government Printing Office.

U.S. Department of Health and Human Services. (1992). *Child abuse: A shared community concern.* Washington, DC: Government Printing Office.

U.S. Department of Health and Human Services. (1995). *Healthy People 2000: Midcourse review and 1995 revisions.* Washington, DC: Government Printing Office.

U.S. Department of Health and Human Services. (1996a). *Health United States, 1995.* Washington, DC: Government Printing Office.

U.S. Department of Health and Human Services. (1996b, November 26). *Healthy people 2000: Progressive review—Violent and abusive behavior.* Washington, DC: Government Printing Office.

Valente, S. (1992). Suicide info missing. *NURSEweek, 5*(21), 6–7.

Warnken, W. J., Rosenbaum, A., Fletcher, K., Hoge, S. K., & Adelman, S. A. (1996). Head-injured males: A population at risk for relationship aggression. In L. K. Hamberger & C. M. Renzetti (Eds.), *Domestic partner abuse* (pp. 103–124). New York: Springer.

Webster, D. W., Vernick, J. S., Ludwig, J., & Lester, K. J. (1997). Flawed gun policy could endanger public safety. *American Journal of Public Health, 876,* 918–921.

Weiler, K. (1989). Financial abuse of the elderly: Recognizing and acting on it. *Journal of Gerontological Nursing, 15*(8), 10–15.

Wonderlich, S. A., Wilsnack, R. W., Wilsnack, S. C., & Harris, T. R. (1996). Childhood sexual abuse and bulimic behavior in a nationally representative sample. *American Journal of Public Health, 86,* 1082–1086.

RESOURCES FOR DEALING WITH FAMILY VIOLENCE

Batterers Anonymous
1850 N. Riverside Avenue, No. 220
Rialto, CA 92376
(909) 355–1100

Child Abuse Listening and Mediation
PO Box 90754
Santa Barbara, CA 93190–0754
(805) 965–2376

Emerge: Counseling and Education
   to Stop Male Violence
2380 Massachusetts Avenue, Ste. 101
Cambridge, MA 02104
(617) 547–9879

National Clearinghouse on Child Abuse
   and Neglect Information
PO Box 1182
Washington, DC 20013–1182
(800) FYI–3366

National Coalition Against Domestic Violence
PO Box 18749
Denver, CO 80218
(303) 839–1852

National Coalition Against Sexual Assault
912 N. 2nd Street
Harrsiburg, PA 17102
(717) 232–6745

National Committee to Prevent Child Abuse
332 South Michigan Avenue, Ste. 1600
Chicago, IL 60604–4357
(312) 663–3520

National Council on Child Abuse
   & Family Violence
1155 Connecticut Avenue, NW, Ste. 400
Washington, DC 20036
(202) 429–6695

National Resource Center
   on Child Abuse and Neglect
63 Inverness Drive East
Englewood, CO 80112–5117
(800) 227–5242

SOURCES OF INFORMATION AND ASSISTANCE IN CONTROLLING SUICIDE

American Association of Suicidology
4201 Connecticut Avenue, NW, Ste. 310
Washington, DC 20008
(202) 237–2280

International Association for Suicide Prevention
Institut fur Medical Psychologie
Severingasse 9
A-1090 Vienna, Austria

Samaritans
500 Commonwealth Avenue
Kenmore Square
Boston, MA 02215
(617) 247–0220

Seasons: Suicide Bereavement
c/o Tina Larsen
PO Box 187
Park City, UT 84060
(801) 649–8327

Youth Suicide Prevention
11 Parkman Way
Needham, MA 02192–2863
(617) 738–0700

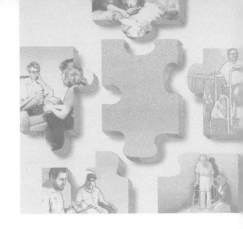

RECOMMENDED READING

CHAPTER 1: THE COMMUNITY CONTEXT

Anderson, R., & Milliner, R. (1990). Assessing the health objectives of the nation. *Health Affairs, 9(2),* 152–162.

> *Critiques the process and result of efforts to create the original set of National Health Objectives for 1990. Also addresses the extent to which objectives were met. Goes on to evaluate the objectives for the year 2000.*

Mason, J. O. (1990). A prevention policy framework for the nation. *Health Affairs, 9(2),* 22–29.

> *Describes the evolution of the national objectives for the year 2000 and addresses their application to local communities. Discusses the differences between the 1990 and year 2000 objectives.*

CHAPTER 2: THE HISTORICAL CONTEXT

Bramadat, I. J., & Saydak, M. I. (1993). Nursing on the Canadian Prairies, 1900–1930: Effects of Immigration. *Nursing History Review, 1,* 105–117.

> *Describes the care provided by community health nurses to early immigrants to the Canadian prairies and the problems encountered in their care.*

Crandall, E. P. (1993). The relation of public health nursing to the public health campaign. *Public Health Nursing, 10,* 204–209. Reprinted from *American Journal of Public Health,* March, 1915.

> *Provides an historical overview of the contributions of community health nurses to the achievement of the goals of public health related to tuberculosis.*

Ecker, M. (1997, April 28). Celebrate the work of a little-known nurse heroine. *NURSEweek,* 13.

> *Describes the work of Mary Seacole, a Jamaican healer who provided health care during the Crimean War.*

Hitchcock, J. E. (1993). Five hundred cases of pneumonia. *Public Health Nursing, 10,* 170–172. Reprinted from *American Journal of Nursing,* December, 1902.

> *Describes the world of the Henry Street nurses during an epidemic of pneumonia in New York City in 1901.*

Miller, A. F. (1993). Community responsibility with regard to tuberculosis. *Canadian Journal of Public Health, 84,* 293. Reprinted from *The Public Health Journal,* March, 1923.

> *Proposes three steps to identifying patients with tuberculosis in Canada in the 1920s: (1) building of community partnerships through a publicity campaign, (2) inspection and weighing of all school children, and (3) a sanitary survey.*

Mosley, M. O. P., (1996). Satisfied to carry the bag: Three black community health nurses' contribution to health-care reform, 1900–1937. *Nursing History Review, 4,* 65–82.

Describes the contributions made by three of the first African American public health nurses to the early development of community health nursing and their efforts to improve the health status of the black population of New York City at the beginning of the 20th century.

Ruffing-Rahal, M. A. (1995). The Navajo experience of Elizabeth Foster, public health nurse. *Nursing History Review, 3*, 173–188.

Presents an overview of the public health nursing practice of Elizabeth Foster, one of the first public health field nurses of the Bureau of Indian Affairs. Describes her collaboration with a noted photographer in capturing the way of life of the Navajo.

Smith, S. L. (1994). White nurses, black midwives, and public health in Mississippi, 1920–1950. *Nursing History Review, 2*, 29–49.

Describes a collaborative effort by public health nurses and black lay midwives to improve the health of pregnant women in the Southeast. What began as an effort to coopt the practice of lay midwives ended in creating a sound, culturally sensitive infrastructure for the delivery of public health services in Mississippi.

Shore, H. L. (1993). Frances Redmond: A pioneer in community health in Vancouver. *Canadian Journal of Public Health, 84*, 13.

Provides a brief description of the practice of Frances Redmond, the first community health nurse in Vancouver, British Columbia.

CHAPTER 3: THE HEALTH CARE CONTEXT

Le Faou, A., & Jolly, D. (1995). Health promotion in France: Toward a new way of giving medical care. *Hospital Topics, 73*(2), 17–21.

Provides a description of France's health care system and efforts to increase the national emphasis on health promotion.

Hurrelmann, K., & Laaser, U. (Eds.). (1996). *International handbook of public health*. Westport, CT: Greenwood Press.

Provides a brief overview of the health care system, including the public health infrastructure, in several countries throughout the world.

Pozanti, M. S., & Bruder, P. (1995). The Turkish healthcare system: Can the United States learn from the Ottoman legacy? *Hospital Topics, 73*(2), 28–34.

Presents a picture of the health care system in Turkey, including both the preventive and curative aspects of care. Also describes similarities and differences between the U.S. and Turkish health care systems.

Swanson, J. (1987). Nursing in Cuba: Population-focused practice. *Public Health Nursing, 4*, 183–191.

Describes the Cuban health care system and its use of

community health nurses as primary care providers in population-based health care.

UNICEF. (1995). *The State of the World's Children*. Oxford: Oxford University Press.

Provides a good overview of concerted international action to resolve health problems. Examines goals for worldwide child health and progress made toward achieving those goals.

CHAPTER 4: COMMUNITY HEALTH NURSING

Bryans, A., & McIntosh, J. (1996). Decision making in community health nursing: An analysis of the stages of decision making as they relate to community nursing assessment practice. *Journal of Advanced Nursing, 24*, 24–30.

Applies decision theory to the types of decisions made in community health nursing.

Kelly, A. (1996). The concept of the specialist community nurse. *Journal of Advanced Nursing, 24*, 42–52.

Presents arguments for classification of community health nursing as an area of specialization based on the characteristics of specialization.

Jezewski, M. A. (1993). Culture brokering as a model for advocacy. *Nursing & Health Care, 14*, 78–85.

Discusses the concept of culture brokering as a model for client advocacy. Maintains that advocacy is essentially a process of mediating between the health professional culture and the culture of the lay community.

Making a difference: Public health nursing. (1993). Edmonton, Alberta: Family Health Services

Describes ten core themes in public health nurses' descriptions of their practice. Provides several anecdotes from nurses to support the themes identified. Presents an interesting view of community health nursing from the perspective of practicing community health nurses.

McMurray, A. (1992). Expertise in community health nursing. *Journal of Community Health Nursing, 9*(2), 65–75.

Reports findings of a study to identify characteristics of expert community health nurses and factors influencing the development of clinical expertise in community health nursing.

Reutter, L. I., & Ford, J. S. (1996). Perceptions of public health nursing: Views from the field. *Journal of Advanced Nursing, 24*, 7–15.

Presents findings of a study of public health nurses' perceptions of the valuable elements of their practice.

Zerwekh, J. V. (1991). At the expense of their souls. *Nursing Outlook, 39*, 58–61.

Describes the results of interviews with practicing community health nurses and the struggles and frustration of practice with multiproblem clients.

Zerwekh, J. V., Young, B., Primo, J., & Deal, L. (1993). *Opening doors: Stories of public health nursing.* Olympia, WA: Washington State Department of Health.

A collection of stories describing the practice of community health nursing derived from the experience of practicing community health nurses.

CHAPTER 5: THE DIMENSIONS MODEL OF COMMUNITY HEALTH NURSING

Baker, J. E. L. (1992). Primary, secondary, and tertiary prevention in reducing pesticide-related illness in farmers. *Journal of Community Health Nursing, 9*(4), 245–254.

Provides a good example of the use of all three levels of prevention in addressing a specific health problem.

Martin, K. J. (1995). Workers' compensation: Case management strategies. *AAOHN Journal, 43,* 245–250.

Applies the concepts of primary, secondary, and tertiary prevention to the care of work injuries by occupational health nurses.

CHAPTER 6: OTHER MODELS FOR COMMUNITY HEALTH NURSING

Barnum B. S. (1994). *Nursing theory: Analysis, application, evaluation* (4th ed.). Philadelphia: Lippincott.

Examines several nursing theories, critiques them, and evaluates their applicability to nursing practice.

Fawcett, J. (1993). *Analysis and evaluation of conceptual models of nursing* (3rd ed.). Philadelphia: F. A. Davis.

Presents an overview of several nursing models and evaluates them in light of their utility for practice.

Fitzpatrick, J. L., & Whall, A. L. (Eds.). (1996). *Conceptual models of nursing: Analysis and application* (3rd ed.). Stamford, CT: Appleton & Lange.

Examines the theoretical models of several nurse theorists. Presents an overview of nursing theory.

CHAPTER 7: THE NURSING PROCESS

Bowles, K. H., & Naylor, M. D. (1996). Nursing intervention classification systems. *Image: Journal of Nursing Scholarship, 28,* 303–308.

Describes several systems for classifying nursing interventions including the Omaha System, the Iowa Nursing Intervention Classification, and the Home Health Care Classification. Also discusses the need for classification systems and their implications for nursing.

Hansten, R. I., & Washburn, M. J. (1994). *Clinical delegation skills: A handbook for nurses.* Gaithersburg, MD: Aspen.

Describes aspects of delegation by nurses. Addresses a variety of considerations in making delegation decisions as well as how to promote acceptance of delegated activities.

Marek, K. D. (1996). Nursing diagnoses and home care nursing utilization. *Public Health Nursing, 13,* 195–200.

Presents the findings of a study to identify nursing diagnoses predictive of the utilization of home nursing services. Uses the Omaha System as the basis for nursing diagnoses in a home health setting.

Neufeld, A., & Harrison, M. J. (1990). The development of nursing diagnoses for aggregates and groups. *Public Health Nursing, 7,* 251–255.

Discusses the process of developing nursing diagnoses related to population groups. Addresses some of the considerations in diagnoses at this level.

CHAPTER 8: THE EPIDEMIOLOGIC PROCESS

Ashton, J. (Ed.). (1994). *The epidemiological imagination: A reader.* Philadelphia: Open University Press.

A series of current and historical essays on epidemiology.

Brubacher, B. H. (1983). Health promotion: A linguistic analysis. *Advances in Nursing Science, 5*(3), 1–14.

Analyzes the meaning of the term "health promotion" as used in community health, medical, and wellness literature. Identifies common themes in the definition of health promotion to create an encompassing definition of the term.

Harkness, G. A. (1995). *Epidemiology in nursing practice.* St. Louis: Mosby.

Provides an overview of epidemiology from a nursing perspective. Relates the epidemiologic process to the nursing process.

Pender, N. J. (1996). *Health promotion in nursing practice* (3rd ed.). Stamford, CT: Appleton & Lange.

Describes nursing strategies for promotion of clients' health. Presents a model of health promotion for nursing practice.

CHAPTER 9: THE HEALTH EDUCATION PROCESS

Bastable, S. B. (1997). Teaching strategies specific to developmental stages of life. In S. B. Bastable (Ed.), *Nurse as educator: Principles of teaching and learning* (pp. 91–123). Boston: Jones & Bartlett.

Examines the utility of specific teaching strategies in health education for specific age groups based on developmental level.

Bloom, B. S., Englehart, M. D., Furst, E. J., Hill, W. F., & Krathwohl, D. R. (1956). *Taxonomy of educational objectives: The classification of educational goals: Handbook 1: The cognitive domain.* New York: David McKay.

Describes early work on the taxonomy of learning objectives for the cognitive domain. Describes, in detail, each level within the domain, as well as subheadings within each level.

Braungart, M. M., & Braungart, R. G. (1997). Learning theory and nursing practice. In S. B. Bastable (Ed.), *Nurse as educator: Principles of teaching and learning* (pp. 31–52). Boston: Jones & Bartlett.

Presents an overview of theoretical perspectives on learning.

Green, L. W., & Kreuter, M. W. (1991). *Health promotion planning: An educational and environmental approach* (2nd ed.). Mountain View, CA: Mayfield.

Describes the PRECEDE and PROCEED models and the levels of educational diagnosis. Addresses the application of the models in practice.

Kitchie, S. (1997). Determinants of learning. In S. B. Bastable (Ed.), *Nurse as educator: Principles of teaching and learning* (pp. 55–89). Boston: Jones & Bartlett.

Presents a PEEK model for assessing readiness to learn that encompasses Physical readiness, Emotional readiness, Experiential readiness, Knowledge readiness. Also discusses principles of learning related to learning style.

Krathwohl, D. R., Bloom, B. S., & Masia, B. B. (1964). *Taxonomy of educational objectives: The classification of educational goals: Handbook 1: The affective domain.* New York: David McKay.

CHAPTER 10: THE HOME VISIT PROCESS AND HOME HEALTH NURSING

Brady, J. (1995). Branching out into home care. *American Journal of Nursing, 85*(6), 34–35.

Describes the experiences of a nurse in the transition from hospital nursing to home health nursing.

Braveman, P., Miller, C., Egerten, S., Bennett, T., English, P., Katz, P., & Showstack, J. (1996). Health service use among low-risk newborns after early discharge with and without nurse home visiting. *Journal of the American Board of Family Practice, 9,* 254–260.

Presents findings of a study of the effects of nursing home visits on newborns after early discharge. Home visits resulted in fewer hospital admissions and acute care visits, as well as fewer missed well-child appointments.

Byrd, M. E. (1995). A concept analysis of home visiting. *Public Health Nursing, 12,* 83–89.

Analyzes the concept of home visiting from historical and current literature. Presents the historical foundation for home visiting and delineates phases in the current home visiting process.

Close, P., Burkey, E., Kazak, A., Danz, P., & Lange, B. (1995). A prospective, controlled evaluation of home chemotherapy for children with cancer. *Pediatrics, 95,* 896–900.

Discusses findings of a study of the effects of home chemotherapy for children with cancer. Home therapy resulted in lower costs and better client outcomes than inpatient therapy.

Josten, L. E., Mullett, S. E., Savik, K., Campbell, R., & Vincent, P. (1995). Client characteristics associated with not keeping appointments for public health nursing home visits. *Public Health Nursing, 12,* 305–311.

Presents findings of a study of factors related to missed appointments with public health nurses making home visits.

Rice, R. (Ed.), *Home health nursing practice: Concepts and application* (2nd ed.). St. Louis: Mosby.

Presents an excellent overview of home health nursing practice.

Stewart, C. J., Blaha, A. J., Weissfield, L., & Yuan, W. (1995). Discharge planning from home health care and patient status post discharge. *Public Health Nursing, 12,* 90–98.

Describes findings of a study of community health nurse activities related to discharge planning. Presents a model for home health care.

CHAPTER 11: THE CASE MANAGEMENT PROCESS

Case Management Society of America. (1995). *Standards of practice for case management.* Little Rock, AR: Case Management Society of America.

Describes standards of care and standards of performance for case management. Also presents measurement criteria related to the standards.

Daly, G. M., & Mitchell, R. D. (1996). Case management in the community setting. *Advanced Practice Nursing, 31,* 527–534.

Describes a nurse managed community health organization in which community health nurses provide case management services for a group of elderly clients.

Flarey, D. L., & Blancett, S. S. (Eds.), *Handbook of nursing case management: Health care delivery in a world of managed care.* Gaithersburg, MD: Aspen.

Presents an overview of case management practice by nurses. Addresses a number of issues related to case management.

St. Couer, M. (1996). *Case management practice guidelines.* St. Louis: Mosby.

Briefly discusses basic principles and concepts of case

management. Then provides case management guidelines for clients with specific health problems.

CHAPTER 12: THE CHANGE, LEADERSHIP, AND GROUP PROCESSES

Misener, T. R., Alexander, J. W., Blaha, A. J., et al. (1997). National Delphi study to determine competencies for nursing leadership in public health. *Image: Journal of Nursing Scholarship, 29*, 47–51.

Describes the findings of a study to determine the leadership competencies needed by nurse leaders in public health.

Pointer, D. D., & Sanchez, J. P. (1997). Leadership in public health practice. In F. D. Scutchfield & C. W. Keck (Eds.), *Principles of public health practice,* (pp. 87–100). Albany, NY: Delmar.

Provides an overview of contingency leadership theories and their application in public health practice.

Porter-O'Grady, T. (1995). *The leadership revolution in health care: Altering systems, changing behaviors.* Gaithersburg, MD: Aspen.

Describes competencies required in nursing leadership in health care systems. Also presents an overview of the leadership process.

Taccetta-Chapnick, M. (1996). Transformational leadership. *Nursing Administration Quarterly, 21*(1), 60–66.

Discusses transformational leadership. Also addresses elements of the change and group processes.

Wiles, R., & Robinson, J. (1994). Teamwork in primary care: The views and experiences of nurses, midwives, and health visitors. *Journal of Advanced Nursing, 20,* 324–330.

Describes the findings of a study of nurses' perceptions of teamwork in primary care teams. Findings are described in terms of three subject groups: primary care nurses, midwives, and health visitors.

CHAPTER 13: THE POLITICAL PROCESS

Betts, V. T. (1996). Nursing's agenda for health care reform: Policy, politics, and power through professional leadership. *Nursing Administration Quarterly, 20*(3), 1–8.

Describes the participation of nursing as a professional group in the debate over health care reform that took place from 1991 to 1994 and the gains that nursing achieved through that participation.

Boykin, A. (Ed.). (1994). *Power, politics, and public policy: A matter of caring.* New York: National League for Nursing.

Presents the need for nursing to engage in political activity to maintain the caring focus of the profession.

Gebbie, K. M. (1996). National health policy: Lessons from a hot seat. *Nursing Administration Quarterly, 20*(3), 9–18.

Describes the experiences of one nurse policy maker in the development of national policies for HIV/AIDS, including the lessons learned for the nursing profession.

Helms, L. B., Anderson, M. A., & Hanson, K. (1996). "Doin' politics": Linking policy and politics in nursing. *Nursing Administration Quarterly, 20*(3), 32–41.

Discusses the influence of the policy environment on the development of health care policy and on participation by nurses in that process.

Longest, B. B. Jr. (1994). *Health policy making in the United States.* Ann Arbor, MI: AUPHA Press.

Presents an excellent overview of the political process.

Meyer, C. (1992). Nursing on the political front. *American Journal of Nursing, 82*(10), 56–64.

Describes the experiences of several nurse leaders in their attempts to influence health care policy.

Roberts, J. I., & Group, T. M. (1995). *Feminism and nursing: An historical perspective on power, status, and political activism in the nursing profession.* Westport, CT: Praeger.

Presents an historical perspective on political activism by nurses from the days of Henry Street to the present. Relates this participation to women's issues as well as to health.

Schneider, J. K., Shawver, M. M., & Martin, A. (1993). Applying a political model to program development. *Nursing Management, 24*(10), 52–55.

Discusses the application of Baldridge's political model to the development of a discharge planning program.

CHAPTER 14: ECONOMIC INFLUENCES ON COMMUNITY HEALTH

Melillo, K. D. (1996). Medicare and Medicaid: Similarities and differences. *Journal of Gerontological Nursing, 22*(7), 12–21.

Presents an excellent overview of the provisions of Medicare. Also discusses Medicaid as it existed prior to the Medigrant proposal.

Pauly, M. V. (1993). U.S. health care costs: The untold true story. *Health Affairs, 12,* 152–159.

Discusses the cost of health care in terms of lost opportunity costs, lost opportunities to address other societal needs.

Shamansky, S. L. (1996). Yet another treatise on managed care. *Public Health Nursing, 13,* 161–162.

Describes a true managed care system and contrasts it with the current situation in health care delivery.

Wyld, D. C. (1996). The capitation revolution in health care: Implications for the field of nursing. *Nursing Administration Quarterly, 20*(2), 1–12.

Explores the implications of a capitated health care delivery system for nursing.

CHAPTER 15: ETHICAL INFLUENCES ON COMMUNITY HEALTH

Aroskar, M. (1989). Community health nurses: Their most significant ethical decision-making problems. *Nursing Clinics of North America, 24,* 967–975.

Presents findings of a research study of ethical problems encountered by community health nurses and the typical values conflicts that arise in practice.

Bayer, R., Dubler, N. N., & Landesman, S. (1993). The dual epidemics of tuberculosis and AIDS: Ethical and policy issues in screening and treatment. *American Journal of Public Health, 83,* 649–653.

Addresses ethical problems inherent in mandatory screening for HIV infection and tuberculosis and the practice of involuntary isolation of clients who refuse tuberculosis therapy.

Kerrige, I. H., & Mitchell, K. R. (1996). The legislation of active voluntary euthanasia in Australia: Will the slippery slope prove fatal? *Journal of Medical Ethics, 22,* 273–278.

Describes the current status of euthanasia in The Netherlands.

Monagle, J. E., & Thomasma, D. C. (Eds.). (1994). *Health care ethics: Critical issues.* Gaithersburg, MD: Aspen.

Presents a good explication of a variety of ethical issues facing health care providers.

O'Neil, T. (Ed.). (1994). *Biomedical ethics: Opposing viewpoints.* San Diego: Greenhaven Press.

Presents opposing views of several controversial issues in biomedical ethics including human subjects research, organ transplants, reproductive technology, and genetic research.

CHAPTER 16: CULTURAL INFLUENCES ON COMMUNITY HEALTH

Abel, E. K. (1996). "We are left so much alone to work out our own problems": Nurses on American Indian Reservations during the 1930s. *Nursing History Review, 4,* 43–64.

Presents an historical look at nursing among Native Americans and the barriers to providing culturally competent care.

The American Indian patient. (1992). *The Crib Sheet, 6*(1), 2, 4.

Discusses cultural practices related to pregnancy and birth among Native Americans.

American Indian Tobacco Education Network. (1996). *Tobacco and the American Indian.* Sacramento, CA: California Rural Indian Health Board.

Discusses the symbolic and ritual uses of tobacco in Native American cultures.

Andrews, M. M. (1989). Culture and nutrition. In J. S. Boyle & M. M. Andrews (Eds.), *Transcultural perspectives in nursing* (pp. 333–355). Glenview, IL: Scott, Foresman.

Provides an overview of nutritional considerations related to culture.

Berry, J. W. (1991). Refugee adaptation in settlement countries: An overview with an emphasis on primary prevention. In F. L. Ahearn & J. L. Athey (Eds.), *Refugee children: Theory, research, and services* (pp. 287–313). Baltimore: Johns Hopkins University Press.

Addresses cultural implications in the care of refugee populations.

Boyle, J. S., & Counts, M. M. (1988). Toward healthy aging: A theory for community health nursing. *Public Health Nursing, 5,* 45–51.

Presents cultural considerations in the care of the elderly.

Camazine, S. (1986). Zuni medicine: Folklore or pharmacy, science or sorcery. In R. P. Steiner (Ed.), *Folk medicine: The art and the science* (pp. 23–40). Washington, DC: American Chemical Society.

Describes folk healing practices and practitioners among the Zuni Indian tribe.

Caudle, P. W. (1992). *How Latinas come to know about AIDS.* Unpublished doctoral dissertation, University of San Diego.

Addresses cultural considerations in the prevention of HIV infection among Latinas.

Chang, K. (1991). Chinese Americans. In J. N. Giger & R. E. Davidhizar (Eds.), *Transcultural nursing: Assessment and intervention* (pp. 359–377). St. Louis: Mosby Year Book.

Provides an overview of Chinese American culture.

Cooper, R. M. (1992). *The impact of child care on the socialization of African American children.* Pasadena, CA: Pacific Oaks College.

Examines family values and child socialization among African Americans.

Daly, E. B. (1995). Health meanings of Saudi women. *Journal of Advanced Nursing, 21,* 853–857.

Explores the definitions of health and health practices among Saudi women.

Dicharry, E. K. (1986). Delivering home health care to the elderly in Zuni pueblo. *Journal of Gerontological Nursing, 12*(7), 25–29.

Addresses cultural considerations in the care of the elderly among the Zuni.

Fontenot, W. L. (1994). *Secret doctors: Ethnomedicine of African Americans.* Westport, CT: Bergin & Garvey.

Describes folk health practitioners and practices in African American society. Presents both an historical and current perspective on folk healing in this cultural group.

Gagne, P. L. (1992). Appalachian women: Violence and social control. *Journal of Contemporary Ethnography*, 20, 387–415.

Discusses cultural influences in the abuse of Appalachian women.

Guendelman, S., & Abrams, B. (1995). Dietary intake among Mexican-American women: Generational differences and a comparison with white non-Hispanic women. *American Journal of Public Health*, 85, 20–25.

Examines dietary changes in Mexican American women with increasing acculturation.

Gwinn, E. R., & Gwinn, D. (1994). Food and dietary adaptation among Hispanics in the United States. In T. Weaver (Ed.), *Handbook of Hispanic cultures in the United States: Anthropology* (pp. 339–366). Houston: Arte Publico Press.

Discusses changing dietary patterns among Latinos in the United States.

Kay, M. A. (1977). Health and illness in a Mexican American barrio. In E. H. Spicer (Ed.), *Ethnic medicine in the southwest.* Tucson: University of Arizona.

Provides an early and detailed qualitative study of cultural health practices among Mexican Americans.

Keefe, S. E. (1986). Southern Appalachia: Analytical models, social services, and natural support systems. *American Journal of Community Psychology*, 14, 479–498.

Discusses the cultural context of social support in Appalachia.

Laderman, C., & Van Esterik, P. (1988). Techniques of healing in Southeast Asia. *Social Science and Medicine*, 27, 747–750.

Provides an overview of folk health practitioners and practices among Southeast Asians.

Lantz, J. E., & Harper, K. (1989). Network intervention, existential depression, and the relocated Appalachian family. *Contemporary Family Therapy*, 11, 213–223.

Addresses cultural considerations in mental health among Appalachians.

McCauley, D. V. (1995). *Appalachian mountain religion: A history.* Urbana, IL: University of Illinois Press.

Presents an historical review of the development and influence of religion in Appalachia.

McCormack, C. P. (Ed.). (1994). *Ethnology of fertility and birth* (2nd ed.). Prospect Heights, IL: Waveland.

Describes birthing practices, maturational events, and related issues in several developing nations and cultural groups. Also addresses the scientific birthing culture in developed countries.

McKenna, M. A. (1990). Transcultural perspectives in the nursing care of the elderly. In J. S. Boyle & M. M. Andrews (Eds.), *Transcultural concepts in nursing* (pp. 189–220). Philadelphia: Lippincott.

Addresses cultural considerations in the care of elderly clients.

Meleis, A. I., Douglas, M. K., Eribes, C., Shih, F., & Messias, D. K. (1996). Employed Mexican women as mothers and partners: Valued, empowered, and overloaded. *Journal of Advanced Nursing*, 23, 82–90.

Examines changes in the traditional role of Mexican American women and their implications for health.

Mellinger, M. B. (1977). The spirit is strong in the root. *Appalachian Journal*, 4, 242–253.

Provides an overview of herbal therapies in Appalachian culture.

Morales, B. (1994). Latino religion, ritual, and culture. In T. Weaver (Ed.), *Handbook of Hispanic cultures in the United States: Anthropology* (pp. 191–208). Houston: Arte Publico Press.

Discusses the influence of religion in Latino culture.

Raczynski, J. M., Taylor, H., Cutter, G., Hardin, M., Rappoport, N., & Oberman, A. (1994). Diagnoses, symptoms, and attribution of symptoms among black and white inpatients admitted for coronary heart disease. *American Journal of Public Health*, 84, 951–956.

Examines cultural influences on symptom interpretation in coronary heart disease among African Americans.

Ruffing-Rahal, M. A. (1995). The Navajo experience of Elizabeth Foster, public health nurse. *Nursing History Review*, 3, 173–188.

Describes the practice of one public health nurse in the Bureau of Indian Affairs and her attempts to provide culturally sensitive care to Native Americans.

Sanjur, D. (1995). *Hispanic foodways, nutrition, and health.* Boston: Allyn and Bacon.

Provides an overview of dietary patterns in several Latino cultural groups.

Simmon, J. M. (1987). Health care of the elderly in Appalachia. *Journal of Gerontological Nursing*, 13(7), 32–35.

Discusses cultural considerations in the care of elderly clients in Appalachia.

Smith, S. (1994). White nurses, black midwives, and public health in Mississippi, 1920–1950. *Nursing History Review*, 2, 29–49.

Discusses the advantages of incorporating traditional health care providers into the scientific health care system. Describes the collaborative efforts between white public health nurses and African American midwives.

Strickland, C. J., Chrisman, N. J., Yallup, M., Powell, K., & Squeoch, M. D. (1996). Walking the journey of womanhood: Yakama Indian women and Papanicolaou (pap) test screening. *Public Health Nursing*, 13, 141–150.

Describes the development of a culturally relevant program to promote Pap smears among Yakama Indians.

Van Esterik, P. (1988). To strengthen and refresh: Herbal therapy in Southeast Asia. *Social Science and Medicine, 27,* 751–759.

> *Describes the use of herbal therapies in Southeast Asian cultural groups.*

Vogel, V. J. (1991). What has American Indian medicine given us? *National Forum, 71*(2), 28–30.

> *Discusses the contributions of Native American medicine to modern medicine. Also addresses some common Native American health practices.*

CHAPTER 17: ENVIRONMENTAL INFLUENCES ON COMMUNITY HEALTH

Kleffel, D. (1996). Environmental paradigms: Moving toward an ecocentric perspective. *Advances in Nursing Science, 18*(4), 1–10.

> *Describes perspectives on environment in nursing theory. Discusses the egocentric, homocentric, and ecocentric perspectives on environment as espoused by nursing.*

Kotchian, S. B. (1995). Environmental health services are prerequisites to health care. *Family and Community Health, 18*(3), 45–53.

> *Discusses the importance of environmental health and protection interventions as a foundation for health promotion, disease prevention, and health care.*

Lum, M. R. (1995). Environmental public health: Future direction, future skills. *Family and Community Health, 18*(1), 24–35.

> *Addresses the importance of ecological factors in determining human health status.*

Pope, A. M., Snyder, M. A., & Mood, L. H. (Eds.). (1995). *Nursing, health, and environment: Strengthening the relationship to improve the public's health.* Washington, DC: National Academy Press.

> *Provides recommendations for incorporating environmental health principles in nursing. Addresses actions needed with respect to nursing practice, education, and research.*

CHAPTER 18: CARE OF THE FAMILY CLIENT

Johnson, S. K., Craft, M., Titler, M., et al. (1995). Perceived changes in adult family members' roles and responsibilities during critical illness. *Image, 27,* 238–243.

> *Reports findings of a study of role changes within families when a family member is hospitalized.*

National Forum: The Phi Kappa Phi Journal. (1995, Fall). 75(3).

> *Contains several articles addressing the call for a return to family values from several different perspectives.*

Nolan, M., Keady, J., & Grant, G. (1995). Developing a typology of family care: Implications for nurses and other service providers. *Journal of Advanced Nursing, 21,* 256–265.

> *Describes conceptualizations of caring as applied to family health nursing.*

Whall, A. L. (1986). The family as the unit of care in nursing: An historical review. *Public Health Nursing, 3,* 240–249.

> *Examines historical perspectives on the family as the unit of nursing care.*

Zerwehk, J. V. (1991). A family caregiving model for public health nursing. *Nursing Outlook, 39,* 213–217.

> *Describes findings of a study on the competencies of expert public health nurses. Presents a model for encouraging family self-help.*

Zerwehk, J. V. (1992). Laying the groundwork for family self-help: Locating families, building trust, and building strength. *Public Health Nursing, 9,* 15–21.

> *Describes three family caregiving competencies derived from a qualitative study of the practice of expert community health nurses.*

CHAPTER 19: CARE OF THE COMMUNITY OR TARGET GROUP

Billings, J. R., & Cowley, S. (1995). Approaches to community needs assessment: A literature review. *Journal of Advanced Nursing, 22,* 721–730.

> *Examines and critically analyzes approaches to community assessment found in the literature.*

Glick, D. F., Hale, P. J., Kulbok, P. A., & Shettig, J. (1996). Community development theory: Planning a community nursing center. *Journal of Nursing Administration, 26*(7/8), 44–50.

> *Describes the use of community development theory as a basis for conducting a needs assessment and planning for a community nursing center.*

Jossens, M. O. R., & Ferjancsik, P. (1996). Of Lillian Wald, community health nursing education, and health care reform. *Public Health Nursing, 13,* 97–103.

> *Describes a pilot project in which students planned and implemented health education presentations in local elementary schools and the use of the projects as a basis for discussion of community reform tactics.*

CHAPTER 20: CARE OF CHILDREN

Fox, J. A. (Ed.). (1997). *Primary health care of children.* St. Louis: Mosby-Year Book.

> *Provides a comprehensive overview of ambulatory health care for children. Addresses epidemiology and risk fac-*

tors for a variety of child health problems as well as interventions.

Hewison, J., & Downswell, T. (1994). *Child health care and the working mother: The juggling act.* London: Chapman & Hall.

Addresses the problem of child care for working parents. Discusses the relevance of child care to child health.

Luepker, R. V., Perry, C. L., McKinlay, S. M., et al. (1996). Outcomes of a field trial to improve children's dietary patterns and physical activity. *JAMA, 275,* 768–776.

Describes the results of a school-based community health program to enhance the dietary and exercise practices of school-age children.

Rains, J. W. (1995). Policy-relevant research in infant mortality: Rhetorical criticism of mass media. *Nursing Outlook, 43,* 158–163.

Presents the results of a review of popular press depictions of the problem of infant mortality. Examines themes and their effects on policy makers. Presents implications for communicating with policy makers regarding the health needs of children and other vulnerable populations.

CHAPTER 21: CARE OF WOMEN

Dudley, W. (Ed.). (1993). *Homosexuality: Opposing viewpoints.* San Diego: Greenhaven Press.

Presents opposing viewpoints on a variety of issues related to homosexuality, including theories of causation, societal responses, appropriate interventions, and so on.

Jay, K. (1995). *Dyke life.* New York: Basic.

Describes the experiences of lesbians in living a gay lifestyle. Provides lesbians' personal insights on family relationships, coming out, and legal issues.

Sargent, C. F. (1996). *Gender and health: An international perspective.* Upper Saddle River, NJ: Prentice Hall.

Addresses a variety of women's issues at the international level, including work, violence, reproductive health, and research needs.

CHAPTER 22: CARE OF MEN

Donovan, J. (1995). The process of analysis during a grounded theory study of men during their partners' pregnancies. *Journal of Advanced Nursing, 21,* 708–715.

Describes stages in men's response to their partners' pregnancies. Suggests that current antenatal care for men is not designed to meet their needs.

Dudley, W. (Ed.). (1993). *Homosexuality: Opposing viewpoints.* San Diego: Greenhaven Press.

Presents opposing viewpoints on a variety of issues re-

lated to homosexuality, including theories of causation, societal responses, appropriate interventions, and so on.

McNaught, B. (1996). *Gay issues in the workplace.* New York: St. Martin's Press.

Discusses the issues facing homosexuals and their families in the work setting. Addresses sources of homophobia and desirable working conditions for gay and lesbian employees.

Sabo, D., & Gordon, D. F. (Eds.). (1995). *Men's health and illness: Gender, power, and the body.* Thousand Oaks, CA: Sage.

Discusses a variety of issues related to men's health, including mortality risks, role expectations, sports injuries, HIV/AIDS, physical disability, and cancer.

CHAPTER 23: CARE OF OLDER CLIENTS

Gibson, H. B. (1992). *The emotional and sexual lives of older people: A manual for professionals.* London: Chapman & Hall.

Provides an excellent overview of sexuality concerns and issues for older individuals. Addresses both the normal effects of aging on sexual activity and problems with sexuality.

Gill, T. M., Williams, C. S., & Tinetti, M. E. (1995). Assessing risk for the onset of functional dependence among older adults: The role of physical performance. *Journal of the American Geriatrics Society, 43,* 603–609.

Describes several simple tests of physical performance that can be used to assess the potential for functional limitations in older clients. Four tests of ability were associated with the onset of physical limitations: standing from a chair, rapid gait, turning 360 degrees, and bending over.

Haber, D. (1996). Strategies to promote the health of older people: An alternative to readiness strategies. *Family and Community Health, 19*(2), 1–10.

Presents several strategies designed to promote the health of older clients including health education, social support, behavioral management, and referral.

Rathbone-McCuan, E., & Fabian, D. R. (Eds.). (1994). *Self-neglecting elders: A clinical dilemma.* New York: Auburn House.

Discusses the problem of self-neglect by elderly persons in terms of contributing factors, ethical issues, family issues, and special groups at risk for self-neglect.

Spector, W. D. (1996). Functional disability scales. In B. Spilker (Ed.), *Quality of life and pharmacoeconomics in clinical trials* (2nd ed.) (pp. 133–143). Philadelphia: Lippincott-Raven.

Discusses several tools for assessing functional disability including measures of activities of daily living and in-

strumental activities of daily living. Also addresses methodology issues in measuring functional disability.

CHAPTER 24: CARE OF HOMELESS CLIENTS

May, K. M., & Evans, G. G. (1994). Health education for homeless populations. *Journal of Community Health Nursing, 11,* 229–237.

Describes a health education program designed especially for homeless clients. Also addresses the findings of an evaluation of the program.

Mayo, K., White, S., Oates, S. K., & Franklin, F. (1996). Community collaboration: Prevention and control of tuberculosis in a homeless shelter. *Public Health Nursing, 13,* 120–127.

Describes a collaborative effort between a clinic for the homeless and a school of nursing to provide TB screening and case finding for residents of a homeless shelter. Also addresses the policies and procedures developed for TB control in the shelter.

Montgomery, C. (1994). Swimming upstream: The strengths of women who survive homelessness. *Advances in Nursing Science, 16*(3), 34–45.

Presents the findings of a qualitative study of strengths and personal resources of women who experienced homelessness as a first step out of abusive or addictive situations.

Norton, D., & Ridenour, N. (1995). Homeless women and children: The challenge of health promotion. *Nurse Practitioner Forum, 6*(1), 29–33.

Provides an overview of barriers to obtaining health care for homeless women and their children. Also discusses the difficulty of promoting health in a crisis and survival-oriented population.

CHAPTER 25: CARE OF CLIENTS IN THE SCHOOL SETTING

Koenning, G. M., Benjamin, J. E., Todaro, A. W., Warren, R. W., & Burns, M. L. (1995). Bridging the "med–ed gap" for students with special care needs: A model school liaison program. *Journal of School Health, 65,* 207–212.

Describes an educational liaison program between a large hospital and a local school system designed to meet the needs of children with special health problems.

Landis, S. E., & Janes, C. L. (1995). The Claxton Elementary School health program: Merging perceptions and behaviors to identify problems. *Journal of School Health, 65,* 250–254.

Describes the use of community-oriented primary care (COPC) principles to identify and prioritize community health problems to be addressed by the school system. Discusses the process of advisory board formation, needs

assessment, prioritization, and program development and implementation. Provides recommendations for using a COPC approach to health promotion in schools.

While, A. E., & Barriball, K. L. (1993). School nursing: History, present practice and possibilities reviewed. *Journal of Advanced Nursing, 18,* 1202–1211.

Provides an historical overview of school nursing and legislative influences on this practice area. Addresses current practice and directions for the future.

CHAPTER 26: CARE OF CLIENTS IN THE WORK SETTING

Dembe, A. E. (1996). *Occupation and disease: How social factors affect the conception of work-related disorders.* New Haven, CT: Yale University Press.

Provides an analysis of factors that have influenced the designation of certain conditions as work-related and compensable. Maintains that health provider determinations are only one of many social factors in such designations.

Parillo, V. L. (1993). Systems analysis of an occupational health department: Recommendations to increase effectiveness. *AAOHN Journal, 41,* 220–227.

Describes a systems approach to assessing and improving occupational health care delivery systems. Discusses occupational health system inputs, throughputs, and expected outputs.

CHAPTER 27: CARE OF CLIENTS IN RURAL SETTINGS

National Institute of Nursing Research. (1995). *Community-based health care: Nursing strategies.* Bethesda, MD: National Institute of Nursing Research.

Describes concepts of community-based care and their application to both rural and urban populations. Outlines nursing research needs related to each area of practice.

Thornton, C. L. (1996). Nurse practitioner in a rural setting. *Nursing Clinics of North America, 31,* 495–505.

Provides a description of rural practice by a nurse practitioner. Addresses some of challenges and rewards of advanced nursing practice in a rural area.

CHAPTER 28: CARE OF CLIENTS IN CORRECTIONAL SETTINGS

American Nurses Association. (1995). *Scope and standards of nursing practice in correctional facilities.* Washington, DC: American Nurses Publishing.

Presents the standards for nursing practice in correctional settings with rationale and measurement criteria.

Kay, S. L. (1991). *The constitutional dimensions of an in-*

mate's right to health care. Chicago: National Commission on Correctional Health Care.

Provides an overview of the constitutional basis for inmates' rights to health care while incarcerated. Examines issues of medical, dental, and mental health care as well as considerations related to personnel, facilities, records, and so on.

CHAPTER 29: CARE OF CLIENTS IN DISASTER SETTINGS

Meyer, M. U., & Graeter, C. J. (1995). Health professionals' role in disaster planning: A strategic management approach. *AAOHN Journal, 43,* 251–262.

Provides an overview of disaster planning by health professionals, particularly nurses, in occupational settings. Reviews the OSHA requirements for disaster planning as well as the process of developing a disaster plan.

Noji, E. K. (Ed). (1997). *The public health consequences of disasters.* New York: Oxford University Press.

Presents a general overview of disasters and their consequences for the health of the public. Then addresses specific health considerations in disaster settings as well as specific types of disasters.

CHAPTER 30: COMMUNICABLE DISEASES

Bayer, R., Dubler, N. N., & Landesman, S. (1993). The dual epidemics of tuberculosis and AIDS: Ethical and policy issues in screening and treatment. *American Journal of Public Health, 83,* 649–653.

Discusses the ethical implications of mandatory HIV testing as a means of controlling the tuberculosis epidemic.

Bryan, R. T., Pinner, R. W., Gaynes, R. P., Peters, C. J., Aguilar, J. R., & Berkelman, R. L. (1994). Addressing emerging infectious disease threats: A prevention strategy for the United States. *MMWR, 43*(RR-5), 1–18.

Provides an overview of control strategies for emerging and reemerging diseases.

Mortimer, E. A. (1994). Communicable diseases. In I. B. Pless (Ed.), *The epidemiology of childhood disorders* (pp. 229–274). New York: Oxford University Press.

Provides an overview of communicable diseases in children.

Rothenberg, K. H., & Paskey, S. J. (1995). The risk of domestic violence and women with HIV infection: Implications for partner notification, public policy, and the law. *American Journal of Public Health, 85,* 1569–1576.

Discusses the ethical implications of partner notification of HIV exposure when there is a risk for domestic violence as a result.

CHAPTER 31: CHRONIC PHYSICAL HEALTH PROBLEMS

Bigel, D. E., Sales, E., & Schulz, R. (1991). *Family caregiving in chronic illness.* Newbury Park, CA: Sage.

Provides insights into the care needed by families with members suffering from Alzheimer's disease, cancer, stroke, chronic mental illness, and heart disease.

Fraley, A. M. (1992). *Nursing the disabled across the lifespan.* Boston: Jones and Bartlett.

Discusses specific nursing interventions for a variety of chronic and disabling conditions.

Morse, J. M., & Johnson, J. L. (1991). *The illness experience: Dimensions of suffering.* Newbury Park, CA: Sage.

Presents insights into the human experience of chronic illness.

CHAPTER 32: CHRONIC MENTAL HEALTH PROBLEMS: SCHIZOPHRENIA AND MOOD DISORDERS

Gournay, K. (1996). Schizophrenia: A review of the contemporary literature and implications for mental health nursing theory, practice, and education. *Journal of Psychiatric and Mental Health Nursing, 3,* 7–12.

Discusses the implications of new information on the possible biological etiology of schizophrenia for nursing practice.

Spitzer, V. M. (1995). Biological aspects of schizophrenia. *Journal of the American Psychiatric Nurses Association, 1,* 204–207.

Presents an overview of biological theories of causation in schizophrenia.

CHAPTER 33: SUBSTANCE ABUSE

Akers, R. L. (1992). *Drugs, alcohol, and society: Social structure, process, and policy.* Belmont, CA: Wadsworth.

Presents an overview of theories of substance abuse as well as a discussion of the most commonly abused psychoactive substances.

Bennet, G. A. (Ed.). (1991). *Substance abuse: Pharmacological, developmental, and clinical perspectives.* New York: Wiley.

Addresses the role of the nurse in preventing and treating substance abuse. Examines the effects of abuse and its treatment on the individual and the family.

Brown, L. P. (1995). *National drug control strategy: Executive summary.* Washington, DC: Office of National Drug Control Policy.

Discusses the strategies for control of drug abuse in the United States. Addresses strategies directed toward minimizing the use of and controlling access to drugs.

CHAPTER 34: VIOLENCE

American Psychological Association. (1996). *Violence and the family: Report of the American Psychological Association Presidential Task Force on Violence and the Family.* Washington, DC: American Psychological Association.

Presents an overview of all forms of family violence. Addresses contributing factors as well as treatment issues.

Hamberger, L. K., & Renzetti, C. M. (Eds.). (1996). *Domestic partner abuse.* New York: Springer.

Discusses partner abuse in both homosexual and heterosexual couples. Addresses epidemiology and treatment issues.

Shepherd, J. (Ed.). (1994). *Violence in health care: A practical guide to coping with violence and caring for victims.* Oxford: Oxford University Press.

Discusses violence in health care and other settings. Addresses prevention strategies as well as care for victims of violence.

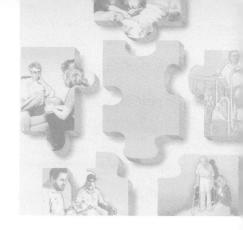

Poems written by Veneta Masson introduce the six units in this textbook. Because the poems were excerpted, they are presented for the reader in their entirety on the following pages.

THE ARITHMETIC OF NURSES

S-s-s, S-s-s, S-s-s
Bennie Smith is trying to speak.
I am counting out cookies
from a faded blue tin.

S-s-s, S-s-s, S-s-s
Twelve!
Are twelve cookies enough to hold
a sick old man for thirty-six hours?
Twelve cookies and one can of
    juice?
Twelve cookies wrapped in a
    towel
tucked under a pillow where
    roaches
ply a brisk trade in crumbs?

Six!
He blurts it out
face lit up by the restless flicker
of the television screen.
No, twelve, I muse.
Unless someone comes
that's all he'll have
till I get back again.

S-s-s-six thousand!
He strains under the weight of the
    words.
Clearly he has something impor-
    tant to say
but I am caught up with my own
    calculations—

The number of minutes
it will take a rivulet of urine
to reach the screaming bedsores
on his back

The number of degrees
his temperature will rise
as infection sets in

the number of days
it will take him
to let me call the ambulance

The number of times
I must walk the long hall
to this dim little room
the width of a bed.

His stiff body straddles the low
    bed
like a piece of plywood on a
    sawhorse.
Push down on the feet, up comes
    the head.
I tilt my ear toward his mouth
to catch the stutterings

S-s-s-six thousand nurses . . .
on strike today . . .
Meh- Meh- Meh- Minnesota!

Half his face breaks into a grin
for if there's one thing Bennie
    understands
it's the arithmetic of nurses
and old, abandoned men.

LADY JANE JACKSON RECEIVES
THE VISITING NURSE

Sweetheart, come up.
I'm up here in my chair.
But first take a look
around my house.
Do you see the pictures
hung in the stairwell
every one framed?
There's me as a school girl
me on the arm of one of my beaus
me posing in my wedding dress
me at the church giving a concert
me at my job in the government
me as Grand Matron
me at a banquet giving a speech
me with Joe at the home
before he died.
Now look in the parlor
and see my diplomas
every one framed.
I'm a certified graduate
practical nurse
and doctor of divinity.
There's Christmas cards
tacked on the door
photos of all the Presidents
all the Mayors
and Dr. King
miniature crosses
fifty at least
verses I painted
on the walls
and that's not all.
Go into the kitchen

and look at my pill nook—
medicine boxes and
cups full of capsules
stacked up in little pyramids
there on the table.
Now go on into the bathroom
and see my collection
of towels and soaps
every color there is.
I love pretty things
and lots of them.
And then on the dresser
there in the bedroom
you'll see my bottles
of perfumes and creams—
the closet won't shut
for all of my gowns.
The bed is arranged
with pillows and dolls.
I haven't slept there
since I don't know when.
I suffered a terrible stroke
you know and I can't
get around like I used to.
But I've been in this house
for thirty years
and everything
is just the way
I want it.

Ms Jackson, excuse me
but why are you
sitting there naked?

Do you find it less trouble
than dressing these days?
And you seem to be slipping
out of your chair.
What is that squeaking
under the bed
and those wet stains
on the ceiling?
There are papers and dishes
all over the floor—
aren't you afraid of falling?
Who do you have
to help you clean up?
I can see you were
very particular, once.
I'm a nurse, you know
and only one person.
You said on the phone
you wanted someone to
check your pressure
once a month.
I wonder somehow
if that's going
to be enough.

I'll have a key made
so you **can get in**
anytime, night or day
and you don't have
to think about money.
A dollar a visit
is what I pay.

MAGGIE JONES

Just
who do you think you are, Maggie
    Jones
following me home from work
insinuating yourself into my
    evening
shading my thoughts?

Just
who do you think you are
lying flat as a pancake in the mid-
    dle of your bed
your world ranged around you in
    brown paper bags?

(Rather like a dead Pharaoh in his
    tomb, I'd say
buried with all his treasure.)

So you fell one day and had to be
    taken to the hospital.
You didn't break any bones, after
    all.
You came home in a taxi
climbed the steep flight of stairs to
    your room
took to your bed and stayed there.
That was three years ago, Maggie
Three years with only one thing to
    look forward to—livin'.

I'm here by the hand of the Lord,
    you always say
        when I come
though the hand of the Lord didn't
    smite the rat
        that bit your foot
        that cold winter day last year
        as it foraged in your sheets for
            bread and jelly.
I guess it'll be all right
        you said in your genteel way
        looking up at me with soft doe
        eyes as I dressed the wound
        that brought us together.

Why don't you go to a home? we
    ask, shocked
to see the condition you're in
(the church ladies, the social
    worker
your niece, your nephew
    and I).
Because I still have my right mind
    you say simply.
        A nursing home is no place
        for someone who still has
        their mind.

But it's not safe here, we say
    (the church ladies, the social
        worker
    your niece, your nephew
        and I)
Don't you know they shoot drugs
    and people in this
        neighborhood?
I've never been bothered
    you say, matter-of-factly.

What about fire? we say
    (the church ladies, the social
        worker
    your niece, your nephew
        and I).
You'd be burned alive in your bed.
There was a fire once, and the
    fireman carried me out.
I own my home and I own my
    grave plot
        and I plan to go from one to
        the other
        when the Lord calls me
        you say quietly, clutching a
        packet
        of long, white envelopes.

But now your gas is cut off
        until you come up with $700
You're lucky it's not freezing and
    there's an electric
        coffeemaker we can use
        to heat water to wash you.
I guess the money will come from
    somewhere
        you say, looking at me
        steadily.

And Meals on Wheels has cut you
    off because it's a bad
        neighborhood to begin with
        and then
        the front door fell off its hinges
        onto the Meals on Wheels
        delivery lady.
I guess there's enough food in the
    United States
        to feed me
        you say, looking at me
        knowingly.

And they've taken away your
    homemaker because they say
        you need more care
        than the agency can give.
I guess things will work out
        you say, looking at me
        trustingly.

How can you lie there and say,
    serenely, you guess
        things will work out?
        Your room is cold
        your sheets are soaked with
            urine
        your skin is bleeding from
            bedsores
        You don't know where your
            next meal is coming from
        you're a poor old lady
            hidden away
            in a falling-down house
            in a no-good
                neighborhood
        And you have expectations?

You told your niece not to worry
    about you
        the nurse was coming
Hey, Maggie Jones, don't wait for
    me, don't count on me
        I'll bathe you
        dress your wounds
        treat your minor ailments
        even do your laundry and
(continued)

bring you food
once in a while.

But save you?
God alone—the hand of the
Lord—can save you.

I see you now in my mind's eye
and wonder
as I sit
after dinner
in my warm house
on a safe street

in a good neighborhood

Just
who do you think you are, Maggie
Jones?

WIDOW

Alma Brown
sits alone
one alone
where yesterday
there were two
Alma and Jesse.
Two alone
passing the years
in a boarding house basement
with flowers on the bookcase
and clocks for Jesse to fix.

"Sometimes he'd drink
and then we'd fight
but come the next morning
I'd always go lean over
his chair and ask him
if he still loved me.
The answer was yes
I could tell by his eyes.

"He died easy
I'm glad for that.
I didn't even believe
he was dead, his toes
stayed warm so long.
He woke up in the night
and started coughing up blood
didn't struggle or nothing
just held my hand tight
like he did that night
we met the first time
drinking beers at the Derby Bar.

Then he lay back
and closed his eyes
and that was it."

The old iron bed is made up now.
Fresh sheets stretch smooth and
    tight

across the mattress.
His chair is empty except
for the cushion she made
to protect him from bedsores
and there is a pack
of cigarettes, one smoked
next to his glasses.

"I come in and look
at the empty bed
I say to myself, well
he must've got up.
Then I look at the chair
and he's not there . . .
Oh, it's all right
I haven't broke down yet.

"Last week he told me
he didn't want me
to see him again
after they took him away.
He wanted to be buried here
not sent to Carolina
to his kin. Said he didn't
want to ride on a train
in a box all alone."

She sits straight
on a straight-back chair
feet planted firm on the floor
hands on her knees
head erect on broad shoulders.

"The ambulance came first.
They were nice but they said
it was no use taking
a dead man. The police
came next. They called
the doctor and helped me
phone the undertaker.
The undertaker said
not to worry, just leave it

all in his hands.
The only thing I'd need to do
is pay him on Monday
so they can start
digging the grave.

"I don't know if I can stay
in this place alone
or not. Jesse wants me to
but I don't know . . .
        We lived here twenty
            years"

She sits straight
on a straight-back chair.
Behind her is the double
bed, one pillow now
and mended sheets
pulled tight
across the mattress.

"The doctor said the cancer
had prob'ly ate into
a vein somewhere and that's
what made him bleed so.
I told him Jesse asked me
for a whiskey late last night
so I gave him two or three
    poured 'em myself.
I told the doctor
I hope that didn't
have nothing to do
with what happened.
He said no, it didn't.

"The ambulance left
and then the police.
The undertaker sent his helper
out to the car, then he
took me out to the kitchen
and when I came back
Jesse was gone."

TICKET TO CHRISTMAS

That day, that Christmas Eve last
  year
I went to work as usual, but full of
  expectation.
I went to the clinic expecting
  Christmas
to happen to me. I thought I knew
  what it would be—
most probably a patient and a
  poignant interruption
in the flow of everyday. There
  might be merriment
or tears. There would be touch. I'd
  touch
and let myself be touched by
  Christmas.

All morning patients came and
  went.
Some laughed. One wept.
I touched them and was touched
  in turn.
But none of them was Christmas.
By afternoon, I knew there was
  something more
I needed to do. I'd go to the market
across the street, buy cookies and
  punch
and set them out in the waiting
  room
like a child making ready for
  Santa.

There wasn't much time, patients
  were waiting.
I threw on my coat and ran out the
  door
just in time to catch a green light.
But a voice called out from the P
  Street side
of the liquor store. Christmas had
  been there
waiting for me. Startled, I stopped
missed the light, stepped
  backwards
up, onto the curb. There wasn't
  much time.

Patients were waiting. I deeply re-
  sented
the interruption even though I
knew who it was.

Christmas was black, fifty or so,
  wearing
an Oriole's baseball cap. He
  swayed a little
but didn't reek and started to
  speak as if
he had something to say I needed
  to hear.
I'm homeless, he said, and then he
  told
how long ago he'd prayed to God
  to show him
how it was to live on the streets,
  but just today
he'd been telling God he'd had
  enough.
Where will you spend the night? I
  asked.
In the shelter at Second and D, he
  said.

He wanted to give me a present. I
  wanted
to make the light. I knew he was
  Christmas
but I was uneasy and wanted to be
  on my way.
Wait! He said and started to empty
  his
pockets into my hands: a red and
  green bag
with a pair of white socks, a lottery
  ticket
he made me scratch while he
  halted the search
(we didn't win), folded papers, a
  tattered
social security card and so on
  down to the lint
in the seams until at last he found
  it.

"Admit One" is what it said. A
  ticket to
the Christmas gala the city puts on
  for
down and outs. Take it, he said.
  I've seen
it all—the stars, the food, the fancy
  decorations.
But don't go dressed like you are
  right now.
Go home and change into
  something a homeless
person might wear so you can feel
  just what
it's like. You get my meaning,
  don't you, Miss?

I waited for the hustle. It never
  came.
He never asked for money or a
  date.
I put the ticket into my pocket and
  left him
when the light turned green. As I
  made my way
to the grocery store I heard his
  voice
behind me once more. Miss! he
  called
Remember that's my ticket.
  Remember
that ticket's my Christmas gift to
  you.

ON HEARING THE NEWS
OF A PATIENT'S DEATH

Morning light glances off the
   chrome
of a stripped down car in the alley
slices through window panes
along the edges of drawn shades
opens fire on sheets pulled up
to shield the eyes of sleepers.

This summer sun won't light your
   eyes.
Not even the cries of the baby
   reach you.
It's too late, for you went early
just as we thought you might
but not like this
manacled to a bed
in the maternity ward
of D.C. General Hospital.

Hearing the news, I call up your
   face
a wide-open face with a slow shy
   smile
as if the shock of life had somehow
   dazed you.
You took each day
   each man
   each child
   each welfare check
   each jail cell
   as it came.
It just wasn't in you to ask why or
   why not
to look ahead or behind.

Since when does someone like you
   get to choose?
Since when do poor ignorant
   women take charge of their
   lives?

The world for you was
   your mother's house, teeming
     with kin
   the street
   the welfare office
   hospital &
   jail.
A heroin high was the only place
   you ever had
     to call your own
and a fix was the only way
   you knew
     to get there.

The judge decided to keep you in
   jail
those last few months of your
   pregnancy—
the best he could do for your
   unborn child.
Why bring another addict into the
   world?

Oh, it isn't that you never tried to
   kick.
You'd come to us in pain
   with abscesses from dirty needles.
You'd come when the drug supply
   dried up.
You'd come when there was no
   money to buy.
You'd come when you felt too
   tired to sell.

I can do it alone, you said
   I can kick.
Just give me a few Valiums.
A little help is all I need.

I suppose we'll never know just
   how you died.
It was after the baby was born
after they'd taken you back to the
   ward.
Some people said they heard calls
   for help.
When they found you, you were
   hanging
   over the side of the bed
   danglin by the foot
   they'd shackled to the
     bedframe.
Your family set up a wail that
   went on for days
   alleged foul play
   hinted at revenge.
There was gunfire at the wake,
   they say
and eight motherless children
   destined for
   your mother's house
   the street
   the welfare office
   hospital &
   jail.

The last light you saw in the blank
   night
   of your life
was your newborn girl.
Is that why you named her Star?

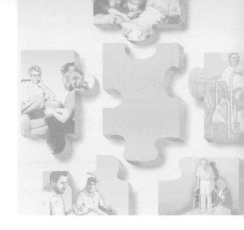

APPENDICES

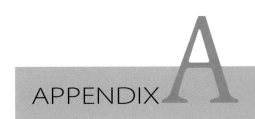
SUMMARY OF HEALTHY PEOPLE 2000: NATIONAL HEALTH OBJECTIVES

In 1991, the National Health Objectives for the year 2000 were published by the Department of Health and Human Services. These objectives were revised, with additional objectives added and some targets changed, in 1995. Presently, national objectives for the year 2010 are being developed. The National Health Objectives most relevant to community health nursing are summarized on the following pages. The objectives are summarized in terms of the minimum requirement for their achievement. Year 2000 targets for certain subpopulations are also included. For a complete listing of all of the year 2000 objectives see *Healthy People 2000: Midcourse Review and 1995 Revisions,* a 1995 publication of the U.S. Department of Health and Human Services.

Category: Physical Activity and Fitness

Number	Objective
1.1	See objective 15.1
1.2	Reduce overweight prevalence to 20% in those age 20 years and older and 15% in adolescents (12–19 years).

	a. Low-income women	25%
	b. Black women	30%
	c. Hispanic women	25%
	d. Native Americans	30%
	e. People with disabilities	25%
	f. Women with hypertension	41%
	g. Men with hypertension	35%
	h. Mexican American men	25%

Number	Objective
1.3	Increase to 30% those over age 6 who exercise regularly (at least 30 minutes per day).

	a. Hispanics	25%

Number	Objective
1.4	Increase vigorous physical activity (3 or more times a week) to 20% of those over age 18 and 75% of children and adolescents.

	a. Low-income adults	12%
	b. Black adults	17%
	c. Hispanic adults	17%

Number	Objective
1.5	Reduce to 15% those over age 6 who have no leisure time physical activity.

	a. People over 65	22%
	b. People with disabilities	20%
	c. Low-income people	17%
	d. Black adults	20%
	e. Hispanic adults	25%
	f. Native Americans	21%

Number	Objective
1.6	Increase those over age 6 engaging in activity to enhance muscle strength to 40%.
1.7	Increase to 50% the proportion of overweight people aged 12 and older who combine sound dietary practices and exercise to attain an appropriate body weight.

	a. Hispanic adult males	24%
	b. Hispanic adult females	22%

Number	Objective
1.8	Increase to 50% the proportion of schoolchildren with daily school physical education.
1.9	Increase to 50% the proportion of school physical education time spent in physical activity.
1.10	Increase the proportion of worksites offering physical fitness programs as follows:

	a. 50–99 employees	20%
	b. 100–149 employees	35%
	c. 250–749 employees	50%
	d. > 750 employees	80%

Number	Objective
1.11	Increase community facilities for physical activity as follows:

	a. hiking, biking, and fitness trails	1 per 10,000 people
	b. public swimming pools	1 per 25,000 people
	c. acres of park and open space	4 per 1000 people

Number	Objective
1.12	Increase to 50% the proportion of health care providers who counsel clients regarding physical activity.
1.13	See objective 17.3

Category: Nutrition

Number	Objective
2.1	See objective 15.1
2.2	See objective 16.1
2.3	See objective 1.2

2.4	Reduce growth retardation in low-income children under age 5 to 10%.	
	a. Black children under age 1	10%
	b. Hispanic children under age 1	10%
	c. Hispanic children aged 1 year	10%
	d. Asian children aged 1 year	10%
	e. Asian children aged 2–4 years	10%
2.5	Reduce dietary fat intake to an average of 30% of calories and saturated fat intake to less than 10% of calories in 50% of the population aged 2 years and older.	
2.6	Increase consumption of fruits and vegetables to five per day and grain products to six per day in 50% of those aged 2 years and older.	
2.7	See objective 1.7	
2.8	Increase consumption of calcium-rich foods to three or more servings per day in 50% of pregnant and lactating women and people aged 11–24 years and in 75% of children aged 2–10 years. Increase consumption to two or more servings per day in 50% of persons aged 25 and older.	
2.9	Increase to:	
	50%, home meal preparers who cook without salt	
	80%, those who do not add salt at the table	
	40%, those who purchase lower sodium foods	
2.10	Reduce iron-deficiency anemia to 3% of children aged 1–4 years and women of childbearing age.	
2.11	Increase to 75% the proportion of women who breastfeed their infants and to 50% those who breastfeed until 5–6 months of age.	
2.12	Increase to 75% the proportion of child caregivers who use feeding practices that prevent baby bottle tooth decay.	
2.13	Increase to 85% those who use food labels to make nutritious food selections.	
2.14	Achieve food nutrition labeling on all processed foods and 40% of carry-away foods.	
2.15	Increase to 5000 the brand items with reduced fat and saturated fat content.	
2.16	Increase to 90% the restaurants and institutional food service operations that offer identifiable low-fat, low-calorie choices.	
2.17	Increase to 90% the proportion of school lunch and breakfast menus consistent with dietary recommendations.	
2.18	Increase to 80% the proportion of those aged 65 and older with difficulty preparing meals who receive home food services.	
2.19	Increase to 75% the proportion of schools that offer nutrition education.	
2.20	Increase to 50% the proportion of worksites with 50 or more employees that offer nutrition education.	
2.21	Increase to 75% the proportion of primary care providers who provide nutrition assessment and counseling.	
2.22	See objective 15.2	
2.23	See objective 16.5	
2.24	See objective 17.11	
2.25	See objective 15.7	
2.26	See objective 15.4	
2.27	See objective 15.6	

Category: Tobacco

Number	Objective	
3.1	See objective 15.1	
3.2	See objective 16.2	
3.3	Slow deaths from chronic obstructive pulmonary disease (COPD) to 25 per 100,000 people.	
3.4	Reduce cigarette smoking prevalence to 15% of those aged 18 years and older.	
	a. People with high school education or less	20%

	b. Blue collar workers	20%
	c. Military personnel	20%
	d. Black adults	18%
	e. Hispanic adults	15%
	f. Native Americans	20%
	g. Southeast Asian men	20%
	h. Women of reproductive age	12%
	i. Pregnant women	10%
	j. Women using oral contraceptives	10%

3.5   Reduce initiation of cigarette smoking by children and youth to 15% by age 20.
       a. Lower socioeconomic status youth   18%

3.6   Increase to 50% adults who smoke who stop for at least 1 day during the year.

3.7   Increase smoking cessation during pregnancy to 60% of pregnant smokers.

3.8   Reduce to 20% the proportion of children under age 6 exposed to tobacco smoke at home.

3.9   Reduce prevalence of smokeless tobacco use among men aged 12–24 years to 4%.
       a. Native American   10%

3.10   Establish tobacco-free environments and include tobacco use education in the curricula of all elementary, middle, and secondary schools.

3.11   Increase to 100% the proportion of worksites with no-smoking policies.

3.12   Enact legislation in 50 states to prohibit or limit smoking in workplaces and enclosed public places.

3.13   Enact legislation in 50 states prohibiting tobacco sales to minors.

3.14   Establish plans in 50 states to reduce tobacco use, especially among youth.

3.15   Eliminate tobacco advertising aimed at youth.

3.16   Increase to 75% the proportion of health care providers who recommend smoking cessation.

3.17   See objective 16.17

3.18   See objective 15.2

3.19   See objective 4.5

3.20   See objective 4.6

3.21   See objective 4.9

3.22   See objective 4.10

3.23   Increase the average tobacco tax to 50% of the retail price of tobacco products.

3.24   Increase to 100% the health insurance plans that cover tobacco use cessation services.

3.25   See objective 10.20

3.26   Enact legislation in 50 states prohibiting tobacco vending machines in areas accessible to youth.

Category: Substance Abuse: Alcohol and Other Drugs

Number	Objective
4.1	Reduce deaths due to alcohol-related motor vehicle accidents to 5.5 per 100,000 people.

       a. Native Americans   35
       b. People aged 15–24   12.5

4.2   Reduce cirrhosis deaths to 6 per 100,000 people
       a. Black men   12
       b. Native Americans   10
       c. Hispanics   10

4.3   Reduce drug-related deaths to 3 per 100,000 people.

4.4   Reduce drug-related hospital emergency department visits by 20%.

4.5   Increase by at least 1 year the average age of first use of cigarettes, alcohol, and marijuana by people aged 12–17.

4.6   Reduce the proportion of young people who have used alcohol, marijuana, cocaine, or cigarettes in the past month as follows:
       Alcohol (age 12–17)   12.6%
       Alcohol (age 18–20)   29%

Marijuana (age 12–17)	3.2%
Marijuana (age 18–25)	7.8%
Cocaine (age 12–17)	0.6%
Cocaine (age 18–25)	2.3%
Cigarettes (age 12–17)	6%

4.7	Reduce the proportion of recent heavy drinking to 28% of high school seniors and 32% of college students.
4.8	Reduce average annual per person alcohol consumption to 2 gallons in people aged 14 years and older.
4.9	Increase the proportion of high school seniors who perceive social disapproval of:

heavy alcohol use	70%
occasional marijuana use	85%
regular tobacco use	95%
experimentation with cocaine	95%

4.10	Increase the proportion of high school seniors who associate physical or psychological harm with:

heavy alcohol use	70%
occasional marijuana use	90%
regular tobacco use	95%
experimentation with cocaine	95%

4.11	Reduce the proportion of high school seniors who use anabolic steroids to 3%.
4.12	Establish and monitor in 50 states plans to ensure access to alcohol and drug treatment for underserved people.
4.13	Provide alcohol and drug education to all schoolchildren.
4.14	Extend to 60% of worksites with 50 or more employees adoption of alcohol and drug policies.
4.15	Extend to all 50 states provisions for drivers license revocation for driving under the influence of intoxicants.
4.16	Increase to 50 the number of states that have and enforce policies to reduce access to alcoholic beverages by minors.
4.17	Increase to 20 the number of states that restrict promotion of alcoholic beverages to young audiences.
4.18	Extend to 50 states blood alcohol tolerance levels of 0.08% for drivers over age 21 and zero tolerance for younger drivers.
4.19	Increase to 75% the proportion of health care providers who screen for alcohol and drug use problems and provide counseling and referral as needed.
4.20	Increase to 30 the number of states with hospitality resource panels to ensure management and server training in the hospitality industry to promote responsible drinking.

Category: Family Planning

Number	Objective
5.1	Reduce pregnancies among females aged 15–17 to 50 per 1000 girls.

a. Black adolescent girls	120
b. Hispanic adolescent girls	105

5.2	Reduce to 30% the proportion of pregnancies that are unintended.

a. Black females	40%
b. Hispanic females	30%

5.3	Reduce the prevalence of infertility to 6.5%.

a. Black couples	9%
b. Hispanic couples	9%

5.4	Reduce to 15% the proportion of adolescents who have had sexual intercourse by age 15 (40% by age 17).

a. Black males (age 15)	15%
b. Black males (age 17)	40%

	c. Black females (age 17)	40%
5.5	Increase to 40% the proportion of ever sexually active adolescents under age 18 who have not had sexual intercourse in the previous 3 months.	
5.6	Increase to 90% the proportion of sexually active, unmarried people aged 15–24 who use contraception.	
5.7	Decrease to 7% the proportion of women who become pregnant while using contraception.	
	a. Black females	8%
	b. Hispanic females	8%
5.8	Increase to 85% the proportion of people aged 10–18 who have received sex education from parents, schools, or other youth programs.	
5.9	Increase to 90% the proportion of family planning counselors who offer education about all options to patients with unintended pregnancies.	
5.10	Increase to 60% the proportion of health care providers who give age-appropriate preconception care and counseling.	
5.11	Increase to 50% the proportion of health care agencies that provide primary prevention and refer for secondary prevention services for HIV infection and other STDs.	
5.12	Increase to 95% the proportion of females aged 15–44 at risk for unintended pregnancies who use contraception.	

Category: Mental Health and Mental Disorders

Number	**Objective**	
6.1	Reduce suicides to 10.5 per 100,000 people.	
	a. Youth aged 15–19	8.2
	b. Men aged 20–34	21.4
	c. White men over 65	39.2
	d. Native American men	17.0
6.2	Reduce the incidence of injurious suicide attempts among adolescents aged 14–17 to 1.8%.	
	a. Adolescent females	2%
6.3	Reduce the prevalence of mental disorder among children and adolescents to 17%.	
6.4	Reduce the prevalence of mental disorders among adults to 10.7%.	
6.5	Reduce the proportion of people aged 18 and older who report adverse health effects from stress to 35%.	
	a. People with disabilities	40%
6.6	Increase the proportion of people aged 18 and older with severe mental disorders who use community support programs to 30%.	
6.7	Increase the proportion of people with major depressive disorder who received treatment to 30%.	
6.8	Increase the proportion of people aged 18 and over who seek help with personal and emotional problems to 20%.	
	a. People with disabilities	30%
6.9	Decrease the proportion of people aged 18 and older who report significant levels of stress who do not seek help to 5%.	
6.10	See objective 7.18	
6.11	Increase the proportion of worksites with 50 or more employees that provide stress reduction programs to 40%.	
6.12	Establish a network to facilitate information access for persons experiencing stress.	
6.13	Increase the proportion of primary care providers who assess clients' cognitive, emotional, and behavioral function and make referrals as needed.	
6.14	Increase the proportion of children's primary care providers who routinely assess their emotional needs and status.	
6.15	Reduce the prevalence of depressive disorders among adults to 4.3%.	
	a. Women	5.5%

Category: Violent and Abusive Behavior

Number	**Objective**	
7.1	Reduce homicides to 7.2 per 100,000 people.	
	a. Children (age 3 and under)	3.1
	b. Spouses (age 15–34)	1.4
	c. Black men (age 15–34)	72.4
	d. Hispanic men (age 14–34)	33.0
	e. Black women (age 15–34)	16.0
	f. Native Americans	9.0
7.2	Reduce suicides to 10.5 per 100,000 people.	
	a. Youth (age 15–19)	8.2
	b. Men (age 20–34)	21.4
	c. White men (age 65 and older)	39.2
	d. Native American men	17.0
7.3	Reduce firearm-related deaths to 11.6 per 100,000 people.	
	a. Blacks	30
7.4	Reverse the incidence of maltreatment of children under age 18 to 22.6 per 100,000 children.	
	a. Physical abuse	4.9
	b. Sexual abuse	2.1
	c. Emotional abuse	3.0
	d. Neglect	14.6
7.5	Reduce physical abuse of women by male partners to 27 per 1000 couples.	
7.6	Reduce assault injuries among people age 12 and older to 8.7 per 1000 people.	
7.7	Reduce rape and attempted rape of women age 12 and older to 108 per 100,000 women.	
	a. Women aged 12–34	225
7.8	Reduce the incidence of injurious suicide attempts among adolescents aged 14–17 by 15%.	
7.9	Reduce the incidence of physical fighting among adolescents aged 14–17 to 110 per 1000.	
	a. Black males	160
7.10	Reduce weapon carrying by adolescents to 86 per 1000.	
	a. Blacks	105
7.11	Reduce the inappropriate storage of weapons by 20%.	
7.12	Develop protocols for handling suicide attempts, sexual assault, and abuse in 90% of emergency departments.	
7.13	Extend unexplained child death review systems to 45 states.	
7.14	Increase the number of states in which 50% of abused or neglected children receive mental health follow up to 30.	
7.15	Reduce the proportion of battered women and their children turned away from shelter to 10%.	
7.16	Increase the proportion of schools that teach nonviolent conflict resolution to 50%.	
7.17	Extend comprehensive violence prevention programs to 80% of jurisdictions with populations over 100,000.	
7.18	Increase to 50 the number of states with established protocols to coordinate mental health, substance abuse, public health, and correctional efforts to prevent suicide by inmates.	
7.19	See objective 9.25	

Category: Educational and Community-based Programs

Number	**Objective**
8.1	See objective 17.1
8.2	Increase the high school completion rate to 90%.
8.3	Provide access to high quality, developmentally appropriate preschool programs to all disadvantaged and disabled children to help prepare them for school entry.

8.4	Increase the proportion of elementary and secondary schools that provide comprehensive health education to 75%.
8.5	Increase the proportion of postsecondary institutions that have institution-wide health promotion programs for students to 50%.
8.6	Increase the proportion of worksites with 50 or more employees that provide employee health promotion programs to 85%.
8.7	Increase the proportion of hourly workers who regularly take part in employer-sponsored health promotion activities to 20%.
8.8	Increase the proportion of people over age 65 who had opportunities to participate in at least one health promotion activity in the last year to 90%.
8.9	Increase the proportion of people under 10 years of age who have discussed nutrition, physical activity, sexual behavior, alcohol and drug use, or safety with family members at least once in the last month to 75%.
8.10	Establish community health programs that address at least three Healthy People 2000 priorities and reach at least 40% of each state's population.
8.11	Increase the proportion of counties with culturally appropriate health promotion programs to 50%.
8.12	Increase the proportion of hospitals, HMOs, and group practices that provide health education programs to 90% and community hospitals offering health promotion programs in local priority areas to 90%.
8.13	Increase the proportion of local television network affiliates in the top 20 markets that have developed partnerships with community agencies to address health problems related to Healthy People 2000 to 75%.
8.14	Increase the proportion of people served by a local health department effectively carrying out the core public health functions to 90%.

Category: Unintentional Injury

Number	Objective
9.1	Reduce deaths due to unintentional injury to 29.3 per 100,000 people.
	a. Native Americans 53.0
	b. Black males 51.9
	c. White males 42.9
	d. Mexican American males 43.0
9.2	Reduce hospitalizations for nonfatal unintentional injuries to 754 per 100,000 people.
	a. Black males 856
9.3	Reduce deaths due to motor vehicle accidents to 1.5 per 100 million miles traveled and 14.2 per 100,000 people.
	a. Children under age 14 4.4
	b. Youth (age 15–24) 26.8
	c. People 70 and over 20.0
	d. Native Americans 32.0
	e. Motorcyclists 0.9
	f. Pedestrians 2.0
	g. Mexican Americans 18.0
9.4	Reduce deaths from falls and fall-related injuries to 2.3 per 100,000 people.
	a. People aged 65–84 14.4
	b. People 85 and older 105.0
	c. Black men aged 30–69 5.6
	d. Native Americans 2.8
9.5	Reduce drowning deaths to 1.3 per 100,000 people.
	a. Children under 5 2.3
	b. Men aged 15–34 2.5
	c. Black males 3.6
	d. Native Americans 2.0

9.6	Reduce residential fire deaths to 1.2 per 100,000 people.	
	a. Children 5 and under	3.3
	b. People aged 65 and over	3.3
	c. Black males	4.3
	d. Black females	2.6
	e. Due to smoking	8%
	f. Native Americans	1.4
	g. Puerto Ricans	2.0
9.7	Reduce hospitalizations for hip fracture in people 65 and older to 607 per 100,000 people.	
	a. White women 85 and older	2177
9.8	Reduce nonfatal poisoning to 88 emergency department treatments per 100,000 people.	
	a. Children under 5	520
9.9	Reduce hospitalization for nonfatal head injury to 106 per 100,000 people.	
9.10	Reduce hospitalizations for nonfatal spinal cord injury to 5 per 100,000 people.	
9.11	Reduce secondary conditions due to spinal cord injury by 20%.	
9.12	Increase use of safety belts and child safety seats to 85% of motor vehicle occupants.	
9.13	Increase use of helmets to 80% of motorcyclists and 50% of bicyclists.	
9.14	Establish laws in all 50 states requiring seat belt and motorcycle helmet use by all age groups.	
9.15	Enact laws in all 50 states requiring new handguns to be designed to minimize discharge by children.	
9.16	Extend the number of jurisdictions with codes addressing installation of sprinkler systems in residences at risk for fire to 2000.	
9.17	Increase the presence of functional smoke alarms to one per floor of inhabited residences.	
9.18	Provide injury prevention education in 50% of public school systems.	
9.19	Extend use of protective equipment to all organizations sponsoring sports or recreational events with risk of injury.	
9.20	Increase the number of states with roadway markings and signs to protect the safety of older drivers and pedestrians to 50.	
9.21	Increase the proportion of primary care providers who provide age-appropriate safety counseling to 50%.	
9.22	Extend the capability to link emergency services, trauma systems, and hospital data to 20 states.	
9.23	See objective 4.1	
9.24	Extend to 50 states laws requiring helmets for all bicycle riders.	
9.25	Enact laws in all 50 states requiring proper storage of firearms to minimize access to minors.	
9.26	Increase the number of states with graduated driver licensing programs for novice drivers and those under 18 to 35.	

Category: Occupational Safety and Health

Number	**Objective**	
10.1	Reduce work-related injuries to 4 per 100,000 full-time workers.	
	a. Mine workers	21.0
	b. Construction workers	17.0
	c. Transportation workers	10.0
	d. Farm workers	9.4
10.2	Reduce work-related injuries resulting in medical treatment, lost work time, or restricted work activity to 6 per 100 full-time workers.	
	a. Construction workers	10.0
	b. Nursing and personal care workers	9.0
	c. Farm workers	8.0
	d. Transportation workers	6.0
	e. Mine workers	6.0
	f. Adolescent workers	3.8

10.3	Reduce cumulative trauma disorders to 60 per 100,000 full-time workers.
	a. Manufacturing workers
	150
	b. Meat product workers
	2000

10.3   Reduce cumulative trauma disorders to 60 per 100,000 full-time workers.
    a. Manufacturing workers   150
    b. Meat product workers   2000

10.4   Reduce occupational skin disorders to 55 per 100,000 full-time workers.

10.5   Reduce hepatitis B incidence among occupationally exposed workers to 623 cases.

10.6   Increase the number of worksites with 50 or more employees that mandate use of occupant protection systems.

10.7   Reduce the proportion of workers exposed to noise levels above 85 dBA to 15%.

10.8   Eliminate work-related exposures that cause blood lead concentrations greater than 25 µg/dL.

10.9   Increase hepatitis B immunization levels among occupationally exposed workers to 90%.

10.10   Implement occupational safety and health plans in 50 states.

10.11   Establish standards for occupational exposures to prevent lung disease in 50 states.

10.12   Increase the proportion of worksites with 50 or more employees that have implemented worker health and safety programs to 70%.

10.13   Increase the proportion of worksites with 50 or more employees that offer back injury prevention and rehabilitation programs to 50%.

10.14   Establish small business health and safety consultation services in 50 states.

10.15   Increase the proportion of health care providers who elicit occupational exposures to 75%.

10.16   Reduce work-related homicides to 0.5 per 100,000 full-time workers.

10.17   Reduce age-adjusted mortality due to occupational lung diseases to 7.7 per 100,000.

10.18   See objective 3.11

10.19   See objective 3.12

10.20   Reduce to 0 the number of states with laws related to clean indoor air that preempt stronger local laws.

Category: Environmental Health

Number	Objective
11.1	Reduce hospitalization for asthma to 160 per 100,000 people.
	a. Nonwhites 265
	b. Children 225
	c. Women 183
11.2	Reduce the prevalence of serious mental retardation in school children to 2 per 1000 children.
11.3	Reduce outbreaks of waterborne diseases to 11 per year.
11.4	Reduce the prevalence of blood lead levels exceeding 15 µg/dL and 25 µg/dL in children aged 6 months to 5 years to 300,000 and zero, respectively.
11.5	Increase the proportion of people who live in counties that have not exceeded air pollution standards in the last year to 85%.
11.6	Increase the proportion of homes tested for radon and found to pose minimal risk or have been modified to reduce risk to 40%.
	a. Homes with smokers and former smokers 50%
	b. Homes with children 50%
11.7	Decrease the release of substances on the Department of Health and Human Services list of carcinogens by 65% and substances on the Agency for Toxic Substances and Disease Registry priority list by 50%.
11.8	Reduce average production of solid waste per person per day to 4.3 pounds before recovery and 3.2 pounds after recovery (recycling and composting).
11.9	Increase the proportion of people who have a safe drinking water supply to 85%.
11.10	Increase the proportion of bodies of water that support beneficial use as follows:

Rivers supporting
    consumable fish   94%
    recreational activities   85%
Lakes supporting
    consumable fish   82%
    recreational activities   88%

	Estuaries supporting	
	consumable fish	97%
	recreational activities	91%
11.11	Perform lead testing in 50% of homes built before 1950.	
11.12	Expand the number of states where at least 75% of jurisdictions have construction standards that minimize indoor radon to 35%.	
11.13	Increase the number of states requiring buyers to be informed of lead-based paint and radon in all buildings for sale to 30.	
11.14	Clean up all hazardous waste sites on the National Priority List.	
11.15	Establish curbside recycling programs that serve 50% of the population.	
11.16	Establish and monitor plans to define and track sentinel environmental diseases in 35 states.	
11.17	See objective 3.8	

Category: Food and Drug Safety (see *Healthy People 2000: Midcourse Review and 1995 Revisions* for related objectives)

Category: Oral Health (see *Healthy People 2000: Midcourse Review and 1995 Revisions* for related objectives)

Category: Maternal and Infant Health

Number	**Objective**	
14.1	Reduce infant mortality to 7 per 1000 live births.	
	a. Blacks	11.0
	b. Native Americans	8.5
	c. Puerto Ricans	8.0
14.2	Reduce the fetal death rate to 5 per 1000 live births plus fetal deaths	
	a. Blacks	7.5
14.3	Reduce maternal mortality to 3.3 per 100,000 live births.	
	a. Blacks	5.0
14.4	Reduce the incidence of fetal alcohol syndrome to 0.12 per 1000 live births.	
	a. Native Americans	2.0
	b. Blacks	0.4
14.5	Reduce the incidence of low birth weight to 5% of live births and very low birth weight to 1%.	
	a. Blacks—low birth weight	9%
	b. Blacks—very low birth weight	2%
	c. Puerto Ricans—low birth weight	6%
	d. Puerto Ricans—very low birth weight	1%
14.6	Increase the proportion of mothers who achieve the minimum recommended weight gain during pregnancy to 85%.	
14.7	Reduce severe complications of pregnancy to 15 per 100 deliveries.	
14.8	Reduce the cesarean delivery rate to 15 per 100 deliveries.	
	a. First time cesarean delivery	12
	b. Repeat cesarean deliveries	65
14.9	See objective 2.11	
14.10	Increase abstinence from tobacco use during pregnancy to 90% and increase abstinence from alcohol, cocaine, and marijuana by 20%.	
14.11	Increase the proportion of pregnant women who receive prenatal care in the first trimester of pregnancy to 90%.	
14.12	See objective 5.10	
14.13	Increase the proportion of women in prenatal care who are offered screening and counseling on detection of fetal abnormalities to 90%.	
14.14	Increase the proportion of pregnant women and infants who receive risk-appropriate care to 90%.	

14.15	Increase the proportion of newborns screened for genetic disorders and other disabling conditions to 95% and increase the proportion of infants testing positive who receive treatment to 90%.
14.16	Increase the proportion of babies under 19 months who receive primary care services to 90%.
14.17	Reduce the incidence of spina bifida and other neural tube defects to 3 per 10,000 live births.

Category: Heart Disease and Stroke

Number	Objective
15.1	Reduce coronary heart disease to 100 per 100,000 people.
	a. Blacks 115 per 100,000
15.2	Reduce stroke deaths to 20 per 100,000 people.
	a. Blacks 27
15.3	Reduce the incidence of end-stage renal disease to 13 per 100,000 people.
	a. Blacks 30
15.4	Increase to 50% the proportion of people with high blood pressure whose blood pressure is under control.
	a. Men 40%
	b. Mexican Americans 50%
	c. Women over age 70 50%
15.5	Increase the proportion of people with high blood pressure who are taking steps to control their blood pressure to 90%.
	a. White men aged 18–34 80%
	b. Black men aged 18–34 80%
15.6	Reduce mean serum cholesterol levels in adults to 200 mg/dL.
15.7	Reduce prevalence of blood cholesterol levels greater than 240 mg/dL to 20% of adults.
15.8	Increase the proportion of adults with high blood cholesterol levels who are taking action to reduce their cholesterol to 60%.
15.9	See objective 2.5
15.10	See objective 1.2
15.11	See objective 1.3
15.12	See objective 3.4
15.13	Increase the proportion of adults who have had their blood pressure checked in the past 2 years and who know whether it was normal or abnormal to 90%.
15.14	Increase the proportion of adults who have had their cholesterol level checked in the last 5 years to 75%.
15.15	Increase the proportion of primary care providers who initiate diet and, if needed, drug therapy for hypercholesterolemia to 75%.
15.16	Increase the proportion of worksites with 50 or more employees that offer blood pressure and cholesterol education and control programs to 50%.
15.17	Increase the proportion of clinical laboratories that meet standards for cholesterol testing to 90%.

Category: Cancer

Number	Objective
16.1	Reduce cancer deaths to 130 per 100,000 people.
	a. Blacks 175
16.2	Slow lung cancer deaths to 42 per 100,000 people.
	a. Females 27
	b. Black males 91
16.3	Reduce breast cancer deaths to 20.6 per 100,000 women.
	a. Black females 25

16.4	Reduce deaths from cancer of the uterine cervix to 1.3 per 100,000 women.	
	a. Black females	3
	b. Hispanic females	2
16.5	Reduce colorectal cancer deaths to 13.2 per 100,000 people.	
	a. Blacks	16.5
16.6	See objective 3.4	
16.7	See objective 2.5	
16.8	See objective 2.6	
16.9	Increase the proportion of people who limit sun exposure, use sunscreen, and avoid sources of artificial ultraviolet light to 60%.	
16.10	Increase the proportion of primary care providers who counsel clients about tobacco use cessation, cancer screening, and diet modification to 75%.	
16.11	Increase the proportion of women aged 50 and over who have received a clinical breast examination in the last 1–2 years to 60%.	
16.12	Increase the proportion of women over age 17 who have ever received a Pap test to 95% and those who have received a Pap test in the last 1–3 years to 85%.	
16.13	Increase the proportion of people who have received fecal occult blood testing in the last 2–3 years to 50%.	
16.14	Increase the proportion of people age 50 and older seen by primary care providers in the last year who received oral, skin, and digital rectal examinations to 40%.	
16.15	Monitor and certify all cytology laboratories.	
16.16	Ensure that 100% of mammograms meet quality standards.	
16.17	Reduce oral cavity and pharyngeal cancer deaths to 10.5 per 100,000 men and 4.1 per 100,000 women aged 45–74.	
	a. Black males	26.0
	b. Black females	6.9

Category: Diabetes and Chronic Disabling Conditions

Number	Objective	
17.1	Increase years of healthy life to 65.	
17.2	Reduce the proportion of people who experience major activity limitation due to chronic conditions to 8%.	
	a. Low-income people	15%
	b. Native Americans	11%
	c. Blacks	9%
	d. Puerto Ricans	10%
17.3	Reduce to 90 per 1000 people the proportion of those over age 65 with difficulty in two or more personal care activities.	
	a. Persons over age 85	325
	b. Blacks over age 65	98
17.4	Reduce the proportion of people with asthma who experience activity limitation to 10%.	
	a. Blacks	19%
	b. Puerto Ricans	22%
17.5	Reduce the prevalence of activity limitation due to chronic back conditions to 19 per 1000 people.	
17.6	Reduce the prevalence of significant hearing impairment to 82 per 1000 people.	
	a. People age 45 and older	180
17.7	Reduce the prevalence of significant vision impairment to 30 per 100 people.	
	a. People age 45 and older	70
17.8	See objective 11.2	
17.9	Reduce diabetes-related deaths to 34 per 100,000 people.	
	a. Blacks	58
	b. Native Americans	41
	c. Mexican Americans	50
	d. Puerto Ricans	42

17.10	Reduce the most severe complications of diabetes as follows:	
	End-stage renal disease	1.4 per 1000 people
	Blindness	1.4 per 1000 people
	Lower extremity amputation	4.9 per 1000 people
	Perinatal mortality	2%
	Major congenital malformation	4%

17.11	Reduce diabetes prevelence to 25 per 1000 people.	
	a. Native Americans	62
	b. Puerto Ricans	49
	c. Mexican Americans	49
	d. Cuban Americans	32
	e. Blacks	32

17.12   See objective 1.2

17.13   See objective 1.3

17.14   Increase the proportion of people with chronic and disabling conditions who receive education and information about resources to 40%.

	a. People with diabetes	75%
	b. People with asthma	50%
	c. Blacks with diabetes	75%
	d. Hispanics with diabetes	75%

17.15   Increase the proportion of primary care providers who routinely screen infants and children for vision, speech, hearing, language, and developmental problems to 80%.

17.16   Reduce the age at which significant hearing impairment is identified in children to 1 year.

17.17   Increase the proportion of primary care providers who routinely screen elderly clients for urinary incontinence and hearing, vision, cognitive, and functional impairments to 60%.

17.18   Increase the proportion of perimenopausal women counseled about the risks and benefits of estrogen therapy to 90%.

17.19   Increase the proportion of worksites with 50 or more employees that hire people with disabilities to 75%.

17.20   Increase the number of states with service systems for disabled or chronically ill children to 50.

17.21   Reduce the prevalence of peptic ulcer disease to 18 per 1000 people.

17.22   Develop and implement a process to identify gaps in disease prevention and health promotion data.

17.23   Increase the proportion of people with diabetes who have a dilated eye examination yearly to 70%.

Category: HIV Infection

Number	Objective	
18.1	Confine annual incidence of diagnosed cases of AIDS to 43 per 100,000 people.	
	a. Men who have sex with men	48,000 cases
	b. Blacks	136 per 100,000
	c. Hispanics	76 per 100,000
	d. Women	13 per 100,000
	e. Injecting drug users	25,000 cases
18.2	Confine the prevalence of HIV infection to 400 per 100,000 people.	
18.3	See objective 5.4	
18.4	Increase the proportion of sexually active unmarried people who used a condom at last intercourse to 50%.	
	a. Sexually active women aged 15–19	60%
	b. Sexually active men aged 15–19	75%
	c. Injecting drug users	75%
	d. Black women aged 15–44	74%

18.5	Increase the proportion of injecting drug users in treatment to 50%.
18.6	Increase the proportion of active injecting drug users who use new or properly decontaminated paraphernalia to 75%.
18.7	Reduce the risk of HIV transmission via transfusion to 1 per 250,000 units.
18.8	Increase the proportion of HIV-infected persons aware of their status to 80%.
18.9	Increase the proportion of primary care and mental health providers who counsel on HIV and other STD prevention to 75%.
18.10	Increase the proportion of schools that have HIV and other STD education programs in grades 4–12 to 95%.
18.11	Increase the proportion of college students who receive on-campus HIV and STD education to 90%.
18.12	Increase the proportion of cities with populations over 100,000 that have outreach programs for injecting drug users to 90%.
18.13	See objective 5.11
18.14	Extend regulations to protect workers from exposure to bloodborne infections to all facilities where workers are at risk.
18.15	See objective 5.5
18.16	Increase the proportion of large businesses that provide HIV/AIDS workplace programs to 50% and the proportion of small businesses to 10%.
18.17	Increase the number of federally funded primary care clinics with linkages to substance abuse treatment programs to 40%.

Category: Sexually Transmitted Diseases

Number	Objective
19.1	Reduce gonorrhea incidence to 100 per 100,000 people.
	a. Blacks 650
	b. Adolescents (age 15–19) 375
	c. Women (age 15–44) 175
19.2	Reduce the prevalence of *Chlamydia trachomatis* infections in women under 25 to 5%.
19.3	Reduce the incidence of primary and secondary syphilis to 4 per 100,000 people.
	a. Blacks 30
19.4	Reduce the incidence of congenital syphilis to 40 per 100,000 live births.
	a. Blacks 175
	b. Hispanics 50
19.5	Reduce first time consultations for genital herpes and genital warts to 138,500 and 246,500, respectively.
19.6	Reduce hospitalization for pelvic inflammatory disease to 100 per 100,000 women aged 15–44 and initial physician visits to 290,000.
19.7	Reduce sexually transmitted hepatitis B to 30,500 cases.
19.8	Reduce the rate of repeat gonorrhea infection to 15%.
19.9	See objective 5.4
19.10	See objective 18.4
19.11	See objective 5.11
19.12	See objective 18.10
19.13	Increase the proportion of primary care providers who correctly manage cases of STD to 90%.
19.14	See objective 18.9
19.15	Increase the proportion of clients with STDs who are offered provider referral services (contact follow-up) to 50%.
19.16	See objective 5.5
19.17	See objective 18.11

Category: Immunization and Infectious Diseases

Number	Objective

20.1   Reduce indigenous cases of vaccine-preventable diseases as follows:

Diphtheria in people under 25	0
Tetanus in people under 25	0
Polio (wild virus type)	0
Measles	0
Rubella	0
Congenital rubella syndrome	0
Mumps	500
Pertussis	1000

20.2   Reduce epidemic pneumonia and influenza deaths in people over 65 to 15.9 per 100,000 people.

20.3   Reduce viral hepatitis (per 100,000 people) as follows:

Hepatitis A	16.0
Hepatitis B	40.0
Hepatitis C	13.7

20.4   Reduce tuberculosis incidence to 3.5 per 100,000 people.

a. Asians	15
b. Blacks	10
c. Hispanics	5
d. Native Americans	5

20.5   Reduce surgical wound infections in intensive care patients by 10%.

20.6   Reduce cases of illness among international travelers as follows:

Typhoid fever	140
Hepatitis A	1119
Malaria	750

20.7   Reduce bacterial meningitis incidence to 4.7 cases per 100,000 people.

a. Alaskan Natives	8

20.8   Reduce infectious diarrhea in children in licensed day care centers by 25%.

20.9   Reduce restricted activity or school absenteeism due to middle ear infection in children under 5 to 105 days per 100 children.

20.10   Reduce pneumonia-related restricted activity days as follows:

People over 65	15.1 days
Children under 5	24.0 days

20.11   Increase basic immunization levels as follows:

Children under age 3	90%
a. Blacks over 65	60%
b. Hispanics over 65	60%

20.12   Reduce postexposure rabies treatment to 9000 per year.

20.13   Expand immunization laws to all antigens in all states.

20.14   Increase the proportion of primary care providers who counsel regarding and provide immunizations to 90%.

20.15   Improve financing and delivery of immunizations so no one has barriers to access.

20.16   Increase the proportion of public health departments that provide adult immunizations to 90%.

20.17   Increase the proportion of local health departments that have TB identification programs for high-risk populations to 90%.

20.18   Increase the proportion of people with TB infection who complete a course of preventive therapy to 85%.

20.19   Increase the proportion of tertiary care hospital laboratories capable of rapid influenza diagnosis to 85% and the proportion of secondary care hospitals and HMO laboratories to 50%.

Category: Clinical Preventive Services

Number	Objective
21.1	See objective 17.1
21.2	Increase the proportion of people who have received selected clinical preventive screening, immunization, and counseling services as recommended by the U.S. Preventive Services Task Force as follows:

Routine check-up	91%
Cholesterol check (last 2 years)	75%
Tetanus booster (last 10 years)	62%
Pneumococcal vaccine (lifetime)	60%
Influenza vaccine (in last year)	60%
Pap test (last 3 years)	85%
Breast examination and mammogram (last 2 years)	60%
Counseling services	80%

Number	Objective
21.3	Increase the proportion of people with a consistent source of primary care to 95%.
21.4	Improve funding and delivery of care so all have access to minimum screening, counseling, and immunization services.
21.5	Increase the proportion of people receiving care from publicly funded services who receive minimum screening, counseling, and immunization services to 90%.
21.6	Increase the proportion of primary care providers who provide basic screening, counseling, and immunization services to 50%.
21.7	Increase the proportion of people served by local health departments that assure essential clinical preventive services to 90%.
21.8	Increase the proportion of degrees in the health professions awarded to minority group members as follows:

Blacks	8.0%
Hispanics	6.4%
Native Americans	0.6%

Increase the proportion of minority individuals enrolled in nursing schools:

Blacks	10%
Hispanics	4%
Asians	5%
Native Americans	1%

Category: Surveillance and Data Systems

Number	Objective
22.1	Develop a set of health status indicators for use at national, state, and local levels and implement their use in 40 states.
22.2	Identify or create data sources to measure progress toward each of the year 2000 objectives.
22.3	Develop and disseminate procedures for collecting data related to year 2000 objectives.
22.4	See objective 17.22
22.5	Implement in all states periodic analysis and publication of data regarding achievement of year 2000 objectives for at least 10 priority areas.
22.6	Expand to all states capabilities for health information transfer among federal, state, and local agencies.
22.7	Achieve timely release of national surveillance and survey data needed by health professionals and agencies.

HEALTH RISK APPRAISAL TOOLS

There are a variety of tools available to community health nurses to identify health risks among individual clients. Community health nurses can use the information derived from the health risk appraisal to assist clients to minimize their risk of developing selected health problems. Data on health risks among individuals can also be aggregated to identify priorities for risk factor modification at the community level. Health risk appraisals have been developed for different populations and the results may or may not be applicable to other population groups, so health risk appraisal tools should be selected carefully for use with appropriate clients and population groups. Information about several health risk appraisal tools is presented here. Information provided includes the title of the tool, its source, appropriate populations, and a brief description of the tool itself. Age groups used are as follows: adolescent (12–18 years), adult (19–64 years), college age (18–22 years), and senior (65 years and older). Particular racial and ethnic groups are indicated for appraisal tools specifically normed for them.

Title: *Adolescent Wellness Appraisal*

Source: University of Michigan Fitness Research Center, 401 Washtenaw Ave., Ann Arbor, MI 48109–2214
(313) 763–2462

Appropriate population: Adolescent

Description: Provides 55 questions addressing health knowledge and behaviors common to adolescents that most influence their health status. Identifies positive as well as negative behaviors and recommendations for behavior change. Allows for simulated situations to assess the impact of specific behaviors.

Title: *AVIVA*

Source: Cleveland State University, 2121 Euclid Ave. UC532, Cleveland, OH 44115
(216) 687–5243

Appropriate population: Appropriate for adults, general population, African Americans, men, women

Description: A computerized appraisal accessed by calling (216) 687–9217 and entering an access code. Poses questions about the caller's lifestyle and derives an evaluation of hospitalization risk. Provides information on access to additional resources such as videotapes.

Title: *Health Logic*

Source: HMC Software, 3001 LBJ Freeway, Suite 224, Dallas, TX 75234
(214) 247–4080

Appropriate population: Adult

Description: CDC-based risk appraisal addressing medical history, preventive care, heart disease risk, cholesterol, blood pressure, smoking, exercise, stress, osteoporosis, nutrition, cancer, motor vehicle accidents, back injury, and home safety. User-defined questions can be added to the database. Also provides human resources data on leave, claims, job satisfaction, and productivity.

Title: *Health Potential Assessment Program*

Source: Health Examinetics, Inc., 15330 Avenue of Science, San Diego, CA 92128
(800) 232–2332

Appropriate population: Adolescent, college age, adult, senior

Description: Combines a self-administered lifestyle questionnaire with physiologic data to derive an overall evaluation of health behavior and risk. Tests are conducted by Health Examinetics staff and include blood pressure, lipid screen, liver function tests, blood sugar, visual acuity, tonometry, fecal occult blood, frame size, and body fat determination.

Title: *Health Profile 500*

Source: Johnson & Johnson Health Management, Inc., 410 George St., New Brunswick, NJ 08901
(908) 524–2144

Appropriate population: College age, adult, senior

Description: Addresses health behaviors that have the greatest impact on health as well as five self-reported biometric measures (height, weight, blood pressure, cholesterol, and percent body fat). Data are used to determine health status and risks. Useful for health education. (*900* version includes biometric data entered by a health professional rather than self-reported data.)

Title: *Health Risk Appraisal*

Source: Queue, Inc., 338 Commerce Dr., Fairfield, CT 06432
(203) 335–0908

Appropriate population: People aged 10 to 75 years, white, black, and Native American men and women

Description: A computerized health risk appraisal. Identifies the top ten causes of death for the individual's age, race, and sex. Then presents a series of risk appraisal questions related to those causes of death. Addresses both genetic inheritance and health-related behaviors. Compares the individual's risk of death to the average risk for someone of his or her age, race, and sex, based on reported health risks. Provides suggestions for behavior change to reduce risk. Only addresses risk for mortality, not for nonfatal morbidity.

Title: *The Healthier People Network Health Risk Appraisal*

Source: The Healthier People Network, Inc., 1549 N. Clairmont Rd., Suite 205, Decatur, GA 30033
(404) 636–3127

Appropriate population: Adult, senior, general population, African Americans, Native Americans

Description: Computerized appraisal. Provides 10-year estimates of the probability of dying of 42 causes of death based on the presence or absence of 23 risk factors. Useful for counseling behavior change.

Title: *HealthMax*

Source: Health Examinetics, Inc., 15330 Avenue of Science, San Diego, CA 92128
(800) 232–2332

Appropriate population: College age, adult, senior

Description: Calculates potential health costs based on risk behaviors. Provides suggestions for behavior change and risk reduction. Useful to employers to calculate potential health plan costs.

Title: *Healthstyle*
Source: National Information Clearinghouse (Office of Disease Prevention and Health Promotion), P.O. Box 1133, Washington, DC 20013
(202) 245–7611
Appropriate population: College age, adult
Description: Self-scored health risk appraisal. Addresses six areas of health. Provides a basis for health education related to behavioral risks.

Title: *Hope Health Appraisal*
Source: Hope Publications, 350 Michigan Ave., Kalamazoo, MI 49007
(616) 343–6260
Appropriate population: Adult
Description: Self-administered 12-section appraisal accompanied by a booklet that suggests lifestyle changes to improve health and longevity.

Title: *Lifestyle Assessment Questionnaire*
Source: National Wellness Institute, 1045 Clark St., Suite 210, Stevens Point, WI 54481–2962
(715) 346–2172
Appropriate population: College age, adult, senior
Description: Available as interactive computer program or mailed questionnaire to be returned for analysis. Assesses lifestyle behaviors and identifies positive lifestyle behaviors as well as risk behaviors and suggestions for changes. Provides strategies to promote behavior change.

Title: *Personal Risk Analysis*
Source: Eris, 4548 Scotts Valley Dr., Scotts Valley, CA 95066
Appropriate population: Adult, Native Americans, Latinos
Description: Provides several computerized modules to conduct basic health risk assessment, nutrition assessment, cardiac risk analysis, and clinical systems review. Available in Spanish, Portugese, and UK English versions. Returns computerized personalized analyses. Data can be scanned in or entered on keyboard.

Title: *Test Well: Health Risk Appraisal*
Source: National Wellness Institute, Inc., 1045 Clark St., Suite 210, Stevens Point, WI 54481–2962
(715) 346–2172
Appropriate population: Adults with minimum of 10th grade education
Description: Analyzes the respondent's risk of death from the leading causes of death for his or her age group. Calculates an appraised health age and an achievable health age if recommended behavior changes are made. Also identifies positive health behaviors.

Title: *Test Well: Wellness Inventory*
Source: National Wellness Institute, Inc., 1045 Clark St., Suite 210, Stevens Point, WI 54481–2962
(715) 346–2172
Appropriate population: Adults with minimum of 10th grade education (also a college-age version)
Description: Assess self-care behaviors related to physical fitness, nutrition, social interaction, self-care, spiritual wellness and values, emotional wellness, intellectual wellness, environmental health, safety, occupational wellness, sexuality, and emotional awareness.

Title: *Wellness Inventory*
Source: Wellness Associates, 12347 Dupont Rd., Sebastopol, CA 95472
(707) 874–1466
Appropriate population: Healthy individuals or those with chronic illness
Description: Computerized appraisal tool. Examines underlying beliefs and values related to health. Intended for use with other health risk appraisals that focus only on risk behaviors. Addresses 12 areas of wellness: breathing, eating, feeling, finding meaning, moving, playing/working, sensing, thinking, transcending, community, self-responsibility, and sex. Concludes with areas of concern derived from answers to questions in each area.

EDUCATIONAL PLANNING AND IMPLEMENTATION GUIDE

The tool presented here is designed to assist the community health nurse to plan health education for individual clients, families, or groups. It is based on the Dimensions Model and can be used by the community health nurse to assess and diagnose client education needs as well as to plan, implement, and evaluate a health education encounter.

The first and second pages of the tool address assessment of the learner and the learning situation. Nursing diagnoses of learning needs and the intervention plan for the health education encounter are documented on the third page of the tool. The intervention plan includes identification and classification of learning objectives, teaching strategies to be used, and plans for evaluation. On the final page of the tool space is provided to document evaluation of the health education encounter and to enter any recommendations for revisions for future encounters.

Educational Planning and Implementation Guide

Client: _____   Phone: _____

Address: _____

Contact person (for group encounters): _____

Assessment of Learning Situation

Biophysical Dimension

Client age(s): _____   Sex: _____   Race: _____

Possible influence of physical maturation on learning: _____

_____

Physical conditions giving rise to health education needs: _____

_____

Physical conditions that might influence ability to learn: _____

_____

Psychological Dimension

- Readiness and motivation to learn: _____

  _____

- Psychological factors that may impede learning (*stress, anxiety, depression, confusion, disorientation*):

  _____

  _____

- Coping abilities: _____

  _____

Physical Dimension

- Physical environment conditions giving rise to health education needs: _____

  _____

- Physical environment for learning (*noise, light levels, distractions*): _____

  _____

Social Dimension

- Education level: _____
- Socioeconomic level: _____
- Religion: _____
- Ethnicity: _____
- Primary language: _____
- Facility with English: _____
- Cultural influences on the learning situation: _____
- Social support for healthy behavior (*peer interactions, role models*): _____

  _____

- Occupation(s): _____

Behavioral Dimension

Nutrition (*food consumption, preferences, preparation*): _____

_____

Other consumption patterns: _____

_____

Health-related behaviors: _____

- Immunizations: _____
- Exercise: _____
- Dental hygiene: _____
- Seat belt use: _____
- Other safety precautions: _____
- Contraceptive use: _____
- Sexual activity: _____

Health Care System

Access to health care: _____

Knowledge of health care resources: _____

Use of health-promotive services: _____

Use of restorative/rehabilitative services: _____

Attitudes to health and health care: _____

Planning and Implementing the Health Education Encounter

Education Diagnoses	Learning Objectives	Classification of Learning Objectives	Teaching Strategies	Plan for Evaluation

Evaluation of Health Education Encounter
Evaluation of Learning Outcomes:

Learning Objective	Status Met/Unmet	Evidence

Process evaluation: _____
_____
_____
_____
_____
_____
_____

Revisions needed: _____
_____
_____
_____
_____
_____
_____

HOME SAFETY INVENTORY

The two tools included in this appendix are designed to help assess home safety for families with children and where older adults live. Relevant portions of the tools may also be used to assess the safety of the home for other clients. The results of either inventory can be used to educate individual clients or families regarding home safety issues. The inventories can also be completed by groups of people and the results used to initiate safety education.

Home Safety Inventory—Child

Age	Safety Consideration	Yes	No
Infant	1. Safe sleeping arrangements made for infant?	☐	☐
	2. Parents aware of bathing safety (not leaving child unattended, water temperature)?	☐	☐
	3. No loose parts on toys?	☐	☐
	4. Approved car restraint used consistently?	☐	☐
	5. Infant seat left on elevated surfaces?	☐	☐
	6. Infant restraint straps consistently used in infant seat, stroller, high chair, car seat?	☐	☐
	7. Small objects kept out of reach?	☐	☐
Toddler/preschool child	1. Poisons, sharp objects, etc., kept locked away?	☐	☐
	2. Poisonous substances stored in appropriate containers?	☐	☐
	3. Childproof lids correctly placed on medications and other toxins?	☐	☐
	4. Medications stored in locked area?	☐	☐
	5. Gates/barriers placed on stairs?	☐	☐
	6. Safety locks present on doors and upstairs windows?	☐	☐
	7. Child closely supervised at play?	☐	☐
	8. Child supervised at all times during bath?	☐	☐
	9. Toys have no small parts?	☐	☐
	10. Electrical outlets covered?	☐	☐
	11. Electrical cords left dangling?	☐	☐
	12. Pots and pans placed toward back of stove with handles turned toward rear?	☐	☐
	13. Play equipment in good repair?	☐	☐
	14. Outdoor play area is fenced and gates locked?	☐	☐
	15. Outdoor play area has resilient surface?	☐	☐
	16. Poisonous plants present in home or yard?	☐	☐
	17. Car seat belt used consistently?	☐	☐
	18. Caution used and taught in crossing streets?	☐	☐
School-age child	1. Child supervised in sports and outdoor play?	☐	☐
	2. Play equipment free of safety hazards?	☐	☐
	3. Outdoor play area floored with sand, shavings, or wood chips?	☐	☐
	4. Firearms kept locked with key inaccessible?	☐	☐
	5. Bicycle helmet worn consistently?	☐	☐
	6. Children taught not to open door to strangers?	☐	☐
	7. Car seat belt used consistently?	☐	☐
Adolescent	1. Firearms safety taught?	☐	☐
	2. Firearms stored unloaded with safety lock on?	☐	☐
	3. Teen cautioned not to admit being home alone?	☐	☐
	4. Car seat belt used consistently?	☐	☐

Home Safety Inventory—Older Person

Safety Consideration	Yes	No
1. Lighting adequate on stairs?	☐	☐
2. Stair rails present and in good repair?	☐	☐
3. Nonskid surfaces on stairs?	☐	☐
4. Throw rugs present safety hazard?	☐	☐
5. Crowded living area presents safety hazard?	☐	☐
6. Tub rails installed?	☐	☐
7. Tub has nonslip surface?	☐	☐
8. Space heaters present safety hazard?	☐	☐
9. Adequate provision made for refrigeration of food?	☐	☐
10. Medications kept in appropriately labeled containers with readable print?	☐	☐
11. Toxic substances have labels with readable print and are stored well away from food?	☐	☐
12. Home is adequately ventilated and heated?	☐	☐
13. Neighborhood is safe?	☐	☐
14. Fire and police notified of older person in home?	☐	☐

SAMPLE FORMS FOR DOCUMENTING HOME NURSING CARE

The four forms included here are examples of the types of forms that may be used to document home nursing care. The first form is a two-page Home Health Nursing Assessment that can be used by the community health nurse to identify the health care needs of the client seen in the home setting. The second form, Patient Progress Notes, can be used to record subsequent observations of the client's status and progress toward desired outcomes. The final two forms are the Home Health Certification and Plan of Treatment form (HCFA-485) and the Medical Update and Patient Information form (HCFA-486). Both are required to document home nursing care for reimbursement under Medicare.

Home Health Nursing Assessment

Patient name: _____   Birth date: _____   Record #: _____

Address: _____

Phone number: _____

Biophysical Dimension

Male _____   Female _____

Primary medical diagnosis: _____

Past medical history: _____

_____

_____

General appearance: _____

_____

Vital signs: Temp _____   Pulse: Apical_____   Radial _____   Respirations: _____

Weight: _____   Height: _____

Blood pressure: (1) Right arm—Supine _____   Sitting _____   Standing _____

(2) Left arm—Supine _____   Sitting _____   Standing _____

Hearing: Normal _____   Hearing impaired: _____   Deaf: _____   Uses hearing aid: R ____   L ____

Vision: Normal _____   Blind: _____   Limited _____   Uses glasses: Sometimes ____   Always ____

Developmental level: _____

Allergies: _____

Functional abilities: No problems: _____   Difficulty with: Bathing: ____   Dressing: ____   Toileting: ____

Mobility/transfer: ____   Eating: ____   Bowel control: ____   Bladder control: ____   Communication: ____

Meal preparation: ____   Housekeeping: ____   Shopping: ____

Use of assistive devices: _____

Describe any limitations noted: _____

_____

Immunization status: _____

Review of Systems

Neurological: No problems ___   Oriented x ___   Headache ___   Vertigo ___   Tremors ___   Seizures ___

Syncope ___   Parasthesias ___   Weakness ___   LOC (describe): _____

Cardiovascular: No problems ___   Palpitations ___   Fainting ___   Dizziness ___   Edema ___

Cyanosis: ____   Neck vein distention ____   Chest pain ____   Pulse irregularity ____   Syncope ____

Circumoral pallor ____

Respiratory: No problems ___   Dyspnea ___   SOB ___   SOBOE ___   Orthopnea ___   Cough ___

Cyanosis ____   Pain ____   Sputum ____   IPPB ____   O$_2$ ____

Lung sounds (describe): _____

_____

Gastrointestinal: No problems ____   Nausea ____   Vomiting ____   Anorexia ____   Bleeding ____

Pain ____   Diarrhea ____   Constipation ____   Incontinent ____   Distention ____   Aphagia ____

NGT ____   GT ____   JT ____

Bowel sounds (describe): _____

Genitourinary: No problems ____   Frequency ____   Urgency ____   Pain ____   Burning ____

Nocturia ____   Hematuria ____   Difficulty urinating ____   Incontinent ____   Retention ____   Catheter ____

Integumentary: No problems ____   Cool ____   Warm ____   Diaphoresis ____   Pallor ____

Cyanosis ____   Flushing ____   Mottling ____   Jaundice ____   Pruritis ____   Petechiae ____   Dry ____

Decubitus ____   Pressure areas ____

Wound/incision (describe): _____

Rash (describe): _____   Bruises (describe): _____

Turgor (describe): _____

Musculoskeletal: No problems ____   Joint swelling ____   Decreased ROM ____   Back pain ____

Reproductive: No problems ____   Impotence ____   Prostatitis ____   Discharge ____   Breast mass ____

Testicular mass ____   Decreased libido ____   Dysmenorrhea ____   Dyspareunia ____

Date of last Pap smear: _____

Hematopoetic: No problems ____   Anemia ____   Epistaxis ____   Bruising ____

Venous access: Good ____   Fair ____   Poor ____

Immunologic: Frequent infection ____   Diminished immune status ____   HIV infection ____

Pain: None ____   Description: _____

Intensity: 1+ (mild) ____   2+ (discomfort) ____   3+ (distressing) ____   4+ (severe) ____   5+ (excruciating) ____

Analgesics taken: _____   Dose: _____   Frequency: _____

Effectiveness: _____

Degree of limitation due to pain: _____

Psychological Dimension

Mood: No problems ____   Depressed ____   Anxious ____   Restless ____   Uncooperative ____

Mentation: Alert ____   Confused ____   Disoriented ____

Coping: Adequate ____   Minimal ____   Inadequate ____

History of mental illness: _____   Recent loss: _____

Life satisfaction: _____

History of family violence: _____

Sources of stress: _____

Physical Dimension

Type of residence: House ____   Apartment ____   Institution ____   Shelter ____   None ____

Ease of access: Stairs to climb ____   Ramp ____

Space: Adequate ____   Inadequate ____

Distance to bathroom: _____

Home safety: Adequate ____   Safety hazards present: _____

Safety features in home: Childproof latches ____   Tub rail ____   Grounded outlets ____   Stair lights ____

Stair rails ____   Smoke alarm ____

Infection control hazards: _____

Inadequate: Lighting ____   Heat ____   Ventilation ____   Air conditioning ____   Refrigeration ____

Cooking facilities ____   Plumbing ____   Waste disposal ____   Electricity ____

Use of space heaters: ____

Storage of hazardous materials: _____

Firearms in home: _____

Home maintenance/repair: Adequate ____   Inadequate ____   Describe problems noted: _____

Pets: Type _____   Indoor ____   Outdoor ____

Neighborhood safety: _____

Environmental pollutants: _____

Social Dimension

Education level: _____   Income: _____

Primary language: _____   Interpreter: _____

Religious affiliation: _____   Ethnicity: _____

Employed ____   Unemployed ____   Retired ____   Occupation(s): _____

Single ____   Married ____   Divorced ____   Widowed ____

Other persons in home: (include ages, health problems, etc.) _____

_____

Quality of family interactions: _____

_____

Opportunity for social interaction: _____

_____

Social support network: _____

_____

Cultural influences: _____

Availability of transportation: _____

Behavioral Dimension

Diet: Inadequate in: Calories ____   Protein ____   Iron ____   Potassium ____   Calcium ____

Vitamin A ____   Vitamin B complex ____   C ____   D ____   K ____   Fluid ____   Fiber ____

Excessive Fat ____   Calories ____   Sodium ____

Method of food preparation: _____

Typical meal pattern: _____

Other substances: Alcohol use ____   Amount: _____

Illicit drug use ____   Type _____   Amount: _____   Route _____

Tobacco use _____   Type _____   Amount: _____   Length of use _____

Medications (include prescription and over-the-counter medications):

Medication	Dose	Frequency	Route	Purpose	Length of Use
1.					
2.					
3.					
4.					
5.					

Sleep patterns: _____

Exercise: _____

Leisure activities: _____

Sexually active: ____ Orientation: _____ Satisfaction: _____

Unsafe sexual practices: _____

Other behaviors: Seat belt use ____ Contraceptive use ____ BSE/TSE ____

Use of other safety equipment _____

Health System Dimension

Usual source of health care: _____

Source of health care funding: _____

Use of preventive services: _____

Attitudes to health and health care: _____

Barriers to access: _____

Patient Progress Notes

Circle All Applicable:

1. Nursing assessment
2. Medication
   a. administration
   b. instruction
   c. review compliance
   d. review side effects
3. Infusion device
   a. instruction
   b. insertion

   c. maintenance care
   d. discontinue
4. IV hydration
   a. instruction
   b. review compliance
   c. review side effects
5. Chemotherapy
   a. administration
   b. instruction

   c. review compliance
   d. review side effects
6. TPN
   a. instruction
   b. administration
   c. review compliance
   d. review side effects
7. Enteral feedings
   a. insert tube

   b. instruction
   c. review compliance
   d. review side effects
8. Pain management
   a. instruction
   b. review compliance
   c. review side effects
9. Lab specimen drawn
10. Nutrition assessment

11. Instruction
    a. patient
    b. caregiver
    c. staff-informal
12. Equipment
    a. delivered
    b. returned
    c. inventoried

OBSERVATIONS:	TEMPERATURE	APICAL PULSE	RADIAL PULSE	RESPIRATIONS	BLOOD PRESSURE	WEIGHT

NEUROLOGICAL: ☐ Oriented x _____ ☐ Level of Alertness ☐ Headache ☐ Vertigo ☐ Tremors ☐ Seizures ☐ Syncope ☐ Coordination ☐ Parathesias ☐ Weakness ☐ Mobility ☐ No Problems
Comments:

CARDIOVASCULAR: ☐ Palpitations ☐ Fainting ☐ Dizziness ☐ Edema ☐ Cyanosis ☐ Neck Vein Distention ☐ Chest Pain ☐ Peripheral Pulses ☐ Pulse Irregularity ☐ Syncope ☐ Circumoral Pallor ☐ No Problems
Comments:

RESPIRATORY: ☐ Dyspnea ☐ SOB ☐ SOBOE ☐ Orthopnea ☐ Cough ☐ Cyanosis ☐ Pain ☐ Lung Sounds ☐ Sputum ☐ Used IPPB ☐ O_2 Used ☐ No Problems
Comments:

GASTROINTESTINAL: ☐ Nausea ☐ Vomiting ☐ Anorexia ☐ Bleeding ☐ Pain ☐ Diarrhea ☐ Incontinent ☐ Nutritional Problem ☐ Bowel Sounds ☐ Distention ☐ Aphagia ☐ NGT ☐ GT ☐ JT ☐ No Problems
Comments:

GENITO/URINARY: ☐ Frequency ☐ Urgency ☐ Pain ☐ Burning ☐ Nocturia ☐ Hematuria ☐ Difficulty Urinating ☐ Incontinent ☐ Retention ☐ Catheter Plugged ☐ No Problems
Comments:

SKIN: ☐ Rash ☐ Bruises ☐ Diaphoresis ☐ Pallor ☐ Cyanotic ☐ Flushing ☐ Jaundice ☐ Pruritis ☐ Petechiae ☐ Dry ☐ Pressure Areas ☐ Wound/Incision ☐ Cool ☐ Warm ☐ Decubitus ☐ No Problems
Comments:

PAIN: No Problems _____ Description _____ Location _____
Intensity: 1+ mild _____ 2+ discomfort _____ 3+ distressing _____ 4+ severe _____ 5+ excruciating _____
Analgesics taken: _____ Frequency _____ Effectiveness _____
Comments:

INFUSION: ☐ Peripheral ☐ Sub Q ☐ Central Line ☐ VAD Type _____ ☐ Intermittant ☐ Continuous ☐ Pump Type _____
Comments:

PSYCHOSOCIAL: ☐ Depressed ☐ Uncooperative ☐ Anxious ☐ Restless ☐ Forgetful ☐ Dependent ☐ Other (Specify) ☐ No Problems
Comments:

Narrative

_____

_____

_____

_____

_____

SIGNATURE

NAME: _____ MR # _____ DATE _____ TIME _____

Department of Health and Human Services
Health Care Financing Administration

Form Approved
OMB No. 0938-0357

HOME HEALTH CERTIFICATION AND PLAN OF TREATMENT

1. Patient's HI Claim No.	2. SOC Date	3. Certification Period		4. Medical Record No.	5. Provider No.
		From:	To:		

6. Patient's Name and Address

7. Provider's Name and Address

8. Date of Birth:	9. Sex	M	F	10. Medications: Dose/Frequency/Route (N)ew (C)hanged

11. ICD-9-CM Principal Diagnosis	Date

12. ICD-9-CM Surgical Procedure	Date

13. ICD-9-CM Other Pertinent Diagnoses	Date

14. DME and Supplies	15. Safety Measures:

16. Nutritional Req.	17. Allergies:

18.A. Functional Limitations

1	Amputation	5	Paralysis	9	Legally Blind
2	Bowel/Bladder (Incontinence)	6	Endurance	A	Dyspnea With Minimal Exertion
3	Contracture	7	Ambulation	B	Other (Specify)
4	Hearing	8	Speech		

18.B. Activities Permitted

1	Complete Bedrest	6	Partial Weight Bearing	A	Wheelchair
2	Bedrest BRP	7	Independent At Home	B	Walker
3	Up As Tolerated	8	Crutches	C	No Restrictions
4	Transfer Bed/Chair	9	Cane	D	Other (Specify)
5	Exercises Prescribed				

19. Mental Status:

1	Oriented	3	Forgetful	5	Disoriented	7	Agitated
2	Comatose	4	Depressed	6	Lethargic	8	Other

20. Prognosis:

1	Poor	2	Guarded	3	Fair	4	Good	5	Excellent

21. Orders for Discipline and Treatments (Specify Amount/Frequency/Duration)

22. Goals/Rehabilitation Potential/Discharge Plans

23. Verbal Start of Care and Nurse's Signature and Date Where Applicable:

24. Physician's Name and Address	25. Date HHA Received Signed POT	26. I ☐ certify ☐ recertify that the above home health services are required and are authorized by me with a written plan for treatment which will be periodically reviewed by me. This patient is under my care, is confined to his home, and is in need of intermittent skilled nursing care and/or physical or speech therapy or has been furnished home health services based on such a need and no longer has a need for such care or therapy, but continues to need occupational therapy.
27. Attending Physician's Signature (Required on 485 Kept on File in Medical Records of HHA)	Date Signed	

Form HCFA-485 (U4) (4-87)

PROVIDER

Department of Health and Human Services
Health Care Financing Administration

Form Approved
OMB No. 0938-0357

MEDICAL UPDATE AND PATIENT INFORMATION

1. Patient's HI Claim No.	2. SOC Date	3. Certification Period From: To:	4. Medical Record No.	5. Provider No.

6. Patient's Name	7. Provider's Name

8. Medicare Covered: ☐ Y ☐ N	9. Date Physician Last Saw Patient:	10. Date Last Contacted Physician:

11. Is the Patient Receiving Care in an 1861 (J)(1) Skilled Nursing Facility or Equivalent? ☐ Y ☐ N ☐ Do Not Know	12. ☐ Certification ☐ Recertification ☐ Modified

13. Specific Services and Treatments

Discipline	Visits (This Bill) Rel. to Prior Cert.	Frequency and Duration	Treatment Codes	Total Visits Projected This Cert.

14. Dates of Last Inpatient Stay: Admission Discharge	15. Type of Facility:

16. Updated Information: New Orders/Treatments/Clinical Facts/Summary from Each Discipline

17. Functional Limitations (Expand From 485 and Level of ADL) Reason Homebound/Prior Functional Status

18. Supplementary Plan of Treatment on File from Physician Other than Referring Physician: ☐ Y ☐ N
(If Yes, Please Specify Giving Goals/Rehab. Potential/Discharge Plan)

19. Unusual Home/Social Environment

20. Indicate Any Time When the Home Health Agency Made a Visit and Patient was Not Home and Reason Why if Ascertainable	21. Specify Any Known Medical and/or Non-Medical Reasons the Patient Regularly Leaves Home and Frequency of Occurrence

22. Nurse or Therapist Completing or Reviewing Form	Date (Mo., Day, Yr.)

Form HCFA-486 (C3) (4-87)

PROVIDER

RESOURCE FILE ENTRY FORM

The form presented here is for community health nurses exploring the available resources of a community. Information contained in the entry will allow the nurse to identify resources that will best meet clients' needs. Information about community agencies will also allow the community health nurse to make appropriate referrals for services. Information obtained about a particular agency or referral resource should be updated frequently.

Resource File Entry Form

Resource category: _____   Funding source: _____

Agency name: _____

Address: _____

Phone number: _____   Business hours: _____

Contact person: _____   Title: _____

Source of referral: _____

Eligibility: _____

_____

Fee: _____

Services: _____

_____

_____

_____

_____

_____

_____

Access: _____

Other comments: _____

_____

_____

_____

_____

_____

_____

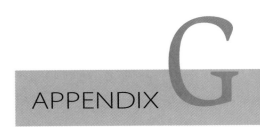

POLITICAL ASTUTENESS INVENTORY*

Place a check mark next to those items for which your answer is "yes." Then give yourself one point for each check mark. After completing the inventory, compare your total score with the scoring criteria at the end of the inventory.

---

*Adapted with permission from Clark, P. E. (1984). Political astuteness inventory. In Clark, M. J. D. *Community nursing: Health care for today and tomorrow*. Reston, VA: Reston.

_____ 1. I am registered to vote.
_____ 2. I know where my voting precinct is located.
_____ 3. I voted in the last general election.
_____ 4. I voted in the last two elections.
_____ 5. I recognized the names of the majority of candidates on the ballot at the last election.
_____ 6. I was acquainted with the majority of issues on the ballot at the last election.
_____ 7. I stay abreast of current health issues.
_____ 8. I belong to the state professional or student nurses' organization.
_____ 9. I participate (committee member, officer, etc) in that organization.
_____ 10. I attended the most recent meeting of my district nurses' association.
_____ 11. I attended the last state or national convention held by my organization.
_____ 12. I am aware of at least two issues discussed and the stands taken at that convention.
_____ 13. I read literature published by my state nurses' association, professional magazines, or other literature on a regular basis to stay abreast of current health issues.
_____ 14. I know the names of my state's senators in Washington, DC.
_____ 15. I know the names of my congressional district's representatives in Washington, DC.
_____ 16. I know the name of the state senator from my district.
_____ 17. I know the name of the state assembly member from my district.
_____ 18. I am acquainted with the voting record of at least one of the above in relation to a specific health issue.
_____ 19. I am aware of the stand taken by at least one of the above on one current health issue.
_____ 20. I know whom to contact for information about health-related policy issues at the state or federal level.
_____ 21. I know whether my professional organization employs lobbyists at the state or federal level.
_____ 22. I know how to contact that lobbyist.
_____ 23. I support my state professional organization's political arm.
_____ 24. I actively supported a candidate for the Senate or House of Representatives (Assembly) (campaign contribution, campaigning service, wore a button, or other) during the last election.
_____ 25. I have written regarding a health issue to one of my state or national representatives in the last year.
_____ 26. I am personally acquainted with a senator or representative or a member of his or her staff.
_____ 27. I serve as a resource person for one of my representatives or his or her staff.
_____ 28. I know the process by which a bill is introduced in my state legislature.
_____ 29. I know which senators or representatives are supportive of nursing.
_____ 30. I know which House and Senate committees usually deal with health-related issues.
_____ 31. I know the committees on which my representatives hold membership.
_____ 32. I know of at least two issues related to my profession that are currently under discussion at the state or national level.
_____ 33. I know of at least two health-related issues that are currently under discussion at the state or national level.
_____ 34. I am aware of the composition of the state board that regulates the practice of my profession.
_____ 35. I know the process whereby one becomes a member of the state board that regulates my profession.
_____ 36. I attend public hearings related to health issues.
_____ 37. I find myself more interested in public issues now than in the past.
_____ 38. I have provided testimony at a public hearing on an issue related to health.
_____ 39. I know where the local headquarters of my political party are located.
_____ 40. I have written a letter to the editor or other piece for the lay press speaking out on a health-related issue.

Scoring

0–9 points	Totally politically unaware
10–19 points	Slightly aware of the implications of political activity for nursing
20–29 points	Shows a beginning political awareness
30–40 points	Politically astute and an asset to the profession

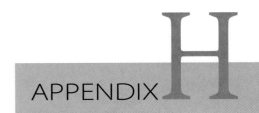

HEALTH ASSESSMENT AND INTERVENTION PLANNING GUIDE—FAMILY CLIENT

The tool presented in this appendix is designed to assist the community health nurse to apply the Dimensions Model to the care of families. The initial sections of the tool address family assessment from the epidemiologic perspective of the model. Later portions guide the learner in developing relevant nursing diagnoses and in planning, implementing, and evaluating appropriate nursing care for the family client. The diagnostic segment of the tool encourages the development of both positive and negative nursing diagnoses, an important feature of community health nursing, and the planning segment facilitates the development of specific outcome objectives to guide the planning, implementation, and evaluation of interventions. Completion of the implementation portion of the tool enhances delegation skills in determining those responsible for implementing the plan of care and allows the user to monitor the extent to which plan interventions are completed. Finally, the evaluation segment of the guide fosters the development and use of specific evidential criteria for evaluating the outcome of nursing care.

Health Assessment and Intervention Planning Guide—Family Client
Assessment

Family surname(s): _____   Phone: _____

Address: _____

_____

Biophysical Dimension

Name	Age	Sex	Physical Health Status

Maturation and Aging

Individual family members' developmental tasks met? _____

_____

Effects of individual development on family health: _____

_____

Significant past health problems of family members: _____

_____

Physiologic Function

Treatment for family members' current health problems (*type, effects, source*): _____

_____

Significant family history of hereditary conditions: _____

_____

Immunization status of family members: _____

_____

Psychological Dimension

Family strengths and weaknesses: _____

_____

Family communication (*typical patterns, effectiveness, purposes, tone, rules*): _____

_____

Family stage of development: _____

_____

Status of developmental tasks of this and previous stages: _____

_____

Extent of emotional support for family members: _____

_____

Coping strategies used (*type, effectiveness*): _____

_____

Discipline (*type, source, consistency, appropriateness*): _____

_____

History of mental illness in family members: _____

_____

Family Roles

Role	Performed by	Adequacy	Role Model
Leader			
Child care			
Sexual			
Breadwinner			
Confidant			
Disciplinarian			
Homemaker			
Repairperson			
Financial manager			

Presence of role conflict or role overload: _____

_____

Family goals (*congruence with individual and societal goals*): _____

_____

Sources of stress for family members: _____

_____

Physical Dimension

Family home (*location, adequacy for family size*): _____

_____

Safety hazards present in home: _____

_____

Neighborhood (*safety, services and facilities available, pollutants*): _____

_____

Social Dimension
Religious affiliations of family members and their influence on health: _____

_____

Family cultural affiliations and influences on health: _____

_____

Family income (*source, adequacy, effectiveness of management*): _____

_____

Education level of family members: _____

_____

External resources available to family: _____

_____

Occupation

Family Member	Occupation	Employer

Occupational health hazards for family members: _____

_____

Behavioral Dimension
Consumption Patterns
Family dietary patterns (*amount, food preferences, preparation, adequacy, special needs*): _____

_____

Use of other substances (*tobacco, alcohol, other drugs*): _____

_____

Use of prescription and nonprescription medications: _____

_____

Rest and exercise patterns: _____

_____

Leisure Activity
Typical leisure activities of family members: _____

_____

Health hazards posed by family leisure pursuits: _____

_____

Use of recreational activities to enhance family cohesion: _____

_____

Other Behaviors

Use of safety devices and practices: _____

_____

Family planning (*need for, type, effectiveness*): _____

_____

Health System Dimension

Family attitudes toward health: _____

_____

Family response toward illness: _____

_____

Use of folk remedies and self-care practices: _____

_____

Usual source of health care: _____

_____

Means of financing health care: _____

_____

Barriers to obtaining health care: _____

_____

Diagnosis

Biophysical Dimension

Positive Nursing Diagnoses	Negative Nursing Diagnoses

Psychological Dimension

Positive Nursing Diagnoses	Negative Nursing Diagnoses

Physical Dimension

Positive Nursing Diagnoses	Negative Nursing Diagnoses

Social Dimension

Positive Nursing Diagnoses	Negative Nursing Diagnoses

Behavioral Dimension

Positive Nursing Diagnoses	Negative Nursing Diagnoses

Health System Dimension

Positive Nursing Diagnoses	Negative Nursing Diagnoses

Planning

Planned Interventions	Outcome Objectives

Implementation

Intervention	Responsible Party/Expected Completion Date	Status

Evaluation

Expected Outcome	Status: Met/Unmet	Supporting Evidence

HEALTH ASSESSMENT AND INTERVENTION PLANNING GUIDE—COMMUNITY CLIENT

The tool presented here can be used by the community health nurse to apply the Dimensions Model to the care of communities as clients. In the assessment portion of the tool, the user is guided in using the model to assess the health status of a community. The diagnostic segment of the tool is framed in terms of the two stages of community nursing diagnoses, identification of a vulnerable population, and diagnosis of the adequacy of community health resources and services for meeting the identified needs of vulnerable populations. Correct use of this portion of the tool will create a set of community nursing diagnoses that reflect both positive and negative diagnoses. In completing the diagnostic segment of the tool, the user should include data supporting the identification of vulnerable populations and the designation of need—service match or mismatch.

Health Assessment and Intervention Planning Guide—Community Client

Assessment

Biophysical Dimension

Births (*annual rate, extent of illegitimacy, abortion*): _____

_____

Composition of population:

Age	Total	Male	Female	White	Black	Hispanic	Asian	Native American
<1 year								
1–5 years								
6–12 years								
13–20 years								
21–30 years								
31–50 years								
51–65 years								
66–80 years								
>80 years								

Mortality rates (*overall, age specific, cause specific*): _____

_____

Morbidity:

Disease	Incidence	Prevalence

Disease	Incidence	Prevalence

How do morbidity and mortality rates compare with previous years? With state and national rates?

_____

_____

What is the immunization status of the population? _____

_____

Psychological Dimension

Future prospects for the community: _____

_____

Significant events in community history: _____

_____

Interaction of groups within the community (*racial tension, etc*): _____

_____

Protective services (*adequacy, local crime rate, insurance rates*): _____

_____

Communication network (*media, informal channels, links to outside world*): _____

_____

Sources of stress in the community: _____

_____

Extent of mental illness in the community: _____

_____

Physical Dimension
Community location (*boundaries, urban/rural*): _____

_____

Size and density: _____

_____

Prominent topographical features: _____

_____

Housing (*type, condition, adequacy, number of persons per dwelling, sanitation*): _____

_____

Safety hazards present in the environment: _____

_____

Source of community water supply: _____

_____

Sewage and waste disposal: _____

_____

Nuisance factors: _____

_____

Potential for disaster: _____

_____

Social Dimension
Government (*type, effectiveness, community officials*): _____

_____

Unofficial leaders (*significant informants*): _____

_____

Political affiliations of community members: _____

_____

Status of minority groups (*influence, length of residence*): _____

_____

Languages spoken by community members: _____

_____

Community income levels (*poverty, coverage by assistance programs*): _____

_____

Education (*prevailing levels, attitudes, facilities*): _____

_____

Religion (*major affiliations, programs and services, influence on health*): _____

_____

Culture (*affiliation, influence on health*): _____

_____

Employment level: _____

_____

Transportation (*type, availability, cost, adequacy*): _____

_____

Shopping facilities (*type, availability, cost, use*): _____

_____

Social services (*type, availability, adequacy, use*): _____

_____

Primary occupations of community members: _____

_____

Major employers (*occupational health programs*): _____

_____

Occupational hazards: _____

_____

Behavioral Dimension

Consumption Patterns
Nutrition (*general levels, preferences, preparation, special needs, prevalence of anemia, obesity*): _____

_____

Alcohol (*consumption patterns, extent of abuse*): _____

_____

Drug use (*licit and illicit*): _____

_____

Smoking (*extent, cessation program availability*): _____

_____

Exercise (*extent, type*): _____

_____

Leisure Activities
Primary leisure activities of community members: _____

_____

Recreational facilities (*availability, adequacy, cost*): _____

_____

Health hazards posed by recreation: _____

_____

Other Behaviors
Use of safety devices: _____

_____

Contraceptive use: _____

_____

Health System Dimension
Community attitudes toward health (*definitions, support of services*): _____

_____

Health services and resources (*type, availability, cost, adequacy, utilization*): _____

_____

Prenatal care (*availability, use*): _____

_____

Emergency services (*availability, adequacy*): _____

_____

Health education services (*availability, adequacy*): _____

_____

Health care financing (*extent of insurance coverage, Medicaid, Medicare, tax support*): _____

_____

Diagnosis
Biophysical Dimension

Community Health Need/Risk	Need–Service Match/Mismatch

Psychological Dimension

Community Health Need/Risk	Need–Service Match/Mismatch

Physical Dimension

Community Health Need/Risk	Need–Service Match/Mismatch

Social Dimension

Community Health Need/Risk	Need–Service Match/Mismatch

Behavioral Dimension

Community Health Need/Risk	Need–Service Match/Mismatch

Health System Dimension

Community Health Need/Risk	Need–Service Match/Mismatch

Planning

Planned Interventions	Outcome Objectives

Implementation

Intervention	Responsible Party/Expected Completion Date	Status

Evaluation

Expected Outcome	Status: Met/Unmet	Supporting Evidence

HEALTH ASSESSMENT AND INTERVENTION PLANNING GUIDE—TARGET GROUP

For the most part, assessing the health needs of a target group from the perspective of the Dimensions Model is similar to assessing a community. For most of the information needed, the community health nurse can use the assessment guide provided in Appendix I, Health Assessment and Intervention Planning Guide—Community Client. Some specific assessment considerations for a target group, however, differ from those for a community. The special considerations are presented here. This tool addresses only the assessment component of the Dimensions Model. For guidance with other portions of the model, use pages 999 to 1001 of Appendix I.

Health Assessment and Intervention Planning Guide—Target Group

Target group: _____

Biophysical Dimension

What is the age, sex, and racial or ethnic composition of the target group? _____

_____

Are there any special maturational or developmental concerns for group members? _____

_____

What health problems are commonly experienced by group members? _____

_____

Are group members particularly vulnerable to any particular illnesses? _____

_____

Are there any special immunization concerns for group members? _____

_____

Psychological Dimension

What effect does group membership have on members' self-image? _____

_____

What coping skills do group members display? Are they adequate? _____

_____

What is the incidence and prevalence of psychological problems among group members? _____

_____

What psychological stressors are experienced by group members? _____

_____

Physical Dimension

Where is the target group located? _____

_____

Are there any special environmental considerations for group members (*wheelchair access, ramps*)? _____

_____

Are group members particularly vulnerable to environmental conditions (*pollutants, temperature changes*)? _____

_____

Do group members have special housing needs? _____

_____

_____

Social Environment

What are the attitudes of the larger society toward group members? _____

_____

What is the extent of group members' social status and influence? _____

_____

Are there special economic concerns for group members? _____

_____

Are there special educational concerns for group members? _____

_____

Does the group have an official spokesperson or group to represent its interests? _____

_____

Do group members have particular protective services needs? _____

_____

Do group members have unique transportation needs? _____

_____

Are group members employable? _____

_____

Are there particular occupational concerns for group members? _____

_____

Behavioral Dimension

Consumption Patterns

Do group members have special nutritional needs? _____

_____

What is the extent of drug or alcohol abuse among group members? _____

_____

Does smoking pose any special problems for group members? _____

_____

Does exercise pose any special problems for group members? _____

_____

Leisure Activities

Do certain leisure activities pose problems for group members? _____

_____

Do group members have access to recreational opportunities open to other members of society? _____

_____

Other Behaviors

Are special safety precautions warranted for group members? _____

_____

Does contraception pose special problems for group members? _____

_____

Health System Dimension

What health services are needed by group members? Are they available and accessible? _____

_____

What is the attitude of health care professionals toward group members? _____

_____

How do group members finance health care? Are there problems with financing such care? _____

_____

Do group members experience barriers to obtaining health care? _____

_____

_____

RECOMMENDED SCREENING PROCEDURES

Over the years a number of screening procedures have been recommended for routine use with various population groups. However, research has shown that some of these recommended procedures were of little actual value in the early identification and resolution of health problems and so were not cost-effective. The U.S. Preventive Services Task Force undertook a major project to review the available research related to both screening procedures and health promotion practices. The findings and recommendations of the task force were first published in 1989. Since then, ongoing work has further refined the recommendations for routine screening and health promotion contained in the second edition of the *Guide to Clinical Preventive Services* published in 1996. Some of those recommendations are presented here. It should be noted that these recommendations address only routine screening procedures for the general population and for selected high-risk groups. Other screening practices are certainly warranted for clients who exhibit certain risk factors for disease. For example, although fecal occult blood testing is not routinely recommended for persons under 50 years of age, it would be a perfectly appropriate screening test for a client with persistent anemia who is not yet 50 years old. The screening procedures addressed here are divided into those appropriate to the general population, those recommended for pregnant women, and those recommended for persons who fall into certain high-risk groups. Only those tests for which there is fair to good evidence of efficacy are included.

Routine Screening Recommendations

Screening Test	Population	Age	Frequency
Amblyopia	Male/Female	3–4 years	Once
Blood pressure	Male/Female	Over 20 years	q 2 years with diastolic pressure < 85 mm
			Annually with diastolic pressure 85–89
	Male/Female	Children and adolescents	During routine visits
Fecal occult blood	Male/Female	Over 50 years	Annually
Gross hearing	Male/Female	Elderly	Periodic[a]
Height and weight	Male/Female	All	Periodic
Mammogram	Female	50–69 years	q 1–2 years
Pap smear	Sexually active females with cervix	All	q 3 years
Phenylketonuria (PKU)	Male/Female	Newborn	Birth and 2 weeks
Problem drinking	Male/Female	Adolescents and adults	Periodic
Rubella titer	Female	Childbearing age	First clinical encounter
Sickle cell hemoglobinopathy	Male/Female	Newborn	Birth
Sigmoidoscopy	Male/Female	Over 50 years	q 3–5 years
Snellen vision testing	Male/Female	Elderly	Periodic
T_4 or TSH	Male/Female	Newborn	Birth
Total blood cholesterol	Male	35–65 years	q 5 years
	Female	45–64 years	q 5 years

[a]Optimal frequency or timing of screening has not been determined and is left to the discretion of the clinician.

Routine Screening—Pregnant Women

Screening Test	Population	Age	Frequency
Amniocentesis	High-risk women	Over 35 years	15–18 weeks gestation
Blood pressure	All	All	Each prenatal visit
Chlamydia	High-risk women	All	Unknown
Gonorrhea	High-risk women	All	First prenatal visit and third trimester
Hepatitis B infection	All	All	First prenatal visit
Hemoglobin/hematocrit	All	All	First prenatal visit
HIV infection	High-risk women	All	First prenatal visit and third trimester
Neural tube defects	All women living in areas with available counseling services	All	16–18 weeks gestation
Problem drinking	All	All	First prenatal visit
Rh incompatibility	All	All	First prenatal visit
Sickle cell hemoglobinopathy	All	All	First prenatal visit
Rubella titer or vaccination status	All	All	First prenatal visit
Syphilis	All	All	First prenatal visit, third trimester, and at delivery
Urine culture	All	All	12–16 weeks gestation

Screening for High-Risk Populations

Screening Test	Population at Risk	Frequency
Blood lead level	Children living in communities with high prevalence of elevated blood lead levels, low-income children, children in central city areas, children in families of low education levels, children of color	12 months of age
Chlamydia	Sexually active adolescent females; sexually active women with prior STD history, new or multiple partners, under 25 years of age, unmarried, inconsistent use of barrier contraceptives, cervical ectopy	At each pelvic examination
Gonorrhea	Commercial sex workers, women under age 25 with two or more partners, persons with repeat history of gonorrhea infection, all sexually active women in communities with high gonorrhea prevalence	Periodic[a]
Hemoglobin/hematocrit	Low-income children, African Americans, Native Americans, Alaskan Natives, and immigrant children Preterm and low birthweight infants, infants on cow's milk	12 months 6–12 months
HIV infection	Persons with other STDs; men who have sex with men; injecting drug users (IDUs); persons who have sex for money or drugs; persons who have sex with HIV-infected partners, IDUs, or men who have sex with men; persons transfused between 1978 and 1985	Periodic
	Infants born to HIV-infected women	Birth and 6 months
Syphilis	Commercial sex workers, persons who exchange sex for money or drugs, those with other STDs, sexual contacts of persons with active syphilis	Periodic
Tuberculosis	HIV-infected persons, contacts to known cases of TB, immigrants from endemic countries, alcoholics, IDUs, residents of long-term care facilities (including jails)	Periodic

[a]Optimal frequency or timing of screening has not been determined and is left to the discretion of the clinician.

CHILD HEALTH ASSESSMENT GUIDE

The assessment guide included here is a basic assessment tool framed in the epidemiologic format of the Dimensions Model. Where appropriate, the guide has been modified to address assessment considerations unique to the child client. Use of the diagnostic, planning, implementation, and evaluation components of the model would involve application of these segments of Appendix H, Health Assessment and Intervention Planning Guide—Family Client.

Child Health Assessment Guide

Client's name: _____   Phone: _____

Address: _____

Assessment

Biophysical Dimension

Maturation and Aging

Age: _____   Date of birth: _____   Sex: _____   Race/ethnic group: _____

Birth weight and length: _____

Pattern of growth (*compared with norms and previous pattern*): _____

_____

Accomplishment of developmental milestones (*DDST or other appropriate test*): _____

_____

Parental knowledge of child development and its implications: _____

_____

Significant family health history (*include genogram*): _____

_____

Physiologic Function

Significant events during pregnancy: _____

_____

Significant events during delivery: _____

_____

Congenital defects: _____

_____

Current acute or chronic illnesses (*describe problem, status, treatment, if any*): _____

_____

Current signs or symptoms of physical health problems: _____

_____

Areas of physical disability or limitation of function: _____

_____

Significant past illnesses, injuries, hospitalizations (*what, when, outcomes*): _____

_____

Review of Systems

Head (*headache* [how often, quality, treatment outcome], *syncope, trauma*): _____

_____

Eyes (*vision problems, burning eyes, glasses, last eye exam, blocked tear duct, discharge, tearing, itching*): _____

_____

Ears (*difficulty hearing, discharge, earache, frequent otitis*): _____

_____

Mouth and throat (*sore throat, lesions, toothache, caries, last dental visit*): _____

_____

Respiratory system (*frequent colds, nosebleeds, cough, pneumonia, asthma, shortness of breath, sinusitis, hayfever*): _____

_____

Cardiovascular system (*heart problems, hypertension, chest pain, cyanosis* [especially when crying], *shortness of breath, murmurs, edema*): _____

_____

Gastrointestinal system (*nausea, vomiting, diarrhea, constipation, flatulence, abdominal pain, loss of appetite, weight loss or gain, rectal pain or bleeding, quality of stool, frequency*): _____

_____

Urinary tract (*dysuria, urinary frequency, nocturia, difficulty voiding, urinary retention, CVA pain, odor, strength of urinary stream, number of wet diapers in infant*): _____

_____

Reproductive system (*vaginal or penile discharge, development of secondary sex characteristics, menarche, wet dreams, extent of sex education, history of STD*): _____

_____

Musculoskeletal system (*joint pain, swelling, tremor, history of trauma, muscle weakness*): _____

_____

Integumentary system (*eczema, diaper rash, lesions* [describe character, locale, color], *changes in skin color, itching, hair loss, discoloration or pitting of nails, clubbing of nails, birthmarks, swollen glands*): _____

_____

Neurological system (*seizures, tics, tremors, paralysis*): _____

_____

Hematopoietic system (*anemia, bleeding tendencies, bruise easily, transfusions* [when, why]): _____

_____

Immunologic system (*frequent infections, HIV infection, use of immunosuppressives*): _____

_____

Immunization status (*up-to-date for age*): _____

_____

Physical Examination
Height, weight, head and chest circumference: _____

_____

Vital signs (*T, P, R, B/P*): _____

_____

General appearance (*posture, gait, deformities, hygiene*): _____

_____

Skin (*diaper rash, eczema, acne, milia, bruises, burns, hygiene*): _____

_____

Head and neck (*lymph nodes, face*): _____

_____

Eyes (*ability to focus and follow objects*): _____

_____

Ears (*ability to localize sound*): _____

_____

Nose and sinuses: _____

_____

Mouth and throat (*monilial patches, number of teeth, dental hygiene, caries*): _____

_____

Chest:

- Breast examination (*newborn engorgement, precocious puberty*): _____

    _____

- Heart (*murmurs, split heart sounds*): _____

    _____

- Lungs: _____

    _____

Abdomen: _____

_____

Genitalia (*undescended testes, vaginal tears, discharge, imperforate anus*): _____

_____

Musculoskeletal system (*symmetry of extremities, spina bifida, scoliosis, congenital hip dislocation*): _____

_____

Nervous system (*cranial nerves, DTRs, temperature, kinesthetic sense, newborn reflexes*): _____

_____

Screening test results (*PKU, T_4, hematocrit, sickle cell, serum lead, TB, urinalysis as appropriate*): _____

_____

Psychological Dimension
Reactivity patterns and parental responses: _____

_____

Parental expectations (*appropriateness*): _____

_____

Discipline (*type, consistency, appropriateness*): _____

_____

Parental coping skills: _____

_____

Parent–child interactions: _____

_____

Self-image: _____

_____

Emotional state or mood (*usual, recent changes*): _____

_____

Evidence of abuse or neglect: _____

_____

Recent experience of significant loss (*death, divorce, move*): _____

_____

Suicide ideation: _____

_____

Level of social or parental pressure to perform: _____

_____

Physical Dimension
Where does the client live? Is there adequate space and privacy in the home? _____

_____

Are safety hazards present in the home? (*see Appendix D, Home Safety Inventory*) _____

_____

Are there pets in the home? (*What kind? How many? Inside or outside?*) _____

_____

What is the neighborhood like? (*safety, pollutants, etc.*) _____

_____

Social Dimension
Education (*grade, performance*): _____

_____

Interaction with peers: _____

_____

Interaction with others: _____

_____

Cultural childrearing attitudes/practices: _____

_____

Child care outside the home (*where, by whom, adequacy*): _____

_____

Behavioral Dimension
Consumption Patterns
Infant (*formula, breast, amount, formula preparation, feeding and burping techniques*): _____

_____

Other age groups (*well-balanced diet, amount of "junk food," food allergies*): _____

_____

Parental knowledge of nutrition needs: _____

_____

Exposure to drugs/alcohol/tobacco: _____

_____

Rest and Exercise
Sleep patterns: _____

_____

Type and amount of exercise: _____

_____

Use of safety precautions, equipment: _____

_____

Other
Sexual activity (*frequency, use of contraceptives, condoms*): _____

_____

Use of seat belts, other safety devices: _____

_____

Health System Dimension
Use of primary prevention services (*general and dental*): _____

_____

Source of illness care: _____

_____

Parental knowledge of illness care and need for medical assistance: _____

_____

NURSING INTERVENTIONS FOR COMMON HEALTH PROBLEMS IN CHILDREN

The interventions presented here are general guidelines that the community health nurse can use to educate parents for home care of health problems commonly encountered among young children.

Nursing Interventions for Common Health Problems in Children

Organ System	Problem	Interventions
Gastrointestinal	Spitting up	Burp baby more frequently.
		Keep infant upright for short time after feeding.
		Check size of nipple hole.
		Change to soy formula.
	Colic	Give small amounts of warm water.
		Exert gentle pressure on abdomen with infant's legs and thighs bent.
	Mild diarrhea or vomiting	Begin oral rehydration to prevent dehydration.
		Do not discontinue feedings.
		Seek medical help if condition continues or worsens.
	Constipation	Increase fluid intake.
		Add bulk to diet.
		Encourage regular toileting habits.
		Discourage postponing defecation.
		Avoid use of laxatives or enemas.
Respiratory	Mild respiratory infection	Increase fluid intake.
		Use a cold mist humidifier to ease breathing.
		Do not use Vicks or other aromatic substances.
		Seek medical help for severe or persistent cough, difficulty breathing, stridor, or nasal flaring.
Integumentary	Diaper rash	Wash diapers with mild soaps and rinse thoroughly.
		Add 3/4 cup vinegar to last rinse to remove ammonia.
		If using disposable diapers, use ones that allow air circulation.
		Frequent diaper change and cleansing of diaper area.
		Do not use powders or lotion in diaper area.
		Leave diaper area exposed when possible.
	Allergic dermatitis	Explore changes in foods or soaps.
		Eliminate possible causative substances.
		Seek medical help for severe rashes or secondary infection.
	Cradle cap	Scrub scalp with soap and soft washcloth during bath.
		Brush scalp with soft brush after bath.
		Do not use oil or lotion on scalp.
	Abrasions and lacerations	Wash with soap and water.
		Keep clean.
Urinary	Urinary tract infection	Seek medical assistance.
	Bedwetting	Limit fluid intake after dinner.
		Empty bladder before bed.
		Awaken child to urinate before parents go to bed.
		Do not make an issue of the problem.
		If problem is severe or continues beyond age 6, seek medical attention.
Musculoskeletal	Sprains and fractures	Perform basic first aid and immobilize injured area.
		Seek medical attention.
	Leg cramps	Increase calcium intake.
		If severe or persistent, seek medical attention.
Neurological	Headache	Give nonaspirin analgesic according to child's age and size.
		If severe or recurrent, seek medical attention.
	Hearing problem	Seek medical attention.
	Vision problem	Seek medical attention.
	Delayed speech	Discourage older children and parents from talking for child.
		Encourage child to verbalize needs before meeting them.
		Seek medical attention for prolonged delay.
	Speech defect	Seek medical attention.
Other	Fever	For temperature over 102°F, give nonaspirin antipyretic.
		For high or persistent fever, seek medical attention.
	Suspected abuse	Refer to child protective services.
	Night terrors	Use a night light or leave bedroom door open.
		Use bedtime rituals of checking for "monsters" if helpful.
		Use a "guardian" stuffed animal to scare away monsters.
		Comfort the child after waking and stay until child returns to sleep.
		Seek assistance for persistent terrors or those related to a real traumatic event.

Nursing Interventions for Common Health Problems in Children (*Continued*)

Organ System	Problem	Interventions
	Jealousy of new baby	Prepare siblings for birth of another child.
		Have child assist with care of newborn.
		Emphasize positive aspects of being older.
		Accept regressive behavior and do not belittle.
		Spend time with just the older child.
		Encourage friends and relatives to pay attention to older child as well as new baby.
	Sibling rivalry	Mediate arguments.
		Encourage children to work out own differences.
		Encourage compromise.
		Give reasons for differences in privileges.
		Use role-play with older children to give insight into feelings and behaviors of others.
	Tantrums	Ignore behavior if possible.
		Remove child to bedroom if disturbing others.
		Do not give in to child's demands.
	Bedtime	Complete bedtime rituals and put child in bed.
		Ignore crying for 15 to 20 minutes. If the child does not stop, see what is wrong.
		If child gets up, put him or her back to bed.
		Place several safe toys in bed with child and allow play until the child falls asleep.
	Poor self-esteem	Praise child for accomplishments.
		Correct mistakes without denigrating child.
		Help child identify and strengthen talents.
		Assist child to accept limitations.
		Seek assistance for severe depression or low self-esteem on the part of the child.

HEALTH ASSESSMENT GUIDE—ADULT CLIENT

Assessment of the health needs of adult clients can be undertaken using this assessment tool. In many respects this tool is similar to the Child Health Assessment Guide presented in Appendix L; however, there are some differences in the degree of emphasis given to aspects of child and adult assessment as well as in specific content addressed.

Only adult client assessment is covered in this tool. Guidelines for diagnostic, planning, implementation, and evaluation components of the Dimensions Model are included in Appendix H, Health Assessment and Intervention Planning Guide—Family Client, and are equally applicable to the care of individual adult clients.

Health Assessment Guide—Adult Client

Client's name: _____   Phone: _____

Address: _____

Assessment
Biophysical Dimension

Maturation and Aging

Age: _____   Date of birth: _____   Sex: _____   Race/ethnic group: _____

Accomplishment of adult developmental tasks: _____

_____

Significant family health history (*include genogram*): _____

_____

Physiologic Function

Current acute or chronic illnesses (*describe problem, status, treatment, if any*): _____

_____

Current signs or symptoms of physical health problems: _____

_____

Areas of physical disability or limitation of function: _____

_____

Significant past illnesses, injuries, hospitalizations (*what, when, outcomes*): _____

_____

Review of Systems

Head (*headache* [how often, quality, treatment outcome], *syncope, trauma*): _____

_____

Eyes (*vision problems, burning eyes, glasses, last eye exam, blocked tear duct, discharge, tearing, itching*): _____

_____

Ears (*difficulty hearing, discharge, earache*): _____

_____

Mouth and throat (*sore throat, lesions, toothache, caries, last dental visit*): _____

_____

Respiratory system (*frequent colds, nosebleeds, cough, pneumonia, asthma, shortness of breath, sinusitis, hayfever*): _____

_____

_____

Cardiovascular system (*heart problems, hypertension, chest pain, cyanosis, shortness of breath, murmurs, edema*): _____

_____

Gastrointestinal system (*nausea, vomiting, diarrhea, constipation, flatulence, abdominal pain, loss of appetite, weight loss or gain, rectal pain or bleeding*): _____

_____

Urinary tract (*dysuria, urinary frequency, urgency, nocturia, difficulty voiding, urinary retention, CVA pain*): _____

_____

Reproductive system (*sexual satisfaction, history of STD*): _____

_____

- Female (*edema of labia or vulva, vaginal discharge* [color, character, odor], *use of oral or other contraceptives, pregnancies* [past or current] *and outcome, age at menarche, LMP, dysmenorrhea, irregular menses, breast discharge, breast self-exam, breast lumps, changes in breast contour, dyspareunia*): _____

  _____

- Male (*prostatitis, penile discharge* [color, character, amount], *lesions on penis, testicular self-exam, testicular pain, lumps, impotence, dysuria, scrotal swelling*): _____

  _____

Musculoskeletal system (*joint pain, swelling, tremor, history of trauma, muscle weakness*): _____

_____

Integumentary system (*lesions* [describe character, locale, color], *changes in skin color, itching, hair loss, discoloration or pitting of nails, birthmarks, swollen glands*): _____

_____

Neurological system (*seizures, ataxia, tics, tremors, paralysis*): _____

_____

Hematopoietic system (*anemia, bleeding tendencies, bruise easily, transfusions* [when, why]): _____

_____

Immunologic system (*frequent infections, HIV infection, use of immunosuppressives*): _____

_____

Immunization status: _____

_____

Physical Examination
Height and weight: _____
Vital signs (*T, P, R, B/P*): _____
General appearance (*posture, gait, deformities, hygiene*): _____

_____

Skin (*include hair and nails*): _____

_____

Head and neck (*lymph nodes, face*): _____

_____

Eyes: _____
Ears: _____
Nose and sinuses: _____
Mouth and throat (*lips, gums, palate, pharynx, tongue, teeth*): _____

_____

Chest:

- Breast examination: _____
- Heart: _____
- Lungs: _____

Abdomen: _____

Genitalia (*including anus and rectum, prostate in male, ovaries in female*): _____

_____

Musculoskeletal system (*extremities, spine, joints, muscles*): _____

_____

Nervous system (*cranial nerves, DTRs, temperature, kinesthetic sense*): _____

_____

Results of screening and other tests: _____

_____

_____

Psychological Dimension

Self-image, level of self-esteem: _____

_____

History of mental illness: _____

_____

Emotional mood or state (*current and recent changes*): _____

_____

Level of orientation: _____

_____

Coping (*strategies used, effectiveness*): _____

_____

Recent experience of significant loss (*death, divorce, move, effects*): _____

_____

Suicide ideation: _____

_____

Communication with others (*extent, effectiveness*): _____

_____

Interpersonal relationships (*satisfaction, extent*): _____

_____

Stress (*sources, coping skills, support*): _____

_____

Evidence of physical or emotional abuse: _____

_____

Physical Dimension

Where does the client live? Is there adequate space and privacy in the home? _____

_____

Are safety hazards present in the home? (*see Appendix D, Home Safety Inventory*) _____

_____

Are there pets in the home? (*What kind? How many? Inside or outside?*) _____

_____

What is the neighborhood like? (*Describe safety, pollutants, etc.*) _____

_____

Social Dimension

Education (*formal education, health knowledge, special learning needs*): _____

_____

Income (*source, adequacy, budgeting skills*): _____

_____

Social support network (*components, adequacy, use*): _____

_____

Cultural practices influencing health: _____

_____

Extent of social support for healthy behavior: _____

_____

Religious affiliation (*importance/influence on health*): _____

_____

Adequacy of adult role models: _____

_____

Employment (*current and past, hazards, job change pattern*): _____

_____

Behavioral Dimension

Consumption Patterns

Usual diet (*meal pattern, preferences, preparation, nutritional adequacy, special needs, cultural restrictions*): _____

_____

Use of alcohol, tobacco, other drugs: _____

_____

Use of caffeine: _____

_____

Use of medications (*type, appropriateness*): _____

_____

Rest and Exercise

Sleep patterns: _____

_____

Type and amount of exercise: _____

_____

Leisure (*type of activity, hazards posed*): _____

_____

Other

Sexual activity (*frequency, use of contraceptives, condoms, sexual orientation, multiple partners, sexual practices*): _____

_____

Use of seat belts, other safety devices: _____

_____

Health System Dimension

Use of primary prevention services (*general and dental*): _____

_____

Attitudes toward health and health care: _____

_____

Usual source of health care: _____

_____

Health care financing (*type, adequacy*): _____

_____

Barriers to care: _____

_____

Use of health care services (*appropriateness*): _____

_____

HEALTH ASSESSMENT GUIDE FOR THE OLDER CLIENT

Generally speaking, Appendix N, Health Assessment Guide—Adult Client, can be used to assess the health care needs of older clients as well as those of persons in other age groups. Remember, though, some assessment considerations are unique to older clients. They are presented here.

Health Assessment Guide for the Older Client
Biophysical Dimension
Physiologic Function
Perceptions of personal health: _____

_____

Review of Systems (include effects of aging)
Eyes (*visual impairment, use of glasses*): _____

_____

Ears (*hearing impairment, use of hearing aid*): _____

_____

Mouth and throat (*dentures* [fit, use], *dry mouth, bleeding gums*): _____

_____

Integumentary (*skin integrity, fragility, dryness, itching, lesions, bruises, bleeding, skin color changes, hair distribution, thickened nails; hair, nail, and skin care practices; temperature of extremities, decreased perspiration*): _____

_____

Respiratory (*shortness of breath with exertion, cyanosis, emphysema, cough*): _____

_____

Cardiovascular (*history of heart disease, palpitations, hypertension, effect of activity on heart rate, edema, fatigue, orthostatic hypotension, varicosities, venous ulcers*): _____

_____

Gastrointestinal (*flatulence, constipation, heartburn, rectal bleeding, incontinence, dysphagia, appetite, ability to chew*): ___

_____

Musculoskeletal (*mobility, joint swelling, pain, use of cane or other device, history of fractures, kyphosis*): _____

_____

Neurological (*seizures, ataxia, tics, tremors, paralysis, diminished sense of smell, touch, heat sensation, taste, numbness or tingling*): _____

_____

Reproductive (*decreased libido*): _____

_____

- Male (*difficulty in achieving erection, prostatitis, impotence*): _____

    _____

- Female (*onset of menopause, last Pap smear, mammogram, breast self-exam*): _____

    _____

Urinary (*frequency, urgency, incontinence, color, odor, nocturia*): _____

_____

Hematopoietic (*anemia, epistaxis, bleeding tendencies*): _____

_____

Immunologic (*frequent infections, HIV infection, use of immunosuppressives*): _____

_____

Existence of acute and chronic health problems (*diagnosis, status, treatment, effects*): _____
_____

Functional abilities related to:
   Bathing: _____
_____

   Dressing: _____
_____

   Toileting: _____
_____

   Mobility: _____
_____

   Eating: _____
_____

   Bowel and bladder function: _____
_____

   Communicating: _____
_____

Immunization status (*tetanus, diphtheria, pneumonia, influenza*): _____
_____

Psychological Dimension
Mental status/orientation: _____
_____

Changes in self-image due to aging, retirement: _____
_____

Adjustment to retirement: _____
_____

Coping abilities: _____
_____

History of mental illness: _____
_____

Provision for privacy: _____
_____

Loss of loved ones: _____
_____

Life satisfaction: _____
_____

Preparation for death: _____
_____

Evidence of depression: _____
_____

Evidence of abuse or neglect: _____
_____

Physical Dimension

Safety hazards in home? (*See Appendix D, Home Safety Inventory*): _____
_____

Presence of safety features in home: _____
_____

Availability of resources in neighborhood: _____
_____

Neighborhood safety: _____
_____

Driving: _____
_____

Home maintenance and repair: _____
_____

Pets: _____
_____

Adequacy of heating, lighting, ventilation: _____
_____

Social Dimension

Social interaction and support network: _____
_____

Income (*source, adequacy, ability to budget*): _____
_____

Relationships with family: _____
_____

Education level: _____
_____

Religion and importance in client's life: _____
_____

Ethnicity and influence on client's health: _____
_____

Possibility of institutionalization and client response: _____
_____

Current employment: _____
_____

Previous occupation: _____
_____

Behavioral Dimension

Consumption Patterns

Nutrition (*adequacy for needs, special needs, appetite, meal pattern, food preferences and modes of preparation, food supplements, food storage, shopping practices*): _____

_____

Use of alcohol or other drugs: _____

_____

Use of medications (*type, appropriateness, effectiveness*): _____

_____

Exercise: _____

_____

Sleep patterns: _____

_____

Leisure Activities

Preferred leisure pursuits: _____

_____

Opportunity for leisure activities: _____

_____

Sexuality

Opportunity for intimacy: _____

_____

Alternative modes of meeting sexual needs: _____

_____

Independence

Ability to care for self: _____

_____

Ability to make independent decisions: _____

_____

Health System Dimension

Source of health care: _____

_____

Health care financing (*Medicare, insurance*): _____

_____

Use of health care services: _____

_____

Barriers to obtaining health care: _____

_____

SPECIAL ASSESSMENT CONSIDERATIONS IN THE SCHOOL SETTING

Assessing the health needs of groups of people within a school setting requires attention to specific assessment considerations. This tool is designed to assist the community health nurse to apply the Dimensions Model to the care of groups of clients in schools. The tool addresses only the assessment component of the model. For the diagnosis, planning, implementation, and evaluation components of the model, the community health nurse can use Appendix I, Health Assessment and Intervention Planning Guide—Community Client. Appendix L, Child Health Assessment Guide, can be used to address the health needs of individual children in the school setting.

Special Assessment Considerations in the School Setting

Biophysical Dimension

Age, sex, and racial/ethnic composition of the school population: _____

_____

Presence of handicapping conditions: _____

_____

Incidence and prevalence of disease: _____

_____

Immunization status: _____

_____

Psychological Dimension

Organization of the school day (*appropriateness to needs, effects on health*): _____

_____

Aesthetic quality of environment: _____

_____

Relationships among students (*quality, appropriateness of adult monitoring*): _____

_____

Teacher–student relations (*quality, extent*): _____

_____

Teacher–teacher relations: _____

_____

Discipline (*type, extent, appropriateness, consistency, fairness*): _____

_____

Grading practices (*consistency, fairness*): _____

_____

Parent–school relations (*quality, extent*): _____

_____

Physical Dimension

Traffic patterns around the school: _____

_____

Safety hazards in the neighborhood: _____

_____

Use of pesticides and other poisons in the neighborhood: _____

_____

Pollutants in the area of the school: _____

_____

Fire or safety hazards in the school environment: _____

_____

Use of toxic chemicals in labs, art classes, cleaning, and maintenance: _____

_____

Use of hazardous equipment in home economics or "shop" classes: _____

_____

Broken glass in play areas: _____

_____

Play equipment in poor repair: _____

_____

Hard surfaces below play equipment: _____

_____

Animals in the school environment: _____

_____

Plant allergens or poisons in the school environment: _____

_____

Adequacy of heating, lighting, cooling: _____

_____

Noise levels: _____

_____

Food sanitation practices: _____

_____

Toilet facilities (*adequacy, state of repair*): _____

_____

Cleaning of shower facilities: _____

_____

Isolation facilities for students with communicable diseases: _____

_____

Facilities and access for handicapped students or staff: _____

_____

Social Dimension

Community attitudes toward education and toward school: _____

_____

Community support of school program: _____

_____

Crime in neighborhood (*extent, effect on school and student health*): _____

_____

Funding (*extent, adequacy, priorities*): _____

_____

Home environment of students: _____

_____

Availability of before- and after-school care: _____

_____

Socioeconomic status of students, staff: _____

_____

Presence of intergroup conflicts: _____

_____

Cultural background of staff, students: _____

_____

Education level of families and extent of health knowledge: _____

_____

Behavioral Dimension

Consumption Patterns

Quality of school meal programs: _____

_____

Student/staff nutrition levels: _____

_____

Special nutritional needs (*students or staff*): _____

_____

Nutrition knowledge (*extent among students, staff, parents*): _____

_____

Extent of alcohol or drug use by students, staff, family members: _____

_____

Extent of smoking by students, staff, family members: _____

_____

Rest and exercise patterns of school population: _____

_____

Leisure Activities

Recreational opportunities (*type, age-appropriateness*): _____

_____

Use of appropriate safety equipment: _____

_____

Other

Sexual activity by students (*extent, use of contraceptives, use of condoms and other barrier devices*): _____

_____   _____

Use of safety devices (*seat belts*): _____

_____

Health System Dimension

Health care services offered by school: _____

_____

Availability of other health care services: _____

_____

Use of health care services by school population: _____

_____

Financing of health care services: _____

_____

Support of school health program by health care professionals in the community: _____

_____

School and community attitudes toward health and health care: _____

_____

SPECIAL ASSESSMENT CONSIDERATIONS IN THE WORK SETTING

Several specific considerations apply to the assessment of population groups in the work setting. These considerations are addressed in the assessment tool presented here. This tool applies the Dimensions Model to the task of assessing health needs in the work setting and is intended to be used with groups of employees. Appendix N, Health Assessment Guide—Adult Client, can be used to assess the health status of individual employees. The tool presented here addresses only the assessment component of the Dimensions Model. Guidance in planning, implementing, and evaluating health care programs in the work setting can be found in Appendix I, Health Assessment and Intervention Planning Guide—Community Client.

Special Assessment Considerations in the Work Setting

Biophysical Dimension

Age, sex, and racial/ethnic composition of the employee population: _____

_____

Presence of handicapping conditions in the employee population: _____

_____

Incidence and prevalence of disease (*communicable and chronic*): _____

_____

Prevalence of genetic predisposition to disease: _____

_____

Extent of absenteeism: _____

_____

Number and type of workers' compensation claims: _____

_____

Immunization status (*diphtheria, tetanus, influenza, pneumonia*): _____

_____

Results of periodic screening tests: _____

_____

Psychological Dimension

Organization of the work day (*shift work, breaks, overtime*): _____

_____

Aesthetic quality of environment: _____

_____

Relationships among employees: _____

_____

Relationships between employees and management: _____

_____

Employee morale: _____

_____

Supervisor leadership styles: _____

_____

Employee evaluation practices (*consistency, fairness*): _____

_____

Job satisfaction: _____

_____

Extent of employee control of job: _____

_____

Extent and sources of stress in the workplace: _____

_____

Extent of work/home role conflict: _____

_____

Availability of stress management programs: _____

_____

Prevalence of emotional problems in the employee population: _____

_____

Availability of employee assistance programs: _____

_____

Physical Dimension
Typical commute (*distance, traffic*): _____

_____

Safety of parking areas: _____

_____

Use of pesticides and other poisons in the work environment: _____

_____

Pollutants in the work environment: _____

_____

Fire or safety hazards: _____

_____

Potential for toxic substance exposures: _____

_____

Use of hazardous equipment: _____

_____

Extent of exposure to extreme weather conditions: _____

_____

Potential for falls: _____

_____

Need for heavy lifting: _____

_____

Ergonomics of workstations: _____

_____

Animals/insects in the work environment: _____

_____

Plant allergens or poisons in the work environment: _____

_____

Adequacy of heating, lighting, cooling, ventilation: _____

_____

Noise levels: _____

_____

Sanitation of food preparation and storage areas: _____

_____

Toilet facilities (*adequacy, state of repair*): _____

_____

Availability of shower facilities for dealing with external toxic substance exposures: _____

_____

Facilities and access for handicapped employees: _____

_____

Potential for disaster: _____

_____

Social Dimension

Economic stability of employing organization: _____

_____

Salary levels (*adequacy, equity*): _____

_____

Health benefits available: _____

_____

Community attitudes to employing organization: _____

_____

Crime in neighborhood: _____

_____

Potential for violence in the work setting: _____

_____

Child care availability: _____

_____

Family leave policies: _____

_____

Intergroup conflicts/discrimination: _____

_____

Cultural background of employees: _____

_____

Languages spoken by employees: _____

_____

Education level of employees and extent of health knowledge: _____

_____

Coworker support for healthy behaviors: _____

_____

Management support for healthy behaviors: _____

_____

Implementation of safety legislation, regulations, policies: _____

_____

Implementation of health-related policies: _____

_____

Types of work performed and health effects: _____

_____

Extent of sexual harassment: _____

_____

Behavioral Dimension
Consumption Patterns
Quality of food services: _____

_____

Employee nutritional levels: _____

_____

Special nutritional needs: _____

_____

Nutrition knowledge: _____

_____

Extent of alcohol or drug use by employees: _____

_____

Smoking (*extent, policies, cessation programs*): _____

_____

Medication use by employees: _____

_____

Leisure Activities
Rest and activity patterns of employees: _____

_____

Opportunity for physical activity: _____

_____

Other
Adequacy of safety policies and procedures: _____

_____

Use of appropriate safety equipment and procedures: _____

_____

Health System Dimension
Health care services offered in work setting: _____

_____

Availability of other health care services: _____

_____

Use of health care services by employee population: _____

_____

Funding of health care services (*adequacy, source*): _____

_____

Employee attitudes to health and health services: _____

_____

Availability of health promotion programs: _____

_____

Procedures to control and monitor toxic exposures: _____

_____

SPECIAL ASSESSMENT CONSIDERATIONS IN THE CORRECTIONAL SETTING

Assessing the health needs of groups of people within a correctional setting requires attention to specific assessment considerations. These considerations are addressed in the assessment tool presented here which applies the Dimensions Model to the task of assessing health needs in the correctional setting. The tool is intended to be used with groups of inmates and corrections personnel. Appendix N, Health Assessment Guide—Adult Client, can be used to assess the health status of individual staff or inmates. The tool presented here addresses only the assessment component of the Dimensions Model. Guidance in planning, implementing, and evaluating health care programs in the correctional setting can be found in Appendix I, Health Assessment and Intervention Planning Guide—Community Client.

Special Assessment Considerations in the Correctional Setting

Biophysical Dimension

Age, sex, and racial/ethnic composition of inmates and staff: _____

_____

Presence of handicapping conditions in the correctional population (*type, effects*): _____

_____

Incidence and prevalence of disease (*communicable and chronic*): _____

_____

Prevalence of genetic predisposition to disease: _____

_____

Immunization status (*diphtheria, tetanus, influenza, pneumonia*): _____

_____

Results of periodic screening tests: _____

_____

Prevalence of TB, HIV infection, hepatitis B: _____

_____

Prevalence of pregnancy in the population: _____

_____

Psychological Dimension

Psychological effects of incarceration: _____

_____

Potential for suicide attempts: _____

_____

Adequacy of suicide prevention procedures: _____

_____

Relationships among inmates: _____

_____

Relationships between inmates and corrections staff: _____

_____

Inmate control practices: _____

_____

Extent of inmate self-determination: _____

_____

Extent and sources of stress in the setting: _____

_____

Prevalence of mental illness among inmates (*type, manifestations*): _____

_____

Incidence of sexual assault of inmates: _____

_____

Prevalence of death sentence (*number, psychological effects*): _____

_____

Physical Dimension

Location of facility (*hazards posed by location*): _____

_____

Adequacy of housing space: _____

_____

Use of pesticides and other poisons in the environment: _____

_____

Pollutants in the environment: _____

_____

Fire or safety hazards: _____

_____

Potential for toxic substance exposures: _____

_____

Safety and repair of recreational facilities/equipment: _____

_____

Animals/insects in the environment: _____

_____

Plant allergens or poisons in the environment: _____

_____

Use of hazardous equipment: _____

_____

Adequacy of heating, lighting, cooling, ventilation: _____

_____

Noise levels: _____

_____

Sanitation of food preparation and storage areas: _____

_____

Toilet facilities/plumbing (*adequacy, state of repair*): _____

_____

Water supply (*source, safety, availability*): _____

_____

Disposal of wastes (*procedures, health hazards posed*): _____

_____

Facilities and access for handicapped staff and inmates: _____

_____

Potential for disaster (*communicable and chronic*): _____

_____

Social Dimension

Attitudes of personnel to inmates: _____

_____

Sanctions employed against inmates: _____

_____

Attitudes of surrounding community to facility and inmates: _____

_____

Crime in facility (*type, prevalence*): _____

_____

Family visitation policies: _____

_____

Intergroup conflicts/discrimination: _____

_____

Cultural background of inmates and staff: _____

_____

Socioeconomic status of inmates: _____

_____

Education level of inmates and extent of health knowledge: _____

_____

Extent of staff and inmate mobility within system (*typical length of stay, transfer policies*): _____

_____

Compliance with correctional standards: _____

_____

Implementation of health-related policies: _____

_____

Types of work performed and health effects: _____

_____

Extent of sexual harassment: _____

_____

Adequacy of security measures (*effects on health and health care*): _____

_____

Transportation availability: _____

_____

Behavioral Dimension

Consumption Patterns

Quality of food services: _____

_____

Inmate nutritional status: _____

_____

Special nutritional needs: _____

_____

Nutrition knowledge: _____

_____

Extent of alcohol or drug use (*inmates and staff*): _____

_____

Ease of access to alcohol or other drugs: _____

_____

Smoking (*extent, availability of tobacco, policies, cessation programs*): _____

_____

Medications (*types used, dispensing policies and procedures*): _____

_____

Rest and Exercise
Recreational opportunities available: _____

_____

Rest and exercise patterns of population: _____

_____

Sexual Activity
Prior history of prostitution among inmates: _____

_____

Extent of sexual activity among inmates: _____

_____

Use of unsafe sexual practices: _____

_____

Availability of condoms to inmates: _____

_____

Other
Use of appropriate safety equipment and procedures: _____

_____

Health System Dimension
Health care services offered in correctional setting (*type, adequacy*): _____

_____

Access to outside health care services: _____

_____

Use of health care services by inmate population: _____

_____

Funding of health care services (*adequacy, source, inmate fees*): _____

_____

Inmate attitudes to health and health services: _____

_____

Availability of health promotion programs: _____

_____

Availability of drug and alcohol treatment services: _____

_____

Emergency response capability of health care staff: _____

_____

Provisions for continuity of care after release: _____

_____

Attitudes of health care providers to inmates: _____

_____

INFORMATION ON SELECTED COMMUNICABLE DISEASES

Chlamydia

Agent: Chlamydia trachomatis
Reservoir: humans
Incubation: probably 7–14 days
Communicability: unknown, relapse possible
Modes of transmission: sexual contact
Immunization: none
Prophylaxis: antibiotics following sexual exposure or for infants born to infected mothers
Treatment: tetracycline, doxycycline, erythromycin, or azithromycin
Contact notification: sexual contacts
Symptoms: frequently asymptomatic; *males* may have urethritis with burning on urination, urethral itching, penile discharge; *females* may have purulent vaginal discharge
Prevention: monogamy, condom use

Coccidioidomycosis

Agent: Coccidioides immitis (fungus)
Reservoir: soil
Incubation: 1–4 weeks
Communicability: no person-to-person transmission
Modes of transmission: inhalation of contaminated dust
Immunization: none

Prophylaxis: none
Treatment: usually self-limiting, amphotericin B for severe infection, fluconazole for meningeal infection, ketoconazole or itraconazole for chronic infection
Contact notification: none
Symptoms: asymptomatic or fever, cough, chills
Prevention: dust control measures

Diphtheria (pharyngotonsillar, laryngeal)

Agent: Corynebacterium diphtheriae
Reservoir: humans
Incubation: 2–5 days
Communicability: usually 2 weeks or less, reduced by antibiotic therapy
Modes of transmission: airborne, raw milk, contact with articles soiled with discharge from lesions (rare)
Immunization: routine use of DTP vaccine (Td for persons over age 7)
Prophylaxis: penicillin or erythromycin and booster dose of diphtheria toxoid or full immunization series
Treatment: diphtheria antitoxin and penicillin or erythromycin
Contact notification: none
Symptoms: sore throat with patchy, grayish membrane

over pharynx, tonsils, uvula, and soft palate; cervical lymphadenopathy
Prevention: immunization of susceptible individuals

Gonorrhea

Agent: Neisseria gonorrhoeae
Reservoir: humans
Incubation: usually 2–7 days
Communicability: until treated
Modes of transmission: sexual contact
Immunization: none
Prophylaxis: antibiotics after exposure
Treatment: ceftriaxone and doxycycline
Contact notification: sexual contacts
Symptoms: vary with site of infection; usually associated with penile discharge and burning on urination in urethritis in males or with anal discharge, tenesmus, and pruritis in rectal infection; may be associated with vaginal discharge and foul odor in females; sore throat in oral infection
Prevention: monogamy, use of condoms

Hantavirus (pulmonary)

Agent: hantavirus (multiple strains)
Reservoir: rodents
Incubation: 2 weeks
Communicability: no person-to-person transmission
Modes of transmission: inhalation of dust contaminated with urine, feces, saliva of infected rodents
Immunization: none
Prophylaxis: none
Treatment: symptomatic
Contact notification: none
Symptoms: fever, myalgias, chills, nonproductive cough, headache, nausea, vomiting, diarrhea, malaise; may progress to fulminant adult respiratory distress syndrome (ARDS) in severe cases
Prevention: rodent control, proper cleaning and disposal of rodent excreta

Hepatitis A

Agent: hepatitis A virus (HAV)
Reservoir: humans, nonhuman primates
Incubation: average 28–30 days
Communicability: latter half of incubation period to a few days after onset of jaundice
Modes of transmission: fecal–oral, sexual contact (homosexual males), contaminated food or water, direct inoculation (rare)
Immunization: hepatitis A vaccine
Prophylaxis: immunoglobulin (IG)
Treatment: symptomatic

Contact notification: household and sexual contacts, day care center classroom contacts
Symptoms: abrupt onset of fever, malaise, anorexia, nausea and vomiting, abdominal discomfort followed by jaundice; adults more likely to be symptomatic than children
Prevention: sanitation, personal hygiene (handwashing), adequate cooking of contaminated foods

Hepatitis B

Agent: hepatitis B (HBV)
Reservoir: humans
Incubation: average 60–90 days
Communicability: several weeks before and after symptom onset; may be lifelong carrier
Modes of transmission: sexual contact, direct inoculation, transplacental
Immunization: hepatitis B vaccine
Prophylaxis: hepatitis B immunoglobulin and/or immunization
Treatment: symptomatic, alfa interferon for chronic infection
Contact notification: household or sexual contacts, drug partners
Symptoms: insidious onset of anorexia, abdominal discomfort, nausea and vomiting, followed by jaundice
Prevention: immunization of infants and persons in high-risk groups; monogamy, condom use, blood donor screening, drug abuse treatment; avoid needle sharing; blood and body fluid precautions

Hepatitis C

Agent: hepatitis C virus (HCV)
Reservoir: humans
Incubation: average 6–9 weeks
Communicability: 1 or more weeks prior to onset through acute clinical phase
Modes of transmission: direct inoculation, sexual contact
Immunization: none
Prophylaxis: none
Treatment: symptomatic, alfa interferon for chronic infection
Contact notification: drug partners
Symptoms: insidious onset of anorexia, vague abdominal discomfort, nausea and vomiting, jaundice
Prevention: same as for hepatitis B

Hepatitis D (Delta)

Agent: hepatitis D virus (HDV)
Reservoir: humans
Incubation: 2–8 weeks

Communicability: prior to onset through acute clinical phase
Modes of transmission: direct inoculation, sexual contact
Immunization: none
Prophylaxis: none
Treatment: symptomatic
Contact notification: none
Symptoms: abrupt onset of symptoms similar to HBV; always associated with coexistent HBV infection
Prevention: same as for hepatitis B

Hepatitis E

Agent: hepatitis E virus (HEV)
Reservoir: humans
Incubation: 26–42 days
Communicability: unknown
Modes of transmission: fecal–oral, contaminated water
Immunization: none
Prophylaxis: none
Treatment: symptomatic
Contact notification: none
Symptoms: similar to HAV
Prevention: sanitation, hygiene

HIV Infection

Agent: human immunodeficiency virus (HIV)
Reservoir: humans
Incubation: 2 months to 10 years
Communicability: unknown; presumed lifelong
Modes of transmission: sexual contact, direct inoculation, transplacental inoculation, breast feeding
Immunization: none
Prophylaxis: antiviral agents
Treatment: antiviral agents
Contact notification: sexual partners, drug use partners who share needles, clients of infected health care professionals, recipients of blood or tissue from infected donors
Symptoms: fatigue, malaise, recurrent and sustained opportunistic infections
Prevention: monogamy, condom use, drug treatment; avoid needle sharing; screen blood and organ donors

HSV Infection

Agent: herpes simplex virus (HSV) type 2
Reservoir: humans
Incubation: 2–12 days
Communicability: 7–12 days, initial lesion; 4–7 days, recurrent lesions
Modes of transmission: sexual contact
Immunization: none

Prophylaxis: none
Treatment: symptomatic, acyclovir
Contact notification: pregnant women
Symptoms: painful genital lesions
Prevention: monogamy, condom use

Influenza

Agent: influenza viruses, A, B, C
Reservoir: humans (animals for new subtypes)
Incubation: 1–3 days
Communicability: 3–7 days after onset of symptoms
Modes of transmission: airborne
Immunization: annual use of influenza vaccine for high-risk individuals
Prophylaxis: amantadine or rimantadine in high-risk persons (type A only)
Treatment: symptomatic, amantadine or rimantidine within 48 hours of onset
Contact notification: none
Symptoms: fever, headache, myalgia, prostration, coryza, sore throat, cough, nausea, vomiting, diarrhea
Prevention: immunization of persons at risk; general health promotion

Lyme Disease

Agent: Borrelia burgdorferi
Reservoir: wild rodents, deer ticks
Incubation: 3–32 days
Communicability: no person-to-person transmission
Modes of transmission: bite of infected tick
Immunization: none
Prophylaxis: none
Treatment: doxycycline, amoxicillin
Contact notification: source case finding if outside endemic areas
Symptoms: distinctive skin lesion, followed by malaise, fatigue, fever, headache, stiff neck, myalgias, migratory arthralgia, lymphadenopathy
Prevention: use insect repellent, wear long-sleeved light-colored clothes, check for ticks regularly, tick control measures

Measles

Agent: measles virus
Reservoir: humans
Incubation: average 10 days
Communicability: beginning of prodrome to 4 days after onset of rash
Modes of transmission: airborne
Immunization: routine use of measles, mumps, rubella (MMR) vaccine
Prophylaxis: MMR within 72 hours of exposure;

measles immunoglobulin for children under 1 year within 6 days of exposure
Treatment: symptomatic
Contact notification: none
Symptoms: prodrome of fever, conjunctivitis, cough, coryza, and Koplik's spots, followed by rash on face and spreading downward
Prevention: routine immunization of all susceptible individuals

Mumps

Agent: mumps virus
Reservoir: humans
Incubation: usually 18 days
Communicability: 6–7 days before swelling to 9 days after
Modes of transmission: airborne
Immunization: routine use of measles, mumps, rubella (MMR) vaccine
Prophylaxis: none
Treatment: symptomatic
Contact notification: none
Symptoms: pain and swelling in parotid area accompanied by difficulty swallowing; redness and swelling around Stensen's duct
Prevention: immunization of susceptible individuals

Pertussis

Agent: Bordetella pertussis
Reservoir: humans
Incubation: 7–10 days
Communicability: early catarrhal stage to 3 weeks after cough begins
Modes of transmission: airborne
Immunization: routine use of diphtheria/tetanus/pertussis (DTP) vaccine
Prophylaxis: DTP booster and erythromycin
Treatment: erythromycin may reduce communicability
Contact notification: nonimmune children
Symptoms: initial catarrhal stage followed by paroxysmal whooping cough
Prevention: immunization of susceptible individuals

Poliomyelitis

Agent: poliovirus, types 1, 2, 3
Reservoir: humans
Incubation: 7–14 days
Communicability: unknown, possible 36–72 hours after exposure to 10 days after symptoms occur
Modes of transmission: airborne, contaminated milk and food
Immunization: routine use of trivalent oral polio vaccine (OPV)

Prophylaxis: none
Treatment: symptomatic
Contact notification: close contacts
Symptoms: fever, headache, gastrointestinal disturbance, stiffness of neck and back with or without paralysis
Prevention: immunization of susceptible children; sanitation

Rubella

Agent: rubella virus
Reservoir: humans
Incubation: 16–18 days
Communicability: 1 week before to 4 days after onset of rash
Modes of transmission: airborne, transplacental inoculation
Immunization: routine use of measles, mumps, rubella (MMR) vaccine
Prophylaxis: immunoglobulin (IG) for pregnant women (value questionable)
Treatment: symptomatic
Contact notification: pregnant women
Symptoms: prodrome of mild fever, headache, and malaise, followed by discrete maculopapular rash, occipital node enlargement
Prevention: immunization of susceptible individuals, especially women of childbearing age

Syphilis

Agent: Treponema pallidum
Reservoir: humans
Incubation: 10–90 days (usually 3 weeks)
Communicability: in stages with lesions
Modes of transmission: sexual contact, direct inoculation, transplacental inoculation
Immunization: none
Prophylaxis: antibiotics after exposure
Treatment: penicillin
Contact notification: sexual contacts to primary, secondary, and early latent syphilis; persons sharing needles
Symptoms: vary with stage of disease
  Primary: painless chancre or lesion at site of infection (usually genitalia, lips, etc); may be accompanied by localized lymphadenopathy in the area of the lesion
  Secondary: coppery, macular rash (may be found in all areas but particularly on palms and soles); may be accompanied by malaise and generalized lymphadenopathy
Latent: asymptomatic
Late: depends on organ system affected

Congenital: Hutchinson's teeth and raspberry molars, saddle nose, snuffles, rash if in secondary stage

Prevention: monogamy, condom use, drug abuse treatment; avoid needle sharing; screening of blood donors

Tetanus

Agent: Clostridium tetani
Reservoir: humans and animals, soil
Incubation: 3–21 days
Communicability: not directly communicable
Modes of transmission: introduction via wound in skin or unhealed umbilicus
Immunization: routine use of diphtheria/tetanus/pertussis (DTP) vaccine
Prophylaxis: tetanus/diphtheria (Td) booster for immunized persons; tetanus immunoglobulin (TIG) or tetanus antitoxin and Td for unimmunized individuals
Treatment: tetanus immunoglobulin (TIG) or antitoxin and penicillin
Contact notification: none
Symptoms: painful muscular contractions with pro-gressive rigidity, especially in muscles of neck and shoulders

Prevention: immunization of susceptible individuals, prevent injury, cleanse injuries thoroughly, control animal feces; asepsis during deliveries

Tuberculosis

Agent: Mycobacterium tuberculosis
Reservoir: humans, cattle, other animals
Incubation: 4–12 weeks
Communicability: during periods of respiratory expulsion of bacteria
Modes of transmission: airborne, contaminated milk
Immunization: bacille Calmette–Guérin (BCG) for selected individuals
Prophylaxis: isoniazid
Treatment: antituberculin agents (multidrug regimen)
Contact notification: close contacts
Symptoms: cough, hemoptysis, unexplained weight loss, night sweats
Prevention: improve social conditions, promote general health

FACTORS IN THE EPIDEMIOLOGY OF SELECTED CHRONIC PHYSICAL HEALTH PROBLEMS

Information presented here includes epidemiologic factors associated with the incidence of selected chronic physical health problems. The health problems addressed are arthritis, cancer, cardiovascular and cerebrovascular disease, chronic obstructive pulmonary disease (COPD), diabetes mellitus, obesity, and conditions resulting from accidental trauma. Factors related to each condition are organized in terms of the Dimensions Model.

Epidemiologic Factors Associated with Arthritis
Biophysical Dimension
- There may be a genetic predisposition to arthritis. Asians and Native Americans have low incidence rates for arthritis.
- The onset of arthritis usually begins in the fourth decade of life.
- Older persons usually have greater disability from arthritis.
- Women are more likely than men to develop arthritis.
- Previous injury to bones and joints may predispose one to arthritis.
- Obesity increases stress on joints and may exacerbate arthritis.

- Pregnancy may cause a temporary remission in arthritis symptoms.

Behavioral Dimension
- Occupational or recreational factors that contribute to injury may lead to arthritis in later life.
- Overeating may lead to obesity and increased severity of arthritis.

Health System Dimension
- Many people with arthritis engage in self-care rather than seek medical help.
- Medical treatment for arthritis has limited effects.

Epidemiologic Factors Associated with Cancers
Biophysical Dimension
- Genetic inheritance may predispose one to cancer.
- Incidence and survival rates for cancer vary among ethnic and racial groups.
- Males have higher mortality rates for most forms of cancer than females.
- Genital HSV infection may contribute to cervical cancer.

Physical Dimension

- Exposure to sunlight increases the risk of skin cancer.
- Cancer incidence is higher in urban than in rural areas.
- Environmental pollutants can contribute to cancer incidence.

Social Dimension

- Occupational exposures can contribute to cancer.

Behavioral Dimension

- Smoking increases one's risk of several forms of cancer.
- Lack of dietary fiber and increased fat in the diet have been linked to increased risk of colon cancer.
- Alcohol consumption may be associated with increased cancer risk (especially liver cancer).
- Self-screening health practices such as breast self-examination and testicular self-examination increase one's chances of cancer survival.

Health System Dimension

- Lack of emphasis on screening has contributed to cancer mortality.
- Aggressiveness of treatment influences cancer survival rates.

Epidemiologic Factors Associated with Cardiovascular and Cerebrovascular Disease

Biophysical Dimension

- Genetic inheritance may predispose one to cardiovascular or cerebrovascular disease.
- Cardiovascular disease is more common in young African Americans and older whites.
- Females have lower mortality rates for cardiovascular and cerebrovascular disease than do males.
- Racial differences in incidence of cardiovascular and cerebrovascular disease probably reflect differences in the prevalence of other biological risk factors such as hypertension, increased serum cholesterol, and diabetes.
- Infection with *Chlamydia pneumoniae* may increase risk of coronary heart disease.

Psychological Dimension

- Stress in the environment can contribute to cardiovascular and cerebrovascular disease.
- Major depressive disorder may increase the risk of heart attack.
- Anger and anxiety contribute to hypertension and heart attack.

Physical Dimension

- Cumulative lead exposure may contribute to hypertension as a risk factor for coronary heart disease.

Social Dimension

- High income and education levels are associated with decreased mortality due to cardiovascular and cerebrovascular disease.

Behavioral Dimension

- Sedentary lifestyle increases the risk of cardiovascular and cerebrovascular disease.
- Smoking increases the risk of cardiovascular and cerebrovascular disease.
- Overeating and increased fat and cholesterol consumption contribute to cardiovascular and cerebrovascular disease.
- Moderate alcohol use may reduce the risk of cardiovascular disease.

Health System Dimension

- Attention to elimination of risk factors has decreased the incidence of cardiovascular and cerebrovascular disease.
- Access to emergency services reduces mortality due to cardiovascular and cerebrovascular disease.

Epidemiologic Factors Associated with COPD

Biophysical Dimension

- Some evidence supports a genetic predisposition to COPD.
- Recurrent respiratory infections early in life can contribute to COPD later in life.
- Respiratory allergies and asthma can increase the risk of COPD.

Physical Dimension

- Environmental pollution can contribute to or exacerbate COPD.
- COPD is more prevalent in highly industrialized urban areas than in rural areas.
- Exposure of nonsmokers to tobacco smoke exacerbates COPD.

Social Dimension

- Occupational exposure to dusts or gases increases the risk of COPD.

Behavioral Dimension

- Smoking increases the risk of COPD and interacts with other contributing factors to increase the risk still more.

Health System Dimension

- Lack of emphasis on primary prevention contributes to COPD.
- Treatment of COPD is minimally effective.
- Overuse of inhaled β-agonists and underuse of corticosteroids contribute to asthma mortality.

Epidemiologic Factors Associated with Diabetes Mellitus

Biophysical Dimension

- Genetic predisposition is a contributing factor in diabetes.
- Native Americans and African Americans have higher incidence rates of diabetes than do other racial groups.
- The presence of hypertension complicates diabetes.
- Diabetes is a risk factor for heart disease and stroke.
- Viral infection may increase the risk of diabetes.
- Pregnancy complicates diabetes control.

Physical Dimension

- Diabetes is more prevalent in industrialized countries.

Behavioral Dimension

- Affluence increases incidence rates of diabetes.
- Smoking may be a risk factor in the development of diabetes.
- Smoking interacts with diabetes to increase the risk of heart disease and stroke.
- Overeating and consequent overweight contribute to diabetes.
- Moderate alcohol use may have a protective effective for development of diabetes.
- Excessive alcohol use contributes to diabetes mortality.
- Exercise can contribute to diabetes control.

Health System Dimension

- Lack of emphasis on screening leads to later diagnosis and poor control of diabetes.
- Lack of access to health care influences diabetes control.
- Failure to monitor treatment effects can contribute to increased diabetes mortality.

Epidemiologic Factors Associated with Obesity

Biophysical Dimension

- There may be a slight genetic predisposition to obesity.
- Obesity occurs in all age groups, both sexes, and all ethnic groups.

Social Dimension

- Prevalence of junk food contributes to obesity.
- Fast-paced life leads to poor nutrition and obesity.
- Occupations that contribute to a sedentary lifestyle also contribute to obesity.

Behavioral Dimension

- Consumption of excess calories, especially fats, contributes to obesity.
- Sedentary lifestyle and lack of exercise contribute to obesity.

Health System Dimension

- Lack of emphasis on nutrition education contributes to poor dietary habits and obesity.
- Treatment of obesity is less effective than it might be because of high rates of noncompliance.

Epidemiologic Factors Associated with Trauma Due to Accidents

Biophysical Dimension

- Drowning, poisoning, and suffocation are common accidents among young children.
- Firearms injuries are common among preadolescents and adolescents.
- Motor vehicle accidents affect all age groups, but occur most often among adolescents and young adults.
- The elderly are particularly susceptible to the effects of falls and fires.
- The presence of physical disability increases the risk of accidental injury.

Psychological Dimension

- Depression or worry may contribute to lack of attentiveness and subsequent accidents.

Physical Dimension

- Improper storage of hazardous materials increases accident risk.
- Use of space heaters contributes to fires and burn injuries.
- Absence of smoke detectors in buildings contributes to fire injuries.
- Road conditions and automobile crashworthiness influence motor vehicle accidents and their effects.

Social Dimension

- Easy access to firearms contributes to accidental injuries.
- Occupations involving heavy labor or motor vehicle operation increase the risk of accidents.

Behavioral Dimension

- Alcohol and drug use and abuse contribute to accidents.
- Recreational activities pose a variety of accident hazards.
- Failure to use safety devices increases the risk of injury.
- Common use and improper storage of medications contribute to poisoning.

Health System Dimension

- Lack of emphasis on safety education has contributed to accidental injuries.
- Access to emergency services influences accident survival rates.
- Long-term consequences of accidents are affected by the availability of rehabilitation services.

SUSPECTED ABUSE REPORT FORMS

The forms included here are examples of the type used to report suspected abuse and violence. Generally, cases of suspected or confirmed abuse are reported immediately by telephone and followed with a completed reporting form within 24 hours. Whenever feasible, specific events leading to suspicion of abuse should be described as fully as possible, including information about specific behavior observed or exact words of those describing events. Community health nurses should become familiar with specific reporting forms used in their local jurisdiction, including forms for reporting spouse and elder abuse if required.

MEDICAL SERVICES
DOMESTIC VIOLENCE AND VIOLENT INJURY REPORT

California Penal Code sections 11160 and 11161 require hospitals and physicians to report immediately, both by telephone and in writing, all injuries resulting from the use of a gun or knife or other deadly weapon, or otherwise inflicted in violation of the criminal law, whether by act of the patient or of another person.
EXCEPTION: Any physical or psychological condition brought about solely by the voluntary self administration of any narcotic or restricted dangerous drug is not reportable.

Time of call to police _____   By _____
                                                                                        print name

REASON FOR REPORT

_____ Gunshot

_____ Knife wound (or from other deadly weapon)

_____ Injury from other criminal law violation

PATIENT'S NAME: _____

PATIENT'S ADDRESS: _____

PATIENT'S WHEREABOUTS: _____

_____
(Facility Name and Address)

_____ Other (specify) _____

NATURE AND EXTENT OF INJURY: _____

_____

_____

_____

_____   _____
       Date/Time   Signature of Attending Physician
                                                            (or other reporting party)

TELEPHONE REPORT GIVEN TO _____   of _____
                                        Name/ID # of Officer   Agency

                                 _____   by _____
                                            Date/Time   ED Staff

Original: Law Enforcement Agency
Yellow: Patient's Chart
Pink: District Attorney, Domestic Violence Unit

If officer does not respond, mail yellow and pink copies to the District Attorney, Domestic Violence Unit, 101 W. Broadway, San Diego, California 92101. Mail original to appropriate law enforcement agency with jurisdiction where the battery occurred.

SUSPECTED CHILD ABUSE REPORT
To Be Completed by Reporting Party
Pursuant to Penal Code Section 11166

A. CASE IDENTIFICATION

TO BE COMPLETED BY INVESTIGATING CPA

VICTIM NAME: _____

REPORT NO./CASE NAME: _____

DATE OF REPORT: _____

B. REPORTING PARTY

NAME/TITLE

ADDRESS

PHONE ( )   DATE OF REPORT   SIGNATURE OF REPORTING PARTY

C. REPORT SENT TO

☐ POLICE DEPARTMENT   ☐ SHERIFF'S OFFICE   ☐ COUNTY WELFARE   ☐ COUNTY PROBATION

AGENCY   ADDRESS

OFFICIAL CONTACTED   PHONE ( )   DATE/TIME

D. INVOLVED PARTIES

VICTIM

NAME (LAST, FIRST, MIDDLE)   ADDRESS   BIRTHDATE   SEX   RACE

PRESENT LOCATION OF CHILD   PHONE ( )

SIBLINGS

NAME	BIRTHDATE	SEX	RACE	NAME	BIRTHDATE	SEX	RACE
1.				4.			
2.				5.			
3.				6.			

PARENTS

NAME (LAST, FIRST, MIDDLE)	BIRTHDATE	SEX	RACE	NAME (LAST, FIRST, MIDDLE)	BIRTHDATE	SEX	RACE

ADDRESS   ADDRESS

HOME PHONE ( )   BUSINESS PHONE ( )   HOME PHONE ( )   BUSINESS PHONE ( )

E. INCIDENT INFORMATION

IF NECESSARY, ATTACH EXTRA SHEET OR OTHER FORM AND CHECK THIS BOX. ☐

1. DATE/TIME OF INCIDENT   PLACE OF INCIDENT   *(CHECK ONE)*   ☐ OCCURRED   ☐ OBSERVED

IF CHILD WAS IN OUT-OF-HOME CARE AT TIME OF INCIDENT, CHECK TYPE OF CARE:
☐ FAMILY DAY CARE   ☐ CHILD CARE CENTER   ☐ FOSTER FAMILY HOME   ☐ SMALL FAMILY HOME   ☐ GROUP HOME OR INSTITUTION

2. TYPE OF ABUSE: *(CHECK ONE OR MORE)* ☐ PHYSICAL   ☐ MENTAL   ☐ SEXUAL ASSAULT   ☐ NEGLECT   ☐ OTHER

3. NARRATIVE DESCRIPTION:

4. SUMMARIZE WHAT THE ABUSED CHILD OR PERSON ACCOMPANYING THE CHILD SAID HAPPENED:

5. EXPLAIN KNOWN HISTORY OF SIMILAR INCIDENT(S) FOR THIS CHILD:

SS 8572 (REV.7/87)   ***INSTRUCTIONS AND DISTRIBUTION ON REVERSE***

DO NOT submit a copy of this form to the Department of Justice (DOJ). A CPA is required under Penal Code Section 11169 to submit to DOJ a Child Abuse Investigation Report Form SS-8583 if (1) an active investigation has been conducted and (2) the incident is **not** unfounded.

Blue and Green Copies to: Social Services Dept.
P.O. Box 11341
San Diego, CA 92111

Police or Sheriff-WHITE Copy; County Welfare or Probation- BLUE Copy; District Attorney-GREEN Copy; Reporting Party-YELLOW Copy

INDEX

LICENSE AGREEMENT AND LIMITED WARRANTY

READ THE FOLLOWING TERMS AND CONDITIONS CAREFULLY BEFORE OPENING THIS DISK PACKAGE. THIS IS AN AGREEMENT BETWEEN YOU AND APPLETON & LANGE (THE "COMPANY"). BY OPENING THIS SEALED PACKAGE, YOU ARE AGREEING TO BE BOUND BY THESE TERMS AND CONDITIONS. IF YOU DO NOT AGREE WITH THESE TERMS AND CONDTIONS, DO NOT OPEN THE DISK PACKAGE, PROMPTLY RETURN THE DISK PACKAGE AND ALL ACCOMPANYING ITEMS TO THE COMPANY.

1. GRANT OF LICENSE: In consideration of your purchase of this book and/or other materials published by the Company, and your agreement to abide by the terms and conditions of this Agreement, the Company grants to you a nonexclusive right to use and display the copy of the enclosed software program (hereinafter the "SOFTWARE") so long as you comply with the terms of this Agreement. The company reserves all rights not expressly granted to you under this Agreement. This license is not a sale of the original SOFTWARE or any copy to you.

2. USE RESTRICTIONS: You may not sell, license, transfer or distribute copies of the SOFTWARE or Documentation to others. You may not reverse engineer, disassemble, decompile, modify, adapt, translate or otherwise reproduce the SOFTWARE or any part of it, or create derivative works based on the SOFTWARE or the Documentation without the prior written consent of the Company.

3. MISCELLANEOUS: This Agreement shall be construed in accordance with the laws of the United States of America and the State of New York, except for that body of law dealing with conflicts of law, and shall benefit the Company, its affiliates and assignees. If any provision of this Agreement is found void or unenforceable, the remainder will remain valid and enforceable according to its terms. Use, duplication or disclosure of the SOFTWARE by the U.S. Government is subject to the restricted rights applicable to commercial computer software under FAR 52.227.19 and DFARS 252.277-7013.

4. LIMITED WARRANTY AND DISCLAIMER OF WARRANTY: Because this SOFTWARE is being given to you without charge, the Company makes no warranties about the SOFTWARE, which is provided "AS-IS." **THE COMPANY DISCLAIMS ALL WARRANTIES, EXPRESS OR IMPLIED, INCLUDING WITHOUT LIMITATION, THE IMPLIED WARRANTIES OF MERCHANTABILITY AND FITNESS FOR A PARTICULAR PURPOSE, THE COMPANY DOES NOT WARRANT, GUARANTEE OR MAKE ANY REPRESENTATION REGARDING THE USE OR THE RESULTS OF THE USE OF THE SOFTWARE. IN NO EVENT, SHALL THE COMPANY, ITS PARENTS, SUBSIDIARIES, AFFILIATES, LICENSORS, DIRECTORS, OFFICERS, EMPLOYEES, AGENTS, SUPPLIERS OR CONTRACTORS BE LIABLE FOR ANY INCIDENTAL, INDIRECT, SPECIAL OR CONSEQUENTIAL DAMAGES ARISING OUT OF OR IN CONNECTION WITH THE LICENSE GRANTED UNDER THIS AGREEMENT INCLUDING, WITHOUT LIMITATION, LOSS OF USE, LOSS OF DATA, LOSS OF INCOME OR PROFIT, OR OTHER LOSSES SUSTAINED AS RESULT OF INJURY TO ANY PERSON, OR LOSS OF OR DAMAGE TO PROPERTY, OR CLAIMS OF THIRD PARTIES, EVEN IF THE COMPANY OR AN AUTHORIZED REPRESENTATIVE OF THE COMPANY HAS BEEN ADVISED OF THE POSSIBILITY OF SUCH DAMAGES.**

SOME JURISDICTIONS DO NOT ALLOW THE EXCLUSION OF IMPLIED WARRANTIES OR THE LIMITATION ON LIABILITY FOR INCIDENTAL, INDIRECT, SPECIAL OR CONSEQUENTIAL DAMAGES, SO THE ABOVE LIMITATIONS MAY NOT ALWAYS APPLY. THE WARRANTIES IN THIS AGREEMENT GIVE YOU SPECIFIC LEGAL RIGHTS AND YOU MAY ALSO HAVE OTHER RIGHTS WHICH VARY IN ACCORDANCE WITH LOCAL LAW.

No sales personnel or other representative of any party involved in the distribution of the software is authorized by the Company to make any warranties with respect to the software beyond what is contained in this agreement. Oral statements do not constitute warranties, shall not be relied upon by you and are not part of this agreement. The entire agreement between you and the Company is embodied herein.

ACKNOWLEDGMENT

YOU ACKNOWLEDGE THAT YOU HAVE READ THIS AGREEMENT, UNDERSTAND IT AND AGREE TO BE BOUND BY ITS TERMS AND CONDITIONS. YOU ALSO AGREE THAT THIS AGREEMENT IS THE COMPLETE AND EXCLUSIVE AGREEMENT BETWEEN YOU AND THE COMPANY.

Should you have any questions concerning this agreement or if you wish to contact the Company for any reason, please contact in writing: Simon & Schuster, c/o StarTek, 237 22nd Street, Greeley, CO 80631. (800) 991-0077

NOTE

If you encounter difficulty using this software in a Windows®-based word processing program after having read the "README.TXT" file on the disk, please contact: Simon & Schuster, c/o StarTek, 237 22nd Street, Greeley, CO 80631. (800) 991-0077